Pediatric Nutrition

8th Edition

Ronald E. Kleinman, MD, FAAP
Editor

Frank R. Greer, MD, FAAP
Editor

Suggested Citation:
American Academy of Pediatrics
Committee on Nutrition.
[chapter title]. In: Kleinman RE,
Greer FR, eds. *Pediatric Nutrition*.
8th ed. Itasca, IL:
American Academy of Pediatrics;
2019:[page numbers]

Policy of the American Academy of Pediatrics

American Academy of Pediatrics
345 Park Blvd
Itasca, IL 60143

Library of Congress Control Number: 2018968584
ISBN: 978-1-61002-360-3
eBook: 978-1-61002-361-0
MA0939

The recommendations in this publication do not indicate an exclusive course of treatment or serve as a standard of care. Variations, taking into account individual circumstances, may be appropriate.

The book has been developed by the American Academy of Pediatrics. The authors, editors, and contributors are expert authorities in the field of pediatrics. No commercial involvement of any kind has been solicited or accepted in the development of the content of this publication.

Products are mentioned for informational purposes only. Inclusion in the publication does not imply endorsement by the American Academy of Pediatrics.

The publishers have made every effort to trace the copyright holders for borrowed material. If they have inadvertently overlooked any, they will be pleased to make the necessary arrangements at first opportunity.

3-337/1019

1 2 3 4 5 6 7 8 9 10

Committee on Nutrition
2018-2019

Steven A. Abrams, MD, FAAP, Chairperson
George J. Fuchs III, MD, FAAP
Praveen S. Goday, MD, FAAP
Tamara S. Hannon, MD, FAAP
Jae H. Kim, MD, PhD, FAAP
C. Wesley Lindsey, MD, FAAP
Ellen S. Rome, MD, MPH, FAAP

Former Committee Members
Stephen R. Daniels, MD, PhD, FAAP, Immediate Past Chairperson
Mark R. Corkins, MD, FAAP
Sarah D. de Ferranti, MD, FAAP
Neville H. Golden, MD, FAAP
Sheela N. Magge, MD, FAAP
Sarah Jane Schwarzenberg, MD, FAAP

Liaison Representatives
Andrew Bremer, MD, PhD, FAAP, *National Institutes of Health*
Andrea Lotze, MD, FAAP, *US Food and Drug Administration*
Cria G. Perrine, PhD, *Centers for Disease Control and Prevention*
Catherine M. Pound, MD, *Canadian Paediatric Society*
Valery Soto, MS, RD, LD, *US Department of Food and Agriculture*

AAP Staff
Debra L. Burrowes, MHA
Madeline Curtis, JD
Tamar Magarik Haro
Katherine Matlin, MPP

Preface

Inadequate nutrition and, more recently, overnutrition in infants and children have immediate consequences for health and well-being, growth, and development and can lead to long-term, intergenerational effects on health, reproduction, cognition, and chronic disease. Overweight affects a significant proportion of the pediatric population in countries that span the levels of the United Nations Human Development Index. In some communities, as many as 60% of school-aged children are overweight. At the same time, undernutrition, stunting, and food insecurity remain major public health issues for infants and children across the globe. With the projected increase in population over the coming decades and the effects of climate change on arable land, farming, and food production, it is critical to understand how to best support the nutritional needs of growing infants and children and how to sustainably provide safe and affordable nutrition. This 8th edition of *Pediatric Nutrition* is meant to serve as a current and integrated resource for the practicing clinician to provide an understanding of the fundamental role of nutrients in human metabolism, the role of nutrition in the prevention and treatment of acute and chronic illnesses, and the interaction between nutrients, the microbiome, and gene function. Every attempt has been made to provide additional resources within each of the chapters that include references to printed materials, links to web-based resources and tools, and contacts for both government and private organizations that will be useful for both clinicians and patients. This edition of the handbook is the work of more than 100 authors and editors, all of whom are recognized experts for the topics on which they have written. All chapters are intended to reflect the current evidence base for each topic and the current policy statements and recommendations of the American Academy of Pediatrics. Our most sincere thanks go to the Chair of the Committee on Nutrition, Dr. Steve Abrams, and the current and past members of the committee who have contributed to the preparation of this book.

Ronald E. Kleinman, MD, FAAP, and Frank R. Greer, MD, FAAP, Editors

Contributors

The American Academy of Pediatrics (AAP) gratefully acknowledges the invaluable assistance provided by the following individuals who contributed to the preparation of this edition of *Pediatric Nutrition*. Their expertise, critical review, and cooperation were essential to the development of this book. Every attempt has been made to recognize all who have contributed to this effort; the AAP regrets any omissions that may have occurred.

Steven A. Abrams, MD, FAAP

Richard C. Adams, MD, FAAP

Banu Aygun, MD, FAAP

Robert Bandsma, MD, PhD

Donna Belcher, MS, RD, LDN, CDE

Carol Brunzell, RD, LD, CDE

Nancy F. Butte, PhD

Cheryl A. Callen

Kathryn Camp, MS, RD

Kevin Chatham-Stephens, MD, MPH, FAAP

Mark R. Corkins, MD, FAAP

Stephen R. Daniels, MD, PhD, MPH, FAAP

Sarah de Ferranti, MD, MPH

Christopher P. Duggan, MD, MPH

Robert Dunn, RD, LDN

Andrew Feranchak, MD

Marta L. Fiorotta, PhD

Jennifer Fischer, RDN, LD

Jennifer O. Fisher, PhD

George J. Fuchs III, MD, FAAP

Kriston Ganguli, MD

Laura B. Gieraltowski, PhD, MPH

Praveen Goday, MBBS, FAAP

Neville H. Golden, MD, FAAP

Annie G. Goodwin, MD, FAAP

Carol L. Greene, MD, FAAP

Frank R. Greer, MD, FAAP

Ian J. Griffin, MD

Ann P. Guillot, MD, FAAP

Laura Hamilton, MA, RD, LD

Lyndsay A. Harshman, MD

Craig L. Jensen, MD, FAAP

Susan L. Johnson, PhD

Daniel S. Kamin, MD

Jess L. Kaplan, MD

Jeffrey M. Karp, DMD

Jae Kim, MD, PhD, FAAP

Ronald E. Kleinman, MD, FAAP

Pamela J. Kling, MD, FAAP

Nancy F. Krebs, MD, FAAP

David M. Krol, MD, MPH, FAAP

Michele LaBotz, MD, FAAP

Elena Ladas, PhD, RD

Anna M. Larson, MD

Maureen M. Leonard, MD

Lynne L. Levitsky, MD, FAAP

C. Wesley Lindsey, MD, FAAP

Alejandro Llanos-Chea, MD

Jennifer A. Lowry, MD, FAAP

Julie C. Lumeng, MD

Sheela N. Magge, MD, FAAP

Maria Makrides, PhD

Martin G. Martin, MD, MPP

Joan Younger Meek, MD, RD, FAAP

Nilesh M. Mehta, MD

Russell J. Merritt, MD, PhD, FAAP

Aeri Moon, MD

Kathleen J. Motil, MD, PhD, FAAP

Marialena Mouzaki, MD, MSc

Robert D. Murray, MD, FAAP

Shweta Namjoshi, MD, MPH

Brandon M. Nathan, MD

Josef Neu, MD, FAAP

Theresa A. Nicklas, DrPH

Rachelle F. Nuss, MD, FAAP

Beth Ogata, MS, RD, CSP

Irene E. Olsen, PhD, RD

Carol O'Neil, PhD, MPH, RD

Cria Perrine, PhD

Heidi H. Pfeifer, RD, LDN

Sarah B. Phillips, MS, RD, LD

Jacquelyn M. Powers, MD, MS, FAAP

Debra S. Regier, MD

Sue J. Rhee, MD

Paul Rogers, MBA, FRCPC, MB

Ellen S. Rome, MD, MPH, FAAP

Daniel E. Roth, MD, FAAP

Meghana N. Sathe, MD

Kelley Scanlon, PhD, RD

Sarah Jane Schwarzenberg, MD, FAAP

Robert J. Shulman, MD, FAAP

Scott H. Sicherer, MD, FAAP

Valery Soto, MS, RD

Jay R. Thiagarajah, MD

Elizabeth A. Thiele, MD, PhD

Vasundhara D. Tolia, MD

Carol C. Wagner, MD

Cassandra Walia, CD, CNS, CMS, RD

Wendy Wittenbrook, MA, RD, LD

Robert Young, RPh

Babette S. Zemel, PhD

Table of Contents

V NUTRIENT DELIVERY SYSTEMS

VI NUTRITION IN ACUTE AND CHRONIC ILLNESS

VII NUTRITION AND PUBLIC HEALTH

APPENDICES

Chapter 1

Nutrition for the 21st Century—Integrating Nutrigenetics, Nutrigenomics, and Microbiomics

Introduction

The importance of nutrition influences on human health and disease at the genetic and molecular levels are becoming increasingly clear. Interactions between diet and the genome can affect health and disease via many interconnected pathways including RNA expression (the transcriptome), epigenetics modification (the epigenome), intermediary metabolites (the metabolome including the lipidome and the proteome), and resident microbiological communities in the gastrointestinal tract—the microbiome[1] (see Fig 1.1). Some may even include among these interconnective pathways the so called "inflammasome," beyond the scope of this chapter, which consists of the functional responses receptors and sensors that regulate the activation of the innate immune system in response to infectious microbes and molecules derived from host proteins.[2] Current information and recommendations are largely based on epidemiologic studies of populations in the absence of specific knowledge of the individual's genetics and the individual metabolic response to nutrients, which may result in erroneous nutritional recommendations. One example is the concept "milk, it does the body good," which applies appropriately to all the population during infancy but to half or less of the world's population after infancy and early childhood, when symptoms of lactose intolerance may preclude ingesting dairy products in significant quantities.

Before the sequencing of genomes was completed, the research community was unable to take an integrative approach to explore the role of the diet in disease and well-being. Most experimental designs (including epidemiologic studies) used common, well characterized, but relatively uninformative biomarkers to advance understanding of various disease states. For example, studies aimed at elucidating the molecular mechanisms promoting cardiovascular diseases have primarily used classical biomarkers, such as plasma cholesterol, triglycerides, or C-reactive protein, rather than ones that provide a more accurate and highly predictable assessment of an individual's response to a nutrient or diet over time. The traditional paradigm has been based on epidemiologic and interventional studies, which did not include family history and environmental exposure. This focus resulted in dietary recommendations using the MyPyramid or MyPlate approach for an entire population rather than an 'n=1' (one's self) approach.[3]

Revolutionary developments in genome sequencing (genomics, epigenomics) and high-throughput omics technologies now allow for simultaneous examination of thousands of genes, gene transcripts, proteins, and intermediate metabolites, as well as the genome of gut microorganisms. Advances in computer technology (bioinformatics) permit the analysis of this massive database, enabling the research community to take an integrative approach to explore the role of diet in health and disease.[1] Individual nutrient-gene-environmental interactions have become critical in this regard and may eventually supplant the traditional dietary guidelines approach. This includes knowledge of an individual nutrient's contributions to phenotypic and epigenetic interactions through various molecular targets, including DNA, RNA, proteins, and various metabolites. The schema in Fig 1.1 leads to the obvious conclusion that gene-nutrient interactions can follow different but interrelated pathways that lead to different phenotypes on the basis of individual variations and environmental stimuli. Accordingly, closely related fields that include nutrigenetics, nutrigenomics,

Fig 1.1.

The environment and the diet interact via nutrigenetics with the human genome and its closely related epigenome and microbiome to influence health and disease via nutrigenomics effects.

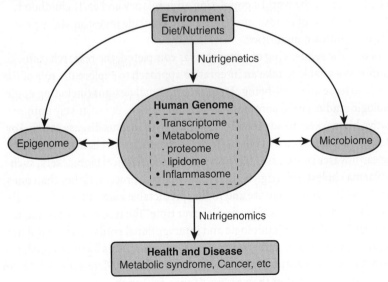

metabolomics, and microbiomics have a common goal, to elucidate the interaction between diet and genes to optimize health through the personalization of diet.[1]

Nutrigenetics

Human beings are not genetically identical and live in different environments. Thus, each person's response to diet would not be expected to be equivalent. Nutrigenetics refers to gene-nutrient interactions and how an individual responds to a certain diet on the basis of one's genome and, thus, considers many underlying genetic polymorphisms.[4]

The following are examples of gene-nutrient interactions:

1. For decades, dietary interventions have been required of individuals with phenylketonuria or galactosemia. These "inborn errors of metabolism" are caused by a single-gene defect that responds to dietary treatment with a low-phenylalanine or low-galactose diet. Phenylketonuria is characterized by the defective phenylalanine hydroxylase (PAH) enzyme, resulting in the accumulation of phenylalanine in the blood, which drastically increases the risk of neurologic damage. Galactosemia is caused by a rare recessive trait in galactose-1-phosphate uridyltransferase (GALT), leading to the accumulation of galactose in the blood and increasing the risk of mental retardation. Galactose-free or phenylalanine-restricted tyrosine-supplemented diets are a means to treat these monogenic diseases nutritionally.

2. Individuals with certain mutations in the enzyme 5,10-methylenetetrahydrofolate reductase (MHTFR) respond idiosyncratically to folate if they consume the recommended intakes of folate established by the dietary guidelines. A specific thermolabile variant of this enzyme, which elevates blood homocysteine levels, has been described in 5% to 15% of the population. This variant is associated with a hypercoagulable state and an increased risk of pregnancy loss and birth defects. Using red cell and plasma folate concentrations, it has been found that folate concentrations are low in nonpregnant women and even lower in pregnant women with a homozygous variant of this gene.[5] Dietary intervention with methlyfolate supplementation requires closer observation of pregnant women with this variant.

3. Intestinal fatty acid binding protein (IFABP) is exclusively expressed in the small intestine. IFABP is believed to bind and transport long-chain fatty acids (LCFAs) in the cytoplasm of columnar absorptive epithelial

small intestine.[6] A polymorphism at codon 54 of the IFABP gene (Ala54Thr), resulting in a change from alanine to threonine, has been associated with a heightened affinity to bind LCFAs with increase secretion into the circulation. The AlaThr54 allele has also been associated with impaired insulin action and increased fat oxidation in several populations. Healthy Pima Indian people homozygous for the gene AlaThr54 have higher plasma concentrations of nonesterified fatty acids (NEFAs) and an increased insulin response after the consumption of a meal with high fat content.[7] This suggests that the effects of IFABP polymorphisms on LCFA transport may compromise health by modulating the bioavailability of dietary components.

These examples of single-gene disorders tend to be relatively rare, with an incidence of less than 1 in 1000 births. On the other hand, chronic health disorders that affect very large segments of the population are associated with polygenetic and multifactorial behavioral and environmental causes that are now being examined using genome-wide association studies. Examples of such chronic health conditions include obesity, coronary heart disease, diabetes mellitus, various cancers, and autoimmune diseases. The high prevalence of these conditions emphasizes the need to better understand their genetic-environmental-dietary determinants. Ultimately, it is possible that this information will move policy away from whole population-based dietary reference intakes and toward a more tailored approach. Dietary intervention to prevent the onset of such diseases is complex and will require not only knowledge of how a single nutrient may affect a biological system but also how a complex mixture of nutrients (ie, diet) will interact to modulate biological functions.[1]

Nutrigenomics

Nutrigenomics refers to the study of the effects of how diet (food and food constituents) may alter an individual's gene expression and encompasses nutritional factors that protect the genome from damage.[8] Interactions between the diet and the genome can effect health and disease via many interconnected pathways including RNA expression (transcriptome), epigenetics modification (epigenome), intermediary metabolites (metabolome), lipids (lipidome), proteins (proteome), and resident microbiological communities in the gastrointestinal tract (microbiome).[1] Nutrigenomics uses functional omics technology (high pass-through technology) to probe a biological system following a nutritional stimulus, which permits a better

Pediatric Nutrition, 8th Edition

understanding of how nutritional molecules affect multiple metabolic pathways and homeostatic control.[8] High-throughput screening tools, as in "arrayed" functional genomic libraries, are being used in nutrigenomics studies that enable millions of genetic screening tests to be conducted at a single time. These libraries include genomic, epigenomic, transcriptomic, nutrimetabolomic (including lipidomic and proteomic), and microbiomic data.[1] Nutrigenomics has the potential to identify genetic predictors of disease from relevant responses to diet. Examples include: (1) how an individual will adapt to increased dietary cholesterol intake by increasing 3-hydroxy-3-methylglutaryl coenzyme A (HMG-CoA) reductase concentrations; (2) how different levels of carbohydrate intake in early life might predispose an individual to metabolic syndrome in adulthood; and (3) how caloric restriction might result in an increased lifespan. All of this should be applicable to the concept of personalized nutrition, although at the present time, this potential is largely unrealized and the evidence base is very limited (see subsequent discussion).[9] As recently pointed out, more than one third of the searchable articles on PubMed on nutrigenomics are review articles.[1]

Transcriptomics

A first step in understanding the health implications of diet-related gene expression is measuring changes related to nutrient exposure. Transcriptomics is a very important part of nutrigenomics that applies omics technology to the transcriptases of messenger RNA emanating from multiple tissues. This technology includes characterizing messenger RNA, important in identifying functional pathways for various proteins, as well as identifying functional clustering of related genes and gene products. A large part of the transcriptome is noncoding RNA, which is not translated into functional proteins. These small RNAs have important signaling functions to regulate gene expression.[1]

Epigenomics

Although much emphasis is being placed directly on nutrient-gene interactions, epigenetic mechanisms mediate many of the effects of diet on gene expression and regulation as well as overall nutritional status. Dietary exposures can have consequences for health years or decades later, as seen in various epidemiologic studies. Epigenetics has raised questions about the mechanisms through which such exposures are "remembered" as pathogenic factors for common complex and chronic diseases, not only in the individual but also for subsequent generations. Epigenetics encompasses changes that may alter gene expression but do not involve changes in the primary DNA sequence. These include 3 distinct but closely interacting mechanisms—DNA methylation, histone modifications, and noncoding microRNAs (miRNAs) (Fig 1.2).[10,11]

Epigenetic mechanisms have been implicated in early nutritional programming in utero or by early life environmental stimuli that cause adaptations, such as a "thrifty phenotype" as a response to nutritional deprivation. These adaptations may persist into childhood and adult years even though

Fig 1.2.

Epigenetic mechanisms: 3 major mechanisms for epigenetic alterations in gene expression have been described. Reproduced with permission from Zaid SK, Young DW, Montecino MA, et al. Mitotic bookmarking of genes: a novel dimension to epigenetic control. *Nature Rev Genet.* **2010;11(8):583-589.**[11]

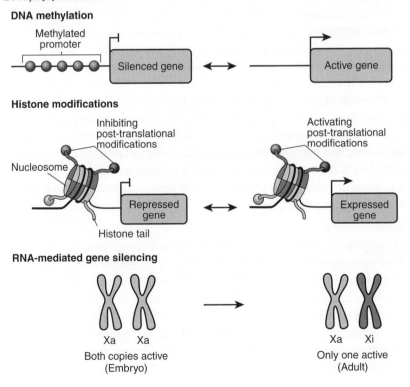

they are no longer needed (eg, when there is an abundance of food). The persistence of this adaptation is thought to contribute to the development of the metabolic syndrome in some adults. Similarly, changes in the nutritional status of pregnant women in The Gambia in dry versus wet seasons have been associated not only with changes in circulating maternal methyl donor metabolites but also effect changes in DNA methylation patterns in the genome of the exposed offspring.[12]

There is growing evidence that numerous dietary factors, including micronutrients and nonnutrient dietary components, can modify epigenetic markers. As noted previously, in cases in which the altered dietary supply of methyl donors effects DNA methylation, there are plausible explanations for the observed epigenetic changes; however, to a large extent, the mechanisms responsible for diet-epigenome-health relationships remain to be discovered. Because there are approximately 1 million sites within the human genome for DNA methylation to occur,[13] specific epigenetic biomarkers that cause disease versus those that are a consequence of disease are hard to identify, even with high-passthrough technology.[10]

Nutrimetabolomics
Metabolomics offers great potential to understand how different dietary nutrients affect metabolic pathways. Importantly, metabolomics can be used to identify patterns of metabolic profiles among individuals that reflect differences in dietary intake or identify individual metabolic activities that explain variation in dietary responses. Some have speculated the metabolomics can be used to identify biomarkers of dietary intake that overcome some of the shortcomings of dietary assessment tools, such as dietary recalls or intake surveys.[14] Characterizing the metabolome relies on nuclear magnetic resonance (NMR) and mass spectrometry, coupled with other separation techniques. Both lipids and proteins contribute significantly to the metabolome.

Lipidomics uses mass spectrometry-based profiling to characterize comprehensive lipid profiles. It is known that there is a strong relationship between dietary fat intake, circulating lipids, and cardiometabolic outcomes and the host's genetically determined metabolism. Proteomics, characterizing the post-translational modification of proteins with dietary exposure, is very complex. Applications of proteomic technologies, including mass spectroscopy with liquid chromatography, are necessary to understand the relationships between dietary and genetic factors affecting health and disease.[1]

Microbiomics

It is not possible to consider nutrigenetics and nutrigenomics without a consideration of the microbiome. As a contributor to systems biology (see below), the trillions of microorganisms that inhabit the gastrointestinal tract represent a reservoir of genetic material that is significantly greater than that of the human genome, with great interindividual variability. As many as 9.9 million genes have been identified from a database of microbiota.[15] Changes in the microbiome are greatly affected by diet, which appears to be a major short- and long-term regulator of structure and function of the gut. Thus, it is not surprising that the microbial population in each person is unique, although significant similarities can be found among individuals living in the same environment or with similar dietary and behavioral characteristics. Its functional capacity is relatively consistent in healthy people with pathways involved in metabolism, fermentation, methanogenesis, oxidative phosphorylation, and lipopolysaccharide biosynthesis.[15]

Microbiomics and omics technology allow for study of the complex interactions between the human genome, the genome of the gut bacteria, and functional consequences such as the response of the gut immune system (the inflammasome[2]). The gut microbiome performs many metabolic activities not encoded by the human genome, including producing energy from "nondigestible" carbohydrates, producing a number of water-soluble B vitamins, modulating the immune system, influencing lipid metabolism (small-chain fatty acids) including adipogenesis, and affecting the coagulation system via the synthesis of vitamin K_2 (menaquinones). The study of interaction of the diet and the microbiota is an intense area of investigation, and the effect of the microbiome on nutritional health will, without a doubt, prove to be of great importance.[16]

Systems Biology, Personalized Nutrition, and the Future

Along with the various "omics" approaches, another new paradigm is the use of "systems biology" to understand biological phenomena. This all-encompassing approach is being used to further advance the understanding of complete sets of circumstances rather than the more limited classic approach. In the classic or reductionist approach, as many variables as possible are controlled, while altering one stimulus and determining its effect on a dependent variable. This provides limited information as to how complex systems relate to one another. The integration of all information at the different levels of genomic expression (transcriptomics, metabolomics [see Fig 1.1]) provides the capacity to measure perturbations of the pathways resulting from nutritional influences. Systems approaches accomplish this in that they model, analyze, and attempt to relate complex biological and chemical systems at multiple levels.[14] Systems approaches integrate data from a variety of experimental platforms to provide insight into the molecular and chemical interactions and cellular phenotypes and disease processes. These approaches incorporate the ability to obtain, integrate, and analyze complex data from multiple experimental sources using interdisciplinary tools. The experimental techniques that most suit systems biology are those that are system wide and attempt to be as complete as possible. Therefore, transcriptomics, metabolomics, proteomics, lipomics, microbiomics, and high-throughput screening techniques are used to collect quantitative data for the construction and validation of models. These technologies are still emerging, and many face the problem in that the larger the quantity of data produced, the lower the quality of the data. Computational biologists, statisticians, mathematicians, computer scientists, engineers, and physicists are working to improve the quality of these approaches.[14] Systems biology has the potential to increase our knowledge of the nutritional influences on metabolic pathways and homeostasis and how this regulation is disturbed in diet-related disease, as well as to what extent individual genotypes contribute to such diseases.[17]

The prevalence of food-related diseases such as obesity, type 2 diabetes mellitus, and coronary heart disease, are on the rise in industrialized nations. A primary reason for the increase in these diseases is thought be changes in lifestyle—an abundance of food coupled with low levels of physical activity. The observed differences in an individual's response to diet have been attributed to differences in the underlying genetic makeup, prompting exploration into the role of nutrient-gene interactions in the determination of a healthy phenotype. An important goal of nutrigenetics, nutrigenomics, microbiomics, and the understanding of systems biology is referred to as "personalized nutrition." Personalized nutrition will lead to an understanding of physiology and disease by integrating and considering molecular pathways, regulatory networks, cells, tissues, organs, the microbiome, and ultimately, the whole organism.[18,19] Personalized nutrition should have the potential to improve quality of life and to reduce morbidity and mortality. Such an integrated approach should result in the ability to identify important relationships between diet and health with targeted modification of an individual's dietary intake. Although this is a worthy health care goal with great potential, it remains elusive at the present time. Current evidence does not yet demonstrate that personalized nutritional advice leads to an improved health outcomes compared with just following the current, more widely based dietary guidelines.[1,16] The technical and ethical challenges of this goal are daunting. Equally as difficult will be the storage, management, and interpretation of the vast quantity of individualized "omics" data required. Working toward this ultimate of goals, the study of human nutrition will continue to be exciting and rewarding.

References

1. Ferguson JF, Allayee H, Gerszten RE, et al. Nutrigenomics, the microbiome, and gene-environment interactions: new directions in cardiovascular disease research, prevention, and treatment. *Circ Cardiovasc Genet.* 2016;9(3):291–313

2. Kanneganti T-D. The inflammasome: firing up innate immunity. *Immunol Rev.* 2015;265(1):1–5

3. van der Greef J, Hankemeier T, McBurney RN. Metabolomics-based systems biology and personalized medicine: moving towards n = 1 clinical trials? *Pharmacogenomics.* 2006;7(7):1087–1094

4. Simopoulos AP. Nutrigenetics/nutrigenomics. *Ann Rev Public Health.* 2010;31 (1):53–68

5. Lucock MD. Synergy of genes and nutrients: the case of homocysteine. *Curr Opin Clin Nutr Metab Care.* 2006;9(6):748–756

6. Pratley RE, Baier L, Pan DA, et al. Effects of an Ala54Thr polymorphism in the intestinal fatty acid-binding protein on responses to dietary fat in humans. *J Lipid Res.* 2000;41(12):2002–2008

7. Ågren JJ, Vidgren HM, Valve RS, Laakso M, Uusitupa MI. Postprandial responses of individual fatty acids in subjects homozygous for the threonine- or alanine-encoding allele in codon 54 of the intestinal fatty acid binding protein 2 gene. *Am J Clin Nutr.* 2001;73(1):31–35

8. Mead MN. Nutrigenomics: the genome–food interface. *Environ Health Perspect.* 2007;115(12):A582–A589

9. Arab L. Individualized nutritional recommendations: do we have the measurements needed to assess risk and make dietary recommendations? *Proc Nutr Soc.* 2004;63(01):167–172

10. McKay JA, Mathers JC. Diet induced epigenetic changes and their implications for health. *Acta Physiol.* 2011;202(2):103–118

11. Zaidi SK, Young DW, Montecino MA, et al. Mitotic bookmarking of genes: a novel dimension to epigenetic control. *Nature Rev Genet.* 2010;11(8):583–589

12. Dominguez-Salas P, Moore SE, Baker MS, et al. Maternal nutrition at conception modulates DNA methylation of human metastable epialleles. *Nature Commun.* 2014;5:3746

13. Greally JM, Drake AJ. The current state of epigenetic research in humans. *JAMA Pediatr.* 2017;171(2):103–104

14. Claus SP, Swann JR. Nutrimetabonomics: applications for nutritional sciences, with specific reference to gut microbial interactions. *Ann Rev Food Sci Technol.* 2013;4(1):381–399

15. Lynch SV, Pedersen O. The human intestinal microbiome in health and disease. *N Engl J Med.* 2016;375(24):2369–2379

16. O'Connor EM. The role of gut microbiota in nutritional status. *Curr Opin Clin Nutr Metab Care.* 2013;16(5):509–516

17. Panagiotou G, Nielsen J. Nutritional Systems biology: definitions and approaches. *Ann Rev Nutr.* 2009;29(1):329–339

18. Butcher EC, Berg EL, Kunkel EJ. Systems biology in drug discovery. *Nat Biotechnol.* 2004;22:1253–1259

19. Desiere F. Towards a systems biology understanding of human health: Interplay between genotype, environment and nutrition. *Biotechnol Annu Rev.* 2004; 10:51–84

Feeding The Infant

Chapter 2

Development of Gastrointestinal Function

The gastrointestinal tract assimilates environmental nutrients for the purposes of homeostasis, growth, and development through its intricate physiological and mechanical design. The absorptive capacity of the gut is determined by multiple variables, including its surface area, transport ability, perfusion, motility, and microbiome.

Development of the Gastrointestinal Tract

Gastrulation begins in the third week of gestation and establishes the 3 germ layers: ectoderm, mesoderm, and endoderm.[1] The mammalian digestive tract forms soon after the embryo undergoes cephalocaudal and lateral folding, incorporating a portion of the endoderm-lined yolk sac cavity into the embryo. This forms the primitive gut and its 3 parts: foregut, midgut, and hindgut.[2] Throughout embryogenesis, the gut lumen seals and recanalizes several times for the purpose of elongation.

The lining of the digestive tube and its glands is generated by endodermal cells. Endodermal cells also derive the parenchyma of the liver, gallbladder, and pancreas.[3] Anterior (cranial) and posterior (caudal) patterning of the gut tube occurs through the expression of several genes (eg, sonic hedgehog [SHH]) that regulate development, and endodermal and mesodermal layers coordinate their differentiation via paracrine signaling between cells of adjacent tissues.[4] Patterning of the human gut endoderm has been recapitulated ex vivo using tissue and stem cell derived organoids, improving our understanding of gut development and disease.[5]

The foregut differentiates into the pharynx, esophagus, and stomach up to the second part of the duodenum and gives rise to the liver and pancreas. Organs of the foregut ingest food and initiate digestion. The midgut is largely responsible for nutrient absorption and gives rise to structures from the third part of the duodenum to the first two thirds of the large intestine. The hindgut gives rise to the remaining third of the large intestine down to the cloaca and urorectal septum, which divides the cloaca into the ventral urogenital sinus and the dorsal anorectal canal. Hindgut structures are responsible for the resorption of water and ions as well expulsion of relatively dehydrated digestive waste.[3]

An intricate network of muscle, nerves, and specialized cells form the gut's motility network.[6,7] These cells together are responsible for propagating a bolus of food from the esophagus to the anus in preparation for excretion. The enteric smooth muscle derives from mesoderm and is layered into the longitudinal muscularis mucosa and circular and longitudinal

muscularis propria. This enteric smooth muscle is dependent on SHH
signaling from the endoderm. The enteric nervous system develops between
gestational weeks 4 and 11 from neural crest-derived cells. These ganglia
migrate in the wall of the bowel rostrocaudally from the foregut to hindgut,
from the outer myenteric plexus to the inner submucosal plexus. Interstitial
cells of Cajal—thought to be the pacemaker of the gut and responsible for
initiating electromechanical coupling—are derived from the mesenchyme
and can be identified as early as week 9 of gestation.[8-11]

The glandular epithelium of the liver and the biliary drainage system,
including the gallbladder, are all formed from the hepatic diverticulum, a
tube of endoderm that extends out from the foregut into the surrounding
mesenchyme.[12] The pancreas develops from the fusion of 2 distinct dorsal
and ventral diverticula, both derived from endodermal cells immediately
caudal to the stomach.[13] Portions of the gut tube and its derivatives are designated intraperitoneal if they are suspended from the dorsal and ventral
body wall by a double layer of peritoneum that enclose and connect them to
the body wall. Organs and portions of the intestinal tube that lie up against
the posterior body wall, covered by peritoneum on their anterior surface
only, are called retroperitoneal. Most of the gut lies intraperitoneally and is
free floating—the exceptions being the majority of the duodenum and parts
of the colon.[14,15]

Developmental Disorders

Complications of embryogenesis constitute a significant portion of the
barriers to oral and enteral feeding seen in neonates and infants, yet their
molecular basis has been infrequently defined. Esophageal abnormalities
include esophageal atresia, stenosis, tracheoesophageal fistula, and laryn-
gotracheal clefts. These disorders complicate infant feeding and respiration
as they result in dysphagia. Stomach malformations include duplication
and prepyloric septum. Less commonly, gastric atresia, gastric volvulus,
and gastric diverticula can occur, resulting in recurrent emesis, reflux, or
obstruction. Duodenal atresia and stenosis are believed to be the result of
incomplete recanalization of the intestinal lumen. Less commonly, duodenal stenosis or obstruction may result from compressive lesions such vascular malformations, webs, or the annular pancreas. Normally, the primary
intestinal loop rotates 270° counterclockwise during embryogenesis. Failure
of the gut to rotate fully, or its reverse rotation, results in malrotation and
predisposes the child to volvulus.[14-16] Jejunal and ileal atresias are generally thought to result from vasoconstrictive or thrombotic accidents in the
mesenteric blood supply, although genetic causes have been identified,

including an association with cystic fibrosis.[17] Herniation of abdominal contents is categorized into 2 forms—gastroschisis, which results in bowel in the amniotic cavity; and omphalocele, in which abdominal contents are located in an enlarged umbilical ring—and both may result in atresia. Anorectal atresias and congenital fistulas are caused by abnormalities in formation of the cloaca and ectopic positioning of the anal opening. Imperforate anus occurs because of improper recanalization of the lower portion of the anal canal.[14-16]

Disordered development of motility, including congenital aganglionosis (or Hirschsprung disease), can also present a barrier to enteral feeding and result in dependency on intravenous nutrition support. Hirschsprung disease is caused by abnormal migration of neural crest cells in the bowel wall and is the most common developmental disorder of motility. Disordered development of smooth muscle, enteric neurons, or interstitial cells of Cajal can also lead to dysmotility and congenital chronic intestinal pseudoobstruction. Aerodigestive reflexes and the migrating motor complex can be delayed in premature and asphyxiated infants, increasing the preterm infant's risk of both primary aspiration and secondary aspiration.[6]

A variety of developmental disorders of the biliary tract may lead to fat malabsorption and malnutrition, including biliary atresia and biliary duct hypoplasia. The lack of fusion of the 2 pancreatic ducts is called pancreatic divisum. Anatomic abnormalities of the pancreas in children, unlike in adults, may be associated with an increased risk of pancreatitis and insufficiency, leading to malabsorption and recurrent and chronic pancreatitis.[18-20]

Development of the Intestinal Epithelium

The rapid epithelial cell turnover of the gastrointestinal tract continues throughout life. This process is maintained and regulated by stem cells that give rise to both absorptive and secretory epithelial cell lineages.[21] These cells form a clonal population toward the base of crypts, and their activity is regulated by paracrine secretion of growth factors from an array of surrounding cells that comprise the niche. Stem cell division is usually asymmetric, with the production of an identical stem cell and a committed progenitor cell that terminally differentiates into the mature cells of the gut epithelium. Symmetric division may result in either 2 daughter cells, with loss of stem cell function, or formation of 2 stem cells and eventual clonal dominance. The apparent stochastic extinction of some stem cell lines with eventual dominance of a single cell line is called niche succession.[22]

The active intestinal stem cell (aISC) population has been identified, residing within the crypt base. The aISC is surrounded by Paneth and other niche cells that provide a canonical Wnt signal to sustain the proliferative capacity of the ISC.[23] In contrast, quiescent intestinal stem cells (qISCs) transform to aISCs following destruction of the aISC after various types of injury (ie, radiation, medication, or immune mediated). These qISCs have a critical role in the repair of the injured gut.[24] aISCs produce proliferating transit-amplifying and progenitor cells that differentiate and form all of the mature cells along the crypt-villus axis.

The epithelial cell lineages derived from the intestinal stem cells include the abundant columnar enterocytes that are specialized for absorption and secretion nutrients and electrolytes; goblet cells, for mucin production; and sensory enteroendocrine cells that secrete hormones influencing satiety, nutrient absorption, and motility in response to lumenal carbohydrates and fat.[25] Hormones produced in these cells affect the contraction of the gallbladder, pancreas, enteric smooth muscle, enteric nervous system, and stomach while also affecting satiety via hormone signaling to the brain. Paneth cells have an immune function, secreting lysozymes and antibacterial defensins at the crypt base, keeping the crypt sterile.[26,27] The rarer taste-chemosensory Tuft cells also expand in response to parasite exposure, in an IL-25–dependent process.[28] The M cells, found near Peyer patches, are involved in antigen and microbial passage across an otherwise tight epithelial barrier.[29]

The lamina propria forms the basement membrane, providing a supporting network for the epithelium and regulating epithelial cell function. It contains numerous kinds of cells, including fibroblasts, myofibroblasts, fibrocytes, vascular endothelial, smooth muscle cells, and various immune lineages, including macrophages and lymphocytes. Some of these cells secrete growth factors and cytokines, essential for stem cell proliferation, epithelial cell differentiation, and intestinal immunity.[30,31]

Infant Nutrient Assimilation

The neonatal gut has several major functions. It is obviously an organ of nutrition, with digestive, absorptive, secretory, and motile functions adapted to a milk diet. However, it also has a resident immune system, containing both humoral and cellular elements of the gut-associated lymphoid tissue (GALT). It is a large endocrine organ that secretes local and distally acting gut hormones and paracrine factors to help regulate intestinal growth and metabolic adaptation during extrauterine life.[32] It plays a role in water conservation and electrolyte homeostasis and maintains a symbiotic relationship with microbial flora, which assists in the digestion and absorption of certain nutrients. The intestinal microbiota also plays a vital role in the development of the gut and peripheral immune system.[33]

The neonatal intestine replaces the role of the placenta as a source of nutrients quite abruptly at birth, which is possible because the majority the processes required for nutrient assimilation are intact well before parturition. The neonatal intestine is uniquely capable of absorbing intact macromolecules via endocytosis, a function utilized for the transport of various maternal growth factors imperative for intestinal development.[34,35]

Dietary Fats *(see also Chapter 17: Fats and Fatty Acids)*

Lipids vary considerably in size and polarity, ranging from hydrophobic triglycerides and sterol esters to the more water-soluble phospholipids and cardiolipins. These compounds are distinguished from other dietary macronutrients in that they must undergo specialized processing during digestion, absorption, transport, and storage prior to utilization in cellular metabolism.[36]

Triglycerides (TGs) make up the largest proportion of stored dietary lipids and are either consumed in the diet or made in the liver during anabolism of other macronutrients. TGs are composed of 3 fatty acids esterified onto a glycerol molecule.[37] These fatty acids are generally nonbranched and have an even number of carbons, from 4 to 26. Double bonds are identified relative to the methyl end by the designation "n" or "ω" to indicate the distance from the first bond. For example, ω-6 indicates that the initial double bond is situated between the sixth and seventh carbon atom from the methyl group end. The human biosynthetic process can only insert double bonds at the ω-9 position or higher, thus *essential fatty acids* (EFAs) are those with double bonds at the ω-6 and ω-3 positions. These EFAs include linoleic acid and linolenic acid, which serve as precursors to the polyunsaturated long-chain fatty acids (LCPUFAs), arachidonic acid and docosahexaenoic acid (DHA). Developmentally critical DHA and ecosapentaenoic acid (EPA) are inefficiently derived from the EFAs, and some have suggested a need to supplement them prenatally.[37-39]

Phospholipids are distinct from TGs in that they contain polar head groups that make them amphipathic and, therefore, capable of forming micelles in water. They include glycerol, choline, serine, inositol, and ethanolamine. Sterols, such as cholesterol, are also amphipathic molecules made up of a steroid nucleus and a branched hydrocarbon tail. Although cholesterol is found only in food of animal origin, plants do contain phytosterols that are chemically related to cholesterol.[36]

Fat Digestion

Catabolism of dietary fat begins in the oral and gastric cavity. Lingual and gastric lipases begin preferentially hydrolyzing short-chain fatty acids (SCFAs) and medium-chain fatty acids from TGs, which can be absorbed directly from the stomach.[40,41] Monoglycerides, however, are poorly hydrolyzed in the stomach. The release of long-chain fatty acids (LCFAs) and very long-chain FAs (VLCFAs) requires the presence of bile and pancreatic lipases.

Pancreatic lipase requires the presence of colipase to remove the inhibitory effect of bile salts that are encountered in the proximal small bowel, where it is more active against insoluble, emulsified substrates. A second pancreatic lipase, carboxylase esterase, is more active against micellar (ie, soluble) substrates and is strongly stimulated by bile salts. Bile is composed of bile salts, phospholipids, and sterols. It emulsifies dietary lipids, allows pancreatic lipase to hydrolyze glycerol's ester bonds, and increases the surface area available to enzymes and protects enzymes from proteolysis themselves.

Infant bile differs from the bile of older children and adults in that it has a higher ratio of cholic acid to chenodeoxycholic acid,[42] has a slower synthetic rate, and is primarily conjugated with taurine instead of glycine.[43] The ileal mechanism for transport of cholyltaurine (ie, the expression of the apical sodium-dependent bile acid transporter [ASBT]) is not well-developed in the newborn infant, resulting in poor recycling of bile acids.[44,45] These patterns may not apply to preterm infants, and ongoing research may clarify bile metabolism throughout gestation.[46]

Fat Absorption

Lipids are absorbed in the brush border of the small intestine as free fatty acids, sterols, and monoacylglycerides. This absorption occurs by passive and active transport mechanisms. Recently, CD36, a transporter found in muscle, vascular endothelium, adipose tissue, and the duodenal and jejunal brush border, has been found to be important in the transport and regulation of fatty acids.[47] Once within the enterocyte, fatty acids are resynthesized into TGs in the enterocyte endoplasmic reticulum in preparation for basolateral secretion into chylomicrons. The resultant release of LCFAs into circulation provides the signaling needed to induce satiety and anabolism in the lingual, cerebral, hepatic, pancreatic, and gastric systems.[48]

Fat Assimilation in the Newborn Infant

The lipid content of human milk can vary with maternal diet and postnatal age. On average, human milk consists of approximately 4% fat, mostly in the form of medium-chain triglycerides (MCTs) and long-chain triglycerides (LCTs).[49] Because almost half of the total calories in an infant's diet is derived from fat, the digestion and absorption of fat must be very efficient.[50,51] Both salivary and gastric lipases are produced early in fetal development. Gastric lipase is detectable in the developing fetus as early as 10 weeks' gestation and reaches adult levels by early infancy[52]; yet, neonatal pancreatic and biliary excretion is generally low in early infancy.[53,54] The importance of human milk factors to aid in infant fat digestion is well documented, as hydrolysis of fat has been shown to be more than twice as efficient in breastfed infants compared with formula-fed infants[55] (see also Chapter 3: Breastfeeding).

Dietary Carbohydrates *(see also Chapter 16: Carbohydrate and Dietary Fiber)*

Carbohydrates are a class of substances with a molar ratio of carbon to hydrogen to oxygen of 1:2:1 $[C_n(H_2O)_n]$, plus oligosaccharides, polysaccharides, and the sugar alcohols (sorbitol, maltitol, mannitol, galactitol, and lactitol). Complex carbohydrates include plant starch, animal glycogen, pectin, cellulose, and gum. Simple carbohydrates include the hexose monosaccharides glucose, galactose, and fructose, the disaccharides maltose (glucose-glucose), sucrose (glucose-fructose), and lactose (glucose-galactose), as well as sporadic trioses, tetroses, and pentoses. Pentoses are important constituents of nucleic acids.[56]

Oligosaccharides are generally defined as yielding 3 to 10 monosaccharides at the time of hydrolysis (eg, maltose, isomaltose, maltotriose, maltodextrin), whereas polysaccharides yield more than 10.[57] Starch, by far the most common dietary polysaccharide, consists of only glucose units and is thus designated a glucosan. Starch is composed of 2 homopolymers of glucose: amylose (linear 1-4 linkages) and amylopectin (branched 1-6 and 1-4 linkages).

Carbohydrate Digestion

The digestion of dietary carbohydrates requires complete hydrolysis of poly-, oligo-, and disaccharides, because absorption of carbohydrates in the intestine is limited to the monosaccharides glucose, galactose, and fructose. Digestion begins with salivary *amylase*, which acts only on the interior (1-4) linkages of polysaccharides, not the outer (1-6) linkages, releasing α-disaccharides (eg, maltose) and trisaccharides (eg, maltotriose), and creating large oligosaccharides (eg, dextrins). Dextrins are sugar molecules containing an average of 8 glucose units with one or more outer links, requiring further digestion by glucoamylase. Pancreatic amylase, similar to salivary amylase, cleaves only interior links. The disaccharidases (eg, lactase, and sucrase-isomaltase) are necessary to ultimately yield free monosaccharide molecules.

Carbohydrate Absorption

Glucose is the major source of metabolic energy. As a hydrophilic polar molecule, it relies on transport across the relatively impermeable hydrophobic intestinal brush-border membrane. Transport occurs via both a family of facilitative glucose transporters (GLUTs) as well as active symporters, such as the sodium-glucose cotransporters (SGLTs).[58] GLUTs are membrane integral proteins found on the surface of all cells. They transport glucose down its concentration gradient, and the energy for the transfer comes from dissipation of the concentration difference. The SGLTs allow for glucose transport against the concentration gradient and are expressed mostly in enterocytes of the small intestine and epithelial cells of the kidney's proximal tubule.[59] The transport of glucose up its concentration gradient occurs in the presence of sodium and results in the passive resorption of water.[60] This concept explains the rationale behind oral rehydration solutions (see also Chapter 28: Oral Therapy for Acute Diarrhea).

Galactose shares the same transport mechanisms as glucose in the enterocytes—namely, apical SGLT cotransporters and the basolateral GLUT2. Once it enters the portal blood circulation, it is cleared in its first passage through the liver, where it is converted by galactokinase into galactose-1-phosphate. The latter is then transformed enzymatically into glucose-1-phosphate and converted into glycogen. Lactose is the sole dietary source of galactose in humans, although glucose can be converted into galactose for supply of cellular needs (eg, glycoproteins and mucopolysaccharides).

Fructose is transported across the brush border membrane by the facilitated transporter GLUT5. Fructose malabsorption (hereditary fructose intolerance) is well-documented in infants and toddlers and is associated with diarrhea and abdominal pain.[61] GLUT5 expression is up-regulated with increased dietary intake of fructose. Once absorbed, fructose is delivered to the liver via the portal circulation and is metabolized by the enzyme fructokinase and then cleaved by aldolase to produce glyceraldehyde and dihydroxyacetone phosphate. This catabolism occurs independent of regulation by insulin or feedback from glycolysis.[62] The metabolites ultimately enter the glycolytic pathway and produce glycogen. Small amounts of fructose act catalytically to enhance glucose metabolism, perhaps via activation of glucokinase.[63]

Carbohydrate Assimilation in the Newborn Infant

The concentrations of salivary and pancreatic amylase as well as brush border glucoamylase and disaccharidases (eg, lactase) are low in the neonatal period but increase to mature levels quite rapidly in the postnatal period.[64] Approximately 25% of term neonates exhibit some lactose malabsorption, and lactase activity in the neonatal period appears to be inducible by lactose intake.[65] Lactose malabsorption in the neonate is generally mild and asymptomatic, with malabsorbed lactose salvaged in the colon with bacterial fermentation and production of short-chain fatty acids (SCFAs). Thus, the finite capacity of the neonatal intestine to absorb lactose may serve to promote the growth of intestinal microflora and provide colonocytes with an important nutrient for growth (ie, butyric acid).[66]

Starch digestion is limited in newborn infants, and pancreatic secretion of a-amylase may remain insufficient for several months.[67] Thus, carbohydrate needs in infancy are met largely via the digestion of lactose into glucose and galactose, and the need for α-amylase digestion is minimal until weaning. Weaning is also the time at which all studied nonhuman mammals, and most humans, begin to experience a decline in lactase concentrations.[68] People with lactase persistence are generally of Western European descent. Hypolactasia occurs in most other individuals, as early as 2 years of age in children from Thailand and Bangladesh and 10 years of age for other Asian, African-American, and Latin-American people. For many white people (eg, Finnish, Irish), hypolactasia occurs as a steady and slow decrease.[69,70] Single nucleotide polymorphisms in noncoding regulatory regions of the lactase-phlorizin hydrolase gene modulate binding of transcription factors that mediate lactase expression in an age-dependent manner.[71,72]

Dietary Protein (see also Chapter 15: Protein)

Made of amino acids, proteins direct and facilitate the biochemical reactions of life. Proteins include enzymes, transporters, signaling peptides, and muscle fiber. Protein differs from carbohydrates and fat in that it contains nitrogen—on average, approximately 16% by weight. When amino acids are oxidized in the citric acid (ie, Krebs or tricarboxylic acid) cycle to carbon dioxide and water to produce energy, nitrogen is produced as a waste product and must be metabolized and removed from the body. The body can also use dietary protein for energy, muscle incorporation, or incorporation into other nitrogen-containing compounds.

Amino acids can be converted to glucose via gluconeogenesis to provide a continuous supply of glucose after glycogen stores are consumed. Similar to carbohydrates, oxidation of amino acids produces approximately 4 kcal/g of protein. The carbon skeletons may also be used for formation of fat via elongation of acetyl units and carbohydrates through the conversion of alanine into pyruvate. Amino acids are also incorporated into various products, such as creatine, nitric oxide, purines and pyrimidines, glutathione, porphyrins, histamine, serotonin, nicotinic acid, thyroid hormone, catecholamines, and carnitine, among many others. The inability to use or break down various amino acids has been implicated in congenital metabolic diseases, such as tyrosinemia and maple syrup urine disease.

Consensus on protein requirements in infancy is lacking, with slight variation being seen among the Recommended Dietary Allowance (RDA), the Dietary Reference Intake (DRI), and the American Society for Parenteral and Enteral Nutrition (ASPEN) guidelines for ill children and infants.[73-75] However, all of these guidelines suggest that protein requirements in infancy (approximately 2 g/kg/day) diminish after the first year of life, as the rate of accretion of new protein is reduced. Protein requirements increase during accelerated growth phases, as observed in prematurity (2–3.5 g/kg/day), early childhood (1.8–3 g/kg/day), and adolescence (1.5–2 g/kg/day), as well as in athletes.[76] The metabolic rate of conversion and utilization of individual amino acids differs in the body depending on age, gender, nutrient exposure, and level of activity.[77] Essential amino acids, or amino acids that must be consumed from food as they cannot be anabolized, constitute approximately one third of the protein requirement in infancy, but only about a fifth later in childhood and a tenth in adulthood.[78] The need for high-quality protein, defined by the protein's ability to support growth, also decreases with age to a minimum of 0.8 g/kg/day in late adolescence and adulthood.[79] High-quality proteins characteristically have an abundance of indispensable amino acids, are easily digestible, and lack contaminating molecules such as inhibitors of digestive enzymes (eg, trypsin inhibitors).

Protein Digestion

Digestion of protein begins in the stomach with pepsin secretion in gastric juice. Pepsin output and parietal cell activity are believed to be lower in the neonate than in older infants.[80] Yet, secretion of gastric acid, intrinsic factor, and gastrin is noted as early as the middle of the second gestational trimester, and infants are in fact able to maintain a gastric pH well below 4 from the first day of life.[81-84]

Proteolytic enzymes secreted from the pancreas and intestinal mucosa break down proteins into smaller peptides. Pancreatic excretion begins in utero at about the fifth month of gestation.[85] Although trypsin activity may be lower in the preterm infant,[86] a substantial difference in trypsin concentration in duodenal fluid between 2 days and 7 weeks of age is not observed,[87] and a physiologic trypsin concentration is attained by 1 to 3 months of age.[88] Chymotrypsin activity may also be low in the newborn infant but increases rapidly, approaching the levels of older children at about 6 months of age and adult levels by 3 years of age.[89] Nonetheless, adults can digest protein at a rate approximately 60% faster than children.[90]

Pancreatic digestive enzymes are secreted in the form of zymogens, precursors that are converted into active proteolytic enzymes in the intestinal lumen. Their activity is largely dependent on the amino acid residue composition of the protein ingested. Trypsin is activated from trypsinogen by enterokinase, a brush border enzyme, and it cleaves the C-terminal of positively charged amino acids. It also activates chymotrypsin from chymotrypsinogen. Chymotrypsin cleaves the same bonds as pepsin (the C-terminus of tyrosine, phenylalanine, and tryptophan), which is inactivated by the increased pH of duodenal content. Carboxypeptidase cleaves the amide bond at the C-terminus of aromatic and branched-chain amino acids. Elastase preferentially cleaves peptide bonds at the C-terminal of small, hydrophobic amino acids as well as elastin, found in connective tissue. Nucleases hydrolyze ingested nucleic acids (RNA and DNA) into their component nucleotides.

The oligopeptide products of gastric and pancreatic proteolysis undergo further hydrolysis in the brush border membrane of the small intestine by carboxypeptidase and aminopeptidase. These enzymes hydrolyze the carboxyl and amino terminals of oligopeptides, respectively, releasing tripeptides, dipeptides, and individual amino acids. Tri- and dipeptides can cross the brush border membrane to be hydrolyzed intracellularly by tri- and dipeptidases. Activity of carboxypeptidase, aminopeptidase, tripeptidase, and dipeptidase is detectable in fetal intestine as early as the second trimester of gestation.[91]

Protein Absorption
Free amino acids are absorbed by amino-acid specific active transporters into the mucosa. Several transport systems are ubiquitously expressed and exhibit preference for certain amino acids. Systems *A* and *ASC*, for example, prefer amino acids with small side chains (eg, glycine, alanine, serine). System *L* transports amino acids with bulky side chains (eg, tyrosine, arginine, valine, asparagine, glutamine). The *B* system (eg, $B^{O,+}$, b^+), which has broad specificity for neutral amino acids, is produced in the small intestine.[92] Other specific amino acid transport systems in the intestine include *IMINO* (proline and glycine) and *rBAT* (cystine and dibasic amino acids). The transport of amino acids across the mucosa of the small intestine has been shown in fetuses as young as 12 weeks.[93]

Protein Assimilation in the Newborn Infant
Larger peptides and proteins can enter the gut intact. The adult intestine absorbs about a quarter of its dietary protein as dipeptides and tripeptides, utilizing intracellular hydrolases to liberate amino acids into the portal blood, but the neonate relies on the transfer of macromolecules to a much greater extent. Macromolecules from maternal milk include enzymes, growth factors, and immunoglobulins that help shape the neonate's digestive, immunologic, and barrier function. Macromolecules can cross the intestinal epithelium either transcellularly or paracellularly. Endocytosis, a transcellular pathway, is the major pathway for macromolecules to cross the mucosal brush border.[94] The paracellular passage of macromolecules across "leaks" between epithelial cell junctions (ie, tight junctions) remains controversial.

The uptake of macromolecules by the neonatal gut may represent the persistence of intrauterine absorptive processes, as the amniotic fluid is known to contain a number of types of protein macromolecules, including immunoglobulins, hormones, enzymes, and growth factors. The small intestine is noted to be more permeable to intact proteins in the neonatal period, and infant serum often contains higher titers of antibodies to food antigens than the serum of adults.[95] Evidence suggests that the epithelial IgG receptor (FCGRT) facilitates the recycling of IgG in the intestinal lumen and systemic endothelial cells, including antigen-immunoglobulin complexes, and accounts for the extraordinary half-life of IgG and albumin in the serum.[96]

Micronutrients *(see also Chapter 18: Calcium, Phosphorus, and Magnesium; Chapter 20: Trace Elements; and Chapters 21.I And 21.II: Vitamins)*

Fat-soluble micronutrients such as prostaglandins and vitamins A, D, E, and K are emulsified within lipid and cross the mucosal brush border membrane as lipophilic molecules. Water-soluble vitamins cross the intestinal brush border membrane by the action of specific carrier-mediated transport. These include the sodium-dependent multivitamin transporter (SMVT), which is produced by enterocytes and transports vitamins such as B complex and pantothenate.[97] Vitamin C (L-ascorbic acid) transport occurs via a sodium-dependent L-ascorbic acid transporter (SVCT1). Thought to be essential in diminishing oxidant injury in rapidly growing tissue, vitamin C serum concentrations decline rapidly postpartum. Thus, SVCT1 expression in neonates may be of vital importance for vitamin C regulation.[98,99]

Most mineral absorption depends on specific carrier-mediated transport as well. Mineral accretion in the fetus occurs exponentially during the last trimester of gestation, increasing the risk of mineral deficiencies in the preterm infant. The transport of calcium is sensitive to the presence and abundance of other nutrients, such as lactose and fatty acids.[100-102] The impact of calcium on newborn bone mineral content (BMC) depends on several factors, including maternal vitamin D levels, gestational age, fetal size, and maternal glucose homeostasis.[103] Infants of mothers with diabetes have low BMC at birth, implying that factors in pregnancy have an effect on fetal BMC or that decreased transplacental mineral transfer may occur, because otherwise BMC is consistently increased with increased newborn weight and length. Moreover, although race and gender differences in BMC appear early in life, they do not appear to exist at birth.

Young animals absorb iron, lead, and calcium much better than do adults.[104,105] Iron is absorbed in the stomach and duodenum by a divalent cation metal transporter, DMT1.[106] The specificity of this apical enterocyte transporter is limited to the reduced or ferrous form of iron. However, it can transport other divalent cationic minerals, such as zinc, copper, manganese, nickel, lead, cobalt, and cadmium. Its affinity for lead makes human infants at greater risk than adults for lead toxicity.[107]

Human Milk *(see also Chapter 3: Breastfeeding)*

The relationship between lactating mammary function and neonatal gastrointestinal function is an example of the parallel evolution of 2 organs that, after birth, together undertake functions previously performed by the placenta.[108] Human milk contains nutrients required by the newborn infant for energy and metabolism as well as nonnutritional components that promote infant health, growth, and development. Nonnutritional components of human milk include antimicrobial factors, digestive enzymes, hormones, trophic factors, immune factors, probiotics, microbial substrate, and growth modulators. Energy nutrients include metabolic fuel (eg, fat, protein, and carbohydrates), free water, micronutrients, and other raw materials required for development. With the exception of vitamin D, which should be supplemented for all exclusively breastfed infants,[109] the nutrient content of human milk is complete and serves the nutrient needs of healthy full-term infants as an exclusive feeding for the first 4 to 6 months of life.

More than 98% of the fat in human milk is in the form of triglycerides, made within the mammary glands from medium- and long-chain fatty acids. Oleic acid (18:1) and palmitic acid (16:0) are the most abundant fatty acids, with palmitic acid occupying the central position of the glycerol molecule in most human milk TGs, a property that increases its overall digestibility.[110] Similarly high proportions of EFAs, including ARA and DHA, are also present.[111] These LCPUFAs are constituents of brain and neural tissue and are needed in early life for mental and visual development.[112] Studies have established that plasma and red blood cell LCPUFA levels of infants fed formulas supplemented with both ω-6 and ω-3 LCPUFA was closer to the status of breastfed infants than to that of infants fed formulas containing no LCPUFA.[113,114] The prebiotic and antimicrobial roles of uniquely paired human milk oligosaccharides (HMOs) are also currently being explored, with complex variation and incredible diversity being noted among mother-infant pairs and throughout lactation. Additionally, it is believed that fucosylation of lactose at the reducing end of HMOs may determine the HMO's antimicrobial or prebiotic properties and may be genetically determined.[115]

Proteins account for approximately 75% of the nitrogen-containing compounds in human milk. Nonprotein nitrogen substances include urea, nucleotides, peptides, free amino acids, and DNA. The proteins of human milk can be divided into 2 categories: micellar caseins and aqueous whey proteins, present in the ratio of approximately 20:80. Proteomic studies show great diversity in the function of these predominant whey proteins, including distributed roles for immunity and metabolism throughout the first year of lactation.[116]

The predominant casein forms micelles of relatively small volume and produces a soft, flocculent curd in the infant's stomach. Certain human milk proteases, such as plasmin, which is highly active against casein, increase infant capacity for protein digestion.

Other important proteins found in human milk are lactalbumin, lacto-ferrin, and secretory immunoglobulin A (IgA), with a large number of other proteins present in smaller amounts. Secretory IgA is the principal immu-noglobulin of human milk and, together with lactoferrin, represents about 30% of all milk protein.[117,118] It is synthesized in the mammary epithelial cell when 2 IgA molecules, produced locally by lymphocytes resident in breast tissue, are coupled with 2 proteins, a J-chain, and a secretory component produced from the polymeric IgA receptor. The specificity of human milk secretory IgA antibodies reflects the mother's exposure to various antigens and targets commensal microorganisms.[119,120] Lactoferrin, which transports and promotes the absorption of iron, is also a bacteriostatic agent.[118]

The principal carbohydrate of human milk is lactose, a disaccharide man-ufactured in the mammary epithelial cell from glucose by a reaction involv-ing lactalbumin.[121] In addition, human milk contains significant quantities of oligosaccharides, predominantly lactose-N-tetraose and its monofucosyl-ated derivatives, representing approximately 10% of total milk carbohydrate. Oligosaccharides can escape luminal digestion and are believed to serve as growth factors for intestinal microflora and colonocytes.[122,123] They also alter bacterial adhesion to intestinal epithelial cells.[124,125]

In addition to energy nutrients, human milk contains a wealth of bioactive components that have beneficial yet nonnutritional functions. Nonnutrient factors compensate for the neonate's immature digestive and barrier functions and modulate the transition from intrauterine to extrauterine life. These factors include a wide range of specific and nonspe-cific antimicrobial factors, cytokines and anti-inflammatory substances, as well as hormones, growth modulators, and digestive enzymes. These components may be of particular importance for young infants, because the digestive system and host defense are still immature and susceptible to infection.[125]

Human milk lipases include bile salt-stimulated lipase (BSSL), which is made in the mammary glands and remains inactive until coming in contact with bile salts in the infant's duodenum. BSSL survives the stomach milieu and is activated in the duodenum by bile acids to convert monoglycerides to glycerol and free fatty acids.[126] Without BSSL, the monoglyceride load would likely exceed neonatal absorptive capacity, and much would escape unabsorbed. The importance of BSSL is supported by a study of low birth weight preterm infants who were fed raw versus heat-treated human milk. Fat absorption was significantly higher in the former group compared with the latter.[127] Other lipases are also present in human milk, such as lipoprotein lipase.[128]

Of the trophic factors active in the newborn infant, epidermal growth factor (EGF) is the best studied. A small polypeptide with mitogenic, antisecretory, and cytoprotective properties, EGF is present in amniotic fluid and colostrum, suggesting that it plays an important role in perinatal adaptation to extrauterine nutrition and gut function.[129] Its roles in activating mucosal function, diminishing gastric hydrolysis of potentially useful milk macromolecules, and protecting the gut epithelium from autodigestion are well described.[130,131] EGF has also been implicated in the induction of lactase secretion and the repression of sucrase activity.[132] Glucagon-like peptide 2 (GLP-2) is another trophic factor, thought to derive from L cells in the small bowel, and may have a role in nutrient assimilation and gut growth in infancy.[133]

Pancreatic lipase secretion in the preterm infant is only approximately 10% of an adult's, and the bile salt pool is only about 50% of that found in the mature neonate.[134] The depressed pancreatic exocrine function ensures that the immature microvillus membrane is spared digestion by pancreatic proteolytic enzymes, and permits prolonged activity of essential brush border enzymes and mammary gland factors. The evolutionary advantage of maintaining certain maternal human milk proteins intact is clear. Such infants are able to maintain the function of immunoglobulins and other biologically important peptides, including enzymes such as salivary and human milk amylases and lipases, which are able to continue their activity in the neutral environment of the duodenum even after temporary inactivation in gastric pH.

A sufficient proportion of antimicrobial proteins is known to escape digestion altogether and emerge in the feces, suggesting that antimicrobial activity continues throughout the length of the infant's gastrointestinal tract. Some antimicrobial components are active both within the breast, minimizing the risk of breast infection and mastitis,[135] as well as within the infant's gastrointestinal and respiratory tracts, protecting the mucosal surfaces from infection by bacteria, viruses, and parasites.[117]

Cytokines in human milk also regulate lactation. The site of action of the peptide feedback inhibitor of lactation, for example, is within the breast itself, its function being the autocrine regulation of milk production.[136] Many bioactive substances also become valuable nutrient sources once they are digested and absorbed.

For most infants, nutrient intake from human milk is sufficient through 4 months of age and becomes increasingly insufficient at about 6 months of age,[137-139] and complementary foods need to be added to the diet (see Chapter 6: Complementary Feeding).

Infant Intestinal Microbiota

The infant gastrointestinal tract is believed to be sterile at birth and subsequently colonized by microbes acquired from birth and the environment.[140,141] The colonization of specific phyla is influenced by many exposures, including location within the gut, mode of delivery, type of feeding, and use of antibiotics. The infant microbiome most certainly also changes when studied over time.[142-145] The microbiome's profound influence on immunology, nutrition, and physiology make some consider it the largest metabolically adaptable and renewable organ in the body.[146]

Current methods used to study the microbiome include analysis of 16s ribosomal RNA and shotgun metagenomic sequencing. The α diversity and β diversity of species can then be measured, helping investigators understand which microbiota are most diverse or rich (α diversity) and which microbiota are most strongly correlated with a given exposure (β diversity).[147] Common exposures currently studied include mode of delivery, antibiotic use, and type of feeding.

Studies suggest that mode of delivery shapes differences between infants in early colonization, with vaginally delivered neonates developing a microbiota that mirrors their mother's vaginal flora and neonates delivered by cesarean section developing a microbiota similar to skin flora. Initial colonization seems to be predominated by facultative anaerobe phyla, such as *Enterobacteriaceae*, and then quickly by obligate anaerobes such as *Bifidobacterium*, *Bacteroides*, and *Clostridiales*.[148] These studies recapitulate older studies showing that infants born via cesarean section are less likely to have a flora enriched with *Bacteroides* organisms, compared with vaginally born infants.[149-151]

Antibiotics can cause a decrease in α diversity immediately after birth, although this effect is inconsistently reproduced among individual children and may not extend beyond the first 6 to 12 months of life.[145,148] Still, long-term consequences of antibiotics are of great interest, because diseases such as obesity have been associated with antibiotic use in animal studies.[152]

Type of feeding may also change the microbial signature. Although breastfed infants and formula-fed infants do not have significantly different a diversity before 12 months of life, formula-fed infants have been shown to have less phylogenetic diversity, bacterial richness, and β diversity between 12 and 24 months.[148] After the introduction of solid foods and with an increased portion of formula being consumed, obligate anaerobes increase until a pattern similar to that seen in adults is achieved, normally by the age of 2 to 3 years.

Longitudinal studies with larger sample sizes are ongoing to determine how, if at all, these patterns change or persist past the age of 2 years, and to determine whether changes in microbial diversity can be persistently associated with exposures from early infancy in humans. For example, some vaginally born infants have an innately "low-*Bacteroides*" signature, with varying responses to exposures such as antibiotics and type of delivery and feeding.[145,148]

The dynamic study of exposure and outcome may lend promising insight into the microbiome-based pathophysiology of a variety of pediatric conditions, including atopic, obesogenic, infectious, and inflammatory diseases.[148,153-155] Future studies will certainly evaluate the microbiome as a therapeutic target for disease modulation as well as a source of understanding for the pathologic basis of disease.

References

1. Spence JR, Lauf R, Shroyer NF. Vertebrate intestinal endoderm development. *Dev Dynamics*. 2011;240(3):501–520

2. Sadler TW, Langman J. Third to eight weeks: the embryonic period. In: Sadler TW, Langman J, eds. *Langman's Medical Embryology*. 13t ed. Baltimore, Maryland: Lippincott Williams & Wilkins; 2015:71–92

3. Sadler TW, Langman J. The gut tube and the body cavities. In: Sadler TW, Langman J, eds. *Langman's Medical Embryology*. 13th ed. Baltimore, Maryland: Lippincott Williams & Wilkins; 2015:95–103

4. Stainier DYR. No organ left behind: tales of gut development and evolution. *Science*. 2005;307(5717):1902–1904

5. Dedhia PH, Bertaux-Skeirik N, Zavros Y, Spence JR. Organoid Models of Human Gastrointestinal Development and Disease. *Gastroenterology*. 2016;150(5): 1098–1112

6. Beckett EA, Young HM, Bornstein JC, Jadcherla SR. Development of gut motility. In: Faure C, Thapar N, Di Lorenzo C, eds. *Pediatric Neurogastroenterology: Gastrointestinal Motility and Functional Disorders in Children*. Cham, Switzerland: Springer International Publishing; 2017:21–37

7. Heanue TA, Burns AJ. Development of the enteric neuromuscular system. In: Faure C, Thapar N, Di Lorenzo C, eds. *Pediatric neurogastroenterology: gastrointestinal motility and functional disorders in children*. Cham, Switzerland: Springer International Publishing; 2017:9–19

8. Huizinga JD, Berezin I, Sircar K, et al. Development of interstitial cells of Cajal in a full-term infant without an enteric nervous system. *Gastroenterology*. 2001;120(2):561–567

9. Ward SM, Sanders KM, Hirst* GDS. Role of interstitial cells of Cajal in neural control of gastrointestinal smooth muscles. *Neurogastroenterol Motil*. 2004;16(s1):112–117

10. Young HM, Ciampoli D, Southwell BR, Newgreen DF. Origin of interstitial cells of Cajal in the mouse intestine. *Developmental Biology*. 1996;180(1):97–107

11. Sanders, Ordog, Koh, Torihashi, Ward. Development and plasticity of interstitial cells of Cajal. *Neurogastroenterol Motil*. 1999;11(5):311–338

12. Davenport M. The liver: anatomy and embryology. In: Kleinman RE, Goulet OJ, Miele-Vergani G, Sanderson IR, Sherman P, B.L. S, eds. *Walker's Pediatric Gastrointestinal Disease*. Vol 2. 5th ed. Hamilton, Ontario: BC Decker Inc; 2008:749–756

13. Lowe M, Whitcomb D. Pancreatic function and dysfunction. In: Kleinman RE, Goulet OJ, Miele-Vergani G, Sanderson IR, Sherman P, Shneider BL, eds. *Walker's Pediatric Gastrointestinal Disease*. Vol 2. 5th ed. Hamilton, Ontario: BC Decker Inc; 2008:1185–1196

14. De Santa BP. The intestine: anatomy and embryology. In: Kleinman RE, Goulet OJ, Miele-Vergani G, Sanderson IR, Sherman P, Shneider BL, eds. *Walker's Pediatric Gastrointestinal Disease*. Vol 2. 5th ed. Hamilton, Ontario: BC Decker Inc; 2008:207–216

15. Thapar N, Roberts DJ. The stomach and duodenum: anatomy, embryology and congenital anomalies. In: Kleinman RE, Goulet OJ, Miele-Vergani G, Sanderson IR, Sherman P, Shneider BL, eds. *Walker's Pediatric Gastrointestinal Disease*. Vol 2. 5th ed. Hamilton, Ontario: BC Decker Inc; 2008:117–126

16. Lloyd DA, Kenny SA. The intestine: congenital anomalies including hernias. In: Kleinman RE, Goulet OJ, Miele-Vergani G, Sanderson IR, Sherman P, Shneider BL, eds. *Walker's Pediatric Gastrointestinal Disease*. Vol 2. 5th ed. Hamilton, Ontario: BC Decker Inc; 2008:217–232

17. Adams SD, Stanton MP. Malrotation and intestinal atresias. *Early Human Dev*. 2014;90(12):921–925

18. Husain SZ, Morinville V, Pohl J, et al. Toxic-metabolic risk factors in pediatric pancreatitis. *J Pediatr Gastroenterol Nutr*. 2016;62(4):609–617

19. Schwarzenberg SJ, Bellin M, Husain SZ, et al. Pediatric chronic pancreatitis is associated with genetic risk factors and substantial disease burden. *J Pediatr.* 2015;166(4):890–896.e891

20. Kumar S, Ooi CY, Werlin S, et al. Risk factors associated with pediatric acute recurrent and chronic pancreatitis. *JAMA Pediatr.* 2016;170(6):562

21. Leedham SJ, Brittan M, McDonald SAC, Wright NA. Intestinal stem cells. *J Cell Molec Med.* 2005;9(1):11–24

22. Yatabe Y, Tavare S, Shibata D. Investigating stem cells in human colon by using methylation patterns. *Proc Natl Acad Sci.* 2001;98(19):10839–10844

23. Sato T, van Es JH, Snippert HJ, et al. Paneth cells constitute the niche for Lgr5 stem cells in intestinal crypts. *Nature.* 2010;469(7330):415–418

24. Yan KS, Gevaert O, Zheng GXY, et al. Intestinal Enteroendocrine Lineage Cells Possess Homeostatic and Injury-Inducible Stem Cell Activity. *Cell Stem Cell.* 2017;21(1):78–90.e76

25. Furness JB, Rivera LR, Cho H-J, Bravo DM, Callaghan B. The gut as a sensory organ. *Nature Rev Gastroenterol Hepatol.* 2013;1010(1212):729–740

26. Bevins CL, Salzman NH. Paneth cells, antimicrobial peptides and maintenance of intestinal homeostasis. *Nature Rev Microbiol.* 2011;9(5):356–368

27. Gounder AP, Myers ND, Treuting PM, et al. Defensins Potentiate a Neutralizing Antibody Response to Enteric Viral Infection. *PLoS Pathogens.* 2016;12(3):e1005474

28. Howitt MR, Lavoie S, Michaud M, et al. Tuft cells, taste-chemosensory cells, orchestrate parasite type 2 immunity in the gut. *Science.* 2016;351(6279):1329–1333

29. Rouch JD, Scott A, Lei NY, et al. Development of Functional Microfold (M) Cells from Intestinal Stem Cells in Primary Human Enteroids. *PLoS One.* 2016;11(1):e0148216

30. Powell DW, Pinchuk IV, Saada JI, Chen X, Mifflin RC. Mesenchymal Cells of the Intestinal Lamina Propria. *Ann Rev Physiol.* 2011;73(1):213–237

31. Neurath MF. Cytokines in inflammatory bowel disease. *Nature Reviews Immunology.* 2014;14(5):329–342

32. Aynsley-Green A. Metabolic and endocrine interrelations in the human fetus and neonate. *Am J Clin Nutr.* 1985;41(2):399–417

33. Houghteling PD, Walker WA. Why is initial bacterial colonization of the intestine important to infants' and children's health? *J Pediatr Gastroenterol Nutr.* 2015;60(3):294–307

34. Menard D. *Growth-Promoting Factors and the Development of the Human Gut.* New York, NY: Raven Press; 1989

35. Weaver LT, Laker MF, Nelson R. Intestinal permeability in the newborn. *Archives of Disease in Childhood.* 1984;59(3):236–241

36. Jones PJH, Kubow S. Lipids, sterols, and their metabolites. In: Shils ME, Shike M, Ross AC, Caballero B, Cousins B, eds. *Modern Nutrition in Health and Disease.* Philadelphia, PA: Lippincott, Williams & Wilkins; 2006:92–122

37. Koletzko B, Lien E, Agostoni C, et al. The roles of long-chain polyunsaturated fatty acids in pregnancy, lactation and infancy: review of current knowledge and consensus recommendations. *J Perinat Med.* 2008;36(1):5–14

38. Martin MA, Lassek WD, Gaulin SJC, et al. Fatty acid composition in the mature milk of Bolivian forager-horticulturalists: controlled comparisons with a US sample. *Matern Child Nutr.* 2012;8(3):404–418

39. Valentine CJ, Morrow G, Pennell M, et al. Randomized controlled trial of docosahexaenoic acid supplementation in Midwestern U.S. human milk donors. *Breastfeed Med.* 2013;8(1):86–91

40. Faber J, Goldstein R, Blondheim O, et al. Absorption of Medium Chain Triglycerides in the Stomach of the Human Infant. *J Pediatr Gastroenterol Nutr.* 1988;7(2):189–195

41. Fink CS, Hamosh P, Hamosh M. Fat Digestion in the Stomach: Stability of Lingual Lipase in the Gastric Environment. *Pediatr Res.* 1984;18(3):248–254

42. Encrantz J-C, Sjövall J. On the bile acids in duodenal contents of infants and children bile acids and steroids 72. *Clin Chim Acta.* 1959;4(6):793–799

43. Heubi JE, Balistreri WF, Suchy FJ. Bile salt metabolism in the first year of life. *J Lab Clin Med.* 1982;100(1):127–136

44. de Belle RC, Vaupshas V, Vitullo BB, et al. Intestinal absorption of bile salts: Immature development in the neonate. *J Pediatr.* 1979;94(3):472–476.

45. Wong M, Oelkers P, Craddock A, Dawson P. Expression cloning and characterization of the hamster ileal sodium-dependent bile acid transporter. *J Biol Chem.* 1994;269(2):1340–1347

46. Kumagai M, Kimura A, Takei H, et al. Perinatal bile acid metabolism: bile acid analysis of meconium of preterm and full-term infants. *J Gastroenterol.* 2007;42(11):904–910

47. Abumrad NA, el-Maghrabi MR, Amri EZ, Lopez E, Grimaldi PA. Cloning of a rat adipocyte membrane protein implicated in binding or transport of long-chain fatty acids that is induced during preadipocyte differentiation. Homology with human CD36. *J Biol Chem.* 1993;268(24):17665–17668

48. Abumrad NA, Davidson NO. Role of the gut in lipid homeostasis. *Physiol Rev.* 2012;92(3):1061–1085

49. Bitman J, Wood L, Hamosh M, Hamosh P, Mehta NR. Comparison of the lipid composition of breast milk from mothers of term and preterm infants. *Am J Clin Nutr.* 1983;38(2):300–312

50. Hamosh M, Scanlon JW, Ganot D, Likel M, Scanlon KB, Hamosh P. Fat digestion in the newborn. *J Clin Invest.* 1981;67(3):838–846

51. Tantibhedhyangkul P, Hashim S. Medium-chain triglyceride feeding in premature infants: effects on fat and nitrogen absorption. *Pediatrics.* 1975;55(3):359–370

52. Sarles J, Moreau H, Verger R. Human gastric lipase: ontogeny and variations in children. *Acta Paediatr.* 1992;81(6–7):511–513

53. Zoppi G, Andreotti G, Pajno-Ferrara F, Njai DM, Gaburro D. Exocrine Pancreas Function in Premature and Full Term Neonates. *Pediatr Res.* 1972;6(12):880–886

54. Brueton MJ, Berger HM, Brown GA, Ablitt L, Iyngkaran N, Wharton BA. Duodenal bile acid conjugation patterns and dietary sulphur amino acids in the newborn. *Gut.* 1978;19(2):95–98

55. Armand M, Hamosh M, Mehta NR, et al. Effect of human milk or formula on gastric function and fat digestion in the premature infant. *Pediatric Research.* 1996;40(3):429–437

56. Keim NL, Levin RJ, Havel PJ. Carbohydrates. In: Shils ME, Shike M, Ross AC, Caballero B, Cousins RJ, eds. *Modern Nutrition in Health and Disease.* Philadelphia, PA: Lippincott Williams & Williams; 2006:62–82

57. Eggermont E. The hydrolysis of the naturally occurring alpha-glucosides by the human intestinal mucosa. *Eur J Biochem.* 1969;9(4):483–487

58. Wright EM, Loo DDF. Coupling between Na+, sugar, and water transport across the intestine. *Ann N Y Acad Sci.* 2006;915(1):54–66

59. Lee WS, Kanai Y, Wells RG, Hediger MA. The high affinitiy of the Na+/glucose cotransporter. Re-evaluation of function and distribution of expression. *J Biol Chem.* 1994;269:12032–12039

60. Loo DDF, Hirayama BA, Meinild A-K, Chandy G, Zeuthen T, Wright EM. Passive water and ion transport by cotransporters. *J Physiol.* 1999;518(1):195–202

61. Hoekstra JH. Fructose breath hydrogen tests in infants with chronic non-specific diarrhoea. *Eur J Pediatr.* 1995;154(5):362–364

62. Tappy L, Lê K-A. Metabolic Effects of fructose and the worldwide increase in obesity. *Physiol Rev.* 2010;90(1):23–46

63. Moore MC. Acute fructose administration decreases the glycemic response to an oral glucose tolerance test in normal adults. *J Clin Endocrinol Metab.* 2000;85(12):4515–4519

64. Lebenthal E, Lee PC. Development of functional responses in human exocrine pancreas. *Pediatrics.* 1980;66(4):556–560

65. Shulman RJ, Schanler RJ, Lau C, Heitkemper M, Ou CN, Smith EOB. Early feeding, feeding tolerance, and lactase activity in preterm infants. *J Pediatr.* 1998;133(5):645–649

66. Topping DL, Clifton PM. Short-chain fatty acids and human colonic function: roles of resistant starch and nonstarch polysaccharides. *Physiol Rev.* 2001;81(3):1031–1064

67. Gray GM. Starch digestion and absorption in nonruminants. *J Nutr.* 1992;122(1):172–177

68. Rings EHHM, Grand RJ, Md HABl. Lactose intolerance and lactase deficiency in children. *Curr Opin Pediatr.* 1994;6(5):562–567

69. Northrop-Clewes CA, Lunn PG, Downes RM. Lactose maldigestion in breast-feeding gambian infants. *J Pediatr Gastroenterol Nutr.* 1997;24(3):257–263

70. Koldovsky O. Digestive-absorptive functions in fetuses, infants, and children. In: Polin RA, Fox WW, eds. *Fetal and Neonatal Physiology.* Vol 2. Philadelphia, PA: WB Saunders Co; 1992:1060–1077

71. Enattah NS, Sahi T, Savilahti E, Terwilliger JD, Peltonen L, Järvelä I. Identification of a variant associated with adult-type hypolactasia. *Nature Genet.* 2002;30(2):233–237

72. Jensen TG, Liebert A, Lewinsky R, Swallow DM, Olsen J, Troelsen JT. The 14010C variant associated with lactase persistence is located between an Oct-1 and HNF1α binding site and increases lactase promoter activity. *Hum Genet.* 2011;130(4):483–493.

73. National Research Council. Protein and amino acids. *Recommended Dietary Allowances.* 10th ed. Washington, DC: National Academies Press; 1989

74. Institute of Medicine, Food and Nutrition Board. *Dietary Reference Intakes for Energy, Carbohydrate, Fiber, Fat, Fatty Acids, Cholesterol, Protein, and Amino Acids.* Washington, DC: National Academies Press; 2005

75. Mehta NM, Compher C. A.S.P.E.N. Clinical guidelines: nutrition support of the critically ill child. *J Parenter Enteral Nutr.* 2009;33(3):260–276

76. Joffe A, Anton N, Lequier L, et al. Nutritional support for critically ill children. *Cochrane Database Syst Rev.* 2016(5):CD005144

77. Matthews DE. Proteins and amino acids. In: Shils ME, Shike M, Ross AC, Caballero B, Cousins RJ, eds. *Modern Nutrition in Health and Disease.* Philadelphia, PA: Lippincott Williams & Wilkins; 2006:23–61

78. Young VR. Adult amino acid requirements: the case for a major revision in current recommendations. *J Nutr.* 1994;124(Suppl 8):1517S–1523S

79. Bjelton L, Sandberg G, Wennberg A, et al. Assessment of biological quality of amino acid solutions for intravenous nutrition. In: Kinney JM, Borum P, eds. *Perspectives in Clinical Nutrition.* Baltimore, MD: Urban & Schwarzenberg; 1989:31–41

80. Dallas D. Digestion of protein in premature and term infants. *J Nutr Disord Ther.* 2012;2(3):112

81. Kelly EJ, Brownlee KG. When is the fetus first capable of gastric acid, intrinsic factor and gastrin secretion? *Neonatology.* 1993;63(3):153–156

82. Hyman PE, Clarke DD, Everett SL, et al. Gastric acid secretory function in preterm infants. *J Pediatr.* 1985;106(3):467–471

83. Kelly EJ, Newell SJ, Brownlee KG, Primrose JN, Dear PRF. Gastric acid secretion in preterm infants. *Early Hum Dev.* 1993;35(3):215–220

84. Grahnquist L, Ruuska T, Finkel Y. Early development of human gastric H,K-adenosine triphosphatase. *J Pediatr Gastroenterol Nutr.* 2000;30(5):533–537

85. Lieberman J. Proteolytic enzyme activity in fetal pancreas and meconium: demonstration of plasminogen and trypsinogen activators in pancreatic tissue. *Gastroenterology.* 1966;50:183–190

86. Borgstrom B. Enzyme concentration and absorption of protein and glucose in duodenum of premature infants. *Arch Pediatr Adolesc Med.* 1960;99(3):338

87. Madey S, Dancis J. The premature infant. *Pediatrics*. 1949;4:177–182
88. Liao TH, Hamosh M, Scanlon JW, Hamosh P. Preduodenal fat digestion in the newborn infant: effect of fatty acid chain length on triglyceride hydrolysis. *Clin Res*. 1980;28:820
89. Bujanover Y, Harel A, Geter R, Blau H, Yahav J, Spirer Z. The development of the chymotrypsin activity during postnatal life using the bentiromide test. *Int J Pancreatol*. 1988;3:53–58
90. Lindberg TOR. Proteolytic activity in duodenal juice in infants, children, and adults. *Acta Paediatr*. 1974;63(6):805–808
91. Kushak RI, Winter HS. Regulation of intestinal peptidases by nutrients in human fetuses and children. *Compar Biochem Physiol A: Molec Integr Physiol*. 1999;124(2):191–198
92. Palacin M, Estevez R, Bertran J, Zorzano A. Molecular biology of mammalian plasma membrane amino acid transporters. *Physiol Rev*. 1998;78(4):969–1054
93. Malo C. Multiple pathways for amino acid transport in brush border membrane vesicles isolated from the human fetal small intestine. *Gastroenterology*. 1991;100(6):1644–1652.
94. Weaver LT, Walker WA. Uptake of macromolecules in the neonate. In: Lebenthal E, ed. *Human Gastrointestinal Development*. New York, NY: Raven Press; 1989:731–748
95. Walker WA. Absorption of protein and protein fragments in the developing intestine: role in immunologic/allergic reactions. *Pediatrics*. 1985;75(Suppl):167–171
96. Yoshida M, Kobayashi K, Kuok TT, et al. Neonatal Fc receptor for IgG regulates mucosal immune responses to luminal bacteria. *J Clin Invest*. 2006;116(8):2142–2151
97. Prasad PD, Wang H, Huang W, et al. Molecular and functional characterization of the intestinal Na+-dependent multivitamin transporter. *Arch Biochem Biophys*. 1999;366(1):79–106
98. Bass WT, Malati N, Castle MC, White LE. Evidence for the safety of ascorbic acid administration to the premature infant. *Am J Perinatol*. 1998;15(2):133–140
99. Tsukaguchi H, Tokui T, Mackenzie B, et a. A family of mammalian Na+-dependent L-ascorbic acid transporters. *Nature*. 1999;399(6731):70–75
100. Ziegler EE, Fomon SJ. Lactose enhances mineral absorption in infancy. *J Pediatr Gastroenterol Nutr*. 1983;2(2):288–294
101. Ghishan FK, Stroop S, Meneely R. The effect of lactose on the intestinal absorption of calcium and zinc in the rat during maturation. *Pediatr Res*. 1982;16(7):566–568
102. Barnes LA, Morrow G, III., Silverio J, Finnegan LP, Heitman SE. Calcium and fat absorption from infant formulas with different fat blends. *Pediatrics*. 1974;54(2):217–221
103. Namgung R, Tsang RC. Factors affecting newborn bone mineral content: in utero effects on newborn bone mineralization. *Proc Nutr Soc*. 2000;59(1):55–63

104. Ghishan FK, Parker P, Nichols S, Hoyumpa A. Kinetics of intestinal calcium transport during maturation in rats. *Pediatr Res.* 1984;18(3):235–239

105. Forbes GB, Reina JC. Effect of age on gastrointestinal absorption (Fe, Sr, Pb) in the rat. *J Nutr.* 1972;102(5):647–652

106. Goodnough LT, Nemeth E. Disorders of iron metabolism and heme synthesis: iron deficiency and related disorders. In: Wintrobe MM, ed. *Wintrobe's Clinical Hematology*. Philadelphia, PA: Lippincott, Williams & Wilkins; 2009:810–834

107. Ziegler EE, Edwards BB, Jensen RL, Mahaffey KR, Fomon SJ. Absorption and retention of lead by infants. *Pediatr Res.* 1978;12(1):29–34

108. Weaver LT. Breast and gut: the relationship between lactating mammary function and neonatal gastrointestinal function. *Proc Nutr Soc.* 1992;51(2):155–163

109. Perrine CG, Sharma AJ, Jefferds ME, Serdula MK, Scanlon KS. Adherence to vitamin D recommendations among US infants. *Pediatrics.* 2010;125(4):627–632

110. Carnielli VP, Luijendijk IH, van Goudoever JB, et al. Feeding premature newborn infants palmitic acid in amounts and stereoisomeric position similar to that of human milk: effects on fat and mineral balance. *Am J Clin Nutr.* 1995;61(5): 1037–1042

111. Jensen RG. Lipids in human milk-composition and fat soluble vitamins. In: Lebenthal E, ed. *Textbook of Gastroenterology and Nutrition in Infancy*. New York, NY: Raven Press; 1981:157–208

112. Ballabriga A. Essential fatty acids and human tissue composition. *Acta Paediatrica.* 1994;402:63–68

113. Clandinin MT. Brain development and assessing the supply of polyunsaturated fatty acids. *Lipids.* 1999;34(2):131–137

114. Sala-Vila A, Castellote AI, Campoy C, Rivero M, Rodriquez-Palmero M, Lopez-Sabater MC. The source of long-chain PUFA in formula supplements does not affect the fatty acid composition of plasma lipids in full-term infants. *J Nutr.* 2004;134(4):868–873

115. Bode L, Jantscher-Krenn E. Structure-function relationships of human milk oligosaccharides. *Adv Nutr.* 2012;3(3):383S–391S

116. Liao Y, Alvarado R, Phinney B, Lonnerdal B. Proteomic characterization of human milk whey proteins during a twelve-month lactation period. *J Proteome Res.* 2011;10(4):1746–1754

117. Lonnerdal B. Biochemistry and physiological functions of human milk proteins. *Am J Clin Nutr.* 1985;42(6):1299–1317

118. Prentice A, Ewing G, Roberts SB, et al. The nutritional role of breast milk IgA and lactoferrin. *Acta Paediatr.* 1987;76(4):592–598

119. Kleinman RE, Walker WA. The enteromammary immune system. *Dig Dis Sci.* 1979;24(11):876–882

120. Kubinak JL, Round JL. Do antibodies select a healthy microbiota? *Nature Rev Immunol.* 2016;16(12):767–774

121. Mepham TB. *Physiology of Lactation*. Milton Keynes, UK: Open University Press; 1987

122. Kunz C, Rudloff S. Biological functions of oligosaccharides in human milk. *Acta Paediatr*. 1993;82(11):903–912

123. Drenckpohl D, Hocker J, Shareef M, Vegunta R, Colgan C. Adding dietary green beans resolves the diarrhea associated with bowel surgery in neonates: a case study. *Nutr Clin Pract*. 2005;20(6):674–677

124. Goldman AS, Goldblum RM. Defense agents in human milk. In: Jensen RG, ed. *Handbook of Milk Composition*. New York, NY: Academic Press; 1995:727–745

125. Ballard O, Morrow AL. Human milk composition: nutrients and bioactive factors. *Pediatr Clin North Am*. 2013;60(1):49–74

126. Hernell O, Blackberg L. Digestion of human milk lipids: physiologic significance of sn-2 monoacylglycerol hydrolysis by bile salt-stimulated lipase. *Pediatr Res*. 1982;16(10):882–885

127. Williamson S, Finucane E, Ellis H, Gamsu HR. Effect of heat treatment of human milk on absorption of nitrogen, fat, sodium, calcium, and phosphorus by preterm infants. *Arch Dis Child*. 1978;53(7):555–563

128. Wang CS, Kuksis A, Manganaro F. Studies on the substrate specificity of purified human milk lipoprotein lipase. *Lipids*. 1982;17(4):278–284

129. Weaver LT, Walker WA. Epidermal growth factor and the developing human gut. *Gastroenterology*. 1988;94(3):845–847

130. Weaver LT, Freiberg E, Israel EJ, Walker WA. Epidermal growth factor in human amniotic fluid. *Gastroenterology*. 1989;95(5):1346

131. Weaver LT, Gonnella PA, Israel EJ, Walker WA. Uptake and transport of epidermal growth factor (EGF) by the small intestinal epithelium of the fetal rat. *Gastroenterology*. 1990;98(4):828–837

132. Menard D, Arsenault P, Pothier P. Biologic effects of epidermal growth factor in human fetal jejunum. *Gastroenterology*. 1988;94(3):656–663

133. Sigalet DL, Martin G, Meddings J, Hartman B, Holst JJ. GLP-2 levels in infants with intestinal dysfunction. *Pediatr Res*. 2004;56(3):371–376

134. Watkins JB, Szczepanik P, Gould JP, Klein P, Lester R. Bile salt metabolism in the human premature infant. *Gastroenterology*. 1975;69(3):706–713

135. Prentice A, Prentice AM, Lamb WH. Mastitis in rural Gambian mothers and the protection of the breast by milk antimicrobial factors. *Trans Royal Soc Trop Med Hyg*. 1985;79(1):90–95

136. Wilde CJ, Prentice A, Peaker M. Breastfeeding: matching supply with demand in human lactation. *Proc Nutr Soc*. 1995;54(2):401–406

137. American Academy of Pediatrics, Section on Breastfeeding. Policy statement: Breastfeeding and the use of human milk. *Pediatrics*. 2012;129(3):e827–e841

138. Carletti C, Pani P, Monasta L, Knowles A, Cattaneo A. Introduction of complementary foods in a cohort of infants in northeast Italy: do parents comply with WHO Recommendations? *Nutrients*. 2017;9(1):e34

139. Kramer MS, Kakuma R. Optimal duration of exclusive breastfeeding. *Cochrane Database Syst Rev.* 2012(8):CD003517

140. Aagaard K, Ma J, Antony KM, Ganu R, Petrosino J, Versalovic J. The placenta harbors a unique microbiome. *Sci Transl Med.* 2014;6(237):237ra265

141. Penders J, Thijs C, Vink C, et al. Factors influencing the composition of the intestinal microbiota in early infancy. *Pediatrics.* 2006;118(2):511–521

142. Dominguez-Bello MG, Costello EK, Contreras M, et al. Delivery mode shapes the acquisition and structure of the initial microbiota across multiple body habitats in newborns. *PNAS.* 2010;107(26):11971–11975

143. Palmer C, Bik EM, DiGiulio DB, Relman DA, Brown PO. Development of the human infant intestinal microbiota. *PLoS Biol.* 2007;5(7):e177

144. Turroni F, Peano C, Pass DA, Foroni E, Severgnini M. Diversity of bifidobacteria within the infant gut microbiota. *PLoS One.* 2012;7(5):e36957

145. Yassour M, Vatanen T, Siljander H, Hämäläinen AM, Härkönen T, Ryhänen SJ. Natural history of the infant gut microbiome and impact of antibiotic treatment on bacterial strain diversity and stability. *Sci Transl Med.* 2016;8(343):343ra381

146. Donaldson GP, Lee SM, Mazmanian SK. Gut biogeography of the bacterial microbiota. *Nature Rev Microbiol.* 2016;14(1):20–32

147. Lozupone CA, Stombaugh JI, Gordon JI, Jansson JK, Knight R. Diversity, stability and resilience of the human gut microbiota. *Nature.* 2012;489(7415):220–230

148. Bokulich NA, Chung J, Battaglia T, et al. Antibiotics, birth mode, and diet shape microbiome maturation during early life. *Sci Transl Med.* 2016;8(343):343ra382

149. Jakobsson HE, Abrahamsson TR, Jenmalm MC, et al. Decreased gut microbiota diversity, delayed Bacteroidetes colonisation and reduced Th1 responses in infants delivered by caesarean section. *Gut.* 2014;63(4):559–566

150. Yatsunenko T, Rey FE, Manary MJ, et al. Human gut microbiome viewed across age and geography. *Nature.* 2012;486(7402):222

151. Azad MB, Konya T, Maughan H, et al. Gut microbiota of healthy Canadian infants: profiles by mode of delivery and infant diet at 4 months. *Can Med Assoc J.* 2013;185(5):385–394

152. Cox LM, Yamanishi S, Sohn J, et al. Altering the intestinal microbiota during a critical developmental window has lasting metabolic consequences. *Cell.* 2014;158(4):705–721

153. Ridaura VK, Faith JJ, Rey FE, Cheng J, Duncan AE, Kau AL. Gut microbiota from twins discordant for obesity modulate metabolism in mice. *Science.* 2013;341(6150):124214

154. Carlisle EM, Morowitz MJ. The intestinal microbiome and necrotizing enterocolitis. *Curr Opin Pediatr.* 2013;25(3):382–387

155. Fujimura KE, Lynch SV. Microbiota in allergy and asthma and the emerging relationship with the gut microbiome. *Cell Host Microbe.* 2015;17(5):592–602

Chapter 3

Breastfeeding

Introduction

The American Academy of Pediatrics (AAP) recommends human milk as the sole feeding for healthy, term infants for about the first 6 months of life and supports continued breastfeeding for at least 12 months.[1] The AAP also recommends human milk as the preferred source of enteral nutrition for the preterm infant. Human milk offers specific advantages, and lack of access is associated with disadvantages. This chapter discusses the recent epidemiology of breastfeeding, composition of human milk, duration of breastfeeding, contraindications to breastfeeding, and how to support breastfeeding.

Recent Epidemiology

In the early part of the 20th century, breastfeeding was the norm in the United States, but by the early 1970s, breastfeeding rates had decreased to 24.7%. Since that time, rates have steadily increased.[2] There has been an improvement in the rates of breastfeeding initiation. According to the US National Immunization Survey conducted by the Centers for Disease Control and Prevention (CDC), 82.5% of mothers initiated breastfeeding in 2014 (most recent national data available), 55.3% were still breastfeeding at 6 months, and 33.7% were still breastfeeding at 12 months.[3] Rates of exclusive breastfeeding also increased in 2013 to 46.6% and 24.9% at 3 and 6 months, respectively.[3]

The improvement in breastfeeding rates nationally over the past several decades is not attributable to any one factor. The US Surgeon General issued a "Call to Action to Support Breastfeeding" in 2011, calling on all sectors of society to eliminate barriers to breastfeeding by implementing 20 action steps.[4] There has been an increase in hospitals designated as Baby-Friendly by following recommendations of the World Health Organization (WHO)/United Nations International Children's Emergency Fund (UNICEF) in their Baby-Friendly Hospital Initiative.[5] The number of facilities designated in the United States by Baby-Friendly USA increased from 2.7% in 2007 to 21.8% in 2017 (https://www.cdc.gov/breastfeeding/pdf/2016breastfeedingreportcard.pdf (https://www.babyfriendlyusa.org/find-facilities).[5,6] The number of certified lactation consultants also has continued to increase, with latest rates of certified lactation consultants per 1000 live births of 3.79, up from 2.12 in 2007.[5] Rates of breastfeeding among African American women have increased but are still not as high as among white or Hispanic women. Currently, 85.7% of non-Hispanic white women initiate breastfeeding,

and only 68.0% of non-Hispanic black women breastfeed. Health disparities among women and infants of color are a significant concern. African
American women often lack the social support, cultural acceptance, and
access to appropriate health care support to breastfeed successfully, which
may have an effect on their higher breast cancer rates.[7,8]

In 2007, the CDC administered the first national survey of maternity
practices related to breastfeeding, known as the Maternity Practices in
Infant Nutrition and Care (mPINC) survey. The survey is administered every
2 years to each facility in the United States that routinely provides maternity
care services and is completed by a key informant on behalf of the institution in his or her capacity as the person most knowledgeable about the
relevant practices surveyed by the mPINC. The participation of hospitals in
the survey undoubtedly has led to improved maternity care practices supportive of breastfeeding initiation and has encouraged hospitals to adopt
practices consistent with the Baby-Friendly Hospital Initiative, discussed
below. The CDC has also provided funding support for quality improvement
activities to achieve Baby-Friendly Hospital designation through 2 major
initiatives: Best-Fed Beginnings (http://www.nichq.org/project/best-fed-
beginnings) and EMPower Breastfeeding: Enhancing Maternity Practices
(http://empowerbreastfeeding.org/). In addition, breastfeeding is receiving
more support from state governments, often in conjunction with healthy
weight initiatives, communities, employers, and the health care system.[3] For
example, breastfeeding data cited earlier make use of the CDC's National
Immunization Surveys. With this annual survey, the CDC collects extensive
breastfeeding data that are state specific and stratified nationally by other
demographic and social indicators (https://www.cdc.gov/breastfeeding/
data/nis_data/index.htm).[3,5,9]

Healthy People 2020 aims for 81.9% of mothers to breastfeed in the early
postpartum period (a goal that has essentially been exceeded at 82.5%,
according to the 2016 CDC Breastfeeding Report Card).[5,9] Other goals not
yet met include 60.6% of mothers to be breastfeeding at 6 months, 34.1%
to be breastfeeding at 1 year, and 25.5% to be exclusively breastfeeding at
6 months; the goal of 46.2% of mothers to be exclusively breastfeeding at
3 months has been achieved. Additional Healthy People 2020 objectives
include increasing the proportion of employers that have worksite lactation
support, reducing the proportion of breastfed newborn infants who receive
formula supplementation within the first 2 days of life, and increasing the
proportion of live births that occur in facilities that provide recommended
care for lactating mothers and their newborn infants. Currently, 15.5% of

US breastfed infants are supplemented with infant formula within the first 2 days of life.[5]

The US Department of Health and Human Services Office on Women's Health initiative, Business Case for Breastfeeding, provides innovative solutions for employers and mothers regarding breastfeeding and milk expression in the workplace (https://www.womenshealth.gov/breastfeeding/breastfeeding-home-work-and-public/breastfeeding-and-going-back-work/business-case).[10] Federal law under the Patient Protection and Affordable Care Act provides coverage for breastfeeding mothers to access breastfeeding counseling and supplies, such as breast pumps and attachments. In addition, most women are entitled to breaks to express milk during the work day until the child is 1 year of age (https://www.dol.gov/whd/nursingmothers/).[11]

On average, mothers who breastfeed have higher educational levels, are older, are more likely to be white, have a middle-level income, and have a higher employment rate than the overall US female population.[12-14] Gains made in breastfeeding rates are impressive, despite continued racial, ethnic, socioeconomic, and geographic disparities. As noted, breastfeeding initiation rates for African American infants was 68% in 2014, lagging behind rates for Hispanic and white infants at 85% and 86%, respectively.

Economic disparities include differences in breastfeeding rates among mothers receiving benefits in the Special Supplemental Nutrition Program for Women, Infants, and Children (WIC) program, which in 2014 were 75.5%, compared with a 91.7% rate among mothers who were WIC ineligible. Education also is a factor: mothers who have graduated from college had breastfeeding initiation rates almost 25% higher than those among mothers who did not graduate from high school.[3]

Regional geographical differences also exist throughout the United States, with higher rates of breastfeeding initiation in the more western states and lowest rates in the southeastern regions. For example, in 2014, fewer than 58% of mothers initiated breastfeeding in Mississippi, compared with 92% of women in Washington state.[3] In the past, women living in rural areas were more likely never to have breastfed than were those living in urban areas.[8,9] A secondary analysis by Wiener et al of the US National Survey of Children's Health showed an urban national vs Appalachian urban breastfeeding prevalence of 0.770 (95% confidence interval [CI], 0.757-0.784) versus 0.715 (95% CI, 0.702-0.728), respectively.[15] Similar trends were reported by Lynch et al in their secondary analysis of the North Carolina Pregnancy Nutrition Surveillance System.[16] More recent data using the

National Immunization Survey shows lower rates of breastfeeding among states with greater rural populations.[3,8]

Although disparities in breastfeeding initiation rates have improved overall, sustained breastfeeding rates at 6 and 12 months still reflect racial, ethnic, socioeconomic, and geographic disparities, which suggests that there are differential factors affecting a woman's ability to continue to breastfeed during the first year after birth.[8] Groups with low breastfeeding rates merit additional support, including education on the benefits and mechanics of breastfeeding. This support requires an increase in the availability of local resources. Guidance is available for cultural- and ethnic-based approaches to breastfeeding in the United States.[17]

Human Milk: Composition, Nutrients, and Bioactive Factors

Human milk is a complex bioactive fluid that consists of various compartments, including a true solution, colloidal dispersions of casein molecules, emulsions of milk fat globules and milk fat globule membranes, and live cells, including stem cells. Appendix A provides the approximate concentrations of some of the constituents of human milk and a list of some important bioactive factors. The concentration of human milk constituents varies over the course of lactation, whether during a single feed, over a 24-hour period, or over weeks and months. There are also differences among women. The first milk, colostrum, is produced in very small amounts (15 ± 11 g in the first 24 hours of life)[11] and has high concentrations of proteins, fat-soluble vitamins, minerals, electrolytes, and antibodies. More yellow in color than mature human milk, colostrum contains significant beta-carotene. The protein content of colostrum is 70% to 80% whey and 20% to 30% casein, and this ratio decreases over time to approximately 55% whey and 44% casein in mature milk. Transitional milk, milk from approximately 5 to 14 days postpartum, is characterized by a decrease in the concentration of immunoglobulins and total proteins and an increase in lactose, fat, and total calories. Mature milk, milk produced after about 2 weeks postpartum, is the fully developed milk that supports healthy term infants exclusively for the first months of life. The milk produced by mothers who continue to lactate beyond 6 to 7 months, extended lactation milk, is characterized by continuing declining concentrations of vitamins, minerals, and some macronutrients like protein.[18,19] By this time, appropriate complementary foods should be part of the infant's diet in addition to human milk.

As noted, the volume and content of major nutrients in mature milk from individual mothers is highly variable, as shown in Appendix A. Most mothers are able to breastfeed successfully, as infants adapt their intake to achieve normal growth despite this nutrient variability, especially those of protein and energy.[20] Although the concentration of calcium in milk decreases slightly during the first months of lactation, the infant's intake of milk increases, and therefore, the total intake of dietary calcium in milk remains stable.[21] The concentrations of some nutrients, such as iron and vitamin D, are low in human milk, and deficiency in the infant can occur.[22] Therefore, the AAP recommends supplementation of breastfed infants with these nutrients. All infants should begin supplementation of vitamin D with 400 IU/day in the first few days of life and continue until the infant is weaned to at least 1 L/day or 1 quart/day of vitamin D-fortified formula or whole milk.[23] Alternatively, some mothers, in consultation with their physician, may elect to consume larger quantities of vitamin D (up to 6400 IU/day) to improve the vitamin D content in their milk transferred to their infants.[22,24–26] Iron supplementation should begin at 4 months of age with 1 mg/kg/day of oral iron or until the infant consumes adequate oral iron from foods or iron-fortified formula.[27] One way to improve iron intake during weaning is to introduce meats as the first complementary food (see Chapter 6). Although meats provide a highly bioavailable source of iron and zinc, this may not be a desirable solution for all families, especially those who do not eat meat, and therefore prefer a vegetarian diet. Oral iron and zinc (given as part of a multivitamin) supplementation in this situation may be more in keeping with cultural beliefs and practices.

Fetuses receive immunoglobulin (IgG) through placental transfer, mainly in the last trimester of gestation. Immunoglobulin A (IgA) is the predominant antibody isotype in human milk and provides passive protection against enteric pathogens to which the infant is exposed.[16–19] Colostrum also contains viable cells and other bioactive proteins, such as lysozymes, lactoferrin, haptocorrin, alpha-1 antitrypsin, insulin,[28] epidermal growth factor[29] and the related compound transforming growth factor-alpha,[30,31] transforming growth factor-beta,[18] vasoactive endothelial growth factor,[32] and various cytokines and chemokines (such as interleukin-5, -7, -8, and -10, growth-related oncogene-α, macrophage-monocyte chemoattractant protein-1, and macrophage inflammatory protein 1-β), to name just a few (Table 3.1).[33] These factors are found to vary in response to the gestational age of the infant at the time of delivery[34] and when there is an active infection in the nursing infant.[35]

Table 3.1.
Selected Bioactive Factors in Human Milk

Substance	Function
Secretory IgA	Specific antigen-targeted anti-infection action
Lactoferrin	Immunomodulation, iron chelation, anti-adhesive, trophic for intestinal growth
Lysozyme	Bacterial lysis, immunomodulation
κ-Casein	Anti-adhesive, bacterial flora
Oligosaccharides (prebiotics)	Block bacterial attachment
Cytokines (eg, IL-5, 7, 8, 10; tumor necrosis factor [TNF]-α)	Anti-inflammatory, epithelial barrier function
Nucleotides	Enhance antibody responses, bacterial flora
Vitamins A, E, C	Antioxidants
Amino acids (including glutamine)	Intestinal cell fuel, immune responses
Lipids	Anti-infective properties
Milk fat globule membrane	Cell signaling capacity
Insulin	Growth modulator
Leptin	Involved in appetite control
Progenitor/stem cells	Further study required
Exosomes	Source of MicroRNAs related to immune responses

Growth Factors	
Epidermal growth factor (EGF)	Luminal surveillance, repair of intestines
Transforming growth factor-alpha (TGF-α)	Stimulates epithelial growth and gut repair; properties similar to EGF
Transforming growth factor-beta (TGF-β)	Involved in regulation of inflammatory processes, particularly in the gut
	Promotes stem cell and T-lymphocyte differentiation and regulation
Vasoactive endothelial growth factor (VEGF)	Promotes angiogenesis
Interleukin-10 (IL-10)	Potent anti-inflammatory properties; plays a central role in limiting host immune response to pathogens
Nerve growth factor	Growth
Enzymes	
Platelet-activating factor (PAF)-acetyl hydrolase	Blocks action of platelet-activating factor
Glutathione peroxidase	Prevents lipid oxidation

The milk fat globule membrane (MFGM), which surrounds the milk fat globule, allows the delivery of fat into a predominately water-based fluid. The MFGM itself is derived from the apical aspect of the mammary epithelial cell and has the surface markers of those cells, including those for growth factors and cytokines, imparting a signaling mechanism between mother and her recipient infant. Hamosh and others in the 1990s provided evidence of the protective properties of the MFGM,[36,37] the second most abundant component of human milk, through membrane-associated glycoproteins, preventing the attachment of pathogens to the intestinal mucosa.[37] More recently, on the basis of animal and human studies, bovine milk fat globule membranes have been added to commercial formula.[38]

An exciting new area of research focuses on human milk exosomes, first identified by Admyre et al in 2007.[39] Exosomes are nanovesicles (30-100 nm) with an endosome-derived limiting membrane secreted by a diverse range of cells. In vitro studies suggest that human milk exosomes have the capacity to influence immune responses[39] and may influence allergy development and risk in the child.[40] In addition, immune-related microRNAs packaged in exosomes may be an additional mechanism by which the mother provides immunologic and epigenetic factors to the breastfeeding infant.[41,42]

Another bioactive factor are the milk leukocytes, first identified in human milk in the 1960s, that have been studied extensively. Leukocytes are believed to also play a role in infant immunity and immunocompetence, enhancing immune function against pathogens in the gastrointestinal tract.[43,44] Leukocytes are believed to exert these functions via phagocytosis, secretion of antimicrobial factors and/or antigen presentation in both the mammary gland and the infant's gastrointestinal tract. Recently, it has been demonstrated that human milk leukocytes respond dynamically to maternal as well as infant infections and are increased with increasing human milk exposure of the infant.[45] Progenitor and stem cells have also been identified in human milk, and their bioactivity is under study.[46-52]

Also present in human milk are milk glycans that are energetically costly for the mammary gland to produce, yet indigestible by infants.[53,54] Milk glycans comprise free oligosaccharides, glycoproteins, glycopeptides, and glycolipids.[55] Human milk oligosaccharides (HMOs), unconjugated complex carbohydrates, are abundant in human milk, providing 1% to 2% weight/volume. Because the human intestine lacks the various glycolytic enzymes that break down HMOs and other glycans, they reach the colon intact as prebiotics.[56] HMOs are believed to play an important role in infant immune function, specifically interacting with gut microbes.[56] They have been shown to be a selective growth substrate for intestinal bifidobacteria, making them the dominant microbiota of breastfed infants. At least 41 different *Bifidobacterium* species have been identified, which include *Bifidobacterium longum, Bifidobacterium bifidum,* and *Bifidobacterium breve.* HMOs have been shown to interact with the surface of pathogenic bacteria and inhibit the binding of pathogens and toxins to host cell receptors.[54,56–59] Certain commercial infant formulas now have added oligosaccharides, but these do not come close to mimicking the abundance of those naturally occurring in human milk.[56]

Human milk offers many nutritional advantages for the healthy term infant, including a clean, safe source of nutrition and a bioactive medium that facilitates development of the infant's immune system, affecting overall health status. A review performed by the Agency for Healthcare Research and Quality (AHRQ) found that in the industrialized world, a history of breastfeeding is associated with a reduced risk of acute otitis media, nonspecific gastroenteritis, severe lower respiratory tract infections, atopic dermatitis, asthma in young children, obesity, type 1 and 2 diabetes mellitus, childhood leukemia, sudden infant death, and necrotizing enterocolitis.[60] No relationship was found between cognitive performance and a history of breastfeeding, and the relationship between breastfeeding and cardiovascular diseases and infant mortality was unclear. A second recent review by the AHRQ found low strength of evidence that ever breastfeeding or longer durations may be associated with lower rates of maternal breast cancer, epithelial ovarian cancer, hypertension, and type 2 diabetes mellitus in industrialized countries.[61] The AHRQ cautions, however, that almost all the available data in these reports were from observational studies, and there was a wide range of quality and heterogeneity among the studies. It is not possible to conduct randomized controlled trials in breastfed infants and their mothers that might account for all the variables that would affect the outcomes. However, carefully conducted cohort studies, particularly intrafamilial studies that control for inherited and environmental factors that are known to affect many of these outcomes, question the causal relationship between breastfeeding/human milk and many of these long-term health outcomes. Thus, causality between breastfeeding and these long-term health outcomes cannot be inferred.

Breastfeeding and Safe Sleep

Important steps of the Ten Steps to Successful Breastfeeding include mothers and newborn infants initiating skin-to-skin contact in the immediate postpartum period and practicing rooming-in and exclusive breastfeeding during the postpartum stay. There have been reports of falls in the neonatal period when mothers drop their babies and of cases of sudden unexpected postnatal collapse (SUPC), although it is unclear whether the incidence of SUPC has actually increased. SUPC occurs most commonly in cases of neonatal infection, congenital heart disease, persistent pulmonary hypertension, metabolic defects, and anemia. It is associated with prone positioning and lack of adequate surveillance of the infant when in skin-to-skin contact.[61] Preventive measures include parent education about maintaining airway patency with proper positioning and surveillance of the newborn infant by staff aware of SUPC. At-risk mothers, such as those who are primiparous, alone, or exhausted, should have continuous clinical supervision of themselves and their infants. Medical supervision is indicated for mothers who are sedated or infected and infants with any signs of distress or concerns for infection. Parents are encouraged to avoid bed sharing, prone sleep positions, soft bedding, and covering the infant's head.

The AAP Committee on Fetus and Newborn and Task Force on Sudden Infant Death Syndrome advocated for continuous monitoring of infants in the immediate postpartum period, with risk stratification of mother-infant pairs.[62] The AAP indicated that the infant's face should be visualized and maintained in a neutral, sniffing position, with the head uncovered, the neck straight, and legs flexed. The Association for Women's Health, Obstetric and Neonatal Nurses (AWHONN) recommend that trained health care professionals should be in attendance during the first 2 hours after birth to monitor proper positioning and ensure maternal and newborn safety through physiologic indicators.[63]

Ludington-Hoe and Morgan published assessment criteria using the acronym RAPP, indicating respiratory effort, activity, perfusion, and position.[64] They recommend that staff should assess respiratory effort, expecting a rate of 40 to 60 breaths/minute, with regular respirations and no increased work of breathing. The newborn infant's state should be documented. Any newborn infant found to be unresponsive should be resuscitated. Assessment of perfusion should determine whether the infant is pink, with acrocyanosis being normal with central perfusion. Any pallor, grayness, or dusky color, or central cyanosis requires evaluation. Tachypnea and abnormal thermal regulation also require evaluation. Finally, the position should be assessed for flexed body position and neck in midline.

The AAP updated its policy statement on sudden infant death syndrome by publishing "SIDS and Other Sleep-Related Infant Deaths: Updated 2016

Recommendations for a Safe Infant Sleeping Environment."[65] The statement recommends breastfeeding, because it reduces risk of sudden infant death syndrome (SIDS). The AAP advocated for room sharing, but not bed sharing. The infant should sleep on his or her back on a separate firm sleep surface, without other loose bedding. Caregivers should avoid use of tobacco, alcohol, and illicit drugs. Because pacifier use has been associated with a decreased incidence of SIDS, the AAP recommended that pacifier use be considered, although advised that parents may delay the introduction of a pacifier in breastfed infants until breastfeeding is established.

Duration of Breastfeeding

For approximately the past decade, there has been an effort to increase the prevalence and duration of time that infants are exclusively breastfed. Table 3.2 lists definitions for breastfeeding. Of note, the definition of exclusive breastfeeding encompasses the administration of supplements, such as vitamins. The AAP recommends exclusive breastfeeding for about the first 6 months of life and continuation after complementary foods have been introduced for at least the first year of life and beyond, as long as mutually desired by mother and child.[1] This approach acknowledges the need for flexibility in that mothers may introduce complementary foods for personal, social, and economic reasons. In addition, a flexible approach also acknowledges the variations in human development that occur.

Initiation of Complementary Foods During Breastfeeding: When Is the Optimal Time?

The optimal time to introduce complementary foods has been an ongoing debate for many years and the subject of much controversy (also see Chapter 6: Complementary Feeding). There is new evidence that avoiding maternal intake of potential allergens during the first year of life has not resulted in decreased risk of allergy and that a diversified diet including common food allergens may be beneficial during both pregnancy and lactation.[66] There is also evidence that earlier exposure to potential food allergens by 4 and 6 months of age in breastfed, mixed-fed, and formula fed infants may result in greater tolerance of allergenic foods without increasing the risk of atopic disease.[67-70] This phenomenon is particularly true for peanuts[67] and perhaps whole egg in infants considered to be at high risk,[68] and it is now recommended by the AAP that for infants with severe eczema or egg allergy (even those who are exclusively breastfeeding), peanut should be introduced between 4 and 6 months of age (see also Chapter 3: Complementary

Table 3.2.

Definitions of Breastfeeding

Type	Description
Exclusive	Human milk is the only food provided. Medicines, minerals, and vitamins may also be given under this definition but no water, juice, or other preparations. Infants fed expressed human milk from their own mothers or from a milk bank by gavage tube, cup, or bottle also can be included in this definition if they have received no nonhuman milk or foods.
Almost exclusive	Human milk is the predominant food provided with very rare feedings of other milk or food. The infant may have been given 1 or 2 formula bottles during the first few days of life but none after that.
Partial or mixed	This may vary from mostly human milk with small amounts of infrequent feedings of nonhuman milk or food *(high partial)*, to infants receiving significant amounts of nonhuman milk or food as well as human milk *(medium partial)*, to infants receiving predominantly nonhuman milk or food with some human milk *(low partial)*.
Token	The infant is fed almost entirely with nonhuman milk and food but either had some human milk shortly after birth or continues to have occasional human milk. This type of breastfeeding may be seen late in the weaning process.
Any breastfeeding	This definition includes all of the above.
Never breastfed	This infant has *never* received *any* human milk, either by direct breastfeeding or expressed milk with artificial means of delivery.

Reproduced with permission from Schanler RJ, Dooley S, Gartner LM, Krebs NF, Mass SB, eds. 2nd edition. *Breastfeeding Handbook for Physicians.* Elk Grove Village, IL: American Academy of Pediatrics; 2012

Feeding, and Chapter 34: Food Allergy).[66] Controversy remains regarding optimal timing and dosing of allergenic foods for infants with moderate or low allergy risk before 6 months of age, particularly in exclusively breastfed infants.[71–73]

In a 2010 report, Fewtrell et al assessed the impact of the 2003 changes in the breastfeeding policy in the United Kingdom by the Health Minister without input from the British Department of Health's Scientific Advisory

Committee on Nutrition.[74] The 2003 United Kingdom policy recommended that infants be breastfed exclusively for 6 months, in concert with WHO recommendations. Fewtrell et al noted that the definition of exclusive breastfeeding varied among the studies supporting the WHO guidelines (see Table 3.2), and their review of the literature noted few advantages for exclusive breastfeeding beyond 4 months from a disease standpoint, including the risk of atopic disease. However, Fewtrell et al raised concerns that prolonged exclusive breastfeeding is associated with a higher risk of iron deficiency anemia, in addition to a higher incidence of food allergies.[74] The risk of iron deficiency is also a concern, and the AAP recommends iron supplementation after 4 months of age for exclusively breastfed infants.[27]

In response to some of the aforementioned concerns, the Robert Wood Johnson Foundation conducted a detailed analysis of factors that affect infant and young toddler feeding behaviors and health outcomes.[66] The report established new feeding guidelines to address the problem of childhood obesity and allergy. In the executive summary, it was noted there was a general consensus that complementary foods (solids) should be introduced once the infant is able to sit without support with good head and neck control and has the ability to chew and use the tongue to move pureed foods to the back of the mouth for swallowing. Equally important is that the infant no longer have the extrusion reflex, pushing solids out of his or her mouth with the tongue automatically, and that the infant shows interest in food at mealtimes. The loss of this reflex occurs somewhere between 4 and 6 months of age but not before 4 months. The new Robert Wood Johnson Foundation guidelines recommended introduction of complementary foods when the infant is developmentally ready, somewhere between 4 and 6 months of age. The guidelines apply to infants who are breastfeeding, formula feeding, or mixed feeding.[66] Although the report noted that breastfeeding may protect children against the development of childhood obesity, this remains controversial. In addition, infants born to mothers who consumed fruits and vegetables during pregnancy and who were breastfed were more likely to learn to accept these foods, compared with formula-fed infants.[66] The report also noted that the risk of allergy does not decrease if an infant's exposure to potential allergies is delayed beyond 6 months of age. Current evidence supports that earlier exposure to a potential allergen may induce tolerance and that it may be preferable to introduce allergenic foods when the infant is developmentally ready for complementary foods. The report also concludes there is no need for pregnant and lactating women to avoid the consumption of common allergens such as eggs, milk, peanuts, tree nuts, fish, shellfish, and wheat, because doing so does not decrease the risk of food allergies in children.[66]

Contraindications to Breastfeeding

Although most women can successfully breastfeed their infants, some cannot and some should not. In the United States, women who are infected with human immunodeficiency virus (HIV) or human T-cell lymphotropic virus (HTLV type 1 and 2) should not breastfeed.[75] Women with untreated active pulmonary tuberculosis should not breastfeed until the mother has completed at least 2 weeks of treatment and has a negative sputum cultures. During this 2-week interval, the mother should be encouraged to express her milk to establish and maintain her milk supply. The expressed milk may be fed to her infant by another caregiver.[75] Infants with certain inborn errors of metabolism, such as the classic form of galactosemia, should not be breastfed. In other circumstances, such as phenylketonuria, partial breast-feeding may be considered with careful monitoring under the supervision of a metabolic specialist.

Although there remains concern for the effect of maternal drugs on nursing infants, the majority of both prescribed and over-the-counter medications are compatible with breastfeeding, so risks of medication exposure should be weighed with benefits of breastfeeding. Only a small amount of a medication ingested orally by a breastfeeding mother is transmitted into human milk and then absorbed by the infant. Transfer of drugs via human milk varies depending on the pharmacokinetics of the drugs and also the age of the child. The AAP lists drugs and therapeutics that may be transferred into human milk by various categories.[67] If a medication is routinely prescribed to infants, then it can be generally considered as safe for the mother to take the drug as well. Even though most drugs and therapeutics are safe for breastfeeding mothers and infants, the AAP advises all physicians to obtain the most up-to-date information on drugs and lactation. In addition to information on the AAP Web site, the National Institutes of Health (NIH)/US National Library of Medicine provides an online database on prescribed medications and recreational drugs available at LactMed (http://toxnet.nlm.nih.gov) and also available as a mobile device application. LactMed is the preferred source for information on medications for nursing mothers, which can aid physicians in obtaining current information on specific drugs to help guide their advice to breastfeeding women.

Perhaps most problematic is the increasing use by lactating mothers of a wide variety psychotropic agents, including selective serotonin-reuptake inhibitors, with many taking multiple medications. In general, there are limited pharmacologic data and information on short- and long-term neurobehavioral effects from infant exposure to these psychotropic agents. There are some data that suggest exposed infants have greater irritability during the newborn period and may need to be monitored and treated, but risk of drug exposure versus the benefits of breastfeeding should be considered.

A growing problem in the United States has been the use of opioids and the resulting epidemic of addiction that includes pregnant and lactating mothers. When a mother is enrolled in a rehabilitation program or on chronically prescribed opioid treatment(s) during pregnancy, the likelihood of neonatal abstinence syndrome (NAS) is high in her neonate, developing hours to days after birth as the opioid concentrations in her neonate decrease. Provision of human milk to her infant can lessen the severity of neonatal abstinence and has been shown to decrease hospital length of stay for that infant.[68,69] Methadone doses of 25 to 180 mg/day produce concentrations in human milk that range from 27 to 260 ng/mL, leading to an average daily methadone ingestion of 0.05 mg (based on an infant's estimated milk intake of approximately 500 mL/day).[68] With maternal methadone intakes between 40 and 180 mg/day, even after correcting for the slower clearance rate of methadone in neonates as compared with adults, the relative infant dose would not exceed 5% of the maternal weight–adjusted dose.[68] Nonpharmacologic management, such as environmental control and rooming-in, have been shown to decrease NAS scores and length of stay for treatment of NAS.[70–73] A knowledgeable health care team must be involved to guide the treatment of the infant in conjunction with breastfeeding support and advice about maternal treatment options affecting the breastfeeding dyad.

How To Support Breastfeeding

The Process Begins During Pregnancy

To begin to meet the goals of Healthy People 2020, families require support to initiate and continue breastfeeding. For initiation, it is helpful to have the obstetric health care provider acknowledge support for breastfeeding early in the pregnancy so families can begin to put into place the necessary

support systems (https://www.acog.org/About-ACOG/ACOG-Departments/
Toolkits-for-Health-Care-Providers/Breastfeeding-Toolkit).[76] Unless there
is a medical condition that prevents early initiation of breastfeeding, the
infant should be placed skin-to-skin on the mother's abdomen or chest
immediately after delivery and remain with the mother continuously, especially through the first breastfeeding, ideally within the first hour of life.
Routine assessment and vital signs should be obtained while the infant is
skin-to-skin. Most infants will find the nipple, but some may need assistance by labor and delivery nurses or lactation consultants. Although breastfeeding is natural, it is a learned skill, and mothers benefit from bedside
teaching of positioning, latching on, and sucking. Follow-up with committed personnel while mother and infant are in the hospital is essential to
provide answers to questions, offer suggestions, and support and problem
solve. During this time, the hospital is very important in terms of attitudes,
support systems, and policies.

Importance of Breastfeeding National, State, and Local Support Infrastructure

All hospitals are encouraged to adopt the Ten Steps for Successful
Breastfeeding recommended by the WHO and endorsed by the AAP.[1,77] The
Ten Steps are listed in Table 3.3 and are an important part of being des-
ignated as a Baby-Friendly Hospital. In some studies, greater likelihood
of initiation and longer duration of breastfeeding have been shown when
hospitals have implemented the Tens Steps to Successful Breastfeeding.[78,79]
However, the recent report and systematic review by the US Preventive
Services Task Force (USPSTF) of the effectiveness of the Ten Steps of the
Baby-Friendly Hospital initiative did not show a benefit for these outcomes
in the United States, even though there have been very significant increases
in breastfeeding initiation in some of the Baby-Friendly certified hospitals.
It is not clear whether the intensified attention to breastfeeding support in
these hospitals is responsible for the increases or if implementation of all
Ten Steps is necessary. The USPSTF conclusions suggest the former may
be the case.[80] However, a recent AHRQ report found that Baby-Friendly
Hospital interventions are effective for improving rates of breastfeeding
initiation and duration, though the evidence from the one large randomized
controlled trial (PROBIT[77]) had limited applicability and the observational
studies do no clearly establish the magnitude of the benefit.[81] They also concluded that low evidence supports the conclusion that implementation of
four or more Baby-Friendly Hospital Initiative steps is associated with lower

Table 3.3.

Ten Steps to Successful Breastfeeding

Step	Activity
Step 1	Have a written breastfeeding policy that is routinely communicated to all health care staff.
Step 2	Train all health care staff in skills necessary to implement this policy.
Step 3	Inform all pregnant women about the benefits and management of breastfeeding.
Step 4	Help mothers initiate breastfeeding within 1 hour of birth.
Step 5	Show mothers how to breastfeed and how to maintain lactation, even if they should be separated from their infants.
Step 6	Give breastfeeding newborn infants no food or drink other than human milk, unless medically indicated.
Step7	Rooming-in—all mothers and infants to remain together 24 hours a day.
Step 8	Encourage breastfeeding on demand.
Step 9	Give no artificial teats or pacifiers to breastfeeding infants.[a]
Step 10	Foster the establishment of breastfeeding support groups and refer mothers to them on discharge from the hospital

Reproduced with permission from Baby-Friendly USA.

[a] The AAP does not support a categorical ban on pacifiers because of their role in SIDS risk reduction and their analgesic benefit during painful procedures when breastfeeding cannot provide the analgesia. Pacifier use in the hospital in the neonatal periods should be limited to specific medical indications, including pain reduction, calming in a drug-exposed infant, nonnutritive sucking in preterm infants, etc. Mothers of healthy term infants should be instructed to delay pacifier use until breastfeeding is well established, usually about 3 to 4 weeks after birth.

rates of weaning than implementation of fewer than 4 steps.[81] An additional consideration is that Baby-Friendly status can be costly for smaller hospitals that cannot afford the certification costs.

Importance of Family Support of the Breastfeeding Dyad

Maintenance of breastfeeding involves challenges for both the infant and mother. Most importantly, a supportive partner and family and access to good information are needed for new mothers. Women often have concerns about their ability to produce adequate milk.[82] There are many possible and manageable causes for inadequate milk intake and subsequent malnutrition and failure to gain weight and length in some breastfed infants. These include preterm birth, illness in the mother or child, mother-baby separation, cessation of lactation for a period of time, maternal diabetes and obesity, as well as anxiety, fatigue, and emotional stress.[83] Most often, milk production can be increased by increasing the frequency of breastfeeding, using relaxation techniques, including skin-to-skin contact (but not cobedding with the newborn infant), having psychosocial support from family and partners, and having an experienced lactation expert, such as a certified lactation consultant, postpartum nurse, or NICU nurse to help with the mechanics of breastfeeding.[84–86]

Insufficient Milk Production and/or Transfer

If an infant does not receive sufficient human milk, the infant will have delayed gut motility and fewer bowel movements, decreased urinary output, early jaundice, hunger, and lethargy and will lose more than 7% of his or her birth weight. Serial weights before and after a feeding will identify whether the infant is getting adequate milk volume. Infants born to mothers who receive high rates of intravenous fluid administration during the intrapartum period have been shown to have more weight loss.[87] Nomograms are available to calculate acceptable weight loss patterns in exclusively breastfed infants.[88,89] As mentioned, allowing the infant to have access to the breast early on with frequent feedings is an important approach to excessive weight loss or failure to gain weight appropriately. Corrective steps must be taken early on to ensure adequate nutrition and hydration to the newborn infant, which may include temporary supplementation of pumped milk, donor human milk, or infant formula until the infant-mother dyad has improved lactation success.

If the infant fails to gain weight, the infant most likely is receiving insufficient milk. At times, this can be overcome by increasing the frequency of feedings. For example, an infant who sleeps for long intervals during the night can be awakened and breastfed. If maternal anxiety or exhaustion are contributing, then more support for the mother can be sought. The AAP and American College of Obstetricians and Gynecologists suggest an organized approach to assessment of inadequate human milk intake that considers infant and maternal factors.[90] However, if objective measures, such as inadequate weight gain, persist despite all efforts, the mother most likely has insufficient milk syndrome, the most common cause of breastfeeding failure.[91] Insufficient milk syndrome occurs in approximately 5% of women. Maternal history can suggest insufficient milk syndrome. Lack of breast enlargement during pregnancy, lack of breast fullness by 5 days after birth, or a history of breast reduction surgery are predictive of insufficient milk syndrome. Maternal history should include questions about pituitary or thyroid disease; in addition, the breasts should be examined for hypoplasia as well as morphology (an abnormal hollow or tubular breast shape, with a wide intermammary space). Maternal hemorrhage and anemia also have been associated with insufficient milk syndrome.[92] In addition, a careful assessment of the infant's oral structures may reveal problems, such as ankyloglossia, poor oral motor tone, or a dysfunctional or weak suck, which may be contributing to poor milk removal and subsequent decreased milk production. Close monitoring of the infant's weight and evaluation of breastfeeding technique to ensure that the infant is transferring enough milk while feeding should occur.

Additional maternal milk expression between feedings can stimulate milk production and provide a human milk supplement to provide to the infant until the infant is gaining adequately with direct breastfeeding. Infants with ankyloglossia, which is causing maternal pain or interfering with milk transfer, may benefit from a frenotomy procedure.[93] Frenotomy procedures have increased significantly in recent years, but there is limited evidence to support their use, other than short-term pain relief and improved latch. The infant and breastfeeding should be evaluated carefully by a qualified provider before frenotomy is recommended or performed.

Women with poor milk production may request galactogogues, substances that induce, maintain, and increase human milk production. The currently available galactogogues were reviewed by the Academy of Breastfeeding Medicine in 2011.[94] The recommendation is for caution in the use of substances to enhance milk production, limited to those women who have no treatable cause for the reduced milk production. Supplementation is often necessary for infants receiving insufficient human milk.

Supplementation

Appropriate supplementation includes expressed human milk, donor human milk, or infant formula. The recommendation that donor milk be used must be approached with caution to be sure that the milk comes from a bank that abides by the protocols recommended by the Human Milk Banking Association of North America (HMBANA)[95,96] and that follows the recommendations of the US Food and Drug Administration and CDC standards for cleanliness and storage of human milk. The milk from these banks is tested for HIV-1 and -2, hepatitis B and C, and syphilis, and donors and their physician must verify that they are healthy, that their infants are thriving, and that they are taking no medications. The donors must undergo serologic testing to screen for potential infectious diseases that could be transmitted via human milk. All HMBANA certified milk banks are nonprofit. In contrast, there are many Web sites that offer human milk that may or may not follow the protocols of the HMBANA, and the use of human milk from these sources should be approached with great caution, including commercially available "'for-profit" sources of banked human milk that are not HMBANA certified, which may vary in their processing guidelines. There are no government standards or oversight currently of donor milk, including nutrient content, whether offered online or via established human milk banks.

Common Breastfeeding Issues
Regular concerns of mothers with regard to breastfeeding include nipple pain, engorgement, and mastitis. Nipple pain is common in the first week or so of breastfeeding. During a feeding, nipple pain typically occurs when the baby first latches on, but it subsequently eases during the course of the feeding. If it persists, the mother's breasts and nipples, as well as the feeding technique, should be observed by a lactation expert. Poor positioning and improper latch are common causes of nipple pain, as is trauma caused by vigorous sucking on the nipple and not suckling with the mouth widely opened on the areola. This may result in nipple cracking and ultimately bleeding if unrelieved. Application of human milk to the nipple after a feed may be helpful to aid in healing. Manual expression for a day or 2 to allow the cracks to heal may ease the pain. Engorgement is usually caused by infrequent or ineffective milk removal. Engorgement is treated by increasing the frequency of breastfeeding.[97] Judicious pumping to relieve pain caused by excessive engorgement may be helpful, as well as gentle hand expression before a feeding to soften the nipple-areolar complex to enhance latch-on. Repeated milk expression may exacerbate the engorgement. Engorgement should be a temporary phenomenon, but if unrelieved, may cause persistent decrease in milk production.

A clogged duct occurs when the breast is incompletely emptied, milk remains in the duct, and inflammation develops. It is diagnosed by palpating a lump in the breast. Treatment consists of gentle massage of the plugged duct with increased nursing to drain the breast. Anecdotally, some mothers report relief in using oral lecithin capsules, especially if plugged ducts persist or recur. It is speculated to decrease the viscosity of the milk and increase its emulsification, but there is no published evidence to support this practice. Mastitis typically presents after the 10th postpartum day as a localized area of warmth, tenderness, edema, and erythema in a breast. It may also present with systemic signs such as fever, malaise, and intense breast pain. It generally starts as a localized inflammatory process but may proceed to a more generalized infectious one. Stasis of milk is considered a significant risk factor, and it is treated by increasing the frequency of breastfeeding to drain the breast, rest, and analgesics. Antibiotics may be prescribed to treat the infection and prevent a breast milk abscess. It is not necessary to stop breastfeeding, but the need for effective treatment is essential.[98,99]

Jaundice

Jaundice associated with breastfeeding falls into 2 distinct entities: breast milk jaundice and breastfeeding jaundice. Breast milk jaundice occurs in many breastfed infants and is characterized by jaundice that persists beyond the second week of life and may last as long as 12 weeks. High serum concentrations of unconjugated bilirubin is a hallmark of breast milk jaundice. Infants with breast milk jaundice are generally healthy, gain weight appropriately, and are developing normally, and in most circumstances, the family can be reassured. The factor in human milk that is responsible for prolonged unconjugated hyperbilirubinemia has not been identified. All infants with the presumptive diagnosis of breast milk jaundice should have a total and conjugated serum bilirubin determination after the third week of life to evaluate for other causes of hyperbilirubinemia and cholestasis. If the conjugated bilirubin concentration is greater than 1.5 mg/dL or 20% of the total bilirubin, an evaluation for liver disease must be performed.

Severe jaundice may occur with the second entity, breastfeeding jaundice. This is also referred to as nonbreastfeeding jaundice, lack of breastfeeding jaundice, or more recently, suboptimal intake or dehydration jaundice.[100] Severe jaundice is the most common reason for readmission for term or near-term infants to the hospital after delivery, and in one very large study, almost all the infants admitted for severe jaundice were breastfed.[101] Thus, poor breastfeeding management is often a contributing factor. Breastfeeding jaundice occurs in the first week of life and can be associated with inadequate milk intake and dehydration. It is similar to starvation jaundice. Other medical factors, such as ABO incompatibility or urinary tract infection, may contribute to the severity of the jaundice. Generally, concentrations of total bilirubin in severe jaundice are 25 mg/dL or greater. These infants should be managed according the AAP policy on neonatal jaundice.[102] A more recent clinical protocol has been published that addresses management of jaundice in the breastfeeding infant.[103] In addition, the various causes of insufficient milk syndrome must be ruled out, as discussed above.

Nutrition of the Lactating Mother

Dietary reference intakes for breastfeeding mothers are similar to or greater than those during pregnancy. The lactating mother has an increased daily energy need of 450 to 500 kcal/day that can be met by modest increases in a normally balanced diet. Mothers should be encouraged to eat a well-balanced diet that includes vegetables and fruits. As was recommended in the Robert Wood Johnson Foundation "Executive Summary on Healthy Eating Research," a diversified maternal diet including foods that are considered allergenic will translate into a more diversified diet in the breast-feeding infant through food flavors in her milk.[66] Although most clinicians recommend the continued use of prenatal vitamins during lactation, there is no specific recommendation or rationale for these supplements.[104] The recommended dietary allowance for vitamin D in lactating women is 600 IU per day, with an upper limit of 4000 IU per day.[23] The results of a randomized controlled trial showed that an intake of 6400 IU per day in lactating women significantly increases the vitamin D content of maternal milk and thus in their recipient infants, although this intake exceeds the upper limit for lactating women recommended by the National Academy of Medicine, as noted above.[22]

Consumption of 1 to 2 servings of ocean-going fish per week is recommended to meet the need for an average daily intake of 200 to 300 mg of omega-3 long-chain fatty acids (docosahexaenoic acid [DHA]). Although there is concern for the risk of intake of excessive mercury or other contaminants, the risk may be offset by the potential neurobehavioral benefits of additional DHA intake beyond what is endogenously synthesized[105] (see Chapter 17: Fats and Fatty Acids). Other sources of DHA for the breastfeeding mother include kelp and seaweed products.

Growth of the Breastfed Infant

Until the 2006 publication of the World Health Organization (WHO) growth charts,[106] the CDC growth charts published in 2000 for infants and children were used by most pediatric health care providers in the United States.[107,108] The CDC charts are a growth reference and describe how US children grow across a wide range of social, ethnic, and economic conditions (see Chapter 24: Assessment of Nutritional Status, and Appendix Q). The CDC charts used data from infants that approximated the mix of feedings that infants received in the 1970s and 1980s. During this period, one third of US infants were breastfed up to 3 months of age, and the other two thirds were predominantly formula fed. Since then, feeding patterns in the United States have changed, as noted previously. The need for alternative growth charts was warranted.

The 2006 WHO charts met the need for how breastfed infants "should" grow, under ideal conditions not subject to economic restraints. They are considered a growth "standard." The charts from birth to 2 years of age are based on 903 infants who were exclusively/predominantly breastfed for 4 to 6 months and who continued breastfeeding for at least 12 months.[106] The median duration of breastfeeding was 17.8 months, and complementary foods were introduced at a mean age of 5.1 months. After comparison of the growth curves, in 2010 the CDC recommended the use of the WHO Multicenter Growth Reference Study growth charts for children younger than 24 months (regardless of diet) in place of the 2000 CDC growth charts[109] (see Chapter 24 and Appendix Q). These charts include weight for age, length for age, head circumference for age, weight for length, body mass index for age, and growth velocity standards. These standards are endorsed by the AAP.

Expressing and Storing Milk

At times, mothers cannot breastfeed directly, and having a supply of milk available to the infant is desirable. There are many books and online resources on the expression of human milk. How a particular mother expresses her milk is a matter of choice. Milk can be hand expressed or expressed using any one of a variety of manual or electric pumps. Before expressing milk, the mother should wash her hands with warm, soapy water. For frequent or sustained milk pumping, a dual chamber pump, or double pump, is recommended. This allows the mother to express milk from both breasts at the same time. This causes a greater increase in the mother's prolactin levels and allows for greater efficiency in pumping. There are many styles of breast pumps available on the market. A hospital-grade pump is available for rental if the mother is pumping for an infant in the neonatal intensive care unit, but commercial pumps work well for most women for occasional use, assuming they are able to breastfeed directly for most feeds, which helps to maintain the milk supply. If using a pump, the mother should wash all components of the pump with warm, soapy water, as soon as possible after using and discard any tubing that has mold visible or milk that cannot be removed and cleaned safely. A spare set of tubing is recommended. The CDC issued guidance in 2017 on cleaning of breast pump kits to minimize the risk of infectious contamination of the expressed milk in response to reports of *Cronobacter sakazakii* transmitted from a breast pump kit (https://www.cdc.gov/healthywater/pdf/hygiene/breast-pump-fact-sheet.pdf).[110]

The expressed milk should be placed in a glass or hard plastic container. Milk should be stored as individual feedings so the same milk is not frozen and thawed numerous times. The milk should be labeled with the date it was collected. When needed, it can be thawed in the refrigerator overnight or more rapidly by holding the container under running tepid water.

Guidelines for storing expressed human milk vary according to the source and differ for milk expressed to be fed to preterm or ill infants. In general milk, for expressed for home use, the rule of "4's" will suffice: 4 hours at room temperature and 4 days in the refrigerator. These are conservative guidelines, and as indicated in the AAP recommendations for freezing and refrigeration of human milk, it may be stored safely for longer periods (https://www.healthychildren.org/English/ages-stages/baby/breastfeeding/Pages/Storing-and-Preparing-Expressed-Breast-Milk.aspx).[111] Newer data suggest that human milk can be stored at refrigerator temperature (4°C) in a neonatal intensive care unit for as long as 96 hours after thawing.[112] Human milk should never be refrozen.

Special Situations, Including Preterm Infants

Infants who are ill, who have developmental delay, or who are born preterm present special challenges for breastfeeding. These infants must be carefully followed by an experienced neonatology and nutrition team. Human milk is the preferred feeding for preterm infants, and the body of evidence is growing that preterm infants who weigh less than 1500 g at birth should only receive human milk (see Chapter 5: Nutritional Needs of the Preterm Infant). Mother's own milk is preferred, and many neonatal intensive care units begin by swabbing the neonate's mouth soon after birth with expressed maternal colostrum. Mothers should express milk for ill or very small preterm infants. If maternal milk is not available, pasteurized donor milk can be used.[113] Preterm infants who weigh less than 1500 g at birth require a human milk fortifier, whether derived from human milk or from cow milk products, to provide adequate nutrients to support growth. If tube feedings are utilized, the length of tubing should be minimized and the milk should be placed in syringes properly positioned with the opening pointed upward. This will prevent loss of the fat and subsequent caloric intake from adherence of fat to the tubing.

The Pediatrician's Role in Breastfeeding Support

The US Surgeon General called for greater education and training in breast-feeding for all health care providers.[4] Many pediatricians have had limited education during their training on assessing breastfeeding and providing appropriate anticipatory guidance, as recently confirmed.[114] Pediatricians must be well informed about breastfeeding and its benefits and under-stand the importance of supporting breastfeeding and the breastfeeding mother from birth and the effect of this support on successful breastfeed-ing initiation and continuation. Pediatricians must be advocates for the institution of policies, either the Baby-Friendly Hospital Initiative or others, designed to provide support for initiation and continuation of breastfeed-ing. Pediatric care providers should be competent in evaluating breastfeed-ing mother-baby dyads in each mother's hospital room. Pediatricians who care for breastfed infants, especially late preterm infants, should know how to assess the infant's latch and transfer of milk. Providers must ensure that infants are breastfeeding adequately, latching on, and transferring milk well in the maternity unit. All infants should be assessed at the time of discharge for excessive weight loss or poor weight gain, which may result in extended hospital stay or a more intensive postdischarge follow-up plan.

Pediatricians should advocate for the availability of certified lactation consultants to evaluate mothers having difficulty with lactation, experi-encing pain, or concerned about milk supply. Timely medical follow-up, generally within 24 to 48 hours after hospital discharge, is essential. Formal observation and evaluation of breastfeeding should occur at the first office visit and any subsequent visit during which the mother expresses concerns. According to the AAP clinical report "The Breastfeeding-Friendly Pediatric Office Practice," training of the office staff, especially nurses who provide telephone triage or assessment of breastfeeding mothers and infants, is important.[115]

Conclusions

Breastfeeding is a natural extension of pregnancy and is important in the early life of the infant. If positive attitudes exist in the family, community, workplace, and health care system, 95% of mothers can breastfeed successfully. Breastfeeding confers benefits to the infant, and lack of access to human milk can be disadvantageous for the infant. The duration of breastfeeding depends on the desires of the mother and the needs of her infant and her family, especially if she is working. Given the emerging evidence that avoiding maternal intake of potential allergens during the first year of life has not resulted in decreased risk of allergy and that a diversified diet including food allergens may be beneficial during both pregnancy and lactation, earlier exposure to potential allergens (such as peanuts and eggs) may result in greater tolerance of allergenic foods without increasing the risk of atopic disease. It is recommended by the AAP that exclusive breastfeeding, supplemented with iron and vitamin D, be continued for about 6 months. Continuing breastfeeding through at least the first year of life, or as long as mutually desired by mother and infant, with continued support for breastfeeding mothers, is also recommended by the AAP.

Care must be taken to assess the infant's growth using either the WHO or the 2010 CDC growth curves that are specific for the breastfeeding infant. Early identification of lactation issues is essential for sustained lactation, with the help of a breastfeeding medicine expert or lactation consultant allowing prompt action and remedy. Although infants with special needs, such as preterm infants, may require additional supplements to ensure adequate growth, the goal is to achieve breastfeeding through the first year.

References

1. American Academy of Pediatrics, Section on Breastfeeding. Breastfeeding and the use of human milk. *Pediatrics.* 2012;129(3):e827–e841
2. American Academy of Pediatrics, Committee on Nutrition. *Pediatric Nutrition Handbook.* 7th ed. Elk Grove Village, IL: American Academy of Pediatrics; 2013
3. Centers for Disease Control and Prevention, National Center for Chronic Disease Prevention and Health Promotion. CDC National Immunization Survey (NIS) Breastfeeding Among US Children Born 2002–2014, CDC National Immunization Survey. Available at: https://www.cdc.gov/breastfeeding/data/nis_data/index.htm. Accessed November 21, 2018
4. US Department of Health and Human Services. *Executive Summary. The Surgeon General's Call to Action to Support Breastfeeding.* Washington, DC: US Department of Health and Human Services, Office of the Surgeon General; 2011

5. Centers for Disease Control and Prevention. Breastfeeding Report Card, Progressing Toward National Breastfeeding Goals. 2016. Available at: https://www.cdc.gov/breastfeeding/pdf/2016breastfeedingreportcard.pdf. Accessed November 21, 2018

6. Centers for Disease Control and Prevention. *Centers for Disease Control and Prevention. South Carolina 2015 Report, CDC Survey of Maternity Practices in Infant Nutrition and Care.* Atlanta, GA: Centers for Disease Control and Prevention; 2016

7. Anstey EH, Shoemaker ML, Barrera CM, O'Neil ME, Verma AB, Holman DM. Breastfeeding and breast cancer risk reduction: implications for black mothers. *Am J Prev Med.* 2017;53(3 Suppl 1):S40–S46

8. Anstey EH, Chen J, Elam-Evans LD, Perrine CG. Racial and Geographic Differences in Breastfeeding - United States, 2011–2015. *MMWR Morb Mortal Wkly Rep.* 2017;66(27):723–727

9. US Department of Health and Human Services, Public Health Service. Healthy People 2020. National Health Promotion and Disease Prevention Objectives. Maternal, Infant, and Child Health. 2010; Available at: https://www.healthypeople.gov/2020/topics-objectives/topic/maternal-infant-and-child-health/objectives. Accessed November 21, 2018

10. Womenshealth.gov. Business Case for Breastfeeding. Available at: https://www.womenshealth.gov/breastfeeding/breastfeeding-home-work-and-public/breastfeeding-and-going-back-work/business-case. Accessed October 18, 2017, 2017

11. US Department of Labor. Break Time for Nursing Mothers. Available at: https://www.dol.gov/whd/nursingmothers/. Accessed October 18, 2017

12. Wagner CL, Wagner MT. The breast or the bottle? Determinants of infant feeding behaviors. *Clin Perinatol.* 1999;26(2):505–526

13. Fein SB, Labiner-Wolfe J, Shealy KR, Li R, Chen J, Grummer-Strawn LM. Infant Feeding Practices Study II: study methods. *Pediatrics.* 2008;122(Suppl 2):S28–S35

14. Fein SB, Grummer-Strawn LM, Raju TN. Infant feeding and care practices in the United States: results from the Infant Feeding Practices Study II. *Pediatrics.* 2008;122(Suppl 2):S25–S27

15. Wiener RC, Wiener MA. Breastfeeding prevalence and distribution in the USA and Appalachia by rural and urban setting. *Rural Remote Health.* 2011;11(2):1713

16. Lynch S, Bethel J, Chowdhury N, Moore JB. Rural and urban breastfeeding initiation trends in low-income women in North Carolina from 2003 to 2007. *J Hum Lact.* May 2012;28(2):226–232.

17. Pak-Gorstein S, Haq A, Graham EA. Cultural influences on infant feeding practices. *Pediatr Rev.* 2009;30(3):e11–e21

18. Karra MV, Udipi SA, Kirksey A, Roepke JL. Changes in specific nutrients in breast milk during extended lactation. *Am J Clin Nutr.* 1986;43(4):495–503

19. Jensen R, ed. *Handbook of Milk Composition.* San Diego: Academic Press; 1995

20. Motil KJ, Sheng HP, Montandon CM, Wong WW. Human milk protein does not limit growth of breast-fed infants. *J Pediatr Gastroenterol Nutr.* 1997;24(1):10–17

21. Basile LA, Taylor SN, Wagner CL, Horst RL, Hollis BW. The effect of high-dose vitamin D supplementation on serum vitamin D levels and milk calcium concentration in lactating women and their infants. *Breastfeed Med.* 2006;1(1):27–35

22. Hollis BW, Wagner CL, Howard CR, et al. Maternal Versus infant vitamin d supplementation during lactation: a randomized controlled trial. *Pediatrics.* 2015;136(4):625–634

23. Institute of Medicine, Food and Nutrition Board, Standing Committee on the Scientific Evaluation of Dietary Reference Intakes. *Dietary Reference Intakes for Vitamin D and Calcium.* Washington, DC: National Academies Press; 2010

24. Saadi H, Dawodu A, Afandi B, Zayed R, Benedict S, Nagelkerke N. Efficacy of daily and monthly high-dose calciferol in vitamin D-deficient nulliparous and lactating women. *Am J Clin Nutr.* 2007;85(6):1565–1571

25. Vieth Streym S, Hojskov CS, Moller UK, et al. Vitamin D content in human breast milk: a 9-mo follow-up study. *Am J Clin Nutr.* 2016;103(1):107–114

26. March KM, Chen NN, Karakochuk CD, et al. Maternal vitamin D(3) supplementation at 50 mug/d protects against low serum 25-hydroxyvitamin D in infants at 8 wk of age: a randomized controlled trial of 3 doses of vitamin D beginning in gestation and continued in lactation. *Am J Clin Nutr.* 2015;102(2):402–410

27. Baker RD, Greer FR, American Academy of Pediatrics, Committee on Nutrition. Diagnosis and prevention of iron deficiency and iron-deficiency anemia in infants and young children (0–3 years of age). *Pediatrics.* 2010;126(5):1040–1050

28. Whitmore TJ, Trengove NJ, Graham DF, Hartmann PE. Analysis of insulin in human breast milk in mothers with type 1 and type 2 diabetes mellitus. *Int J Endocrinol.* 2012;2012:296368

29. Guillet S, Baatz J, Forsythe D, Wagner CL. Establishing the presence of EGF and EGFr in human milk's compartments. Paper presented at: Pediatric Academic Society Meeting; Baltimore, MD; 2002

30. Wagner CL, Baatz JE. TGFalpha within compartments of human milk. *Adv Exp Med Biol.* 2004;554:417–421

31. Wagner CL, Baatz JE. Higher molecular mass forms of TGFalpha in human milk. *Adv Exp Med Biol.* 2004;554:411–415

32. Siafakas C, Anatolitou F, Fusunyan R, Walker W, Sanderson I. Vascular endothelial growth factor (VEGF) is present in human breast milk and its receptor is present on intestinal epithelial cells. *Pediatr Res.* 1999;45(5 Pt 1):652–657

33. Ruiz L, Espinosa-Martos I, Garcia-Carral C, et al. What's normal? Immune profiling of human milk from healthy women living in different geographical and socioeconomic settings. *Front Immunol.* 2017;8:696

34. Zambruni M, Villalobos A, Somasunderam A, et al. Maternal and pregnancy-related factors affecting human milk cytokines among Peruvian mothers bearing low-birth-weight neonates. *J Reprod Immunol.* 2017;120:20–26

35. Riskin A, Almog M, Peri R, Halasz K, Srugo I, Kessel A. Changes in immunomodulatory constituents of human milk in response to active infection in the nursing infant. *Pediatr Res.* 2012;71(2):220–225

36. Peterson JA, Hamosh M, Scallan CD, et al. Milk fat globule glycoproteins in human milk and in gastric aspirates of mother's milk-fed preterm infants. *Pediatr Res.* 1998;44(4):499–506

37. Hamosh M, Peterson JA, Henderson TR, et al. Protective function of human milk: the milk fat globule. *Semin Perinatol.* 1999;23(3):242–249

38. Gallier S, Vocking K, Post JA, et al. A novel infant milk formula concept: mimicking the human milk fat globule structure. *Colloids Surf B Biointerfaces.* 2015;136:329–339

39. Admyre C, Johansson SM, Qazi KR, et al. Exosomes with immune modulatory features are present in human breast milk. *J Immunol.* 2007;179(3):1969–1978

40. Torregrosa Paredes P, Gutzeit C, Johansson S, et al. Differences in exosome populations in human breast milk in relation to allergic sensitization and lifestyle. *Allergy.* 2014;69(4):463–471

41. Zhou Q, Li M, Wang X, et al. Immune-related microRNAs are abundant in breast milk exosomes. *Int J Biol Sci.* 2012;8(1):118–123

42. Kosaka N, Izumi H, Sekine K, Ochiya T. microRNA as a new immune-regulatory agent in breast milk. *Silence.* 2010;1(1):7

43. Wagner CL, Forsythe DW, Pittard WB. Variation in the biochemical forms of transforming growth factor-alpha present in human milk and secreted by human milk macrophages. *Biol Neonate.* 1995;68(5):325–333

44. Ichikawa M, Sugita M, Takahashi M, et al. Breast milk macrophages spontaneously produce granulocyte-macrophage colony-stimulating factor and differentiate into dendritic cells in the presence of exogenous interleukin-4 alone. *Immunology.* 2003;108(2):189–195

45. Hassiotou F, Geddes DT. Immune cell-mediated protection of the mammary gland and the infant during breastfeeding. *Adv Nutr.* 2015;6(3):267–275

46. Cregan MD, Fan Y, Appelbee A, et al. Identification of nestin-positive putative mammary stem cells in human breastmilk. *Cell Tissue Res.* 2007;329(1):129–136

47. Fan Y, Chong YS, Choolani MA, Cregan MD, Chan JK. Unravelling the mystery of stem/progenitor cells in human breast milk. *PLoS One.* 2010;5(12):e14421

48. Hassiotou F, Beltran A, Chetwynd E, et al. Breastmilk is a novel source of stem cells with multilineage differentiation potential. *Stem Cells.* 2012;30(10):2164–2174

49. Hassiotou F, Hepworth AR, Williams TM, et al. Breastmilk cell and fat contents respond similarly to removal of breastmilk by the infant. *PLoS One.* 2013;8(11):e78232

50. Hosseini SM, Talaei-Khozani T, Sani M, Owrangi B. Differentiation of human breast-milk stem cells to neural stem cells and neurons. *Neurol Res Int.* 2014;2014:807896

51. Hassiotou F, Hartmann PE. At the dawn of a new discovery: the potential of breast milk stem cells. *Adv Nutr.* 2014;5(6):770–778

52. Sani M, Hosseini SM, Salmannejad M, et al. Origins of the breast milk-derived cells; an endeavor to find the cell sources. *Cell Biol Int.* 2015;39(5):611–618

53. Donovan SM. Human milk oligosaccharides - the plot thickens. *Br J Nutr.* 2009;101(9):1267–1269

54. Donovan SM, Comstock SS. Human Milk Oligosaccharides Influence Neonatal Mucosal and Systemic Immunity. *Ann Nutr Metab.* 2016;69(Suppl 2):42–51

55. Newburg D. Oligosaccharides in human milk and bacterial colonization. *J Pediatr Gastroenterol Nutr.* 2000;30:S8–S17

56. Musilova S, Rada V, Vlkova E, Bunesova V. Beneficial effects of human milk oligosaccharides on gut microbiota. *Benef Microbes.* 2014;5(3):273–283

57. Wang M, Li M, Wu S, et al. Fecal microbiota composition of breast-fed infants is correlated with human milk oligosaccharides consumed. *J Pediatr Gastroenterol Nutr.* 2015;60(6):825–833

58. Donovan SM. Human Milk Oligosaccharides: Potent Weapons in the Battle against Rotavirus Infection. *J Nutr.* 2017;147(9):1605–1606

59. Comstock SS, Li M, Wang M, et al. Dietary Human milk oligosaccharides but not prebiotic oligosaccharides increase circulating natural killer cell and mesenteric lymph node memory T cell populations in noninfected and rotavirus-infected neonatal piglets. *J Nutr.* 2017;147(6):1041–1047

60. Ip S, Chung M, Raman G, et al. *Breastfeeding and Maternal and Infant Health Outcomes in Developed Countries. Evidence Report/Technology Assessment No. 153.* Prepared by Tufts-New England Medical Center Evidence-based Practice Center, under Contract No. 290-02-0022. Rockville, MD: Agency for Healthcare Research and Quality; 2007

61. Herlenius E, Kuhn P. Sudden unexpected postnatal collapse of newborn infants: a review of cases, definitions, risks, and preventive measures. *Transl Stroke Res.* 2013;4(2):236–247

62. Feldman-Winter L, Goldsmith JP, Committee on Fetus and Newborn, Task Force on Sudden Infant Death Syndrome. Safe sleep and skin-to-skin care in the neonatal period for healthy term newborns. *Pediatrics.* 2016;138(3):e20161889

63. Association for Women's Health, Obstetric and Neonatal Nurses. Immediate and sustained skin-to-skin contact for the healthy term newborn after birth: AWHONN Practice Brief Number 5. *J Obstet Gynecol Neonatal Nurs.* 2016;45(6):842–844

64. Ludington-Hoe S, Morgan K. Infant Assessment and Reduction of Sudden Unexpected Postnatal Collapse Risk During Skin-to-Skin Contact. *NAINR.* 2014;14(1):28–33

65. American Academy of Pediatrics, Task Force on Sudden Infant Death Syndrome. SIDS and other sleep-related infant deaths: updated 2016 recommendations for a safe infant sleeping environment. *Pediatrics.* 2016;138(5):e20162938

66. Pérez-Escamilla R, Segura-Pérez S, Lott M. *RWJF HER Expert Panel on Best Practices for Promoting Healthy Nutrition, Feeding Patterns, and Weight Status for Infants and Toddlers from Birth to 24 Months. Feeding Guidelines for Infants and Young Toddlers: A Responsive Parenting Approach. Guidelines for Health Professionals.* Durham, NC: Healthy Eating Research; 2017

67. Sachs HC, Committee on Drugs. The transfer of drugs and therapeutics into human breast milk: an update on selected topics. *Pediatrics.* Sep 2013;132(3): e796–e809

68. Meites E. Opiate exposure in breastfeeding newborns. *J Hum Lact.* 2007;23(1):13

69. Glatstein MM, Garcia-Bournissen F, Finkelstein Y, Koren G. Methadone exposure during lactation. *Can Fam Physician.* 2008;54(12):1689–1690

70. Whalen BL, Holmes AV. Neonatal abstinence syndrome and the pediatric hospitalist. *Hosp Pediatr.* 2013;3(4):324–325

71. Newman A, Davies GA, Dow K, et al. Rooming-in care for infants of opioid-dependent mothers: Implementation and evaluation at a tertiary care hospital. *Can Fam Physician.* Dec 2015;61(12):e555–e561

72. Jones HE, Seashore C, Johnson E, et al. Psychometric assessment of the Neonatal Abstinence Scoring System and the MOTHER NAS Scale. *Am J Addict.* 2016;25(5):370–373

73. Holmes AV, Atwood EC, Whalen B, et al. Rooming-in to treat neonatal abstinence syndrome: improved family-centered care at lower cost. *Pediatrics.* 2016;137(6):e20152929

74. Fewtrell M, Wilson D, Booth I, Lucas A. Six months of exclusive breast feeding: how good is the evidence? *BMJ.* 2010;342:c5955

75. American Academy of Pediatrics, American College of Obstetricians and Gynecologists. *Breastfeeding Handbook for Physicians.* 2nd ed. Elk Grove Village, IL: American Academy of Pediatrics; 2013

76. American College of Obstetricians and Gynecologists. ACOG Breastfeeding Toolkit. Available at: https://www.acog.org/About-ACOG/ACOG-Departments/Toolkits-for-Health-Care-Providers/Breastfeeding-Toolkit. Accessed October 18, 2017

77. UNICEF. *Ten Steps to Successful Breastfeeding.* Geneva, Switzerland: UNICEF; 1991

78. Kramer MS, Chalmers B, Hodnett ED, et al. Promotion of Breastfeeding Intervention Trial (PROBIT): a randomized trial in the Republic of Belarus. *JAMA.* 2001;285(4):413–420

79. Spaeth A, Zemp E, Merten S, Dratva J. Baby-Friendly Hospital designation has a sustained impact on continued breastfeeding. *Matern Child Nutr.* 2018;14(1). doi: 10.1111/mcn.12497

80. Patnode CD, Henninger ML, Senger CA, Perdue LA, Whitlock EP. Primary care interventions to support breastfeeding: an updated systematic review for the US Preventative Services Task Force. Evidence Synthesis No. 143. AHRQ publication 15-05218-EF-1. Rockville, MD: Agency for Healthcare Research and Quality; 2016

81. Feltner C, Weber RP, Stuebe A. *Breastfeeding Programs and Policies, Breastfeeding Uptake, and Maternal Health Outcomes in Developed Countries. Comparative Effectiveness Review No. 210.* Rockville, MD: Agency for Healthcare Research and Quality, US Department of Health and Human Services; 2015

82. Dewey KG, Nommsen-Rivers LA, Heinig MJ, Cohen RJ. Risk factors for suboptimal infant breastfeeding behavior, delayed onset of lactation, and excess neonatal weight loss. *Pediatrics.* 2003;112(3 Pt 1):607–619

83. Nommsen-Rivers LA, Chantry CJ, Peerson JM, Cohen RJ, Dewey KG. Delayed onset of lactogenesis among first-time mothers is related to maternal obesity and factors associated with ineffective breastfeeding. *Am J Clin Nutr.* 2010;92(3):574–584

84. Yamauchi Y, Yamanouchi I. The relationship between rooming-in/not rooming-in and breast-feeding variables. *Acta Paediatr Scand.* 1990;79(11):1017–1022

85. Yamauchi Y, Yamanouchi I. Breast-feeding frequency during the first 24 hours after birth in full-term neonates. *Pediatrics.* 1990;86(2):171–175

86. DiGirolamo AM, Grummer-Strawn LM, Fein SB. Effect of maternity-care practices on breastfeeding. *Pediatrics.* 2008;122(Suppl 2):S43–S49

87. Chantry CJ, Nommsen-Rivers LA, Peerson JM, Cohen RJ, Dewey KG. Excess weight loss in first-born breastfed newborns relates to maternal intrapartum fluid balance. *Pediatrics.* 2011;127(1):e171–e179

88. Schaefer EW, Flaherman VJ, Kuzniewicz MW, Li SX, Walsh EM, Paul IM. External validation of early weight loss nomograms for exclusively breastfed newborns. *Breastfeed Med.* 2015;10(10):458–463

89. Flaherman VJ, Schaefer EW, Kuzniewicz MW, Li SX, Walsh EM, Paul IM. Early weight loss nomograms for exclusively breastfed newborns. *Pediatrics.* 2015;135(1):e16–e23

90. American Academy of Pediatrics, American College of Obstetricians and Gynecologists. Maintenance of breastfeeding. In: Schanler RJ, ed. *Breastfeeding Handbook for Physicians.* 2nd ed. Elk Grove Village, IL: American Academy of Pediatrics; 2013:107–110

91. Sjolin S, Hofvander Y, Hillervik C. Factors related to early termination of breast feeding. A retrospective study in Sweden. *Acta Paediatr Scand.* 1977;66(4):505–511

92. Willis CE, Livingstone V. Infant insufficient milk syndrome associated with maternal postpartum hemorrhage. *J Hum Lact.* 1995;11:123–126

93. Bin-Nun A, Kasirer YM, Mimouni FB. A dramatic increase in tongue tie-related articles: a 67 years systematic review. *Breastfeed Med.* 2017;12(7):410–414

94. Academy of Breastfeeding Medicine Protocol Committee. ABM Clinical Protocol #9: Use of galactogogues in initiating or augmenting the rate of maternal milk secretion (First revision January 2011). *Breastfeed Med.* 2011;6(1):41–46

95. Eitenmiller R. An overview of human milk pasteurization. Paper presented at: Sixth Annual Conference HMBANA. Human Milk Banking: Scanning the Future. Lexington, KY: Human Milk Banking Association of North America; 1990.

96. Human Milk Banking Association of North America. *Guidelines for the Establishment and Operation of a Donor Human Milk Bank.* Fort Worth, TX: Human Milk Banking Association of North America; 1994

97. Mangesi L, Zakarija-Grkovic I. Treatments for breast engorgement during lactation. *Cochrane Database Syst Rev.* 2016(6):CD006946

98. Chambers AH, Wagner CL. History: a lesson from the past: excerpts from a clinical lecture on the treatment of a breast abscess, by Dr. Gunning S. Bedford (c. 1855). *Breastfeed Med.* 2007;2(2):105–111

99. Amir LH, Academy of Breastfeeding Medicine Protocol Committee. ABM clinical protocol #4: Mastitis, revised March 2014. *Breastfeed Med.* 2014;9(5):239–243

100. Flaherman VJ, Maisels MJ, Academy of Breastfeeding Medicine. ABM Clinical Protocol #22: Guidelines for Management of Jaundice in the Breastfeeding Infant 35 Weeks or More of Gestation—Revised 2017. *Breastfeeding Medicine.* 2017;12(5):250–257

101. Newman TB, Liljestrand P, Escobar GJ. Infants with bilirubin levels of 30 mg/dL or more in a large managed care organization. *Pediatrics.* 2003;111(6 Pt 1): 1303–1311

102. American Academy of Pediatrics, Subcommittee on Hyperbilirubinemia. Management of hyperbilirubinemia in the newborn infant 35 or more weeks of gestation. *Pediatrics.* 2004;114(1):297–316

103. Flaherman VJ, Maisels MJ, Brodribb W, et al; Academy of Breastfeeding Medicine. ABM clinical protocol #22: Guidelines for management of jaundice in breastfeeding infant 35 weeks or more of gestation-revised 2017. *Breastfeed Med.* 2017;12(5):250–257

104. Picciano MF, McGuire MK. Use of dietary supplements by pregnant and lactating women in North America. *Am J Clin Nutr.* 2009;89(2):663S–667S

105. Carlson SE. Docosahexaenoic acid supplementation in pregnancy and lactation. *Am J Clin Nutr.* 2009;89(2):678S–684S

106. WHO Multicentre Growth Reference Study Group. WHO Child Growth Standards based on length/height, weight and age. *Acta Paediatr Suppl.* 2006;450:76–85

107. Kuczmarski RJ, Ogden CL, Guo SS, et al. 2000 CDC Growth Charts for the United States: methods and development. *Vital Health Stat 11.* 2002(246):1–190

108. Ogden CL, Kuczmarski RJ, Flegal KM, et al. Centers for Disease Control and Prevention 2000 growth charts for the United States: improvements to the 1977 National Center for Health Statistics version. *Pediatrics.* 2002;109(1):45–60

109. Centers for Disease Control and Prevention. Use of World Health Organization and CDC growth charts for children aged 0–59 months in the United States. *MMWR Recomm Rep.* 2010;59(RR-9):1–15

110. Centers for Disease Control and Prevention, National Center for Emerging and Zoonotic Infectious Diseases. How to Keep Your Breast Pump Kit Clean. Available at: https://www.cdc.gov/healthywater/pdf/hygiene/breast-pump-fact-sheet.pdf. Accessed October 18, 2017

111. DiMaggio D. Tips for Freezing & Refrigerating Breast Milk. 2016; https://www. healthychildren.org/English/ages-stages/baby/breastfeeding/Pages/Storing-and-Preparing-Expressed-Breast-Milk.aspx. Accessed October 18, 2017

112. Slutzah M, Codipilly CN, Potak D, Clark RM, Schanler RJ. Refrigerator storage of expressed human milk in the neonatal intensive care unit. *J Pediatr.* 2010;156(1):26–28

113. Abrams SA, Landers S, Noble LM, Poindexter BB. American Academy of Pediatrics, Committee on Nutrition, Section on Breastfeeding, Committee on Fetus and Newborn. Donor human milk for the high-risk infant: preparation, safety, and usage options in the United States. *Pediatrics.* 2017;139(1):e20163440

114. Meek JY. Pediatric competency in breastfeeding support has room for improvement. *Pediatrics.* 2017;140(4):e20172509

115. Meek JY, Hatcher AJ, American Academy of Pediatrics, Section on Breastfeeding. The breastfeeding-friendly pediatric office practice. *Pediatrics.* 2017;2017(139):5

Chapter 4

Formula Feeding of Term Infants

General Considerations and Historical Perspective

The American Academy of Pediatrics (AAP) seeks to support the optimal physical, mental, and social health and well-being of all infants and children.[1] Largely because of its health benefits, the preferred method of feeding for achieving these goals for almost all young infants is exclusive breastfeeding for about the first 6 months and continued breastfeeding until at least 12 months of age.[2] The growth pattern of breastfed infants defines normal growth in infancy. Prior to the advent of safe drinking water, refrigeration, techniques for food preservation, and curd-reducing milk technologies, breastfeeding by mother or wet nurse was necessary for infant survival, although the previously common practice of wet nursing was associated with its own medical and social liabilities.[3]

> Infants in 1900 whose mothers, for one reason or other, did not nurse them were given either milk from some other women or a poorly devised concoction of which cow milk was usually the basis. The milk was almost always dirty and unsterilized and was put into dirty bottles and fed through dirty nipples. Proprietary foods, which had become very popular, were usually deficient in most elements except carbohydrates.[4]

In the 1940s, approximately 65% of infants were being breastfed, but by 1958, with safer infant foods, improved hygiene, and changed attitudes toward breastfeeding and maternal adaptations to modern life, the percentage of 7-day-old infants who were breastfed had decreased to just 25%. The breastfeeding rate remained at that level for more than a decade.[4,5] Despite major swings in breastfeeding initiation and duration, mortality in the United States decreased rapidly throughout the 20th century.[6]

Medical professional, government, and lay group enthusiasm for, and promotion of, breastfeeding since the early 1970s has been associated with increased breastfeeding initiation, exclusivity, and duration.[7] The most recent Centers for Disease Control and Prevention Breastfeeding Report Card (2015 data) cites the US breastfeeding initiation rate at 83%, exclusive breastfeeding for 3 months at 47%, and any breastfeeding at 1 year of age at 36%,[8] achieving the Healthy Children 2020 goals.[9] Women in southeastern states, those of lower socioeconomic status, those younger than 20 years, those who are employed, those receiving WIC benefits, and African American women are less likely to breastfeed.[10-12]

With their advocacy for breastfeeding, children's health care professionals and other advocates for children's health have been variably successful in enacting and enforcing constraints on the marketing of infant formula directly to mothers, and even to health care professionals. The AAP expressed its disapproval of direct advertising of infant formula to the general public in 1989 and reaffirmed that stance in 1993.[13] Such advertising runs counter to the World Health Organization (WHO) "International Code of Marketing of Breastmilk Substitutes," of which the United States is not a signatory.[14] Another development that has reduced some forms of promotion of infant formula in the United States has been the Baby-Friendly Hospital Initiative of the WHO and United Nations International Children's Emergency Fund (UNICEF). Attaining certification as a Baby-Friendly Hospital requires documentation of hospital practices that are believed to support of breastfeeding, including a requirement that hospitals not distribute infant formula "discharge packs" and do not accept free formula samples for hospital use.[15] Initiation of breastfeeding is higher in Baby-Friendly Hospitals, and use of discharge packs has been decreasing.[16,17]

Despite decades of domestic and international promotion of the advantages of breastfeeding, not all infants are partially or exclusively breastfed for the first 6 months. For those infants, the AAP recommends use of an iron-fortified infant formula as the best and safest alternative for the first year of life.[18]

At some point during their first year, most US infants receive infant formula,[19] and for many infants, most of their nutrition in the first year of life comes from infant formula. The mean age of introduction of infant formula has increased slowly. As of 2015, 29% of infants received some infant formula before 3 months of age[20] (see Fig 4.1), and despite recommendations to the contrary, as of 2008, 16.6% of infants received cow milk before 1 year of age.[19] Given the widespread use of commercial infant formula and its advantages for infants relative to cow milk and other human milk alternatives, it is important for pediatric health care providers to have a practical understanding of its use and the nutrition that it provides, even in this era of increasing breastfeeding.[21,22] This chapter reviews the development, composition, and safe feeding of infant formulas for term infants.

In the first year of life, infant formula fills the gaps left by noninitiation of breastfeeding, partial breastfeeding, and termination of breastfeeding. Consequently, as with human milk in breastfed infants, formula makes up a progressively smaller percentage of energy and nutrient consumption in the second 6 months of life. Early formula supplementation generally reduces the duration of breastfeeding, although this phenomenon was not observed in African American and Hispanic mothers.[23]

Fig 4.1.

Percent of infants receiving formula supplementation by age 2009-2015.
From: Centers for Disease Control and Prevention, National Center for Chronic Disease Prevention and Health Promotion. CDC National Immunization Survey (NIS) Breastfeeding Among US Children Born 2002-2015, CDC National Immunization Survey. Available at: https://www.cdc.gov/breastfeeding/data/nis_data/index.htm. Accessed December 19, 2018

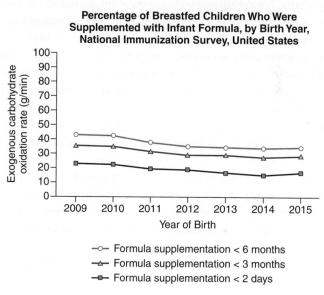

Percentage of Breastfed Children Who Were Supplemented with Infant Formula, by Birth Year, National Immunization Survey, United States

—○— Formula supplementation < 6 months
—▲— Formula supplementation < 3 months
—■— Formula supplementation < 2 days

Complementary foods may be introduced at 4 to 6 months of age on the basis of developmental readiness (eg, oromotor coordination, head control) and nutritional needs of the growing infant. After 6 months, in addition to solid foods, either breastfeeding or iron-fortified infant formula should be used for the remainder of first year of life rather than feeding cow milk. The composition of cow milk does not match the nutritional requirements of infants, and its early introduction can increase blood loss from the gastrointestinal tract and contribute to iron-deficiency anemia.[24] Avoidance of cow milk until 1 year of age reduces the risk of inadequate intakes of nutrients such as iron, zinc, vitamin E, essential fatty acids, and long-chain polyunsaturated fatty acids and prevents excessive intakes of protein and electrolytes. Similarly, there is no role for fruit juice in the diet in the first year of life.[25]

The development of modern infant formulas became possible with advances in knowledge and practice of chemistry, nutritional analysis of foods, nutritional requirements, and food preservation technologies that began in earnest in the 19th century. Initially, the goal for developing microbiologically safe, shelf-stable infant feeding products was to provide energy and protein and only later to better match the macro- and micronutrient composition of human milk. Early efforts focused largely on preserving and modifying cow milk and grains to make them more suitable for feeding infants. Both shelf-stable concentrated milk products and milk and carbohydrate powders were commercialized. By 1919, a detailed report was published related to a feeding mixture, in many ways close to modern infant formulas, that was well tolerated and supported infant growth.[26] Until the middle of the 20th century, infant formulas were mostly made at home, largely from canned milk products, corn syrup, and powdered sugars with guidance from physicians on their preparation. Dietary vitamin sources, especially orange juice for ascorbic acid and cod liver oil for vitamin D, were fed separately or incorporated into formula ingredients and reduced the high prevalence of scurvy and rickets. Nearly complete infant formulas were available by the 1920s, and most were milk or milk/whey concentrate based.[27] The initial use of milk fat gave way to the use of vegetable oils as the lipid components, which were better absorbed and eliminated the foul smell of spit-up containing butyric acid from partially digested milk fat.[28,29]

The goal of nutritionally imitating human milk was gradually shown to be quantitatively possible but not qualitatively feasible. Most commercial infant formulas are based on cow milk, and although the amounts of macronutrients delivered can be quantitatively modified by food technology to approach those of human milk, the biochemical composition does not match that of human milk. For example, the whey-casein ratios of cow milk and human milk are different (and the ratio changes over the period of lactation in human milk), and the protein and amino acid compositions of the whey and casein protein fractions differ. The human milk fatty acid profile is unlike that of butterfat or vegetable oils used in formulas. Human milk, with its low content of iron and vitamins D and K, is a problematic model for a complete infant formula. For some nutrients, bioavailability and utilization also differ between infant formulas and human milk. In addition, there are largely nonnutritional constituents of human milk, including hormones, growth factors, antibodies, immune modulating factors, enzymes, and leukocytes, with functional properties that cannot be readily incorporated into infant formula. As a result, the human milk composition model for infant formula has broadened to include the important functional perspective of imitating the growth, development, physiology, and health of breastfed infants.[30] The history of early infant foods and subsequent commercial infant formulas, as well as the people and the science behind them, make for fascinating reading and are described elsewhere.[27,31-34,35,3,36-38,39-41]

The first US infant formulas were manufactured as powders. These were followed by liquid concentrates and, ultimately, ready-to-feed formulas. All 3 forms remain marketed today for use by healthy infants. In addition, "exempt" infant formulas are manufactured for use by infants with medical conditions that benefit from a modified formula and are typically exempted from the guidelines for one or more ingredients, as designated by the Infant Formula Act (IFA) of 1980.

The evolution of infant formula regulations has contributed to the safety of US formulas (see Chapter 50.I for formula ingredient requirements and additional regulatory information). Federal regulation of infant feeding mixtures dates to 1941, when initial composition and labeling requirements were first adapted as an amendment to the Food and Drug Act. Expert groups have provided guidance to the US Food and Drug Administration (FDA) regarding US infant formula ingredient levels.[42-44] The AAP Committee on Nutrition developed recommendations for minimum nutrient levels for complete infant formulas in 1967, and these were largely adopted by the FDA in 1971, and at FDA's request, these were updated in 1983.[7] Micronutrient deficiencies (eg, ascorbic acid, vitamin D, thiamine, pyridoxine, and chloride) continued to be reported sporadically in the United States with specific (mostly "milk-free") formulas before implementation of the IFA and its 1986 amendments with its provisions that ensure the nutritional composition of formulas.[33,45] Lower and upper limits for selenium were most recently added in 2016. Infant formula manufacturers must document bacteriologic safety and nutrient content within the ranges set forth in the IFA and keep detailed records of each batch of infant formula. The labeling of infant formulas must follow a specific format and include a list of ingredients and nutrient content. All US infant formulas must be manufactured according to Good Manufacturing Practices, and all production facilities are inspected at least annually by the FDA. The agency is authorized to initiate a mandatory recall if it determines that an adulterated or misbranded infant formula presents a risk to human health. With these safeguards in place, the bacteriologic and nutritional quality of infant formula can be assured, and recalls related to nutritional composition have become largely of historical importance. As of 2016, there were only 5 manufacturers registered with FDA to manufacture infant formula under the Infant Formula Act.[46]

All currently available standard infant formulas manufactured under the IFA meet the energy and nutrient requirements for healthy term infants during the first 4 to 6 months of life. If human milk or formula intake is adequate, healthy infants do not need additional water, except when the environmental temperature is extremely high. When formula feeding is used, bottles should be offered ad libitum, the goal being to allow the infant to regulate intake to meet his or her energy needs. The infant should not be encouraged to empty a bottle when fed infant formula.[47] Typical intakes of human milk or formula will be 140 to 200 mL/kg per day for the first 3 months of life. This intake provides approximately 90 to 135 kcal/kg of body weight per day and should result in an initial weight gain of 25 to 30 g/day. Between 3 and 6 months of age, weight gain decreases to 15 to 20 g/day, and between 6 and 12 months of age, weight gain decreases to 10 to 15 g/day.

The late Dr. Samuel Fomon described breastfeeding as an evolutionary compromise between the nutritional needs of the infant and the nutritional needs of the mother.[48] This concept implies that human milk is unlikely to provide much nutritional surfeit and that infants are likely to consume more than what is provided by breastfeeding, given the opportunity. Increasing milk volume or milk nutrient density in early life above that usually consumed by breastfed infants can increase growth rates beyond that typical of exclusively breastfed infants. Both of these concepts have been demonstrated in clinical studies. When feeding was compared in infants receiving human milk by bottle versus by breast, infants feeding by bottle consumed greater quantities of human milk and experienced greater weight gain.[49] Increasing the nutrient density of a formula also accelerates growth in early infancy.[50,51] Thus, to the extent that achieving the growth rate and pattern of exclusively breastfed infants is an important goal of formula feeding, one not universally embraced,[48] there are both compositional and behavioral challenges.

Growth of US infants, including those who are formula fed, approximates, but is not identical to, that of breastfed infants as depicted in the 2006 WHO growth charts, which are based on anthropometric measurements from a study of mostly breastfed infants.[52] In 2010, the Centers for Disease Control and Prevention and the AAP recommended the use of the WHO growth charts for the first 24 months of life.[52] US infants tend to grow a little faster than the reference data after the first few months of life. It is worth noting that milk sources other than human milk consumed by infants in the largely international WHO growth study did not include infant formula for many of the study sites.[53]

In the United States, the Special Supplemental Nutrition Program for Women, Infants, and Children (WIC) was adopted as a permanent national nutrition program in 1975 to combat poverty and malnutrition that had been well documented. The WIC program has substantial influence and impact on US infant feeding practices. More than half of US infant formulas are powdered and concentrated liquid formulas sold through state WIC programs. As of 2014, more than 2.1 million US infants were enrolled in the WIC program.[54] WIC recipients receive monthly vouchers for infant formula that are redeemed in food stores to meet most, but not necessarily all, of an infant's formula usage. In 2007, monthly per capita WIC formula allotments were decreased. Subsequently, concerns were expressed that food-insecure households may "stretch" infant formula, with the potential for the feeding diluted formula.[55]

Breastfeeding rates are lower among WIC participants, consistent with the demographic profile of this population and some WIC practices, if not policies, that promote formula feeding.[11] Attempts to promote more breast-feeding have been made, in part, by more generous WIC food packages being provided to mothers who breastfeed relative to those feeding infant formula.[56]

Before WIC mandated iron fortification of at least 10 mg/L in infant formula, iron deficiency in the first year of life and iron deficiency anemia in the second year of life were common in the United States.[7,33] Nutritional calculations of infant iron requirements and clinical experience from feeding iron-fortified formula to high-risk populations had both indicated that a milk-based formula providing about 12 mg/L could prevent iron deficiency and iron-deficiency anemia.[57,58] After WIC mandated that formulas provided through its program contain at least 10 mg of iron/L and began providing infant formula through the first year of life, both iron deficiency and iron-deficiency anemia decreased dramatically.[59]

Safe Handling, Preparation, and Storage of Infant Formula

Careful preparation and handling of infant formulas are important to ensure their safety. Despite label instructions covering their use, some parents fail to follow basic hygienic practices.[60] Parents should be instructed to use proper hand-washing techniques whenever preparing infant formula or feeding their infant, and to use a clean surface for formula preparation. They also should be given guidance on (1) proper storage of formula product remaining in the original container that will be used or mixed later; and

(2) proper storage of formula that has been prepared, if it is not to be fed immediately. All formulas should be prepared in clean containers and fed from clean bottles with clean nipples. In most cases, it is not necessary to sterilize bottles (or nipples) before mixing formula in them, especially if they have been washed in a dishwasher.[61] Detailed pictorial information on the preparation of standard infant formulas is available on the WIC Web site.[62]

Once opened, cans of ready-to-feed and concentrated liquid product can generally be stored covered (with a plastic over-cap or aluminum foil) in the refrigerator for no longer than 48 hours. Powdered formula (both unopened and opened cans) should be stored in a cool, dry place, not in the refrigerator. Once opened, cans of powder should be covered with the overcap. Opened powder product can be used for up to 4 weeks with no loss of quality, if proper precautions are taken to avoid microbiologic contamination.

Ready-to-feed formula should be shaken before use to re-suspend any mineral sediment and can be poured directly into the bottle and fed immediately. Formula from concentrated liquid or powder can be prepared in individual bottles just before each feeding or in a larger clean container before transferring the desired amount to individual bottles. For mixing, use of a blender is specifically advised against, because of the risk of bacterial contamination. If multiple feeds are prepared at a time, bottles for later use should be refrigerated immediately. Immediate refrigeration is especially important for powder products prepared with hot water (see below), because they take longer to cool to reach a safe storage temperature. All prepared bottles should be used within 24 hours. "Unopened" bottles of prepared formula should be taken out of the refrigerator no more than 2 hours before being fed. After this time, any remaining contents should be discarded.

Concentrated liquids should also be shaken before use. The normal preparation of formula from concentrated liquid products requires dilution with an equal volume of water. Most concentrated liquid products contain 38 to 40 kcal/fl oz and are diluted with an equal volume of water for feeding. Mixing instructions are shown in Appendix C.

In preparing formula from powder products, it is important to adhere closely to the manufacturer's instructions on the label; most powders of standard formulas are mixed using 1 level, unpacked scoop of powder per 2 fl oz of water. It is important to use the scoop provided by the manufacturer with the specific product and not to use standard measuring spoons or scoops from other products, because powders from different manufacturers provide slightly different amounts of nutrients per unit of volume, and scoop sizes vary accordingly.

For special feeding situations, both powders and concentrated liquids can be reconstituted to provide formulas with more than the standard energy (calorie) concentration, which is 19 kcal/fl oz or 20 kcal/fl oz (Appendix C). Instructions for preparation of more-concentrated formulas from powder should be obtained from the manufacturer for the specific product in question. In some instances, instructions may be available on the manufacturers' Web sites listed at the end of this chapter.

In the early months of life especially, infants prefer warm infant formula. This warming can be accomplished by putting the unopened bottle in a bowl of warm water for 5 to 10 minutes prior to feeding. Bottles of infant formula should not be warmed in a microwave oven. Microwave ovens can create "hot spots" in the formula in the bottle, and burns to the infant's mouth can occur, despite the formula seeming to be at the right temperature when tested by the mother before feeding.

Ready-to-feed and concentrated liquid products are commercially sterile—that is, they contain no pathogenic organisms. Liquid products may contain small numbers of nonpathogenic spores that are capable of growing only at very high temperatures, so-called thermophiles. These organisms may spoil the formula if it has not been stored properly.

Powdered formula products are heat-treated during manufacture and must meet strict standards regarding the allowable amounts and types of bacteria they may contain. However, they are not completely sterile and, in rare cases, may contain pathogenic organisms. Of ongoing concern has been the occasional presence of *Cronobacter sakazakii* (formerly *Enterobacter sakazakii*) in some powdered infant formulas and in the environment, including other foods, water, and kitchen surfaces.[63-66] This opportunistic organism has been the sporadic cause of rare, severe infections (sepsis and meningitis) mostly in preterm infants in the early months of life and in other immunocompromised infants. For this reason, powdered infant formulas generally are not recommended for these infants. As of 2014, the FDA mandated prerelease testing of all batches of powdered infant formula specifically for *Cronobacter* and *Salmonella*.[67]

"Safe, potable water" should be used to prepare infant formula. This means that the water is both free of microorganisms capable of causing disease and low in minerals and other contaminants that may be detrimental. In some instances, the use of bottled water may be the best choice.

Municipal water supplies are generally free of pathogenic microorganisms but may contain variable concentrations of minerals, including fluoride, depending on the source. Some experts recommend running the cold water tap for 2 minutes before using the water to prepare infant formula.[62] Well water needs to be tested for pathogens regularly and may contain high concentrations of fluoride as well as other minerals, such as copper or arsenic. High levels of water copper have been reported to cause gastrointestinal symptoms and possible hepatotoxicity. Arsenic is a carcinogen.

It has been recommended that the concentration of fluoride in formula be less than 60 to 100 μg/100 kcal (400–670 μg/L). Infant formulas are produced with defluoridated water. Fluoride is not added during production, but some of the ingredients naturally contain fluoride. There is no need to supplement the diet of the formula-fed infant with fluoride during the first 6 months of life. After 6 months of age, the need for additional fluoride depends principally on the fluoride content of the water (for recommendations, see Chapter 48: Diet, Nutrition, and Oral Health). Health care professionals should ascertain the fluoride concentrations in the local water supplies of the communities in which their patients live. If the fluoride content of the municipal or well water used to prepare infant formula is high, bottled water that has been defluoridated should be used.

If there is any doubt about bacterial contamination, water to be used for formula preparation should be brought to a rolling boil for 1 minute; longer boiling may concentrate minerals to an undesirable degree. Instructions from most manufacturers are to cool the water to *at least* 38°C (approximately 100°F) and using this lukewarm water to prepare formula. Water for diluting concentrated liquid formula can be allowed to cool before mixing formula. Varying temperature recommendations have been made for water used to reconstitute infant formula powder. Historically, the recommendation was for water to be allowed to cool, as for concentrated liquid. In 2004, an expert group convened by the Food and Agriculture Organization (FAO) of the United Nations and the WHO recommended that powder formula be prepared with water that is at least 70°C (approximately 158°F) to decrease the risk of infection with *C sakazakii*.[68] Their data suggested that this approach could result in as much as a 4-log decrease in the concentrations of *C sakazakii*.[69] A temperature of 70°C implies that after boiling, water is allowed to cool at room temperature for no more than 30 minutes before it is used. This recommendation has since been adopted and promulgated by some authorities,[61] but not by others.[62,70] US manufacturers do not recommend powder formula reconstitution with 70°C water in part because of

Formula Preparation

Water used for mixing infant formula must be from a safe water source, as defined by the state or local health department. If there are concerns or uncertainties about the safety of tap water, bottled water may be used, or cold tap water may be brought to a rolling boil for 1 minute (no longer), then cooled to room temperature for no more than 30 minutes before it is used.

Warmed water should be tested in advance to make sure it is not too hot for the infant. The easiest way to test the temperature is to shake a few drops on the inside of the caregiver's wrist. Otherwise, a bottle can be prepared by adding powdered formula and room temperature water from the tap just before feeding. Bottles made in this way from powdered formula can be ready for feeding, as no additional refrigeration or warming would be required.

Prepared formula must be discarded within 1 hour after serving an infant. Prepared formula that has not been given to an infant may be stored in the refrigerator for 24 hours to prevent bacterial contamination. An open container of ready-to-feed formula, concentrated liquid formula, or formula prepared from concentrated liquid formula should be covered, refrigerated, and discarded after 48 hours if not used.

concerns about the potential risks of burns, labile nutrient loss (notably vitamin C), and formula clumping.[71]

Formula Composition and Labeling

At the broadest level in the United States, there are standard infant formulas, as described in the IFA, including cow milk- and soy-based formulas for general use, and "exempt" formulas for use by infants who have inborn errors of metabolism (see Appendix B) or low birth weight infants (see Chapter 5: Nutritional Needs of the Preterm Infant) or who otherwise have unusual medical or dietary problems.[72] In the United States, most standard infant formulas are recommended for use at any time in the first year of life, although formulas designed for use in the second 6 months of life are available. In other parts of the world, different formulas are routinely recommended for the first and second 6 months of life, and some experts have advocated even more age- and development-specific stages of formulas.[73] To date, evidence for benefit from such an approach has not been demonstrated.[21]

US infant formulas must be demonstrated to meet "the two quality factors of normal physical growth and sufficient biological quality of the protein component of the formula." In practice, the growth requirement is generally met with a 4-month growth study conducted in young infants showing growth equivalent to breastfed infants or an existing infant formula, and the protein quality factor by a protein efficiency ratio (PER) rat growth bioassay. All ingredients in infant formulas must be either "generally recognized as safe" (GRAS) or FDA-approved safe food additives. "Exempt" infant formulas are only exempt from provisions of the IFA that are inconsistent with the specific modifications needed to make the formula suitable for the disease state managed, for example cow milk allergy or phenylketonuria. Feeding experience with a growth study including blood biochemical testing is important to assess the performance of a new formula, because unanticipated nutritional issues may arise with new formulations.[74] The AAP has provided extensive guidance to the FDA regarding recommended clinical testing of infant formulas,[75] and more recently a committee for the Institute of Medicine provided guidance on evaluating the safety of new ingredients for infant formulas.[76]

Infant formulas are available in 3 forms: ready-to-feed, concentrated liquid, and powder. The different forms of a given product are nearly identical in nutrient composition, but small differences may exist for technical reasons. Ready-to-feed formulas for healthy, full-term infants are available principally in 32-fl oz containers and also in smaller volume containers (2, 3, 6, and 8 fl oz), depending on the product and manufacturer. Concentrated liquid products are available in 13-fl oz and 1-quart containers. When diluted with equal amounts of water, concentrated liquids yield formula with nutrient levels that are the same as the corresponding ready-to-feed product. Powder products are available in a number of different sizes of containers that have anywhere from the amount needed to prepare a single serving to as high as 2.2 lb of powder.

There is a standardized FDA format for labeling infant formulas (see Chapter 50.I). For nutrient content in the United States, "label claim" for the amount of each nutrient is the *minimum* amount of the nutrient that must be present in the formula at the end of shelf life.[a] It is not the average amount of the nutrient in the formula, as is the case in many other countries. A survey of actual nutrient levels in infant formulas produced between 2000 and 2005 and sold in the United States and other countries revealed that although all formulas met label claim requirements, there was wide variability of actual levels of many nutrients from batch to batch.[77] Among

---

[a] This is especially important for some vitamins. Although some vitamins degrade very little over shelf life (eg, vitamin K), others, such as riboflavin, vitamin B_{12}, and vitamin C, are subject to considerable loss. This means that early in shelf life, the levels of those vitamins that degrade are higher than at the end of shelf life, although in all cases, the final actual levels will be above the amount claimed on the label.

other requirements of the IFA, all labels must have detailed mixing instructions, which may differ among manufacturers' products and should be followed for the specific formula being used.

Standard infant formulas vary in composition. These variations include differing milk or soy protein, carbohydrate and lipid levels and sources, and added ingredients not specifically required by the IFA (Table 4.1). Some of these formula variations and their structure function claims have been associated with various clinical symptoms including gastrointestinal tolerance (spit-up, stool frequency, consistency and odor, and gassiness, constipation/ colic), fussiness and crying, and illness symptom incidence and prevalence (Table 4.2). In addition, specific ingredients are used or added because they are present in human milk and/or are thought to positively affect brain, eye, immune, bone, behavior and/or intestinal microbiome development (Table 4.2). According to FDA draft guidance in this sphere, any structure-function label claims regarding ingredients in infant formula are held to the standard of "truthful and not misleading" and should be supported by "competent and reliable scientific evidence."[78]

Protein sources for standard infant formulas provide approximately 7% to 12% of calories and come in many different forms. The protein source determines the amino acid profile and protein efficiency ratio of an infant formula. These sources include nonfat milk protein, milk protein concentrate, partially hydrolyzed nonfat milk protein, the acid soluble whey protein concentrate fraction of milk, casein, partially hydrolyzed whey protein, soy protein isolate, and hydrolyzed soy protein isolate. Soy protein isolate requires a higher level of protein plus *l*-methionine supplementation to ensure protein adequacy and quality.

Carbohydrate sources in standard formulas provide approximately 35% to 40% of calories and include lactose, corn syrup solids, sucrose, modified starch, or other complex carbohydrates such as maltodextrins. Lactose is the major carbohydrate source of energy in human milk and in most standard cow milk-based infant formulas. Lactose is hydrolyzed in the small intestine by the action of lactase, which is located on the brush border of the intestinal villus epithelial cell. Lactase appears later than other brush-border disaccharidases in the developing fetal intestine but is present in maximal amounts in full-term infants. Nevertheless, even in full-term infants, some unabsorbed lactose enters the large intestine, where it is fermented by bacteria. The end-products of fermentation are short-chain fatty acids and several gases, among them carbon dioxide and hydrogen. This fermentation helps to maintain an acidic environment in the colon, which in turn

Table 4.1.

Changes to Formula That May Address Common Feeding Problems/Concerns

	Vegetarian Option	Loose Stools	Spit-up	Cow Milk Allergy	High Allergy Risk	Cry/Fuss/ Gas/Sleep	High Atopic Dermatitis Risk	Excess Energy Density
Soy protein isolate	X			X		X		
Reduced lactose		X				X		
Rice starch thickener			X					
Extensive milk protein hydrolysates				X	X		X	
Partial milk protein hydrolysates					X	X	X	
Amino acid protein source				X	X			
Soy fiber		X						
Lactobacillus reuteri						X		
19 kcal/oz								X

Table 4.2.
Rationale for Addition of Ingredients to Infant Formula Not Required by the Infant Formula Act

Ingredient	Brain Development	Eye Development	Immune Support	GI Tolerance	Cry/Fuss	Decreased Illness	Microbiome Health
Taurine	X	X					
Nucleotides			X			X	
DHA	X	X					
ARA	X						
Prebiotics[a]			X	X			X
Lutein/lycopene	X	X					
Probiotics			X	X	X	X	X
Lactoferrin			X				
MFGM	X						

DHA indicates docosahexaenoic acid; ARA, arachidonic acid; MFGM, milk fat globule membrane.
[a] Includes fructo-oligosaccharides (FOS), galacto-oligosaccharides, and 2'fucosyllactose.

fosters normal and beneficial bacterial flora including lactobacilli, bifido-bacteria, and other organisms that suppress the growth of more pathogenic organisms.

Fat calorie sources (which provide about half the calories in infant formula, as in human milk) include a blend of any of the following: soy oil, sunflower oil, safflower oil, high-oleic safflower or sunflower oils, palm olein oil, and coconut oil. The oil blend determines the fatty acid profile of the formula. Determination of the ideal fatty acid composition for infant formulas is challenging. Human milk fatty acid profiles are highly variable and dependent on maternal diet. Some oil blends reduce calcium absorption because of formation of calcium fatty acid soaps, which may increase stool firmness.[79,80]

Total calories in infant formulas may now be 19 or 20 kcal/fl oz, based on the differing estimates of the energy content in human milk. This is a complex issue related to the volume of milk collected, collection method, and approach to determining milk caloric density (estimates based on measured milk macronutrients, bomb calorimetry of human milk or the doubly labeled water method for determining energy expenditure, and indirectly energy intake, in breastfed infants).[81-84]

Current IFA regulations set minimum levels for 30 macro- and micronutrients and maximums for 11 that appear to lead to satisfactory infant nutritional status (see Appendix B). The industry has an excellent safety record under the IFA in terms of protecting infants from nutritional deficiencies related to infant formulas. Two of the micronutrients regulated under the IFA (iron and vitamin D) and 1 additional micronutrient, fluoride, warrant specific comments.

Although iron nutrition is covered in greater detail later in this book (Chapter 19: Iron), it is important to note here that iron-deficiency anemia can impair infant mental development, and achieving adequate iron status is important in infant nutrition. Although fetal iron accumulation in healthy term pregnancies along with delayed cord clamping is generally sufficient to meet infant needs of term infants for the first 4 to 6 months of life (irrespective of maternal diet), between 4 and 6 months of age, another dietary source of iron is needed to prevent iron deficiency, because iron levels in human milk are low. Dietary iron may come from iron-fortified formula, iron-fortified cereal, or early introduction of meat as a complementary food (see Chapter 6: Complementary Feeding). The AAP recommends the use of iron-fortified infant formulas throughout the first year of life, when formula is used. Formulas with iron content of 10 to 12 mg/L have been highly effective in controlling iron-deficiency anemia in the context of US feeding practices, but lower levels may suffice in some circumstances.[85] Currently, all standard US infant formulas provide the 10 to 12 mg of iron/L recommended by the AAP. Concerns regarding gastrointestinal intolerance with these levels of iron fortification appear unfounded,[86,87] but recent interest in the microbiome has led to speculation about possible effects of supplemental iron on the microbiome.[88]

Rickets has become rare in term US infants, but low levels of vitamin D are not uncommon, defined by serum 25-OH vitamin D concentrations less than 50 nmol/L or 20 ng/mL (see Chapter 21.I). Concern for infant vitamin D status relates primarily to the central role of vitamin D for bone development, but low vitamin D status is associated with increased risks for infections and a number of chronic diseases.

The AAP-endorsed infant vitamin D Recommended Dietary Allowance is 400 IU per day.[89,90] Vitamin D content in human milk is inadequate to meet this need, unless mothers are taking high-dose supplements of vitamin D.[91-93] The intake from formula depends on the volume of formula consumed and the level of vitamin D in the formula. The IFA allowable range for vitamin D of 40 to 100 IU/100 kcal has proven too narrow. Given manufacturing variability, shelf life losses, and the requirement that the stated label value (currently 60 or 75 IU/100 kcal) be maintained to the end of shelf life without ever exceeding the maximum, it has proven difficult to meet the full infant RDA with typical intakes of formula. For infants to obtain 400 IU of vitamin D solely from current infant formulas, they need to consume 800 to 1000 mL/day (27–33 fl oz).

Advisable fluoride intakes are targeted to minimize dental carries risk and avoid all but mild fluorosis (see Chapter 48: Diet, Nutrition, and Oral Health). Beneficial effects of fluoride are believed to come from topical, rather than systemic, effects. Regardless of the fluoride content of the water supply, no supplementation is advised in the first 6 months of life, because the teeth have not erupted. Human milk fluoride content tends to be low, and reports on the relationship of human milk fluoride to local water fluoride content are inconsistent. Infant formula is manufactured with defluoridated water, and the fluoride content of water used to dilute concentrated liquid or powder formula will largely determine the fluoride content. Because of the inherent fluoride content of the ingredients, soy formulas have higher fluoride content than cow milk formulas. Many home water filtration systems, including those using ion-exchange resins, activated alumina, and reverse osmosis, reduce water fluoride content. Filtered water or low-fluoride bottled water can be used for mixing infant formula when there is concern about possible fluorosis, especially during the first 6 months of life.

Uses of Infant Formulas

Iron-fortified cow milk-based infant formulas, labeled as "infant formula with iron" are preferred for feeding healthy term infants, when human milk is not available or the mother chooses to feed infant formula.[94] The choice of formula is determined by preferred features, infant tolerance, cost, packaging, and whether or not infants are WIC eligible. Multiple similar formulas from the same manufacturer, the proliferation of store-brand formulas, and frequent changes in product or feature/ingredient names make it challenging for the pediatrician to remain current with commercial formula offerings, although this is not unique to the current era.[3] Formulas not regulated under the IFA may also be available via Internet purchasing or in markets with packaging and labels that make them difficult to distinguish from formulas manufactured under IFA regulations. A number of formulas are certified organic or made without genetically modified organisms for parents who prefer and can afford such products. In a clinical report, the AAP did not identify health outcome benefits to individuals related to consumption of organic food.[95] Kosher and Halal formulas are available. Less expensive, private-label store brands largely adopt existing formulations already in the market and do not participate in the WIC program.

Infant formulas have been manufactured to address common feeding concerns and problems. For example, rice starch has been added to thicken feeds to reduce symptoms of gastroesophageal reflux,[96,97] prebiotics have been added to make stools more like those of breastfed infants,[98-101] soy fiber has been added to firm loose stools,[102] and *Lactobacillus reuteri* has been added to reduce symptoms of colic, with inconsistent reports of benefit.[103-106]

Soy formula may be recommended when parents want a vegetarian infant formula feeding option, and this is the only use of soy formula for the healthy term infant recommended by the AAP[107] (see text box, p 97). Historically, soy formulas provided a way to avoid both cow milk protein and lactose when a change in formula was desired.[107]

Soy formula has also been used in the management of galactosemia, because it does not contain lactose or free galactose. It can also be used in the very rare condition of congenital lactase deficiency. Although lactose-free (soy) formulas may slightly reduce the duration of diarrhea in some situations, soy formula is not generally recommended to accelerate recovery from acute gastroenteritis. Soy formulas are not recommended for the feeding of preterm infants because of concerns about protein quality and mineral absorption.[107] Caution should also be used in feeding soy formula to infants with congenital hypothyroidism treated with thyroxin. Soy formulas reduce thyroid hormone absorption. Higher doses of thyroxin may be needed.

Concerns have been raised about possible adverse hormonal effects of phytoestrogens absorbed from soy protein formulas,[108] particularly in regard to sexual development. A large study retrospectively compared adult subjects who had been prospectively fed soy- or cow milk-based infant formulas. The investigators found an association of more menstrual discomfort and a tendency to longer menstrual flow in females and no other health effects.[109] Subsequent studies found heavier menstrual flow and larger uterine fibroids but no difference in fibroid prevalence in young African American women who had been exposed to soy protein infant formula,[110,111] although a comprehensive meta-analysis of available clinical studies supported soy safety.[112] An expert committee explored animal and human studies of soy phytoestrogens for the National Toxicology Program in great detail and concluded that soy was of "minimal" developmental

---

AAP

The American Academy of Pediatrics finds that isolated soy protein-based formulas are a safe and nutritionally equivalent alternative to cow milk-based formula for term infants whose nutritional needs are not met from human milk. **The AAP specifically recommends the use of soy formulas for the following:**
1. Term infants with galactosemia or hereditary lactase deficiency.
2. Term infants with documented transient lactase deficiency.
3. Infants with documented immunoglobulin E-associated allergy to cow milk who are not also allergic to soy protein.
4. Patients seeking a vegetarian-based diet for a term infant.

The use of soy protein-based formula is not recommended for the following:
1. Preterm infants with birth weights less than 1800 g.
2. Prevention of colic or allergy.
3. Infants with cow milk protein-induced enterocolitis or enteropathy.

Pediatrics. 2008:121;1062-1068

concern.[113] The federally sponsored Beginnings study subsequently examined concerns regarding soy infant formulas. The results were reassuring in regard to reproductive organ and brain development.[114,115] Recently, changes of unknown significance have been observed in vaginal cell maturation index and methylation of an estrogen-responsive gene in the vaginal epithelial cells of girls who had been fed soy formula.[116,117] The interpretation of findings of differences in soy formula-fed infants is particularly difficult, given health benefits of soy foods in the diet after infancy, as succinctly summarized by Vandenplas.[112]

Follow-up Formulas

Referred to variously as "follow-up" or "follow-on formulas," these formulas are directed at infants older than 6 months who are consuming solid food and, in many countries, are seen as a normal step in the progression of an infant's diet. Codex Alimentarius, the WHO/FAO food standards organization, defined follow-on formula in 1987 as "a food intended for use as a liquid part of the weaning diet for the infant from the 6th month on and for young children."[118] These products are used less the in the United States than in other parts of the world. Follow-up formulas and formulas for older babies, which are directed at children at the end of the first and into the second year of life and sometimes referred to as "growing up milks," are available in the United States in milk-based and soy-based forms. Their compositions, by convention, differ from those of standard formulas (increased minerals and sometimes protein, among other differences), but unlike other countries, the United States does not have separate regulatory requirements for their nutrient levels. They are nutritionally adequate. They offer no clear advantage over standard infant formula during the first year of life, although the iron fortification and balance of nutrients they contain may be an advantage for toddlers receiving inadequate amounts in their solid feedings.

Newer Ingredients

Many new ingredients have been added to infant formulas beyond those mandated by the IFA that have largely contributed to the many variations of infant formulas currently on the market (Table 4.1, Table 4.2). Clinical evidence in support of the addition of such ingredients are not required other than for growth and tolerance studies, and all of these formulas must meet the requirements of the IFA (also see Chapter 50.I, Federal Regulation of Food and Infant Formulas). To date, clinical studies and meta-analyses evaluating the clinical impact of these ingredients have provide limited support for most of them (eg, improved visual acuity for long-chain polyunsaturated fatty acids and reduced early eczema for pre- and probiotics).[119-121]

Long-Chain Polyunsaturated Fatty Acids

In recent decades, there has been intense interest in the very long-chain, polyunsaturated fatty acid derivatives docosahexaenoic acid (DHA) and arachidonic acid (ARA), because they are important for brain and eye structure and their accretion rate in the brain of the fetus and neonate has been documented[122] (see Chapter 17: Fats and Fatty Acids). ARA, and especially DHA, are present in a wide range of concentrations in human milk, depending on maternal diet. These very long-chain fatty acids can also be synthesized to a limited extent from their precursor essential fatty acids by mothers and in both term and preterm infants. Animal and clinical studies have explored whether natural variations of DHA content in human milk and varying levels added to term and preterm infant formulas could influence brain and eye development. On the basis of this research, sources of DHA and ARA are now added to infant formula.

Clinical studies have found inconsistent improvements in short- and long-term performance of tests of visual and cognitive functions in preterm and term infants fed supplemented formulas. Recent meta-analyses have not found consistent benefits, although a 2012 meta-analysis of studies of visual acuity in both term and preterm infants did find some support for improved visual acuity.[119] Challenges faced by such research comparing formula-fed infants with breastfed infants include how similar the development of breastfed and formula-fed infants already was prior to addition of long-chain polyunsaturated fatty acids, the tools available for such clinical studies, and the need to control for confounding variables such as sociodemographic differences between mothers who choose to breastfeed and those who do not.[43,123-125] Some investigators believe that by looking at more specific developmental outcomes and by using more refined statistical techniques, differences attributable to supplementation may be more readily identified.[126-128]

ARA and DHA derived from single-cell microfungi and microalgae, respectively, have been classified as "generally recognized as safe" (GRAS) for use in infant formula when added over a narrow range of GRAS concentrations and ratios. (For more details of the GRAS process, see Chapter 50.) Although there is no regulatory requirement for the inclusion of ARA and DHA in infant formulas, formulas in the United States now provide them. Since 1994, several international groups have made recommendations regarding appropriate levels for infant formulas that have ranged from 0.2% to 0.5% fatty acids from DHA and 0.5% to 1% fatty acids from ARA,[129-132] with the most recent WHO/FAO guidance at 0.2% to 0.36% fatty acids from DHA and 0.4% to 0.6% fatty acids from ARA.[131] Most US term infant formulas provide 0.15% to 0.35% fatty acids from DHA and 0.35% to 0.64% fatty acids from ARA.

Prebiotics

In addition to lactose, human milk contains more complex carbohydrates, oligosaccharides, which account for approximately 10% of the carbohydrate. These oligosaccharides are indigestible in the small intestine but are fermented in the large intestine and help maintain an acidic environment in the colon, which favors growth of nonpathogenic, acidophilic flora. The majority of US formula manufacturers now offer at least one formula with added indigestible, complex carbohydrates that, like the oligosaccharides in human milk, can be fermented in the colon. Prebiotics in use include galacto-oligosaccharides, fructo-oligosaccharides, and the oligosaccharide 2-fucosyllactose. The goal of such additions is to foster the growth of those bacteria more typical of those found in the colonic microbiome of a healthy breastfed infant.[133] However, in its most recent review in 2010, the AAP did not find that the available evidence supported benefits to adding prebiotics to infant formula.[133]

Probiotics

Although not nutrients, probiotics—nonpathogenic microorganisms, especially strains of some bacteria that ferment lactose and prebiotics and that may affect the colonic microflora and immune system—have also been added to some infant formulas. Because these are viable organisms, their addition has been limited to powder products, which do not undergo the stringent heat treatment involved in sterilization of liquid products. The AAP believes that, although the addition of probiotics to infant formulas appears to be safe for healthy infants, such formulas should not be fed to children who are immunocompromised or seriously ill. Furthermore, the evidence of clinical efficacy for probiotics "is insufficient to recommend the routine use of these formulas."[133] Formulas containing both pre- and probiotics (synbiotics) have more recently also become available.

Infant Formula Allergy-Related Issues *(see also Chapter 34: Food Allergy)*

It is unclear to what extent breastfeeding reduces the risk of milk or other allergies,[134,135] but breastfeeding is recommended for all children, including those infants at high risk with a family history of allergy. One study found that use of an extensive casein hydrolysate formula was effective in reducing the risk of infant eczema when used as sole feeding or when used with or after breastfeeding.[136] Other studies have compared partial hydrolysates to other types of formulas.[137] In 2009, the FDA permitted a qualified health claim for reduction of infant eczema risk for a partial whey hydrolysate formula on the basis of what they perceived as weak evidence.[138] A recent meta-analysis based on 37 studies concluded that neither extensively nor partially hydrolyzed formulas have demonstrated consistent efficacy for allergy prevention.[139,140] Other ingredients added to infant formula that potentially contribute to the reduction of risk for early eczema include pre- and probiotics, but evidence is not convincing at this time.[120,121]

A hypoallergenic formula containing an extensive cow milk protein hydrolysate or free amino acid-based protein source is currently recommended for the treatment of cow milk allergy. For infants who developed intolerance or allergy to cow milk-based formula in the past, soy was the next formula choice. However, in patients with cow milk protein sensitivity manifesting with gastrointestinal symptoms—colitis, enterocolitis, or food protein-induced enterocolitis—there is a high likelihood of a cross-reaction to soy. This is much less true for immunoglobulin E (IgE)-mediated cow milk allergy presenting with rash, wheezing, or anaphylaxis, but 10% to 14% of cases may still react.[107] There is recent evidence that addition of the probiotic *L reuteri* to an extensive casein hydrolysate formula may accelerate recovery in infants with cow milk-related hematochezia, accelerate cow milk tolerance in milk-allergic infants, and reduce the likelihood of other allergic symptoms.[141-143] Soy is no longer the first choice of formula for infants with IgE-mediated cow milk allergy, despite its lower cost and improved taste relative to hypoallergenic formulas.[107] Although some children with milk allergy have tolerated a partial whey hydrolysate formula, these formulas are specifically not recommended for infants with milk allergy. Most forms of milk allergy resolve over time, but usually not during the period of infant formula use.

Hypoallergenic formulas, the current formulas of choice for cow milk allergy, must be clinically documented to have a 95% probability of being tolerated by 90% of milk-allergic children[144] and include both extensive hydrolysates of milk proteins and formulas with amino acids as the protein source. Partial protein hydrolysate formulas do not meet this definition. Amino acid formulas may be especially effective in the nutritional management of eosinophilic esophagitis/gastroenteritis and the food protein-induced enterocolitis syndrome form of protein allergy in infants.[145-147]

Exempt hypoallergenic infant formulas based on extensive hydrolysates of milk proteins or made with free amino acids have features that extend their use beyond the management of allergic disorders. These formulas are lactose free and provide a substantial percentage of fat from medium-chain triglycerides. As a result, they are useful in the management of macronutrient malabsorption in conditions such as short gut syndrome, intestinal lymphangiectasia, protein-losing enteropathies, congenital enteropathies, and cholestatic diseases. In formula-fed infants with cystic fibrosis (and other forms of infantile pancreatic insufficiency), such formulas are not generally recommended, and cow milk-based infant formulas with pancreatic enzyme supplementation appear to suffice for most infants.[148]

Manufacturers' Information for Product Compostion and Other Resources

Similac® formulas: www.abbott.com/our-products/for-professionals/nutrition.html
Gerber® formulas: https://medical.gerber.com/products
Enfamil® formulas: www.meadjohnson.com/pediatrics/us-en/
Nutricia formulas: www.nutricialearningcenter.com/globalassets/pdfs/prg-jul2016_us.pdf
Private label formulas (most store brands): www.perigonutritionals.com/infant-formulas.aspx

References

1. American Academy of Pediatrics. Mission Statement. Available at: https://healthychildren,org/english/pages/about-aap.aspx. Accessed June 29, 2017
2. American Academy of Pediatrics, Section on Breastfeeding. Breastfeeding and the use of human milk. *Pediatrics*. 2012;129(3):e827–e841
3. Wickes JG. A history of infant feeding. IV. Nineteenth century continued. *Arch Dis Child*. 1953;28(141):416–422
4. American Academy of Pediatrics, Committee on Nutrition; Canadian Paediatric Society, Nutrition Committee. Breast-feeding. A commentary in celebration of the International Year of the Child, 1979. *Pediatrics*. 1978;62(4):591–601

5. Fomon S. *Infant Nutrition*. Philadelphia, PA: WB Saunders; 1974

6. Centers for Disease Control and Prevention. Healthier mothers and babies. *MMWR Morb Mortal Wkly Rep*. 1999;48(38):849–858

7. Fomon SJ. Reflections on infant feeding in the 1970s and 1980s. *Am J Clin Nutr*. 1987;46(1 Suppl):171–182

8. American Academy of Pediatrics, National Center for Chronic Disease Prevention and Health Promotion. Breastfeeding Report Card. 2016. Available at: https://www.cdc.gov/breastfeeding/pdf/2016breastfeedingreportcard.pdf. Accessed June 29, 2017

9. US Department of Health and Human Services. Office of Disease Prevention and Health Promotion. Maternal infant and Child Health Objectives. Available at: https://www.healthypeople.gov/2020/topics-objectives/topic/maternal-infant-and-child-health/objectives. Accessed June 29, 2017

10. Kozhimannil KB, Jou J, Gjerdingen DK, McGovern PM. Access to workplace accommodations to support breastfeeding after passage of the Affordable Care Act. *Womens Health Issues*. 2016;26(1):6–13

11. Deming DM, Briefel RR, Reidy KC. Infant feeding practices and food consumption patterns of children participating in WIC. *J Nutr Educ Behav*. 2014;46(3 Suppl):S29–S37

12. Ryan AS, Zhou W, Gaston MH. Regional and sociodemographic variation of breastfeeding in the United States, 2002. *Clin Pediatr* (Phila). 2004;43(9):815–824

13. American Academy of Pediatrics, Board of Directors. The AAP re-examines its policy on direct advertisng of infant formula to the public. *AAP News* 1993;9(4)2. Available at: http://www.aappublications.org/content/aapnews/9/4/2.3.full.pdf. Accessed November 27, 2018

14. Abrams E. The US Position on Infant Feeding. *Nutrition Today*. 1981;16(4)

15. Baby Friendly USA Initiative. Guidelines and Evaluation Criteria. 2016. Guideline 111. Available at: www.babyfriendlyusa.org. Accessed June 29, 2017

16. Nelson JM, Li R, Perrine CG. Trends of US hospitals distributing infant formula packs to breastfeeding mothers, 2007 to 2013. *Pediatrics*. 2015;135(6):1051–1056

17. Hawkins SS, Stern AD, Baum CF, Gillman MW. Compliance with the Baby-Friendly Hospital Initiative and impact on breastfeeding rates. *Arch Dis Child Fetal Neonatal Ed*. 2014;99(2):F138–F143

18. American Academy of Pediatrics, Work Group on Breastfeeding. Breastfeeding and the use of human milk. *Pediatrics*. 1997;100(6):1035–1039

19. Siega-Riz AM, Deming DM, Reidy KC, Fox MK, Condon E, Briefel RR. Food consumption patterns of infants and toddlers: where are we now? *J Am Diet Assoc*. 2010;110(12 Suppl):S38–S51

20. Centers for Disease Control and Prevention. National Immunization Survey, Breastfeeding. 2017. Available at: https://www.cdc.gov/breastfeeding/data/nis_data/. Accessed June 29, 2017

21. Baker RD, Baker SS. Need for infant formula. *J Pediatr Gastroenterol Nutr*. 2016;62(1):2–4

22. American Academy of Pediatrics, Committee on Practice and Ambulatory Medicine. Pediatrician's responsibility for infant nutrition. *Pediatrics.* 1997;99(5):749–750

23. Holmes AV, Auinger P, Howard CR. Combination feeding of breast milk and formula: evidence for shorter breast-feeding duration from the National Health and Nutrition Examination Survey. *J Pediatr.* 2011;159(2):186–191

24. Ziegler EE, Fomon SJ, Nelson SE, et al. Cow milk feeding in infancy: further observations on blood loss from the gastrointestinal tract. *J Pediatr.* 1990;116 (1):11–18

25. Heyman MB, Abrams SA; American Academy of Pediatrics, Section on Gastroenterology, Hepatology, and Nutrition; Committee on Nutrition. Fruit juice in infants, children, and adolescents: current recommendations. *Pediatrics.* 2017;139(6):e20170967

26. Gerstenberger HJ Ruh HO, Brickman MJ, et al. Studies in the adaptation of an artificial food to human milk. II A report of three years' experience with the feeding of S.M.A. (synthetic milk adapted). *Am J Dis Child.* 1919;45(1):1–37

27. Obladen M. Historic records on the commercial production of infant formula. *Neonatology.* 2014;106(3):173–180

28. Fomon SJ. Fat. In: Fomon SJ, ed. *Infant Nutrition.* 2nd ed. Philadelphia, PA: WB Saunders Co; 1974:152–181

29. Fomon SJ. Infant feeding in the 20th century: formula and beikost. *J Nutr.* 2001;131(2):409S–420S

30. Benson JD, Masor ML. Infant formula development: past, present and future. *Endocr Regul.* 1994;28(1):9–16

31. Tsang RC, Zlotkin SH. Preface. In: Tsang RC, Zlotkin SH, Nichols BL, Hansen JW, eds. *Nutrition During Infancy: Principles and Practice.* 2nd ed. Cincinnati, OH: Digital Educational Publishing, Inc; 1997:vii–xii

32. Cone TE Jr. *200 Years of Feeding Infants in America.* Columbus. OH: Ross Laboratories; 1976

33. Anderson SA, Chinn HI, Fisher KD. History and current status of infant formulas. *Am J Clin Nutr.* 1982;35(2):381–397

34. Wargo WF. The history of infant formula: quality, safety, and standard methods. *J AOAC Int.* 2016;99(1):7–11

35. Stevens EE, Patrick TE, Pickler R. A history of infant feeding. *J Perinat Educ.* 2009;18(2):32–39

36. Wickes IG. A history of infant feeding. II. Seventeenth and eighteenth centuries. *Arch Dis Child.* 1953;28(139):232–240

37. Wickes IG. A history of infant feeding. III. Eighteenth and nineteenth century writers. *Arch Dis Child.* 1953;28(140):332–340

38. Wickes IG. A history of infant feeding. V. Nineteenth century concluded and twentieth century. *Arch Dis Child.* 1953;28(142):495–502

39. Weinberg F. Infant feeding through the ages. *Can Fam Physician.* 1993;39:2016–2020

40. Radbill SX. Infant feeding through the ages. *Clin Pediatr* (Phila). 1981;20(10): 613–621

41. Wickes IG. A history of infant feeding. I. Primitive peoples; ancient works; Renaissance writers. *Arch Dis Child*. 1953;28(138):151–158

42. Proposed changes in Food and Drug Administration regulations concerning formula products and vitamin-mineral dietary supplements for infants. *Pediatrics*. 1967;40(5):916–922

43. Raiten DJ TJ, Waters JH. Assessment of nutrient requirements for infant formulas. *J Nutr*. 1998;128(11S):2059S–2293S

44. Fomon SJ ZE. Upper limits of nutrients in infant formulas. *J Nutr*. 1989;119(12 Suppl A):1762–1873

45. Fomon SJ. Infant formulas. In: Fomon SJ, ed. *Nutrition of Normal Infants*. St Louis, MO: Mosby; 1993:424–442

46. Rhode Island Department of Health. Infant formula manufacturers that are currently (updated 10/20/2016) registered with the FDA and are marketing infant formulas in the U.S. 2016. Available at: http://www.health.ri.gov/ publications/lists/InfantFormulaManufacturers.pdf. Accessed June 29, 2017

47. Li R, Scanlon KS, May A, Rose C, Birch L. Bottle-feeding practices during early infancy and eating behaviors at 6 years of age. *Pediatrics*. 2014;134(Suppl 1):S70–S77

48. Fomon SJ. Assessment of growth of formula-fed infants: evolutionary considerations. *Pediatrics*. 2004;113(2):389–393

49. Li R, Magadia J, Fein SB, Grummer-Strawn LM. Risk of bottle-feeding for rapid weight gain during the first year of life. *Arch Pediatr Adolesc Med*. 2012;166(5): 431–436

50. Raiha N, Minoli I, Moro G. Milk protein intake in the term infant. I. Metabolic responses and effects on growth. *Acta Paediatr Scand*. 1986;75(6):881–886

51. Fomon SJ. Voluntary food intake and its regulation. In: Fomon SJ, ed. *Infant Nutrition*. 2nd ed. Philadelphia, PA: WB Saunders Co; 1974:20–33

52. Grummer-Strawn LM, Reinold C, Krebs NF; Centers for Disease Control and Prevention. Use of World Health Organization and CDC growth charts for children aged 0–59 months in the United States. *MMWR Recomm Rep*. 2010;59(RR-9):1–15

53. WHO Multicentre Growth Reference Study Group. Breastfeeding in the WHO Multicentre Growth Reference Study. *Acta Paediatr Suppl*. 2006;450:16–26

54. Patlan KL, Mendelson M. WIC Participant Program Characteristics 2014. Arlington, VA: Insight Policy Research; 2015. Available at: https://fns-prod. azureedge.net/sites/default/files/ops/WICPCFoodPackage2014.pdf. Accessed June 29, 2017

55. Burkhardt MC, Beck AF, Kahn RS, Klein MD. Are our babies hungry? Food insecurity among infants in urban clinics. *Clin Pediatr (Phila)*. 2012;51(3):238–243

56. US Department of Agriculture, Food and Nutrition Service. Breastfeeding Promotion in WIC: Current Federal Requirements. 2013. Available at: https://www.fns.usda.gov/wic/breastfeeding-promotion-wic-current-federal-requirements. Accessed June 29, 2017

57. Fomon SJ. Iron. In: Fomon SJ, ed. *Infant Nutrition*. 2nd ed. Philadelphia, PA: WB Saunders Co; 1974:298–319

58. American Academy of Pediatrics. Iron balance and requirements in infancy. *Pediatrics*. 1969;43(1):134–142

59. Miller V, Swaney S, Deinard A. Impact of the WIC program on the iron status of infants. *Pediatrics*. 1985;75(1):100–105

60. Labiner-Wolfe J, Fein SB, Shealy KR. Infant formula-handling education and safety. *Pediatrics*. 2008;122(Suppl 2):S85–S90

61. Centers for Disease Control and Prevention. Cronobacter Prevention and Control. 2016. Available at: https://www.cdc.gov/cronobacter/prevention.html. Accessed June 29, 2017

62. US Department of Agriculture, Food and Nutrition Service. Infant formula feeding. In: *Infant Nutrition and Feeding: A Guide for Use in the WIC and CSF Programs*. Washington, DC: US Department of Agriculture; 2009:81–99. Available at: https://wicworks.fns.usda.gov/wicworks/Topics/FG/Chapter4_InfantFormulaFeeding.pdf. Accessed June 29, 2017

63. Baumgartner A, Grand M, Liniger M, Iversen C. Detection and frequency of Cronobacter spp. (Enterobacter sakazakii) in different categories of ready-to-eat foods other than infant formula. *Int J Food Microbiol*. Dec 31 2009;136(2):189–192.

64. Garbowska M, Berthold-Pluta A, Stasiak-Rozanska L. Microbiological quality of selected spices and herbs including the presence of Cronobacter spp. *Food Microbiol*. Aug 2015;49:1–5.

65. Killer J, Skrivanova E, Hochel I, Marounek M. Multilocus sequence typing of cronobacter strains isolated from retail foods and environmental samples. *Foodborne Pathog Dis*. 2015;12(6):514–521

66. Kilonzo-Nthenge A, Rotich E, Godwin S, Nahashon S, Chen F. Prevalence and antimicrobial resistance of Cronobacter sakazakii isolated from domestic kitchens in middle Tennessee, United States. *J Food Prot*. 2012;75(8):1512–1517

67. FDA Issues Final Rule Setting Manufacturing Standards for Infant Formula. 2014. CFSAN Constituent Update. Available at: https://www.fda.gov/Food/NewsEvents/ConstituentUpdates/ucm400182.htm. Accessed June 29, 2017

68. World Health Organization, Food and Agriculture Organization of the United Nations. *Safe preparation, storage and handling of powdered infant formula Guidelines*. Geneva, Switzerland: World Health Organization; 2007

69. World Health Organization, Food and Agriculture Organization of the United Nations. *Enterobacter sakazakii and Other Microorganisms in Powdered Infant Formula: Meeting Report*. Geneva, Switzerland: World Health Organization; 2004

70. US Food and Drug Administration. FDA Takes Final Step on Infant Formula Protections. 2014. Consumer Updates. Available at: https://www.fda.gov/ForConsumers/ConsumerUpdates/ucm048694.htm. Accessed June 29, 2017

71. Infant Nutrition Council of America. NCA Infant Formula Preparation Position: Powdered Infant Formula Preparation Recommendations. 2017. Available at: https://infantnutrition.org/infant-formula-preparation/. Accessed November 27, 2018

72. US Food and Drug Administration. Exempt Infant Formulas Marketed in the United States By Manufacturer and Category. Guidance Documents and Regulatory Information. Available at: https://www.fda.gov/Food/GuidanceRegulation/GuidanceDocumentsRegulatoryInformation/InfantFormula/ucm106456.htm.

73. Lonnerdal B, Hernell O. An opinion on "staging" of infant formula: a developmental perspective on infant feeding. *J Pediatr Gastroenterol Nutr.* 2016;62(1):9–21

74. Gonzalez Ballesteros LF, Ma NS, Gordon RJ, et al. Unexpected widespread hypophosphatemia and bone disease associated with elemental formula use in infants and children. *Bone.* 2017;97:287–292

75. US Food and Drug Administration. Clinical Testing of Infant Formulas With Respect to Suitability for Term Infants. 1988. FDA contract 223-286-2117. Available at: https://www.fda.gov/Food/GuidanceRegulation/GuidanceDocumentsRegulatoryInformation/InfantFormula/ucm170649.htm. Accessed June 29, 2017

76. Institute of Medicine. *Infant Formula: Evaluating the Safety of New Ingredients.* Washington, DC: National Academies Press; 2004

77. Maclean WC Jr, Van Dael P, Clemens R, et al. Upper levels of nutrients in infant formulas: comparison of analytical data with the revised Codex infant formula standard. *J Food Comp Analysis.* 2010;23(1):44–53

78. US Food and Drug Administration. Substantiation for Structure/Function Claims Made in Infant Formula Labels and Labeling: Guidance for Industry. 2016; Draft Guidance. Available at: https://www.fda.gov/downloads/Food/GuidanceRegulation/GuidanceDocumentsREegulatoryInformation/UCM514642.pdf. Accessed June 29, 2017

79. Koo WW, Hockman EM, Dow M. Palm olein in the fat blend of infant formulas: effect on the intestinal absorption of calcium and fat, and bone mineralization. *J Am Coll Nutr.* 2006;25(2):117–122

80. Lloyd B, Halter RJ, Kuchan MJ, Baggs GE, Ryan AS, Masor ML. Formula tolerance in postbreastfed and exclusively formula-fed infants. *Pediatrics.* 1999;103(1):E7

81. Gidrewicz DA, Fenton TR. A systematic review and meta-analysis of the nutrient content of preterm and term breast milk. *BMC Pediatr.* 2014;14:216

82. Khan S, Prime DK, Hepworth AR, Lai CT, Trengove NJ, Hartmann PE. Investigation of short-term variations in term breast milk composition during repeated breast expression sessions. *J Hum Lact.* 2013;29(2):196–204

83. Hosoi S, Honma K, Daimatsu T, Kiyokawa M, Aikawa T, Watanabe S. Lower energy content of human milk than calculated using conversion factors. *Pediatr Int.* 2005;47(1):7–9

84. Lucas A, Ewing G, Roberts SB, Coward WA. How much energy does the breast fed infant consume and expend? *Br Med J (Clin Res Ed).* 1987;295(6590):75–77

85. Hernell O, Fewtrell MS, Georgieff MK, Krebs NF, Lonnerdal B. Summary of current recommendations on iron provision and monitoring of iron status for breastfed and formula-fed infants in resource-rich and resource-constrained countries. *J Pediatr.* 2015;167(4 Suppl):S40–S47

86. Nelson SE, Ziegler EE, Copeland AM, Edwards BB, Fomon SJ. Lack of adverse reactions to iron-fortified formula. *Pediatrics.* 1988;81(3):360–364

87. Iron-fortified formulas and gastrointestinal symptoms in infants: a controlled study, With the cooperation of The Syracuse Consortium for Pediatric Clinical Studies. *Pediatrics.* 1980;66(2):168–170

88. Krebs NF, Domellof M, Ziegler E. Balancing Benefits and Risks of Iron Fortification in Resource-Rich Countries. *J Pediatr.* 2015;167(4 Suppl):S20–S25

89. Institute of Medicine. *Dietary Reference Intakes for Calcium and Vitamin D.* Washington, DC: National Academies Press; 2011

90. Golden NH, Abrams SA; American Academy of Pediatrics, Committee on Nutrition. Optimizing bone health in children and adolescents. *Pediatrics.* 2014;134(4):e1229–e1243

91. Wagner CL, Hulsey TC, Fanning D, Ebeling M, Hollis BW. High-dose vitamin D3 supplementation in a cohort of breastfeeding mothers and their infants: a 6-month follow-up pilot study. *Breastfeed Med.* 2006;1(2):59–70

92. Wheeler BJ, Taylor BJ, Herbison P, et al. High-dose monthly maternal cholecalciferol supplementation during breastfeeding affects maternal and infant vitamin D status at 5 months postpartum: a randomized controlled trial. *J Nutr.* 2016;146(10):1999–2006

93. Oberhelman SS, Meekins ME, Fischer PR, et al. Maternal vitamin D supplementation to improve the vitamin D status of breast-fed infants: a randomized controlled trial. *Mayo Clin Proc.* 2013;88(12):1378–1387

94. Baker RD, Greer FR; American Academy of Pediatrics, Committee on Nutrition. Diagnosis and prevention of iron deficiency and iron-deficiency anemia in infants and young children (0–3 years of age). *Pediatrics.* 2010;126(5):1040–1050

95. Forman J, Silverstein J; American Academy of Pediatrics, Committee on Nutrition, Council on Environmental Health. Organic foods: health and environmental advantages and disadvantages. *Pediatrics.* 2012;130(5):e1406–e1415

96. Lasekan JB, Linke HK, Oliver JS, et al. Milk protein-based infant formula containing rice starch and low lactose reduces common regurgitation in healthy term infants: a randomized, blinded, and prospective trial. *J Am Coll Nutr.* 2014;33(2):136–146

97. Vanderhoof JA, Moran JR, Harris CL, Merkel KL, Orenstein SR. Efficacy of a pre-thickened infant formula: a multicenter, double-blind, randomized, placebo-controlled parallel group trial in 104 infants with symptomatic gastroesophageal reflux. *Clin Pediatr (Phila).* 2003;42(6):483–495

98. Ziegler E, Vanderhoof JA, Petschow B, et al. Term infants fed formula supplemented with selected blends of prebiotics grow normally and have soft stools similar to those reported for breast-fed infants. *J Pediatr Gastroenterol Nutr.* 2007;44(3):359–364

99. Williams T, Choe Y, Price P, et al. Tolerance of formulas containing prebiotics in healthy, term infants. *J Pediatr Gastroenterol Nutr.* 2014;59(5):653–658

100. Ashley C, Johnston WH, Harris CL, Stolz SI, Wampler JL, Berseth CL. Growth and tolerance of infants fed formula supplemented with polydextrose (PDX) and/or galactooligosaccharides (GOS): double-blind, randomized, controlled trial. *Nutr J.* 2012;11:38

101. Vandenplas Y, Zakharova I, Dmitrieva Y. Oligosaccharides in infant formula: more evidence to validate the role of prebiotics. *Br J Nutr.* 2015;113(9):1339–1344

102. Burks AW, Vanderhoof JA, Mehra S, Ostrom KM, Baggs G. Randomized clinical trial of soy formula with and without added fiber in antibiotic-induced diarrhea. *J Pediatr.* 2001;139(4):578–582

103. Chau K, Lau E, Greenberg S, et al. Probiotics for infantile colic: a randomized, double-blind, placebo-controlled trial investigating Lactobacillus reuteri DSM 17938. *J Pediatr.* 2015;166(1):74–78

104. Xu M, Wang J, Wang N, Sun F, Wang L, Liu XH. The efficacy and safety of the probiotic bacterium *Lactobacillus reuteri* DSM 17938 for infantile colic: a meta-analysis of randomized controlled trials. *PLoS One.* 2015;10(10):e0141445

105. Sung V, Hiscock H, Tang ML, et al. Treating infant colic with the probiotic Lactobacillus reuteri: double blind, placebo controlled randomised trial. *BMJ.* 2014;348:G2107

106. Szajewska H, Dryl R. Probiotics for the Management of Infantile Colic. *J Pediatr Gastroenterol Nutr.* 2016;63(Suppl 1):S22–S24

107. Bhatia J, Greer F; American Academy of Pediatrics, Committee on Nutrition. Use of soy protein-based formulas in infant feeding. *Pediatrics.* 2008;121(5):1062–1068

108. Cao Y, Calafat AM, Doerge DR, et al. Isoflavones in urine, saliva, and blood of infants: data from a pilot study on the estrogenic activity of soy formula. *J Expo Sci Environ Epidemiol.* 2009;19(2):223–234

109. Strom BL, Schinnar R, Ziegler EE, et al. Exposure to soy-based formula in infancy and endocrinological and reproductive outcomes in young adulthood. *JAMA.* 2001;286(7):807–814

110. Upson K, Harmon QE, Baird DD. Soy-based infant formula feeding and ultrasound-detected uterine fibroids among young African-American women with no prior clinical diagnosis of fibroids. *Environ Health Perspect.* 2016;124(6):769–775

111. Upson K, Harmon QE, Laughlin-Tommaso SK, Umbach DM, Baird DD. Soy-based infant formula feeding and heavy menstrual bleeding among young African American women. *Epidemiology.* 2016;27(5):716–725

112. Vandenplas Y, De Greef E, Devreker T, Hauser B. Soy infant formula: is it that bad? *Acta Paediatr.* 2011;100(2):162–166

113. National Toxicology Program. NTP-CERHR monograph on soy infant formula. NTP-CERHR MON. 2010;(23):i–661

114. Andres A, Cleves MA, Bellando JB, Pivik RT, Casey PH, Badger TM. Developmental status of 1-year-old infants fed breast milk, cow's milk formula, or soy formula. *Pediatrics.* 2012;129(6):1134–1140

115. Andres A, Moore MB, Linam LE, Casey PH, Cleves MA, Badger TM. Compared with feeding infants breast milk or cow-milk formula, soy formula feeding does not affect subsequent reproductive organ size at 5 years of age. *J Nutr.* 2015;145(5):871–875

116. Bernbaum JC, Umbach DM, Ragan NB, et al. Pilot studies of estrogen-related physical findings in infants. *Environ Health Perspect.* 2008;116(3):416–420

117. Harlid S, Adgent M, Jefferson WN, et al. Soy formula and epigenetic modifications: analysis of vaginal epithelial cells from infant girls in the IFED Study. *Environ Health Perspect.* 2017;125(3):447–452

118. Alimentarius C. CODEX standard for follow-up formula CODEX STAN 156-1987. 1987. Available at: www.fao.org/input/download/standards/293/CXS_156e.pdf. Accessed August 15, 2017

119. Qawasmi A, Landeros-Weisenberger A, Bloch MH. Meta-analysis of LCPUFA supplementation of infant formula and visual acuity. *Pediatrics.* 2013;131(1): e262–e272

120. Osborn DA, Sinn JK. Prebiotics in infants for prevention of allergy. *Cochrane Database Syst Rev.* 2013(3):CD006474

121. Cuello-Garcia CA, Brozek JL, Fiocchi A, et al. Probiotics for the prevention of allergy: A systematic review and meta-analysis of randomized controlled trials. *J Allergy Clin Immunol.* 2015;136(4):952–961

122. Clandinin MT, Chappell JE, Heim T, Swyer PR, Chance GW. Fatty acid utilization in perinatal de novo synthesis of tissues. *Early Hum Dev.* 1981;5(4):355–366

123. Der G, Batty GD, Deary IJ. Effect of breast feeding on intelligence in children: prospective study, sibling pairs analysis, and meta-analysis. *BMJ.* 2006;333(7575):945

124. Anderson JW, Johnstone BM, Remley DT. Breast-feeding and cognitive development: a meta-analysis. *Am J Clin Nutr.* 1999;70(4):525–535

125. von Stumm S, Plomin R. Breastfeeding and IQ Growth from Toddlerhood through Adolescence. *PLoS One.* 2015;10(9):e0138676

126. Mulder KA, King DJ, Innis SM. Omega-3 fatty acid deficiency in infants before birth identified using a randomized trial of maternal DHA supplementation in pregnancy. *PLoS One.* 2014;9(1):e83764

127. Colombo J, Carlson SE, Cheatham CL, et al. Long-term effects of LCPUFA supplementation on childhood cognitive outcomes. *Am J Clin Nutr.* 2013;98(2):403–412

128. Cai S, Pang WW, Low YL, et al. Infant feeding effects on early neurocognitive development in Asian children. *Am J Clin Nutr.* 2015;101(2):326–336

129. Uauy R, Dangour AD. Fat and fatty acid requirements and recommendations for infants of 0–2 years and children of 2–18 years. *Ann Nutr Metab.* 2009;55(1–3): 76–96

130. Briend A, Legrand P, Bocquet A, et al. Lipid intake in children under 3 years of age in France. A position paper by the Committee on Nutrition of the French Society of Paediatrics. *Arch Pediatr.* 2014;21(4):424–438

131. Food and Agriculture Organization of the United Nations. *Fats and Fatty Acids in Human Nutrition. Report of an Expert Consultation.* Geneva, Switzerland: World Health Organization; 2010. Available at: https://www.who.int/nutrition/publications/nutrientrequirements/fatsandfattyacids_humannutrition/en/. Accessed November 27, 2018

132. Koletzko B, Baker S, Cleghorn G, et al. Global standard for the composition of infant formula: recommendations of an ESPGHAN coordinated international expert group. *J Pediatr Gastroenterol Nutr.* 2005;41(5):584–599

133. Thomas DW, Greer FR, American Academy of Pediatrics Committee on N, American Academy of Pediatrics Section on Gastroenterology H, Nutrition. Probiotics and prebiotics in pediatrics. *Pediatrics.* 2010;126(6):1217–1231

134. Kramer MS, Matush L, Vanilovich I, et al. Effects of prolonged and exclusive breastfeeding on child height, weight, adiposity, and blood pressure at age 6.5 y: evidence from a large randomized trial. *Am J Clin Nutr.* 2007;86(6):1717–1721

135. Lodge CJ, Tan DJ, Lau MX, et al. Breastfeeding and asthma and allergies: a systematic review and meta-analysis. *Acta Paediatr.* 2015;104(467):38–53

136. Zeiger RS, Heller S, Mellon MH, et al. Effect of combined maternal and infant food-allergen avoidance on development of atopy in early infancy: a randomized study. *J Allergy Clin Immunol.* 1989;84(1):72–89

137. Halken S, Hansen KS, Jacobsen HP, et al. Comparison of a partially hydrolyzed infant formula with two extensively hydrolyzed formulas for allergy prevention: a prospective, randomized study. *Pediatr Allergy Immunol.* 2000;11(3):149–161

138. Chung CS, Yamini S, Trumbo PR. FDA's health claim review: whey-protein partially hydrolyzed infant formula and atopic dermatitis. *Pediatrics.* 2012;130(2):e408–e414

139. Boyle RJ, Ierodiakonou D, Khan T, et al. Hydrolysed formula and risk of allergic or autoimmune disease: systematic review and meta-analysis. *BMJ.* 2016;352:i974

140. Lodge CJ, Lowe AJ, Dharmage SC. Do hydrolysed infant formulas reduce the risk of allergic disease? *BMJ.* 2016;352:i1143

141. Baldassarre ME, Laforgia N, Fanelli M, Laneve A, Grosso R, Lifschitz C. Lactobacillus GG improves recovery in infants with blood in the stools and presumptive allergic colitis compared with extensively hydrolyzed formula alone. *J Pediatr.* 2010;156(3):397–401

142. Berni Canani R, Di Costanzo M, Bedogni G, et al. Extensively hydrolyzed casein formula containing Lactobacillus rhamnosus GG reduces the occurrence of other allergic manifestations in children with cow's milk allergy: 3-year randomized controlled trial. *J Allergy Clin Immunol.* 2017;139(6):1906–1913.e1904

143. Berni Canani R, Nocerino R, Terrin G, et al. Formula selection for management of children with cow's milk allergy influences the rate of acquisition of tolerance: a prospective multicenter study. *J Pediatr.* 2013;163(3):771–777.e771

144. American Academy of Pediatrics. Committee on Nutrition. Hypoallergenic infant formulas. *Pediatrics.* 2000;106(2 Pt 1):346–349

145. Koletzko S, Niggemann B, Arato A, et al. Diagnostic approach and management of cow's-milk protein allergy in infants and children: ESPGHAN GI Committee practical guidelines. *J Pediatr Gastroenterol Nutr.* 2012;55(2):221–229

146. Venter C, Groetch M. Nutritional management of food protein-induced enterocolitis syndrome. *Curr Opin Allergy Clin Immunol.* 2014;14(3):255–262

147. Furuta GT, Liacouras CA, Collins MH, et al. Eosinophilic esophagitis in children and adults: a systematic review and consensus recommendations for diagnosis and treatment. *Gastroenterology.* 2007;133(4):1342–1363

148. Stallings VA, Stark LJ, Robinson KA, et al. Evidence-based practice recommendations for nutrition-related management of children and adults with cystic fibrosis and pancreatic insufficiency: results of a systematic review. *J Am Diet Assoc.* 2008;108(5):832–839

Chapter 5

Nutritional Needs of the Preterm Infant

Introduction

The provision of optimal nutrition is critical in the management of preterm infants. Optimal nutrition improves survival while decreasing the potential for both short- and long-term morbidities. Current nutritional goals for the preterm infant are to provide nutrients to approximate the rate of growth and composition of weight gain for a normal fetus of the same postmenstrual age while maintaining normal concentrations of nutrients in blood and other tissues.[1,2] In the very low birth weight infant, considerable efforts have been made over the past 2 decades to reduce the degree of extrauterine or postnatal growth restriction that typically occurs by the time of hospital discharge. Although progress has been made, it was reported as late as 2013 that among preterm infants in the United States (birth weights between 500 and 1500 g), up to 50% of infants still demonstrated postnatal growth failure and 25% demonstrated severe growth failure.[3] Presumably, much of the progress can be attributed to changes in practice that include very early introduction of parenteral nutrition within hours of birth, early initiation of enteral feedings in the first few days after birth, adoption of standardized feeding guidelines, and improved nutrient fortification strategies.[1,4] However, the ideal rate of growth and optimal nutritional support regimens for the preterm infant have yet to be defined.[5] Postnatal growth restriction in preterm infants is largely attributable to the interaction of acute neonatal illnesses and nutritional practices, in which inadequate parenteral and enteral nutrition support lead to the development of energy, protein, and mineral deficits.[5] Both adequate growth (including head growth) as well as improved nutritional support have been associated with improved long-term neurodevelopmental outcomes.[6] Although the evidence is compelling, the effects may not be large, and any direct relationship between growth and optimal nutritional regimens on neurodevelopmental outcomes remains unclear. Concerns have also been raised that the differences in early postnatal growth in preterm infants, including rate of catch-up growth, may predispose to later development of the metabolic syndrome. However, recent reviews have concluded that the evidence is relatively poor that preterm birth, low birth weight, early postnatal growth failure, and subsequent catch-up growth have a negative effect on metabolic outcomes in preterm infants.[7] These effects include increased adiposity, blood pressure, insulin resistance, and dyslipidemia. On balance, the evidence that the postnatal catch-up growth of the very low birth weight (VLBW) infant after hospital discharge supports the beneficial effects of improved nutritional support on neurodevelopmental outcomes, is more convincing than long-term negative effects on metabolic outcomes.[7]

Two sets of intauterine curves are now available to assess preterm infant growth (ee Chapter 24: Assessement of Nutritional Status, and Appendix Q). The 2013 Fenton gowth curves are sex-specific and combine intratuter-ine and postnatal curves from 22 to 50 weeks. They include data on 35 000 infants born at <30 weeks' gestation between 1991 and 2007 in multiple countries, including the United States.[8] The 2010 Olsen growth curves include data on 250 000 infants at 21 to 41 weeks' gestation delivered at hospitals in the United States between 1998 and 2006.[9] In addition to curves for weight, length, and head circumference, the Olson curves also include body mass index (BMI)[10] (see Appendix Q). The Olsen and Fenton curves are similar between approximately 23 and 36 weeks (Olsen data included in Fenton dataset; see Chapter 24: Assessment of Nutritional Status). Currently, there are no widely used reference data for growth velocity, arm and leg circumferences, or skinfold measurements for preterm infants. However, a 2017 report described cross-sectional body composition refer-ence charts (fat mass, fat-free mas, percentage of body fat) in 223 stable preterm infants between 30 and 36 weeks' gestation.[11] Fenton et al recently reported on the variability of methods used to evaluate preterm infant growth velocity in a systematic review of 373 studies in which growth veloc-ity was reported. Using the Fenton and Olsen growth curves, their goal was to assess the frequently quoted growth velocity recommendation of 15 g/kg/day of weight and 1 cm/week gain in length and head circumfer-ence.[12] They concluded that a rate of weight gain of 15 to 20 g/kg per day was a reasonable goal for infants 23 to 36 weeks' gestational age, but not beyond. They also concluded that 1 cm/week increase in head circumference fit the Fenton and Olsen growth curves well from 24 to 33 weeks' gestational age, but the 1 cm/week in length dropped to the third percentile by 32 weeks and remained there.

Specific Nutrient Recommendations

Since 1993, specific nutrient recommendations for very low birth weight preterm infants have been based on series of "consensus reports" most recently updated in 2014.[13-15] These are based on acceptable ranges of intakes (ARs), defined as the range of intake derived from observational studies or evaluated under controlled conditions, that appear to sustain adequate nutrition on the basis of the absence of abnormal clinical signs/symptoms or evidence that these levels preserve biochemical and functional normalcy. For most nutrients, the AR for preterm infants is the best "guestimate" made by expert opinion with careful analysis of the available data. Therefore, it is not surprising that the recommended range of intakes in Table 5.1 and Table 5.2 for many nutrients is based on limited evidence. Individual needs for preterm infants may differ depending on disease state, level of tolerance of nutritional support, and other factors.[16,17]

Parenteral Nutrition

Parenteral administration of glucose, fat, and amino acids is an important aspect of the nutritional care of preterm infants, particularly those who weigh less than 1500 g (Table 5.1). Feeding intolerance is a common problem as a result of gastric dysmotility, intestinal hypomotility, and complicating illnesses in small preterm infants. These factors dictate the slow advancement of the volume of enteral feeding and delays in achieving full enteral feeding. Parenteral nutrition is, therefore, an essential supplement to enteral feedings so that total daily intake by both means of nutrition support meets the infant's nutritional needs. When necessary, basic nutritional needs can be met for considerable periods by the parenteral route alone. There have been no new general recommendations for parenteral nutrition requirements for infants with birth weight <1500 g since the consensus report of 2005 (Table 5.1).

Parenteral nutrition for preterm infants weighing greater than 1500 g and for late preterm infants (born at 34–36 weeks' gestation) has not been well studied, despite the need for increased nutritional support compared with those of term infants.[18] Advancement of enteral feeding for moderate preterm infants (≥29 weeks' gestation) may take at least 5 to 10 days to reach full fortified feeding, and therefore, parenteral nutrition support remains necessary during this transitional period. Parenteral nutrition support is particularly important for late preterm infants with intrauterine growth restriction who require special nutritional considerations.[19]

Fluid therapy is designed to avoid dehydration or overhydration, to provide stable electrolyte and glucose concentrations, and to avoid abnormal acid-base balance. Because insensible water losses occurring primarily through the skin vary tremendously depending on gestational age at birth, birth weight, and postnatal age, emphasis is placed on individualized fluid management. For preterm infants with birth weight ≥1000 g, fluid

Table 5.1.

Comparison of Parenteral Intake Recommendations for Growing Preterm Infants in Stable Clinical Condition

	Consensus Recommendations		Consensus Recommendations	
	<1000 g Birth Weight/kg/day	<1000 g Birth Weight/100 kcal	1000–1500 g Birth Weight/kg/day	1000–1500 g Birth Weight/100 kcal
Water/fluids, mL	140–180	122–171	120–160	120–178
Energy, kcal	105–115	100	90–100	100
Protein, g	3.5–4.0	3.0–3.8	3.2–3.8	3.2–4.2
Carbohydrate, g	13–17	11.3–16.2	9.7–15	9.7–16.7
Fat, g	3–4	2.6–3.8	3–4	3.0–4.4
Linoleic acid, mg	340–800	296–762	340–800	
Linoleate:linolenate = C18:2/C18:3	5–15	5–15	5–15	5–15
Vitamin A, IU	700–1500	609–1429	700–1500	700–1667
Vitamin D, IU	40–160		40–160	
Vitamin E, IU	2.8–3.5	2.4–3.3	2.8–3.5	2.8–3.9
Vitamin K₁, µg	10	8.7–9.5	10	10.0–11.1
Ascorbate, mg	15–25	13.0–23.8	15–25	15.0–27.8
Thiamine, µg	200–350	174–333	200–350	200–389
Riboflavin, µg	150–200	130–190	150–200	150–222
Pyridoxine, µg	150–200	130–190	150–200	150–222
Niacin, mg	4–6.8	3.5–6.5	4–6.8	4.0–7.6
Pantothenate, mg	1–2	0.9–1.9	1.2	1.0–2.2

Biotin, µg	5–8	1.3–7.6	5–8	5.0–8.9
Folate, µg	56	49–53	56	56–62
Vitamin B$_{12}$, µg	0.3	0.26–0.29	0.3	0.30–0.33
Sodium, mg	69–115	60–110	69–115	69–128
Potassium, mg	78–117	68–111	78–117	78–130
Chloride, mg	107–249	93–237	107–249	107–277
Calcium, mg	60–80	52–76	60–80	60–89
Phosphorus, mg	45–60	39–57	45–60	45–67
Magnesium, mg	4.3–7.2	3.7–6.9	4.3–7.2	4.3–8.0
Iron, µg	100–200	87–190	100–200	100–222
Zinc, µg	400	348–381	400	400–444
Copper, µg	20	17–19	20	20–22
Selenium, µg	1.5–4.5	1.3–4.3	1.5–4.5	1.5–5.0
Chromium, µg	0.05–0.3	0.04–0.29	0.05–0.3	0.05–0.33
Manganese, µg	1	0.87–0.95	1	1.00–1.11
Molybdenum, µg	0.25	0.22–0.24	0.25	0.25–0.28
Iodine, µg	1	0.87–0.95	1	1.00–1.11
Taurine, mg	1.88–3.75	1.6–3.6	1.88–3.75	1.9–4.2
Carnitine, mg	≈2.9	≈2.5–2.8	≈2.9	≈2.9–3.2
Inositol, mg	54	47–51	54	54–60
Choline, mg	14.4–28	12.5–26.7	14.4–28	14.4–31.1

Reprinted with permission from Tsang RC, Uauy R, Koletzko B, Zlotkin SH, eds. *Nutrition of the Preterm Infant: Scientific Basis and Practical Guidelines*. Cincinnati, OH: Digital Educational Publishing; 2005

Table 5.2.
Current Recommendations of Advisable Nutrient Intakes for Fully Enterally Fed Preterm VLBW Infants per kg per Day, and per 100 kcal Energy Intake, Compared With Previous Intake Recommendations

Nutrient	Current Recommendation (per kg/day)	Current Recommendation (per 100 kcal)	LSRO, 2002 (formula-fed infants only, per kg/day)[74,136]	Tsang et al, 2005 (per kg/day)[14]	ESPGHAN, 2010 (per kg/day)[2]
Fluids	135–200	—	NS	150–200	135–200
Energy, kcal	110–130 (85–95 IV)	—	100–141	110–120	110–135
Protein, g	3.5–4.5	3.2–4.1	3.0–4.3	3.0–3.6	4.0–4.5 (<1 kg) 3.5–4.0 (1–1.8 kg)
Lipids, g	4.8–6.6	4.4–6	5.3–6.8		4.8–6.6 (<40% MCT)
Linoleic acid, mg	385–1540	350–1400	420–1700	(4–15 E%)	385–1540
a-Linolenic acid, mg	>55	>50	90–270	(1–4 E%)	>55
DHA, mg	(18–) 55–60	(16.4–) 50–55	NS	NS	12–30
EPA, mg	<20	<18	NS	NS	(<30% of DHA)
ARA, mg	(18–) 35–45	(16.4–) 32–41	NS	NS	18–42
Carbohydrate, g	11.6–13.2	10.5–12	11.5–15.0 lactose 4.8–15.0	lactose: 3.8–11.8 oligomers: 0–8.4	11.6–13.2
Sodium, mg[a]	69–115	63–105	46.8–75.6	0–23	69–115

Potassium, mg[b]	78–195	71–177	72–192	0–39	66–132
Chloride, mg	105–177	95–161	72–192	0–35	105–177
Calcium, mg	120–200	109–182	148–222	120–230	120–140
Phosphate, mg	60–140	55–127	98–131	60–140	60–90
Magnesium, mg	8–15	7.3–13.6	8.2–20.4	7.9–15	8–15
Iron, mg	2–3	1.8–2.7	2–3.6	0–2	2–3
Zinc, mg	1.4–2.5	1.3–2.3	1.32–1.8	0.5–0.8	1.1–2.0
Copper, µg	100–230	90–210	120–300	120	100–132
Selenium, µg	5–10	4.5–9	2.2–6.0	1.3	5–10
Manganese, µg	1–15	0.9–13.6	7.6–30	0.75	<27.5
Fluoride, µg	1.5–60	1.4–55	NS	NS	1.5–60
Iodine, µg	10–55	9–50	7.2–42	11–27	11–55
Chromium, ng	30–2250	27–2045	NS	50	30–1230
Molybdenum, µg	0.3–5	0.27–4.5	NS	0.3	0.3–5

Reprinted with permission from Koletzko B, Poindexter B, Uauy R. Recommended nutrient intake levels fo stable, fully enterally fed very low birth weight infants. In Koletzko B, Poindexter B, Uauy R, eds. *Nutritional Care of Preterm Infants. Scientific Basis and Practical Guidelines.* New York, NY: Karger; 2014: 297–299.

ARA indicates arachidonic acid; DHA, docosahexaenoic acid; EPA, eicosapentaenoic acid; IV, intravenous; LSRO, Life Sciences Research Office; MCT, medium-chain triglyceride; RE, retinol equivalents; αTE, α-tocopherol equivalents.

[a] 1 mEq Na = 23 mg.

[b] 1 mEq K = 39 g.

Continued

Table 5.2. *Continued*

Current Recommendations of Advisable Nutrient Intakes for Fully Enterally Fed Preterm VLBW Infants per kg per Day, and per 100 kcal Energy Intake, Compared With Previous Intake Recommendations

Nutrient	Current Recommendation (per kg/day)	Current Recommendation (per 100 kcal)	LSRO, 2002 (formula-fed infants only, per kg/day)[74,136]	Tsang et al, 2005 (per kg/day)[14]	ESPGHAN, 2010 (per kg/day)[2]
Thiamin, μg	140–300	127–273	36–300	180–240	140–300
Riboflavin, μg	200–400	181–364	96–744	250–360	200–400
Niacin, mg	1–5.5	0.9–5	660–6000	3.6–4.8	0.38–5.5
Pantothenic acid, mg	0.5–2.1	0.45–1.9	360–2280	1.2–1.7	0.33–2.1
Pyridoxine, μg	50–300	45–273	36–300	150–210	45–300
Cobalamin, μg	0.1–0.8	0.09–0.73	0.096–0.84	0.3	0.1–077
Folic acid, μg	35–100	32–91	36–54	25–50	35–100
L-Ascorbic acid, mg	20–55	18–50	10–45	18–24	11–46

Biotin, µg	1.7-16.5	1.5-15	1.2-44.4	3.6-6	1.7-16.5
Vitamin A, µg RE	400-1100	365-1000	245-456	700	400-1000
Vitamin D, IU	(400-1000 per day, from milk + supplement)	100-350 from milk only	90-324	150-400	(800-1000 per day) (100-350 per 100 kcal from milk only)
Vitamin E, mg α-TE	2.2-11	2-10	2.4-9.6	6-12	2.2-11
Vitamin K1, µg	4.4-28	4-25	4.8-30	(300 bolus injection)	4.4-28
Nucleotides, mg	NS	NS	NS	NS	<5
Choline, mg	8-55	7.3-50	8.4-27.6	14.4-28	8-55
Inositol, mg	4.4-53	4-48	4.8-52.8	32-81	4.4-53

Reprinted with permission from Koletzko B, Poindexter B, Uauy R. Recommended nutrient intake levels for stable, fully enterally fed very low birth weight infants. In Koletzko B, Poindexter B, Uauy R, eds. *Nutritional Care of Preterm Infants. Scientific Basis and Practical Guidelines.* New York, NY: Karger; 2014: 297-299.

ARA indicates arachidonic acid; DHA, docosahexaenoic acid; EPA, eicosapentaenoic acid; IV, intravenous; LSRO, Life Sciences Research Office; MCT, medium-chain triglyceride; RE, retinol equivalents; αTE, α-tocopherol equivalents.

[a] 1 mEq Na = 23 mg.
[b] 1 mEq K = 39 g.

requirements approximate 60 to 80 mL/kg on the first day, increasing by 20 mL/kg/day, to a total of 140 to 160 mL/kg/day by day 5 of life. Parenteral sodium intake is restricted until the physiological postnatal loss of extracellular fluid is underway.[20] Sodium should be added after serum sodium concentration falls below 140 mg/dL with around 2 to 4 mEq/kg/day of sodium as an appropriate mixture of chloride and acetate to correct both sodium losses and metabolic acidosis.[20-22]

For infants weighing less than 1000 g at birth, fluid intake should start higher at 80 to 100 mL/kg/day and then rise in the first 5 days largely in accord with urine output and insensible water losses, which may be 5 to 7 mL/kg/hour in extreme cases.[20-22] Water losses are significantly minimized through the use of modern incubators that can achieve dynamic thermal, air, and humidity control. Eventually, if total parenteral nutrition (TPN) is used exclusively for nutritional support, fluid rates of up to 140 to 160 mL/kg/day can be attained for most infants to achieve a weight gain of 15 to 20 g/kg/day. Higher intakes of sodium and chloride may be required in extremely preterm infants with high urinary excretion of electrolytes. The sodium and chloride need in the first week of life may reach 4 to 8 mEq (92–184 mg)/kg/day before settling closer to 2 to 4 mEq (46–92 mg)/kg/day by 1 month postnatal age.[22] Hyponatremia (serum sodium concentration less than 135 mg/dL) is a potentially growth-limiting state and should be corrected when identified. The addition of 1.5 to 2 mEq (58–78 mg)/kg/day of potassium will be needed for this period of active growth.[21]

Protein (Including Early Parenteral Administration of Amino Acids)

It has been established that the protein requirement for the growing preterm infant receiving parenteral solutions is between 3 and 4 g/kg day. Glucose infusions without amino acids provide energy but do not address the need for a minimum intake of 1.2 g/kg/day of amino acids just to match protein breakdown and urinary losses.[23,24] However, VLBW infants can be provided 3 g/kg/day of amino acids within the first few hours of life to support anabolism.[25] This can be achieved through the provision of prepared stock dextrose (5% or 10%) and amino acid solutions (2%–4%) before full parenteral nutrition is instituted.[26] Studies have continued to document no significant increases in metabolic acidosis, serum ammonia concentration. or adverse effects of increased blood urea nitrogen concentrations with early amino acid administration.[27-29] Thus, there has been optimism that this strategy would improve growth and lower morbidity, including neurodevelopmental outcomes. However, studies have demonstrated mixed results for improvement of growth including head circumference, particularly from randomized controlled trials (RCTs).[27,28] Two meta-analyses have addressed this issue. The first included 7 RCTs and found that early administration of amino acids has no impact on mortality, early and late growth, and neurodevelopment but was associated with a positive nitrogen balance and did not affect acid base status or ammonia levels.[30] The second report determined that administering a high dose (>3.0 g/kg/day) and an early dose (≤24 hours) is safe and well tolerated but does not offer significant benefits in growth and morbidity.[31]

Glucose

The preterm infant has high energy requirements because of very metabolically active organs, most importantly the brain. Glucose is the major source of energy for most metabolic processes in the preterm infant, especially the brain and heart. It is also the major source of carbon for de novo synthesis of fatty acids and some nonessential amino acids. Because glycogen stores are limited, hypoglycemia commonly develops in VLBW infants without an early and continuous intravenous glucose supply. It can be extrapolated from existing data that 54 mg/dL is the lower limit for blood sugar in preterm infants born at a gestational age of 24 to 32 weeks, considerably higher than the current definition of neonatal hypoglycemia.[32] Paradoxically, despite adequate glucose infusion rates in the preterm infant, endogenous glucose production is sustained, frequently resulting in hyperglycemia particularly in the first few weeks of life.[32,33] The degree of hyperglycemia increases with decreasing gestation, particularly between 22 and 24 weeks. Intravenous infusion rates greater than 10 to 11 minutes/kg nearly always result in hyperglycemia. The upper limit of a normal glucose range has not been defined, but many references use a glucose concentration of up to 120 mg/dL in very preterm infants. There is some evidence that higher glucose concentrations are associated with adverse effects, and insulin infusion, with its own complications, has been used to treat hyperglycemia in very low birth weight infants.[34] However, further studies are needed to show that that insulin, beyond reduction in serum glucose concentrations, is of efficacy in reducing any associated morbidity before generally recommending insulin therapy.

A generally accepted recommendation is to begin glucose infusions at 5 to 7 mg/kg/minute beginning at birth, gradually increasing to 10 to 11 mg/kg/minute (38–42 kcal/kg/day) for full intravenous nutrition. As noted previously, these rates may even be too high for the most preterm and sickest of preterm infants. Blood glucose concentration should be checked frequently to keep plasma glucose concentrations between 60 and 120 mg/dL.[32] In addition, early initiation and advancement of protein infusions has resulted in less hyperglycemia.

Intravenous Lipids

Intravenous lipid emulsions allow the provision of a dense energy source critical for the rapidly growing preterm infant. A 20% phospholipid preparation (as opposed to 10%), allowing for a more efficient triglyceride clearance, is preferred in preterm infants.[35] A minimum provision of 0.5 g/kg/day protects against essential fatty acid deficiency.[32] Lipid intolerance (serum triglyceride concentration >200 mg/dL) is seen more frequently in infants of lower birth weight, born at lower gestational age, with lipid infusions greater than 2.6 g/kg/day, and with sepsis.[36] Unlike the need for amino acids very soon after birth, the benefits of very early lipid administration are less clear. When infused at a similar amount (g/kg/day) of amino acids, a dose of 2 to 3 g/kg/day of parenteral lipids can be safely used from birth onward.[37] That this improves nitrogen balance and also improves conditions for anabolism has been demonstrated in an RCT.[38] Fat tolerance can be assessed indirectly by measuring serum triglyceride concentrations. The maximum value is poorly defined but generally between 200 to 250 mg/mL. Lipid intake should usually provide 25% to 40% of nonprotein calories in fully parenterally fed patients.[35]

It has been suggested by some that the addition of carnitine to parenteral nutrition may enhance the preterm infant's ability to use exogenous fat for energy. However, the available studies are contradictory, and to date there is no evidence to support the routine supplementation of parenterally fed preterm infants with carnitine.[37,39]

In the past, there have been concerns for adverse effects of intravenous lipids in preterm infants including hyperglycemia, potential interference with immune function including increased rates of infection, impaired bilirubin metabolism, adverse effects on pulmonary function, and cholestasis. However, there is no recent evidence supporting these concerns at the currently recommended infusion rates of lipid.[32] The exception is the potential for long-term parenteral lipid infusion adversely affecting cholestatic disease, but it is still not clear to what extent lipid emulsions are involved in the development of cholestasis.[35,37] Lipid emulsions may be reduced (down to 1 g/kg/day) or held entirely to assist in slowing the cholestatic process, especially in infants with intestinal dysfunction that requires long-term TPN. Cycling lipids alone has not been shown to reduce parenteral nutrition-associated cholestasis.[40]

Currently, there are no lipid emulsions approved by the US Food and Drug Administration (FDA) specifically for preterm infants. The 2 predominant lipid emulsions used in the United States are soy based and, as such, contain omega-6 fatty acids without omega-3 oils. Thus, there is the potential for intralipid infusions to lead to greater amounts of vasoactive, prostaglandin-derived products and lesser amounts of critical central nervous system membrane-producing products. This issue needs further study given the potential for docosahexaenoic acid (DHA) deficiency in preterm infants maintained long-term on parenteral nutrition. Newer lipid emulsions containing improved fatty acid blends (olive oil, medium-chain triglycerides [MCTs], fish oil, etc) are now available in North America but still have only have FDA approval for adults. There are not yet enough data to recommend these emulsions in preterm infants, but they may prove to cause less parenteral nutrition-associated cholestasis in preterm infants in the future.[37,41]

Calcium, Phosphorus, and Trace Minerals

Levels of fetal calcium and phosphorus accretion cannot generally be met with parenteral nutrition, but severe metabolic bone disease in preterm infants can be minimized by adding calcium and phosphorus to parenteral amino acid solutions containing at least 2.5 g/dL amino acids and by administering calcium- and phosphorus-containing solution at 120 to 150 mL/kg per day.[42] Each institution should establish calcium and phosphorus solubility curves for their own parenteral nutrition solutions. The provision of calcium and phosphorus intravenously is optimized by the addition of cysteine to amino acid mixtures, as cysteine lowers the pH of the solution permitting a higher amount of calcium and phosphorus to solubilize in the parenteral nutrition solution. Goals for calcium intake are 60 to 80 mg/kg/day, and goals for phosphorous intake are 39 to 67 mg/kg/day.[42]

Although some have recommended beginning parental calcium at 24 to 35 mg/kg/day on the first day of life to treat the early hypocalcemia of prematurity, the efficacy of this "traditional" therapy has not been demonstrated and is controversial.[43] This hypocalcemia is typically asymptomatic and occurs mostly in the first 72 hours of life. It responds readily to the calcium and phosphorus added to standard TPN solutions as the amount of parenteral nutrition is increased in the first week of life.

When TPN supplements are limited to 1 to 2 weeks, zinc is the only trace mineral that needs to be added at approximately 400 μg/kg/day[44,45] (Table 5.1). If TPN is required for a longer period, the other trace minerals may be added; however, manganese and copper should be omitted in patients with cholestasis.[44] Removal of copper will depend on copper concentrations, because copper is necessary for antioxidant synthesis and is variably accumulated in the presence of cholestasis secondary to prolonged parenteral nutrition therapy. Current recommendations for copper are 20 to 40 µg/kg/day.[44,45] Selenium and chromium should be omitted in patients with renal dysfunction. Supplemental iron is not usually required during parenteral nutrition in preterm infants unless it is the sole source of nutrition (including absence of red cell transfusions) for more than 2 months.[44,45]

Multivitamins

Recommended parental doses of fat-soluble and water-soluble vitamins are given in Table 5.1 and are unchanged since the previous edition of this text.[46,47] Several parenteral vitamin solutions are available for use in preterm infants in the United States. From a practical standpoint, the recommended daily dose of parenteral vitamins for preterm infants is 40% of the currently available reconstituted single dose (5 mL) of the multivitamin mixture (Table 5.3).[47,48] Vitamin mixtures given at this dosage provide the recommended amounts of vitamins E and K, low levels of vitamin A and D, and excess levels of most B vitamins. However, a more appropriate mixture is not available, and individual vitamins are not available for parenteral use.

In summary, despite some positive short-term outcomes, particularly for early introduction of parenteral nutrition, the absence of long term-data makes it difficult to determine the optimal strategy for parenteral nutrition in the preterm infants. Although there is no doubt that early nutrition modulates morbidity including neurodevelopment, long-term functional outcomes need to be demonstrated in adequately powered RCTs. The practice and details of delivering parenteral nutrition in VLBW infants is beyond the scope of this chapter and has been reviewed elsewhere[48] (see also Chapter 22: Parenteral Nutrition).

Transition From Parenteral to Enteral Nutrition

The transition from parenteral nutrition to complete enteral nutrition is a critical period when total nutrient requirements may fluctuate as parenteral nutrition is weaned and enteral intake is insufficient. In most cases, this generates a gap in nutrient provision that requires care in calculating concentrations of each nutrient in parenteral nutrition to minimize excessive reductions in nutrient delivery during this period. This gap is particularly important for protein. Thus, in general, tapering of parenteral amino acid intake should not start before at least 75 mL/kg of enteral nutrition has been reached.[49] For most infants, parenteral nutrition can generally be

Table 5.3.
Vitamins Provided With PN Solutions[a]

Vitamin	Amount Provided Per 5 mL
Ascorbic acid (vitamin C)	80 mg
Vitamin A (retinol)[b]	2300 USP units
Vitamin D[b]	400 USP units
Thiamine (vitamin B₁) (as the hydrochloride)	1.20 mg
Riboflavin (vitamin B₂) (as riboflavin-5-phosphate sodium)	1.4 mg
Pyridoxine (vitamin B₆) (as the hydrochloride)	1.0 mg
Niacinamide	17.0 mg
Dexpanthenol (pantothenyl alcohol)	5 mg
Vitamin E (d-α-tocopheryl acetate)	7.0 USP units
Biotin	20 g
Folic acid	140 g
Vitamin B₁₂ (cyanocobalamine)	1.0 g
Vitamin K₁ (phylloquinone)[b]	200 g

[a] MVI Pediatric is a lyophilized, sterile powder intended for reconstitution and dilution in intravenous infusions. INFUVITE Pediatric is provided as a 4-mL and 1-mL vial that can be combined for administration. For each vitamin mixture, 5 mL of reconstituted product provides the indicated amounts of the vitamins. The recommended dose is 40% (2 mL) of the currently available reconstituted single dose (5 mL) of the MVI mixture.

[b] Fat-soluble vitamins solubilized with polysorbate 80.

discontinued when enteral feeds are at least 120 mL/kg/day, because basic fluid requirements will be met. Some approaches to reducing this potential parenteral to enteral nutrient gap, include excluding early enteral feeds from the total fluid requirements and introducing fortified human milk earlier if preterm infant formula is not used.

Enteral Feeding

Standard infant formula intended for full-term infants or unfortified human milk is not sufficient for optimal growth of preterm infants. The use of preterm infant formulas and preterm human milk fortifiers results in a composition of weight gain and bone mineralization closer to that of the reference fetus, as compared with infants fed standard term formulas or unfortified human milk. Randomized prospective trials of preterm infant formulas have shown significant improvements in growth and cognitive development compared with standard formulas for term infants.[50] Preterm infants fed standard infant formulas gain a higher percentage of their weight as fat when compared with a fetus of the same maturity.[32] These findings underscore the need for the health care professional to carefully plan and monitor the nutritional care of preterm infants during hospitalization and after discharge.

The following review of recommended nutrient requirements is based on the 2014 "consensus report" for stable, fully enterally fed very low birth weight infants[15] (Table 5.2).

Energy and Water Requirements

Energy is required for body maintenance and growth. VLBW infants are particularly sensitive to energy fluctuations because of their exceptionally high growth demands that are more than double those of a term infant. Energy requirements of the low birth weight infant are estimated in Table 5.4.[51] The estimated resting metabolic rate of preterm infants, with minimal physical activity, is lower during the first week after birth. In a

Table 5.4.
Estimation of the Energy Requirement of the Low-Birth-Weight Infant[a]

	Average Estimation, kcal/kg per day
Energy expended	40–60
Resting metabolic rate	40–50[b]
Activity	0–5[b]
Thermoregulation	0–5[b]
Synthesis	15[c]
Energy stored	20–30[c]
Energy excreted	15
Energy intake	90–120

[a] Adapted from the Committee on Nutrition of the Preterm Infant, European Society of Paediatric Gastroenterology and Nutrition.[51]

[b] Energy for maintenance.

[c] Energy cost of growth.

thermoneutral environment, the resting metabolic rate is approximately 40 kcal/kg/day when the infant is parenterally fed and 50 kcal/kg/day by 2 to 3 weeks of age when the infant is fed orally. By 6 weeks, most preterm infants have a baseline energy expenditure of 80 kcal/kg/day.[52] Each gram of weight gain, including the stored energy and the energy cost of synthesis, requires between 3 and 4.5 kcal. Thus, a daily weight gain of 15 g/kg requires a caloric expenditure of 45 to 67 kcal/kg above the 50 kcal/kg/day for the resting metabolic rate.

The energy needs for activity, basal energy expenditure at thermoneutrality, nutrient absorption, and new tissue synthesis (growth) vary among infants. These variations may be more pronounced in growth-restricted or small-for-gestational-age infants. In practice, energy intake by the enteral route of 110 to 130 kcal/kg/day enables most preterm infants to achieve satisfactory rates of growth.[17] More calories may be given if growth is unsatisfactory at these intakes, particularly with the increased energy requirements such as in infants with chronic lung disease.

Minimum water requirements are set to match ongoing measurable (urine and stool) and insensible (skin, respiratory) losses. After initial stabilization in the first 2 weeks of life, the minimum water requirements approximate 120 to 150 mL/kg/day. However, this volume of formula or fortified human milk may not be sufficient for adequate growth. A higher density feeding (24–30 kcal/oz) may be needed.

The energy density of preterm and term human milk is approximately 65 to 67 kcal/dL or about 20 kcal/oz at 21 days of lactation. It is important recognize that energy density in human milk varies largely between mothers and by time of day, time of lactation, and fraction of milk pumped (foremilk vs hind milk, the latter containing more fat).[53,54] Fortification of human milk to 24 kcal/oz is required and sufficient for most infants; current fortifiers achieve this level. Preterm formulas (81 kcal/dL or 24 kcal/oz) are designed to achieve this caloric density. The increased caloric density allows smaller feeding volumes, an advantage when the gastric capacity is limited. The volume of these feedings is in excess of water requirements and is sufficient for the excretion of protein metabolic products and electrolytes. In some cases, further fluid restriction is required, and then higher caloric densities between 24 and 30 kcal/oz will be necessary to achieve optimal growth.

Protein
Recent research has concluded that enteral protein intakes between 3.5 and 4.5 g/kg per day are safe and support growth and development.[49] These intakes take into account the need for catch-up growth (Table 5.2).

The type and quantity of protein in infant formulas most suitable for preterm infants has been examined in multiple studies.[49] In general, term infants fed whey-predominant formulas had metabolic indices and plasma amino acid concentrations closer to those of infants fed pooled, mature human milk. However, bovine whey does not have the same amino acid composition as human milk whey, and the amino acid profiles differ significantly from those of human milk. Some have argued that the gold standard for protein quality should reflect the plasma amino acid patterns of optimally growing low birth weight infants only fed human milk proteins. Others have argued that the standard should take into account functional outcomes such as growth and neurodevelopment.[49] Soy-based formulas are not recommended for preterm infants, because optimal carbohydrate, protein, and mineral absorption and utilization are not well documented for soy-based formulas.[55]

Fat

With very little new evidence, the recommended total fat intake has not changed significantly over time.[1,14] However, the recommendations for DHA and alpha-linoleic acid (ALA) intakes have increased (Table 5.2).

Fat is a major source of energy for growing preterm infants. In human milk, approximately 50% of the energy is from fat; in commercial formulas, fat provides 40% to 50% of the energy. These feedings provide 5 to 7 g/kg of fat per day. The saturated fat of human milk is well absorbed by the preterm infant, in part because of the distribution pattern of fatty acids on the triglyceride molecule. Palmitic acid is present in the beta position in human milk fat and is more easily absorbed than palmitic acid in the alpha position, which occurs in cow milk as well as most other animal fats, and vegetable oils.[37] Gastric lipase and enzymes found in human milk (pancreatic lipase-related 2 and bile salt-stimulated lipase) facilitate the digestion of triglycerides into fatty acids and glycerol digestion in the gastrointestinal tract. However, in preterm infants, as much as 20% to 30% (or more) of the dietary lipid is excreted in the stool.[56] There are many reasons for this high rate of lipid excretion, including low levels of intestinal lipase secretion (gastric, pancreatic, and bile-salt stimulated lipase) and low luminal bile salt concentrations. Additionally, pasteurization of donor human milk inactivates bile salt-stimulated lipase and changes the structure and function of milk fat globules.

Preterm infant formulas contain a mixture of MCTs and vegetable oils rich in polyunsaturated long-chain polyunsaturated fatty acids (LCPUFAs), both of which are well absorbed by preterm infants, despite the presence of low intraluminal bile salts and pancreatic lipases.[37] With carnitine-independent transport of MCTs into the mitochondria, essential fatty acids can be spared from oxidation. This fat blend meets the estimated essential fatty acid requirement of at least 3% of energy in the form of linoleic acid with additional small amounts of ALA. Human milk, on the other hand, contains relatively small amounts of DHA and arachidonic acid (ARA), varying widely according to maternal diet, with the North American diet on the lower end of the spectrum. DHA and ALA are the major omega-3 and omega-6 fatty acids of neural tissue and are a major component of the photoreceptor membranes. For a more detailed review of the importance of DHA and ALA in the diet of both term and preterm infants, see Chapter 17: Fats and Fatty Acids.

Stable isotope studies have shown that endogenous synthesis of both DHA and ARA occurs in both term and preterm infants.[57] The need for LCPUFAs in the preterm infant is believed to be larger than that of the term infant, given the significant needs during the third trimester of pregnancy primarily supplied from maternal plasma, the low fat reserves at the time of birth, and the minimal LCPUFA content of early feeding regimens, including TPN (see previous discussion). Thus, infants born preterm are thought to be at significant risk for dietary LCPUFA insufficiency. However, this hypothesis has not been consistently demonstrated in numerous studies, either for visual acuity or neurodevelopmental outcomes (see Chapter 17: Fats and Fatty Acids). The relevant RCTs for visual acuity (n=8) have been summarized in a recent Cochrane systematic review.[58] This review also found no overall effects of LCPUFA supplementation on Bayley mental or psychomotor scores, confirming the results of a previous review of the same studies.[58,59] Two newer trials in which DHA total dose reflected more closely the in utero accretion rate of DHA also included human milk-fed preterm infants.[60,61] Both trials reported no differences in mental developmental scores at 18 to 20 months of age. However, the largest and more robust of the 2 trials demonstrated that girls only had a 4.5 point (approximately 0.3 SD) improvement in mental developmental scores (95% confidence interval [CI], 0.5–8.5) and that significant mental delay (mental development scores <70) was reduced from 10.5% in the control group compared with 5% in the higher DHA group (relative risk 0.50; 95% CI, 0.26–0.93). However, this trial recently reported no differences at 7 years' corrected age for preterm infants born at <33 weeks' gestation.[62]

Carbohydrates

Carbohydrates contribute a readily usable energy source and protect against tissue catabolism. Once the preterm infant's condition is stabilized, the requirement for carbohydrate is estimated at 40% to 50% of calories, or approximately 11.6 to 13.2 g/kg per day (Table 5.2). By 34 weeks' postconceptional age, preterm infants have intestinal lactase activities that are only 30% of those of term infants.[33] However, in clinical settings, lactose intolerance is rarely a problem with formula and human milk, which may be attributable to the fact that preterm infants acquire a relatively efficient capacity to hydrolyze lactose in the small intestine at an earlier developmental stage than do fetuses in utero.[63] Glycosidase enzymes for glucose polymers are active in small preterm infants, and these polymers are well tolerated by preterm infants. Because glucose polymers add fewer osmotic particles to the formula per unit weight than does lactose, they permit the use of a high-carbohydrate formula with an osmolality below 300 mOsm/kg of water. Lactose enhances calcium absorption. Carbohydrates in formulas designed for preterm infants contain approximately 40% to 50% lactose and 50% to 60% glucose polymers, a ratio that does not impair mineral absorption.[64] It is unclear whether the addition of glucose polymers in formula for preterm infants is necessary over a fully lactose-based feeding such as found in human milk, as this not has not been the focus of any RCTs.

Oligosaccharides (Prebiotics)

Human milk oligosaccharides play an important role as bioactive factors that provide immunologic protection to the growing term infant by promoting the growth of an age appropriate microflora in the colon. For more information on the importance of oligosaccharides, see Chapter 3: Breastfeeding. Although some oligosaccharides have been added to term infant formula, their function and benefits have not been studied in preterm infants.[65,66] Therefore, there are no preterm formulas that contain added oligosaccharides at this time.

Minerals

Sodium, Potassium, and Chloride

Preterm infants, particularly VLBW infants, have high fractional excretion rates of sodium for at least the first 10 to 14 days after birth, although urinary loss of sodium is also related to total fluid intake. The low sodium concentrations of human milk and human milk fortifiers designed for the feeding of preterm infants may lead to hyponatremia. Special formulas for preterm infants provide 1.7 to 2.2 mEq/kg per day of sodium at full feeding levels (Appendix D).[21] During the stable and growing period, sodium requirements are usually met with a daily intake of 3 to 5 mEq/kg per day. Current potassium requirement of preterm infants is 2 to 5 mEq/kg per day (see Table 5.2).

Calcium, Phosphorus

During the last trimester of pregnancy, the human fetus accrues approximately 80% of the calcium, phosphorus, and magnesium present at term. To achieve similar rates of accretion for normal growth and bone mineralization, small preterm infants require higher intakes of these minerals per kilogram of body weight than do term infants. The American Academy of Pediatrics (AAP) has reviewed this topic and made specific recommendations for intakes and monitoring for adequacy of calcium, phosphorus, and vitamin D status. Current recommendations include a calcium intake of 150 to 220 mg/kg day for VLBW preterm infants who are fully enterally fed and a phosphorus intake of 75 to 140 mg/kg/day.[67] These are similar to the current consensus recommendations (Table 5.2) and reflect the high daily intake requirements for these minerals.[68] However, providing adequate amounts of these nutrients, particularly calcium and phosphorus, to VLBW infants during the first few weeks of life is not always possible because of solubility limits of parenteral nutrition solutions, delayed fortification of human milk, and delays in advancement of enteral feedings. As a result, 10% to 20% of hospitalized infants with a birth weight <1000 g have radiologically defined rickets (metaphyseal changes), and fractures develop in some.[67]

The AAP has recommended assessment of VLBW infants for rickets and adequacy of calcium and phosphorus intakes beginning at 4 to 5 weeks after birth (see AAP text box on next page).[67]

The use of powdered or liquid human milk fortifiers and special formulas for preterm infants has significantly improved mineral balance and bone mineralization VLBW infants.[67,68] Fortified human milk provides 165 to 180 mg of calcium per 100 kcal and 82 to 100 mg of phosphorus per 100 kcal. Preterm infant formulas contain 165 to 180 mg of calcium per 100 kcal and 82 to 100 mg of phosphorus per 100 kcal (see Appendices D-1 and D-2: Formulas for Low Birth Weight Infants).

Iron (see also Chapter 19: Iron)

Because most of the iron accumulation in the human fetus also occurs during the last trimester of pregnancy, preterm infants are at high risk

---

AAP

The AAP recommends[67]:

- Preterm infants, especially those born at <27 weeks' gestation or with birth weight <1000 g with a history of multiple medical problems, are at high-risk of rickets.
- Routine evaluation of bone mineral status by using biochemical testing indicted for infants with birth weight <1500 g but not those with birth weight >1500 g. Biochemical testing should usually be started 4 to 5 weeks after birth.
- Serum alkaline phosphatase activity >800 to 1000 IU/L or clinical evidence of fractures should lead to a radiographic evaluation for rickets and management focusing on maximizing calcium and phosphorus intake and minimizing factors leading to bone mineral loss.
- A persistent serum phosphorus concentration less than approximately 4.0 mg/dL should be followed, and consideration should be given for phosphorus supplementation.
- Routine management of preterm infants, especially those with birth weight <1800 to 2000 g, should include human milk fortified with minerals or formulas designed for preterm infants (see Appendix D).
- At the time of discharge from the hospital, VLBW infants will usually be provided higher intakes of minerals than are provided by human milk or formulas intended for term infants with the use of transitional formulas. If exclusively breastfed, a follow-up serum alkaline phosphatase activity at 2 to 4 weeks after discharge from the hospital may be considered.
- When infants reach a body weight >1500 g and tolerate full enteral feeds, vitamin D intake should generally be approximately 400 IU/day, up to a maximum of 1000 IU/day.

Pediatrics. 2013;131(5):e1676–e1683

---

of depletion of iron stores within the first 2 months of life as well as iron deficiency later during the first year of life. On a weight basis, the iron stores of preterm infants at birth (75 mg/kg) are lower than those of term infants.[43] Preterm infants who are growth restricted have lower iron stores than their appropriately grown preterm counterparts.[69] Approximately 75% of the iron is present in circulating hemoglobin, and the frequent blood sampling that occurs with many preterm infants often depletes the amount of iron available for erythropoiesis.[43] The rapid restoration of iron stores with transfusions of packed red blood cells that supply 1 mg/mL of elemental iron is countered by the exposure risk to blood products. The use of human recombinant erythropoietin (hrEPO) to avoid blood transfusions, along with its requirement for additional enteral or parenteral iron, remains a controversial practice and is not generally recommended.[70] Successful efforts to reduce blood sampling in the neonatal intensive care unit (NICU) and the practice of delayed cord clamping in the preterm infant have further decreased the use of hrEPO.[70,71] Currently, starting iron supplements before 2 weeks of age is not recommended.[43,45]

After 2 weeks of age, there is general agreement that iron supplements to provide up to 2 to 3 mg/kg day of total enteral iron should be provided to VLBW preterm infants, to support their iron needs and sustain normal ferritin levels, an indicator of iron stores. Iron supplements should be continued until 6 to 12 months of age, depending on diet.[43,45,72] It has also been recommended to follow VLBW infants with regular measurements of ferritin concentrations to assess iron status. The normal range of ferritin concentrations in VLBW preterm infants is 35 to 300 µg/L. If ferritin level is <35 µg/L, the iron dose should be increased. If ferritin level is >300 µg/L, commonly occurring after red blood cell transfusions, iron fortification should be discontinued.[45]

Trace Minerals (see also Chapter 20, Trace Elements)

Zinc

Zinc is essential for normal growth and development because of its ubiquitous role in enzymatic functions.[45,73] During the last trimester of pregnancy, the estimated fetal accretion rate for zinc is 400 µg/kg/day.[74] On the basis of data from 14 metabolic balance studies, it has been calculated that an enteral zinc intake of 2.0 to 2.25 mg/kg/day is needed to achieve this zinc retention rate.[75] Despite the fact preterm infants are at risk of low zinc status because of missed accretion, increased losses, and poor intake, there are few randomized trials of zinc intake in preterm infants. The zinc concentration of colostrum is high (5.4 mg/L), but its concentration in human milk rapidly declines to concentrations of 2.5 mg/L by 1 month and 1.1 mg/L by 3 months postpartum.[76] These concentrations of zinc are inadequate to meet the requirements of the stable growing preterm infant, as demonstrated by reports of clinical zinc deficiency among human milk-fed preterm infants.[45] Estimated enteral recommendations for zinc are 1.4 to 2.5 mg/kg/day (Table 5.2).[45] The added zinc to human milk fortifiers and preterm formulas will provide the zinc needed to meet these recommendations (see Appendix D).

Copper

Copper plays critical roles in supporting enzymatic functions, especially those that are part of the antioxidant defense system. Copper retention by the fetus has been estimated to be about 50 µg/kg/day.[45] Human milk from mothers of preterm infants contains 58 to 72 μg/dL during the first month after birth and drops to 22 μg/dL by 5 months postpartum.[76] Preterm infants absorb copper at rates of 57% from fortified human milk to 27% from standard cow milk-based formula.[77] Current recommendations for daily enteral copper intake are 100 to 230 μg/kg/day (Table 5.2). These intakes are achievable with fortified human milk or preterm infant formula (Appendix D).

Iodine

Preterm infants have lower iodine and thyroid hormone stores compared with term infants.[78] Transient hypothyroidism has been reported among preterm infants receiving 10 to 30 μg/kg per day of iodine, although the recommended iodine intake is 10 to 60 μg/kg/day.[44] All formulas for preterm infants will supply this amount. Currently available powdered human milk fortifiers do not contain added iodine. Because the iodine content of human milk is dependent on maternal diet and highly variable, it may not supply enough iodine by itself if the preterm infant is maintained for extended periods on human milk. A recent small study in the United States showed the content of iodine in maternal milk fed to preterm infants ranged from 33 to 177 μg/L.[78] Given these low-iodine food sources, the need for iodine supplementation in this population needs further study, and an RCT investigating the effect of 30 μg/kg/day of iodine in preterm infants with a 2-year follow-up is underway in the United Kingdom.[45] A Cochrane review has determined that there is insufficient evidence to determine whether iodine supplements improve health outcomes in preterm infants.[79] Current recommended enteral intakes for healthy preterm infants are 10 to 55 μg/kg/day (Table 5.2).

Other Trace Elements

Deficiencies of selenium, chromium, molybdenum, or manganese have not been reported for healthy preterm infants fed human milk.[44] Current minimum recommended intakes for these trace minerals are based on their concentrations in human milk (see Table 5.2 and Appendix D).

Water-Soluble Vitamins (see also Chapter 21.II: Water-Soluble Vitamins)

The recommended intakes of water-soluble vitamins are based on number of factors, including the estimated amount provided by human milk and current feeding regimens, an understanding of their physiologic functions and excretion rates, stability during storage, and the very limited amount of research data on the water-soluble vitamin needs of preterm infants

(Table 5.2).[47,80] As a group, the body's reserves (stores) of water-soluble vitamins is limited, and a continuing supply of these nutrients is essential for normal metabolism. The higher recommended intakes for preterm infants compared with those for term infants are based on their higher protein requirements and limited vitamin reserves. The recommended enteral intakes of water-soluble vitamins for preterm infants fed human milk may be achieved by using a vitamin-containing human milk fortifier, as relatively few of these vitamins are provided by standard, oral multivitamin supplements. In formula-fed preterm infants, recommendations may be met by feeding formulas designed for preterm infants that contain higher levels of water-soluble vitamins than standard formulas for term infants. There are no guidelines for supplementing preterm infants with water-soluble vitamins after hospital discharge, and no published studies are available.

The ascorbic acid (vitamin C) content of human milk is approximately 8 mg/100 kcal, and that of formulas for preterm infants ranges from 20 to 40 mg/100 kcal. Although no reports of deficiency among preterm infants receiving these feedings have occurred, no published studies have assessed the ascorbic acid status of enterally fed preterm infants. Because ascorbic acid is essential for the metabolism of several amino acids, its requirement may be increased because of the high level of protein metabolism in the growing preterm infant. Enteral supplementation of ascorbic acid has not shown net benefit for any neonatal morbidity, including bronchopulmonary dysplasia.[81] Loss of ascorbic acid can occur during handling and storage of human milk, but ascorbic acid supplementation of human milk with a human milk fortifier or multivitamins can offset this. Current guidelines for ascorbic acid intake are 20 to 55 mg/kg/day[17,80] (Table 5.2).

Thiamine (vitamin B_1) is a cofactor for 3 enzyme complexes required for carbohydrate metabolism as well as for the decarboxylation of branched-chain amino acids. The thiamine content of human milk is 29 μg/100 kcal, and thiamine content of formulas for preterm infants is 200 to 250 μg/100 kcal (see Appendix D). Commercially available human milk fortifiers provide an equivalent amount of thiamine when used to fortify human milk to 24 kcal/oz. Recommendations for thiamine intake range from 140 to 300 μg/kg/day.[17,80]

Riboflavin (vitamin B_2) is a primary component of flavoproteins that serve as hydrogen carriers in numerous oxidation-reduction reactions. Infants with a negative nitrogen balance may have increased urinary losses of riboflavin, and those requiring phototherapy may use their reserves of riboflavin in the photocatabolism of bilirubin. The riboflavin content is 49 µg/100 kcal in human milk and 150 to 620 µg/100 kcal in formulas for preterm infants (Appendix D). Commercially available human milk fortifiers provide 250 to 500 µg/100 kcal when used to fortify human milk to 24 kcal/oz. Because of the photosensitivity of riboflavin, its content in human milk decreases during storage and handling. Guidelines for riboflavin intake range from 200 to 400 µg/kg/day.[17,80] The higher intake allows for increased losses of riboflavin associated with medical problems commonly found among preterm infants.

Pyridoxine (vitamin B_6) is a cofactor for numerous reactions involved in amino acid synthesis and catabolism. The requirement for pyridoxine is directly related to protein intake. The pyridoxine content of human milk is 28 µg/100 kcal, and pyridoxine content of formula for preterm infants is 150 to 250 µg/100 kcal (Appendix D). Human milk fortifiers contain the equivalent amount when used as directed. Current recommendations for pyridoxine intake range from 50 to 300 µg/kg/day.[17,80]

Niacin (vitamin B_3) is a primary component of cofactors that function in numerous oxidation-reduction reactions, including glycolysis, electron transport, and fatty acid synthesis. Human milk contains 210 µg of niacin/100 kcal, and formulas for preterm infants contain 3.9 to 5.0 mg of niacin/100 kcal (Appendix D). Human milk fortifiers contain the equivalent amount when used as directed. No cases of niacin deficiency have been reported among healthy preterm infants using current feeding regimens; however, no studies of niacin status among enterally fed infants are available. Recommended intake ranges from 1 to 5.5 mg/kg/day.[17,80]

Biotin is a cofactor for 4 carboxylation reactions and is active in folate metabolism. The only reports of biotin deficiency have occurred among infants supported on biotin-free parenteral nutrition for several weeks.[82] The biotin content of human milk is 0.56 µg/100 kcal, and the content of formulas for preterm infants is 3.9 to 37 µg/100 kcal (Appendix D). Biotin deficiency may be a risk for preterm infants receiving human milk alone.[82] Powdered human milk fortifiers contain the equivalent amount when used as directed. The recommended daily intake ranges from 1.7 to 16.5 µg/kg/day.[17,80]

Pantothenic acid (vitamin B_5) is a component of the acyl transfer group coenzyme A that is essential for fat, carbohydrate, and protein metabolism. Human milk provides 250 µg of pantothenic acid/100 kcal, and formulas for preterm infants contain 1.2 to 1.9 mg of pantothenic acid/100 kcal (Appendix D), which will easily provide the recommended daily intake of 0.5 to 2.1 mg/kg/day.[17,80] Powdered human milk fortifiers contain the equivalent amount when used as directed (Appendix D).

Folic acid (vitamin B$_9$) is a cofactor that serves as an acceptor and donor of one-carbon units in amino acid and nucleotide metabolism. Deficiency alters cell division, particularly in tissues with rapid cell turnover, such as the intestine and bone marrow. Preterm infants are at increased risk of folate deficiency because of limited hepatic stores and rapid postnatal growth. Studies of preterm infants have shown improved folate status, assessed by red blood cell folate concentrations, among those provided supplemental folic acid.[17,47,80] Current recommendations for folic acid intake range from 35 to 100 μg/kg.[80] Human milk provides approximately 7 μg/100 kcal of folic acid. Formulas for preterm infants contain 20 to 37 μg folic acid/100 kcal. Powdered human milk fortifiers will supply up to 30 μg folic acid/100 kcal when used as directed (Appendix D).

Vitamin B$_{12}$ (cobalamine) is a cofactor involved in the synthesis of DNA and the transfer of methyl groups. Clinical symptoms of deficiency have been reported among infants who were exclusively breastfed by vegetarian mothers.[47,80] Deficiency has not been reported among term or preterm infants born to well-nourished mothers. Vitamin B$_{12}$ is well absorbed from human milk and infant formula. Human milk provides 0.07 μg of vitamin B$_{12}$/100 kcal, and preterm infant formulas provide 0.25 to 0.55 μg of vitamin B$_{12}$/100 kcal. Powdered human milk fortifiers will provide 0.22 to 0.79 μg of vitamin B$_{12}$/100 kcal when used as directed (Appendix D). The recommended intake is 0.1 to 0.8 μg/kg/day.[17,80]

Fat-Soluble Vitamins (see also Chapter 21.I: Fat-Soluble Vitamins)

There are 4 fat-soluble vitamins: A, D, E and K. Levels of fat-soluble vitamins in human milk vary depending on maternal diet. The intestinal absorption of fat-soluble vitamins is subject to the limitations of fat digestion (lower pancreatic lipases and bile acids) in preterm infants.

Vitamin A

Vitamin A is a collective term for several fat-soluble retinoids including retinol, beta-carotene, and carotenoids, which promote normal growth and differentiation of epithelial tissues. Specific functions include the effects on visual acuity, growth, healing, reproduction, cell differentiation, and immune function. Vitamin A is required in the fetal lung for cellular differentiation and surfactant synthesis and the individual surfactant proteins, which interact with retinoic acid nuclear receptors in regulating gene expression.[80] The preterm infant is at high risk of low vitamin A stores. The liver is the primary storage site for vitamin A, and at birth, the hepatic vitamin A content of preterm infants is low. Measured concentrations have indicated limited reserves and, in some cases, depletion. In addition, the plasma retinol, retinol-binding protein (RBP), and retinol-to-RBP molar ratios of preterm infants are less than those of infants born at term.[46] The low vitamin A reserves, in conjunction with impaired absorption, attributable to reduced hydrolysis of fats and low levels of intestinal carrier proteins for retinol, place the preterm infant at risk of developing vitamin A deficiency. This includes increased risk for bronchopulmonary dysplasia and respiratory infections.

Several studies have indicated that sufficient vitamin A status reduces the incidence and severity of lung disease in the preterm infant.[83] The largest study to date demonstrated a reduction in bronchopulmonary dysplasia, defined as the need for oxygen treatment at 36 weeks' postmenstrual age.[84] Although additional supplementation may be beneficial for preterm infants at risk of lung disease, clinicians must weigh the modest benefits against necessity for repeated intramuscular injections.[85] Postdischarge blood concentrations of vitamin A in preterm infants do not reach those of term infants and may not be sufficient with current supplemental approaches using supplemental vitamins.[85] There is no benefit or harm on long-term neurodevelopmental outcomes.[84]

The recommendations for vitamin A intake range from 400 to 1100 µg /kg/day /kg/day.[17,80] Given their high vitamin A content (3045 µg /L, 375 µg /100 kcal), special formulas for preterm infants will supply this amount (Appendix D). Human milk, with a vitamin A concentration of 670 µg /L (100 µg /100 kcal), will not supply the recommended intake. Human milk fortifiers, when used as directed, will provide an additional 1860 to 2850 µg /L.

Vitamin E is another collective group of compounds that function as antioxidants that actively inhibit fatty acid peroxidation in cell membranes. The very preterm infant should receive 2.2 to 11 mg/kg/day of vitamin E enterally (Table 5.2).[17,80] Preterm infant formulas supply 2.7 to 4 mg of vitamin E/100 kcal (Appendix D). The vitamin E content of mature human milk is quite variable and generally low, but current human milk fortifiers support more than the recommended amount per 100 kcal/day (Appendix D). Pharmacologic doses of vitamin E for the prevention or treatment of retinopathy of prematurity, bronchopulmonary dysplasia, and intraventricular hemorrhage are not recommended.[86]

Vitamin D

Vitamin D is a pluripotent steroid prohormone that, in addition to having a pivotal role in maintaining bone health, may be increasingly important in numerous health conditions. Most tissues and cells in the body have a vitamin D receptor. Vitamin D has been associated with improved cardio-vascular health, stimulation of the immune system, and cancer prevention as well as prevention of other chronic diseases. However, there are no studies in preterm infants that document functional outcomes. Even data documenting the role of vitamin D in maintaining serum calcium and bone health is sparse particularly in the first weeks of life in preterm infants.[67,68] Maternal vitamin D status is highly variable, and many mothers may be unknowingly insufficient or deficient in vitamin D stores and may put their fetus at risk of having low vitamin D concentrations.[87,88] Because measuring vitamin D status is not routinely recommended, there may be some preterm infants who are deficient at birth (25-OH-D concentrations <20 ng/mL) because of poor maternal vitamin D status. In fact, a recent study found infants born at less than 32 weeks' gestation (n=72) had increased odds of 25-OH-D concentrations <20 ng/mL (50 nmol/L) compared with more mature infants (odds ratio [OR], 2.4; 95% CI, 1.2–5.3)[89] This is corrected by the addition of vitamin D to parenteral nutrition and to formulas and human milk fortifiers for preterm infants. Preterm infants with birth weight <1250 g and gestational age <32 weeks who receive a high mineral-containing bovine milk-based formula and a daily vitamin D intake of approximately 400 IU maintain normal serum 25-hydroxyvitamin D and appropriately elevated 1,25-dihydroxyvitamin D for many months.[90]

The AAP recommends, on the basis of limited data, that for infants who weigh <1500 g, 400 IU/kg/day of vitamin D is sufficient, although 200 IU per day is acceptable.[67] This intake should be increased to 400 IU/day when the weight exceeds 1500 g and the infant is tolerating full enteral nutrition.[67] In Europe, guidelines suggest higher intakes of vitamin D of 800 to 1000 IU/day[68] (Table 5.2), but there is no direct comparison of this approach compared with the recommendations by the AAP. No data are available for VLBW infants with birth weight <1000 g to assess the safety of providing these vitamin D intakes, which, on a body-weight basis, may be 5 to 10 times the amount recommended for full-term neonates.[67]

Vitamin K

Vitamin K is poorly stored, and therefore, daily intake is important. Hemorrhagic disease of the newborn infant, most commonly seen in exclusively breastfed infants, results from vitamin K deficiency.[91] Unless vitamin K is given at birth, most preterm infants will develop at least subclinical deficiency within 7 to 10 days after birth.[92] As a preventive measure, an intramuscular injection of vitamin K is routinely provided after birth. In preterm infants who weigh more than 1 kg at birth, the standard prophylactic dose of 1 mg of phylloquinone is appropriate. For infants weighing less than 1 kg, a dose of 0.2 mg of phylloquinone is recommended.[93] Formulas for preterm infants provide sufficient vitamin K to meet daily needs thereafter. Human milk has a low vitamin K content, but the use of human milk fortifiers that contain additional vitamin K meet the recommended intake of 4.4 to 28 µg/kg per day (Table 5.2).

Human Milk *(see also Chapter 3: Breastfeeding)*

Fortified human milk from the infant's own mother is the ideal enteral feeding for the preterm infant. Human milk contains living cells including stem cells and many bioactive factors that contribute positively to the infant's health and development (see Appendix A). Human milk is generally well tolerated by preterm infants and promotes earlier achievement of full enteral feeding compared with infant formula.[94] Milk from mothers of preterm infants, especially during the first 2 weeks of lactation, contains higher levels of energy, fat, protein, and sodium, but slightly lower concentrations of lactose, calcium, and phosphorus compared with milk from mothers of term infants.[95] Nevertheless, once full feeds are established, all nutrients are present in inadequate concentrations to meet the nutritional needs of the preterm infant, with shortfalls ranging from small to very large. Shortfalls are particularly high for protein, calcium, phosphorus, and zinc.[96] In VLBW preterm infants, this necessitates the addition of a human milk fortifier, which may be necessary even after hospital discharge (see below). Preterm infants with intrauterine growth restriction (IUGR) are at additional risk of not meeting their nutrient requirements and may need additional fortification, especially when receiving human milk.

Human Milk Fortification

Both powder and liquid human milk fortifiers (HMFs) that provide additional protein, minerals, and vitamins are available for supplementing human milk for the preterm infant (Appendix D).[97] These HMFs are well balanced and contain similar amounts of protein, minerals, and vitamins and can be used to supplement human milk for the preterm infant up to 24 kcal/oz. The newer cow milk-based liquid HMFs provide higher amounts of protein than the powder fortifiers and have protein hydrolysates instead of intact protein. These cow milk-based liquid fortifiers have been shown to support improved growth comparable to the powder HMFs.[98,99] The human milk-based liquid fortifiers do require vitamin D supplementation. They are designed for mixing with human milk at the bedside.

Human milk intake is associated with a reduction in the incidence of necrotizing enterocolitis (NEC) compared with preterm infant formula, likely because of immunologic and antimicrobial components in human milk.[100,101] A dose-dependent effect of human milk on survival without NEC has been observed in a retrospective analysis of a national neonatal database.[102] Thus, VLBW infants should be encouraged to consume as much human milk (mother's own or donor human milk) within the period when NEC occurs most often—before 34 weeks' postconceptional age.

The use of an exclusive human milk feeding regimen that includes pasteurized human milk and human milk-derived milk fortifier has also been shown to decrease NEC and surgical NEC in infants born weighing less than 1250 g.[103] However, in that study, the control group was fed mother's own milk fortified with bovine human milk fortifier and received cow milk-based preterm formula when mother's milk was not available. No donor human milk was used. Thus, at the present time, there is no definitive evidence in preterm infants of any adverse effect from the addition of intact bovine milk protein to human milk nor any advantage of using human milk-derived milk fortifier over bovine-based human milk fortifiers for the prevention of NEC.[97,101] There is no question that fortification of human milk improves growth, although there are no data from RCTs that this growth is optimal. Similarly, evidence that neurodevelopmental function is improved in preterm infants fed fortified human milk, compared with those fed preterm infant formula, is not available.[97,101] A recent review also found no evidence for any effect of human milk intake on neurodevelopmental outcomes in preterm infants through 18 months' corrected age, but these studies were underpowered for this outcome.[104]

Facilitating Lactation and Human Milk Handling

Mothers of preterm infants should be encouraged to provide their milk for feeding their infants. Mothers should be supported to start expressing their milk within the first few hours after delivery (see also Chapter 3: Breastfeeding). Because many mothers of preterm infants deliver by Cesarean section, coordinating lactation support with labor, delivery, and neonatal staff is crucial. Mothers should be encouraged to express their milk for their infants even if they had no intention of ever breastfeeding. It is important that mothers receive information on the value of their milk prenatally and postnatally. Mothers should be given verbal and written instructions about appropriate methods for collection, storage, and handling of their milk and assisted in locating a supplier for breast pumping equipment needed to establish and maintain a milk supply.[105] Individual counseling from certified lactation consultants about lactation management issues, such as pumping frequency, methods to facilitate milk letdown, and breast and nipple care, should be readily available.

Fresh milk from an infant's mother may be fed immediately or refrigerated at approximately 4°C. Refrigerated milk can be safely fed up to 96 hours after expression.[106] Any milk that will not be fed within 48 to 96 hours should be frozen at −20°C immediately after it has been expressed. Freezing and heat treatment of human milk alter such labile factors as cellular elements, immunoglobulin (Ig) A, IgM, lactoferrin, lysozyme, and C3 complement. Freezing is generally preferred, because human milk that has been frozen retains most of its immunologic properties (except for cellular elements) and vitamin content when fed within 3 months of expression. Routine bacteriologic testing and pasteurization of human milk is not necessary when it is fed to the mother's own infant.[105]

Frozen milk should be thawed gradually in the refrigerator or in lukewarm water (running tap water or standing basin). Commercial milk warmers are also available to thaw and warm milk to body temperature at steady rates. Care should be taken to avoid contaminating the lids of the milk containers while warming. Thawing in a microwave is not recommended, because it reduces the levels of IgA and lysozyme activity and may produce hot spots in the milk.[105] Thawed human milk should be stored in a refrigerator and used within 24 hours.

Donor Human Milk for the Preterm Infant

The use of donor human milk is an established practice in North America. Donor human milk was used frequently for term and preterm infants until the concerns for HIV transmission in the 1980s, at which time the use of donor milk decreased dramatically. With appropriate screening and preparation standards, however, the use of donor milk is now particularly targeted for the needs of the preterm infant. There are no federal regulations of donor human milk banks or for the use of donor milk. The more than 24 North American nonprofit milk banks are all members of the Human Milk Banking Association of North America (HMBANA), which has established practice and safety guidelines.[107] Each bank follows specific procedures set by HMBANA for screening potential donors for infectious diseases, medical history, and lifestyle behaviors that could affect the quality of donated milk.

Commercial human milk banking is also growing and is available from several entities in the United States. Pooled donor human milk is made available to hospitals through physician prescription. Although there are no federal regulations or guidelines for banking human milk, the FDA has endorsed the use of human milk banking and deemed the informal sharing of human milk to be unsafe. Donor milk is pooled, pasteurized, tested for bacteria and HIV, and frozen for storage.[a] Donor milk consists primarily of human milk from mothers of term infants several months into lactation.

In 2017, the AAP published a policy statement on the use of donor milk for the high-risk infant, while acknowledging that the principal goal for VLBW infants is the provision of mother's own milk. Donor milk should be used as a bridge until the mother's milk is available and volume is sufficient.[108] Like mother's own milk, donor milk requires fortification when used as a feeding for preterm infants.

Both pasteurization and freezing of donor milk destroys cells (neutrophils and stem cells), and affects the levels of macronutrients, micronutrients, and many bioactive factors. Donor human milk generally has lower protein, lactoferrin, immunoglobulins, inactive lipase, and vitamin and electrolyte content.[108] It is also of note that pasteurization of human milk results in a 30% reduction in fat absorption and may account for some of the decreased growth rates seen in preterm infants receiving donor human milk.[37] Overall, only 70% to 80% of ARA and DHA in pasteurized human milk is absorbed by VLBW preterm infants.[37]

There are no clear guidelines for discontinuing the use of donor milk in VLBW infants when mother's own milk is not available. A range of postmenstrual ages from 32 to 36 weeks is commonly used. Breastfeeding should be encouraged during hospitalization to enhance the likelihood that successful breastfeeding will occur after hospital discharge.[108]

A recent randomized, double-blind trial confirmed that NEC occurred less frequently among infants fed donor milk supplemented with bovine human milk fortifiers compared with those fed preterm infant formula (1.7% vs 6.6%, risk ratio [RR], −4.9%, 95% CI, −9.0% to −0.9%; $P = .02$).[109] In this largest study to date in 363 VLBW infants, all infants were fed mother's own milk when available, but then were randomized to donor milk plus bovine milk fortifiers or preterm infant formula only, when mother's milk was insufficient or no longer available. About 25% of the infants in each group

---

[a] Information about donor human milk banks in the United States and Canada is available from the Human Milk Banking Association of North America Web site (www.hmbana.org).

AAP

AAP Recommendations for Donor Human Milk for the High-Risk Infant: Preparation, Safety, and Usage Options in the United States[108]:

- Although a mother's own milk is always preferred, donor human milk may be used for high-risk infants when the mother's milk is not available or the mother cannot provide milk. Priority should be given to providing donor human milk to infants <1500 g birth weight.
- Human milk donors should be identified and screened by using methods such as those currently used by HMBANA milk banks or other established commercial milk banks.
- Donor milk should be pasteurized according to accepted standards. Postpasteurization testing should be performed according to internal quality-control guidelines.
- Health care providers should discourage families from direct human milk sharing or purchasing human milk from the Internet because of the increased risks of bacterial or viral contamination of nonpasteurized milk and the possibility of exposure to medication, drugs, or other substances, including cow milk protein.
- The use of donor milk in appropriate high-risk infants should not be limited by an individual's ability to pay. Policies are needed to provide high-risk infants access to donor human milk on the basis of documented medical necessity, not financial status.

Pediatrics. 2017;139(1):e20163440

---

received only mother's own milk, and the remainder received, on average, 60% maternal milk. There was no difference in growth between the groups. In addition, when infants were assessed at 18 to 22 months, the cognitive composite scores of the Bayley-III (the primary outcome) were not significantly different between the donor milk group (92.9) and the formula group (94.5), with a fully adjusted mean difference of −2.0 (95% CI, −5.8 to 1.8).

Commercial Formulas for Preterm Infants

Preterm infants may require infant formula when mother's or donor milk is unavailable. Infant formulas for preterm infants (Appendix D) have been developed to meet the unique nutritional needs of the growing preterm infant. Preterm infant formulas have a nutrient composition comparable to fortified human milk and produce growth rates similar to that of fortified human milk.[110]

Characteristics of this group of formulas compared with standard formulas for term infants include increased amounts of protein (whey predominant) and minerals, carbohydrate blends of lactose and glucose polymers, and fat blends containing a large portion of fat as MCT oils[110] (see Appendix D).

The higher intake of calcium and phosphorus provided by formulas for preterm infants increases net mineral retention and improves bone mineral content compared with standard formulas for term infants.[67,68] The vitamin content of these formulas is generally sufficient once intake volumes of at least 600 mL per day are achieved. Prior to this, vitamin D may be given to meet the recommended 400 IU/day target.[67]

Following a series of infections in preterm infants with *Cronobacter sakazakii* attributed to the use of contaminated powdered formulas, the FDA recommended against the use of these powdered formulas in preterm infants in 2002, because they cannot be sterilized.[111,112] Only sterile liquid formula preparations are now used in preterm infants in the United States, and a number of human milk sterile liquid human milk fortifiers have also become available.[98,99] Infant formula preparation guidelines established by the Academy of Nutrition and Dietetics are a practical resource to minimize contamination risks during the preparation and delivery of enteral nutrition in preterm infants (http://www.eatright.org).

There are currently no available infant formulas for preterm infants containing probiotics in the United States, primarily for safety and efficacy concerns. There are also no enteral supplements of probiotics with FDA approval for use in preterm infants. However, 2 recent systematic reviews have more or less concluded that there are protective effects of probiotics against NEC and all-cause mortality in preterm infants, largely on the basis of data collected outside of North America.[113,114] Yet, controversy and disagreement on their use continues,[115] and they may be indicated in settings where there is a very high prevalence of NEC. On the other hand, in the United States, with the growing use of fortified human milk in the NICU, NEC is less of a concern, as noted previously. Even so, given the myriad of choices of probiotics available worldwide, which ones should be used? Ideally, these would be the best studied, with the highest effect size and best safety profile.[115] Clearly, much more data from randomized controlled trials are needed.

Methods of Enteral Feeding

Enteral feeding of VLBW infants is a fundamental part of clinical care. The method of enteral feeding chosen for each infant should be based on gestational age, birth weight, clinical condition, and experience of the hospital nursing personnel. Therefore, there is a great deal of heterogeneity among care providers for the management of enteral feedings. Specific feeding decisions that must be made by the clinician include age to initiate feeding, type of feeding (mother's milk, donor human milk, formula), method of delivery, feeding frequency, rate of advancement, and timing of fortification or supplementation. Adoption of a NICU-specific standardized feeding guideline for preterm infants results in earlier attainment of full enteral feeding, improved growth, and a reduction in neonatal morbidities, including NEC.[96,116] Additional information on many other aspects of the topic of enteral feeding of the preterm infant can be found in a recent detailed review.[117]

Growth Target Objectives

All preterm and term infants lose some weight after birth that represents an adaptation to extrauterine life. The primary loss of weight is attributable to a contraction of the extracellular water compartment; however, for the preterm infant, the ability to provide adequate nutrients and energy in the first week of life can be challenging, and some of the initial weight loss represents loss of lean body mass. This loss is reflected in decreased weight percentiles within the first week of life following birth, and as such, a deviation from anticipated intrauterine rates. Growth thereafter, for the most part, can be targeted at 15 to 20 g/kg/day, but because the growth is curvilinear and changes over time, it is important to graph weight and length on a growth chart to determine whether the infant is meeting reference standards.[12]

Oral Colostrum Care

The earliest oral feedings of human milk to preterm infants can be delivered as "priming doses" of colostrum. This may support the biologic need for early passive immunologic protection in a premature newborn infant. Oral colostrum care involves the addition of very small amounts of colostrum (0.2–0.5 mL) every 2 to 6 hours starting within hours after birth. In a very small study, it has been shown that oral colostrum care may reduce the incidence of sepsis and transfers measurable quantities of some bioactive compounds such as IgA and lactoferrin to the infant.[118] There are also microorganisms in colostrum that may contribute to the seeding of the infant's developing microbiome.[119]

Trophic Feeding

Small initial feedings without increasing volumes over time are called "trophic," "priming," or "minimal" enteral feedings and range anywhere from 1 to 25 mL/kg/day. Proponents of trophic feedings of colostrum and transitional milk start them as soon as possible after birth. Because of the greater enrichment of bioactive components in colostrum, feeding the earliest milk sequentially may be of benefit. However, a 2013 Cochrane review of 9 trials in 754 VLBW infants found that there was no evidence that early trophic feedings affected feeding tolerance or growth rates. There was no evidence of harm, however, including no increased risk of NEC.[120] However, this review could not rule out that there may be differences in human milk versus formula trophic feedings, given the information that feeding human milk versus formula reduces the risk of NEC in VLBW infants (see previous discussion).

Route of Feeding

The route (gavage vs nipple) for enteral feeding is determined by the infant's ability to coordinate sucking, swallowing, and breathing, which appear at approximately 32 to 34 weeks of gestation but do not become efficient until after 34 to 35 weeks. More mature preterm infants who appear alert and vigorous may be fed by nipple or offered the breast. Infants who are more preterm or critically ill require feeding by a gavage tube. The use of the stomach maximizes the digestive capability of the gastrointestinal tract. The gavage tube may be nasogastric or orogastric, with insufficient data available to inform this practice.[121] Infants who receive tube feedings may be fed on an intermittent bolus or continuous drip feeding schedule. At the present time, available data does not support one route over the other. No differences in time to achieve full feedings in VLBW infants with continuous feedings (over 10 to 20 minutes) versus bolus feedings every 2 to 3 hours have been observed.[122] On the other hand, nutrient losses in the tubing of continuous feedings, especially those of human milk, have been consistently observed.[123,124]

Transpyloric feedings provide no improvement in energy intake or growth and may be associated with significant risks.[125] This method of feeding should be undertaken only in rare instances (ie, prolonged gastroparesis, severe gastroesophageal reflux, or aspiration risk) and gastric feedings should be resumed as soon as possible. Gastrostomy tube feeding should be considered for infants unable to nipple feed for long periods of time to decrease negative oral stimulation associated with feeding tubes and other complications, such as aspiration.

Advancement of Enteral Feedings

Slower advancement with smaller volume of enteral feedings have historically been considered modifiable risk factors for NEC, although clearly delaying the time to achieve full enteral feeds. A recent review of 10 RCTs with a total of 3753 infants found no evidence that advancing enteral feed volumes at daily increments of 15 to 20 mL/kg versus 30 to 40 mL/kg reduces the risk of NEC or death in preterm VLBW infants.[126]

Feeding the Preterm Infant After Discharge

The nutrition of preterm infants after discharge has assumed new importance and is of growing concern. Infants are typically discharged weeks before their due dates, and there is an increasing use of human milk for feedings after discharge. The heterogeneity of "relative healthiness" is large, and infants are typically followed after discharge by care providers who were not part of the NICU team and who have variable experience for providing care for VLBW infants after discharge. Even though the rate of intrauterine weight gain may be achieved prior to discharge with intensive dietary management, catch-up growth itself does not occur until later.[18,127,128] Thus, the postdischarge VLBW infant is at high risk of developing significant nutritional deficits.

In general, there is a paucity of data on what to feed the preterm infant after hospital discharge, especially if the goal is to achieve "catch-up" growth. How fast these preterm infants (and especially those born growth restricted) should demonstrate catch-up growth is an area of critical research need, given the potential for increased risk for developing obesity and the consequences later in life from rapid weight gain during this period.[7,127,128] However, the evidence supporting these adverse outcomes is weak, as discussed at the beginning of this chapter. On balance, the evidence that the catch-up growth of the VLBW infant after hospital discharge supports improved neurodevelopmental outcomes is more convincing than the evidence for possible long-term negative effects on metabolic outcomes such as increased adiposity, blood pressure, insulin resistance, and dyslipidemia.[7,127,128]

The preferred milk feeding at discharge is now fortified human milk, although evidence supporting this recommendation is limited and conflicting.[128,129] A recent cross-sectional analysis from Vermont Oxford Network found fewer than half (42%) of all VLBW infants are receiving any human milk by the time of discharge.[130] The high variability in the nutrient content of human milk, as well as the gradual decline in its protein content over time, place exclusively human milk-fed infants at higher risk of nutritional deficiencies.[128,131] Human milk feeding alone at discharge for VLBW infants will typically not provide an adequate amount of calories, protein, minerals, and vitamins without additional fortification and supplementation. The existing data on the need for postdischarge fortification for human milk-fed preterm infants are conflicting and limited.[129,132–134] In one study, infants weighing less than 1800 g were given human milk fortified to 22 kcal/oz with human milk fortifier powder for 12 weeks after discharge. These infants had better growth and bone mineral density at 18 months' corrected age than did controls but did not demonstrate improved short-term neurodevelopmental outcomes.[132,133] In another study with a larger sample size but lower amounts of supplementation until 4 months' corrected age, no differences in growth were noted at 12 months' corrected age.[134] A meta-analysis of 14 studies that included the above studies concluded that these studies provided inconsistent evidence of fortified human milk on longer-term growth and development in preterm infants.[129]

When human milk is not available, a nutrient-enriched formula for preterm infants may be used. However, as with fortification of human milk, evidence supporting this practice is sparse. A recent Cochrane review identified 16 good-quality studies that examined the efficacy of feeding preterm infants after hospital discharge with nutrient-enriched formulas (3 different preparations) compared with a standard formula for term infants.[135] This review concluded that there is moderate quality evidence that unrestricted feeding with nutrient-enriched (vs standard) formula has no important effects on growth and development up to 18 months of age follow-up. There were not enough data to make any assessment of effect on neurodevelopmental outcomes. In interpreting these data, it is noted that preterm infants at the highest nutritional risk were either excluded or underrepresented in this meta-analysis. Eight of the included trials included infants with a birth weight >1500 g.[128]

In conclusion, decisions to fortify human milk should be individualized to optimize the growth trajectory of the infant over the first year of life. Expert opinion has concluded that infants born with birth weight less than 1000 g and discharged before a weight of 2000 g will require fortification of both human milk and infant formula.[128] Consideration should be given to fortification of human milk and use of fortified infant formula for a minimum of 12 weeks after discharge. Current practical strategies for preterm infants who are receiving human milk after discharge include: human milk fortification with powdered postdischarge formula (22–24 kcal/oz); the use of several bottle feedings per day of postdischarge formula for human milk-fed preterm infants; or liquid fortification of human milk with high-calorie formula intended for preterm infants (30 kcal/oz). The powder options for fortification are concerning, given the inability to sterilize these products.

There is little information regarding supplementation of fat-soluble vitamins or iron after hospital discharge. For infants fed human milk, supplements of A, D, and E are readily available as oral solutions. None of these contain vitamin K. The bovine-based human milk fortifiers supply added vitamin D when used after discharge. There is no need to supplement noncholestatic preterm infants with more than 400 IU per day of vitamin D after hospital discharge.[67,128] Supplementing formula-fed infants is more problematic, but in general, if preterm infants are discharged on standard term infant formulas, they may not receive the recommended amounts of these vitamins, as discussed previously, until they reach a weight of 3 kg. Therefore, in the "healthy" preterm infant, it is probably not necessary to supplement with fat-soluble vitamins after attaining a weight of 3 kg, except for vitamin D. On the other hand, formulas designed for preterm infants following discharge from the NICU should supply adequate amounts of fat-soluble vitamins (Appendix D).

There is general agreement that iron supplements to provide up to 2 to 3 mg/kg day of total enteral iron should be provided to VLBW preterm infants after hospital discharge to support their iron needs and sustain normal ferritin concentrations as an indicator of iron stores. Iron supplements should be continued until 6 to 12 months of age, depending on diet.[72,128] Preterm infants fed human milk after discharge will likely need iron supplements until weaned to iron-fortified formula, or appropriate iron-containing complementary foods. It has also been recommended to follow VLBW infants with regular measurements of ferritin to assess iron status (see Chapter 19: Iron). The normal range of ferritin concentrations in VLBW preterm infants is 35 to 300 µg/L. If ferritin concentration is <35 µg/L, the iron dose should be increased. If ferritin concentration is >300 µg/L, commonly seen after red blood cell transfusions, iron fortification should be discontinued.[45]

Preterm infants being discharged home need to be followed closely, with nutritional assessment of growth, iron, vitamin, and mineral status by their primary care physician. This can be facilitated by providing the primary care physician with the inpatient growth chart and a set of nutritional recommendations as part of the medical discharge summary. Reliable, cost-effective measures of body composition and bone mineral density are still not readily available, so routine monitoring of these measures cannot be recommended at this time. For infants receiving human milk, appropriate lactation support should be provided to the mother to promote breastfeeding after discharge.

Conclusion

Nutrition plays a critical role in the optimal health and developmental outcomes of the VLBW preterm infant. The impact of potential malnutrition (growth retardation) associated with extreme prematurity is a significant concern. Because of the potential consequences of inadequate nutrition during the early neonatal period, the goal of feeding the preterm infant is to provide nutritional support to ensure optimal growth and development and to prevent nutrition-related morbidity and mortality. The implementation of early optimized nutrition is targeted at reducing the postnatal growth delays seen in many preterm infants that is typically seen at the time of discharge. Further research to determine the optimal postdischarge nutritional strategy for the VLBW preterm infant is an important goal.

References

1. Ehrenkranz RA. Nutrition, growth and clinical outcomes. *Nutritional Care of Preterm Infants: Scientific Basis and Practical Guidelines*. New York, NY: Karger; 2014:11–26

2. Agostoni C, Buonocore G, Carnielli VP, et al. Enteral Nutrient Supply for Preterm Infants: Commentary From the European Society of Paediatric Gastroenterology, Hepatology and Nutrition Committee on Nutrition. *J Pediatr Gastroenterol Nutr.* 2010;50(1):85–91

3. Horbar JD, Ehrenkranz RA, Badger GJ, et al. Weight growth velocity and postnatal growth failure in infants 501 to 1500 grams: 2000–2013. *Pediatrics.* 2015;136(1):e84–e92

4. Su B-H. Optimizing nutrition in preterm infants. *Pediatr Neonatol.* 2014;55(1):5-13

5. Bertino E, Di Nicola P, Occhi L, Prandi G, Gilli G. Causes of postnatal growth failure in preterm infants. In: Griffin IJ, ed. *Perinatal Growth and Nutrition*. Boca Raton, FL: CRC Press; 2014:41–59

6. Chan SHT, Johnson MJ, Leaf AA, Vollmer B. Nutrition and neurodevelopmental outcomes in preterm infants: a systematic review. *Acta Paediatr.* 2016;105(6): 587–599

7. Cooke RJ, Griffin I. Postnatal growth failure in preterm infants metabolic outcomes. In: Griffin IJ, ed. *Perinatal Growth and Nutrition*. Boca Raton, FL: CRC Press; 2014:149–184

8.   Fenton TR, Kim JH. A systematic review and meta-analysis to revise the Fenton growth chart for preterm infants. *BMC Pediatr.* 2013;13(1):59

9.   Olsen IE, Groveman SA, Lawson ML, Clark RH, Zemel BS. New intrauterine growth curves based on United States data. *Pediatrics.* 2010;125(2):e214–e224

10. Olsen IE, Lawson ML, Ferguson AN, et al. BMI curves for preterm infants. *Pediatrics.* 2015;135(3):e572–e581

11. Demerath EW, Johnson W, Davern BA, et al. New body composition reference charts for preterm infants. *Am J Clin Nutr.* 2016;105(1):70–77

12. Fenton TR, Anderson D, Groh-Wargo S, Hoyos A, Ehrenkranz RA, Senterre T. An attempt to standardize the calculation of growth velocity of preterm infants—evaluation of practical bedside methods. *J Pediatr.* 2018;196:77–83

13. Tsang RC, Lucas A, Uauy R, Zlotkin S, eds. *Nutritional Needs of the Preterm Infant: Scientific Basis and Practical Guidelines.* Philadelphia, PA: Williams & Wilkins; 1993

14. Tsang RC, Uauy R, Koletzko B, Zlotkin S, eds. *Nutrition of the Preterm Infant: Scientific Basis and Practical Guidelines.* Cincinnati, OH: Digital Education Publishing Inc; 2005

15. Koletzko B, Piondexter B, Uauy R, eds. *Nutritional Care of Preterm Infants: Scientific Basis and Practical Guidelines.* New York, NY: Karger; 2014

16. Uauy R, Koletzko B. Defining the nutritional needs of preterm infants. In: Koletzko B, Piondexter B, Uauy R, eds. *Nutritional Care of Preterm Infants: Scientific Basis and Practical Guidelines.* New York, NY: Karger; 2014:4-10

17. Koletzko B, Poindexter B, Uauy R. Recommended nutrient intake levels for stable, fully enterally fed very low birth weight infants. In: Koletzko B, Poindexter B, Uauy R, eds. *Nutritional Care of Preterm Infants: Scientific Basis and Practical Guidelines.* New York, NY: Karger; 2014:297–299

18. Lapillonne A, O'Connor DL, Wang D, Rigo J. Nutritional recommendations for the late-preterm infant and the preterm infant after hospital discharge. *J Pediatr.* 2013;162(3):S90–S100

19. Tudehope D, Vento M, Bhutta Z, Pachi P. Nutritional requirements and feeding recommendations for small for gestational age Infants. *J Pediatr.* 2013;162(3): S81–S89

20. Modi N. Management of fluid balance in the very immature neonate. *Arch Dis Child Fetal Neonat Ed.* 2004;89(2):108F–111F

21. Fusch CH, Jochum F. Water, sodium, potassium and chloride. In: Tsang RC, Uauy R, Koletzko B, Zlotkin SH, eds. *Nutrition of the Preterm Infant: Scientific Basis and Practical Guidelines.* Cincinnati, OH: Digital Educational Publishing; 2005:201–244

22. Bischoff AR, Tomlinson C, Belik J. Sodium intake requirements for preterm neonates. *J Pediatr Gastroenterol Nutr.* 2016;63(6):e123–e129

23. Denne SC. Early nutritional support for extremely premature infants: what amino acid amount should be given? *Am J Clin Nutr.* 2016;103(6):1383–1384

24. Hay WW, Thureen P. Protein for preterm infants: How much is needed? How much is enough? How much is too much? *Pediatr Neonatol.* 2010;51(4):198–207

25. Blanco CL, Gong AK, Green BK, Falck A, Schoolfield J, Liechty EA. Early changes in plasma amino acid concentrations during aggressive nutritional therapy in extremely low birth weight infants. *J Pediatr.* 2011;158(4):543–548.e541

26. Van Goudoever JB, Colen T, Wattimena JLD, Huijmans JGM, Carnielli VP, Sauer PJJ. Immediate commencement of amino acid supplementation in preterm infants: Effect on serum amino acid concentrations and protein kinetics on the first day of life. *J Pediatr.* 1995;127(3):458–465

27. Thureen PJ, Melara D, Fennessey PV, Hay WW. Effect of low versus high intravenous amino acid intake on very low birth weight infants in the early neonatal period. *Pediatr Res.* 2003;53(1):24–32

28. Uthaya S, Liu X, Babalis D, et al. Nutritional evaluation and optimisation in neonates: a randomized, double-blind controlled trial of amino acid regimen and intravenous lipid composition in preterm parenteral nutrition. *Am J Clin Nutr.* 2016;103(6):1443–1452

29. Balakrishnan M, Jennings A, Przystac L, et al. Growth and neurodevelopmental outcomes of early, high-dose parenteral amino acid intake in very low birth weight infants. *J Parent Enteral Nutr.* 2017:014860711769633

30. Trivedi A, Sinn JK. Early versus late administration of amino acids in preterm infants receiving parenteral nutrition. *Cochrane Database Syst Rev.* 2013;(7):CD008771

31. Leenders EKSM, de Waard M, van Goudoever JB. low- versus high-dose and early versus late parenteral amino-acid administration in very-low-birth-weight infants: a systematic review and meta-analysis. *Neonatology.* 2017;113(3):187–205

32. Thureen PJ, Hay WW. Nutritional requirements of the very-low birth weight infant. In: Neu J, Polin RA, eds. *Gastroenterology and Nutrition: Neonatology Questions and Controversies.* 2nd ed. Philadelphia, PA: Elsevier Saunders; 2012:107–128

33. Hay WW, Brown LD, Denne SC. Energy requirements, protein-energy metablolism and balances, and carbohydrates in preterm infants. In: Koletzko B, Piondexter B, Uauy R, eds. *Nutritional Care of Preterm Infants: Scientific Basis and Practical Guidelines.* New York, NY: Karger; 2014:64–81

34. Beardsall K, Vanhaesebrouck S, Ogilvy-Stuart AL, et al. Early insulin therapy in very-low-birth-weight infants. *N Engl J Med.* 2008;359(18):1873–1884

35. Koletzko B, Goulet O, Hunt J, Krohn K, Shamir R. Guidelines on Paediatric Parenteral Nutrition of the European Society of Paediatric Gastroenterology, Hepatology and Nutrition (ESPGHAN) and the European Society for Clinical Nutrition and Metabolism (ESPEN), Supported by the European Society of Paediatric Research (ESPR). *J Pediatr Gastroenterol Nutr.* 2005;41(Supplement 2): S1-S87

36. Choi Y-j, Bae H-j, Lee J-Y, et al. Analysis of risk factors for lipid intolerance of intravenous fat emulsion in very low birth weight infants. *Arch Pharmacol Res.* 2014;38(5):914–920

37. Lapillone A. Enteral and parenteral lipid requirements of preterm infants. In: Koletzko B, Poindexter B, Uauy R, eds. *Nutritional Care of Preterm Infants: Scientific Basis and Practical Guidelines*. New York, NY: Karger; 2014:82–98

38. Vlaardingerbroek H, Vermeulen MJ, Rook D, et al. Safety and efficacy of early parenteral lipid and high-dose amino acid administration to very low birth weight infants. *J Pediatr*. 2013;163(3):638–644.e635

39. Cairns PA, Stalker DJ. Carnitine supplementation of parenterally fed neonates. *Cochrane Database Syst Rev*. 2000(4):CD000950

40. Salvador A, Janeczko M, Porat R, Sekhon R, Moewes A, Schutzman D. Randomized controlled trial of early parenteral nutrition cycling to prevent cholestasis in very low birth weight infants. *J Pediatr*. 2012;161(2):229–233.e221

41. Diamond IR, Grant RC, Pencharz PB, et al. Preventing the progression of intestinal failure-associated liver disease in infants using a composite lipid emulsion: a pilot randomized controlled trial of SMOFlipid. *J Parent Enteral Nutr*. 2016;41(5):866–877

42. Atkinson S, Tsang RC. Calcium, magnesium, phosphorus, and vitamin D. In: Tsang RC, Uauy R, Koletzko B, Zlotkin SH, eds. *Nutrition of the Preterm Infant: Scientific Basis and Practical Guidelines*. Cincinnati, OH: Digital Education Publishing Inc; 2005:135–155

43. Greer F. Controversies in neonatal nutrition: macronutrinet and micronutrients. In: Neu J, Polin RA, eds. *Gastroenterology and Nutrition: Neonatology Questions and Controversies*. 2nd ed. Philadelphia, PA: Elsevier Saunders; 2012:129–155

44. Rao R, Georgieff MK. Microminerals. In: Tsang RC, Uauy R, Koletzko B, Zlotkin SH, eds. *Nutrition of the Preterm Infant: Scientific Basis and Practical Guidelines*. Cincinnati, OH: Digital Educational Publishing Inc; 2005:277–310

45. Domellof M. Nutritional care of premature infants: microminerals. In: Koletzko B, Poindexter B, Uauy R, eds. *Nutritional Care of Preterm Infants: Scientific Basis and Practical Guidelines*. New York, NY: Karger; 2014:121–139

46. Greer FR. Vitamins A, E, and K. In: Tsang RC UR, Koletzko B, Zlotkin SH, ed. *Nutrition of the Preterm Infant: Scienific Basis and Practical Guidelines*. Cincinnati, OH: Digital Educational Publishing Inc; 2005:141–172

47. Schanler RJ. Water soluble vitamins. In: Tsang RC, Uauy R, Koletzko B, Zlotkin SH, eds. *Nutrition of the Preterm Infant: Scientific Basis and Practical Guidelines*. Cincinnati, OH: Digital Educational Publishing Inc; 2005:173–200

48. Embleton ND, Simmer K. Practice of parenteral nutrition in VLBW and ELBW infants. In: Koletzko B, Poindexter B, Uauy R, eds. *Nutritional Care of Preterm Infants: Scientific Basis and Practical Guidelines*. New York, NY: Karger; 2014:177–189

49. Goudoever J, Vlaardingerbroek H, van den Akker CH, de Groof F, van der Schoor SRD. Amino acids and proteins. In: Koletzko B, Poindexter B, Uauy R, eds. *Nutritional Care of Preterm Infants: Scientific Basis and Practical Guidelines*. New York, NY: Karger; 2014:49–63

50. Morley R, Lucas A. Influence of early diet on outcome in preterm infants. *Acta Paediatr*. 1994;83(S405):123–126

51. European Society for Paediatric Gastroenterology Hepatology and Nutrition, Committee on Nutrition. Nutrition and Feeding of Preterm Infants. Oxford, England: Blackwell Scientific Publications; 1987

52. Bauer J, Werner C, Gerss J. Metabolic rate analysis of healthy preterm and full-term infants during the first weeks of life. *Am J Clin Nutr.* 2009;90(6):1517–1524

53. Daly SE, Di Rosso A, Owens RA, Hartmann PE. Degree of breast emptying explains changes in the fat content, but not fatty acid composition, of human milk. *Experimental Physiology.* 1993;78(6):741–755

54. Lubetzky R, Littner Y, Mimouni FB, Dollberg S, Mandel D. Circadian variations in fat content of expressed breast milk from mothers of preterm infants. *J Am Coll Nutr.* 2006;25(2):151–154

55. Shenai JP, Jhaveri BM, Reynolds JW, Huston RK, Babson SG. Nutritional balance studies in very-low-birth-weight infants: role of soy formula. *Pediatrics.* 1981;67(5):631–637

56. Lindquist S, Hernell O. Lipid digestion and absorption in early life: an update. *Curr Opin Clin Nutr Metab Care.* 2010;13(3):314–320

57. Sauerwald TU, Hachey DL, Jensen CL, Chen H, Anderson RE, Heird WC. Intermediates in endogenous synthesis of C22:6ω3 and C20:4ω6 by term and preterm infants. *Pediatr Res.* 1997;41(2):183–187

58. Moon K, Rao SC, Schulzke SM, Patole SK, Simmer K. Longchain polyunsaturated fatty acid supplementation in preterm infants. *Cochrane Database Syst Rev.* 2016;(12):CD000375

59. Smithers LG, Gibson RA, McPhee A, Makrides M. Effect of long-chain polyunsaturated fatty acid supplementation of preterm infants on disease risk and neurodevelopment: a systematic review of randomized controlled trials. *Am J Clin Nutr.* 2008;87(4):912–920

60. Henriksen C, Haugholt K, Lindgren M, et al. Improved cognitive development among preterm infants attributable to early supplementation of human milk with docosahexaenoic acid and arachidonic acid. *Pediatrics.* 2008;121(6):1137–1145

61. Makrides M, Gibson RA, McPhee AJ, et al. Neurodevelopmental outcomes of preterm infants fed high-dose docosahexaenoic acid. *JAMA.* 2009;301(2):175

62. Collins CT, Gibson RA, Anderson PJ, et al. Neurodevelopmental outcomes at 7 years' corrected age in preterm infants who were fed high-dose docosahexaenoic acid to term equivalent: a follow-up of a randomised controlled trial. *BMJ Open.* 2015;5(3):e007314–e007314

63. Parimi P, Kalhan SC. Carbohydrates including oligosaccharides and inositol. In: Tsang RC, Uauy R, Koletzko B, Zlotkin SH, eds. *Nutrition of the Preterm Infant: Scientific Basis and Practical Guidelines.* Cincinnati, OH: Digital Educational Publishing Inc; 2005:81–96

64. Wirth FH, Numerof B, Pleban P, Neylan MJ. Effect of lactose on mineral absorption in preterm infants. *J Pediatr.* 1990;117(2):283–287

65. Boehm G, Stahl B, Jelinek J, Knol J, Miniello V, Moro G. Prebiotic carbohydrates in human milk and formulas. *Acta Paediatr.* 2005;94(0):18–21

66. Marriage BJ, Buck RH, Goehring KC, Oliver JS, Williams JA. Infants fed a lower calorie formula with 2'FL show growth and 2'FL uptake like breast-fed infants. *J Pediatr Gastroenterol Nutr.* 2015;61(6):649–658

67. Abrams SA, American Academy of Pediatrics, Committee on Nutrition. Calcium and vitamin D requirements of enterally fed preterm infants. *Pediatrics.* 2013;131(5):e1676–e1683

68. Mimouni FB, Mandel D, Lubetzky R, Senterre T. Calcium, phosphorus, and magesium and vitamin D requirements of the preterm infant. In: Koletzko B, Poindexter B, Uauy R, eds. *Nutritional Care of Preterm Infants: Scientific Basis and Practical Guidelines.* New York, NY: Karger; 2014:140–151

69. Mukhopadhyay K, Yadav RK, Kishore SS, Garewal G, Jain V, Narang A. Iron status at birth and at 4 weeks in preterm-SGA infants in comparison with preterm and term-AGA infants. *J Matern Fetal Neonat Med.* 2012;25(8):1474–1478

70. Ohlsson A, Aher SM. Early erythropoiesis-stimulating agents in preterm or low birth weight infants. *Cochrane Database Syst Rev.* 2017(11):CD004863

71. Backes CH, Rivera BK, Haque U, et al. Placental transfusion strategies in very preterm neonates. *Obstet Gynecol.* 2014;124(1):47–56

72. Baker RD, Greer FR. Diagnosis and prevention of iron deficiency and iron-deficiency anemia in infants and young children (0-3 years of age). *Pediatrics.* 2010;126(5):1040–1050

73. Terrin G, Berni Canani R, Di Chiara M, et al. Zinc in early life: a key element in the fetus and preterm neonate. *Nutrients.* 2015;7(12):10427–10446

74. Klein CJ. Nutrient requirements for preterm infant formulas. *J Nutr.* 2002;132(6):1395S-1577S

75. Bhatia J, Griffin I, Anderson D, Kler N, Domellöf M. Selected macro/micronutrient needs of the routine preterm infant. *J Pediatr.* 2013;162(3):S48–S55

76. Casey CE, Neville MC, Hambidge KM. Studies in human lactation: secretion of zinc, copper, and manganese in human milk. *Am J Clin Nutr.* 1989;49(5):773–785

77. Ehrenkranz RA, Gettner PA, Nelli CM, et al. Zinc and copper nutritional studies in very low birth weight infants: comparison of stable isotopic extrinsic tag and chemical balance methods. *Pediatr Res.* 1989;26(4):298–307

78. Belfort MB, Pearce EN, Braverman LE, He X, Brown RS. Low iodine content in the diets of hospitalized preterm infants. *J Clin Endocrinol Metab.* 2012;97(4):E632–E636

79. Ibrahim M, Sinn J, McGuire W. Iodine supplementation for the prevention of mortality and adverse neurodevelopmental outcomes in preterm infants. *Cochrane Database Syst Rev.* 2006(2):CD005253

80. Leaf A, Landsowne Z. Vitamins - conventional uses and new insights. In: Koletzko B, Poindexter B, Uauy R, eds. *Nutritional Care of Preterm Infants: Scientific Basis and Practical Guidelines.* New York, NY: Karger:152–166

81. Darlow BA. Vitamin C supplementation in very preterm infants: a randomised controlled trial. *Arch Dis Child Fetal Neonat Ed.* 2005;90(2):F117–F122

82. Tokuriki S, Hayashi H, Okuno T, et al. Biotin and carnitine profiles in preterm infants in Japan. *Pediatr Int.* 2013;55(3):342–345

83. Darlow BA, Graham PJ. Vitamin A supplementation for preventing morbidity and mortality in very low birthweight infants. *Cochrane Database Syst Rev.* 2002(4):CD000501

84. Tyson JE, Wright LL, Oh W, et al. Vitamin A supplementation for extremely-low-birth-weight infants. National Institute of Child Health and Human Development Neonatal Research Network. *N Engl J Med.* 1999;340(25):1962–1968

85. Salle BL, Delvin E, Claris O, Hascoet JM, Levy E. Est-il légitime d'administrer des vitamines liposolubles (A, E et D) chez le prématuré pendant 6 mois? *Archives de Pédiatrie.* 2007;14(12):1408–1412

86. Brion LP, Bell EF, Raghuveer TS. Vitamin E supplementation for prevention of morbidity and mortality in preterm infants. *Cochrane Database Syst Rev.* 2003(4):CD003665

87. Brannon PM, Picciano MF. Vitamin D in pregnancy and lactation in humans. *Ann Rev Nutr.* 2011;31(1):89–115

88. Nassar N, Halligan GH, Roberts CL, Morris JM, Ashton AW. Systematic review of first-trimester vitamin D normative levels and outcomes of pregnancy. *Am J Obstet Gynecol.* 2011;205(3):208.e201–208.e207

89. Burris HH, Van Marter LJ, McElrath TF, et al. Vitamin D status among preterm and full-term infants at birth. *Pediatr Res.* 2013;75(1):75–80

90. Cooke R, Hollis B, Conner C, Watson D, Werkman S, Chesney R. Vitamin D and mineral metabolism in the very low birth weight infant receiving 400 IU of vitamin D. *J Pediatr.* 1990;116(3):423–428

91. Greer FR. Vitamin K the basics—What's new? *Early Hum Dev.* 2010;86(1):43–47

92. Clarke P. Vitamin K prophylaxis for preterm infants. *Early Human Development.* 2010/07 2010;86(1):17–20

93. Clarke P, Mitchell SJ, Wynn R, et al. Vitamin K prophylaxis for preterm infants: a randomized, controlled trial of 3 regimens. *Pediatrics.* 2006;118(6):e1657–e1666

94. Schanler RJ. Randomized trial of donor human milk versus preterm formula as substitutes for mothers' own milk in the feeding of extremely premature infants. *Pediatrics.* 2005;116(2):400–406

95. Atkinson SA. Effects of gestational age at delivery on human milk components. In: Jensen RG, ed. *Handbook of Milk Composition.* San Diego, CA: Academic Press; 1995:222–237

96. Senterre T. Practice of enteral nutrition in very low birth weight and extremely low birth weight infants. In: Koletzko B, Poindexter B, Uauy R, eds. *Nutritional Care of Preterm Infants: Scientific Basis and Practical Guidelines.* New York, NY: Karger; 2014:201–214

97. Ziegler EE. Human milk and human milk fortifiers. In: Koletzko B, Poindexter B, Uauy R, eds. *Nutritional Care of Preterm Infants: Scientific Basis and Practical Guidelines.* New York, NY: Karger; 2014:215–227

98. Kim JH, Chan G, Schanler R, et al. Growth and tolerance of preterm infants fed a new extensively hydrolyzed liquid human milk fortifier. *J Pediatr Gastroenterol Nutr.* 2015;61(6):665–671

99. Moya F, Sisk PM, Walsh KR, Berseth CL. A new liquid human milk fortifier and linear growth in preterm infants. *Pediatrics.* 2012;130(4):e928–e935

100. Neu J. Necrotizing enterocolitis. In: Koletzko B, Poindexter B, Uauy R, eds. *Nutritional Care of Preterm Infants: Scientific Basis and Practical Guidelines.* New York, NY: Karger; 2014:253–263

101. Quigley M, McGuire W. Formula versus donor breast milk for feeding preterm or low birth weight infants. *Cochrane Database Syst Rev.* 2014(4):CD002971

102. Meinzen-Derr J, Poindexter B, Wrage L, Morrow AL, Stoll B, Donovan EF. Role of human milk in extremely low birth weight infants' risk of necrotizing enterocolitis or death. *J Perinatol.* 2008;29(1):57–62

103. Sullivan S, Schanler RJ, Kim JH, et al. An exclusively human milk-based diet is associated with a lower rate of necrotizing enterocolitis than a diet of human milk and bovine milk-based products. *J Pediatr.* 2010;156(4):562–567.e561

104. Jacobi-Polishook T, Collins CT, Sullivan TR, et al. Human milk intake in preterm infants and neurodevelopment at 18 months corrected age. *Pediatr Res.* 2016;80(4):486–492

105. Jones F. *Best Practice for Expressing, Storing and Handling Human Milk in Hospitals, Homes, and Child Care Settings.* 3rd ed. Fort Worth, TX: Human Milk Banking Association of North America; 2011

106. Slutzah M, Codipilly CN, Potak D, Clark RM, Schanler RJ. Refrigerator storage of expressed human milk in the neonatal intensive care unit. *J Pediatr.* 2010;156(1):26–28

107. Human Milk Banking Association of North America. *Guidelines for the Establishment and Operation of a Donor Human Milk Bank.* Forth Worth, TX: Human Milk Banking Association of North America; 1994

108. American Academy of Pediatrics, Section on Breastfeeding, Committee on Fetus and Newborn. Donor human milk for the high-risk infant: preparation, safety, and usage options in the United States. *Pediatrics.* 2017;139(1):e20163440

109. O'Connor DL, Gibbins S, Kiss A, et al. Effect of supplemental donor human milk compared with preterm formula on neurodevelopment of very low-birth-weight infants at 18 months. *JAMA.* 2016;316(18):1897–1905

110. Yu VYH, Simmer K. Enteral nutrition: practical aspects, strategy, and management. In: Tsang RC, Uauy R, Koletzko B, Zlotkin SH, eds. *Nutrition of the Preterm Infant: Scientific Basis and Practical Guidelines.* Cincinnati, OH: Digital Educational Publishing Inc; 2005:311–322

111. Taylor C. Health professionals letter on *Enterobacter sakazakii* infections associated with the use of powdered (dry) infant formulas in neonatal intensive care units. Silver Spring, MD: US Food and Drug Administration, Center for Food Safety and Applied Nutrition, Office of Nutritional Products, Labeling and Dietary Supplements; 2002

112. World Health Organization. *Enterobacter sakazakii and other microorganisms in powdered infant formula. Meeting report.* Geneva, Switzerland: World Health Organization; 2004

113. Al Faleh K, Anabrees J, Bassler D, Al-Kharfi T. Probiotics for prevention of necrotizing enterocolitis in preterm infants. *Cochrane Database Syst Rev.* 2014(4): CD005496

114. Athalye-Jape G, Deshpande G, Rao S, Patole S. Benefits of probiotics on enteral nutrition in preterm neonates: a systematic review. *Am J Clin Nutr.* 2014;100(6): 1508–1519

115. Szajewska H, van Goudoever JB. To give or not to give probiotics to preterm infants. *Am J Clin Nutr.* 2014;100(6):1411–1412

116. McCallie KR, Lee HC, Mayer O, Cohen RS, Hintz SR, Rhine WD. Improved outcomes with a standardized feeding protocol for very low birth weight infants. *J Perinatol.* 2011;31(S1):S61–S67

117. Dutta S, Singh B, Chessell L, et al. Guidelines for feeding very low birth weight infants. *Nutrients.* 2015;7(1):423–442

118. Lee J, Kim HS, Jung YH, et al. Oropharyngeal colostrum administration in extremely premature infants: an RCT. *Pediatrics.* 2015;135(2):e357–e366

119. Sohn K, Kalanetra KM, Mills DA, Underwood MA. Buccal administration of human colostrum: impact on the oral microbiota of premature infants. *J Perinatol.* 2015;36(2):106–111

120. Morgan J, Bombell S, McGuire W. Early trophic feeding versus enteral fasting for very preterm or very low birth weight infants. *Cochrane Database Syst Rev.* 2013(3):CD000504

121. Watson J, McGuire W. Nasal versus oral route for placing feeding tubes in preterm or low birth weight infants. *Cochrane Database Syst Rev.* 2013(3): CD003952

122. Premji SS, Chessell L. Continuous nasogastric milk feeding versus intermittent bolus milk feeding for premature infants less than 1500 grams. *Cochrane Database Syst Rev.* 2011(2):CD001819

123. Bhatia J. Human milk supplementation. *Am J Dis Child.* 1988;142(4):445

124. Greer FR, McCormick A, Loker J. Changes in fat concentration of human milk during delivery by intermittent bolus and continuous mechanical pump infusion. *J Pediatr.* 1984;105(5):745–749

125. McGuire W, McEwan P. Transpyloric versus gastric tube feeding for preterm infants. *Cochrane Database Syst Rev.* 2002(3):CD003487

126. Oddie SJ, Young L, McGuire W. Slow advancement of enteral feed volumes to prevent necrotising enterocolitis in very low birth weight infants. *Cochrane Database Syst Rev.* 2017(7):CD001241

127. Lapillonne A, Griffin IJ. Feeding preterm infants today for later metabolic and cardiovascular outcomes. *J Pediatr.* 2013;162(3):S7-S16

128. Lapillonne A. Feeding the preterm infant after discharge. In: Koletzko B, Poindexter B, Uauy R, eds. *Nutritional Care of Preterm infants. Scientific basis and Practical Guidelines.* New York, NY: Karger; 2014:264–277

129. Brown JVE, Embleton ND, Harding JE, McGuire W. Multi-nutrient fortification of human milk for preterm infants. *Cochrane Database Syst Rev.* 2016(3):CD000343

130. Hallowell SG, Rogowski JA, Spatz DL, Hanlon AL, Kenny M, Lake ET. Factors associated with infant feeding of human milk at discharge from neonatal intensive care: Cross-sectional analysis of nurse survey and infant outcomes data. *Int J Nurs Stud.* 2016;53:190–203

131. Saarela T, Kokkonen J, Koivisto M. Macronutrient and energy contents of human milk fractions during the first six months of lactation. *Acta Paediatr.* 2007;94(9):1176–1181

132. O'Connor DL, Khan S, Weishuhn K, et al. Growth and nutrient intakes of human milk-fed preterm infants provided with extra energy and nutrients after hospital discharge. *Pediatrics.* 2008;121(4):766–776

133. Aimone A, Rovet J, Ward W, et al. Growth and body composition of human milk–fed premature infants provided with extra energy and nutrients early after hospital discharge: 1-year follow-up. *J Pediatr Gastroenterol Nutr.* 2009;49(4):456–466

134. Zachariassen G, Faerk J, Grytter C, et al. Nutrient enrichment of mother's milk and growth of very preterm infants after hospital discharge. *Pediatrics.* 2011;127(4):e995–e1003

135. Young L, Embleton ND, McGuire W. Nutrient-enriched formula versus standard formula for preterm infants following hospital discharge. *Cochrane Database Syst Rev.* 2016(5):CD004696

136. Klein CJ, Heird WC. *Summary and Comparison of Recommendations for Nutrient Contents in Low-Birth-Weight Infant Formulas.* Princeton, NJ: Life Sciences Research Office; 2005

Chapter 6

Complementary Feeding

Introduction

The importance of complementary feeding has received tremendous recognition in international nutrition circles because of the well-established risk of infectious diseases and malnutrition with premature introduction of complementary food and nonexclusive breastfeeding during early infancy. For older infants, inadequate complementary feeding, either because of delayed introduction and/or reliance on poor-quality foods, is cited as a major cause of preventable mortality in young children.[1,2]

In industrialized nations, however, the high prevalence of nonexclusive breastfeeding and formula feeding as well as the availability of relatively inexpensive, hygienically prepared commercial foods in a wide array of choices designed specifically for infants, has largely mitigated concerns about micronutrient deficiencies, with the possible exception of iron. Rather, the increasing prevalence of overweight and obesity in young children has directed attention to the potential for excessive caloric intake from complementary foods.[3] Such a narrow focus, however, belies the complexity of the nutritional and developmental progression that underlies the complementary feeding process. Despite this importance, remarkably limited data are available for determining "best practices." Rather, much of the advice provided on complementary feeding is based on traditions rather than evidence. This chapter will review biological, nutritional, developmental, and behavioral issues related to successful complementary feeding for the typically developing, healthy older infant and toddler.

Definitions

Complementary foods and beverages refer to nutrient- and energy-containing solid or semi-solid foods or liquids fed to infants in addition to human milk or formula. Importantly, the choice of complementary foods ideally "complements" the nutritional gaps that develop as a result of the dynamic nutritional composition of human milk and the dynamic nutritional needs of the infant. Generally, the progression from the fully liquid diet of the young infant to the mixed diet of "family foods" occurs from mid-way through the first year of life through the second year—that is, approximately 6 to 24 months of age.

Nutritional Considerations

The most important factor affecting an infant's dependence on complementary food choices to meet nutritional requirements is whether he or she has been exclusively breastfed or formula fed (or if mixed, the relative balance between human milk and formula). For simplicity, the following discussion, after first addressing energy and macronutrient needs, will address human milk compared with formula feeding but will not specifically address so-called "mixed feeding," which is very common[4,5] and clearly influences nutritional intake and nutrient utilization. The following subsections discuss general considerations for energy and nutritional requirements of older infants and toddlers up to 24 months of age.

Energy Requirements

Over the first year of life, energy requirements relative to body weight gradually decrease, whereas total calorie needs increase as physical size and activity increase. The proportion of energy required to support growth also steadily decreases, from 25% to 30% between birth and 4 months of age to approximately 5% by the end of the first year[6] (Fig 6.1). Estimated daily energy requirements for infants and toddlers are presented in Table 6.1.[6]

For breastfed infants, the volume of milk intake typically decreases over the first year of life after complementary foods are introduced, in both

Fig 6.1.

Allocation of energy expenditure during the first year of life.[6]

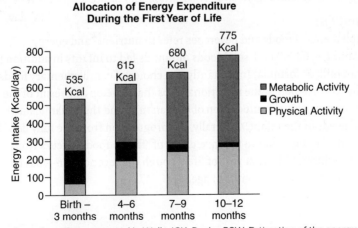

Figure drawn from data presented in Wells JCK, Davies PSW. Estimation of the energy cost of physical activity in infancy. *Arch Dis Child.* 1998;78:131–136, and in Butte et al.[63]

Table 6.1.
Total Energy Requirements in Infants and Toddlers

Age	Energy Requirement (kcal/day) for Boys	Energy Requirement (kcal/day) for Girls
3 mo	535 ± 105	530 ± 100
6 mo	630 ± 110	615 ± 110
9 mo	750 ± 110	680 ± 100
12 mo	830 ± 170	775 ± 125
18 mo	950 ± 115	855 ± 170
24 mo	1000 ± 150	990 ± 170

Adapted from Butte, et al[63]; figures rounded to nearest 5 kcal.

developing and industrialized countries, with the extent being influenced by the availability and intake of calories from other sources. Ideally, the total caloric intake to support normal growth will reflect a decrease in the human milk/formula component as intake of complementary foods increases. According to estimates derived from direct measurements of energy expenditure along with careful growth and body composition measurements, the average total energy requirements for the intervals 6 through 8, 9 through 11, and 12 to 24 months of age are approximately 615, 685, and 895 kcal/day, respectively.[6] Considering the average energy transferred from human milk at each of these age intervals, the average estimated energy intake required from complementary foods is approximately 200, 300, and 550 kcal/day, respectively.[6] A recent small trial reported energy intakes of 9- to 10-month-old breastfed infants that were very similar to these figures. Despite markedly different macronutrient distribution and caloric intake from the complementary foods, the infants adjusted their intakes of human milk and complementary foods to achieve very similar average daily energy intake.[7]

For bottle-fed infants, typically receiving infant formula (or increasingly, expressed human milk), for whom there is more propensity to overfeed, the volume of formula should, likewise, decrease as intake of complementary foods increases.[8,9] However, data from national surveys, including both the Feeding Infants and Toddlers Study (FITS) and National Health and Nutrition Examination Survey (NHANES), indicate that formula-fed infants tend to have total daily energy intakes 20% to 30% greater than the estimated energy requirement of an infant of average weight.[10,11]

Although estimates of caloric needs of infants and young children are useful for programmatic planning and for feeding under controlled conditions (eg, in the hospital or with nutrition support), for a healthy individual child, energy requirements are impossible to gauge precisely. Determining energy requirements is difficult because of the virtual impossibility of accurately estimating calorie requirements for physical activity and for basal metabolic activity, which is influenced by body composition. The daily energy requirements noted previously are, thus, best considered "first approximation" estimates. Therefore, recommendations for specific calorie goals to parents or care providers can be misleading and may result in undue focus on a "number" instead of on healthy/appropriate eating patterns. More appropriately, parents should be encouraged to be guided by an infant or child's hunger cues—that is, follow responsive feeding practices. Ultimately, an infant or toddler's growth should guide energy intake recommendations. For infants gaining weight too rapidly, an emphasis on foods with low caloric density, such as selected vegetables and fruits, is appropriate in combination with other nutrient rich foods. For infants with evidence of faltering weight gain, nutrient-rich foods with higher caloric density, such as those with higher fat and protein content, should be encouraged.[12,13] Careful investigations of the effect of energy density and frequency of feeding have demonstrated that for any frequency of feeding, a higher energy density of complementary foods results in higher total energy intake.[12] Inappropriately rapid or slow weight gain should be explored and addressed in the context of food choices, feeding behaviors, and activity patterns, not by specific calorie intake goals.

Macronutrient Recommendations

Protein

As with energy, protein requirements relative to body weight decrease with age but increase in absolute amounts. The Adequate Intake for infants 0 through 6 months of age is 1.52 g protein/kg/day, and the Recommended Dietary Allowances (RDAs) are 1.2 and 1.05 g/kg/day for children 7 to 12 months and 1 to 3 years, respectively.[14] Additionally, by 6 months of age, the average requirement for protein per kg is about two thirds that for a newborn infant.[15] The concentration of protein in human milk decreases modestly but steadily over the course of lactation.[16] By late infancy, typical protein intakes from human milk alone will be marginally adequate and reflect a moderate dependence on complementary foods to meet the total requirement. For example, an average-weight, 8-month-old breastfed infant weighing 8 kg and consuming 700 mL of human milk (a generous estimate, providing approximately 60 kcal/kg) would receive approximately 6.3 g/day or 0.8 g/kg/day of protein. The quality of protein in human milk is maintained independently of maternal diet. In contrast to breastfed infants, a formula-fed infant weighing 8 kg consuming a similar amount of formula would receive approximately 1.3 g of protein/kg/day. Intake data from NHANES indicated mean total intakes of 2.4 and 4.1 g protein/kg/day for 6- through 11-month-old and 12- through 23-month-old infants and toddlers, respectively.[11] For reference, the estimated average requirements are 1 and 0.87 g protein/kg/day for these respective age intervals.[14] High protein intakes, both from infant formula and from complementary foods, have been identified as a potential risk factor for excessive infant weight gain, and recommendations have been proposed to limit total protein intake to a maximum of 15% of energy intake,[17] although experimental data on the long-term effect of such guidance is limited. Quality, as well as quantity, of protein (eg, meat vs dairy vs vegetable) may also be important, but specific recommendations are not yet warranted.

Fat

Lipids contribute approximately 45% to 50% of the calories in human milk, infant formulas, and whole cow milk. Notably, plant-based so-called "milks" (eg, soy, almond, rice, hemp) tend to be lower in fat and, hence, in calories compared with animal milks and formulas. In contrast to protein, the fatty acid composition of human milk does reflect maternal intake (see Chapter 3, Breastfeeding, and Appendix A). Fats from "milk" products are an important source of concentrated calories to maintain normal growth in older infants and young children. As complementary foods gradually provide a larger percentage of energy intake, they should ideally include sources of "healthy" mono- and polyunsaturated fatty acids, including the long-chain polyunsaturated fatty acids. Recommendations for fat intake for young children are approximately 30% to 40% of daily energy.[14] As noted later in this chapter, the traditional and current emphasis on cereals, vegetables, and fruits results in fat intakes that may be unnecessarily and potentially undesirably low. Data from a survey of US infants and children reported that approximately 28% of 12- through 23-month-olds have fat intakes less than recommended.[11] This has been reinforced by the most recent FITS report, which also indicated that approximately one third of 12- through 48-month-olds had lower-than-recommended intakes of total fats, although saturated fat intake exceeded recommendations for a majority of young children.[18]

However, diets containing less than 30% of calories from fat for older infants and toddlers have been shown to be safe in terms of growth and development,[19] unless total energy intake is suboptimal reflected by underweight and growth faltering, in which case increasing the fat intake of the diet is an efficient and effective intervention.

Carbohydrate

As complementary foods provide increasing amounts of calories and nutrients in the diet, carbohydrates become the major source of energy, providing 45% to 65% of total calorie intake. This is in contrast to the young infant's diet, in which approximately 40% of calories in human milk (or formula) are provided by carbohydrate as lactose. Similar to recommendations for older children and adults, the recommendations for type of carbohydrate in complementary foods emphasize complex, unrefined sources over simple added sugars. Consumption of sugar-sweetened beverages during the first year of life have been reported to be associated with higher rates of childhood obesity, although isolating this factor from other potentially contributory obesogenic behaviors was not possible.[20]

Micronutrient Requirements

Because of the fortification of all standard infant formulas with virtually all essential micronutrients, the risk of micronutrient deficiencies in formula-fed infants is very low. After 12 months of age, when most healthy infants are no longer consuming formula, the risk of certain micronutrient deficiencies gradually increases if the diet is restricted to a few foods. However, 2009–2012 data from the NHANES indicated that the average intakes of most micronutrients, including antioxidants and B vitamins, were adequate for children 6 through 23 months of age.[11]

For breastfed infants, assuming maternal diet is adequate and unrestricted, the gap between typical intake from human milk and the micronutrient requirement is highest for the micronutrients iron, zinc, and vitamin D.[13] In practice, iron and zinc are defined as "problem nutrients" because of the great discrepancy between their content in human milk and traditional complementary foods and the estimated daily requirements.[13,21] These gaps in intakes must be made up from complementary foods (or dietary supplements). As for vitamin D, because human milk, like most complementary foods, contains small amounts, vitamin D supplements or fortified products such as cow milk are the principal means to meet requirements from diet (see Chapter 21.I: Fat-Soluble Vitamins).

Iron (see also Chapter: 19 Iron)

As noted previously, infant formula is fortified with iron (12 mg/L in the United States). However, human milk is distinctly low in iron.[16] Although the relatively favorable bioavailability enhances its absorption, the low iron concentration means that the contribution of human milk to infants' iron needs is very modest. Maternal iron status has no effect on milk iron concentrations, although it affects fetal iron accretion. In general, healthy term infants are born with approximately 75 mg/kg of total body iron. As discussed in Chapter 19 (see Table 19.2), the breastfed infant's need for iron from complementary foods is dictated by gestational age (iron stores are acquired during the third trimester), complications of pregnancy (eg, infants of mothers with diabetes or maternal obesity, infants born small or large for gestational age, or those who have experienced intrauterine growth restriction or have decreased iron stores), whether or not there is delayed or immediate umbilical cord clamping, postnatal growth rate, and duration of exclusive breastfeeding. The healthy term infant who is exclusively breastfed will need an alternate iron source to support erythropoiesis and normal brain development between 4 and 6 months of age. The risk of iron deficiency and iron-deficiency anemia increases progressively the longer complementary foods or other sources of iron, such as supplements, are delayed beyond 6 months.[22] This concept is supported by a large cross-sectional study in Canada that found an association between increasing breastfeeding duration and lower serum ferritin concentration.[23] Limited information about complementary feeding was included, but associations with lower serum ferritin concentration were found with higher volume of cow milk consumption as well as younger age (<2 years) and higher birth weight. The American Academy of Pediatrics (AAP) recommends that exclusively breastfed infants, beginning at 4 months of age, receive 1 mg iron/kg/day until iron-rich foods are consumed.[22]

The common practice of introducing infant cereals as a first complementary food is based on the recognized need for iron; essentially all commercial infant cereals in the United States are iron fortified. Accounting for the low bioavailability of the electrolytic iron fortificant, 1 to 2 servings per day are recommended to meet iron requirements. Indeed, the RDA of 11 mg/day for infants 7 to 12 months of age is based on the assumption that most iron consumed by the older infant will be from cereal and, thus, will be poorly absorbed.[14] Elevated levels of arsenic intake have been reported for young children and infants when rice cereal is a relevant source of iron. To reduce

infants' exposure to arsenic, the US Food and Drug Administration (https://
www.fda.gov/NewsEvents/Newsroom/PressAnnouncements/ucm493740.
htm) and the AAP recommend consumption of a variety of infant cereals,
including oat, barley, and multigrain cereals, all of which have lower arsenic
levels than rice cereal.[24]

Plant foods, including whole grains and most vegetables, are naturally
low in iron and may contain inhibitors of iron absorption, such as phytate,
tannins, or polyphenols. Flesh foods, especially red meats, are naturally rich
in heme iron, which has a much more favorable bioavailability (20%–35%
absorption rate).[22] Numerous studies have reported that iron-rich complementary foods, including meats and/or iron-fortified cereals, support iron
status and help to prevent deficiency in breastfed infants who do not have
another major source of iron in the diet, such as iron-fortified formula.[25]
During the second year of life, when most infants have weaned from infant
formula, choices of iron-rich foods become especially important for all
young children. Indeed, NHANES data from 2007–2010 indicated 13.5% of
1- to 2-year-olds were iron deficient.[26]

Zinc *(see also Chapter 20: Trace Minerals)*

The older fully breastfed infant also is dependent on complementary foods
to provide adequate zinc intake, unlike the formula-fed infant. In contrast to iron, human milk initially contains high concentrations of zinc,
but a sharp physiologic decline in human milk zinc content over the first
several months postpartum (independent of maternal zinc status) results
in inadequate intake if other dietary sources are not consumed by the
infant. As with iron, high absorption efficiency of zinc in human milk does
not compensate for the low concentrations and intakes by approximately 5
to 6 months of age.[27] Zinc fortification of infant cereals has become more
common in the United States, but amounts are quite variable and provide,
on average, the RDA of 3 mg/day for infants between 7 months and 3 years of
age. The zinc content of unfortified plant foods, including cereal grains and
legumes, tends to be low and/or poorly absorbed.[28] As for iron, red meats
(and liver) are the best natural sources of zinc in the diet, with pork and
poultry being medium rich and fish and eggs being lowest in zinc content
of animal products. Zinc needs can typically be met by 1 to 2 oz of pureed
meat/day.[28] Dairy foods, such as cow milk, yogurt, and cheese, are only
moderate sources of zinc. Fruits and vegetables are low in zinc; whole grains
and legumes have moderately high concentrations, but the absorption is
inhibited by intrinsic compounds in the plants (eg, phytate). Commercially
available mixed dinner purees, which combine a vegetable or starch with

a meat source, contain much lower amounts of zinc and iron than "single-ingredient" pureed meats.[29] Notably, formula-fed infants are at low risk for zinc deficiency because of ample fortification of formula; after weaning, the need for consumption of zinc-rich foods is similar to that for iron. National survey data indicate very low rates of zinc intakes below recommended levels,[11,18,30] at least in part because of food fortification. This emphasizes the importance of recognizing clinical scenarios when zinc intake may be inadequate, such as the older breastfed infant or toddlers who do not consume meats or fortified products or who consume diets with overall limited diversity.[27]

Vitamin D

The content of vitamin D in human milk is typically quite low relative to requirements, even with adequate maternal vitamin D status. With the exception of fatty fish, fortified infant formula and cow milk, some other vitamin D-fortified dairy products, and selected calcium/vitamin D-fortified fruit juices, complementary foods are not good sources of vitamin D. Thus, the AAP has recommended routine vitamin D supplements of 400 IU/day for breastfed infants and formula-fed infants up to 12 months of age who are consuming <1 L/day of formula[31] (see Chapter 21.I: Fat-Soluble Vitamins). For toddlers 12 through 23 months of age, national intake data indicate that nearly 75% of children did not meet an estimated average requirement of 400 IU/day from their diets,[11] and this was before the RDA was established at 600 IU/day by the Institute of Medicine and endorsed by the AAP in 2011.[31] These recommendations do not take into account sunshine exposure, although it is noted that use of sunscreen, when applied appropriately, blocks synthesis of vitamin D in the skin.

Other Micronutrients

For well-nourished mothers, the human milk content of vitamins will generally be adequate to meet breastfed infants' nutritional requirements; thus, complementary food choices are less critical to meet requirements for these micronutrients. An important exception to this generalization is vitamin B_{12} for vegan mothers (see Chapter 11: Nutritional Aspects of Vegetarian Diets, and Chapter 21.II: Water-Soluble Vitamins). Vitamin B_{12} is found only in foods of animal origin. If the mother has not consumed foods of animal origin or taken supplements containing B_{12} during pregnancy and lactation, her milk may be low in vitamin B_{12}, and the breastfed infant will be at risk of deficiency. Case reports of vitamin B_{12} deficiency in breastfed infants of mothers who are vegan are readily found in the literature. Recent reports also describe vitamin B_{12} deficiency in infants of mothers who have not received adequate vitamin B_{12} therapy after gastric bypass surgery or who have untreated pernicious anemia.[32] Furthermore, if parents wish to provide a vegan diet for the weaning infant and toddler, the risk of vitamin B_{12} is moderately high (especially if the mother has not used supplements during pregnancy and/or lactation), as are the risks of iron and zinc deficiencies.

Physiologic and Developmental Considerations
The progression of physiologic and motor maturation aligns typically midway through the first year of life. The infant gastrointestinal tract is able to digest and efficiently absorb virtually all nutrients by 2 to 3 months of age. Therefore, it follows that by the time complementary feeding is recommended, no foods need to be avoided on the basis of gastrointestinal tract immaturity. Developmentally, an infant should have truncal strength and stability to allow sitting in an upright position with little or no support, skills typically present between 4 and 7 months of age. The sucking, rooting, and extrusion primitive reflexes will normally have diminished by this time, and oral motor skills to handle nonliquid foods should be emerging. The gag reflex also gradually declines during this period and the infant is able to handle more complex textures.

Oral motor skills needed for greater manipulation of food within the mouth and for handling of more complex textures like thicker purees appear at approximately 6 months of age and include up-down jaw movements, tongue lateralization, and rotary motion of jaws. By the end of the first year, relatively refined chewing jaw motions and incisor teeth allow controlled bites of soft solids.[33]

The ability to transfer objects to and across the midline, exploration of objects and food by bringing them to the mouth, and refinement of pincer grasp all develop progressively after 6 months and support self-feeding skills.[33] Finger-feeding skills and desire are often particularly strong after 9 months of age, and preference to this over being spoon fed by an adult may be quite firm. Because effective handling of a spoon, however, does not typically develop until after 12 months of age, parents may be encouraged to offer as many "finger foods" as possible, to encourage self-feeding and to support the child's emerging autonomy. Cup skills, with assistance, progressively improve between 7 and 8 months of age, and by 12 months of age, most infants are able to hold an open cup with 2 hands and take several swallows without choking.[33] The use of "sippy cups" facilitates cup-drinking skills while minimizing spillage, but the spill-proof designs may also encourage grazing behavior for toddlers allowed to have continuous access to them.

The pace at which infants obtain oral motor skills and accept new tastes and textures varies widely. Parents should be encouraged to respect the pace their infant dictates, and they should be reassured that infants who are otherwise developmentally appropriate will eventually be able and willing to handle a wide variety of textures and tastes. One study found that infantile "feeding disorders" followed a final common pathway, linking an interaction between food refusal and intrusive feeding by care providers. A bidirectional pattern leading to disrupted feeding behaviors was described: either intrusive feeding by parents or caregivers led to food refusal, or an episode of infant feeding refusal was followed by an inappropriate parental or caregiver response, which then was associated with persistent disordered feeding[34] (see Chapter 25: Pediatric Feeding and Swallowing Disorders).

The period from 6 to 8 months of age is often referred to as a critical window for initiating complementary feeding because of the developmental processes that are occurring at this time. As the infant's own desire for autonomy progresses toward the end of the first year and through the second year, the potential for conflict around being fed versus self-feeding increases.

When to Initiate Complementary Feeding (see also Chapter 3: Breastfeeding)

Several organizations, including the World Health Organization (WHO), have recommended exclusive breastfeeding through 6 months of age. The AAP supports this recommendation, stipulating introduction of complementary foods at approximately 6 months of age (see Chapter 3: Breastfeeding). A systematic review on the optimal duration of exclusive breastfeeding concluded that exclusive breastfeeding for 6 months is associated with less morbidity from nonhospitalized gastrointestinal tract disease, and possibly respiratory disease, compared with mixed feeding by 3 to 4 months of age. Growth deficits were not identified with exclusive breastfeeding for 6 months or longer, although sample sizes were rarely adequate to rule out small effects on growth.[35] Two trials that randomized introduction of complementary foods at 4 versus 6 months of age also found no difference in growth at 6 or 12 months or at follow-up at preschool age.[36,37] The evidence, thus, demonstrates no apparent risks for normal growth, as a general recommendation, for exclusive breastfeeding for 6 months in both industrialized and developing nations. Of note, however, is the distinction between recommendations for populations and those for individual infants, all of whom should be monitored for growth faltering or other adverse effects, and appropriate interventions should be undertaken when indicated. Similarly, health care providers should encourage responsive feeding and consider the wide variations in the attainment of oral motor and other critical developmental skills in infants when deciding when to initiate complementary feeding, as noted previously, and recently reconfirmed.[38]

The data supporting an effect of timing of complementary feeding on later obesity are quite limited and are mainly based on observational studies, and findings have provided mixed results.[39] Introduction of complementary foods prior to 4 months of age is most consistently identified as contributing to later overweight.[40-42] One narrative review concluded that timing of the introduction of complementary foods was not associated with later risk of obesity.[43]

Timing of complementary feeding has also been examined in relation to prevention of atopic disease, including food allergies. One evidence review comparing introduction of complementary foods at 3 to 4 months of age versus 6 months of age for exclusively breastfed infants found no protective effect of the later introduction of complementary food and atopic disease.[35] The AAP has, likewise, concluded that evidence does not support a strong relationship between timing of introduction of first complementary feeding and development of atopic disease in exclusively breastfed infants.[44] However, there is evidence that exclusive breastfeeding for the first 3 to 4 months decreases the cumulative incidence of eczema in the first 2 years of life. The AAP has also concluded that any duration of breastfeeding beyond 3 to 4 months is protective of wheezing in the first 2 years of life, and a longer duration of breastfeeding, as opposed to less breastfeeding, protects against childhood asthma ever after 5 years of age.[44] A shift in the recommendations from the AAP and others has occurred in timing of exposure of commonly allergenic foods (eg, peanut, eggs, cow milk, soy, wheat, fish, and seafood) into infant diets. It is now generally recognized that there is no evidence that delaying the introduction of allergenic foods beyond 4 to 6 months prevents atopic disease, including peanut, eggs, and fish.[44] There is also evidence that early introduction of infant-safe forms of peanut between 4 and 6 months of age reduces the risk for peanut allergy, especially in high-risk infants (presence of severe eczema and or egg allergy). Data are less clear for the timing of introduction of egg. See Chapter 34: Food Allergy, and AAP recommendations and the text box for further details.

AAP recommendations for preventing atopic disease and complementary feeding[44]

1. There is lack of evidence to support maternal dietary restrictions either during pregnancy or lactation to prevent atopic disease.
2. The evidence regarding the role of breastfeeding in the prevention of atopic disease can be summarized as follows:
   A. There is evidence that **exclusive** breastfeeding for the first 3 to 4 months decreases the cumulative incidence of eczema in the first 2 years of life.
   B. There are no short- or long-term advantages for **exclusive** breastfeeding beyond 3 to 4 months for prevention of atopic disease.
   C. The evidence suggests that any duration of breastfeeding beyond 3 to 4 months is protective against wheezing in the first 2 years of life. This effect is irrespective of duration of exclusivity.
   D. There is some evidence that longer duration of any breastfeeding, as opposed to less breastfeeding, protects against asthma even after 5 years of age.[64]
   E. No conclusions can be made about the role of any duration of breastfeeding in either preventing or delaying the onset of specific food allergies.
3. There is lack of evidence that partially or extensively hydrolyzed formula prevents atopic disease in infants and children, even in those at high risk for allergic disease.
4. The current evidence for the importance of the timing of introduction of allergenic foods and the prevention of atopic disease can be summarized as follows:
   A. There is no evidence that delaying the introduction of allergenic foods beyond 4 to 6 months prevents atopic disease, including peanut, eggs, and fish.
   B. There is evidence that the early introduction of infant-safe forms of peanut reduces the risk for peanut allergies. Data are less clear for timing of introduction of egg.
   C. The new recommendations for the prevention of peanut allergy are based largely on the LEAP trial and endorsed by the AAP. An Expert Panel has advised peanut introduction as early as 4 to 6 months of age for infants at high risk for peanut allergy (presence of severe eczema and/or egg allergy). The recommendations contain details of implementation for high-risk infants, including appropriate use of testing (specific IgE measurement, skin-prick test, and oral food challenges) and introduction of peanut-containing foods in the health care provider's office versus the home setting, as well as amount and frequency. For infants with mild to moderate eczema, the panel recommended introduction of peanut containing foods around 6 months of age, and for infants at very low risk for peanut allergy (no eczema or any food allergy), the panel recommended introduction of peanut-containing food when age appropriate and depending on family preferences and cultural practices (ie, after 6 months of age if exclusively breastfeeding).

The effect of timing of introduction of complementary foods, including specific components such as gluten, on such autoimmune conditions as celiac disease and type 1 diabetes mellitus, has been of considerable interest.[43] Two different RCTs examined the effect of gluten exposure at 4 versus 6 months of age[45] or at 6 versus 12 months of age[46] in high-risk infants (based on HLA typing and family history) on later development of celiac disease. Neither found an effect of early or delayed exposure on subsequent disease. Breastfeeding at the time of exposure was not protective. Systematic reviews have supported these findings, concluding that no specific recommendations related to gluten introduction or to duration of breastfeeding to prevent celiac disease were possible.[47,48] Regarding type 1 diabetes mellitus, the data have been primarily observational. A systematic review found that available evidence did not support recommendations about infant feeding practices, including breastfeeding or timing of gluten introduction, to alter the risk of developing diabetes.[49] The exception may be that gluten exposure before 3 months may be associated with higher diabetes risk, but after 3 months, neither breastfeeding at the time of gluten introduction nor age of gluten introduction was related to development of type 1 diabetes mellitus.

For reasons described previously, iron and zinc deficiencies are not uncommon in older breastfed infants, with the risk progressively increasing after 6 months if iron- and zinc-rich complementary foods or supplements are not consumed. One study in the United States specifically examined the risk of iron deficiency in toddlers associated with full breastfeeding for 6 versus 4 months by analyzing data from the NHANES III (1988–1994) and from the 1999–2002 NHANES data set. A significantly lower risk of iron deficiency (low serum ferritin concentration) without anemia was found in those who were exclusively breastfed for 4 to 5 months versus those who were exclusively breastfed for 6 months or longer without any dietary supplements of iron.[50] Few trials have been conducted to investigate the effect of timing of complementary feeding on zinc or other micronutrient status.

Current Practices in the United States for Complementary Feedings

Introduction of solid foods before 4 months of age has declined in the United States. Among infants enrolled in the Special Supplemental Nutrition Program for Women, Infants, and Children (WIC), introduction of complementary foods before 4 months has decreased from approximately 60% in 1994–1995 to 20% in 2013–2014 (https://fns-prod.azureedge.net/sites/default/files/ops/WIC-ITFPS2-Infant.pdf). A report based on the NHANES

II

survey provides a rich description of food consumption patterns in infants and toddlers, including changes from 2005–2008 to 2009–2012.[51] In 2009–2012, among infants 6 through 11 months of age, 71% received infant cereal on a given day, while nearly a quarter of consumed noninfant cereals. Additionally, in both periods, consumption of infant (fortified) cereals was reported by approximately 15% of infants in the second year of life. Also relevant to the discussion above for food choices for breastfed infants to meet iron and zinc needs, poultry was the most consumed flesh food, being consumed by 28% of 6- through 11-month-olds, and all other meats were less than 12%. The most popular category for all protein sources was "mixed dishes," which tend to be primarily a starch or vegetable base, less actual meat, and lower amounts of iron and zinc. All protein source categories increased during the second year of life. Yogurt consumption (a good source of calcium but poor source of iron) remains a popular protein source. Fruit and vegetable consumption overall was reported by the majority in both age groups, but in the second year of life, French fries and white potatoes were the most commonly reported vegetable. Consumption of 100% fruit juice in the first year of life has dramatically declined to slightly less than 50% of children (coincident with its reduction in the WIC food packages); in the 2nd year of life, 70% reported consumption. The AAP has recommended against juice in the first year of life, and suggests limiting the amount for toddlers 1 through 3 years of age to 4 oz/day.[52] Although decreased from earlier surveys, more than 40% of 6- to 11-month-olds consumed sweet or salty snacks and desserts, and this doubled to more than 80% for 12- through 23-month-olds. Sugar-sweetened beverages were consumed by more than 50% of toddlers, with fruit-flavored drinks being the predominant type.[51] From other national data and follow-up from the Infant Feeding Practices Study II,[53] consumption of sugar-sweetened beverages during infancy was associated with approximately a twofold higher obesity rate at 6 years of age and was highlighted as a potential modifiable risk factor for early childhood obesity.[20] Consumption of sodium and added sugars by toddlers has also been identified as a concern. In contrast to commercial "infant-only" foods, which are low in sodium, high amounts of sodium and added sugars have been documented in many toddler meals and savory snacks.[54,55] The concerns for potentially high sugar and salt intake in commonly available foods for toddlers are twofold: further accentuating innate taste preferences at a developmental stage when lifelong eating habits are being formed, and raising risk for chronic diseases (eg, obesity, hypertension) by exaggerated early exposures.

In summary, common complementary feeding practices in the United States often are not tailored to the distinctly different risk profiles for micronutrient deficiencies in breastfed infants compared with formula-fed infants. The substantial change in recommendations to mitigate risk of atopic disease—from avoidance to controlled exposure—warrants recognition by pediatricians of those at risk and provision of appropriate, anticipatory guidance around feeding. Furthermore, although improved practices have been implemented, such as less early (before 4 months) introduction of complementary foods and less juice consumption in infants, there remain many opportunities for improvements.

Which Complementary Foods to Feed

In its guidelines for complementary feeding, with an emphasis on resource-limited settings and populations with generally high rates of breastfeeding, the WHO emphasizes the importance of variety in food choices. Specifically, the WHO recommends that flesh foods, including meats, poultry, and fish, as well as eggs be eaten daily or as often as possible. Diets with adequate fat content are recommended. Vegetarian diets are noted to be unlikely to meet nutrient needs at this age unless nutrient supplements or fortified products are used. Recommendations also include avoidance of low-nutrient drinks, such as teas, coffee, and sugary drinks such as soda; limits on juice are also recommended to avoid displacement of more nutritious foods.[56]

In contrast, in industrialized nations such as the United States, emphasis has traditionally been on iron-fortified cereals, followed by fruits or vegetables, with later introduction of meats. The ready availability and common use of infant formulas reduces the reliance on specific choices of complementary foods. As more infants are breastfed in the United States, however, the importance of complementary feeding patterns has gained attention. Data from the Infant Feeding Practices Study II indicate that nearly 20% of 6-month-old breastfed or mixed-fed (human milk and formula fed) infants had received neither iron-fortified cereals nor meat in the past week, and 15% had never received cereal, meat, or supplements. Despite being at the highest risk of iron deficiency, exclusively breastfed infants at 6 months of age had the highest rates of noncompliance with recommendations for iron intake, with 70% having less than 2 servings of infant cereal or meat daily or receiving iron supplements at least 3 times per week.[57]

With the recognition of the potential value of meats as a source of heme iron with enhanced iron absorption and as a source of bioavailable zinc, the AAP also encourages consumption of meats, vegetables with higher iron content, and iron-fortified cereals for infants and toddlers between

6 and 24 months of age.[22] It is appropriate to start with meat, especially if iron-fortified infant cereal is not being provided. Absorption data suggest that 1 to 2 oz/day of meat generally provides the iron requirement for healthy older infants and likely also for toddlers.[28] Although this amount of meat is also appropriate to support iron status, especially if other fortified sources are included, adequacy of intakes of foods is difficult to predict for iron because of the complexity of physiologic factors that influence its absorption—for example, stores at birth, growth rate, gender, inflammatory states, and iron status (see Chapter 19: Iron, for recommendations for screening of iron status).[58]

A good variety of healthy foods generally promotes good nutritional status for infants and toddlers, and repeated exposures is the best way for young children to learn to accept different foods. Because the digestive and absorptive functions are mature well before 6 months of age, there is no reason to introduce whole food groups sequentially. Rather, considering the dynamic changes in infants' nutritional needs in the second half of the first year of life, gradual introduction of foods across all food groups is a better paradigm. To identify adverse reactions, new foods should be introduced singly over several days. For example, an infant cereal may be the first food, followed by meats, fruits, and vegetables. Progression to foods from 4 food groups (grains, meats, fruits, and vegetables) could reasonably be achieved within the first month of complementary feeding. Amounts of each food and variety are expected to gradually increase with the infant's age. Infants have been demonstrated to accept cereals and meats equally well by 5 months of age.[59] Although formula-fed infants are less dependent on specific food choices to avoid micronutrient deficiencies than are predominantly found in breastfed infants, exposure to all food groups in infancy provides important familiarity for the second year of life, when fortified formula will no longer be consumed by most toddlers.

Food choices to be encouraged, whether home or commercially prepared, are those with no added salt or sugar; as detailed above, this is especially important for commercial foods marketed for toddlers. Fats, particularly healthy fats, such as those containing mono- and polyunsaturated fatty acids—for example, avocado, ground nuts, or nut butters—should not be discouraged. Nearly 30% of toddlers have been reported to have intakes of fat below recommended levels.[11,18] Energy intakes of older infants and toddlers are notoriously difficult to measure, and energy requirements are difficult to estimate. Appropriateness of energy intake for an individual child is best judged by appropriateness of growth.

How to Guide Complementary Feeding

The following guiding principles are provided for introduction of complementary foods and for the progression through the second year of life.

1. **Choose first foods that provide key nutrients and help meet energy
   needs.** As discussed in the preceding sections, iron and zinc are the
   micronutrients that become limiting for primarily breastfed infants,
   and they are also the most likely to be low in the diets of older infants.
   To provide these nutrients, iron- and zinc-fortified infant cereals and
   meats are excellent first foods and are equally well accepted by infants.[59]
   The suggested intake is approximately 2 servings/day for cereal
   (2 tablespoons/serving) or meat (1–2 oz/day meat or 1–2 small jars of
   commercially prepared single-ingredient meat/day).

2. **Introduce one "single-ingredient" new food at a time,** from any food
   group. Do not introduce other new foods for several days to observe for
   possible allergic reactions or intolerance. Foods most commonly associated with infant allergies are cow milk, eggs, soy, peanuts, tree nuts
   (and seeds), wheat, fish, and shell fish. There is no current convincing
   evidence that delaying the introduction of solid foods associated with
   infant allergies beyond 4 months has a significant protective effect on
   the development of atopic disease. Introduction of infant-safe peanut
   between 4 and 6 months of age in high-risk infants (those with severe
   eczema and/or egg allergy) is now recommended to reduce the prevalence of peanut allergy by up to 86%.[40] Thus, for those at risk for allergies, "controlled exposure" rather than avoidance or delayed exposure is
   now recommended (see Chapter 34: Food Allergy, for more detail).

3. **Introduce a variety of foods.** By 7 to 8 months of age, infants should be
   consuming foods from all food groups. The food variety should progressively increase over the next several months. Parents should be encouraged to offer foods multiple times over several days (≥8 exposures) for
   infants and toddlers to become accepting of new flavors and textures.[60]

4. **Withhold cow milk and other plant-based "milks" not formulated for
   infants during the first year of life.** Fresh cow milk has been associated with low-grade intestinal blood loss in infants and, thus, is not
   recommended. Liquids, so-called "milks," based on plant foods (eg, soy,
   rice, almond, or hemp) should not be used as a human milk or infant
   formula substitute (ie, when human milk or infant formula provides a
   significant portion of daily energy intake). The caloric density of these
   products is typically lower than that of human milk or infant formula;

protein quality is low and the protein quantity is very low for most such beverages; products are not fortified with micronutrients to levels recommended for infants and young children; and some contain high levels of phytate, which bind iron, zinc, and calcium. Use of such alternative fluids as a major component of the diet has been associated with severe protein energy malnutrition and with growth faltering.[61]

5. **During the second year of life, low-fat milk may be considered** if growth and weight gain are appropriate or especially if weight gain is excessive or family history is positive for obesity, dyslipidemia, or cardiovascular disease (see Chapters 32: Dyslipidemia, and Chapter 33: Pediatric Obesity).[62] Total dairy product intake of 16 to 24 oz is appropriate to meet calcium needs. Intakes greater than 32 oz/day predispose to iron deficiency.

6. **Juice consumption should be limited.** No juice should be offered before 6 months of age, and it is best to avoid juice completely until the infant is at least 12 months of age.[52] If juice is medically indicated for an infant older than 6 months, it should only be served in a cup, not a bottle. After 1 year of age, 100% fruit juice may be served as part of a meal or snack, but total daily volume should not exceed 4 oz/day for children 1 through 3 years of age.[52] Juice drinks, which typically contain added sweeteners, should be discouraged. Dilution of juice with water may encourage excessive fluid consumption and grazing behaviors.

7. **Ensure that complementary foods are prepared in a healthy and safe manner.** Home preparation of pureed or mashed table foods is practical for many families. Practices to encourage include:
   a. Match texture and consistency to infant's oral motor skills.
   b. Use thick purees to enhance caloric density.
   c. Provide healthy "single ingredient" foods, especially while total variety is still limited.
   d. Avoid added sugar or salt.
   e. Avoid foods that could be choking or aspiration risks (hot dogs, nuts, grapes, raisins, raw carrots, popcorn, hard candies).
   f. Use caution when using a microwave to warm foods; check temperature before feeding to infants.

8. **Encourage infant's involvement in feeding process.** By 9 months of age, infants should be presented with finger foods, and an open cup may be introduced. Effective use of utensils develops progressively after approximately 12 months of age.

9. **Encourage routine meal times and "responsive feeding," watching for and responding to infant's hunger and satiety cues.** General feeding practices to encourage include:
   a. Avoid intrusive behaviors (eg, force feeding) by care providers.
   b. Establish routines for meals and snacks in a predictable schedule, typically allowing 2 to 3 hours between eating and drinking opportunities, resulting in eating 5 to 6 times per day (eg, 3 meals, 2–3 snacks).
   c. Avoid "grazing" behaviors with snacks or liquids by allowing constant access to foods and drinks; eat only in a high chair, at a table, or at other designated areas.
   d. Limit meals to 15 to 20 minutes, as appropriate for infants' or toddlers' attention spans.
   e. Praise eating but resist attention for not eating; using food as means of punishment or a reward is not appropriate.
   f. Minimize distractions during meal times (TV, videos, cell phones, other screens, pets, etc).
   g. Resist offering multiple alternative choices of preferred foods if the foods initially offered are refused; calmly encourage tasting, do not force eating, and end meal after appropriate time.
10. **Monitor appropriateness of growth as a guide to adequacy of complementary feeding practices.** Avoid giving calorie goals to parents, which encourages overemphasis on numbers and may lead to intrusive feeding behaviors. The focus should be on the quality of food choices, the feeding environment, and feeding routines and behaviors.

References

1. Katz J, Lee AC, Kozuki N, et al. Mortality risk in preterm and small-for-gestational-age infants in low-income and middle-income countries: a pooled country analysis. *Lancet.* 2013;382(9890):417–425
2. Black RE, Allen LH, Bhutta ZA, et al. Maternal and child undernutrition: global and regional exposures and health consequences. *Lancet.* 2008;371(9608):243–260
3. Ogden CL, Carroll MD, Lawman HG, et al. Trends in Obesity Prevalence Among Children and Adolescents in the United States, 1988–1994 Through 2013–2014. *JAMA.* 2016;315(21):2292–2299
4. Grummer-Strawn LM, Scanlon KS, Fein SB. Infant feeding and feeding transitions during the first year of life. *Pediatrics.* 2008;122(Suppl 2):S36–S42

5. Shealy KR, Scanlon KS, Labiner-Wolfe J, Fein SB, Grummer-Strawn LM. Characteristics of breastfeeding practices among US mothers. *Pediatrics.* 2008;122(Suppl 2):S50–S55

6. Butte NF, Wong WW, Hopkinson JM, Heinz CJ, Mehta NR, Smith EO. Energy requirements derived from total energy expenditure and energy deposition during the first 2 y of life. *Am J Clin Nutr.* 2000;72(6):1558–1569

7. Tang M, Krebs NF. High protein intake from meat as complementary food increases growth but not adiposity in breastfed infants: a randomized trial. *Am J Clin Nutr.* 2014;100(5):1322–1328

8. Li R, Fein SB, Grummer-Strawn LM. Do infants fed from bottles lack self-regulation of milk intake compared with directly breastfed infants? *Pediatrics.* 2010;125(6):e1386–e1393

9. Heinig MJ, Nommsen LA, Peerson JM, Lonnerdal B, Dewey KG. Energy and protein intakes of breast-fed and formula-fed infants during the first year of life and their association with growth velocity: the DARLING Study. *Am J Clin Nutr.* 1993;58(2):152–161

10. Saavedra JM, Deming D, Dattilo A, Reidy K. Lessons from the feeding infants and toddlers study in North America: what children eat, and implications for obesity prevention. *Ann Nutr Metab.* 2013;62(Suppl 3):27–36

11. Ahluwalia N, Herrick KA, Rossen LM, et al. Usual nutrient intakes of US infants and toddlers generally meet or exceed Dietary Reference Intakes: findings from NHANES 2009–2012. *Am J Clin Nutr.* 2016;104(4):1167–1174

12. Brown KH, Sanchez-Grinan M, Perez F, Peerson JM, Ganoza L, Stern JS. Effects of dietary energy density and feeding frequency on total daily energy intakes of recovering malnourished children. *Am J Clin Nutr.* 1995;62(1):13–18

13. Dewey KG, Brown KH. Update on technical issues concerning complementary feeding of young children in developing countries and implications for intervention programs. *Food Nutr Bull.* 2003;24(1):5-28

14. Institute of Medicine. *Dietary Reference Intakes; The Essential Guide to Nutrient Requirements.* Washington, DC: National Academies Press; 2006

15. Fomon SJ. Requirements and recommended dietary intakes of protein during infancy. *Pediatric Res.* 1991;30(5):391–395

16. Schanler RJ, Krebs NF, Mass SB, eds. *Breastfeeding Handbook for Physicians.* 2nd ed. Elk Grove Village, IL/Washington, DC: American Academy of Pediatrics/American College of Obstetricians and Gynecologists; 2014

17. Fewtrell M, Bronsky J, Campoy C, et al. Complementary Feeding: A Position Paper by the European Society for Paediatric Gastroenterology, Hepatology, and Nutrition (ESPGHAN) Committee on Nutrition. *J Pediatr Gastroenterol Nutr.* 2017;64(1):119–132

18. Bailey RL, Catellier DJ, Jun S, et al. Total usual nutrient intakes of US children (under 48 months): findings from the Feeding Infants and Toddlers Study (FITS) 2016. *J Nutr.* 2018; in press

19. Simell O, Niinikoski H, Ronnemaa T, et al. Cohort Profile: the STRIP Study (Special Turku Coronary Risk Factor Intervention Project), an Infancy-onset Dietary and Life-style Intervention Trial. *Int J Epidemiol.* 2009;38(3):650–655

20. Pan L, Li R, Park S, Galuska DA, Sherry B, Freedman DS. A longitudinal analysis of sugar-sweetened beverage intake in infancy and obesity at 6 years. *Pediatrics.* 2014;134(Suppl 1):S29–S35

21. Young BE, Krebs NF. Complementary Feeding: Critical Considerations to Optimize Growth, Nutrition, and Feeding Behavior. *Curr Pediatr Rep.* 2013;1:247–256

22. Baker RD, Greer FR. Diagnosis and prevention of iron deficiency and iron-deficiency anemia in infants and young children (0-3 years of age). *Pediatrics.* 2010;126(5):1040–1050

23. Maguire JL, Salehi L, Birken CS, et al. Association between total duration of breastfeeding and iron deficiency. *Pediatrics.* 2013;131(5):e1530–e1537

24. Lai PY, Cottingham KL, Steinmaus C, Karagas MR, Miller MD. Arsenic and Rice: translating research to address health care providers' needs. *J Pediatr.* 2015;167(4):797–803

25. Krebs NF, Sherlock LG, Westcott J, et al. Effects of different complementary feeding regimens on iron status and enteric microbiota in breastfed infants. *J Pediatr.* 2013;163(2):416–423.e414

26. Gupta PM, Perrine CG, Mei Z, Scanlon KS. Iron, anemia, and iron deficiency anemia among young children in the United States. *Nutrients.* 2016;8(6):E330

27. Krebs NF. Update on zinc deficiency and excess in clinical pediatric practice. *Ann Nutr Metab.* 2013;62(Suppl 1):19–29

28. Krebs NF, Westcott JE, Culbertson DL, Sian L, Miller LV, Hambidge KM. Comparison of complementary feeding strategies to meet zinc requirements of older breastfed infants. *Am J Clin Nutr.* 2012;96(1):30–35

29. Krebs NF, Hambidge KM. Complementary feeding: clinically relevant factors affecting timing and composition. *Am J Clin Nutr.* 2007;85(2):639S-645S

30. Hamner HC, Perrine CG, Scanlon KS. Usual Intake of key minerals among children in the second year of life, NHANES 2003–2012. *Nutrients.* 2016;8(8):E468

31. Wagner CL, Greer FR. Prevention of rickets and vitamin D deficiency in infants, children, and adolescents. *Pediatrics.* 2008;122(5):1142–1152

32. Hinton CF, Ojodu JA, Fernhoff PM, Rasmussen SA, Scanlon KS, Hannon WH. Maternal and neonatal vitamin B12 deficiency detected through expanded newborn screening—United States, 2003–2007. *J Pediatr.* 2010;157(1):162–163

33. Pridham KF. Feeding behavior of 6- to 12-month-old infants: assessment and sources of parental information. *J Pediatr.* 1990;117(2 Pt 2):S174–S180

34. Levine A, Bachar L, Tsangen Z, et al. Screening criteria for diagnosis of infantile feeding disorders as a cause of poor feeding or food refusal. *J Pediatr Gastroenterol Nutr.* 2011;52(5):563–568

35. Kramer MS, Kakuma R. Optimal duration of exclusive breastfeeding. *Cochrane Database Syst Rev.* 2012(8):CD003517

36. Jonsdottir OH, Kleinman RE, Wells JC, et al. Exclusive breastfeeding for 4 versus 6 months and growth in early childhood. *Acta Paediatr.* 2014;103(1):105–111

37. Perkin MR, Logan K, Tseng A, et al. Randomized Trial of Introduction of Allergenic Foods in Breast-Fed Infants. *N Engl J Med.* 2016;374(18):1733–1743.

38. Perez-Escamilla R, Segura-Perez S, Lott M. Feeding guidelines for infants and young toddlers. a responsive parenting approach. *Nutrition Today.* 2017;52: 223–231

39. Burdette HL, Whitaker RC, Hall WC, Daniels SR. Breastfeeding, introduction of complementary foods, and adiposity at 5 y of age. *Am J Clin Nutr.* 2006;83(3): 550–558

40. Taveras EM, Gillman MW, Kleinman K, Rich-Edwards JW, Rifas-Shiman SL. Racial/ethnic differences in early-life risk factors for childhood obesity. *Pediatrics.* 2010;125(4):686–695

41. Huh SY, Rifas-Shiman SL, Taveras EM, Oken E, Gillman MW. Timing of solid food introduction and risk of obesity in preschool-aged children. *Pediatrics.* 2011;127(3):e544–e551

42. Baker JL, Michaelsen KF, Rasmussen KM, Sorensen TI. Maternal prepregnant body mass index, duration of breastfeeding, and timing of complementary food introduction are associated with infant weight gain. *Am J Clin Nutr.* 2004;80(6):1579–1588

43. Daniels L, Mallan KM, Fildes A, Wilson J. The timing of solid introduction in an 'obesogenic' environment: a narrative review of the evidence and methodological issues. *Aust N Z J Public Health.* 2015;39(4):366–373

44. Greer FR, Sicherer SH, Burks AW; American Academy of Pediatrics, Committee on Nutrition, Section on Allergy and Immunology. Effects of early nutritional interventions on the development of atopic disease in infants and children: the role of maternal dietary restriction, breastfeeding, timing of introduction of complementary foods, and hydrolyzed formulas. *Pediatrics.* 2019:in press

45. Vriezinga SL, Auricchio R, Bravi E, et al. Randomized feeding intervention in infants at high risk for celiac disease. *N Engl J Med.* 2014;371(14):1304–1315

46. Lionetti E, Castellaneta S, Francavilla R, et al. Introduction of gluten, HLA status, and the risk of celiac disease in children. *N Engl J Med.* 2014;371(14): 1295–1303

47. Pinto-Sanchez MI, Verdu EF, Liu E, et al. Gluten Introduction to Infant Feeding and Risk of Celiac Disease: Systematic Review and Meta-Analysis. *J Pediatr.* 2016;168:132–143.e133

48. Silano M, Agostoni C, Sanz Y, Guandalini S. Infant feeding and risk of developing celiac disease: a systematic review. *BMJ Open.* 2016;6(1):e009163

49. Piescik-Lech M, Chmielewska A, Shamir R, Szajewska H. Systematic review: early infant feeding and the risk of type 1 diabetes. *J Pediatr Gastroenterol Nutr.* 2017;64(3):454–459

50. Chantry CJ, Howard CR, Auinger P. Full breastfeeding duration and risk for iron deficiency in U.S. infants. *Breastfeed Med.* 2007;2(2):63–73

51. Miles G, Siega-Riz AM. Trends in food and beverage consumption among infants and toddlers: 2005–2012. *Pediatrics.* 2017;139(6):e20163290

52. Heyman MB, Abrams SA; American Academy of Pediatrics, Section on Gastroenterology, Hepatology, and Nutrition, Committee on Nutrition. Policy statement: Fruit juice in infants, children, and adolescents: current recommendations. *Pediatrics.* 2017;139(6):e20170967

53. Fein SB, Li R, Chen J, Scanlon KS, Grummer-Strawn LM. Methods for the year 6 follow-up study of children in the Infant Feeding Practices Study II. *Pediatrics.* 2014;134(Suppl 1):S4-S12

54. Maalouf J, Cogswell ME, Bates M, et al. Sodium, sugar, and fat content of complementary infant and toddler foods sold in the United States, 2015. *Am J Clin Nutr.* 2017;105(6):1443–1452

55. Cogswell ME, Gunn JP, Yuan K, Park S, Merritt R. Sodium and sugar in complementary infant and toddler foods sold in the United States. *Pediatrics.* 2015;135(3):416–423

56. Pan American Health Organization/World Health Organization. *Guiding Principles for Complementary Feeding of the Breastfed Child.* Washington, DC: PAHO/WHO; 2003

57. Dee DL, Sharma AJ, Cogswell ME, Grummer-Strawn LM, Fein SB, Scanlon KS. Sources of supplemental iron among breastfed infants during the first year of life. *Pediatrics.* 2008;122(Suppl 2):S98–S104

58. Food and Nutrition Board, Institute of Medicine. *Dietary Reference Intakes for Vitamin A, Vitamin K, Boron, Chromium, Copper, Iodine, Iron, Manganese, Molybdenum, Nickel, Silicon, Vanadium and Zinc.* Washington, DC: National Academy Press; 2001

59. Krebs NF, Westcott JE, Butler N, Robinson C, Bell M, Hambidge KM. Meat as a first complementary food for breastfed infants: feasibility and impact on zinc intake and status. *J Pediatr Gastroenterol Nutr.* 2006;42(2):207–214

60. Spill MK, Johns K, Callahan EH, et al. Repeated exposure to food and food acceptability in infants and toddlers: a systematic review. *Am J Clin Nutr.* 2019;109(Suppl 1):978S-989S

61. Liu T, Howard RM, Mancini AJ, et al. Kwashiorkor in the United States: fad diets, perceived and true milk allergy, and nutritional ignorance. *Arch Dermatol.* 2001;137(5):630–636

62. Daniels SR, Greer FR; American Academy of Pediatrics, Committee on Nutrition. Clinical report: Lipid screening and cardiovascular health in childhood. *Pediatrics.* 2008;122(1):198–208

63. Butte NF, Hopkinson JM, Wong WW, Smith EO, Ellis KJ. Body composition during the first 2 years of life: an updated reference. *Pediatr Res.* 2000;47(5):578–585

64. Lodge CJ, Tan DJ, Lau MX, et al. Breastfeeding and asthma and allergies: a systematic review and meta-analysis. *Acta Paediatr.* 2015;104(467):38–53

Feeding the Child and Adolescent

Chapter 7

Feeding the Child

Introduction

Following infancy, children experience developmental progress that is fundamentally tied to the evolution and establishment of eating behavior. In contrast to infancy, however, the period from 1 year of age to puberty is a slower period of physical growth. Birth weight is tripled during the first year of life but is not quadrupled until 2 years of age; birth length is increased by 50% during the first year but is not doubled until 4 years of age. Although growth patterns vary in individual children, children from 2 years of age to puberty gain an average of 2 to 3 kg (4.5–6.5 lb) and grow 5 to 8 cm (2.5 –3.5 in) in height per year.[1] As growth rates decline during the preschool years, appetites often decrease, and food intake may appear erratic and unpredictable. Parental confusion and concern are not uncommon. Frequently expressed concerns include the limited variety of foods ingested, dawdling and distractibility, limited consumption of vegetables and meats, and a desire for too many sweets. As children enter the school age years, parental concern about overeating and excessive weight gain often begins to emerge. Parents may begin to seek advice regarding how to adaptively guide children's intake to prevent excessive weight gain while not inadvertently promoting unhealthy weight control behaviors or body image concerns. Parental concern regarding children's eating behaviors, whether warranted or unfounded, should be addressed with developmentally appropriate nutrition information. Anticipatory guidance for parents and caregivers is key to preventing many feeding problems.

An important goal of early childhood nutrition is to ensure children's present and future health by fostering the development of healthy eating behaviors. Parents and caregivers are called on to offer foods that are developmentally appropriate in content, timing, frequency, and portion size. Parents and caregivers are responsible for providing a variety of nutritious foods; limiting the availability of calorically dense, less healthy foods; structuring the timing and frequency of eating occasions (including both meals and snacks); and providing appropriate portion sizes that are not excessively large. Excessive control in the form of pressure to eat or restriction should be avoided. However, sensitive guidance in the form of encouragement to eat healthy foods and imparting healthy norms about foods to eat in moderation are essential elements of food parenting in the current obesogenic environment.

Toddlerhood

Toddler eating patterns are characterized by independence both in terms of
the physical skills that facilitate mobility and self-feeding and the acquisition of language skills that enable the toddler to verbally express eating
preferences and needs. Weaning from the bottle should be accomplished by
18 months of age to prevent the adverse health consequences of prolonged
bottle use, including iron deficiency,[2,3] excessive weight gain,[4] and tooth
decay. Drinking from a cup (either an open cup or a sippy cup) is generally
introduced by age 12 months, with gradual transition off all bottle feeding
by 18 months. More than 1 in 5 US toddlers continue to use a bottle at
24 months.[4] Transition from the bottle to a sippy cup instead of an open cup
is common and may not reduce the risks associated with bottle use[5]; therefore, transition to an open cup is optimal. Avoiding the use of juice in bottles
and any bottles during sleeping, in particular, reduces exposure to sugars
and risk of dental caries (see Chapter 48: Diet, Nutrition, and Oral Health).[6]

Between 12 and 24 months, toddlers develop the motor skills to use
utensils; more than 95% of children can use a spoon by 18 months.[7] Children
learn to spear food and use a fork between 18 and 24 months. Supporting
self-feeding is theorized to encourage self-regulation of energy intake, the
mastery of feeding skills, and the socialization of eating behaviors. Given
earlier opportunities for mastery of self-feeding skills, the older toddler
(2 years) is ready to consume most of the same foods offered to the rest of
the family, with some extra preparation to prevent choking.

Toddlers continually explore cause-and-effect relationships, and eating
is a primary domain for exploration. Toddlers are acculturated into social
norms for eating in their community through structured eating occasions,
supportive social interaction, and sensitive guidance. Toddlerhood represents the transition from allowing free exploration of the environment to
promote learning and development to increasing expectations to adhere to
social rules (ie, manners and mealtime behavior). Guiding caregivers and
parents to make this transition slowly and sensitively will keep eating occasions pleasant and productive.

Preventing Choking

Choking is a significant concern for young children, with more than
12 000 emergency department visits per year for choking among children
and about 70 fatalities.[8,9] The mean age of children treated in emergency
departments for nonfatal food-related choking is 4.5 years.[8] However, about
one third of emergency department visits for choking are among children

<1 year old,[8] and 79% of choking fatalities occur in children younger than 3 years.[10] Incomplete dentition, small airway diameter, immature swallowing coordination, and high activity levels during eating (eg, running) make young children particularly vulnerable to choking. Foods that are small and cylindrical as well as hard, highly elastic, slippery, or crunchy present the greatest risk.[13] Hot dogs are the food most commonly associated with fatal choking in children.[9] Other high-risk foods include meat, bone, peanuts/nuts, seeds, hard candy/chewing gum, carrots, popcorn, and apples.[8,10,11] Anticipatory guidance for caregivers should include selecting appropriate foods, adequately processing foods offered, and supervising children during eating.[13] Toddlers should be given foods that gradually build self-feeding skills—starting with soft, mashed, or ground foods and building to prepared table foods by 12 to 18 months. Soft, round foods, such as hot dogs, grapes, and string cheese, must be cut into very small pieces or avoided entirely.

Children should be seated while eating and parents or caregivers should always be present and able to observe the child (ie, avoid having the child eat in a rear-facing car safety seat). The feeding environment should ideally be free of distractions. Finally, analgesics used to numb the gums during teething may anesthetize the posterior pharynx. Children who receive such medications should be carefully observed during feeding.

Food Acceptance
Preferences for the taste of sweet have been observed shortly after birth,[12] and young children show the capacity to readily form preferences for the flavors of energy-rich foods.[13] In contrast, the response to bitter and sour

---

AAP

The American Academy of Pediatrics policy statement "Prevention of Choking Among Children" states that more than 10 000 emergency department visits annually are attributable to food-related choking for children younger than 14 years.

Risk factors for choking include age younger than 4 years, swallowing and neuromuscular disorders, developmental delay, and traumatic brain injury. Behavioral risk factors, such as walking or running while eating, laughing and talking with food in the mouth, and eating quickly, may also increase risk of choking.

High-risk foods for choking in all young children include: hot dogs, hard candy, peanuts/nuts, seeds, whole grapes, raw carrots, apples, popcorn, chunks of peanut butter, marshmallows, chewing gum, and sausages.
Pediatrics. 2010;125(3):601-607

tastants is reflexively negative.[14] Early experiences in utero and early infant
feeding, via transmission of aromatic compounds from the maternal diet
into amniotic fluid and human milk,[15] also potentially influence flavor and
food acceptance. These flavor experiences are believed to set the stage for
later food preferences and may be important in establishing lifelong food
habits. Acceptance of some foods, like vegetables, is not immediate and may
only occur after as many as 10 exposures to those foods in a noncoercive and
pleasant manner.[16–18] Many parents are not aware of the lengthy but normal
course of food acceptance in young children; approximately 25% of mothers
with toddlers reported offering new foods only 1 or 2 times before deciding
whether the child liked it, and approximately half made similar judgments
after serving new foods 3 to 5 times; thus, sufficient exposure to new foods
may not be attained for most children.[19] Touching, smelling, and playing
with new foods as well as putting them in the mouth and spitting them back
out are normal exploratory behaviors that precede acceptance and even
willingness to taste and swallow foods.[17] Beginning around 2 years of age,
children become characteristically resistant to consuming new foods—and
sometimes, dietary variety seemingly diminishes to a handful of well-
accepted favorites. In a study of 3022 infants and toddlers ranging from 6
to 24 months, half of mothers with 19- to 24-month-old toddlers reported
picky eating, whereas only 19% reported picky eating among 4- to 6-month-
old infants.[19] It should be stressed to families that children's failure to
immediately accept new foods is a normal stage of child development that,
although potentially frustrating, can be dealt with effectively with knowledge, consistency, and patience. Acceptance can be promoted by offering
children very small tastes of new and previously disliked vegetables.[20,21]
Further, whereas pressuring children to eat can produce dislike,[22] noncoercive strategies that emphasize "liking" over "eating" appear to promote food
acceptance. Positive experiences with eating, including enthusiastic modeling by adults,[23–26] praising children for trying new foods, providing small
token rewards (eg, stickers),[27–29] reading books with food-related characters
and themes,[30,31] and offering foods with "dips" or other preferred accompa-
niments may promote better acceptance of new or initially disliked foods.[32]
There is some suggestion that exposure to a variety of healthful foods and
textures during weaning and toddlerhood acts to promote acceptance into
childhood.[33–35] However, particularly for families with limited resources,
concerns about waste of time and finances may override willingness to offer
foods that are rejected more than once.[36]

Although toddlers are in a generally explorative phase, they can go on food "jags," during which certain foods are preferentially consumed to the exclusion of others. Parents who become concerned when a "good eater" in infancy becomes a "fair to poor" or "picky" eater as a toddler should be reassured that this change in acceptance is developmentally normative and, in most cases, lasts for a relatively short duration (<2 years).[37] Continuing to establish routines for mealtimes and snacks as well as offering new or previously rejected foods can help to establish an expectation that food preferences can change.[38] Encouraging caregivers to persist in offering tastes of less preferred, nutrient-dense foods (even as many as 8–10 tries), without expectations that children will consume a full serving, is considered the most effective approach. It is important to emphasize that benefits have been demonstrated when only small tastes are provided at each offering.[20] Encouragement of this strategy should be provided with the recognition that repeatedly offering foods that are rejected by the child may not be seen as feasible by some caregivers, particularly among low-income families with limited resources.

Preschool-Aged Children

Preschool-aged children have more fully developed motor skills, handle utensils and cups efficiently, and can sit at the table for meals.[39] Because growth has slowed, their interest in eating may be unpredictable, with characteristic periods of disinterest in food. Their attention span may limit the amount of time that they can spend in the mealtime setting; however, they should be encouraged to attend and partake in family meals for reasonable periods of time (15–20 minutes)—whether they choose to eat or not.

As children move from toddlerhood to the preschool years, they become increasingly aware of the environment in which eating occurs, particularly the social aspects of eating. By interacting with and observing other children and adults, preschool-aged children become more aware of when and where eating takes place, what types of foods are consumed at specific eating occasions (ie, ice cream is a dessert food), and how much of those foods are consumed at each eating occasion (ie, "finish your vegetables"). Consequently, children's development of norms for food selection and intake patterns are influenced by a variety of environmental cues, including the time of day[40]; energy-dense foods (defined as high amounts of energy per volume of food and drink in grams)[41–43] and large portion sizes[44–46] of foods; the home environment with respect to food and eating[47,48]; parental feeding styles and practices[49,50]; and the preferences and eating behaviors of important others, including family, teachers, and peers.[25,51,52]

During the preschool period, most children have moved from eating on demand to a more adult-like eating pattern, consuming 3 meals each day as well as 1 to 3 smaller snacks. Although children's intake from meal to meal may appear to be erratic, children show the capacity to adjust food intake such that total daily energy intake remains fairly constant.[53] Children show the ability to respond to the energy content of foods by adjusting their intake to reflect the energy density of the diet.[54-57] It is important to note, however, that this ability can be diminished when large food portion sizes of energy dense foods are frequently offered. In contrast to their skills in regulation of food intake, young children do not appear to have the innate ability to choose a well-balanced diet.[58] Rather, they depend on adults to offer them a variety of nutritious and developmentally appropriate foods and to model the consumption of those foods.

School-Aged Children

During the school years, increases in memory and logic abilities are accompanied by reading, writing, and math skills. This developmental period is one in which basic nutrition education concepts can be successfully introduced. Emphasis should be placed on enjoying the taste of fruits and vegetables rather than focusing exclusively on their healthfulness, because young children tend to think of taste and healthfulness as mutually exclusive.[59] Socially, children are learning rules and conventions and also begin to develop friendships. During the period between 8 and 11 years of age, children begin making more peer comparisons, including those pertaining to weight and body shape. An awareness of the physical self begins to emerge, and comparisons with social norms for weight and weight status begin to occur. During this period, children vary greatly in weight, body shape, and growth rate, and teasing of those who fall outside the perceived norms for weight status frequently occurs. Friends and those outside the family can alter food attitudes and choices, which may have either a beneficial or a negative effect on the nutritional status of a given child.

School-aged children have increased freedom over their food choices and, during the school year, eat at least 1 meal per day away from the home. These choices, such as the decision to consume school lunch or a snack bar meal, may affect dietary quality.[60]

Eating Patterns and Nutrient Needs

Toddlers

Toddlers eat, on average, 5 to 6 times each day, with snacks representing approximately one quarter of daily energy intake.[61] Between 15 and 24 months of age, approximately 59% of energy comes from table foods.[62] Milk constitutes the leading source of daily energy (approximately 25%), macronutrients, and many vitamins and minerals, including vitamins A and D, calcium, and zinc.[63] Recent data indicate that a majority of US toddlers' diets contain adequate amounts of protein and carbohydrates, but more than a quarter have total fat intakes below the recommended range.[64–66] Alternatively, vegetable and whole grain intakes are notably low or absent among some toddlers. Although 92% of children 9 through 11 months of age consume some type of vegetable daily, this number drops precipitously during toddlerhood, when close to 30% of children do not consume vegetables on a given day.[67–69] White potatoes remain the most commonly consumed vegetable among toddlers; nonfried forms (eg, baked, mashed) can be encouraged, along with other vegetables, as sources of fiber and potassium, which tend to be low in children's diets.[68,70] Finally, close to one quarter of 2-year-olds consume salty snacks daily and just under one half of children 1 to 2 years of age consume higher than the Tolerable Upper Level of intake for sodium.[64,66,71] Micronutrient-rich animal-source proteins should be encouraged in light of a recent focus on iron deficiency, which remains relatively common in toddlers at 13.5%[72]; 1 in 4 US 2-year-olds have usual iron intakes below the Recommended Dietary Allowance (RDA).[73]

Preschool- and School-Aged Children

Like toddlers, most preschool-aged children fail to meet current recommendations for vegetables and whole grains.[65] Additionally, only approximately 30% of preschoolers meet the 5-a-day recommendation for fruits and vegetables.[74] As such, a majority of preschool-aged children consume less than the recommended amounts of fiber and potassium,[75] with fruits and yeast breads making the greatest food group contributions to daily fiber intake and milk, fruit juice, and white potatoes making the greatest contributions to daily potassium intakes among US children.[76] Alternatively, young children's intakes of "extra" or "empty" calories from solid fats and added sugars exceed recommendations.[75,77,78] On any given day, approximately 90% of US children aged 2 to 4 years of age consume sweetened beverages, desserts, or sweets, which are top sources of added sugars.[76,79] Young children who consume high levels of added sugar (>25% of daily energy) have lower micronutrient intakes and may be at greater risk of inadequate intakes of number of micronutrients, particularly potassium.[80]

Anticipatory Guidance Related to Food and Eating

These findings collectively suggest that anticipatory guidance for toddlers and preschoolers should focus on encouraging intake of fruits, vegetables, and whole grains as well as lower-sodium foods at snacks and meals and should further stress that young children have high nutrient needs and relatively low energy requirements, leaving little room for sugar- and fat-dense foods (Table 7.1).[60]

Energy Needs

Dietary Reference Intakes (DRIs) are a set of nutrient-based reference values that can be used for planning and assessing diets of individuals and groups (see Appendix E).[81] The DRIs also include data on safety and efficacy, reduction of chronic degenerative disease (in addition to the avoidance of nutritional deficiency), and data on upper levels of intake (where available). The Estimated Average Requirement (EAR) refers to the median usual intake value that is estimated to meet the requirements of one half of apparently healthy individuals of a given age and sex over time. The RDA refers to the level of intake that is adequate for nearly all healthy individuals of a given sex and age (97%–98%). When the EAR or RDA has not been established, an Adequate Intake (AI) is provided and is based on average intake of a nutrient

Table 7.1.
Key Eating Recommendations

Nutrients
■ Limit sodium, added sugars
■ Consume adequate potassium, fiber, vitamins D and E, calcium
Foods
■ Chose appropriate weaning foods
■ Avoid sugar-sweetened beverages
■ Avoid energy-dense, nutrient-poor snacks
■ Encourage vegetables, fruits, and whole grains
■ Encourage low-fat dairy or alternatives fortified with calcium and vitamin D
Feeding
■ Establish meal and snack routines, with limits
■ Provide small tastes, repeated exposure to new foods
■ Model healthful eating

on the basis of intakes of healthy people. The Tolerable Upper Intake Level (UL) is the highest level of continuing daily nutrient intake that is likely to pose no risk of adverse health effects in almost all individuals. The UL, however, is *not* intended to be a recommended level of intake nor an expression of "toxicity." Using the age- and sex-specific EAR, it is possible to make a quantitative statistical assessment of the adequacy of an individual's usual intake of a nutrient and to assess the safety of an individual's usual intake by comparison with the UL.

Energy needs are highly variable in children and depend on basal metabolism, rate of growth, physical activity, body size, sex, and onset of puberty (see also Chapter 14: Energy). Many nutrient requirements depend on energy needs and intake. Micronutrients that are most likely to be low or deficient in the diets of young children are vitamin D, vitamin E, and potassium.[64,70,75] Of note, intakes of preformed vitamin A, zinc, and sodium are reported as increasingly exceeding ULs for a significant proportion of toddlers and preschool-aged children.[64] This is likely related to high intakes of fortified foods and use of supplements.[82] Although the ULs for nutrients are not meant to be used as rigid cutoffs or standards for ingestion, nutrients that are consumed in amounts over the ULs merit consideration regarding source (food-based vs supplement sources) and for potential adverse effects resulting from excessive consumption.[83]

Supplements

Parents frequently ask health care providers whether their children need vitamin supplements, and many routinely give supplements to their children, with recent estimates suggesting that approximately 25% of toddlers and 40% preschool-aged children are given a vitamin/mineral supplement daily.[75] The children who receive the supplements are not necessarily the children who need them most, however, and, in some cases, adequate or bioavailable amounts of marginal nutrients in their diets, such as calcium and zinc, are not included in the supplement. Routine supplementation is not necessary for healthy growing children who consume a varied diet as many processed foods that are commonly consumed (eg, ready-to-eat cereals, grain, and milk products) are fortified with additional nutrients. Foods that are fortified supply additional nutrients for which children may be at risk (eg, folate, other B vitamins, and calcium) and the majority of children who consume fortified products meet the reference standards for nutrient intakes.[83] For children and adolescents who cannot or will not consume adequate amounts of micronutrients from any dietary sources, the use of supplements should be considered. Children at nutritional risk who may benefit from supplementation include those:

1. With anorexia or an inadequate appetite or who have extremely selective diets;
2. With chronic disease (eg, cystic fibrosis, inflammatory bowel disease, or hepatic disease);
3. From food-deprived families or who suffer neglect or abuse;
4. Who participate in a dietary/bariatric surgery program for managing obesity;
5. Who consume a vegetarian diet without adequately consuming products with bioavailable minerals for bone deposition and maintenance;
6. With growth faltering (failure to thrive);
7. With developmental disabilities; or
8. From families with limited resources.[84]

Evaluation of dietary intake should be included in any assessment of the need for supplementation.[85–87] If parents wish to give their children supplements, a standard pediatric vitamin-mineral product containing nutrients in amounts no larger than the DRI (EAR or RDA) poses little risk. Levels higher than the DRI should be discouraged and counseling provided about the potential adverse effects, especially of fat-soluble vitamins and synthetic folate. Because the taste, shape, and color of most pediatric preparations are as attractive as candy, parents should be cautioned to keep them out of reach of children (see also Chapter 18: Calcium, Phosphorus, and Magnesium; Chapter 20: Trace Elements; and Chapter 21: Vitamins, for more information on vitamins and minerals).

Dietary Fats

In recent decades, emphasis and educational efforts supporting low-fat, low-cholesterol diets for the general population have increased, and changes in food packages distributed through the Special Supplemental Nutrition Program for Women, Infants, and Children (WIC) have resulted in decreases in children's total and saturated fat intake as well as improvements in overall diet quality.[88] A variety of health organizations, including the AAP, recommend against fat or cholesterol restriction for infants younger than 2 years, when rapid growth and development require high energy intakes.[78] For this reason, nonfat and low-fat milks are not recommended for use during the first 2 years of life, except in the case of children with a history of or concern for obesity and/or a family history of obesity, dyslipidemia, or cardiovascular disease.[89] For children between 12 months and 2 years of age with such a history, the use of reduced-fat milks and dairy products is appropriate. During the toddler years, fat intake should be gradually decreased so that total fat intake is limited to approximately 30% to 40% of total energy intake and saturated fats are limited to about 10% of total energy intake.[90] Parents should be reassured that this level of intake is sufficient for adequate growth[91,92] and does not place children at increased risk of nutritional inadequacy. Concerns have been expressed that some parents and their children may overinterpret the need to restrict their fat intakes. Indeed, 28% of toddlers 12 to 23 months of age and 47% of preschool-aged children 24 to 47 months of age consume less fat than recommended.[64,91] At the same time, mean intakes for consumption of saturated fats in children aged 2 through 11 years of age is higher than the recommended 10% of total energy.[93] Whole milk is a primary source of saturated fats in young children's diets.[65,77] Transitioning children's diets to provide less than 10% energy from saturated fat can be achieved by substituting low-fat milk products and dairy products, fruits, vegetables, beans, lean meat, poultry, fish, and whole-grain foods for those higher in saturated fats.[89] Recent meta-analyses of epidemiologic studies evaluating the relationship between solid fat intake and cardiovascular disease have questioned the relationship between the two and revealed that additional evidence should be collected to support the guidance on saturated fat consumption.[94] Of note, the US Food and Drug Administration determined recently that *trans* fats, or partially hydrogenated oils that were previously added to extend shelf life, were not "generally recognized as safe" (GRAS) as additives to the food supply, and most *trans* fats now are prohibited from being added to commercially produced food products. The Nutrition Facts Label includes the amount of *trans* fats found in a product from naturally occurring and added ingredients.[95] The Dietary Guidelines for Americans 2015–2020 recommend that all Americans, 2 years of age and older, limit ingestion of *trans* fats.[90]

Dietary Guidelines and ChooseMyPlate

The US Department of Agriculture has developed 2 main nutritional guides that can be used in feeding children. Dietary Guidelines for Americans 2015 is intended for children 2 years and older to encourage 5 main concepts: (1) follow a healthy eating pattern across the lifespan; (2) focus on variety, nutrient density, and amount; (3) limit calories from saturated fats and added sugars and reduce sodium intake; (4) shift to healthier food and beverage choices; and (5) support healthier eating patterns for all.[90] The Dietary Guidelines were developed for policy makers and health care providers as a basis for nutrition education materials, health policies, and federal food programs. ChooseMyPlate (see Appendix F)[96] is the consumer-oriented compendium that was introduced with the 2010 Dietary Guidelines to help consumers make better food choices by translating the Dietary Guidelines into food group-based recommendations. Key recommendations are: (1) "building a healthy plate" with a focus on increasing fruit, vegetable, and whole grain consumption; and (2) choosing appropriate portion sizes. These 2 strategies are aimed at increasing nutrient density and balancing energy intakes with energy expenditure. In addition to helping parents understand the amounts that children need from each food group, this tool can be used to convey basic nutrition concepts for feeding young children, such as variety, moderation, the allowance for all types of foods in the diet, and appropriate portion sizes.

Understanding appropriate portions for children is important in light of large food portion sizes that are common in the marketplace,[97] and both adults and children consume more food and beverages when offered larger food portion sizes than when offered smaller sizes.[98] Table 7.2 gives examples of portion sizes that can be offered to children of differing ages to achieve recommended daily food group intakes. One standard for portions that may be followed for young children (2–6 years of age) is to initially offer 1 tablespoon of foods (fruits, vegetables, and protein/main course foods) for every year of age, with more provided according to appetite.[99,100]

On balance, the 2015 Dietary Guidelines urge adults and children to shift to better food choices and eating patterns, eat fewer calories, and be active.[90] Parents are encouraged to: (1) help children to maintain appropriate calorie balance during childhood and adolescence; (2) encourage consumption of fruits, vegetables, and whole grains in everyday food choices with moderate consumption of 100% fruit juice; (3) reduce intakes of refined grain products, sodium, calories from saturated fats and added sugars, particularly from sugar-sweetened beverages; and (4) enable children to achieve at least 60 minutes of physical activity on most, if not all, days of the week and to reduce sedentary pastimes by limiting screen time.

In all settings where children are offered food and beverage, attention to food safety is paramount. Observance of good food safety protocols includes the steps in Table 7.3 (see also Chapter 51: Food Safety: Infectious Disease).

Table 7.2.
Feeding Guide for Children[a]

Food	Age, y						
	2 to 3 (1000–1400 kcal)		4 to 6 (1200–1800 kcal)		7 to 12 (1400–2000 kcal)		Comments
	Portion Size	Daily Amounts	Portion Size	Daily Amounts	Portion Size	Daily Amounts	
Low-fat milk and dairy	½ c (4 oz)	2½ c	½–¾ c (4–6 oz)	2½–3 c	½–1 c (4–8 oz)	2½–3 c	½ c milk equivalents: ½ oz natural cheese, 1 oz processed cheese, ½ c low fat yogurt, 2½ T nonfat dry milk.
Meat, fish, poultry or equivalent	1–2 oz	2–4 oz	1–2 oz	3–5 oz	2 oz	4–5½ oz	1 oz meat equivalents: 1 egg, 1 T peanut butter, ½ cup cooked beans or peas.
Vegetables Cooked, Raw[b]	¼ c Few pieces	1½ c	½ c Few pieces	1½–2½ c	½ c Several pieces	1½–2½ c	Include dark green and orange vegetables for vitamin A, such as carrots, spinach, broccoli, winter squash, or greens. Limit starchy vegetables.
Fruit Canned Raw[b]	¼ c ½–1 small	1½ c	½ c ½–1 small	1–1½ c	½ c 1 medium	1½–2 c	Include vitamin C-rich sources such as citrus juices, orange, grapefruit, strawberries, melon, tomato, or broccoli.
Juice[c]		3–4 oz		4–6 oz		≤8 oz	

[a] Adapted from http://www.choosemyplate.gov/ and the 2015 Dietary Guidelines for Americans.
[b] Do not give to young children until they can chew well.
[c] AAP recommendations.

Continued

Table 72. *Continued*
Feeding Guide for Children[a]

| Food | 2 to 3 (1000–1400 kcal) | | 4 to 6 (1200–1800 kcal) | | 7 to 12 (1400–2000 kcal) | | Comments |
	Portion Size	Daily Amounts	Portion Size	Daily Amounts	Portion Size	Daily Amounts	
Grains Whole grain or enriched bread Cooked cereal Dry cereal	½ slice ½ c ½ c	3–5 oz (1½–2½ oz whole grain)	½–1 slice ½–1 c ½–1 c	4–6 oz (2–3 oz whole grain)	1 slice 1 c 1 c	5–6 oz (2½–3 oz whole grain)	1 slice bread equivalents: ½ c noodles, rice, or corn grits; 5 saltines; ½ English muffin or bagel; 1 tortilla. Make ½ of grain intake *whole grains*.
Oils		4 tsp		4–5 tsp		4–6 tsp	Choose soft margarines. Avoid *trans* fats. Use liquid vegetable oils rather than solid fats.

[a] Adapted from http://www.choosemyplate.gov/ and the 2015 Dietary Guidelines for Americans.
[b] Do not give to young children until they can chew well.
[c] AAP recommendations.

Table 7.3.
Appropriate Food Safety Protocols

- **Clean** hands, food-contact surfaces, and vegetables and fruits.
- **Separate** raw, cooked, and ready-to-eat foods while shopping, storing, and preparing foods.
- **Cook** foods to a safe temperature.
- **Chill** (refrigerate) perishable foods promptly.
- Some foods pose high risk of foodborne illness. These include raw (unpasteurized) milk, cheeses, and juices; raw or undercooked animal foods, such as seafood, meat, poultry, and eggs; and raw sprouts.

Federal Food Safety Gateway: www.foodsafety.gov and http://www.fightbac.org

Parenting and the Feeding Relationship

The parent-child relationship is transactional, meaning that although the child's behavior is influenced by the parent, the parent's behavior is equally influenced by the child. It is always important to recognize that the child is not a "tabula rasa" (ie, a blank slate) but is bringing behaviors to the table that are likely biologically determined and to which the parent is tasked with responding. For example, a substantial proportion of the variance in body weight[101] and both selective eating[102] and propensity for overeating are genetic.[103,104] Thus, the parent of a thin, picky eater will need different parenting skills than the parent of a child with rapid weight gain who frequently asks for food and eats meals quickly and voraciously. The pediatric provider may be most effective if he or she is able to tailor advice to the individual child and family.

Across different types of child eating styles, there are a number of parenting behaviors that should be promoted. Structuring the timing and frequency of eating occasions is important. This is an opportunity to limit snacking and establish eating routines. Likewise, offering a variety of healthy foods in appropriate portion sizes is a valuable strategy for all types of eaters. Using eating occasions to model healthy eating for the child and teach the child about healthy eating and nutrition are also strategies that are likely to be universally beneficial. Ideally, eating should occur in a designated area of the home with a developmentally appropriate seating arrangement for the child. Family meals, with adults present and eating at least some of the same foods as the child, have been linked with a number of positive outcomes. Finally, providing repeated opportunities to taste new foods (up to 8–10) is likely to increase the child's acceptance of a new food and diversify the diet.

In general, behaviors to avoid in parenting around feeding are those that reflect excessive control. Excessive control can take the form of either pressuring children to eat or exerting too much restriction. The manner in which parents approach feeding has important implications for child behavioral, dietary, and weight outcomes.[49,50,105] Authoritative approaches to feeding, characterized by adults encouraging children to eat healthy foods and allowing the child to have limited choices but stopping short of pressuring or forcing, has been associated with increased availability and intake of fruits, vegetables, and dairy and lower intake of "less nutritious" foods.[105,106] In contrast, authoritarian approaches to feeding, characterized by attempts to control children's eating, have been associated with lower intakes of fruit, juices, and vegetables. Highly controlling feeding practices, including the use of bribes, threats, and food restriction, have negative effects on eating behaviors in young children and have been related to the inability to regulate energy intake and weight status in some studies.[22,105,107,108] Alternatively, some parents have difficulty saying "no" to their toddlers' demands and indulge children's wishes rather than establish limits. Indulgent approaches to feeding, characterized by little structure or limit setting in feeding, have been associated with greater intake of fat and sweet foods, more snacks, fewer healthy food choices, and overweight among preschool-aged children.[105,109] Whether excessive pressure or restriction actually cause unhealthy eating behaviors or inadequate or excessive weight gain remains in debate.[105] However, these parenting practices are unlikely to be helpful and are likely to contribute to unnecessary parent-child conflict and stress. As in most domains of parenting, moderation and flexibility are essential. For example, gentle and sensitive encouragement to expand the child's dietary repertoire is appropriate, but pressure is not helpful. Likewise, attentiveness to keeping unhealthy foods out of the home, providing reasonable portion sizes, and ongoing teaching about the how and why to avoid consuming junk food are appropriate, but excessive and punitive restriction is not.

Parents face unique challenges in feeding today. Their child's weight status and eating behaviors are often viewed as entirely a result of the quality of parenting, when in reality children are not simply blank slates. Parents are cautioned against restricting their child's intake for fear of imparting unhealthy weight control behaviors and body image concerns

Table 7.4.
Feeding Guidance for Parents

- Offer a variety of healthy foods and limit unhealthy food availability in the home.
- Promote routines for eating occasions with regard to timing, frequency, and location.
- Create positive eating environments with appropriate physical components (chairs, tables, utensils, cups, etc) that are free of distractions (eg, screen media).
- Offer developmentally appropriate portion sizes.
- Model healthy eating behaviors.
- Regard eating occasions as a time of learning and mastery with respect to eating and social skills and with respect to family and community time.
- Offer foods repeatedly (up to 8–10 times) and patiently to establish children's acceptance.
- Offer 3 meals and 2 snacks per day.
- Avoid excessive control, including pressure, coercion, and extreme restriction.
- Recognize and respect the biologically based contributors to the child's eating behavior and growth patterns.

but are also faced with appropriately limiting their child's intake in a highly obesogenic environment. Weight-related stigma regarding adults is well-documented, and there is an increasing focus in adults to recognize that obesity is largely not a result of poor self-control. Pediatric providers are in a key position to recognize the stigma experienced by parents of children who are both particularly thin and particularly heavy, and to provide parents understanding and support. Sharing with parents the perspective that their child's growth patterns and eating behaviors are driven by both nature and nurture acknowledges the complexity of parenting and the need to tailor feeding practices to the individual child. Basic feeding guidance that can be offered to parents is provided in Table 7.4.

Special Topics

Feeding During Illness
The AAP clinical practice guideline on the management of acute gastroenteritis in young children recommends that only oral electrolyte solutions be used to rehydrate infants and young children and that a normal diet be

continued throughout an episode of gastroenteritis[100,101] (see also Chapter 28: Oral Therapy for Acute Diarrhea). Infants and young children can experience a decrease in nutritional statuos and the illness can be prolonged with a clear liquid diet, especially when it is extended beyond a few days.[102] The practice of withholding food for 24 or more hours is inappropriate.[110] Continuous or early refeeding has been shown to shorten the duration of the diarrhea. Recommendations for toddlers and preschool-aged children include reintroduction of solid foods shortly after rehydration. Foods that are usually well tolerated include rice cereals, bananas, potatoes, eggs, rice, plain pasta, and other similar foods. Dairy products, in recommended amounts, can also be included. Lactose-free formulas and avoiding fat are usually unnecessary.[111] Further, highly restrictive diets such as the "BRAT" diet (bananas, rice, applesauce, and toast) are also unnecessary and do not provide adequate amounts of essential nutrients.[111] During acute childhood illnesses, a variety of foods should be offered according to the child's appetite and tolerance, with extra fluids provided when fever, diarrhea, or vomiting are present.

Obesity

Obesity is among the most pressing nutritional issues facing US children, currently affecting 17.0% of children 2 to 19 years of age, with extreme obesity seen among 5.8% of children.[112] Health consequences of obesity are profound and include elevated risks of social stigmatization, hyperlipidemia, abnormal glucose tolerance, noninsulin-dependent diabetes mellitus, and hypertension.[113,114] The incidence of obesity and its risks during childhood increases with age. During the period of 2011–2014, obesity affected 8.9% of children 2 through 5 years of age, 17.5% of children 6 through 11 years of age, and 20.5% of adolescents 12 to 19 years of age.[112] The most recent prevalence data from 2011–2014 provide evidence of decreases in obesity among preschool-aged children and leveling off among children 6 through 11 years of age. However, increases in obesity prevalence continue to be seen among adolescents[128] (see also Chapter 33: Obesity).

For many children, obesity is established at an early age. A recent nationally representative longitudinal study of children found that 72% of children who were obese in kindergarten and 63% who had even episodic periods of obesity during the subsequent 3 years remained obese in adolescence.[115] Environmental factors are thought to play an important role the development of obesity, given that secular increases have occurred too rapidly to be explained solely by genetic influences alone.[116,117] For children, exposure to environmental influences is filtered through the contexts in which eating routinely occurs, including home, early care and education settings, and school. Parents have a particularly important role in the etiology of childhood overweight, because they provide children with both genes and the environment in which eating and physical activity take place.[118] Evidence of this point is found in the fact that the tracking of childhood overweight into adulthood is particularly strong among children who have one or more overweight parents.[119]

It is recommended that children 6 years or older with body mass index (BMI) $\geq$95th percentile undergo evaluation and referral to an intensive, comprehensive behavioral treatment that includes nutrition, physical activity, and behavioral counseling and active parental involvement.[120] A longitudinal developmental approach by pediatricians is encouraged to help identify children early in the excess weight gain trajectory. Prevention efforts, at a minimum, should include adherence to recommendations to plot and track BMI on growth charts and to discuss obesity-related topics frequently (see Chapter 33: Obesity). When possible, guidance to promote healthful eating patterns in the overweight child should be directed toward modifying the dietary intake patterns and behaviors of the family as a whole rather than focusing only on the overweight child.[121] These discussions should focus on the types of foods that are available in the home, identifying appropriate portion sizes, and incorporating low-energy, nutrient-rich foods into the child and family's diet, as referenced earlier in the discussion of ChooseMyPlate.gov. Helping parents and caregivers to assess their home food and physical activity environments, including foods that should be limited (such as sweetened beverages and high-calorie snacks), and to determine what changes can be made to the environment may be helpful. Parents should also be made aware that highly restrictive approaches to child feeding are not effective but rather appear to promote the intake of restricted foods[108,122] and contribute to low self-appraisal.[123] Further, parents should be encouraged to exhibit the eating behaviors they would like their children to adopt and act as agents of change, because children learn to model their parents' eating and behaviors.[124]

Increased physical activity is a critical component of childhood obesity prevention, because sedentary behavior has been associated with overweight among children.[125,126] Health care providers should inquire about the child's amount of screen time and whether there is access to screen media in the child's bedroom.[127,128] Parents should be encouraged to limit screen time to 1 hour per day for children 2 through 5 years of age and to avoid media exposure for children younger than 18 to 24 months.[129] For children 6 years and older, the recommendation for consistent limits on the amount of all types of media are encouraged, and designating mealtime as "media free" is endorsed.[130] Parents and caregivers have a central responsibility in this area, because they serve as role models for active lifestyles and are children's gatekeepers to opportunities to be physically active. Play and adequate sleep time are essential to children's healthy development and well-being.[131] The establishment of child and family routines for eating, activity, and sleep hygiene are recommended, particularly for the young child. Health care providers should convey the importance of encouraging activity in the entire family as well as among individuals within the family. Children should be encouraged to participate in discussions of modifications of diet and physical activity. Taking into account their preferences will allow them a sense of responsibility for decisions about their behavior.

Beverage Consumption

Consumption of 100% fruit juice is common among young children, and its contribution to diet and growth have been debated. In 2009–2010, approximately 50% of children younger than 1 year through 5 years of age consumed 100% fruit juice on any given day.[132] On one hand, excessive juice consumption has been associated with carbohydrate malabsorption and chronic nonspecific diarrhea in healthy children and the development of dental caries.[133] Additionally, excessive juice consumption has been linked to both malnutrition and nonorganic failure to thrive as well as excessive consumption and obesity. On the other hand, 100% fruit juice consumption has been positively associated with children's intake of vitamin C, folate, magnesium, and potassium.[132,134] Currently, roughly one third of total fruit intake among US children 2 to 19 years of age, which is lower than recommended, comes from 100% fruit juice.[135] Further, when consumed within recommended levels, 100% fruit juice does not appear to be associated with overweight/obesity or childhood dental caries and does not compromise fiber intake.[134]

AAP

AAP Recommendations for Fruit Juice Intake in Children[133]

- Intake of fruit juice should be limited to 4 oz per day for children 1 through 3 years of age and to 4–6 oz for children 4 to 6 years of age. For children 7 through 17 years old, juice intake should be limited to 8 oz per day.
- Children should be encouraged to eat whole fruits to meet their recommended daily fruit intake.
- Children should not consume unpasteurized juice.
- Health care providers should determine the amount of juice consumed by children being evaluated for malnutrition (overnutrition and undernutrition), chronic diarrhea, excessive flatulence, abdominal pain and bloating, and dental caries.
- Pediatricians should routinely discuss fruit juice, fruit drinks, and the difference between the 2 with parents.

Pediatrics. 2017;139(6):e20170967

According to ChooseMyPlate, 1 cup of 100% fruit juice can be considered as 1 cup from the Fruit Group.[96] Preschool-aged children 2 through 5 years of age with 1000 to 1600 kcal daily energy requirements should consume 1 to 1½ cups of fruit per day and may be offered up to ½ cup to ¾ cup (4–6 oz) of 100% fruit juice per day. Fruit punch and fruit drinks contain little or no fruit; these drinks provide calories, but few or no nutrients.

Similarly, the AAP position on fruit juice consumption in children holds that 100% fresh or reconstituted fruit juice can be a healthy part of the diet of children older than 1 year when consumed as part of a well-balanced diet. AAP recommendations for juice intake among children are detailed in the text box.[133] However, children should be encouraged to eat whole fruit as the primary way to meet their recommended daily fruit intake. Parents should be educated regarding the benefit of fiber intake from whole fruit relative to juice and, conversely, the potential concerns about dental caries and excessive energy intake from fruit juice relative to whole fruit.

Sugar-sweetened beverages including fruit-flavored juices, soft drinks, sweetened teas, and sports drinks are also commonly consumed among children and make significant contributions to intakes of added sugars and energy.[78,136] Almost a third of toddlers and 66% of children 2 to 19 years of age consume sweetened beverages daily.[74,137–139] Further, sweetened beverages are one of the top 10 contributors (3.1%) to daily energy among toddlers[140] and in the top 5 contributors to daily energy among older children,[76] currently providing 7.3% of energy in the diets of children 2 to 19 years of age.[139] Between 1977 and 2001, soft drink intake among children 2 to 18 years of age more than doubled, largely because of increases in the average portion size consumed.[141] Since that time, however, decreases in soft drink consumption have been noted among children. Currently, fruit drinks represent the greatest proportion of sugar-sweetened beverage intakes among US children 2 through 11 years of age. Consistent evidence links consumption of sugar-sweetened beverages with weight gain and adiposity among children,[142–144] underscoring the need for anticipatory feeding guidance to parents and caregivers.[163,164]

In the past decade, sports and energy drinks have become a more focal part of children's sugar-sweetened beverage consumption.[158] From 1999–2000 to 2008, consumers of sports and energy drinks increased from 3% to 7% among children and from 4% to 12% among adolescents.[138,145] Although both contain significant calories, a primary distinction between sports and energy drinks is the caffeine content of energy drinks. In 2009–2010, 58% of US children 2 through 5 years of age and 75% of children 6 through 11 years of age consumed caffeine on a given day; the median consumption among consumers in these age groups, however, was relatively low, at 4.7 mg and 9.1 mg, respectively.[146,147] Energy drinks contain large and varied amounts of caffeine, with the total amount of caffeine in some energy drinks exceeding 500 mg (approximately the amount in 15 cans of caffeinated soft drinks).[159] A recent systematic review concluded that no adverse effects were associated with daily caffeine consumption among children of ≤2.5 mg/kg of body weight, although the evidence remains limited for outcomes of interest.[148] Given the absence of health benefits and concerns regarding caffeine consumption and excessive energy intakes from these drinks,[149] the AAP recommends that children do not consume caffeine.[150] Pediatricians should inquire about the use of sports and energy drinks during routine health visits.

AAP

The American Academy of Pediatrics recommends that sports and energy drinks not be consumed by children to avoid excess energy intake and any level of caffeine intake.

Pediatrics. 2017;127(6):1182–1189

In summary, evidence to date suggests that consumption of sugar-sweetened beverages should be limited.[165] For children with either chronic diarrhea or excessive weight gain, obtaining a diet history, including the volume of fruit and soft drinks consumed, is useful for anticipatory guidance. Intake of 100% fruit juice should be monitored and it should be in moderation. Parents should be encouraged to routinely offer plain, unflavored water to children, particularly for fluids consumed outside of meals and snacks.[150]

Snacking

Snacking is nearly universal among young children.[61] Because of smaller and fluctuating appetites, most young children eat several small snacks daily in addition to meals. Nationally representative data from 1977–2014, however, indicate that US children 2 through 5 years of age currently snack more frequently and consume greater energy from snacks than in previous decades, with larger increases seen among children in the lowest poverty and household education groups.[151] Although often considered an accessory to mealtime intake, snacking occasions contribute more energy to young children's diets than any other single meal. In 2013–2014, US children 2 through 5 years of age consumed close to one third of their daily energy intake from snacks. [151] Whether snacking habits of young children contribute to dietary adequacy or excess is debated and the optimal frequency of snacking remains unknown. In 2013–2014, snacks contributed approximately 25% or more to young children's intake of several shortfall nutrients, including vitamin E, vitamin D, and potassium. At the same time, snacks contributed nearly 40% of daily added sugar intakes among preschool-aged children,[152] with greater daily intakes of energy and added sugars seen among children who snacked more frequently.[153,154] Frequent snacking has been suggested to contribute to obesity; however, the evidence is equivocal,[155] limited to studies of older children, and lacking methodologic rigor. An analysis of 2003–2012 NHANES data that adjusted for the accuracy of dietary reporting revealed positive associations of snacking frequency with overweight and abdominal obesity among US children 6 through 11 years of age.[156] There is some suggestion that heavier children with greater eating motivation may also be prone to more frequent snacking and greater energy intakes from snacks.[154] Recent work also highlights the role of parenting in snacking behavior of young children. Qualitative studies reveal that caregivers offer children snacks for both nutritive and nonnutritive purposes including uses as rewards, to manage behavior, and to quiet/calm the child. Offering children snacks for nonnutritive reasons has been associated with lower child adherence to dietary recommendations relevant to obesity prevention.[157] Anticipatory guidance should encourage parents and caregivers to think of snacks as "mini-meals" and planned so they contribute to the total day's nutrient intake. Healthful snacks accepted by many children include fresh fruit, cheese, whole-grain crackers, bread products (eg, bagels, pita, tortillas, and rice crackers), milk, vegetables, 100% fruit juices, sandwiches, peanut butter, and yogurt.

Food Availability in the Home Environment

One approach to improving individuals' dietary patterns, including children's dietary intakes, is to improve the quality of the food that is available in the home eating environment. Interventions targeted at changing the foods that are available and accessible for young children to consume have been effective in promoting increases in fruit and vegetable consumption.[158,159] Further, interventions that have sought to reduce the availability of noncore, less nutritious foods have demonstrated decreases in children's consumption of these foods and modest improvements in child weight status.[160,161] The effects of these interventions have been suggested to be both direct and indirect—that is, increases in availability of healthy foods is likely to give rise to increases in caregivers offering children these foods. It also follows that decreasing home availability of noncore, high-energy/low-nutrient density foods would result in fewer offerings and less intake of highly desirable foods that are associated with power struggles and contentious transactions between caregivers and young children. Moreover, some studies reveal that when healthy foods are more available, caregivers also consume more of them and thereby increase the modeling of healthy eating behaviors for their children—an indirect pathway to improving children's dietary intake and quality.[159,162–164] These associations have been noted across child age and socioeconomic strata as well as in different cultures and countries.

Therefore, it would seem that one strategy to improve the foods that children consume is to focus on the home food environment in addition to the child. By reducing the number of noncore foods and increasing healthy food options, parents can increase children's exposure to healthy foods they desire them to learn to eat, consume and model consumption of these foods for their children, potentially reduce consumption of less healthy options, and avoid some difficult transactions and power struggles with their children over highly palatable foods.

Media Influences on Children's Eating

Among US children 8 through 10 years of age, the average amount of time spent in a variety of media is nearly 8 hours per day and even more in teenagers (>11 hours per day).[165] Children watch more television than any other type of media.[166] One study showed that preschool-aged children spend an average of 1.8 hours each day watching television, and children 6 through 11 years of age were reported to watch about 2.1 hours per day.[167] The more time children spend watching television, the more likely they are to have higher energy intakes and to be overweight compared with children who watch less television.

Exposure to advertisements for foods high in solid fats, added salt, and sugar, including fast foods and carbonated beverages, may contribute to this relationship.[173] In 2009, 48 companies spent $1.8 billion in targeted food marketing to children 2 through 17 years of age.[168] Half of these marketing dollars were focused on media characters and tie-ins with movies, television programs, videogames, and social media targeted at children. Analysis of television advertisements on popular children's television in 11 countries showed that 53% to 87% of foods advertised were high in undesirable nutrients, including added sugars and fats. Children who are exposed to food advertisements are more likely to recall and prefer advertised foods and brands and to request and consume advertised brands.[169,170] In fact, young children prefer and choose foods that have been associated with popular food brands and cartoon characters.[171] In one study, children's knowledge of toys and promotions offered by fast food outlets was positively associated with their consumption of foods from these outlets, even when controlling for parent demographics and parent fast food consumption.[172] In a Canadian study of 9- through 11-year-olds, television viewing was negatively associated with consumption of fruits, vegetables, and green vegetables and positively associated with consumption of sweets, soft drinks, diet soft drinks, French fries, fast food, and other noncore foods.[173] Children who watch more television also have shorter average sleep durations, particularly if there is a television in the bedroom,[174] and this has previously been associated with childhood obesity rates.[175] Anticipatory guidance should strongly encourage parents and caregivers to limit screen time for toddlers and young children or to actively coview television with their children, including dialogue about advertising content. [152,153]

Feeding in the Context of Food Insecurity

As disussed in Chapter 49: Preventing Food Insecurity – Available Community Nutrition Programs, food insecurity is common and substantially affect children's nutrition and well-being. Food insecurity has a signficant effect on parents' ability to implement feeding recommendations and also shapes their feeding behaviors. In addition, mothers in food insecure households have been reported to have more controlling feeding styles, both pressuring and restricting their children's eating.[176] These more controlling feeding behaviors may occur because families cannot afford to waste food, and therefore, even when chidlren may not like what is being offered, they may be pressured to eat it since there may not be other options. Families with limited resoruces for food may also purchase more low-cost, energy-dense foods to "fill the child up."[177] There may also be a greater focus on quantity of intake as opposed to quality.[178] Thus, pediatric health care providers should consider how feasible it is for some families to offer a child a vegatable 8 to 10 times, only to have that vegetable repeatedly rejected and for the child to be hungry later with no other food to offer. In addition, some families living in "food deserts" in which there are few accessible supermarkets and grocery stores may struggle as well to include frequent variety in the child's diet. In summary, the pediatric health care provider should consider the social context in which families attempt to implement feeding recommendations, recognize barriers, and assist families in accessing food-related resources (ie, WIC, food stamps).

The Role of Anticipatory Guidance in Promoting Healthy Eating Behaviors

Prevention is generally much more effective than treatment once a problem has developed. Therefore, the pediatric provider has a key role in delivering anticipatory guidance to parents to promote the development of healthy eating behaviors that could last a lifetime. Parents' primary concern for toddlers and young preschoolers is often selective or picky eating behaviors, and the pediatric provider's role in this developmental stage is generally to provide reassurance and prevent the emergence of inappropriately pressuring feeding behaviors. However, in the current obesogenic environment, parents are also increasingly concerned about how to prevent excessive weight gain in their children in healthy and adaptive ways. The pediatric provider plays a key role in guiding parents regarding creating structure with regard to timing and frequency of eating occasions, appropriate portion sizes and sensitive responding to frequent food requests.

The pediatric health care provider is especially well-positioned to deliver information about developing healthy eating habits timed to the child's specific developmental stage. Each well-child visit provides the opportunity to discuss with the family what they can anticipate to occur in the coming months and to guide the family through these developmental transitions. The pediatric health care provider, who usually has a long-term relationship with the family, is also able to tailor guidance to the unique attributes of the child and family. For example, some children may be thinner and selective or picky eaters with concerned parents, in which case anticipatory guidance may be best focused on alleviating parental concern and reducing pressure to eat. In contrast, other children may be hearty eaters with excessive weight gain, in which case anticipatory guidance may instead best focus on sensitive guidance around preventing early childhood obesity.

In summary, the pediatric provider is in an ideal position to provide anticipatory guidance to achieve optimal health outcomes with regard to growth, feeding, and nutrition. Tailoring this guidance to the developmental stage of the child and unique attributes of the child and family that may confer specific risks can optimize the health and well-being of each child.

References

1. WHO Multicentre Growth Reference Study Group. WHO Child Growth Standards: Length/height-for-age, weight-for-age, weight-for-length, weight-for-height, and body mass index-for-age: Methods and development. Geneva, Switzerland: World Health Organization; 2006

2. Brotanek JM, Halterman JS, Auinger P, Flores G, Weitzman M. Iron deficiency, prolonged bottle-feeding, and racial/ethnic disparities in young children. *Arch Pediatr Adolesc Med.* 2005;159(11):1038–1042

3. Brotanek JM, Schroer D, Valentyn L, Tomany-Korman S, Flores G. Reasons for prolonged bottle-feeding and iron deficiency among Mexican-American toddlers: an ethnographic study. *Acad Pediatr.* 2009;9(1):17–25

4. Gooze RA, Anderson SE, Whitaker RC. Prolonged bottle use and obesity at 5.5 years of age in US children. *J Pediatr.* 2011;159(3):431–436

5. Bonuck K, Avraham SB, Lo Y, Kahn R, Hyden C. Bottle-weaning intervention and toddler overweight. *J Pediatr.* 2014;164(2):306–312 e301–302

6. Section on Pediatric D, Oral H. Preventive oral health intervention for pediatricians. *Pediatrics.* 2008;122(6):1387–1394

7. Carruth BR, Ziegler PJ, Gordon A, Hendricks K. Developmental milestones and self-feeding behaviors in infants and toddlers. *J Am Diet Assoc.* 2004;104 (1 Suppl 1):S51–S56

8. Chapin MM, Rochette LM, Annest JL, Haileyesus T, Conner KA, Smith GA. Nonfatal choking on food among children 14 years or younger in the United States, 2001–2009. *Pediatrics.* 2013;132(2):275–281

9. Committee on Injury V, Poison P. Prevention of choking among children. *Pediatrics.* 2010;125(3):601–607

10. Altkorn R, Chen X, Milkovich S, et al. Fatal and non-fatal food injuries among children (aged 0-14 years). *Int J Pediatr Otorhinolaryngol.* 2008;72(7):1041–1046

11. Centers for Disease C, Prevention. Nonfatal choking-related episodes among children—United States, 2001. *MMWR Morb Mortal Wkly Rep.* 2002;51(42):945–948

12. Desor JA, Maller O, Turner RE. Taste acceptance of sugars by human infants. *J Compar Physiol Psychol.* 1973;84(3):496–501

13. Kern DL, McPhee L, Fisher J, Johnson S, Birch LL. The postingestive consequences of fat condition preferences for flavors associated with high dietary fat. *Physiol Behav.* 1993;54(1):71–76

14. Hayes JE, Johnson SL. Sensory aspects of bitter and sweet tastes during early childhood. *Nutrition Today.* 2017;52(2):S41–S51

15. Beauchamp GK, Mennella JA. Early flavor learning and its impact on later feeding behavior. *J Pediatr Gastroenterol Nutr.* 2009;48(Suppl 1):S25–S30

16. Sullivan S, Birch LL. Pass the sugar, pass the salt; experience dictates preference. *Dev Psychol.* 1990;26(4):546–551

17. Johnson SL, Bellows L, Beckstrom L, Anderson J. Evaluation of a social marketing campaign targeting preschool children. *Am J Health Behav.* 2007;31(1):44–55

18. Wardle J, Cooke LJ, Gibson EL, Sapochnik M, Sheiham A, Lawson M. Increasing children's acceptance of vegetables; a randomized trial of parent-led exposure. *Appetite.* 2003;40(2):155–162

19. Carruth BR, Ziegler PJ, Gordon A, Barr SI. Prevalence of picky eaters among infants and toddlers and their caregivers' decisions about offering a new food. *J Am Diet Assoc.* 2004;104(1 Suppl 1):S57–S64

20. Lakkakula A, Geaghan J, Zanovec M, Pierce S, Tuuri G. Repeated taste exposure increases liking for vegetables by low-income elementary school children. *Appetite.* 2010;55(2):226–231

21. Lakkakula A, Geaghan JP, Wong WP, Zanovec M, Pierce SH, Tuuri G. A cafeteria-based tasting program increased liking of fruits and vegetables by lower, middle and upper elementary school-age children. *Appetite.* 2011;57(1):299–302

22. Birch LL, Birch D, Marlin DW, Kramer L. Effects of instrumental consumption on children's food preference. *Appetite.* 1982;3(2):125–134

23. Hendy HM. Comparison of five teacher actions to encourage children's new food acceptance. *Ann Behav Med.* 1999;21(1):20–26

24. Hendy HM. Effectiveness of trained peer models to encourage food acceptance in preschool children. *Appetite*. 2002;39(3):217–225

25. Hendy HM, Raudenbush B. Effectiveness of teacher modeling to encourage food acceptance in preschool children. *Appetite*. 2000;34(1):61–76

26. Addessi E, Galloway AT, Visalberghi E, Birch LL. Specific social influences on the acceptance of novel foods in 2-5-year-old children. *Appetite*. 2005;45(3):264–271

27. Cooke LJ, Chambers LC, Anez EV, et al. Eating for pleasure or profit: the effect of incentives on children's enjoyment of vegetables. *Psychol Sci*. 2011;22(2):190–196

28. Corsini N, Slater A, Harrison A, Cooke L, Cox DN. Rewards can be used effectively with repeated exposure to increase liking of vegetables in 4-6-year-old children. *Public Health Nutr*. 2013;16(5):942–951

29. Horne PJ, Greenhalgh J, Erjavec M, Lowe CF, Viktor S, Whitaker CJ. Increasing pre-school children's consumption of fruit and vegetables. A modelling and rewards intervention. *Appetite*. 2011;56(2):375–385

30. Health PM, Houston-Price C, Kennedy OB. Can visual exposure impact on children's visual preferences for fruit and vegetables? *Proc Nutr Soc*. 2010;69:e422

31. Houston-Price C, Butler L, Shiba P. Visual exposure impacts on toddlers' willingness to taste fruits and vegetables. *Appetite*. 2009;53(3):450–453

32. Fisher JO, Mennella JA, Hughes SO, Liu Y, Mendoza PM, Patrick H. Offering "dip" promotes intake of a moderately-liked raw vegetable among preschoolers with genetic sensitivity to bitterness. *J Acad Nutr Diet*. 2012;112(2):235–245

33. Cooke LJ, Wardle J, Gibson EL, Sapochnik M, Sheiham A, Lawson M. Demographic, familial and trait predictors of fruit and vegetable consumption by pre-school children. *Public Health Nutr*. 2004;7(2):295–302

34. Northstone K, Emmett P, Nethersole F, Pregnancy ASTALSo, Childhood. The effect of age of introduction to lumpy solids on foods eaten and reported feeding difficulties at 6 and 15 months. *J Hum Nutr Diet*. 2001;14(1):43–54

35. Skinner JD, Carruth BR, Bounds W, Ziegler P, Reidy K. Do food-related experiences in the first 2 years of life predict dietary variety in school-aged children? *J Nutr Educ Behav*. 2002;34(6):310–315

36. Goodell LS, Johnson SL, Antono AC, Power TG, Hughes SO. Strategies low-income parents use to overcome their children's food refusal. *Matern Child Health J*. 2017;21(1):68–76

37. Mascola AJ, Bryson SW, Agras WS. Picky eating during childhood: a longitudinal study to age 11 years. *Eat Behav*. 2010;11(4):253–257

38. Bekelman TA, Bellows LL, Johnson SL. Are family routines modifiable determinants of preschool children's eating, dietary intake, and growth? A review of intervention studies *Current Nutrition Reports*. 2017:1-9

39. Johnson SL, Hayes JE. Developmental readiness, caregiver and child feeding behaviors, and sensory science as a framework for feeding young children. *Nutrition Today*. 2017;52(2):S30–S40

40. Birch LL, Billman J, Richards SS. Time of day influences food acceptability. *Appetite*. 1984;5(2):109–116

41. Leahy KE, Birch LL, Fisher JO, Rolls BJ. Reductions in entree energy density increase children's vegetable intake and reduce energy intake. *Obesity (Silver Spring)*. 2008;16(7):1559–1565

42. Leahy KE, Birch LL, Rolls BJ. Reducing the energy density of multiple meals decreases the energy intake of preschool-age children. *Am J Clin Nutr.* 2008;88(6):1459–1468

43. Leahy KE, Birch LL, Rolls BJ. Reducing the energy density of an entree decreases children's energy intake at lunch. *J Am Diet Assoc.* 2008;108(1):41–48

44. Fisher JO. Effects of age on children's intake of large and self-selected food portions. *Obesity (Silver Spring)*. 2007;15(2):403–412

45. Orlet Fisher J, Rolls BJ, Birch LL. Children's bite size and intake of an entree are greater with large portions than with age-appropriate or self-selected portions. *Am J Clin Nutr.* 2003;77(5):1164–1170

46. Rolls BJ, Engell D, Birch LL. Serving portion size influences 5-year-old but not 3-year-old children's food intakes. *J Am Diet Assoc.* 2000;100(2):232–234

47. De Decker A, Verbeken S, Sioen I, et al. Palatable food consumption in children: interplay between (food) reward motivation and the home food environment. *Eur J Pediatr.* 2017;176(4):465–474

48. Shier V, Nicosia N, Datar A. Neighborhood and home food environment and children's diet and obesity: Evidence from military personnel's installation assignment. *Soc Sci Med.* 2016;158:122–131

49. Hurley KM, Cross MB, Hughes SO. A systematic review of responsive feeding and child obesity in high-income countries. *J Nutr.* 2011;141(3):495–501

50. Ventura AK, Birch LL. Does parenting affect children's eating and weight status? *Int J Behav Nutr Phys Act.* 2008;5:15

51. Birch LL. Effects of peer model's food choices and eating behaviors on preschoolers' food preferences. *Child Dev.* 1980;51:489–496

52. Salvy SJ, Kieffer E, Epstein LH. Effects of social context on overweight and normal-weight children's food selection. *Eat Behav.* 2008;9(2):190–196

53. Birch LL, Johnson SL, Andresen G, Peters JC, Schulte MC. The variability of young children's energy intake. *N Engl J Med.* 1991;324(4):232–235

54. Birch LL, Deysher M. Conditioned and unconditioned caloric compensation: evidence fo self-regulation of food intake by young children. *Learning and Motivation.* 1985;16:341–355

55. Johnson SL, Birch LL. Parents' and children's adiposity and eating style. *Pediatrics.* 1994;94(5):653–661

56. Faith MS, Pietrobelli A, Heo M, et al. A twin study of self-regulatory eating in early childhood: estimates of genetic and environmental influence, and measurement considerations. *Int J Obes (Lond).* 2012;36(7):931–937

57. Savage JS, Fisher JO, Marini M, Birch LL. Serving smaller age-appropriate entree portions to children aged 3-5 y increases fruit and vegetable intake and reduces energy density and energy intake at lunch. *Am J Clin Nutr.* 2012;95(2): 335–341

58. Nutrition classics. American Journal of Diseases of Children, Volume 36 October, 1928: Number 4. Self selection of diet by newly weaned infants: an experimental study. By Clara M. Davis. *Nutr Rev.* 1986;44(3):114–116

59. Wardle J, Huon G. An experimental investigation of the influence of health information on children's taste preferences. *Health Educ Res.* 2000;15(1):39–44

60. Council on School H, Committee on N. Snacks, sweetened beverages, added sugars, and schools. *Pediatrics.* 2015;135(3):575–583

61. Deming DM, Reidy KC, Fox MK, Briefel RR, Jacquier E, Eldridge AL. Cross-sectional analysis of eating patterns and snacking in the US Feeding Infants and Toddlers Study 2008. *Public Health Nutr.* 2017;20(9):1584–1592

62. Briefel RR, Reidy K, Karwe V, Jankowski L, Hendricks K. Toddlers' transition to table foods: Impact on nutrient intakes and food patterns. *J Am Diet Assoc.* 2004;104(1 Suppl 1):S38–S44

63. Fox MK, Reidy K, Novak T, Ziegler P. Sources of energy and nutrients in the diets of infants and toddlers. *J Am Diet Assoc.* 2006;106(1 Suppl 1):S28–42

64. Ahluwalia N, Herrick KA, Rossen LM, et al. Usual nutrient intakes of US infants and toddlers generally meet or exceed Dietary Reference Intakes: findings from NHANES 2009–2012. *Am J Clin Nutr.* 2016;104(4):1167–1174

65. Fox MK, Gearan E, Cannon J, et al. Usual food intakes of 2- and 3-year old U.S. children are not consistent with dietary guidelines. *BMC Nutr.* 2016;2:67

66. Bailey RL, Catellier D, Shinyoung J, Dwyer JT, Jacquier EF, Anater AS, Eldridge AL. Total usual nutrient intakes of US children (under 48 months): findings from the Feeding Infants and Toddlers Study (FITS) 2016. J Nutr. 2018;148 (9 Suppl):1557S-1566S

67. Miles G, Siega-Riz AM. Trends in food and beverage consumption among infants and toddlers: 2005–2012. *Pediatrics.* Jun 2017;139(6).

68. Roess AA, Jacquier EF, Catellier DJ, et al. Food Consumption Patterns of Infants and Toddlers: Findings from the Feeding Infants and Toddlers Study (FITS) 2016. *J Nutr.* 2018;148(Suppl 3):1525S-1535S

69. Denney L, Reidy KC, Eldridge AL. Differences in complementary feeding of 6 to 23 month olds in China, US and Mexico. *J Nutr Health Food Sci.* 2016;4:1-8

70. Storey ML, Anderson PA. Nutrient intakes and vegetable and white potato consumption by children aged 1 to 3 years. *Adv Nutr.* 2016;7(1):241S-246S

71. Tian N, Zhang Z, Loustalot F, Yang Q, Cogswell ME. Sodium and potassium intakes among US infants and preschool children, 2003–2010. *Am J Clin Nutr.* 2013;98(4):1113–1122

72. Baker RD, Greer FR, Committee on Nutrition American Academy of P. Diagnosis and prevention of iron deficiency and iron-deficiency anemia in infants and young children (0-3 years of age). *Pediatrics.* 2010;126(5):1040–1050

73. Hamner HC, Perrine CG, Scanlon KS. Usual intake of key minerals among children in the second year of life, NHANES 2003–2012. *Nutrients.* 2016;8(8)

74. Briefel RR, Deming DM, Reidy KC. Parents' perceptions and adherence to children's diet and activity recommendations: the 2008 Feeding Infants and Toddlers Study. *Prev Chronic Dis.* 2015;12:E159

75. Butte NF, Fox MK, Briefel RR, et al. Nutrient intakes of US infants, toddlers, and preschoolers meet or exceed dietary reference intakes. *J Am Diet Assoc.* 2010;110(12 Suppl):S27–S37

76. Keast DR, Fulgoni VL, 3rd, Nicklas TA, O'Neil CE. Food sources of energy and nutrients among children in the United States: National Health and Nutrition Examination Survey 2003–2006. *Nutrients.* 2013;5(1):283–301

77. Reedy J, Krebs-Smith SM. Dietary sources of energy, solid fats, and added sugars among children and adolescents in the United States. *J Am Diet Assoc.* 2010;110(10):1477–1484

78. Vos MB, Kaar JL, Welsh JA, et al. Added sugars and cardiovascular disease risk in children: A scientific statement from the American Heart Association. *Circulation.* 09 2017;135(19):e1017–e1034

79. Welker EB, Jacquier EF, Catellier DJ, Anater AS, Story MT. Room for improvement remains in food consumption patterns of young children aged 2–4 years. *J Nutr.* 2018;148(9 Suppl):1536S-1546S

80. Marriott BP, Olsho L, Hadden L, Connor P. Intake of added sugars and selected nutrients in the United States, National Health and Nutrition Examination Survey (NHANES) 2003–2006. *Crit Rev Food Sci Nutr.* 2010;50(3):228–258

81. Institute of Medicine. Dietary Reference Intakes: The Essential Guide to Nutrient Requirements. Washington, DC: The National Academies Press; 2006

82. Berner LA, Keast DR, Bailey RL, Dwyer JT. Fortified foods are major contributors to nutrient intakes in diets of US children and adolescents. *J Acad Nutr Diet.* 2014;114(7):1009–1022.e1008

83. Fulgoni VL, 3rd, Keast DR, Bailey RL, Dwyer J. Foods, fortificants, and supplements: Where do Americans get their nutrients? *J Nutr.* 2011;141(10): 1847–1854

84. Kong A, Odoms-Young AM, Schiffer LA, et al. Racial/ethnic differences in dietary intake among WIC families prior to food package revisions. *J Nutr Educ Behav.* 2013;45(1):39–46

85. American Dietetic A. Position of the American Dietetic Association: food fortification and dietary supplements. *J Am Diet Assoc.* 2001;101(1):115–125

86. American Dietetic A. Position of the American Dietetic Association: fortification and nutritional supplements. *J Am Diet Assoc.* 2005;105(8):1300–1311

87. Datta M, Vitolins MZ. Food Fortification and Supplement Use—Are There Health Implications? *Critical Reviews in Food Science and Nutrition.* 2016;56(13): 2149–2159

88. Kong A, Odoms-Young AM, Schiffer LA, et al. The 18-month impact of special supplemental nutrition program for women, infants, and children food package revisions on diets of recipient families. *Am J Prev Med.* 2014;46(6):543–551

89. Daniels SR, Greer FR, Committee on N. Lipid screening and cardiovascular health in childhood. *Pediatrics.* 2008;122(1):198–208

90. US Department of Agriculture. 2015 Dietary Guidelines for Americans, 8th ed. Washington, DC: US Govermentment Printing Office; 2015

91. Butte NF. Fat intake of children in relation to energy requirements. *Am J Clin Nutr.* 2000;72(5 Suppl):1246S-1252S

92. Obarzanek E, Hunsberger SA, Van Horn L, et al. Safety of a fat-reduced diet: the Dietary Intervention Study in Children (DISC). *Pediatrics.* 1997;100(1):51–59

93. Ervin RB, Ogden CL. Trends in intake of energy and macronutrients in children and adolescents from 1999–2000 through 2009–2010. *NCHS Data Brief.* 2013(113):1-8

94. Freeland-Graves JH, Nitzke S, Academy of N, Dietetics. Position of the academy of nutrition and dietetics: total diet approach to healthy eating. *J Acad Nutr Diet.* 2013;113(2):307–317

95. Department of Health and Human Services. Final determination regarding partially hydrogenated oils, Docket No. FDA–2013–N–1317. Rockville, MD: US Food and Drug Administration; 2015

96. US Department of Agriculture. ChooseMyPlate.gov Web site. Available at: https://www.choosemyplate.gov/. Accessed September 5, 2017

97. Young LR, Nestle MS. Portion sizes in dietary assessment: issues and policy implications. *Nutr Rev.* 1995;53(6):149–158

98. Hollands GJ, Shemilt I, Marteau TM, et al. Portion, package or tableware size for changing selection and consumption of food, alcohol and tobacco. *Cochrane Database Syst Rev.* 2015(9):CD011045

99. Ramsay SA, Branen LJ, Johnson SL. How much is enough? Tablespoon per year of age approach meets nutrient needs for children. *Appetite.* 2012;58(1):163–167

100. Satter E. *How to get your kid to eat...but not too much.* Palo Alto, CA: Bull Publishing Company; 1987

101. Maes HH, Neale MC, Eaves LJ. Genetic and environmental factors in relative body weight and human adiposity. *Behav Genet.* 1997;27(4):325–351

102. Dovey TM, Staples PA, Gibson EL, Halford JC. Food neophobia and 'picky/fussy' eating in children: a review. *Appetite.* 2008;50(2-3):181–193

103. Scaglioni S, Arrizza C, Vecchi F, Tedeschi S. Determinants of children's eating behavior. *Am J Clin Nutr.* 2011;94(6 Suppl):2006S-2011S

104. Llewellyn C, Wardle J. Behavioral susceptibility to obesity: Gene-environment interplay in the development of weight. *Physiol Behav.* 2015;152(Pt B):494–501

105. Shloim N, Edelson LR, Martin N, Hetherington MM. Parenting styles, feeding styles, feeding practices, and weight status in 4-12 year-old children: a systematic review of the literature. *Front Psychol.* 2015;6:1849

106. Patrick H, Nicklas TA, Hughes SO, Morales M. The benefits of authoritative feeding style: caregiver feeding styles and children's food consumption patterns. *Appetite.* 2005;44(2):243–249

107. Faith MS, Berkowitz RI, Stallings VA, Kerns J, Storey M, Stunkard AJ. Parental feeding attitudes and styles and child body mass index: prospective analysis of a gene-environment interaction. *Pediatrics.* 2004;114(4):e429–e436

108. Fisher JO, Birch LL. Restricting access to palatable foods affects children's behavioral response, food selection, and intake. *Am J Clin Nutr.* 1999;69(6):1264–1272

109. Hughes SO, Power TG, O'Connor TM, Orlet Fisher J, Chen TA. Maternal feeding styles and food parenting practices as predictors of longitudinal changes in weight status in Hispanic preschoolers from low-income families. *J Obes.* 2016;2016:7201082

110. Sandhu BK, European Society of Pediatric Gastroenterology H, Nutrition Working Group on Acute D. Practical guidelines for the management of gastroenteritis in children. *J Pediatr Gastroenterol Nutr.* 2001;33(Suppl 2):S36–S39

111. Centers for Disease Control and Prevention. Managing acute gastroenteritis among children: oral rehydration, maintenance, and nutritional therapy. *MMWR Morb Mortal Wkly Rep.* 2003;52:1-16

112. Ogden CL, Carroll MD, Lawman HG, et al. Trends in obesity prevalence among children and adolescents in the United States, 1988–1994 through 2013–2014. *JAMA.* 2016;315(21):2292–2299

113. Dietz WH. Health consequences of obesity in youth: childhood predictors of adult disease. *Pediatrics.* 1998;101(3 Pt 2):518–525

114. Reilly JJ, Kelly J. Long-term impact of overweight and obesity in childhood and adolescence on morbidity and premature mortality in adulthood: systematic review. *Int J Obes (Lond).* 2011;35(7):891–898

115. Cunningham SA, Datar A, Narayan KMV, Kramer MR. Entrenched obesity in childhood: findings from a national cohort study. *Ann Epidemiol.* 2017;27(7):435–441

116. Hill JO, Peters JC. Environmental contributions to the obesity epidemic. *Science.* 1998;280(5368):1371–1374

117. Poston WS, 2nd, Foreyt JP. Obesity is an environmental issue. *Atherosclerosis.* 1999;146(2):201–209

118. Davison KK, Birch LL. Childhood overweight: a contextual model and recommendations for future research. *Obes Rev.* 2001;2(3):159–171

119. Whitaker RC, Wright JA, Pepe MS, Seidel KD, Dietz WH. Predicting obesity in young adulthood from childhood and parental obesity. *N Engl J Med.* 1997;337(13):869–873

120. Wilfley DE, Staiano AE, Altman M, et al. Improving access and systems of care for evidence-based childhood obesity treatment: Conference key findings and next steps. *Obesity (Silver Spring).* 2017;25(1):16–29

121. Krebs NF, Himes JH, Jacobson D, Nicklas TA, Guilday P, Styne D. Assessment of child and adolescent overweight and obesity. *Pediatrics.* 2007;120(Suppl 4):S193–228

122. Fisher JO, Birch LL. Restricting access to foods and children's eating. *Appetite.* 1999;32(3):405–419

123. Davison KK, Birch LL. Weight status, parent reaction, and self-concept in five-year-old girls. *Pediatrics.* 2001;107(1):46–53

124. Cutting TM, Fisher JO, Grimm-Thomas K, Birch LL. Like mother, like daughter: familial patterns of overweight are mediated by mothers' dietary disinhibition. *Am J Clin Nutr.* 1999;69(4):608–613

125. American Academy of Pediatrics. Committee on Public E. American Academy of Pediatrics: Children, adolescents, and television. *Pediatrics.* 2001;107(2):423–426

126. Crespo CJ, Smit E, Troiano RP, Bartlett SJ, Macera CA, Andersen RE. Television watching, energy intake, and obesity in US children: results from the third National Health and Nutrition Examination Survey, 1988–1994. *Arch Pediatr Adolesc Med.* 2001;155(3):360–365

127. Council on C, Media, Strasburger VC. Children, adolescents, obesity, and the media. *Pediatrics.* 2011;128(1):201–208

128. Council on C, Media, Brown A. Media use by children younger than 2 years. *Pediatrics.* 2011;128(5):1040–1045

129. American Academy of Pediatrics, Council on Communications and Media. Policy statement: Media and young minds. *Pediatrics.* 2016;138(5):e20162591

130. American Academy of Pediatrics, Council on Communications and Media. Policy statement: Media use in school-aged children and adolescents. *Pediatrics.* 2016;138(5):e20162592

131. Milteer RM, Ginsburg KR; American Academy of Pediatrics, Council on Communications and Media, Committee on Psychosocial Aspects of Child and Family Health. Clinical report: The importance of play in promoting healthy child development and maintaining strong parent-child bond: focus on children in poverty. *Pediatrics.* 2012;129(1):e204–e213

132. Fulgoni VL III, Quann EE. National trends in beverage consumption in children from birth to 5 years: analysis of NHANES across three decades. *Nutr J.* 2012;11:92

133. Heyman MB, Abrams SA; American Academy of Pediatrics, Section on Gastroenterology, Hepatology, and Nutrition, Committee on Nutrition. Policy statement: Fruit juice in infants, children, and adolescents: current recommendations. *Pediatrics.* 2017;139(6)

134. Byrd-Bredbenner C, Ferruzzi MG, Fulgoni VL III, Murray R, Pivonka E, Wallace TC. Satisfying america's fruit gap: Summary of an expert roundtable on the role of 100% fruit juice. *J Food Sci.* 2017;82(7):1523–1534

135. Herrick KA, Rossen LM, Nielsen SJ, Branum AM, Ogden CL. Fruit consumption by youth in the United States. *Pediatrics.* 2015;136(4):664–671

136. Watowicz RP, Anderson SE, Kaye GL, Taylor CA. Energy contribution of beverages in US children by age, weight, and consumer status. *Child Obes.* 2015;11(4):475–483

137. Grimes CA, Szymlek-Gay EA, Nicklas TA. Beverage consumption among U.S. children aged 0-24 Months: National Health and Nutrition Examination Survey (NHANES). *Nutrients.* 2017;9(3):e264

138. Han E, Powell LM. Consumption patterns of sugar-sweetened beverages in the United States. *J Acad Nutr Diet.* 2013;113(1):43–53

139. Rosinger A, Herrick K, Gahche J, Park S. Sugar-sweetened beverage consumption among U.S. youth, 2011–2014. *NCHS Data Brief.* 2017(271):1-8

140. Grimes CA, Szymlek-Gay EA, Campbell KJ, Nicklas TA. Food sources of total energy and nutrients among U.S. infants and toddlers: National Health and Nutrition Examination Survey 2005–2012. *Nutrients.* 2015;7(8):6797–6836

141. Nielsen SJ, Popkin BM. Changes in beverage intake between 1977 and 2001. *Am J Prev Med.* 2004;27(3):205–210

142. Bucher Della Torre S, Keller A, Laure Depeyre J, Kruseman M. Sugar-sweetened beverages and obesity risk in children and adolescents: A systematic analysis on how methodological quality may influence conclusions. *J Acad Nutr Diet.* 2016;116(4):638–659

143. Malik VS, Pan A, Willett WC, Hu FB. Sugar-sweetened beverages and weight gain in children and adults: a systematic review and meta-analysis. *Am J Clin Nutr.* 2013;98(4):1084–1102

144. DeBoer MD, Scharf RJ, Demmer RT. Sugar-sweetened beverages and weight gain in 2- to 5-year-old children. *Pediatrics.* 2013;132(3):413–420

145. Mesirow MS, Welsh JA. Changing beverage consumption patterns have resulted in fewer liquid calories in the diets of US children: National Health and Nutrition Examination Survey 2001–2010. *J Acad Nutr Diet.* 2015;115(4):559–566.e554

146. Ahluwalia N, Herrick K. Caffeine intake from food and beverage sources and trends among children and adolescents in the United States: review of national quantitative studies from 1999 to 2011. *Adv Nutr.* 2015;6(1):102–111

147. Ahluwalia N, Herrick K, Moshfegh A, Rybak M. Caffeine intake in children in the United States and 10-y trends: 2001–2010. *Am J Clin Nutr.* 2014;100(4):1124–1132

148. Wikoff D, Welsh BT, Henderson R, et al. Systematic review of the potential adverse effects of caffeine consumption in healthy adults, pregnant women, adolescents, and children. *Food Chem Toxicol.* 2017;109(Pt 1):585–648

149. Field AE, Sonneville KR, Falbe J, et al. Association of sports drinks with weight gain among adolescents and young adults. *Obesity (Silver Spring).* 2014;22(10):2238–2243

150. Committee on N, the Council on Sports M, Fitness. Sports drinks and energy drinks for children and adolescents: are they appropriate? *Pediatrics.* 2011;127(6):1182–1189

151. Dunford EK, Popkin BM. 37 year snacking trends for US children 1977–2014. *Pediatr Obes.* 2018;13(4):247–255

152. Shriver LH, Marriage BJ, Bloch TD, et al. Contribution of snacks to dietary intakes of young children in the United States. *Matern Child Nutr.* 2018;14(1). doi: 10.1111/mcn.12454

153. Evans EW, Jacques PF, Dallal GE, Sacheck J, Must A. The role of eating frequency on total energy intake and diet quality in a low-income, racially diverse sample of schoolchildren. *Public Health Nutr.* 2015;18(3):474–481

154. Rudy E, Bauer KW, Hughes SO, et al. Interrelationships of child appetite, weight and snacking among Hispanic preschoolers. *Pediatr Obes.* 2018;13(1):38–45

155. Larson N, Story M. A review of snacking patterns among children and adolescents: what are the implications of snacking for weight status? *Child Obes.* 2013;9(2):104–115

156. Murakami K, Livingstone MB. Associations between meal and snack frequency and overweight and abdominal obesity in US children and adolescents from National Health and Nutrition Examination Survey (NHANES) 2003–2012. *Br J Nutr.* 2016;115(10):1819–1829

157. Blaine RE, Fisher JO, Taveras EM, et al. Reasons low-income parents offer snacks to children: How feeding rationale influences snack frequency and adherence to dietary recommendations. *Nutrients.* 2015;7(7):5982–5999

158. Haire-Joshu D, Elliott MB, Caito NM, et al. High 5 for Kids: the impact of a home visiting program on fruit and vegetable intake of parents and their preschool children. *Prev Med.* 2008;47(1):77–82

159. Knowlden A, Sharma M. One-Year efficacy testing of Enabling Mothers to Prevent Pediatric Obesity Through Web-Based Education and Reciprocal Determinism (EMPOWER) randomized control trial. *Health Educ Behav.* 2016;43(1):94–106

160. Stark LJ, Clifford LM, Towner EK, et al. A pilot randomized controlled trial of a behavioral family-based intervention with and without home visits to decrease obesity in preschoolers. *J Pediatr Psychol.* 2014;39(9):1001–1012

161. Wyse R, Wolfenden L, Bisquera A. Characteristics of the home food environment that mediate immediate and sustained increases in child fruit and vegetable consumption: mediation analysis from the Healthy Habits cluster randomised controlled trial. *Int J Phys Activity Behav Nutr.* 2015;12(1):118

162. Goldman RL, Radnitz CL, McGrath RE. The role of family variables in fruit and vegetable consumption in pre-school children. *J Public Health Res.* 2012;1(2): 143–148

163. Patrick H, Nicklas TA. A review of family and social determinants of children's eating patterns and diet quality. *J Am Coll Nutr.* 2005;24(2):83–92

164. van Ansem WJ, Schrijvers CT, Rodenburg G, van de Mheen D. Is there an association between the home food environment, the local food shopping environment and children's fruit and vegetable intake? Results from the Dutch INPACT study. *Public Health Nutr.* 2013;16(7):1206–1214

165. Rideout V. *Generation M2: Media in the lives of 8- to 18-year-olds.* Menlo Park, CA: Kaiser Family Foundation; 2010

166. Nielsen Company. *Television, Internet and Mobile Usage in the U.S.: A2/M2 three screen report.* New York, NY: Nielsen Company; 2009

167. Loprinzi PD, Davis RE. Secular trends in parent-reported television viewing among children in the United States, 2001–2012. *Child: Care, Health and Development.* 2016;42(2):288–291

168. Kraak VI, Story M. Influence of food companies' brand mascots and entertainment companies' cartoon media characters on children's diet and health: a systematic review and research needs. *Obes Rev.* 2015;16(2):107–126

169. Boyland EJ, Whalen R. Food advertising to children and its effects on diet: review of recent prevalence and impact data. *Pediatr Diabetes.* 2015;16(5):331–337

170. Sadeghirad B, Duhaney T, Motaghipisheh S, Campbell NR, Johnston BC. Influence of unhealthy food and beverage marketing on children's dietary intake and preference: a systematic review and meta-analysis of randomized trials. *Obes Rev.* 2016;17(10):945–959

171. Robinson TN, Borzekowski DL, Matheson DM, Kraemer HC. Effects of fast food branding on young children's taste preferences. *Arch Pediatr Adolesc Med.* 2007;161(8):792–797

172. Longacre MR, Drake KM, Titus LJ, et al. A toy story: Association between young children's knowledge of fast food toy premiums and their fast food consumption. *Appetite.* 2016;96:473–480

173. Borghese MM, Tremblay MS, Leduc G, et al. Independent and combined associations of total sedentary time and television viewing time with food intake patterns of 9- to 11-year-old Canadian children. *Appl Physiol Nutr Metab.* 2014;39(8):937–943

174. Cespedes EM, Gillman MW, Kleinman K, Rifas-Shiman SL, Redline S, Taveras EM. Television viewing, bedroom television, and sleep duration from infancy to mid-childhood. *Pediatrics.* 2014;133(5):e1163–e1171

175. Dennison BA, Erb TA, Jenkins PL. Television viewing and television in bedroom associated with overweight risk among low-income preschool children. *Pediatrics.* 2002;109(6):1028–1035

176. Feinberg E, Kavanagh PL, Young RL, Prudent N. Food insecurity and compensatory feeding practices among urban black families. *Pediatrics.* 2008;122(4):e854–e860

177. Drewnowski A, Specter SE. Poverty and obesity: the role of energy density and energy costs. *Am J Clin Nutr.* 2004;79(1):6-16

178. Matheson DM, Robinson TN, Varady A, Killen JD. Do Mexican-American mothers' food-related parenting practices influence their children's weight and dietary intake? *J Am Diet Assoc.* 2006;106(11):1861–1865

Chapter 8

Adolescent Nutrition

Introduction

Approximately 42 million people in the United States, or 14% of the population, are 10 to 19 years old.[1] Outside of the first year of life, adolescence is the period of greatest growth and development across the lifespan. Longitudinal height increases 20%, body weight doubles, 40% to 60% of peak bone mass is accrued, muscle mass increases, blood volume expands, and the heart, brain, lungs, liver, and kidney all increase in size. As a result, nutritional requirements increase dramatically, and many adolescents consume inadequate amounts of vitamins, minerals, and nutrients for their needs (including folic acid; vitamins A, D, E, and B_6; calcium; iron; zinc; magnesium; and fiber) as well as foods from several important groups, such as fruits, vegetables, and whole grains.[2-5] Adolescent diets also frequently exceed recommendations for fat, saturated fat, sodium, and cholesterol. Furthermore, a substantial number of teenagers frequently eat energy-dense foods (such as fast food and sugar-sweetened beverages), are physically inactive,[5,6] and gain an excessive amount of weight during the adolescent years.[7] Special situations, such as pregnancy, chronic disease, and physical conditioning, increase nutritional requirements of the adolescent. Some disorders that develop during adolescence, such as eating disorders, obesity, and chronic illnesses are associated with either insufficient or excessive nutrient intake.

Factors Influencing Nutritional Needs of Adolescents

In contrast to other age groups, nutritional requirements during adolescence depend more on sexual maturity rating (Tanner staging) than on chronologic age.[8] Health care providers should use the sexual maturation rating or Tanner stages to assess the degree of pubertal maturation in the adolescent at each annual health maintenance visit. The stages of sexual maturity rating for boys and girls are shown in Table 8.1. Increased growth rates occur in girls between 10 and 12 years of age and in boys about 2 years later, although substantial individual variability occurs. In girls, peak height velocity occurs early in puberty, usually between Tanner stages 2 and 3 of breast development. Growth in girls is accompanied by a greater increase in the proportion of body fat than in boys, and growth in boys is accompanied by a greater increase in the proportion of lean body mass and blood volume than in girls. In girls, menarche occurs late in puberty, usually

Table 8.1.
Sexual Maturity Rating for Girls and Boys

Girls' Stage	Breast Development	Pubic Hair Growth
1	Prepubertal; nipple elevation only	Prepubertal; no pubic hair
2	Small, raised breast bud	Sparse growth of hair along labia
3	General enlargement of breast extending beyond areola	Pigmentation, coarsening, and curling, with an increase in amount
4	Further enlargement with projection of areola and nipple as secondary mound	Hair resembles adult type, but not spread to medial thighs
5	Mature, adult contour, with areola in same contour as breast, and only nipple projecting	Adult type and quantity, spread to medial thighs
Boys' Stage	Genital Development	Pubic Hair Growth
1	Prepubertal; no change in size or proportion of testes, scrotum, and penis from early childhood	Prepubertal; no pubic hair
2	Enlargement of scrotum and testes; reddening and change in texture in skin of scrotum; little or no penis enlargement	Sparse growth of hair at base of penis
3	Increase first in length, then width of penis; growth of testes and scrotum	Darkening, coarsening, and curling; increase in amount
4	Enlargement of penis with growth in breadth and development of glands; further growth of testes and scrotum, darkening of scrotal skin	Hair resembles adult type, but not spread to medial thighs
5	Adult size and shape genitalia	Adult type and quantity, spread to medial thighs

between Tanner stage 4 and 5 of breast development and 2 to 3 years after onset of breast development. Median age of menarche in the United States is 12.4 years and occurs earlier in black girls (12.06 years) than Hispanic girls (12.25) or white girls (12.55). However, completion of sexual secondary maturation occurs at approximately the same time for all racial groups.[9] Longitudinal growth is usually complete 1 year after menarche.

The onset of puberty in boys typically occurs at 10 to 13 years, and peak height velocity occurs later in puberty, usually between Tanner genital stages 4 and 5. As a result, boys grow, on average, for 2 years longer than girls. Increased muscle mass development occurs during Tanner genital stages 4 and 5, secondary to rising androgen concentrations. In both boys and girls, peak bone mass acquisition occurs approximately 6 to 12 months after peak height velocity.

Dietary Reference Intakes

The Dietary Reference Intakes (DRIs) provide guidelines for normal nutrition for adolescent males and females in 2 age categories—9 to 13 years and 14 to 18 years (Appendix E)—and include Recommended Dietary Allowances (RDAs) for many nutrients, which provide an estimate of the minimum daily average dietary level that meets the nutrient requirements for 97% to 98% of healthy individuals. Although there are no RDAs established for energy intake, estimated energy requirements (EERs) provide guidance on the calorie intakes needed to maintain energy balance on the basis of age, sex, weight, height, and physical activity. Among adolescents, individual variability occurs in the rates of physical growth, timing of pubertal growth spurt, and physiologic maturation, all of which may affect energy needs. In addition, individual physical activity patterns vary widely. For these reasons, assessment of energy needs of adolescents should include consideration of appetite, growth, activity level, and weight gain in relation to deposition of subcutaneous fat. Restricted food intake in the physically active adolescent results in diminished growth and a drop in the basal metabolic rate and, in girls, amenorrhea. The RDAs for micronutrients, including vitamins and minerals, are designed to meet the needs of almost all healthy adolescents; therefore, they exceed the requirements for the average person. A healthy diet for the whole population, including adolescents, should provide approximately 25% to 35% of calories from fat, 45% to 65% of calories from carbohydrate, and 10% to 30% of calories from dietary protein.[10]

Table 8.2.

Daily Increments in Body Content of Minerals and Nitrogen During Adolescent Growth[a]

Mineral	Sex	Average for 10–20 y, mg	Average at Peak of Growth Spurt, mg
Calcium	M	210	400
	F	110	240
Iron	M	0.57	1.1
	F	0.23	0.9
Nitrogen[a]	M	320	610
	F	160	360
Zinc	M	0.27	0.50
	F	0.18	0.31
Magnesium	M	4.4	8.4
	F	2.3	5.0

Adapted from Forbes.[11]
[a] Multiply by 0.00625 to obtain g of protein.

Average caloric intake for moderately active adolescents is approximately 2700 kcal for males and 2300 kcal for females.

During adolescence, increases in requirements for energy and such nutrients as calcium, nitrogen, and iron are determined by increases in lean body mass rather than an increase in body weight, with its variable fat content. Assuming that the lean body contents of calcium, iron, nitrogen, zinc, and magnesium of adolescents are the same as those of adults, the daily increments of body nutrients for the growing adolescent can be estimated (Table 8.2).[11] The increased nutrient needs are not constant throughout adolescence and vary during different stages of pubertal development.

Nutrition Concerns During Adolescence

Many teenagers in the United States, particularly females, consume inadequate amounts of numerous vitamins, minerals, and nutrients including folic acid; vitamins A, D, E, and B_6; calcium; iron; zinc; magnesium; and fiber. In addition, adolescent diets also frequently exceed recommendations for fat, saturated fat, sodium, and cholesterol. Moreover, adolescents

9 to 18 years of age consume inadequate amounts of foods from several important groups, including fruits, vegetables, and whole grains.[4,12] For example, among adolescents 14 to 18 years of age, males consume an average of 1 cup of fruit/day, and females consume 0.8 cups/day, approximately half of recommended levels (2 cups for males of this age, 1.5 cups for females). Vegetables are also frequently underconsumed; males 14 to 18 years of age consume an average of 1.3 cups/day, and females consume 1.1 cups/day, far less than the 3 cups recommended for males and 2.5 cups for females. Furthermore, few adolescents are consuming nutrient-dense vegetables, highlighted by the fact that more than 95% of 9- to 18-year-olds consumed fewer than 0.2 cups of dark-green vegetables daily. In addition, a vast majority (>95%) of adolescents consume an insufficient level of whole grains and a substantial amount of added sugar in their diets.[12]

Food habits of adolescents are characterized by: (1) an increased tendency to skip meals, especially breakfast and lunch; (2) eating more meals outside the home; (3) snacking, especially energy-dense foods and beverages; (4) consumption of fast foods; and (5) dieting.[13] Some adhere to vegetarian diets or to more restrictive dietary regimens, such as Zen macrobiotic diets (see Chapter 11: Nutritional Aspects of Vegetarian Diets, and 13: Fast Foods, Organic Foods, Fad Diets, and Herbs, Herbals, and Botanicals). Although it is very possible for adolescents to maintain healthy dietary intakes when consuming a vegetarian diet, some adolescents may use vegetarian diets as a means of controlling their intake in unhealthy ways. Thus, recent onset of becoming a vegetarian may be a warning sign of an underlying eating disorder (see Chapter 38).[13] It is not unusual for adolescents to follow fad diets and change their eating habits frequently. These dietary patterns can be explained by the adolescents' emerging independence, desire to challenge existing values by engaging in risk-taking behaviors, dissatisfaction with body image, search for self-identification, desire for peer acceptance, and need to conform with peers.

The following describe specific nutrient requirements and concerns during adolescence:

1. **Energy:** Results from the 2011–2012 National Health and Nutrition Examination Survey (NHANES) reveal that 34.5% of individuals between 12 and 19 years of age were overweight or obese.[7] Among adolescents aged 12 to 19 years, obesity prevalence rates have stabilized since 2005–2006,[14] although the prevalence remained alarmingly high (see Chapter 33: Obesity).

2. **Protein:** Protein is required for growth, development, and maintenance of body tissues. The peak in protein intake correlates with the peak in energy intake, and during adolescence, protein needs, like those for energy, correlate more closely with growth pattern than with chronologic age. In the United States, mean protein intake is much greater than the RDAs, so protein deficiency is not common but can occur in strict vegans, in chronic dieters, or in households with food insecurity.

3. **Iron:** The need for iron for males and females is increased during adolescence to sustain the rapidly enlarging muscle mass, expansion of blood volume, and increase in hemoglobin concentration; in females, it is needed to offset menstrual losses, and adolescent girls with menorrhagia are at increased risk of developing iron deficiency.[15]

4. **Zinc:** Zinc is essential for growth and sexual maturation. Growth retardation and hypogonadism have been reported in adolescent males with zinc deficiency. Diets high in phytates can reduce the bioavailability of dietary zinc.

5. **Vegan diets:** Adolescents who consume no animal products may be vulnerable to deficiencies of several nutrients, particularly vitamins D and B_{12}, riboflavin, protein, calcium, iron, zinc, and perhaps other trace elements (see Chapter 11).

6. **Dental caries:** Although dental caries begin in early childhood, they are a highly prevalent nutrition-related problem of adolescence. Caries are associated with low fluoride intake in childhood and frequent consumption of foods containing carbohydrates (see Chapter 48).

7. **Conditioned deficiencies:** A number of medications can interact with the absorption or metabolism of nutrients[16] (Appendix G). Anticonvulsant drugs, especially phenytoin and phenobarbital, interfere with the metabolism of vitamin D and can lead to rickets and/or osteomalacia; therefore, supplementation with vitamin D may be desirable. Isoniazid interferes with pyridoxine metabolism. Oral contraceptives increase serum lipid concentrations, an effect that may have some clinical significance.[17]

8. **Chronic disease:** Adolescents with chronic illnesses such as inflammatory bowel disease, celiac disease, diabetes mellitus, juvenile idiopathic arthritis, or sickle cell disease may develop nutritional deficiencies as a result of a combination of dietary limitations, increased metabolic requirements associated with chronic inflammation, and ongoing nutrient losses through the stools or urine. These chronic diseases can profoundly affect nutritional status. (see appropriate chapters).

9. **Calcium and vitamin D:** see next section on Bone Health.
10. **Pregnancy:** see later section on Pregnancy.

Nutritional Concerns For Adolescent Bone Health *(see also Chapter 18: Calcium, Phosphorus, and Magnesium)*

Adolescence is a critical time for bone mass accretion, and 40% to 60% of adult bone mass is accrued during the adolescent years, with 25% of peak bone mass accrued during the 2-year period around peak height velocity.[18] Maximal bone mineral accretion rates occur at an average of 12.5 years of age for girls and 14.0 years for boys.[19] By the age of 18 years, approximately 90% of peak bone mass has been accrued, but there is some continued net deposition between the ages of 20 and 30 years.[20] Age of peak bone mass accrual lags behind age of peak height velocity by approximately 6 to 12 months in both boys and in girls.[19] This dissociation between linear growth and bone mineral accrual may confer increased vulnerability to bone fragility and may explain, to some degree, the increased rate of forearm fractures in boys 10 through 14 years of age and in girls 8 through 12 years of age.[21,22] Once peak bone mass has been achieved, there is a slow but progressive decline in bone mass. The amount of bone accrued at the end of adolescence, therefore, can affect future fracture risk during adulthood. Factors that influence bone mass during adolescence include genetics, hormonal status, exercise, adequacy of dietary calcium and vitamin D, general nutrition, and health. Although genetic factors account for more than half of the variance in final bone mineral density, the remaining factors are amenable to modification.[18]

There are a number of impediments to the teenager attaining optimal bone health. According to the Institute of Medicine (IOM) and the American Academy of Pediatrics (AAP), the recommended daily allowance of calcium for teenagers is 1300 mg/day,[18,23] but most teenagers in the United States do not consume the recommended daily amount. One of the principal causes is the general decline in dairy intake during these years and the inadequate consumption of calcium-rich dairy alternatives. The AAP recommends that teenagers consume 4 servings of dairy products or equivalent per day.[18] In 2011, only 9.3% of girls in the United States consumed 3 or more servings of milk per day.[24] Teenagers decrease their milk consumption for various reasons. Some are truly lactose intolerant, some do not like the taste, and others consider milk to be a "child's drink." A substantial number of adolescents also may substitute sugar-sweetened beverages (such as soda) for plain milk in their diet. Soda consumption is associated with lower intakes of milk and dairy products.[25] Fortunately, soda consumption by adolescents, although still high, has declined from 2007 to 2015. However, in 2015, 1 in 5 high school students consumed soda daily.[26]

Vitamin D is a fat-soluble vitamin necessary for the absorption and utilization of calcium. In 2011, the IOM increased the RDA for vitamin D to 600 IU/day for adolescents.[23] Vitamin D deficiency is prevalent in northern climates and in those consuming low-fat diets. Vitamin D is synthesized in the skin after exposure to ultraviolet light from sunlight. Dietary sources include cod liver oil; fatty fish such as salmon, sardines, and tuna; and fortified foods and drinks.[18]

The AAP recommends that pediatricians ask about dairy intake, nondairy sources of calcium and vitamin D, use of calcium and/or vitamin D supplements, and soda consumption during the adolescent health maintenance visits. The AAP also recommends encouraging increased dietary intake of calcium and vitamin D-containing foods and beverages.[18] Juices and ready-to-eat cereals fortified with calcium and vitamin D are commercially available. Other nondairy sources of calcium include some types of fish (such as sardines, canned with bones) and fortified soy products. Green, leafy vegetables that are not high in oxalates, such as broccoli, have bioavailable calcium; spinach, because of its high oxalate level, is not an optimal source of calcium. Current data do not support routine calcium or vitamin D supplementation for healthy adolescents,[18] although supplementation may be considered in those with diseases associated with increased bone fragility.[27] Finally, to promote optimal bone health, weight-bearing physical activity should be encouraged.[18] Walking, running, jumping, skipping, and dancing activities are preferable to swimming or cycling to optimize bone health.

Nutritional Considerations During Pregnancy

The rate of pregnancy among US adolescent females was estimated at 22.3 per 1000 teenagers 15 to 19 years of age in 2015.[28] This was a historic low for US teenagers and a drop of 8% from 2014. Nutrient needs are higher during adolescence than at any other time in a female's life, and the additional nutrient needs of pregnancy can make it difficult for teenagers to obtain adequate nutrient intakes. Iron deficiency is likely common among pregnant adolescents, given that during their third trimester of pregnancy a prevalence rate of 29.9% was found in a national sample of all pregnant women.[29] As with iron, calcium intakes are low and requirements are high among adolescents. However, the recent revision of the RDA of 1300 mg of calcium for pregnant and lactating adolescents is the same for nonpregnant and nonlactating adolescents.[23]

Weight gain during pregnancy is an important issue to be addressed by health care providers and was the subject of recent IOM report.[30] Obesity prior to pregnancy is an increasingly common issue that places both the mother and fetus at risk of poor pregnancy outcomes. Higher rates of gestational diabetes, birth defects, preeclampsia, cesarean delivery, post-partum weight retention, large- and small-for-gestational-age infants, and preterm birth have been associated with females who enter pregnancy obese. However, the recent IOM report did not find enough evidence to support the idea that weight gain itself during pregnancy was associated with gestational diabetes and preeclampsia. Prepregnancy obesity status and excessive gestational weight gain have been found to be predictive of the development of obesity within 1 to 9 years postpartum among primiparous adolescent mothers.[31,32]

A review of nutrition interventions among pregnant adolescents found that prenatal care enhanced with intensive nutrition counseling and supple-mental foods has been shown to decrease the rates of low birth weight, very low birth weight, and preterm birth.[33] School-based nutrition education and with home-visit programs by nurses have been shown to lead to modest improvements in dietary intake but no improvements in birth outcomes.[32] A comprehensive health care program for the pregnant adolescent should include proper prenatal care; monitoring of weight gain; nutritional assess-ment, counseling, and support; and family planning. Whenever possible, the parents or other caregiver should be included in counseling sessions.

Assessing and Maintaining Adequate Nutrition in Adolescents

Health guidance for adolescents should begin with an annual screening for indicators of nutritional risk (see Table 8.3). These include overweight and underweight, eating disorders, hyperlipidemia, hypertension, and iron-deficiency anemia. Unhealthy eating practices for which the adolescent should be screened include frequent dieting, meal skipping, food fads, and increased consumption of foods and beverages high in fat and sugar, such as fast foods and soft drinks. Nutrition screening should include a physical

Table 8.3.
Tools for Practice—Adolescent Nutrition

Tool	Description	Reference
CDC Growth Curves 2000	For children 2 to 20 years; includes BMI, height, weight, and head circumference	www.cdc.gov/growthcharts/whocharts.htm
Adolescent Nutritional Questionnaire	Assesses dietary intake with selective questions about nutritional status to be completed prior to the office visit; includes interpretive notes	Tool C: Nutrition Questionnaire for Adolescents. In : American Academy of Pediatrics. *Bright Futures Nutrition*. 3rd ed. Elk Grove Village, IL: American Academy of Pediatrics; 2011:233–238
Assessing Nutrition Risk	Includes screening for food intakes, meeting dietary guidelines, excessive intakes of fats and sweets, poor dietary practices (fast foods, meal skipping, dieting, food fads, eating disorders), obesity, iron deficiency, dental caries, alcohol and tobacco use; includes criteria for further screening and assessment	Tool D: Key Indicators of Nutritional Risk for Children and Adolescents. In : American Academy of Pediatrics. *Bright Futures Nutrition*. 3rd ed. Elk Grove Village, IL: American Academy of Pediatrics; 2011:239–243
Nutrition Counseling	A simplified approach to behavior modification and nutrition counseling for children and adolescents—could be used for obesity and eating disorders	Tool F: Stages of Change—A Model for Nutrition Counseling. In : American Academy of Pediatrics. *Bright Futures Nutrition*. 3rd ed. Elk Grove Village, IL: American Academy of Pediatrics; 2011:249–250

Promotion of Healthy Eating Behavior	Tips for promoting healthy eating behavior at the office visit for adolescents	Tool G: Strategies of Health Professionals to Promote Healthy Eating Behaviors. In : American Academy of Pediatrics. *Bright Futures Nutrition.* 3rd ed. Elk Grove Village, IL: American Academy of Pediatrics; 2011:251–253
Promoting Positive Body Image	Useful for counseling adolescents with a distorted body image	Tool I: Tips for Fostering a Positive Body Image Among Children and Adolescents. In : American Academy of Pediatrics. *Bright Futures Nutrition.* 3rd ed. Elk Grove Village, IL: American Academy of Pediatrics; 2011:257–258
Scoff Questionnaire for Identifying Eating Disorders	Although only validated in adults, provides useful screening questions about eating and body image that should be asked of adolescents	See AAP clinical report[13]
Dietary Guidelines for Americans 2015–2020 and My Plate	Contains specific and detailed information about nutrient requirements for adolescents and food based guidelines for a healthy diet	See Dietary Guidelines for Americans[37]

CDC indicates Centers for Disease Control and Prevention.

examination with measurement of blood pressure, an assessment of sexual maturity rating (Table 8.1), an accurate measurement of height and weight, and a calculation of body mass index (BMI). Nutrition screening should also include a broader dietary assessment of adolescents who are at increased nutritional risk (see Table 8.3) with a food frequency questionnaire, 24-hour dietary recall, or a food diary to further define nutritional problems.

Anthropometric measures should be plotted on the National Center for Health Statistics 2000 growth charts (www.cdc.gov/growthcharts/whocharts.htm). Adolescents below the 5th percentile for weight or BMI are underweight and should undergo additional evaluation. Those with a BMI greater than the 85th percentile but less than the 95th percentile are considered overweight and should also undergo additional evaluation. Adolescents with a BMI greater than or equal to the 95th percentile are obese and should be referred for a full-scale medical evaluation as well as to a weight management program designed to meet the needs of adolescents and their families.

As noted previously, obesity prevention in adolescents is a real concern for the health care professional, and obese adolescents are at risk of becoming obese adults,[34,35] with the associated adverse complication including the metabolic syndrome. Adolescents are very concerned about physical appearance and maintaining a healthy weight. Those engaged in competitive sports can be encouraged to maintain a healthy energy intake as a competitive advantage. The AAP recently published the report from the Expert Panel on Integrated Guidelines for Cardiovascular Health and Risk Reduction in Children and Adolescents sponsored by the National Heart, Lung, and Blood Institute of the National Institutes of Health.[36] This report recommended universal lipid screening between 9 and 11 years of age and again between 17 and 21 years of age with a nonfasting non-high-density lipoprotein (HDL), or fasting lipid panel.[36] Adolescents between 12 and 17 years of age may need additional fasting lipid panels to be performed if significant risk factors for cardiovascular disease develop, such as obesity. Dietary intervention should include avoiding high intakes of saturated fats and trans fats as well as cholesterol. For adolescents, the Expert Panel recommended that energy from fat not exceed 25% to 30% of total energy intake. If lipid screening reveals an abnormality, adolescents will need close follow-up and ongoing dietary management.[36] These adolescents are also at risk of the metabolic syndrome, including type 2 diabetes mellitus.

Relatively few adolescents meet the dietary guidelines for intakes of fruits, vegetables, whole grains, and dairy products, although they often exceed their daily energy requirement—males more so than females.[37] Fast food snacks account for 25% to 33% of daily energy intake and tend to be energy dense and nutrient poor. The physician can advise the adolescent to choose a variety of nutrient-dense foods across and within all food groups in recommended amounts, to limit calories from added sugars and saturated fats, to reduce sodium intake, and to shift to healthier food and beverage choices.[37] Pediatricians can also advocate at the local and state level to continue to improve the quality of food and beverage selections brought into schools for packed lunches and snacks, fundraisers, sporting events, school parties, and school celebrations.[38]

Parents are still the gatekeepers of foods and again serve as important role models for eating behavior. They should be advised to keep a variety of healthy foods in the home, provide fruits and vegetables at every meal, and use whole-grain breads and cereals. Adolescents require 4 servings a day of low-fat (1%) or nonfat milk or other low-fat dairy products to provide adequate amounts of calcium and vitamin D for strong bones.[18] Lean meats, including chicken and fish, should be served. High-fat foods, sweetened beverages, and fast foods low in nutrient density should be avoided. Eating meals as a family has been shown to improve dietary intake, with higher intakes of essential nutrient such as calcium, iron, and vitamins. The intake of fruits and vegetables is also increased with family meals.[39] Adolescents frequently skip breakfast, the meal that has been shown to have a positive effect on school performance.[40] Skipping breakfast also adversely affects dietary intake, because it promotes snacking on less healthy food throughout the day to make up for the loss in energy intake.[41] Dieting and skipping of meals in adolescents has been associated with the development of both obesity and eating disorders 5 to 10 years later.[35,42] Family meals are associated with improved dietary quality and provide opportunities for parents to model healthy eating practices. Improvements in dietary quality are sustained 5 years later, when the adolescents become young adults.[35]

Adolescents engage in significant amounts of screen time, and the influence of the media and the Internet have an increasingly negative effect on dietary intake, with their emphasis on foods with low nutrient density and increased amounts of fat, sugar, and salt.[39] Parents should be encouraged to keep healthy snacks around the home and to encourage adolescents to take breakfast bars or fruit with them to school rather than skipping breakfast.

Encouraging participation in both organized and unorganized physical activity is crucial, because there is often a significant drop in physical activity at adolescence, especially among females.[43] It is recommended that adolescents engage in 60 minutes or more of physical activity per day, with muscle strengthening and bone strengthening activities as part of the 60 minutes or more a day, on at least 3 days a week.[37] Electronic social networking is greatly increased in adolescence, and parents should be encouraged to limit screen time (TV, video, computer) to 2 hours per day and never allow television watching in the bedroom.[39] This intervention can also help prevent obesity.[44] Average caloric intake for moderately active adolescents is approximately 2700 kcal for males and 2000 kcal for females.[37] Individual energy needs will vary greatly depending on age, sex, body size, degree of physical maturation, rate of growth, and level of physical activity (Table 8.4). The assessment of growth rate is key to determining

Table 8.4.
Estimated Calorie Needs per Day by Age, Gender, and Physical Activity Level

Males Age (y)	Activity Level		
	Sedentary	Moderately Active	Active
12	1800	2200	2400
13	2000	2200	2600
14	2000	2400	2800
15	2200	2600	3000
16	2400	2800	3200
17	2400	2800	3200
19–20	2600	2800	3000

Females Age (y)	Activity Level		
	Sedentary	Moderately Active	Active
12	1600	2000	2200
13	1600	2000	2200
14	1800	2000	2400
15	1800	2000	2400
16	1800	2000	2400
17	1800	2000	2400
19–20	2000	2200	2400

Adapted from the US Department of Agriculture and the US Department of Health and Human Services. *Dietary Guidelines for Americans, 2015–2020.*[37]

adequate energy intake. Adolescents also need large amounts of protein, up to 0.5 g/lb of body weight per day. Thus, a 124-lb adolescent will need approximately 60 g of daily protein intake.[37] The RDA for iron is 15 mg/day for females and 12 mg/day for males, the difference being menstrual losses of blood in females.[45] Heme iron from meat (including shellfish) is the best source of iron, given its relatively high absorption rate. Adolescents should be screened for iron deficiency if, by history, they are at risk of iron deficiency.[45]

Other key nutrients for adolescents include adequate calcium and vitamin D for bone growth. The RDA for calcium, according to the IOM, is 1300 mg for adolescents.[23] This RDA can be achieved with 4 servings of dairy products per day. Fortified milk will also supply the daily 600 IU of vitamin D recommended for adolescents.[18] Weight-conscious adolescents should be assured that reduced-fat or nonfat milk contains just as much calcium and vitamin D as does whole milk. Alternative sources of calcium are tofu, fortified soy milk, and dark green, leafy vegetables. Many adolescents fail to achieve the recommended intakes of vitamins and minerals because of their food choices.

References

1. US Census Bureau. *Age and Sex Composition: 2012 Census Briefs*. Available at https://www.census.gov/population/age/data/2012comp.html. Accessed February 14, 2017

2. Stang J, Story MT, Harnack L, Neumark-Sztainer D. Relationships between vitamin and mineral supplement use, dietary intake, and dietary adequacy among adolescents. *J Am Diet Assoc*. 2000;100(8):905–910

3. US Department of Agriculture, Agriculture Research Service. *What we eat in America*. NHANES 2013–2014. Available at: https://www.ars.usda.gov/northeast-area/beltsville-md/beltsville-human-nutrition-research-center/food-surveys-research-group/docs/wweia-data-tables/. Accessed February 14, 2017

4. Nielsen SJ, Rossen LM, Harris DM, Odgen CL. Fruit and vegetable consumption of U.S. Youth, 2009–2010. *NCHS Data Brief*. 2014(156):1-8

5. Centers for Disease Control and Prevention. Fruit and vegetable consumption among high school students—United States, 2010. *MMWR Morb Mortal Wkly Rep*. 2010;60(46):1583–1586

6. Centers for Disease Control and Prevention. Youth Risk Behavior Surveillance — United States, 2015. Available at: https://www.cdc.gov/healthyyouth/data/yrbs/pdf/2015/ss6506_updated.pdf. Accessed February 14, 2017

7. Ogden CL, Carroll MD, Kit BK, Flegal KM. Prevalence of childhood and adult obesity in the United States, 2011–2012. *JAMA*. 2014;311(8):806–814

8. Corkins MR, Daniels SR, de Ferranti SD, et al. Nutrition in children and adolescents. *Med Clin North Am*. 2016;100(6):1217–1235

9. American Academy of Pediatrics, Committee on Adolescence; American College of Obstetricians and Gynecologists, Committee on Adolescent Health Care. Menstruation in girls and adolescents: using the menstrual cycle as a vital sign. *Pediatrics*. 2006;118(5):2245–2250

10. Institute of Medicine Food and Nutrition Board. *Dietary Reference Intakes: The Essential Guide to Nutrient Requirements*. Otten JJ, Hellwig JP, Meyers LD, eds. Washington, DC: National Academies Press; 2006

11. Forbes GB. Nutritional requirements in adolescence. In: Suskind RM, ed. *Textbook of Pediatric Nutrition*. New York, NY: Raven Press; 1981:381–391

12. Usual Dietary Intakes: Food Intakes, U.S. Population, 2007–10. Epidemiology and Genomics Research Program website. National Cancer Institute. Available at: http://epi.grants.cancer.gov/diet/usualintakes/pop/2007–10/index.html. Updated May 20, 2015. Accessed February 14, 2017

13. Rosen DS; American Academy of Pediatrics, Committee on Adolescence. Identification and management of eating disorders in children and adolescents. *Pediatrics*. 2010;126(6):1240–1253

14. Ogden CL, Carroll MD, Lawman HG, et al. Trends in obesity prevalence among children and adolescents in the United States, 1988–1994 Through 2013–2014. *JAMA*. 2016;315(21):2292–2299

15. Cooke AG, McCavit TL, Buchanan GR, Powers JM. Iron deficiency anemia in adolescents who present with heavy menstrual bleeding. *J Pediatr Adolesc Gynecol*. 2017;30(2):247–250

16. Roe DA. Diet-drug interactions and incompatibilities. In: Hathcock JN, Coon J, eds. *Nutrition and Drug Interrelations*. New York, NY: Academic Press; 1978:319–345

17. Webber LS, Hunter SM, Johnson CC, Srinivasan SR, Berenson GS. Smoking, alcohol, and oral contraceptives. Effects on lipids during adolescence and young adulthood—Bogalusa Heart Study. *Ann N Y Acad Sci*. 1991;623:135–154

18. Golden NH, Abrams SA, Committee on Nutrition. Optimizing bone health in children and adolescents. *Pediatrics*. 2014;134(4):e1229–e1243

19. Bailey DA, Martin AD, McKay HA, Whiting S, Mirwald R. Calcium accretion in girls and boys during puberty: a longitudinal analysis. *J Bone Miner Res*. 2000;15(11):2245–2250

20. Bachrach LK. Acquisition of optimal bone mass in childhood and adolescence. *Trends Endocrinol Metab*. 2001;12(1):22–28

21. Khosla S, Melton LJ, 3rd, Dekutoski MB, Achenbach SJ, Oberg AL, Riggs BL. Incidence of childhood distal forearm fractures over 30 years: a population-based study. *JAMA*. 2003;290(11):1479–1485

22. Faulkner RA, Davison KS, Bailey DA, Mirwald RL, Baxter-Jones AD. Size-corrected BMD decreases during peak linear growth: implications for fracture incidence during adolescence. *J Bone Miner Res*. 2006;21(12):1864–1870

23. Institute of Medicine. 2011 *Dietary Reference Intakes for Calcium and Vitamin D.* Washington, DC: The National Academies Press; 2011

24. Centers for Disease Control Prevention. Beverage consumption among high school students—United States, 2010. *MMWR Morb Mortal Wkly Rep.* 2011;60(23):778–780

25. Vartanian LR, Schwartz MB, Brownell KD. Effects of soft drink consumption on nutrition and health: a systematic review and meta-analysis. *Am J Public Health.* 2007;97(4):667–675

26. Miller G, Merlo C, Demissie Z, Sliwa S, Park S. Trends in beverage consumption among high school students—United States, 2007–2015. *MMWR Morb Mortal Wkly Rep.* 2017;66(4):112–116

27. Golden NH, Carey DE. Vitamin D in health and disease in adolescents: when to screen, whom to treat, and how to treat. *Adolesc Med State Art Rev.* 2016;27(1): 125–139

28. Centers for Disease Control and Prevention. Reproductive health: teen pregnancy (2007–2015). Available at: https://www.cdc.gov/teenpregnancy/about/index.htm. Accessed January 13, 2019

29. Mei Z, Cogswell ME, Looker AC, et al. Assessment of iron status in US pregnant women from the National Health and Nutrition Examination Survey (NHANES), 1999–2006. *Am J Clin Nutr.* 2011;93(6):1312–1320

30. Institute of Medicine. *Weight Gain During Pregnancy: Reexamining the Guidelines.* Washington, DC: National Academies Press; 2009

31. Groth SW. The long-term impact of adolescent gestational weight gain. *Res Nurs Health.* 2008;31(2):108–118

32. Nielsen JN, Gittelsohn J, Anliker J, O'Brien K. Interventions to improve diet and weight gain among pregnant adolescents and recommendations for future research. *J Am Diet Assoc.* 2006;106(11):1825–1840

33. Joseph NP, Hunkali KB, Wilson B, Morgan E, Cross M, Freund KM. Pre-pregnancy body mass index among pregnant adolescents: gestational weight gain and long-term post partum weight retention. *J Pediatr Adolesc Gynecol.* 2008;21(4):195–200

34. The NS, Suchindran C, North KE, Popkin BM, Gordon-Larsen P. Association of adolescent obesity with risk of severe obesity in adulthood. *JAMA.* 2010;304(18):2042–2047

35. Golden NH, Schneider M, Wood C, American Academy of Pediatrics, Committee on Nutrition, Committee on Adolescence, Section on Obesity. Preventing obesity and eating disorders in adolescents. *Pediatrics.* 2016;138(3):e20161649

36. Expert Panel on Integrated Guidelines for Cardiovascular Health Risk Reduction in Children and Adolescents, National Heart Lung Blood Institute. Expert panel on integrated guidelines for cardiovascular health and risk reduction in children and adolescents: summary report. *Pediatrics.* 2011;128(Suppl 5):S213–S256

37. US Department of Health and Human Services, US Department of Agriculture. 2015–2020 Dietary Guidelines for Americans. 8th ed. December 2015. Available at: http://health.gov/dietaryguidelines/2015/guidelines/. Accessed February 21, 2017

38. American Academy of Pediatrics, Council on School Health, Committee on Nutrition. Snacks, sweetened beverages, added sugars, and schools. *Pediatrics.* 2015;135(3):575–583

39. Liang T, Kuhle S, Veugelers PJ. Nutrition and body weights of Canadian children watching television and eating while watching television. *Public Health Nutr.* 2009;12(12):2457–2463

40. Hoyland A, Dye L, Lawton CL. A systematic review of the effect of breakfast on the cognitive performance of children and adolescents. *Nutr Res Rev.* 2009;22(2):220–243

41. Szajewska H, Ruszczynski M. Systematic review demonstrating that breakfast consumption influences body weight outcomes in children and adolescents in Europe. *Crit Rev Food Sci Nutr.* 2010;50(2):113–119

42. Neumark-Sztainer DR, Wall MM, Haines JI, Story MT, Sherwood NE, van den Berg PA. Shared risk and protective factors for overweight and disordered eating in adolescents. *Am J Prev Med.* 2007;33(5):359–369

43. Kimm SY, Glynn NW, Kriska AM, et al. Decline in physical activity in black girls and white girls during adolescence. *New Engl J Med.* 2002;347(10):709–715

44. Robinson TN. Reducing children's television viewing to prevent obesity: a randomized controlled trial. *JAMA.* 1999;282(16):1561–1567

45. Institute of Medicine, Food and Nutrition Board. *Dietary Reference Intakes for Vitamin A, Vitamin K, Arsenic, Boron, Chromium, Copper, Iodine, Iron, Manganese, Molybdenum, Nickel, Silicon, Vanadium, and Zinc.* Washington, DC: National Academies Press; 2001

Chapter 9

Nutrition in School, Preschool, and Child Care

Introduction

School food service is complex. It is not simply the provision of school meals but encompasses many components, including nutritional quality, staff training, economics, food safety, provisions for specialized diets, and frequently changing national and state regulations. The topic covers federal meal programs in schools but also food service in child care, preschool, after school, and summer care settings, as well as all foods available in and around schools during the school day. As such, it forms a critical pillar of child nutrition.

Foods in schools are made available to students in 3 different venues: (1) federal school meal programs administered by the US Department of Agriculture (USDA); (2) items vended in schools in competition with federal meal programs; and (3) items brought into school from myriad other sources (packed meals, snacks and beverages, in-class parties, club sales, sporting events, etc).

Recent neurocognitive testing and brain imaging studies have underscored the fact that healthy children are better students, particularly children and adolescents facing economic or social disadvantages.[1] More than 95% of American school-aged children, or 55 million, attend public or private schools. A typical child spends as much as 6 hours per day in school and consumes 35% of his or her daily energy at school, compared with 56% at home. In early life, of the 24 million children 0 through 5 years of age, 60% participate in some form of child-care arrangement supplying meals or snacks that affect dietary patterns.[2] One of the core missions of school meals is to support the needs of children from families facing food insecurity or chronic dietary inadequacy (see Chapter 49: Preventing Food Insecurity).

The US Nutrition Safety Net

Since the Great Depression in the 1930s, governmental nutrition assistance has provided a crucial protection from hunger and malnutrition in the lives of Americans, especially children (Table 9.1)[3] (see also Chapter 49). The largest federal program, the Supplemental Nutrition Assistance Program (SNAP), served an average of 42.2 million people per month at an annual cost of $68 billion in 2017, while the Special Supplemental Nutrition Program

Table 9.1.
Nutrition Safety Net Programs for Preschool and School Children

- The National School Lunch Program (NSLP)
- The School Breakfast Program (SBP)
- After School Snacks
- The Special Milk Program
- The Fresh Fruit and Vegetable Program
- The Child and Adult Care Food Program (CACFP)
- The Summer Food Service Program (SFSP)
- Team Nutrition

for Women, Infants, and Children (WIC) Program served nearly 7.3 million people per month at an annual cost of $5.6 billion in 2017. The federal programs targeting school-aged children represent an additional investment of $18 billion in cash and commodity costs in 2017, serving 30 million in the school lunch program and 14.7 million in the school breakfast program.[4] Collectively, these programs have a profound effect on preventing hunger and preserving diet quality among US children at the highest nutritional risk. However, in 2016 the USDA Economic Research Service (ERS) which tracks US food insecurity, reported a food insecurity rate of 12.3% in US households, or 15.6 million households containing 41.2 million people.[4] The American Academy of Pediatrics (AAP) has issued policy statements discussing the associated threats that food insecurity and family poverty pose for child health and mental health[5,6] (see also Chapter 49).

The Legacy of School Meals

Early models of school meals date back to the late 1800s. Even before Congress passed and President Harry Truman signed the 1946 National School Lunch Act (Pub L No. 79-396), it was recognized that children in poverty needed school meals both for nutritional stability and for academic productivity. The intent of the National School Lunch Program (NSLP) was to provide children with at least 1 nutritious meal every day at school. The lunch was designed to provide one third to one half of the daily requirements for a 10- to 12-year-old child, a benchmark that was sustained for 3 decades. The Child Nutrition Act of 1966 established the School Breakfast Program (SBP) as a pilot for low-income children, especially those traveling long distances to school. In 1975, the SBP became a permanent entitlement alongside the NSLP, administered by the USDA Food and Nutrition Service (FNS). Optimal growth and development and the provision of balanced macro- and micronutrients, as specified by the Recommended Dietary Allowances (RDAs), served as the scientific foundation for program standards. The landmark Healthy, Hunger-Free Kids Act of 2010 (HHFKA [Pub L No. 111-196]) extensively revised school meals to meet the directives of the Dietary Guidelines for Americans (DGAs).[7,8]

The Landmark Healthy, Hunger-Free Kids Act of 2010

The 2010 HHFKA included the most significant changes for the school food program in more than 3 decades.[9] The bill included several new provisions to update school nutrition, including moving to a model based on the number of servings of the 5 food groups per week, aligned with the most recent DGAs. For the first time in a quarter-century, the bill provided some additional funding to schools per meal to help offset rising costs of food purchases. It also authorized higher-quality commodity foods for use by school food service. The bill introduced some new, far-reaching provisions and gave the USDA the authority to set nutritional standards for all foods regularly sold during the school day, including vended and a la carte items, as well as those sold in school stores. The new USDA rules were instituted in 2014. Besides schools, they also established directives to promote new nutrition standards in child care settings through the Child and Adult Care Food Program (CACFP). Further, the law enhanced school food safety, stressed greater educational training opportunities for school food staff, and gave further guidance to each school's wellness committee to help shape food and physical activity policies not covered under the federal nutrition standards.

Adherence to these guidelines, with their emphasis on whole-grain foods, fruits, and vegetables, naturally limits discretionary solid fats and added sugars within school meals. Minimum and maximum calorie recommendations were intended to represent the average daily amount for a 5-day school week and not on a per-meal or per-day basis. For certain age groups, such as adolescent males, achieving the minimum daily calories may be a challenge for the school food service to achieve consistently. To address this, discretionary sources of calories (solid fats and added sugars) may be added to the meal pattern, provided that they remain within the overall specifications for calories, saturated fat, trans fat, and sodium. The law directed that school breakfasts gradually cut sodium by 25% and school lunches by 50% over the ensuing 10 years.

New alternatives for meat servings were introduced to include other protein sources, such as nuts, seeds, or nut butters or flours, yogurt

Table 9.2.
Nondairy Alternative Fortification Requirements

Nutrient	Per cup (8 fl oz)
Calcium	276 mg
Protein	8 g
Vitamin A	500 IU
Vitamin D	100 IU
Magnesium	24 mg
Phosphorus	222 mg
Potassium	349 mg
Riboflavin	0.44 mg
Vitamin B$_{12}$	1.1 µg

products, and enriched macaroni. Forms of meats or meat alternatives may not be repeated more than 3 times weekly. Similarly, fluid milk substitutes may be used if warranted for students with medical, dietary, or cultural needs. However, nondairy substitutes must follow fortification guidelines of the US Food and Drug Administration (Table 9.2).

Standards for Food Sold in Competition to School Meals
One of the most far-reaching provisions in the HHFKA of 2010 was to delegate to the USDA responsibility for *all* foods sold on the school campus during "the school day," which was defined as the period from midnight before to 30 minutes after the end of the school day.[9] This included all snack items sold in competition to the school meal programs. Despite the wide variety of definitions attached to the term "empty calories," studies for more than a decade had found that snack-type foods and beverages high in energy and low in nutritional value represent 30% to 40% of the total energy consumed by children and adolescents.[10] At the request of the USDA, an expert committee of the National Academy of Medicine (NAM; formerly, Institute of Medicine) studied the issue of competitive foods and made recommendations. The committee found that many forms of snack foods and beverages were consumed in schools, made available through snack bars, school stores, a la carte lines, and booster and bake sales. The NAM

committee outlined criteria to ensure that all vended food items contributed to the child's personal dietary pattern without raising the risk of excess daily energy. These recommendations formed the basis for new USDA rules, "Smart Snacks in Schools."[11]

To qualify as a "Smart Snack," a snack or entrée had to meet these nutrition standards (see Table 9.3):

- Be a grain product that contains 50% or more whole grains by weight (have a whole grain as the first ingredient); or
- Have as the first ingredient a fruit, a vegetable, a dairy product, or a protein food; or
- Be a combination food that contains at least ¼ cup of fruit and/or vegetable; *and*
- Meet the nutrient standards for calories, sodium, sugars, and fats.

Within Smart Snacks, an entrée must contain one of the following combinations:

- meat/meat alternate + whole grain-rich food
- vegetable + meat/meat alternate
- fruit + meat/meat alternate
- meat/meat alternate alone, except for meat snacks (eg, beef jerky), yogurt, cheese, nuts, seeds, and nut or seed butters; *and*
- a grain solely, that is, a whole grain-rich entrée that is served as the main dish within the School Breakfast Program reimbursable meal.

Beverages were addressed by the standards as well. Water, with or without carbonation, was not limited. Milk portions were limited to 8 fl oz

Table 9.3.
Smart Snack Guidelines

Nutrient	Snack	Entree
Energy (kcals)	200 kcal or less	350 kcal or less
Sodium	200 mg or less	480 mg or less
Total fat	35% of kcal or less	35% of kcal or less
Saturated fat	Less than 10% of kcal	Less than 10% of kcal
Trans fat	0 g	0 g
Sugar	35% by weight or less	35% by weight or less

for elementary schools, 12 fl oz for middle schools, and 12 fl oz for high schools. Unflavored varieties may be low fat or fat free, but flavored milks had to be fat free, mirroring the standards for federal school meal programs. Portion sizes of 100% fruit or vegetable juices, with or without dilution or carbonation, were the same as those for milk. Low-calorie (12 fl oz or less) and no-calorie (less than 5 kcal/8 fl oz, up to 10 kcal/20 fl oz) beverages, with or without caffeine or carbonation, were made available only in high schools.

School districts had to address several issues surrounding the issue of vended competitive foods, such as planning for a successful transition, communicating with food manufacturers or vendors, identifying compliant food and beverage products, ensuring ongoing support from school leaders, dealing with situations in which foods and beverages were not covered by the law (ie, nonvended foods, class parties, banquets, fundraising sales, etc). Districts also had to deal with any substantial changes in sales that may affect revenue streams.[12] To determine whether a particular product meets the standards, schools have utilized the information available on the Nutrition Facts Panel, along with a calculator, provided by the FNS (Smart Snacks Product Calculator). The FNS, in conjunction with the Alliance for a Healthier Generation, also provided a simple reference that listed qualified products and identified items that were exempted because they contained critical nutrients that help meet requirements, such as fresh, canned, or dried fruits or cheese or nut butters provided in conjunction with fruits or vegetables.[11]

The Basis for New School Nutrition Standards

Optimal nutrition for all Americans older than 2 years is described by the DGAs. The most recent guidelines (2015–2020) were released in December 2015.[13] The Dietary Guidelines for Americans Committee based its recommendations on evidence supporting consumption of healthy eating patterns, which the committee defined this way: "An eating pattern represents the totality of all foods and beverages consumed. All foods consumed as part of a healthy eating pattern fit together like a puzzle to meet nutritional needs without exceeding limits, such as those for saturated fats, added sugars, sodium, and total calories. All forms of foods, including fresh, canned, dried, and frozen, can be included in healthy eating patterns."[13] Dietary patterns are adaptable, meaning that there are many paths for an individual's personal dietary pattern to support health outcomes. The basis

Table 9.4.

Minimum and Maximum Calorie Intakes

Grades	Breakfast Program	Lunch Program
K–5	350–500 kcal	550–650 kcal
6–8	400–550 kcal	600–700 kcal
9–12	450–600 kcal	750–850 kcal

for a healthy personal dietary pattern consists of consumption of nutrient-dense foods within each of the 5 food groups: vegetables (diversity of red, yellow, green items), assorted fruit and 100% fruit juices, grains (in particular whole grains), reduced-fat or no-fat milk and dairy products, and quality protein sources (lean meats, fish, legumes, eggs, nuts, and seeds).

The new DGAs stressed limiting the intake of solid fats, added sugars, and sodium, along with greater physical activity at all ages with an emphasis on achieving energy balance, matching caloric intake with routine activity levels. The DGAs also identified 4 nutrients of public health concern for nearly all Americans: potassium, fiber, vitamin D, and calcium. The NAM provided new recommendations for school meals based on the 2005 DGAs. This report, and the subsequent FNS proposals in 2011, recommended that school meals be based on the provision of the appropriate number servings of food groups per week. To do so, the rules established serving frequency, appropriate serving sizes, and minimum and maximum caloric intake targets by age and grade (Table 9.4). By following their serving-based approach, the NAM determined that students would meet the Dietary Reference Intakes for all nutrients.

Participation in School Meals

Any student can consume school meals if his or her school participates in the federal meal programs. What the student pays depends on family income. Families below 130% of the federal poverty level (FPL) qualify for free school meals, and those between 130% and 185% of the FPL qualify for reduced-price meals and pay $0.30 per breakfast and $0.40 per lunch. Children and adolescents from families above 185% of the FPL pay charges set by the school, which receives a small federal reimbursement to offset costs for each. Most students establish free or reduced-price eligibility through applications to their school district. However, children from households already participating in SNAP, the Temporary Assistance for Needy Families (TANF), or the Food Distribution Program on Indian Reservations (FDPIR), as well as those in Head Start and Early Head Start, migrants, homeless, runaway youth, and foster care children are considered "categorically eligible" without additional application.

USDA meal programs exist in nearly every one of the nation's 105 000 public and nonprofit private schools and residential child care institutions. In 2018, of the total meals served in the NSLP and SBP, 74% and 85%, respectively, qualify for free or reduced-price meals, indicating that the original mission to protect the food-insecure child is being met.[14]

Participation in school meal programs is increasing, reflective of the economic status of US children. Participation rose substantially after the 2007 recession, peaking in 2014, although rates of participation decreased slightly through 2018.[14,15] The recession caused a large influx of children who had not previously qualified for federal meals in the past. Nearly all of them matched criteria for free meals. School meals offered struggling families an extension of their food budget, preventing many from falling below federal poverty thresholds.[15] Increases in the cost of full-pay meals for students who do not qualify for free or reduced-price meal support, along with stringent regulation of vended competitive foods in schools, have decreased participation rates among children from higher-income families.[15]

Participation rates were further stimulated by the USDA's rollout of the Community Eligibility Provision (CEP) in 2015.[16] The CEP is a meal service option for schools and school districts in low-income areas. It was a novel provision of the HHFKA of 2010 intended to make it easier for districts and local educational agencies within the nation's highest poverty areas to serve universal breakfast and lunch to all enrolled students without cost. Participating in the CEP is a voluntary decision made by local school districts on the basis of their specific student population. Participating districts with 40% of students qualifying for free and reduced-price meals are exempt from the burden of collecting individual household applications, saving time and money. However, participating districts must offer a SBP along with the NSLP, a stipulation that has greatly stimulated breakfast access for the nation's poorest children. The ratio of school breakfasts served relative to school lunches is a national measure of improvement toward coverage for all high-risk children, tracked annually for all states by the Food Research and Action Center (FRAC).[17] By raising meal participation rates, the CEP has provided additional financial stability for school food service and has helped ameliorate nutritional risk for children in economic areas with the highest likelihood of temporary, circumstantial food insecurity.

The Summer Food Service Program (SFSP)

Summer recess is 3 months long. For food-insecure children, this represents a very stressful time without the security of school meals. Evidence has shown that during summer, all children consume foods with a lower diet quality, are more sedentary, and are more prone to weight gain than during the school year.[18] The USDA Summer Food Service Program (SFSP) was designed to ensure that low-income children continue to receive nutritious meals by employing the CEP formula to offer universal free meals wherever possible, without individual eligibility applications.[19] Meals are provided by local organizations and agencies, such as libraries, parks and recreation sites, opened school cafeterias, youth sport leagues, camps, and organizations such as the YMCA/YWCA, Big Brothers/Big Sisters, and many others.[20] Each qualified site receives reimbursement for the cost and the administration of the meals. Although the approved SFSP sites served more than 200 million free meals to children 18 years and younger during the summer of 2017, that that number represents a mere fraction of the 44 million school meals served every day throughout the school year in US schools. Championing the creation of approved access sites for summer meals is a simple but powerful way for pediatricians and child health professionals across the country to improve the nutritional stability of children and adolescents within their local community. Furthermore, since being piloted at Arkansas Children's Hospital in 2008, establishing meal programs within children's hospitals across the nation has been a key strategy of the USDA.[21,22]

The Nutritional Effectiveness of the School Meal Programs

An independent research firm contracted by the USDA, the FNS closely monitors school meals nutrition in relation to the recommendations of the DGAs. The School Nutrition Dietary Assessment Studies (SNDAs)—SNDA I 1991–92, SNDA II 1998–99, SNDA III 2004–05, and SNDA IV 2012–13—have each informed changes to federal school nutrition policy for more than 2 decades. As a result, the nutritional quality of school meals has increased steadily. Because of a focus on total, saturated, and trans fats by the DGAs in the 1970s through early 2000s, SNDA I-III aimed to ensure balanced consumption of macro- and micronutrients, especially lowering the contribution of fats within meals. To do so, meals during this phase were designed using standardized menu-planning tools with quantitative goals for nutrient content. This approach successfully limited total and saturated fats, primarily by limiting milks to low-fat and nonfat varieties.[23] The early SNDAs also answered a critical question of whether participation in school meals was a factor in increasing rates of obesity. Data clearly showed neutral or lowered risk for obesity in children consuming school meals regularly.

The advent of the obesity "crisis" shifted the DGA's national nutrition goals away from the risk of individual nutrient concerns toward the benefits of a health-promoting dietary pattern, as first delineated in the DGA 2010. The pivotal HHFKA of 2010, relying on data gathered in SNDA III and IV, attempted to mirror the novel shift in DGA directives, as applied to school meal preparation. Because of its emphasis on increasing whole grains, fruits, and vegetables while limiting sodium and added sugars, concerns were raised about decreased participation and increased food waste. Preliminary research studies suggest that school environments have shown positive changes in diet quality of all foods sold on campus. Students have adjusted well to the substantially altered servings-based menu design, without evidence of significant increases in plate waste.[24] However, the data are indirect, generally. The first comprehensive evaluation of the impact of the HHFKA of 2010 will come from the School Nutrition and Meal Cost Study (SNMCS) for the years 2014–15.[25] It will study the food and nutrient content of school meals as well as the costs of school meals, evaluate the food environments in schools, and contain a 24-hour food recall component to assess the contribution of school meals to children's overall diets.

Nutrition Standards in Preschool and Child Care

Of the 24 million children 5 years and younger in 2012, more than 60% attended some form of nonparental child care. Between ages 3 and 5 years, 75% of children attend child care. Working parents use many different types of care, including center-based care (34%), child care in another family's home (8%), or relative care (26%). A minority used multiple forms of child care (12%).[26] State-level child care statistics are gathered annually by Child Care Aware.[27]

Child care offers a particularly important opportunity for laying a foundation of quality nutrition and routine physical activity in early life.

Experiences in various child-care settings offer the potential for encouraging balanced nutrition and physical activity that could help to shape a child's development, food preferences, and play habits. In the preschool phase from ages 3 to 5 years, only 55% of the children in child care are in a center-based educational service with written policies that cover dietary practices.[28] In higher quality child-care settings, nutrition is an important part of the learning experience. But the cost of higher-quality, center-based child care averaged nearly $7000 annually per child in the period immediately following the recession, with costs ranging widely from $4000 to $18000 across the United States.[26] Informal child care, provided by relatives or paid caregivers in their homes, has lower diet quality compared with the child's home, highlighting the opportunity for improving child nutrition.[29]

In a position statement on nutrition in child care settings, the Academy of Nutrition and Dietetics encouraged all child care providers to align their food offerings with the DGAs and the CACFP meal patterns and portion sizes, although the DGAs do not cover the first 2 years of life.[30] State requirements for nutrition in child care settings most commonly follow the CACFP meal plans.[31] The CACFP serves 4.2 million children and, like the school meal programs for older children, reimburses free or reduced-price meals for very young children on the basis of financial need in child care centers, group homes, and in-home care settings for 3 age categories: 1 through 2 years, 3 through 5 years, and 6 through 12 years. The CACFP designates nutrition quality on the basis of a meal pattern approach, offering portion size guidance and nutrition education. A variety of child care settings are eligible: at-risk after school care centers, child care centers, day care homes, and emergency shelters and Head Start programs. Individual states often augment the CACFP standards with provisions that further limit foods of low nutritional value in child care settings (see also Chapter 49).

In April 2016, the USDA issued revised nutrition standards for CACFP meal patterns to align them with the DGAs, following the mandate of the HHFKA of 2010.[32] Meal patterns stipulate servings for infants and young children for fruits, vegetables, meats, meat alternatives, juices and milks, and cereals and grains along with recommendations for best practices in nutrition and food safety. Importantly, independent child care centers and in-home child care sites are eligible to participate in CACFP with reimbursement for meals and snacks served. This reimbursement not only encourages improved diet quality for the child and education for the child care provider, but also reduces the cost of providing care and supports these sites as small businesses. Some states have organizations that help support CACFP in private child care arrangements.[33] For many preschool-aged children, consumption of breakfast at home is followed by a second breakfast at school or in child care. In one recent study, nearly one third of students in a Head Start preschool consumed double breakfast.[34] Despite concerns about higher risk of obesity, the study failed to show a correlation with obesity, mirroring studies on middle school students consuming 2 breakfasts.[35] Among Hispanic preschool children, double breakfast was associated with a 60% lower likelihood of obesity. Early wake-up time was a significant factor in consumption of breakfast at home before school.[34] Conversely, young children who skipped breakfast show a higher risk of obesity.[36]

The Complex Business of School Food Service

The USDA FNS sets policy that directs how school menus should be designed. The School Food Service (SFS) staff is responsible for producing meals that are palatable, are economical, and can be delivered within a strict time frame set aside within the school day. The SFS generally consists of:

- SFS director (supervisor, coordinator): oversees all aspects of the food service in accordance with local, state, and federal policies, working closely with the district chief financial officer and reporting directly to the superintendent.

- SFS nutrition supervisor (assistant director, specialist, dietitian, executive chef): larger school districts often require greater management for food production, particularly if a central facility produces meals for many schools. The SFS nutrition supervisor often handles procurement, financial budgeting, menu planning, recipe development, personnel, training, catering or vending operations, and warehouse management.

- SFS assistant manager (head cook, lead): is involved in day-to-day operations at an individual feeding site or school, ensuring food safety, sanitation, meal quality, special meal needs (food allergies, celiac disease, etc), supervising employees, and ordering and inventory of foods.

- SFS employee (assistant, technician, cook/cashier, dishwashers): work within individual schools to prepare and serve food, ensure efficiency of meal times, and clean and maintain the facility and equipment.

One of the directives of the HHFKA of 2010 was to improve the professional training and qualifications of the individuals who manage SFS. The School Nutrition Association (SNA) provides training, credentialing, certification, and resources for SFS staff and engages in national advocacy for those in the field.

The most difficult challenge for SFS is balancing limited operating costs with ever-stringent federal nutrition requirements. According to the School Lunch and Breakfast Cost Study II, SFS budgets consist of food (37%), personnel/benefits (48%), supplies (5%), and "other" (including leased equipment, custodial services, etc). Indirect costs, such as equipment maintenance, utilities, transportation, fuel, and waste charges, generally are not included in the reported SFS budget. The cost of producing an NSLP-reimbursable lunch averaged $2.28 and the SBP-reimbursable breakfast averaged $1.92 (Table 9.5). But when total costs were calculated, a school lunch cost well above the current reimbursement rate.[37] The USDA estimated that the stipulations of the HHFKA of 2010 added $0.10 to the cost of each school lunch and $0.27 of each breakfast, on the basis of costs for whole grains, fresh fruits, and vegetables, primarily. But the HHFKA provided only $0.06 additional funds to cover them. Further, these numbers are skewed by larger school districts that are able to maintain relatively low costs per meal by producing a high volume of meals and by efficiencies in centralized production. The ever-increasing expenses of SFS over the past 3 decades have never been fully offset by the annual cost-of-living adjustments that are built into the Child Nutrition Reauthorizations.

A significant hidden expense for the SFS is unpaid meals. Since the recession in 2007, the number of children who receive meals even when

Table 9.5.

Per-Meal Reimbursement Rates for School Meal Programs (2016–17)

Centers	Breakfast	Lunch/Supper	Snack
Contiguous 48 States[a]			
Free	$1.71	$3.16	$0.86
Reduced	$1.41	$2.76	$0.43
Full price	$0.29	$0.30	$0.07

[a] Reimbursement is higher for Alaska and Hawaii.

their parents fail to pay the charges has increased significantly. According to the SNA State of School Nutrition 2016 survey, 76% of districts reported unpaid meal debt at the end of the school year.[38]

Agricultural commodity stores represent a critical supplement to help schools meet nutritional guidelines and maintain a reasonable cost.[39] Commodities provide approximately 15% to 20% of the food items served. More than 180 products are available to schools that cover all 5 food groups, including sauces, meats, canned and frozen vegetables, fruits, juices, and grains. Food purchasing agents, the American Marketing Service, and the and USDA Farm Service Agency must meet the USDA's strict food safety guidelines. Each commodity item is accompanied by a food fact sheet for the SFS staff that lists the food item, the amount, a description of the product, its nutrition fact label, storage information, and tips for preparation. Fruits are packed in extra light sucrose syrup or remain unsweetened, such as applesauce. Vegetable products are limited to 140 mg of sodium per serving or less, many as no-salt varieties. Meats are offered as lean, low-fat servings. Lard and butter have been eliminated altogether as commodity products. In this way, the USDA contributes to the provisions of the DGAs as it helps the nation's 105 000 schools meet the directives of the FNS. In fiscal year 2012, the commodity food service was estimated to have delivered to schools agricultural products valued at more than $1.12 billion dollars.

School Meal Standards, Nutrient Intake, and Plate Waste

The HHFKA of 2010 was a watershed in child nutrition but also represented a high-stakes gamble. By aligning the design of federal school meals with the guidance of the 2010 DGAs, the aim was to strengthen every child's dietary pattern. To achieve this, food group servings per week became the primary benchmark. By mandating more fruits, vegetables, and whole grains while curtailing saturated fats, added sugars, and sodium, the USDA made a number of assumptions about the capabilities of the SFS. New food items required to meet the standards were expensive, yet little accommodation was made to offset costs before the rollout in the new rules in the 2012–13 school year. Standards dramatically altered foods available through a la carte lines and vending machines, a lucrative revenue stream that SFS directors previously had used to counterbalance losses in school meal preparation. Most critically, the HHFKA of 2010 assumed that the cumulative changes to school foods would be accepted by children and adolescents. Maintaining meal participation and increasing food consumption are the most critical measures of success. SFS meal preparation entails fixed costs for personnel, food, equipment, and indirect expenses of the school. Any decrease in participation rapidly drains revenue. In terms of nutrition, mandating the healthier food items is one thing, but getting children to consume it is another. Taste, value, and convenience—the 3 pillars of food choice—made this a risky proposition in terms of student participation and plate waste.

In serving 44 million school meals per day, the nation's SFS has always dealt with extensive food waste. Plate waste is not the same every day, but rather is affected by students' food preferences, convenience, the eating environment, the amount of time allotted for meals, the decision to offer recess before lunch, and the impact of SFS innovations. Even before the HHFKA of 2010, plate waste was consistently recorded as 20% to 50% of all foods served. Fruit and vegetable intake always was poor.[40] In general, younger students consumed significantly fewer calories and wasted more total and red-orange vegetables, fruit, total/whole/refined grains, and total protein foods than older students.[41] In a study published in 2014, using digital photography, researchers quantified plate waste in elementary and middle school populations. Only 45% of elementary and 34% middle school students selected a vegetable. Elementary school students wasted more than a third of grain, fruit, and vegetable menu items. Middle school students left nearly 50% of fresh fruit, 37% of canned fruit, and nearly a third of vegetables unconsumed. Less than half of the students met the national meal standards for vitamins A and C or iron.[40]

Increasing children's fruit and vegetable consumption was a fundamental goal of the HHFKA of 2010. One of the most significant changes, as it pertains to food waste, was that all students were required "to be served" a fruit or vegetable with lunch. Previously, schools were only required "to offer" fruit or vegetable.[24,42] Concern was heightened among the public, school administrators, and elected officials that this change was causing an increase in food waste while adding costs to school budgets. Los Angeles Unified School District reported daily waste to cost $100 000 per day, not only in food value but also in paying for removal of the waste.[43] Initially, of 240 school nutrition directors surveyed, more than 80% subjectively reported an increase in the amount of plate waste by students, particularly of vegetables.[44] Justifiably, SFS directors were concerned that increased waste was a harbinger for decreased participation in meal programs that could have a catastrophic effect on the SFS budget.

Initial research studies quantifying plate waste showed mixed results immediately following implementation of the HHFKA of 2010. Just and Price[45] found that requiring students to take at least 1 serving of fruit or vegetable at 3 elementary schools (kindergarten through 5th grade) in Utah significantly increased the amount of fruits and vegetables wasted. Cohen et al,[46] however, found that after implementation of the new rules at 4 schools within 1 low-income, urban school district in Massachusetts, increases in meal waste for entrées, fruits, or vegetables was not seen. The increase in portion size for vegetables actually resulted in more cups of vegetables consumed. Byker et al[47] measured food waste generated from preschool and kindergarten students, who are the most likely to waste food, after implementation of the new regulations at an elementary school in an urban cluster of a rural county in the southwestern United States. Over the course of a week, overall food wastage was 45.3%, with vegetables discarded in the highest amount (51.4%) and fruit in the lowest amount (33.0%). However, there was significant variability in the amount of food wasted on any given day; vegetables ranged from 26.1% to 80%, for instance. Cullen et al[48] studied both elementary and middle school students in both intervention and control school cafeterias. In intervention cafeterias, the new meal pattern allowed students to select 1 fruit and 2 vegetable servings per reimbursable meal. In control cafeterias, students could only select a total of 2 fruit and vegetable servings per meal. Significantly more intervention elementary and intermediate school students selected and consumed total and starchy vegetables, fruit, legumes, protein foods. In addition, significantly fewer calories were consumed by elementary and intermediate students at the intervention schools.

In 2017, Cullen and Dave[24] reviewed the available studies completed since the introduction of the new meal standards. Two approaches to studying effects of the new standards were used:(1) changes in student dietary outcomes, and(2) changes in the school food environment. The results generally showed improvements over time. However, differences in grade level, ethnicities, geographic locations, and percent of free and reduced-price populations included in the studies made comparisons difficult. In the 3 studies that utilized similar methodologies and evaluated student consumption directly, the evidence suggested that the new meal patterns did not increase plate waste and had improved fruit and/or vegetable consumption. Of note, a large study at 3 high schools and 3 middle schools in Washington state by

Johnson et al[49] not only measured participation rates but also assessed diet quality in the 15 months before and the 16 months after implementation, assessing a central outcome of the HHFKA of 2010. Nutritional quality was calculated using monthly mean adequacy ratios of 6 nutrients (calcium, vitamin C, vitamin A, iron, fiber, and protein), along with energy density of the foods selected by the students. The study showed significant improvements in nutritional quality of foods selected, along with decreased energy density of the meals. Participation was unchanged.

Collectively, the data suggest promising outcomes from the HHFKA of 2010 changes. But as Cullen and Dave pointed out, only 2 national surveys provide consumption data for students in schools, the National Health and Examination Survey (NHANES) and the SNDA.[24] The latter provides information not only on school meal programs but also on the nutrient content of the meals and the effect of school meals on children's diets. The fifth SNDA study, completed following the 2014–15 school year, also performed a dietary assessment of 2500 individual students via a 24-hour dietary recall, which, when published, will provide a definitive look at the nutritional impact of the 2010 guideline changes.

Despite the challenges, SFS adaptations to and innovations around standards of the HHFKA of 2010 helped to stabilize participation rates and plate waste. The USDA conducted a research survey in April 2015 to assess the types of steps SFS directors had utilized to improve consumption.[42] SFS directors in the survey confirmed that plate waste had increased initially but cited several measures that had successfully reduced waste during school year 2013–2014 to levels comparable to those before implementation of the HHFKA. The directors cited 3 main challenges in minimizing plate waste in their districts: (1) accommodating student taste preferences and unfamiliarity with menu items; (2) helping students deal with early meal schedules and insufficient time to eat; and (3) redistributing uneaten, intact items. To address these challenges, SFS directors involved students in menu planning and conducting taste tests, provided more menu choices, served foods with familiar flavors, served ready-to-eat fruit, and invited school staff and teachers to eat meals with students. Further, SFS directors encouraged principals to schedule recess before lunch, encouraged students to keep food items for later snacks, offered grab-and-go items to improve convenience, and began to serve breakfast in classrooms to support consumption and minimize hunger. SFS also initiated several measures to recover food that would otherwise be wasted, such as establishing sharing/trading tables and donating intact items to local food banks. Many of the innovations hinged on better staff training on using well-tested recipes, strategies for marketing school meals to students, and incentivizing student's tasting new items. The USDA and the Environmental Protection Agency, in collaboration with the University of Arkansas, has introduced a strategy to directly involve students in monitoring plate waste in their schools.[50]

One stipulation of the HHFKA of 2010 that caused great concern among SFS staff was the directive to cut sodium levels in meals by 50% over 10 years. Initial cuts up to 20% have not lead to falling participation rates directly, but additional decreases will entail extensive changes in production and manufacturing methods. Children and adolescents consumed far more sodium than recommendations call for during the period before the advent of the new guidelines.[51] Studies showed that nearly 50% of the sodium consumed in schools could be traced to 10 foods: Mexican-mixed dishes, sandwiches, breads, cold cuts, soups, savory snacks, cheese, plain milk, and poultry. With the exception of the inherent sodium in milk, all the other foods add salt during preparation or processing.[52] This suggests that efforts to reformulate a limited set of entrees may help to extensively lower sodium intake among students without requiring substantial changes to the majority of menu items.

Behavioral Economics

The psychology of food choice is a complex mix of cues, some internal and others external. One novel approach to improve the quality of dietary patterns has been to gently "nudge" students toward healthier selections. Called "behavioral economics," this new discipline offers a set of simple, inexpensive, environmental tools for SFS to use by melding research findings about behavior change with decision models grounded in marketing, consumer studies, economics, and social sciences.[53]

There are limited ways to improve the nutritional quality of meals, continue to produce the palatable foods expected by the student, and stay solvent without an infusion of additional revenue. The basic tenets of food choice are taste, value, and convenience. But many additional factors can influence food selection.[54] Psychologists use the term *reactance* to describe typical human rebellion against being coerced. On the other hand, when a choice is freely made, humans tend toward positive ownership of the decision, called *self-attribution*.[53] The aim of behavioral economics is to promote nutritious choices using the physical environment. For instance, clouding the plastic cover over frozen desserts lessens their visual appeal. Placing salad bars early in the food line or directly in the path of students as they enter the cafeteria increases vegetable consumption. Removing snack-type foods from the cashier's waiting line to a less accessible area and replacing them with an array of fruits stimulates fruit consumption. Even more powerful is to use the hassle factor. Allowing use of the meal debit card only for nutritious foods and requiring cash purchases of items with low nutritional quality effectively shapes student choice without restrictions.[53,56] Similarly, increasing plate or bowl size can improve consumption of high-quality foods, whereas decreasing their size can lessen intake of low-quality foods.[55] Kessler[56] compiled interventions from 16 studies to illustrate a wide range of options available for SFS within the cafeteria environment. These strategies have proved effective even in very large, diverse districts, such as Los Angeles Unified Schools.[57]

Several studies also have shown the potential for teaching interventions to improve the eating habits of primary school children.[58] The USDA has endorsed and helped to fund the behavioral economics work of The Smarter Lunchroom movement, designed by the Cornell University Behavioral Economics Nutrition Center, to aid the SFS in the redesign of school cafeterias.[59]

Food Safety

The USDA FNS provides detailed training guides for SFS staff to ensure safe meal provision in a sanitary environment.[60] Several additional safety measures were added in the HHFKA of 2010. Schools participating in the federal SBP and NSLP must obtain 2 inspections yearly, post the inspection report, and release a copy to the public on request. The protocols examine such issues as food handling, hand washing, equipment, food temperature, food storage, and the work environment. Although this rule has been in effect since 2004, fiscal pressures, inadequate inspection personnel, and the lack of tangible punitive measures at the state level may limit compliance by individual schools. Nevertheless, despite serving 42 million meals served daily in US schools, reports of foodborne illnesses are uncommon, probably as a result of careful training, increased requirements for written school policies, better continuing-education programs for SFS personnel, and the commitment of the food service staff to protect the children in their care.

Special Dietary Needs Within the School Environment

The Individuals with Disabilities Education Act (IDEA) specified that children with disabilities must be provided with a free and appropriate public education to prepare them for future employment and independent living. As a result, schools, school nurses, and the SFS have developed policies and practices to address a variety of nutritional challenges, such as for food allergies, celiac disease, lactose intolerance, and special diets for genetic or medical conditions, as well as for religious and lifestyle preferences and vegetarian or vegan diets. Such accommodations can be costly for schools, not only in terms of supplying and preparing unique menus for a variety of different children, but also in personnel time, quality control, and monitoring.

Food Allergies in the School Environment

The most common specific SFS dietary adjustment is for food allergies. Food allergies, especially more severe cases, are increasing in prevalence. A large study of school children with allergies found that 8% (5.9 million) have food allergies, and of that group, 30% have allergies to multiple foods and 39% had severe forms of the reaction.[61] In 90% of the nation's schools, more than 1 child in attendance has a food allergy. Half of these schools have experienced an allergic reaction. Because food allergies are the most common cause of anaphylaxis, representing a sudden, potentially fatal, reaction, parents of children with severe food allergies have concerns about the potential for contact with allergic trigger foods both in the school meals and in packed meals of other students. Although the food service staff is trained to deal with allergy by careful food handling techniques, children who bring in packed lunches or trade foods and contaminate surfaces make the cafeteria environment difficult to control. Misconceptions about food allergy prevalence, definition, and triggers are common. The AAP Section on Allergy and Immunology has issued a clinical report to help clarify the issue for schools and guide pediatricians.[62] Although any food can elicit a reaction, there are 8 foods that account for 90% of all food allergies in children: egg, milk, soy, wheat, peanuts, tree nuts, fish, and shellfish. The most frequent reactions occur in young children but generally are milder. Severe anaphylactic or fatal reactions in children usually are attributable to peanut and tree nuts (eg, walnuts, cashews, etc), milk, and seafood. Anaphylaxis is often associated with adolescence and underlying asthma. In 25% of cases involving anaphylaxis in schools, no prior diagnosis of food allergy existed.[62] A 2017 consensus report updated current thinking on food allergies.[63]

The management of proven food allergy relies on 3 components: strict avoidance of the food, recognition of symptoms (intestinal, respiratory, and neurologic), and the administration of epinephrine as soon as possible. In schools, t eatment is more challenging, although the 3 pillars of management remain the same. Avoidance is the front-line strategy for food allergies. Little is published in the way of controlled studies on approaches to avoidance in schools and child-care centers, but best practice guidelines are available from the AAP. Some basic principles can be applied. Skin contact and routine inhalation, which might occur routinely without heat vaporization, do not induce systemic reactions. Cleaning of hands and surfaces with soap and water or commercial wipes is, effective; antibacterial gels alone are not. Although the concept of an "allergen-safe table" in the cafeteria may be important for some hypersensitive children, they need not be physically separated from their friends or other children, provided that the others at the table are eating safe foods.[62]

The most important approach for schools is to have available the student's Individualized Health Care Plan (IHCP) as a management strategy. To write the IHCP, the school nurse will require documentation of the food allergy from the primary care physician, along with a description of the food allergy, triggers, warning signals noted, and a history of past reactions, including anaphylactic reactions. To make the task more uniform across the country, the AAP Section on Allergy and Immunology created a standardized, customizable written emergency plan for handling allergy and anaphylaxis in schools. The tool offers specific guidance for pediatricians to counsel patients, parents, and schools.[64] Because allergic reactions can be unpredictable, the treatment pathways outlined in the plan emphasized that if there is any uncertainty about the severity of an allergic reaction, epinephrine should be used promptly, because this life-saving medication is the first-line treatment for anaphylaxis. Health care providers were encouraged to develop an IHCP with their patients and families, to be shared with extended family, nonfamily caregivers, and school personnel, particularly the school nurse. The school nurse is the individual responsible for ensuring 2-way communication between the pediatrician and the school staff.[65] The AAP statement on the appropriate utilization of epinephrine for the immediate treatment of anaphylaxis symptoms also has been updated.[66]

The risk of food allergens contaminating the classroom is a warranted concern for parents of an allergic child as well as for school staff. Within the classroom environment, blanket bans of offending allergens may be warranted, particularly for younger children with a higher likelihood of incidental spread and ingestion of the allergen. Eating bans on field trips and school buses also are important means of control. Education is the most effective way to prevent an unforeseen allergic reaction. Many schools have addressed these concerns by having the SFS prepare all foods for use within the schools, including for birthdays, celebrations, banquets, and holiday parties. This solves many problems that may occur when foods are brought into the school and classroom. The SFS already is well-versed in dealing with high-risk food allergens. SFS staff is responsible for maintaining the cleanliness of surfaces in food preparation areas as well as in the cafeteria. Menu ingredients, food preparation, and handling require knowledge of ingredient labels, including any recent manufacturer modifications to food products that may introduce an offending allergen. Cross-contamination of equipment, storage containers, and serving utensils is another common route for exposure that is routinely addressed by the SFS. The protocol of maintaining a list of new food ingredients for a period after first introduction has been a crucial means for alerting the SFS director to new food allergies as they occur within the student population. However school administrators choose to deal with classroom celebrations, their approach should be clearly delineated in policy and made available for the parents, family, teachers, and physicians caring for the child with food allergies.

References

1.   Centers for Disease Control and Prevention. Health and Academic Achievement. Available at: https://www.cdc.gov/healthyyouth/health_and_academics/pdf/health-academic-achievement.pdf. Accessed August 14, 2017

2.   Lauchlan L. Who's Minding the Kids? Child Care Arrangements: Spring 2011. April 2013; Available at: https://www.census.gov/prod/2013pubs/p70–135.pdf. Accessed August 13, 2017

3.   US Department of Agriculture, Food and Nutrition Service. Programs and Services. Available at: https://www.fns.usda.gov/programs-and-services. Accessed August 14, 2017

4.   US Department of Agriculture, Food and Nutrition Service. Estimated fiscal year 2016 expenses. Available at: https://www.fns.usda.gov/sites/default/files/pd/cncost.pdf. Accessed April 4, 2017

5.   American Academy of Pediatrics, Council on Community Pediatrics. Poverty and child health in the United States. *Pediatrics*. 2016;137(4):e20160339

6.   American Academy of Pediatrics, Council on Community Pediatrics, Committee on Nutrition. Promoting food security for all children. *Pediatrics*. 2015;136(5):e1431–e1438

7. Hirschman J, Chriqui JF. School food and nutrition policy, monitoring and evaluation in the USA. *Public Health Nutr.* 2013;16(6):982–988

8. Hopkins LC, Gunther C. A historical review of changes in nutrition standards of USDA child meal programs relative to research findings on the nutritional adequacy of program meals and the diet and nutritional health of participants: implications for future fesearch and the Summer Food Service Program. *Nutrients.* 2015;7(12):10145–10167

9. US Department of Agriculture, Food and Nutrition Service. Final Rule: Local School Wellness Policy Implementation Under the HHFKA of 2010. Available at: https://www.fns.usda.gov/school-meals/fr-072916c. Accessed July 29, 2017

10. Reedy J, Krebs-Smith SM. Dietary sources of energy, solid fats, and added sugars among children and adolescents in the United States. *J Am Diet Assoc.* 2010;110(10):1477–1484

11. US Department of Agriculture, Food and Nutrition Service. A Guide to Smart Snacks in Schools. Available at: https://www.fns.usda.gov/tn/guide-smart-snacks-schools. Accessed July 29, 2017

12. Rosenfeld LE, Cohen JF, Gorski MT, et al. How do we actually put smarter snacks in schools? NOURISH (Nutrition Opportunities to Understand Reforms Involving Student Health) conversations with food-service directors. *Public Health Nutr.* 2017;20(3):556–564

13. US Department of Health and Human Services, US Department of Agriculture. 2015–2020 Dietary Guidelines for Americans. 8th ed. 2015: Available at: https://health.gov/dietaryguidelines/2015/. Accessed July 29, 2017

14. US Department of Agriculture, Food and Nutrition Service. Child nutrition tables. Available at: https://www.fns.usda.gov/pd/child-nutrition-tables. Accessed July 29, 2017

15. Food Research and Action Center. National School Lunch Program: Trends and factors affecting student participation. Available at: http://frac.org/wp-content/uploads/national_school_lunch_report_2015.pdf. Accessed July 29, 2017

16. US Department of Agriculture FaNS. Community Eligibility Provision. Available at: https://www.fns.usda.gov/school-meals/community-eligibility-provision. Accessed July 29, 2017

17. Food Research and Action Center. School Breakfast Scorecard: School year 2015–2016. Available at: http://frac.org/wp-content/uploads/school-breakfast-scorecard-sy-2015–2016.pdf. Accessed July 29, 2017

18. Von Hippel PT, Workman J. From kindergarten through second grade, U.S. children's obesity prevalence grows only during summer vacations. *Obesity.* 2016;24(11):2296–3000

19. US Department of Agriculture, Food and Nutrition Service. Summer food service program. Available at: https://www.fns.usda.gov/sfsp/summer-food-service-program. Accessed July 29, 2017

20. US Department of Agriculture. Best Practices: Model Programs. Available at: https://www.fns.usda.gov/sites/default/files/Model_Programs_Booklet_2005.pdf. Accessed July 29, 2017.

21. ArkansasMatters.com. Food Insecurity Prompts AR Children's Hospital Free Lunch Program. Available at: http://www.arkansasmatters.com/news/news/food-insecurity-prompts-ar-childrens-hospital-free-lunch-program. Accessed July 29, 2017

22. Cahil C. Reaching Children in Hospitals With Summer Meals Feeding America. Hunger in America. Available at: http://www.feedingamerica.org/hunger-in-america/news-and-updates/hunger-blog/reaching-children-in-hospitals-with-summer-meals.html. Accessed July 29, 2017

23. Gordon A, Niland K, Fox MK. *Learning from the Past and Shaping the Future: How School Nutrition Dietary Assessment Studies Helped Change School Meals.* Mathematica Policy Research Issue Brief; 2016

24. Cullen KW, Dave JM. The new federal school nutrition standards and meal patterns: early evidence examining the influence on student dietary behavior and the school food environment. *J Acad Nutr Diet.* 2017;117(2):185–191

25. Mathematica Policy Research. School Nutrition and Meal Cost Study 2013–2017. Available at: https://www.mathematica-mpr.com/our-publications-and-findings/projects/school-nutrition-and-meal-cost-study. Accessed July 29, 2017

26. Redford J, Desrochers D. *The years before school: Children's nonparental care arrangements from 2001–2012. Stats in Brief,* 2017–096. US Department of Education, National Center for Education Statistics; 2017

27. Child-care Aware. Checking In: A Snapshot of the Child-Care Landscape, 2017. Available at: http://usa.childcareaware.org/wp-content/uploads/2017/07/FINAL_SFS_REPORT.pdf Accessed July 29, 2017

28. Sissona SB, Kigera AC, Anundsona KC, et al. Differences in preschool-age children's dietary intake between meals consumed at childcare and at home. *Prev Med Rep.* 2017;6:33–37

29. US Department of Education, National Center for Educational Statistics. Fast Facts. Available at: https://nces.ed.gov/fastfacts/display.asp?id=4. Accessed July 29, 2017

30. Hoelscher DM, Kirk S, Ritchie L, Cunningham-Sabo L, Academy Positions Committee. Position of the Academy of Nutrition and Dietetics: Interventions for the prevention and treatment of pediatric overweight and obesity. *J Acad Nutr Diet.* 2013;113:1375–1394

31. US Department of Agriculture, Food and Nutrition Service. Child and Adult Food Care Program (CACFP). Available at: https://www.fns.usda.gov/cacfp/child-and-adult-care-food-program. Accessed July 29, 2017

32. US Department of Agriculture, Food and Nutrition Service. Child and Adult Care Food Program: Meal Pattern Revisions Related to the Healthy, Hunger-Free Kids Act of 2010. *Federal Register.* 2016;81(79):24347–24383

33. Children's Hunger Alliance Web site. Child care providers. Available at: https://www.childrenshungeralliance.org/provider-services/childcare-providers/. Accessed July 27, 2017

34. Bruening M, Afuso K, Mason M. Associations of eating two breakfasts with childhood overweight status, sociodemographics, and parental factors among preschool students. *Health Educ Behav.* 2016;2016(43):665–673

35. Wang S, Schwartz MB, Shebi FM, Read M, Henderson KE, Ickovics JR. School breakfast and body mass index: a longitudinal observational study of middle school students. *Pediatr Obes.* 2016;12(3):213–220

36. Alsharairi NA, Somerset SM. Skipping breakfast in early childhood and its associations with maternal and child BMI: a study of 2-5-year-old Australian children. *Eur J Clin Nutr.* 2016;70(4):450–455

37. US Department of Agriculture, Food and Nutrition Service. School Lunch and Cost Study II, 2013. Available at: https://www.fns.usda.gov/school-lunch-and-breakfast-cost-study-ii. Accessed July 29, 2017

38. School Nutrition Association. State of School Nutrition 2016. Available at: https://schoolnutrition.org/AboutSchoolMeals/SchoolMealTrendsStats/. Accessed July 29, 2017

39. US Department of Agriculture, Food and Nutrition Service. Food Distribution Programs. Available at: https://www.fns.usda.gov/fdd/food-distribution-programs. Accessed July 29, 2017

40. Smith SL, Cunningham-Sabo L. Food choice, plate waste and nutrient intake of elementary- and middle-school students participating in the US National School Lunch Program. *Public Health Nutr.* 2014;17(6):1255–1263

41. Niaki SF, Moore CE, Chen TA, Weber Cullen K. Younger elementary school students waste more school lunch foods than older elementary school students. *J Acad Nutr Diet.* 2017;117(1):95–101

42. US Department of Agriculture, Food and Nutrition Service. Plate Waste. Available at: https://fns-prod.azureedge.net/sites/default/files/ops/HHFKA-PlateWaste.pdf. Accessed July 29, 2017

43. Watanabe T. Solutions sought to reduce food waste at school. *LA Times.* April 1, 2014. Available at: https://www.latimes.com/local/la-me-lausd-waste-20140402-story.html#page=1. Accessed December 5, 2018

44. School Nutrition Association. School Nutrition Trends Survey 2014. Available at: https://schoolnutrition.org/uploadedFiles/Resources_and_Research/Research/SNA2014TrendsSurvey.pdf. Accessed July 29, 2017

45. Just D, Price J. Default options, incentives and food choices: evidence from elementary-school children. *Pub Health Nutr.* 2013;16(12):2281–2288

46. Cohen JF, Richardson S, Austen SB, Economos CD, Rimm EB. School lunch waste among middle school students: Implications for nutrients consumed and food waste costs. *Am J Prev Med.* 2013;44(2):114–121

47. Byker CJ, Farris AR, Marcanelle M, Davis GC, Serrano EL. Food waste in a school nutrition program after implementation of new lunch program guidelines. *J Nutr Educ Behav.* 2014;46(5):406–411

48. Cullen KW, Chen TA, Dave JM, Jensen H. Differential improvements in student fruit and vegetable selection and consumption in response to the new National School Lunch Program regulations: a pilot study. *J Acad Nutr Diet.* 2015;115(5):743–750

49. Johnson DB, Podrabsky M, Rocha A, Otten JJ. Effect of the Healthy Hunger-Free Kids Act on the nutritional quality of meals selected by students and school lunch participation rates. *JAMA Pediatr.* 2016;17(1):e153918

50. US Department of Agriculture, Food and Nutrition Service. Guide to conducting student food waste audits: a resource for schools. March 2017. Available at: https://www.usda.gov/oce/foodwaste/Student_Food_Waste_Audit_FINAL_4-6-2017.pdf. Accessed July 30, 2017

51. Cogswell ME, Yuan K, Gunn JP, Gillespie C. Vital signs: sodium intake among U.S. school-aged children - 2009–2010. *MMWR Morb Mortal Wkly Rep.* 2014;63(36):789–797

52. Quader ZS, Gillespie C, Sliwa SA, et al. Sodium intake among US school-aged children: National Health and Nutrition Examination Survey, 2011–2012. *J Acad Nutr Diet.* 2017;117(1):39–47

53. Just D, Wankink B. Smarter lunchrooms: Using behavioral economics to improve meal selection. *Choices.* 2009;24(3). Available at: http://www.choicesmagazine.org/UserFiles/file/article_87.pdf. Accessed December 5, 2018

54. Chandon P, Wansink B. Does food marketing need to make us fat? A review and solutions. *Nutr Rev.* 2012;70(10):571–593

55. Wansink B, Van Ittersum K, Payne CR. Larger bowl size increases the amount of cereal children request, consume, and waste. *J Pediatr.* 2014;164(2):323–326

56. Kessler HS. Simple interventions to improve healthy eating behaviors in the school cafeteria. *Nutr Rev.* 2016;74:198–209

57. Williamson DA, Han H, Johnson WD, Martin CK, Newton RL. Modification of the school cafeteria environment can impact childhood nutrition: Results from the Wise Mind and LA Health studies. *Appetite.* 2013;61:77–84

58. Dudley DA, Cotton WG, Peralta LR. Teaching approaches and strategies that promote healthy eating in primary school children: a systematic review and meta-analysis. *Int J Behav Nutr Phys Act.* 2015;12:28–54

59. Cornell University. Smarter Lunchroom Movement. Available at: https://www.smarterlunchrooms.org/. Accessed July 30, 2017

60. US Department of Agriculture, Food and Nutrition Service. Food safe schools action guide: Creating a culture of food safety. 2014. Available at: https://www.fns.usda.gov/sites/default/files/Food-Safe-Schools-Action-Guide.pdf. Accessed July 30, 2017

61. Gupta RS, Springston EE, Warrier MR, et al. The prevalence, severity, and distribution of childhood food allergy in the United States. *Pediatrics.* 2011;128(1):e9–e17

62. Sicherer SH, Mahr T, American Academy of Pediatrics, Section on Allergy and Immunology. Clinical report: Management of food allergy in the school setting. *Pediatrics.* 2010;126(6):1232–1239

63. Sicherer SH, Allen K, Lack G, Taylor SL, Donovan SM, Oria M. Critical issues in food allergy: a National Academies Consensus Report. *Pediatrics.* 2017;140(2):e20170194

64. Wang J, Sicherer SH, American Academy of Pediatrics, Section on Allergy and Immunology. Guidance on completing a written allergy and anaphylaxis emergency plan. *Pediatrics.* 2017;139(3):e20164005

65. Holmes B, Sheetz A, American Academy of Pediatrics, Council on School Health. Role of the school nurse in providing school health services. *Pediatrics.* 2016;137(6):e20160852

66. Sicherer SH, Simons FER, American Academy of Pediatrics, Section on Allergy and Immunology. Epinephrine for first-aid management of anaphylaxis. *Pediatrics.* 2017;139(3):e20164006

III

Chapter 10

Pediatric Global Nutrition

Global Burden of Undernutrition

Undernutrition in Low- or Middle-Income Countries

Nutritional deficits are common among infants, children, and adolescents in low- or middle-income countries (LMICs), particularly in settings of material deprivation, political instability, war, famine, or other humanitarian crises. Nutritional assessment and management of young children is a major focus of child health policies and programs in resource-limited settings, because nutritional status is closely interrelated with physical growth, cognitive development, and the risk of death from acute infectious diseases.[1,2] The spectrum of "undernutrition" encompasses clinically apparent macronutrient malnutrition as well as growth faltering and micronutrient deficiencies. However, overweight and obesity are increasing in prevalence in LMICs,[3] and it is now widely recognized that undernutrition and overweight often coexist within communities and even within households (eg, child with growth faltering whose mother is overweight) and individuals (eg, overweight child with iron deficiency). This chapter focuses on undernutrition in LMICs; the diagnosis and management of overweight and obesity are addressed in Chapter 33: Pediatric Obesity.

Definitions of Undernutrition

Measurement of undernutrition serves to document the overall health status of vulnerable populations. It may also guide the clinical care of individual children within the context of community-based health surveillance and promotion programs as well has hospital management. The most common method of globally quantifying childhood undernutrition is anthropometry—the measurement of a child's physical size and dimensions (see Chapter 24: Assessment of Nutritional Status). Each child's weight and height (or length, if <2 years) may be used to calculate a sex- and age-standardized weight-for-height z-score (WHZ), weight-for-age z-score (WAZ) and height-for-age z-score (HAZ) based on a pediatric growth reference or standard (ie, the "growth chart"). Globally, the World Health Organization (WHO) child growth standards are the most widely used growth charts to generate anthropometric indices for children younger than 5 years (Appendix Q).[4] Using current conventional nomenclature, a child is classified as "stunted" if the HAZ is more than −2 standard deviations (SD) below the mean of the WHO standards or "wasted" if the WHZ is more than

−2 SD below the mean of the WHO standard population (Table 10.1). More specifically, a WHZ <−2 but >−3 is referred to as a moderate acute malnutrition (MAM), whereas severe wasting (marasmus) or severe acute malnutrition (SAM) is defined as WHZ <−3 SD or a mid-upper arm circumference (MUAC) less than 115 mm for children 6 through 59 months of age. Apart from severe wasting, SAM can also present as nutritional edema, which is called kwashiorkor. For infants younger than 6 months, there are no accepted MUAC criteria for SAM. A child may be considered "underweight" if the WAZ is more than 2 SD below the mean, but this index has become less commonly used because of the recognition that WAZ is essentially a composite of HAZ and WHZ.

Causes of Undernutrition
The etiology of stunting (or linear growth faltering) is incompletely understood but is considered to represent the cumulative effect of numerous adverse factors that constrain bone growth, such as fetal growth restriction, inadequate dietary diversity and/or nutrient density, recurrent infections (eg, gastroenteritis), chronic intestinal inflammation, stress, and acute or chronic illnesses.[1] Conversely, wasting is assumed to reflect more specifically inadequacy of the child's diet resulting in reduced fat stores and lean body mass and is, therefore, often considered synonymous with "acute malnutrition," although this can be misleading, because wasting can develop and persist chronically. In addition, chronic systemic illnesses such as tuberculosis can contribute to wasting.

Public and Individual Health Relevance of Undernutrition
The overall proportions of children 0 to 5 years of age who are classified as wasted or stunted are key population indicators of the global burden of child undernutrition.[1] On the basis of recent population-based estimates (from 2015), the worldwide prevalence of stunting is 23% and wasting is 7%.[3] To understand these figures, it is helpful to consider that in a healthy community, the expected proportion of children below −2 SD (for either WHZ or HAZ) is about 2.3%. Therefore, there are approximately 10 times as many stunted children and about 3 times as many wasted children as would be expected under optimal circumstances. Prevalence varies widely across and within countries, but in most settings there have been recent declines in the prevalence of undernutrition.[3] The WHO has established a set of 6 "Global Nutrition Targets" for the year 2025, including a 40% reduction in the number of stunted children and to "reduce and maintain childhood

Table 10.1.
Diagnostic Criteria for Undernutrition

	Severe Acute Malnutrition	Moderate Acute Malnutrition	Stunting	Underweight
Weight-for-age	NA	NA	NA	<–2 SD
Height-for-age (or length-for-age)	NA	NA	<–2 SD	NA
Weight-for-height (or weight-for-length)	<–3 SD	Between –2 SD and –3 SD	NA	NA
Mid-upper arm circumference	<11.5 cm	Between 11.5 and 12.5 cm	NA	NA
Edema	+/–	No	No	NA

NA indicates not applicable.

wasting to less than 5%."[5] These goals have been incorporated into the United Nations Sustainable Development Goals (SDGs) as part of goal No. 2 ("End hunger, achieve food security and improved nutrition, and promote sustainable agriculture").[6]

It is important to distinguish the uses of WHZ and HAZ at the population versus individual (clinical) levels. The indicators "% wasted" and "% stunted" are valuable metrics that enable public health advocates and policy makers to compare countries/regions and quantitatively track progress in reducing undernutrition over time using standardized gauges. However, it may be misleading to use z-score cut-offs to establish clinical diagnoses; for example, it is a misconception that all stunted children are malnourished, whereas all nonstunted children (ie, those with HAZ >-2) are necessarily healthy or adequately nourished. In fact, an increased prevalence of stunting is usually observed in communities in which there is a downward shift in the *entire* HAZ distribution, indicating that most children in the affected community—not just stunted children—are of shorter stature than they would be under optimal conditions.[7] A similar phenomenon has been observed in settings in which the prevalence of wasting is high, whereby the whole WHZ distribution is shifted down toward more negative values.[8] Nonetheless, within LMICs, the lower a child's HAZ or WHZ, the higher his or her relative risk of adverse outcomes, including mortality.[2] The associations between undernutrition and other health outcomes suggest that these indices may enable risk stratification in the clinical context. For example, during a well-child visit or other clinical encounter, the WHZ may be used to screen for children at risk of MAM or SAM. In addition, an MUAC is easy to measure and offers the best index to identify children with a high risk of dying.[9] The detection of MAM or SAM may have implications for the clinical care or referral of the individual child, as described below. In contrast, the classification of an individual child as stunted or not has limited direct clinical implications, primarily because HAZ is a function of cumulative long-term exposures that are challenging (if not impossible) to tackle in the immediate health care context. In most LMICs, population-average HAZ begins to decline early in infancy and progresses throughout at least the first 2 years of life.[10] HAZ in childhood is significantly predicted by size at birth,[11] indicating the importance of fetal or intergenerational determinants of HAZ. The clinical and nutritional care of the child with linear growth faltering in an LMIC may be cautiously guided by the principles that underlie the approach to the child with failure to thrive (see Chapter 26). However, aggressive nutritional rehabilitation is not recommended for the otherwise healthy child who has low HAZ but proportional weight and height (ie, not wasted), given the potential long-term cardiometabolic risks of rapid weight gain out of proportion to linear growth[12] (see Chapter 33: Obesity).

Management of Moderate Acute Malnutrition

MAM in children affects both mortality and morbidity in LMICs, and therefore, targeted interventions for this population are warranted. Adverse outcomes are related to impairments in immune function, increasing the susceptibility to intercurrent infections. MAM might also have long-term effects on cognitive development.[13] Preventive strategies should be focused on infection prevention strategies, continuation of breastfeeding, and complementary feeding practices. Unfortunately, screening for MAM is frequently not performed structurally in either community or hospital settings. Once MAM has developed, it is managed in the community using different nutritional strategies. However, there is no definitive consensus on the most effective way to treat children with MAM. Management is based on the concept that children need to receive nutrient-dense foods to meet their augmented needs for nutritional and functional recovery. For detailed information, see the WHO technical note on nutritional management of MAM at http://www.who.int/nutrition/publications/moderate_malnutrition/9789241504423/en/.

Recommended calorie intakes for moderately malnourished children 6 through 59 months of age have been determined on the basis of data in severely malnourished and healthy children. In communities where the supply of food is not limited, nutritional counseling of caregivers is the main focus of interventions to induce nutritional recovery. In households or communities with food insecurity, nutrient-rich supplemental foods are provided to ensure the provision of the daily recommended dietary allowance for energy and micronutrients in addition to the child's regular diet. Ready-to-use supplementary foods (RUSFs), which are lipid-based nutrient supplements or blended food supplements, are predominantly used for the nutritional recovery of children with MAM, either in full dose (75 kcal/kg/day) or in a lower dose to complement the regular diet. A systematic review indicated that, in general, food supplementation is more effective than nutritional counseling for children with MAM.[14] There does not appear to be a significant difference in mortality of children treated with RUSFs or blended food supplements, although nutritional recovery might be better with RUSFs compared with blended foods.[15]

Management of Severe Acute Malnutrition

General Considerations
Children with SAM can be divided into 2 groups: those with uncomplicated SAM and those with complicated SAM. Uncomplicated SAM is generally managed in the community and is defined by the presence of a good appetite and the absence of general danger signs or medical conditions requiring hospital admission. The flow diagram (Figure 10.1) highlights basic concepts around treatment of SAM and MAM. In addition, uncomplicated SAM is characterized by the absence of edema that warrants hospital management. The WHO recommends treating all cases of SAM with routine antibiotics.[16] There has been debate about the risks of development of antibiotic resistance versus the benefits of treatment of unrecognized infections.[17] A large clinical trial demonstrated improvements in survival of children with uncomplicated SAM treated with antibiotics.[18] Management of uncomplicated SAM further consists of feeding children with lipid-based RUTFs aiming at a calorie intake of 175 kcal/kg/day.[19,20] The advantage of RUTFs is their low water content, allowing for safe storage for long periods of time

Fig 10.1.
Flow diagram for the management of malnutrition

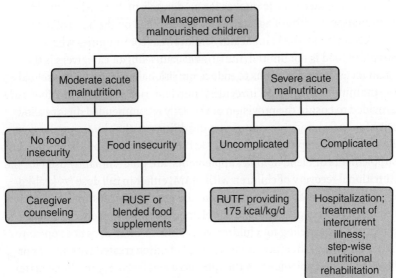

RUSF, ready-to use supplementary food; RUTF, ready-to-use therapeutic food.

and preventing bacterial growth in case of accidental contamination. The advancement of this approach has enabled most severely malnourished children to be treated in the community with low mortality rates.[21]

Children with complicated SAM require hospital treatment. Health care providers treating patients with SAM should be aware of 2 key principles: First, the reason for caregivers to seek medical help is generally not the malnutrition but an intercurrent illness; second, undernutrition markedly increases the risk of mortality secondary to the intercurrent illness, such as pneumonia, malaria, or gastroenteritis, and that risk is closely related to the severity of the wasting.[22] Mortality rates of 10% to more than 20% have been reported for hospitalized children with SAM, with mortality being the highest in children younger than 2 years.[23-25] Treatment of infections with antibiotics and nutritional rehabilitation are the central elements of hospital-based management of SAM. Although the 2 clinical phenotypes of SAM—severe wasting or nutritional edema—can be distinguished, overlap often exists. SAM is associated with multiorgan changes, with some specifically present in children with nutritional edema (Table 10.2).

Interestingly, management guidelines do not distinguish between the 2 distinct phenotypes of SAM, as no studies have focused on specific interventions for edematous malnutrition versus severe wasting. A detailed description of the management can be found in the 2003 WHO guideline (http://www.who.int/nutrition/publications/guide_inpatient_text.pdf) with an update published in 2013 (http://apps.who.int/iris/bitstream/10665/95584/1/9789241506328_eng.pdf).

Nutritional Management of Complicated SAM

Hospital management of SAM consists of different phases. The first phase is focused on clinical stabilization. Feeding is initially started relatively slowly using a specifically designed liquid diet (F-75 [Nutriset, Malaunay, France]; 75 kcal/100 mL), providing up to approximately 95 kcal/kg/day. Infants younger than 6 months with SAM should continue or reestablish exclusive breastfeeding. If not possible to exclusively breastfeed, commercial infant formula or F-75 (75 kcal/100 mL) or diluted F-100 (Nutriset; 100 kcal/100 mL) can be given as a supplementary or complete feed depending on the availability of mother's milk. It is prepared by adding 650 mL instead of 500 mL of water to a 115-g sachet of powdered formula or 2.7 L instead of 2 L of water to a sachet of 460 g of powder. Undiluted F-100 should not be given to infants younger than 6 months because of high renal solute load. Once a child has been stabilized and his or her appetite has increased, he or she

Table 10.2.

Major Multiorgan Changes in Severe Acute Malnutrition

Organ/System	Change
Skin	Loss of integrity
Cardiac	Cardiac muscle atrophy Potentially decreased cardiac output in sepsis
Respiratory	Susceptibility to respiratory tract infections Increased mortality related to respiratory tract infections
Intestine	Susceptibility to intestinal tract infections Reduced macro- and micronutrient absorption Intestinal inflammation Increased mortality related to intestinal tract infections
Hepatobiliary	Impaired hepatic oxidative and synthetic function Reduced biliary bile salt secretion
Endocrine	Impaired endocrine pancreatic function Exocrine pancreas insufficiency Reduced thyroid function
Metabolic	Refeeding syndrome Hypoglycemia Decreased protein metabolism[a]
Renal	Potentially impaired glomerular and tubular function
Central nervous system	Decreased appetite[a] Increased lethargy and irritability[a] Likely long-term effects on development

[a] Specifically associated with edematous malnutrition.

can move to the next phase of treatment, aimed at nutritional rehabilitation with ready-to-use therapeutic foods or a higher energy/protein liquid formulation (F-100; 100 kcal/100 mL). The aim is to provide 150 to 220 kcal/kg/day. Breastfeeding can continue with therapeutic foods, but it is advised that no other foods are consumed. Children are generally discharged from the hospital and referred to outpatient treatment centers after medical complications have resolved and social factors have been addressed as best as possible. Nutritional recovery is not a criterion for discharge, but availability of outpatient feeding programs is essential.

Pathophysiological Considerations and Medical Management of SAM

Hospital management SAM is based on the 10 steps published in the 2003 WHO guidelines (http://www.who.int/nutrition/publications/guide_inpatient_text.pdf).[19] However, the 10 steps do not completely cover the spectrum of pathophysiological changes in SAM. Given the complex pathophysiology, high mortality, and diverse range of comorbidities, hospitalized children with SAM require intense monitoring and individualized medical care. In addition to providing broad-spectrum antibiotics, specific infections should be treated. Hypothermia is often present, which can mask serious infections and should be aggressively treated. Intestinal dysfunction with macronutrient malabsorption, especially carbohydrate malabsorption, can limit enteral tolerance of nutrition as children often develop significant diarrhea and dehydration during hospitalization. Dehydration attributable to diarrhea is managed with rehydration using ReSoMal (Nutriset), a reduced-sodium oral rehydration solution (ORS, sodium 45 mmol/L) with added potassium 40 mmol/L). It is based on the concept that severely malnourished children have higher concentrations of intracellular sodium attributable to impaired function of sodium/potassium pumps. However, the scientific basis for the use of ReSoMal versus standard ORS with 75 mEq of sodium/L is weak.

Refeeding syndrome can occur in the context of rapidly increasing calorie and protein provision, which stimulates insulin secretion and leads to tissue utilization of glucose, shifts of electrolytes such as potassium and phosphate from the extracellular to the intracellular space, and increasing demand for electrolytes (eg, phosphate) for ATP synthesis. As a result, hypoglycemia and severe electrolyte disturbances can ensue, which can lead to generalized weakness, seizures, and impaired cardiac and respiratory function. Electrolytes such as potassium and phosphate are supplemented in F-75 to prevent refeeding syndrome-induced electrolyte disturbances,[26] but its effectiveness has not rigorously been tested.

Minerals and vitamins such as zinc and vitamin A are also included in the therapeutic diet, because deficiencies are likely to be common in children with SAM. In deciding whether a child is ready for hospital discharge, the risk of developing health care-associated infections in the hospital should be weighed against the degree of vulnerability and frailty as well as the access to adequate postdischarge care.

Micronutrient Deficiencies in Children

Infants, children, and adolescents in LMICs are at high risk of inadequate intakes and impaired intestinal absorption of micronutrients (vitamins and minerals).[1] In contrast to macronutrient-related malnutrition, micronutrient deficiencies are often subclinical and have therefore, historically, been referred to as "hidden hunger." Deficits in micronutrient intakes are primarily attributable to inadequate dietary diversity and low consumption of animal-source foods or fortified staples. Impaired absorption of essential nutrients—particularly minerals such as iron, zinc, and calcium—may be attributable to low bioavailability of nutrients from plant sources, excess dietary phytates, nutrient-nutrient interactions, and recurrent infections or inflammation; for example, hepcidin, a key inhibitor of iron absorption, is upregulated in the context of systematic inflammation (see Chapter 19: Iron).[27] In young infants, micronutrient deficiencies may also be attributable to maternal micronutrient deficiencies that prevent adequate transplacental or human milk transfer of nutrients to the fetus/infant.

In the absence of large-scale agricultural and food systems-based strategies to address micronutrient deficiencies, targeted micronutrient supplementation programs have been implemented in many countries.[28] There has been substantial interest and research into the potential public health benefits of routine supplementation of infants and children with specific vitamins or minerals.[1,29] However, the WHO currently only recommends routine supplementation of infants and children with oral vitamin A[30] and iron[31] in certain high-risk settings (Table 10.3). Iron supplementation in young children in regions with endemic malaria came under scrutiny in the wake of research indicating that it increased the risk of adverse events in settings where malaria control was inadequate.[32] However, the WHO currently advises that iron supplementation is safe when undertaken "in conjunction with public health measures to prevent, diagnose and treat malaria."[31] In settings with a prevalence of anemia greater than 20%, the WHO also recommends "point-of-use fortification of complementary foods with iron-containing micronutrient powders" to reduce the risk of iron deficiency and anemia in infants and children 6 months and older.[33] Multimicronutrient powders (MNPs) contain varying combinations of micronutrients other than iron usually at age-appropriate recommended nutrient intake levels; however, beyond the prevention of iron-deficiency anemia, there uncertain additional health benefits. Routine daily oral vitamin D supplementation of all breastfed infants for the prevention of nutritional rickets (see Chapter 3) has been implemented in several countries but is not currently a global WHO recommendation.[34] However, the WHO recommends that very low

Table 10.3.

World Health Organization (WHO) Recommendations for Routine Vitamin A and Iron Supplementation for Infants and Children

Age group	Vitamin A	Iron
Context	Routine supplementation in settings where the prevalence of night blindness is ≥1% in children 24 through 59 months of age or where the prevalence of vitamin A deficiency (serum retinol 0.70 μmol/L or lower) is ≥20% or higher in infants and children 6 through 59 months of age	Routine supplementation in settings of ≥40% prevalence of anemia
0 through 5 months	Not recommended	Not recommended[a]
6 through 11 months	100 000 IU (30 mg RE)[b] as a single dose	10 to 12.5 mg elemental iron, daily, for 3 consecutive months of each year
12 through 23 months	200 000 IU (60 mg RE)[b] every 4 to 6 months	10 to 12.5 mg elemental iron, daily, for 3 consecutive months of each year
24 through 59 months	200 000 IU (60 mg RE)[b] every 4 to 6 months	30 mg elemental iron, daily, for 3 consecutive months of each year
5 through 12 years	Not recommended	30 to 60 mg elemental iron, daily, for 3 consecutive months of each year

RE, retinol equivalents; IU, international units.
[a] WHO guidelines for very low birth weight (VLBW) infants (1 to 1.5 kg) indicate that "VLBW infants fed mother's own milk or donor human milk should be given 2–4 mg/kg per day iron supplementation starting at 2 weeks until 6 months of age."[35]
[b] Retinyl palmitate or retinyl acetate in an oil-based vehicle.

birth weight infants (1 to 1.5 kg at birth) receive daily vitamin D (400 IU to 1000 IU/day) until 6 months of age.[35]

Health care providers practicing in resource-limited settings should be aware of the recommended uses of micronutrients as adjunctive therapies in the treatment of acute pediatric illnesses, particularly because these are practices that are not typically adopted in the United States or other industrialized countries. In addition to the provision of standard oral rehydration therapy to treat acute gastroenteritis (Chapter 28: Oral

Therapy for Acute Diarrhea), zinc supplementation should routinely be prescribed for 10 to 14 days.[36] Vitamin A supplementation is recommended in the treatment of children with measles in settings where measles fatality rates is >1%, regions with established vitamin A deficiency, and in cases of severe complicated measles.[37] Intravenous thiamine (vitamin B₁) should be administered in all suspected cases of infantile beri-beri,[38] and, in settings with known thiamine deficiency or where diets are dominated by polished rice or cassava, consideration should be given to the routine administration of thiamine in the management of all infants with congestive heart failure or other critical illnesses, as the signs and symptoms of severe thiamine deficiency can be protean.[39] Table 10.4 provides recommended doses of zinc,

Table 10.4.

Adjunctive Micronutrient Therapies Recommended for Use in the Treatment of Acute Illness in Resource-Limited Settings

Age Group	Zinc[36]	Vitamin A[30]	Thiamine[38]
Indication	Acute gastroenteritis	Measles	Suspected thiamine deficiency in the context of heart failure, convulsions, or coma
Route	Oral	Oral	Intravenous, intramuscular, then oral
0 through 5 months	10 mg per day for 10 to 14 days	50 000 IU immediately, then 50 000 the next day[a]	25–50 mg as slow intravenous injection, then 10 mg/day intramuscular dose for 1 week, then 3–5 mg/day orally for at least 6 weeks
6 through 11 months	20 mg per day for 10 to 14 days	100 000 IU immediately, then 100 000 the next day[a]	
12 through 59 months		200 000 IU immediately, then 200 000 the next day[a]	

[a] A third dose is given at least 2 weeks after the second dose if there are eye signs indicating vitamin A deficiency.

vitamin A, and thiamine when used as adjunctive therapies in the treatment of acute illnesses.

Specific clinical features of micronutrient deficiencies typically only manifest when the deficiency is severe and protracted. However, micronutrient status assessment through biochemical testing is not generally recommended in the clinical management of children with acute illnesses or malnutrition in resource-limited settings, because specimen collection and laboratory facilities are often unavailable, and the interpretation of many micronutrient biomarkers is complicated in the setting of acute infection or inflammation.[40] Therefore, although individual test-and-treat approaches are commonly used to manage suspected micronutrient deficiencies in the United States and other industrialized countries, indications for routine supplementation in resource-limited countries are intentionally broad, inclusive, and based on clinical and epidemiologic factors.

Environmental Enteric Dysfunction and the Cycle of Undernutrition and Enteric Infection

Apart from repeated clinical infections, there is growing data on the role of a chronic subclinical enteropathy contributing to undernutrition in LMICs. This entity was historically called "tropical sprue" but has been renamed as environmental enteropathy and most recently environmental enteric dysfunction (EED). EED is thought to result from continuous exposure to fecally contaminated food or water or other contaminated substances such as soil.[41] EED is a condition characterized by anatomical (eg, flattened small intestinal villi), functional (eg, increased intestinal permeability), and inflammatory changes in the intestine.[42] HAZ trajectories have proven to be very difficult to ameliorate in response to pre- or postnatal health and diet-related interventions.[28] Recent reports have provided some evidence that EED might be a crucial contributor to the development of undernutrition, including HAZ trajectories.

The enteropathy caused by EED and subsequent undernutrition appears to be related to the intestinal microbial content and composition.[43,44] The term "intestinal microbiota" refers to forms of life, such as bacteria, viruses, eukaryotes, and Archaea (single-cell organisms with no nucleus or other membrane bound organelles), that are inhabitants of the intestinal lumen, and the term "microbiome" refers to the genetic material of these microorganisms.[45] Intestinal microbiota are key determinants of the host's health, as they are heavily involved in nutrient digestion, absorption and metabolism,[46] and immune regulation.[47] Intestinal microbiota composition is, in part, determined by the host's genetic background[48] as well as dietary intake[49] and is largely established during the first 3 years of life.[50] Beyond early childhood, small shifts in microbial composition can occur secondary to environmental pressures (eg, dietary changes, medications, infections, etc).

The interplay between intestinal microbiota and nutrition is bidirectional and can determine the host's nutritional status. Microbiota can affect dietary intake and nutrient handling through effects on appetite regulation, determination of calorie extraction from the diet, involvement in host gene expression, and regulation of insulin sensitivity.[51] In addition, bacteria and Archaea assist in the fermentation of nutrients that are otherwise indigestible by the host, releasing nutrients (eg, short-chain fatty acids) that can subsequently be utilized by the host. Lastly, the release of bacterial products (eg, endotoxin) in the circulation and the inflammation that ensues prevent normal insulin signaling, subsequently limiting the anabolic activities of the host. All these processes are crucial for nutrient metabolism, and as such, it is not surprising that dysbiosis (an imbalance between health- and disease-promoting bacteria) is seen in both stunting and wasting.

In LMICs, dysbiosis has been clearly linked to the development of SAM. This relationship has been shown in studies from Malawi, which investigated twin children discordant for malnutrition,[52] and Bangladesh.[44] Stunting severity was linked to decreased microbial diversity in a larger cohort of children from Malawi and Bangladesh.[53] Furthermore, the studies showed that the severity of malnutrition correlated with the degree of microbial immaturity and that this immaturity was only partly restored during the short period of nutritional rehabilitation that was prescribed. It remains to be seen whether complete reversal of microbiota immaturity during nutritional rehabilitation is associated with improved long-term nutritional outcomes. A shift in treatment focus may be necessary whereby maintenance bacterial diversity will become one of the goals of nutritional rehabilitation. This approach could potentially affect a large number of children. Apart from efforts to modulate the microbiome through specific nutritional interventions, the importance of preventing EED by limiting exposure to microorganisms (eg, ensuring clean household conditions, access to toilets, etc) and the beneficial effect of such an intervention on growth has been suggested in different pediatric cohorts.[54,55]

Nutrition in Humanitarian Crises
Natural and man-made disasters greatly increase the incidence of malnutrition in children in settings with weak or significantly damaged public

health and social infrastructure. Infants are an especially vulnerable group, and weight loss can develop rapidly in the context of a crisis and is associated with significant mortality. Crises are frequently the result of different factors coming together, such as environmental, political, and economic factors and conflicts. It is, therefore, essential that interventions are guided by a holistic approach to address the underlying contributing factors where possible. Emergencies frequently lead to both macronutrient as well as micronutrient deficiencies, which can lead to, for example, neurologic impairments (eg, from vitamin B_{12} or vitamin E deficiencies), blindness (eg, from vitamin A deficiency), or death. Signs and symptoms of specific micronutrient deficiencies are discussed in Chapters 18 through 21. Macronutrient deficiencies are most frequently a direct as well as indirect cause of death, related to a higher susceptibility to severe infections. Infants are the most vulnerable group in humanitarian disasters. A decision tool was developed for children with MAM by the Global Nutrition Cluster, which can be accessed at http://nutritioncluster.net/resources/ma/.

Exclusive breastfeeding should be promoted for sick and healthy infants younger than 6 months, particularly given that clean water is often unavailable in disaster-affected areas and breastfeeding provides protection against infections. Lactating mothers should be provided with fortified blended food commodities and micronutrient supplementation in addition to receiving nutritional counseling. In areas with high HIV prevalence, efforts should be made to offer HIV counseling and testing to allow mothers to make an informed decision around continuation of breastfeeding. Breastfeeding should be continued in all infants younger than 6 months, except for infants of HIV-positive mothers if safe alternatives are available. Efforts should be made to provide safe breastfeeding alternatives for infants of HIV-positive mothers. For infants older than 6 months, complimentary foods that contain adequate energy and micronutrients and can be safely prepared using locally available products should be introduced.

Many disasters occur in resource-limited settings where the prevalence of stunting, wasting, and micronutrient deficiencies including iron, iodine, and vitamin A are already high. It is important to pay special attention to populations from areas where specific nutritional deficiencies are known to be prevalent. In case of preexisting high prevalence rates of specific micronutrient deficiencies, interventions should be aimed at providing foods rich in limiting micronutrients, supplementing these micronutrients and identifying and treating children manifesting signs of specific deficiencies.

For detailed recommendations, refer to specific guidelines and policy papers that have been produced for vulnerable pediatric populations in disaster areas. Guidelines for assessing, estimating, and monitoring the food and nutrition needs of populations in emergencies have been developed by a joint effort of United Nations High Commissioner for Refugees, the United Nations International Children's Emergency Fund, the World Food Programme, and the WHO.[56] For children specifically, a practical guidance document was produced by the Infant and Young Child Feeding in Emergencies Core Group, another interagency collaboration.[57]

References

1. Black RE, Victora CG, Walker SP, Bhutta ZA, Christian P, de Onis M. Maternal and child undernutrition and overweight in low-income and middle-income countries. Child Nutrition Study Group. *Lancet.* 2013;382(9890):427–451

2. Olofin I, McDonald CM, Ezzati M, et al. Associations of suboptimal growth with all-cause and cause-specific mortality in children under five years: a pooled analysis of ten prospective studies. Nutrition Impact Model Study. *PLoS One.* 2013;8(5):e64636

3. UNICEF, WHO, The World Bank Group. Joint child malnutrition estimates - Levels and trends (2016 edition). Available at: http://www.who.int/nutgrowthdb/estimates2015/en/. Accessed December 10, 2018

4. World Health Organization. Child Growth Standards. Available at: http://www.who.int/childgrowth/en/. Accessed December 10, 2018

5. World Health Organization. Global Targets 2025: To improve maternal, infant and young child nutrition. Available at: http://www.who.int/nutrition/global-target-2025/en/. Accessed December 10, 2018.

6. United Nations. Sustainable Development Goals. Available from: https://sustainabledevelopment.un.org/. Accessed December 10, 2018

7. de Onis M, Branca F. Childhood stunting: a global perspective. *Matern Child Nutr.* 2016;12(Suppl 1):12–26

8. Yip R, Scanlon K. The burden of malnutrition: a population perspective. *J Nutr.* 1994;124(10 Suppl):2043S-2046S

9. Briend A, Khara T, Dolan C. Wasting and stunting—similarities and differences: policy and programmatic implications. *Food Nutr Bull.* 2015;36(S15–S23)

10. Victora CG, de Onis M, Hallal PC, Blossner M, Shrimpton R. Worldwide timing of growth faltering: revisiting implications for interventions. *Pediatrics.* 2010;125(3):e473–e480

11. Christian P, Lee SE, Donahue Angel M, Adair LS, Arifeen SE, Ashorn P. Risk of childhood undernutrition related to small-for-gestational age and preterm birth in low- and middle-income countries. *Int J Epidemiol.* 2013;42(5):1340–1355

12. Adair LS, Fall CH, Osmond C, et al. Associations of linear growth and relative weight gain during early life with adult health and human capital in countries of low and middle income: findings from five birth cohort studies. *Lancet.* 2013;382(9891):525–534

13. Nahar B, Hossain MI, Hamadani JD, et al. Effects of a community-based approach of food and psychosocial stimulation on growth and development of severely malnourished children in Bangladesh: a randomised trial. *Eur J Clin Nutr.* 2012;66(6):701–709

14. Lazzerini M, Rubert L, Pani P. Specially formulated foods for treating children with moderate acute malnutrition in low- and middle-income countries. *Cochrane Database Syst Rev.* 2013(6):CD009584

15. Lenters LM, Wazny K, Webb P, Ahmed T, Bhutta ZA. Treatment of severe and moderate acute malnutrition in low- and middle-income settings: a systematic review, meta-analysis and Delphi process. *BMC Public Health.* 2013;13 (Suppl 3):S23

16. World Health Organization. *Management of Severe Malnutrition: A Manual for Physicians and Other Senior Health Workers.* Geneva, Switzerland: World Health Organization; 1999

17. Alcoba G, Kerac M, Breysse S, et al. Do children with uncomplicated severe acute malnutrition need antibiotics? A systematic review and meta-analysis. *PLoS One.* 2013;8(1):e53184

18. Trehan I, Goldbach HS, LaGrone LN, et al. Antibiotics as part of the management of severe acute malnutrition. *N Engl J Med.* 2013;368:425–435

19. Ashworth A, Khanum S, Jackson A, Schofield C. Guidelines for the inpatient treatment of severely malnourished children. Geneva, Switzerland: World Health Organization; 2003: Available at: http://www.who.int/nutrition/publications/guide_inpatient_text.pdf. Accessed December 10, 2018

20. World Health Organization. Updates on the management of severe acute malnutrition in infants and children. Available at: http://apps.who.int/iris/bitstream/10665/95584/1/9789241506328_eng.pdf. Accessed December 10, 2018

21. Maleta K, Amadi B. Community-based management of acute malnutrition (CMAM) in sub-Saharan Africa: case studies from Ghana, Malawi, and Zambia. *Food Nutr Bull.* 2014;35(2 Suppl):S34–S38

22. Man WD, Weber M, Palmer A, et al. Nutritional status of children admitted to hospital with different diseases and its relationship to outcome in The Gambia, West Africa. *Trop Med Int Health.* 1998;3(8):678–686

23. Heikens GT, Bunn J, Amadi B, et al. Case management of HIV-infected severely malnourished children: challenges in the area of highest prevalence. *Lancet.* 2008;371(9620):1305–1307

24. Rytter MJH, Babirekere-Iriso E, Namusoke H, et al. Risk factors for death in children during inpatient treatment of severe acute malnutrition: a prospective cohort study. *Am J Clin Nutr.* 2016;105(2):494–502

25. Talbert A, Thuo N, Karisa J, et al. Diarrhoea complicating severe acute malnutrition in Kenyan children: a prospective descriptive study of risk factors and outcome. *PLoS One.* 2012;7(6):e38321

26. Namusoke H, Hother A-L, Rytter MJH, et al. Changes in plasma phosphate during in-patient treatment of children with severe acute malnutrition: an observational study in Uganda1. *Am J Clin Nutr.* 2016;103(2):551–558

27. Prentice AM, Doherty CP, Abrams SA, et al. Hepcidin is the major predictor of erythrocyte iron incorporation in anemic African children. *Blood.* 2012;119(8):1922–1928

28. World Health Organization. The Global Database on the Implementation of Nutrition Action (GINA). Available at: https://extranet.who.int/nutrition/gina/. Accessed December 10, 2018

29. Bhutta ZA, Das JK, Rizvi A, et al. Evidence-based interventions for improvement of maternal and child nutrition: what can be done and at what cost? Lancet Nutrition Interventions Review Group, the Maternal and Child Nutrition Study Group. *Lancet.* 2013;9890(382):452–477

30. World Health Organization. Vitamin A supplementation in infants and children 6–59 months of age. Available at: http://www.who.int/elena/titles/guidance_summaries/vitamina_children/en/. Accessed December 10, 2018

31. World Health Organization. Daily iron supplementation in infants and children. Available at: http://www.who.int/nutrition/publications/micronutrients/guidelines/daily_iron_supp_childrens/en/. December 10, 2018

32. Sazawal S, Black RE, Ramsan M, Chwaya HM, Stoltzfus RJ, Dutta A. Effects of routine prophylactic supplementation with iron and folic acid on admission to hospital and mortality in preschool children in a high malaria transmission setting: community-based, randomised, placebo-controlled trial. *Lancet.* 2006;367(9505):133–143

33. World Health Organization. Multiple micronutrient powders for point-of-use fortification of foods consumed by infants and children. Available at: http://www.who.int/elena/titles/guidance_summaries/micronutrientpowder_infants/en/. Accessed December 10, 2018

34. World Health Organization. Vitamin D supplementation in infants. Available at: http://www.who.int/elena/titles/vitamind_infants/en/. Accessed December 10, 2018

35. World Health Organization. Micronutrient supplementation in low-birth-weight and very-low-birth-weight infants. Available at: http://www.who.int/elena/titles/supplementation_lbw_infants/en/. Accessed December 10, 2018

36. World Health Organization guidelines. Zinc supplementation in the management of diarrhoea. Available at: http://www.who.int/elena/titles/zinc_diarrhoea/en/. Accessed December 10, 2018.

37. World Health Organization. Treating Measles in Children. Available at: http://www.who.int/immunization/documents/EPI_TRAM_97.02/en/. Accessed December 10, 2018

38. World Health Organization, United Nations High Commissioner for Refugees. Thiamine deficiency and its prevention and control in major emergencies. Available at: http://www.who.int/nutrition/publications/emergencies/WHO_NHD_99.13/en/. Accessed December 10, 2018

39. Hiffler L, Rakotoambinina B, Lafferty N, Martinez Garcia D. Thiamine deficiency in tropical pediatrics: new insights into a neglected but vital metabolic challenge. *Front Nutr.* 2016;3. doi: 10.3389/fnut.2016.00016

40. Thurnham DI, Northrop-Clewes CA. Inflammation and biomarkers of micronutrient status. *Curr Opin Clin Nutr Metab Care.* 2016;19(6):458–463

41. Syed S, Duggan CP. Risk factors for malnutrition and environmental enteric dysfunction—you really are what you eat. *J Pediatr.* 2016;178:7–8.

42. Owino V, Ahmed T, Freemark M, et al. Environmental enteric dysfunction and growth failure/stunting in global child health. *Pediatrics.* 2016;138(6):e20160641

43. Ordiz MI, Stephenson K, Agapova S, et al. Environmental enteric dysfunction and the fecal microbiota in Malawian children. *Am J Trop Med Hyg.* 2016;96(2):473–476

44. Subramanian S, Huq S, Yatsunenko T, et al. Persistent gut microbiota immaturity in malnourished Bangladeshi children. *Nature.* 2014;510(7505): 417–421

45. Subramanian S, Blanton LV, Frese Steven A, Charbonneau M, Mills David A, Gordon Jeffrey I. Cultivating healthy growth and nutrition through the gut microbiota. *Cell.* 2015;161(1):36–48

46. Sonnenburg JL, Bäckhed F. Diet–microbiota interactions as moderators of human metabolism. *Nature.* 2016;535(7610):56–64

47. Planer JD, Peng Y, Kau AL, et al. Development of the gut microbiota and mucosal IgA responses in twins and gnotobiotic mice. *Nature.* 2016;534(7606):263–266

48. Turpin W, Espin-Garcia O, Xu W, et al. Association of host genome with intestinal microbial composition in a large healthy cohort. *Nat Genet.* 2016;48(11):1413–1417

49. Turnbaugh PJ, Ridaura VK, Faith JJ, Rey FE, Knight R, Gordon JI. The effect of diet on the human gut microbiome: a metagenomic analysis in humanized gnotobiotic mice. *Sci Transl Med.* 2009;1(6):6ra14–16ra14

50. Voreades N, Kozil A, Weir TL. Diet and the development of the human intestinal microbiome. *Front Microbiol.* 2014;5

51. Mouzaki M, Bandsma R. Targeting the gut microbiota for the treatment of non-alcoholic fatty liver disease. *Curr Drug Targets.* 2015;16(12):1324–1331

52. Smith MI, Yatsunenko T, Manary MJ, Trehan I, Mkakosya R, Cheng J. Gut microbiomes of Malawian twin pairs discordant for kwashiorkor. *Sci Transl Med.* 2013;339(6119):548–554

53. Gough EK, Stephens DA, Moodie EEM, et al. Linear growth faltering in infants is associated with *Acidaminococcus* sp. and community-level changes in the gut microbiota. *Microbiome.* 2015;3(1). Doi: 10.1186/s40168-015-0089-2

54. Lin A, Huda TMN, Afreen S, et al. Household environmental conditions are associated with enteropathy and impaired growth in rural Bangladesh. *Am J Trop Med Hyg*. 2013;89(1):130–137

55. Pickering AJ, Djebbari H, Lopez C, Coulibaly M, Alzua ML. Effect of a community-led sanitation intervention on child diarrhoea and child growth in rural Mali: a cluster-randomised controlled trial. *Lancet Global Health*. 2015;3(11):e701–e711

56. World Health Organization. Food and Nutrition Needs in Emergencies. Available at: http://files.ennonline.net/attachments/864/food-and-nutrition-needs-in-emergencies.pdf. Accessed December 10, 2018

57. World Health Organization. Operational Guidance on Infant and Young Child Feeding in Emergencies. Available from: http://www.who.int/nutrition/publications/emergencies/operational_guidance/en/. Accessed December 10, 2018

Chapter 11

Nutritional Aspects of Vegetarian Diets

Vegetarian Diets

There are many variations of the vegetarian diet and the practice of vegetarianism. Vegetarianism, according to the Merriam–Webster dictionary, is defined as "the theory or practice of living on a diet made up of vegetables, fruits, grains, nuts, and sometimes eggs or dairy products." Vegetarianism is a way of life for many individuals for various reasons that can provide adequate and balanced nutrition at any age when practiced appropriately.[1] However, there can be potentially serious implications for the growing pediatric and adolescent population because of self-imposed or misguided limitations of the vegetarian diet. Therefore, pediatricians should proactively ask about vegetarianism and assess the nutritional status of their vegetarian patients to ensure optimal health and growth and provide anticipatory guidance to prevent any potential deficits.

A true vegetarian is a person who does not eat meat, fish, or fowl or products containing these foods. Many so-called semivegetarians eat some meat, fish, or seafood products. Thus, vegetarians are a heterogenous group of individuals that may be categorized as shown in Table 11.1. A lacto-ovo-vegetarian eating pattern is based on grains, vegetables, fruits, legumes,

Table 11.1.
Types of Vegetarians

Classic Vegetarians	*New Vegetarians*
Lacto-ovo-vegetarians	Low-meat vegetarians
Lacto-vegetarians	Almost vegetarians
Ovo-vegetarians	Semi-vegetarians
Vegans	Pesco-vegetarians
Raw food eaters	Pollo-vegetarians
Sproutarians	Pudding vegetarians
Fruitarians Nutritarians	
Macrobiotic vegetarians	
Anthroposophic vegetarians	

Adapted from Fuhrman and Ferreri[5] and Leitzmann.[35]

seeds, nuts, dairy products, and eggs. The lacto-vegetarian excludes eggs
but can consume milk products. The eating pattern of a vegan, or total
vegetarian, is similar to the lacto-vegetarian diet, with the exclusion of dairy
and all products of animal origin, including gelatin and honey. A macrobiotic diet is based largely on grains, legumes, and vegetables. Fruits, nuts,
and seeds are consumed to a lesser extent.[2] However, some individuals on
a macrobiotic diet also consume limited amounts of fish. A sproutarian
eats primarily sprouted seeds (eg, bean, wheat, or broccoli sprouts) supplemented with other raw foods. Fruitarianism diets include fruits, berries,
juices, grains, nuts, seeds, legumes, and a few vegetables. Raw foodism
excludes anything cooked above 118°F; this is the temperature at which a
number of enzymes present in foods begin to degrade.[3] People leading an
anthroposophical lifestyle have a diet consisting of vegetables fermented
by lactobacilli and a restriction on antibiotics, antipyretics, and immunizations.[4] A nutritarian diet has increased amounts of unrefined plant food
with high amounts of micronutrients as well as avoidance or minimal intake
of refined grain products.[5] Each of these eating styles has different implications for the nutrition and health of children and adolescents. Therefore,
it is important for the nutrition counselor to determine which groups
of foods are actually consumed and which are avoided and the degree of
conviction and adherence to the dietary pattern, to provide appropriate
recommendations.

Health considerations, concern for the environment, animal welfare
activism, or economic considerations and religious beliefs, alone or in
combination, are often cited as reasons to follow a vegetarian diet pattern.
In the United States, economic reasons alone are usually not prominent,
because a wide variety of both plant and animal foods are widely available
and inexpensive. Immigrants from developing countries (eg, mainland
China, India, Pakistan, and Southeast Asia) may maintain vegetarian eating
patterns from tradition, habit, and religious beliefs.[1,6] Other reasons for
eating vegetarian diets include concerns about the risks of omnivorous diets
and the negative publicity about bacterial foodborne disease from animal
foods.[7] There is a group of moral vegetarians who avoid meat by linking
it to cruelty, environmental degradation, or political reasons.[8] Ecologic
reasons involving views that the environmental impact of meat and poultry
production is an inefficient use of the planet's resources motivate others.
Some have religious beliefs (e.g., Seventh-Day Adventists, some Hindus,

Jains, and Buddhists) or philosophical beliefs (macrobiotics, transcendental meditators, anthroposophists, some yogic groups) that encourage various types of vegetarian diets and/or other food avoidances in their followers. Among the health considerations that lead some to follow a vegetarian diet is the suggestion that children consuming a vegetarian diet have a higher IQ as young adults.[9] This, of course, remains highly speculative and has not been validated.

Trends

A survey conducted by the Vegetarian Resource Group in 2016 showed that approximately 8 million, or 3.3% of US adults, are vegetarians; of which 46% are vegans.[10] A similar poll in 2010 determined that approximately 7% of 8- to 18-year-old children and adolescents in the United States are vegetarians.[11] In Europe, 10% of the population is vegetarian, varying by country. India has the highest proportion of vegetarians at 31% of the population.[12]

Knowledge and perspective on plant-based diets have evolved over the last 5 decades, from such diets being considered unsafe to actually conferring health benefits.[13] As with any dietary pattern, the degree of adherence to vegetarian patterns varies, and thus, overall nutrient intake differs from one vegetarian to the next. Most dietary patterns can be accommodated while fulfilling nutrient needs with appropriate dietary planning on the basis of scientific principles of sound nutrition. Most vegetarian parents welcome such advice. However, when beliefs are zealously pursued and nutrition principles are ignored, the health consequences can be unfortunate, especially for infants and young children. It is very possible to provide a balanced diet to vegetarians and vegans, and it may provide lifelong health benefits when adopted at a young age.[14,15]

The extent and degree of animal food restriction does not always predict either the extent of other food avoidances or the divergences in lifestyle and philosophical beliefs from nonvegetarians, although there is some correspondence. Generally, vegetarians with the most restrictive diets have the largest number of reasons for their eating styles, and their dietary patterns are most closely interwoven into their philosophy and belief systems.[6,8]

Position papers of the Academy of Nutrition and Dietetics and Canadian Paediatric Society state that appropriately planned vegetarian diets are healthful and nutritionally adequate and provide health benefits in the prevention and treatment of certain diseases.[1,14] A vegetarian, including a vegan, diet can also meet current recommended daily requirements for protein, iron, zinc, calcium, vitamin D, riboflavin, vitamin B_{12}, vitamin A, omega-3 fatty acids, and iodine with appropriate supplementation if required.[16] Use of fortified foods or supplements can be helpful in meeting recommendations for individual nutrients. Well-planned vegan and other types of vegetarian diets are appropriate for all stages of the life cycle, including pregnancy, lactation, infancy, childhood, and adolescence.[17] Vegetarian diets, in general, have lower levels of saturated fat and cholesterol and higher levels of complex carbohydrates, fiber, magnesium, vitamins C and E, carotenoids, and phytochemicals.[18,19]

Although vegetarians also can have coronary artery disease, hypertension, type 2 diabetes mellitus, metabolic syndrome, and colon cancer, the incidence of these diseases is lower than in omnivores.[20-29] There may be other advantages of vegetarian diets besides an improved lipid profile.[22] High fruit and vegetable consumption is a marker of a healthy lifestyle, but there is also strong evidence from in vitro studies and clinical trials that micronutrients and other components of fruit and vegetables have beneficial biological effects. A study evaluating circulating E-selectin levels, which include circulating intercellular adhesion molecule and circulating vascular adhesion molecule, in vegetarian and control adults showed that low circulating E-selectin levels of vegetarians may reflect the favorable cardiovascular risk profile of this group.[30] Most attention has focused on antioxidants, B group vitamins, minerals, and fiber, but several strands of evidence now indicate that increased intake of salicylates from fruit and vegetable consumption may be an additional benefit.[31] Urinary excretion of salicyluric acid and salicylic acid is significantly increased in vegetarians compared with nonvegetarians, but they excrete significantly less salicylic acid than do patients consuming 75 mg or 150 mg of aspirin per day.[32,33] The concentrations of salicylic acid in vegetarians have been shown to inhibit cyclooxygenase-2 (COX-2) in vitro.[34] Thus, it is plausible that dietary salicylates may contribute to the beneficial effects of a vegetarian diet.

Additional Implications of Vegetarianism

The lifestyle of vegetarians is different from omnivores in 3 major ways, which may have direct or indirect effects on children. First, they may practice abstinence or moderation in alcohol consumption as well as other stimulating substances, including nicotine. Second, they tend to be engaged in increased physical activities as well. Third, overall, plant foods are less calorie dense and, thus, predispose to lower overall calorie intake. Thus, the overall benefit of a vegetarian diet may derive from a vegetarian lifestyle rather than diet alone.[35]

Families that follow an anthroposophical lifestyle often justify it by claiming overall health benefits for their children. Their diet involves high intake of organically produced food items, including spontaneously fermented vegetables and foods containing probiotics. In addition, these families restrict the use of antibiotics, antipyretics, and immunizations. A study evaluating gut flora in children younger than 2 years with this lifestyle in comparison with those with a traditional lifestyle reported that microflora-associated characteristics were different between the 2 groups,[36] and it has been suggested that this provides a "probiotic" benefit.[37] Others have suggested that potential health benefits may be the result of restriction of antibiotics.[38] In an unmasked study in adults with refractory atopic dermatitis, alternative therapy with a low-energy, vegetarian diet caused a striking improvement in the severity of dermatitis as well as in lactate dehydrogenase-5 activity and in the number of circulating peripheral eosinophils.[39] Some have suggested that vegetarian diets have an effect on the development of allergy as a result of the fatty acid composition of the diet.[40]

There have been concerns that vegetarians, and in particular vegans, have lower-than-adequate intakes of vitamin B_{12}, vitamin D, calcium, zinc, and riboflavin.[41] A Polish study suggested that prepubertal vegetarian children had lower levels of leptin, a polypeptide that plays a role in bone growth, maturation, and weight regulation, in comparison with their omnivore counterparts,[42] which may contribute to reduced bone growth and development in childhood. A vegan diet may also put children at risk of vitamin A deficiency and subsequent keratomalacia, anemia, and protein and zinc deficiency if diet is not monitored and the family is not given appropriate information on the potential dietary deficiencies relevant to the vegetarian diet.[43] However, the overall belief that individuals following vegan or vegetarian diets suffer from nutritional deficiencies may be exaggerated, as reports of specific malnutrition in these populations are rare.[44,45]

Dietary practices among vegetarians are varied; hence, individual assessment of dietary intakes by a trained dietitian is important. Such

Table 11.2.

Tips for Meal Planning

1. Encourage a variety of foods from Fig 11.1–11.3.
2. The number of servings in each group is for minimum daily intakes, as shown in Fig 11.1 and 11.2. Choose more foods from any of the groups to meet energy needs.
3. A serving from the calcium-rich food group provides Approximately 10% of adult daily requirements. Choose 8 or more servings a day. These also count toward servings from other food groups in the guide. For example, ½ cup (125 mL) of fortified fruit juice counts as a calcium rich food and also counts toward servings from the fruit group.
4. Include 2 servings every day of foods that supply omega-3 fats. Foods rich in omega-3 fats are found in the legumes/nuts group and the fats group. A serving is 1 teaspoon (5 mL) of ground flaxseed oil, 3 teaspoons (15 mL) of canola or soybean oil, 1 tablespoon (15 mL) of ground flaxseed, or ¼ cup (60 mL) of walnuts. Olive and canola oil are the best choices for cooking.
5. Equivalent servings of nuts and seeds can replace servings from the fats group.
6. Vitamin D from daily sun exposure or through fortified foods or supplements. Cow milk and some brands of soy milk and breakfast cereals are fortified with vitamin D.
7. Include at least 3 good food sources of vitamin B_{12} in daily diet—for example: 1 tbsp (15 mL) of Red Star Vegetarian support formula nutritional yeast, 1 cup (250 mL) fortified soy milk, ½ cup (125 mL) cow's milk, ¾ cup (185 mL) yogurt, 1 large egg, 1 oz of fortified breakfast cereal, 1 to 1½ oz of fortified meat analog. If these foods are not consumed regularly (at least 3 servings per day) a daily vitamin B_{12} supplement of 5 to 10 µg or a weekly dose of 2000 µg is recommended.
8. Consume sweets or alcohol in moderation. Use foods in the Vegetarian food guide to get most of calories.

Adapted from Messina et al.[47]

assessments can be best made by using a 24- to 72-hour food recall and food frequency questionnaire.[46] Suggestions for balanced meal planning are shown in Table 11.2. A knowledgeable and skilled dietitian or physician can educate vegetarian patients about food sources of specific nutrients, food purchase and preparation, and any dietary modifications that may be necessary to meet individual needs. Menu planning for vegetarians can be simplified by use of a food guide that specifies food groups and serving sizes as shown in Fig 11.1, 11.2, and 11.3. Such guidance is of particular importance in

Fig 11.1.
Vegan Pyramid

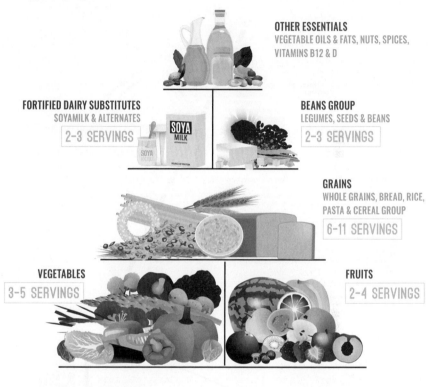

THE VEGAN FOOD PYRAMID

Reproduced with permission from Messina et al.[47]

planning adequate meals for pediatric patients of all ages to ensure proper growth and development.[47] A questionnaire to assess diet quality with special reference to micronutrient adequacy for lacto-vegetarian adolescent girls was reported to be helpful as an assessment tool to suggest dietary intervention.[48] More recently, use of personal mobile phones to report dietary intake via texting and digital images has been reported to be more efficacious among adolescents.[49]

Fig 11.2.
Vegetarian Food Guide Pyramid

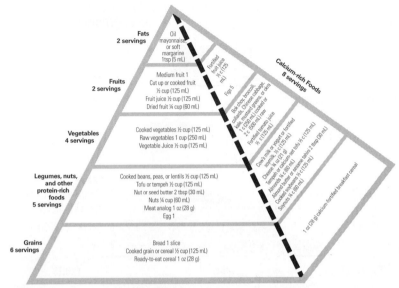

Reproduced with permission from Messina et al.[47]

Fig 11.3.
Vegetarian Food Guide Rainbow

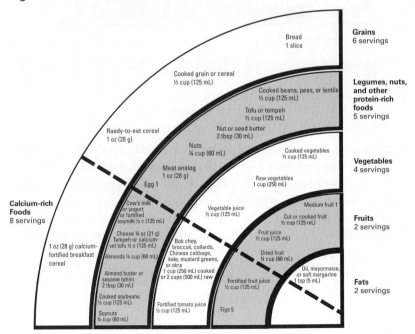

Reproduced with permission from Messina et al.[47]

Nutrient Intake Guidelines

Some basic guidelines are used to determine the daily nutrient requirements for healthy vegetarians. The recommendation for daily calorie intake is the same as for the general population. The recommendations for most other nutrient intakes are increased by 2 standard deviations above the Recommended Dietary Allowance to compensate for potential deficiencies or poor bioavailability of nutrients in the vegetarian diet and, thus, ensure adequacy of nutrient intake.[16,17,47]

Whole Foods Concept

The concept of whole foods as a principle of vegetarian diets relies on the fact that almost any kind of food processing, including freezing, heating, and cooking, can lead to loss of nutrients. Whole-grain products contain an excellent combination of nutrients to meet human needs, although they are deficient in calcium and vitamin C. Processing whole grains to white flour leads to a loss of minerals, vitamins, phytochemicals, and dietary fibers by 75% to 95%.[50] The changes that occur in freezing, baking, boiling, and frying may also be significant. However, the relevance of this concept to overall human nutrition is unclear, because processing has a number of functions, including increasing palatability and digestibility, food preservation, and safety and fortification. Thus, when an appropriate variety and amount of food is consumed over several days, both children and adults can meet their daily nutrient requirements. Furthermore, home cooking using heat, sprouting, fermentation, malting, and addition of acidulants has been shown to improve bioavailability iron, zinc, and beta carotene.[51]

Nutritional Considerations

Energy

Studies of vegan children have indicated that their energy intake is close to the recommended level for nonvegetarian controls.[45,47] During infancy and weaning, the amount of food needed to meet energy needs on vegan diets may exceed gastric capacity; hence, the child should be fed frequently.[47] Concentrated sources of calories that are acceptable for older infants and children include soy products, legumes, oils, nuts, nut butters, and fruit juices.[5,16]

Protein

Despite the low caloric density of strict vegetarian diets, food intakes are usually sufficient to support protein needs even for the weanling infant.[52,53] Plant protein can meet requirements when a variety of plant foods is consumed. Additional protein need not be consumed at the same meal, as long as the protein requirement is consumed over a period of 24 hours. Variations in plant protein quality, quantity, and digestibility are all of potential concern, especially when vegan-vegetarian diets are used during infancy. Compared with children fed a mixed diet, some studies suggest that the lower quality of protein sources in a vegan diet increases the protein requirements of infants by 30% to 35%, those of children 2 to 6 years of age by 20% to 30%, and those of children older than 6 years by 15% to 20%.[16,53]

The 5 major food sources of plant protein are legumes, cereals, nuts and seeds, fruits, and other vegetables. Each of these has nutritional advantages and disadvantages. For example, legumes and cereals provide relatively large amounts of high-quality protein, but they must be cooked or processed to enhance their palatability and to remove substances that decrease digestibility, such as tough skins, amylase inhibitors, lectins, and tannins.[47,53] A standard method for determining protein quality is the protein digestibility-corrected amino acid score.[54] Using this method, isolated soy protein is shown to meet protein needs as effectively as animal protein, unlike wheat protein, which is almost 50% less usable than animal protein.[55,56] Soy foods have been valuable for vegetarians for both their high protein content and versatility. Soybeans are distinct from other legumes in macronutrient content, having much higher fat and protein content and lower carbohydrate content.[57] There is an increasing interest in healthy and good-tasting meat-free foods that enhance the eating experience for vegetarians partly driven by the increasing use of low-cost vegetable protein such as textured soy protein, mushroom, wheat gluten, pulses, etc, as substitutes for animal protein. Simulated meat-like products have a texture, flavor, color, and nutritive value similar to meat and can be substituted for it easily.[58] These products have been reported to be well accepted in school lunch research studies.[59,60] Lysine concentration is lower in all plant foods than in animal foods. The levels of the sulfur-containing amino acids methionine and cysteine are lower in legumes and fruits. The level of the essential amino acid threonine is lower in cereals, and tryptophan content tends to be lower in fruits than in most animal foods.[52] Therefore, if parents feed diets that are adequate in food energy and select a wide variety of plant foods with proteins that complement each other, vegetarian children should be able to receive an adequate amount of protein to grow and thrive.

Fat

Dietary fat intakes of vegetarian children older than 2 years are between 25% and 35% of total calories, which are similar to or slightly lower than those of omnivores; effects on growth appear to be small.[61] However, when dietary fat intake falls below approximately 15% of calories, special care must be taken to ensure that recommended intakes of essential fatty acids are met. At least 3% of energy should be from linoleic acid (an omega-3 fatty acid), and 1% of energy should be from alpha-linolenic acid (an omega-6 fatty acid).[52] The recommended ratio of omega-6 fatty acids to omega-3 fatty acids ranges from 2:1 to 4:1.[61,62] Linoleic acid is found in seeds, nuts, and grains. Alpha-linolenic acid is found in the green leaves of plants, in phytoplankton and algae, and in certain seeds, nuts, and legumes, such as flax seeds, canola seeds, walnuts, hazelnuts, and soybeans. These can be converted into more highly unsaturated fatty acids, including arachidonic acid (ARA), eicosapentaenoic acid (EPA), and docosahexaenoic acid (DHA).[63] ARA and EPA serve as precursors for the eicosanoids. Tentative recommended intakes for these polyunsaturated fatty acids range from 3% to 10% of total energy intakes.[62] ARA is found in animal foods such as meat, poultry, and eggs. EPA and DHA are largely found in fish and seafood. Vegan vegetarians have no direct sources of these long-chain omega-3 fatty acids in their diets and, thus, must convert alpha-linolenic acid to them.[1,16] There is concern that pregnant women who are vegan or vegetarian or who follow a macrobiotic diet and consume little or no fish or other animal foods may not obtain enough of these fatty acids, especially during pregnancy and while breastfeeding.[16,18] Risks may be especially high if infants are born preterm, because their capacity to desaturate alpha-linolenic acid to DHA is limited.[16] Such individuals may need DHA supplements, either from fish oils or from cultured micro algae.[61-63] Algae sources of DHA have been shown to positively affect blood levels of DHA and of EPA through retroconversion.[64,65] However, such supplements for young infants should only be dispensed under a physician's direction, because they are also potent anticoagulants.

Fiber

Recommended daily fiber intake for 1- to 3-year-olds is 19 g/day, for 4 to 8-year-old children is 25 g/day, and for adolescents is up to 38 g/day.[66] In very small children, the sheer bulk and low energy density of such a high-fiber diet may make consumption of sufficient energy difficult for the child and may inhibit absorption of some minerals.[52] The sieving or mashing of cereals, pulses, and vegetables that are fed to infants can increase their digestibility, and partial replacement of whole-grain cereals with more highly refined cereals that are lower in fiber can further increase energy intakes and decrease bulk if this is a problem in small children. Lacto-ovo-vegetarian children usually consume adequate but not excessive amounts of dietary fiber.

Vitamins

Vitamin A/Beta Carotene
Because plant foods contain only dietary carotenoids, vitamin A requirements can be met by 3 servings a day of plant foods rich in beta carotene, such as leafy or deep yellow or orange vegetables and fruits. Absorption of beta carotene can be increased by cooking, chopping, or pureeing or addition of small amounts of fat.[16,19,52,67]

Riboflavin
Intakes of riboflavin appear to be similar in vegetarians and omnivores.[68] Riboflavin deficiency has occasionally occurred in people following severely restricted macrobiotic diets, but it is not a problem in other forms of vegetarianism. Good sources of riboflavin include yeast, wheat germ, soy, fortified cereals, and enriched grains.

Folic Acid
Usually, vegetarians who consume high amounts of vegetables and fruits as well as other plant foods have adequate intakes of folic acid. However, those who consume vegetables that are usually braised or fried at high temperature and who rarely drink fruit juices or eat grain products fortified with folic acid may be at risk of deficiency. Additionally, postmenarcheal adolescent girls who are capable of becoming pregnant should consume 400 µg of folic acid as a supplement or in fortified foods in addition to usual food sources of the nutrient.[16,68]

Vitamin B$_{12}$
No plant foods, except for certain sea vegetables or plant foods that are fortified, contain vitamin B$_{12}$. Cobalamin is only found in animal food sources and, therefore, is absent from a vegetarian diet. Absorption is effective when small amounts of vitamin B$_{12}$ are consumed at regular intervals.[16,19] Lacto-ovo-vegetarians get sufficient amounts of vitamin B$_{12}$ if dairy products are consumed on a regular basis.[68] Studies indicate that some strict vegans are deficient in vitamin B$_{12}$, and vegetarian diets typically high in folic acid mask hematologic symptoms of deficiency, sometimes leading to a delayed diagnosis.[69,70] In such situations, the presentation is often with

neurologic symptoms.[70-72] A case of dietary deficiency of cobalamin presenting only as schizoaffective disorder without hematologic/neurologic manifestations has been reported.[71] In another report, 27 exclusively breastfed infants of vegetarian mothers, aged 6 to 27 months, with vitamin B_{12} deficiency, presented with tremors, developmental delay or regression, pallor, skin hyperpigmentation, and sparse brown hair. All improved with vitamin B_{12} supplementation.[72] Regular intake of vitamin B_{12}-fortified foods or dairy products should be encouraged in vegetarians and especially in mothers of breastfed infants.

Vitamin D

Serum vitamin D concentrations are dependent on sunlight exposure and intake of vitamin D-rich foods or supplements. Infants and children synthesize vitamin D less efficiently than older individuals.[73] Foods such as cow milk, some types of soy milk and rice milk, and breakfast cereals that are enriched with vitamin D_2 (ergocalciferol) and/or vitamin D_3 (cholecalciferol, animal based) should be consumed. Intake of such fortified foods, wherever possible, should be encouraged. Vitamin D_2 may be less biologically active than vitamin D_3, thus raising the requirements for certain types of vegetarians.[73] A recent study reported that deficient consumption of vitamin D and calcium may reduce bone density in vegans by affecting bone turnover rate adversely; hence, vitamin D and calcium intakes should be monitored proactively in the pediatric vegetarian population.[74] If sunlight exposure and intake of fortified foods are insufficient or if sun-protective lotions are used, then supplements are recommended.[15,18,73]

Minerals

Iron

Iron is vital at all ages, and there is a risk of deficiency of this nutrient during infancy, the adolescent growth spurt, and pregnancy.[75-79] The iron status of vegetarian infants and children varies. Although iron deficiency is by far the most common of the micronutrient deficiencies exhibited by vegetarian children, the incidence of iron-deficiency anemia among vegetarians is similar to that among nonvegetarians.[75] Although vegetarians are more likely to have lower iron stores than do omnivores, higher iron stores may be a risk factor for certain noncommunicable disease such as type 2 diabetes mellitus.[78] Iron deficiency is particularly common in children consuming vegan diets, because plant foods contain nonheme iron as opposed to heme iron found in animal sources.[75] Nonheme iron is more sensitive to inhibitors of iron absorption, such as phytates, calcium, herbal teas, cocoa, some spices, and fiber.[75] Vitamin C and other organic acids in fruits and vegetables enhance the absorption of iron.[52,78] Recommended iron intakes for vegetarians are approximately 1.8 to 2 times those of omnivores because of the lower bioavailability of iron in a vegetarian diet.

Zinc

Approximately half of the zinc in the diet comes from meat, poultry, and fish.[75,80,81] The bioavailability of relatively rich plant sources of zinc, such as whole-grain cereals, soy, beans, lentils, peas, and nuts tends to be low, because most of them also contain large amounts of phytate and fiber, which inhibit zinc absorption.[80,82] Because vegetarian diets have ingredients that may enhance as well as inhibit mineral bioavailability, knowledge of prudent cooking practices and use of ideal combinations of food additives that can significantly enhance micronutrient bioavailability is recommended.[51,82] In lacto-ovo-vegetarians, zinc absorption is approximately a third less than in omnivores.[83]

The requirement for zinc may be as much as 50% greater among strict vegetarians.[16,19] Vegetarian diets also tend to be lower in this mineral than are omnivorous diets.[80] When daily requirements for zinc are increased, as they are in infants and children, the risk of suboptimal zinc nutritional status is increased, because the ability to increase zinc absorption is limited. Because the presence of inhibitors is highest in vegan diets, vegans are at special risk. Despite this risk, zinc supplementation is not recommended, because clinical signs of deficiency are rare among vegetarians, even in children younger than 24 months.[84] Good plant sources of zinc are yeast-fermented whole-grain breads (the phytic acid content is reduced) and zinc-fortified infant and adult cereals.

Calcium

Calcium intakes of vegans tend to be lower than those of lacto-vegetarians and nonvegetarians. Although oxalates, phytates, and fiber in plant foods decrease calcium availability, the bioavailability of calcium from plant foods and soy products can be higher than from milk,[85] although in general, this is not the case. Calcium is present in a large number of plant and fortified foods, such as broccoli, Chinese cabbage, collards, kale, okra, and turnip greens. It has been suggested but not substantiated that soy products may have favorable effects on bone health apart from their calcium content.[86] If vegetarian children's diets do not contain adequate sources of dietary calcium, supplements may be advisable.

Iodine

Iodine deficiency is not commonly observed in vegetarian children when iodized salt is readily available. Vegans whose diets are restricted to kosher or sea salts, which are generally not iodized, or who also have a substantial intake of goitrogens, such as broccoli, mustard, kale, turnips, etc, are at risk of iodine deficiency. For these children, especially for those living in iodine-poor areas, iodine-fortified foods are recommended.[87]

Carnitine and Taurine

Serum carnitine and taurine concentrations are decreased in lacto-ovo-vegetarian and vegan diets; however, the functional significance of this is not apparent, and therefore, supplementation does not seem to be warranted.[88,89]

Vegetarian Diets for Special Populations

Infants

Exclusively breastfed infants of omnivorous mothers receive adequate amounts of energy and nutrients during the first 4 to 6 months of life.[90,91] The milk of vegetarian women is similar in nutrient composition to that of nonvegetarians. Vegetarian mothers should be encouraged to breastfeed. Soy formula is the only option for vegan infants who are not being breastfed. Soy and rice beverages and other homemade formulas should not be used to replace human milk or commercial formulas for those infants of vegan mothers who are not being breastfed.[18]

Guidelines for the introduction of complementary foods in infancy are similar for vegetarians and nonvegetarians.[90,91] Infants older than 6 months are potentially at the greatest risk of overt deficiency states related to inappropriate restrictions of the diet, although deficiencies of vitamins B_{12} and essential fatty acids may appear earlier.[91] They are particularly vulnerable during the weaning period if fed a macrobiotic diet and may experience psychomotor delay in some instances.[92] Anticipating these potential problems for vegetarian families by explaining the principles of providing calorie-dense foods at the time of weaning is important so the increased bulk of vegetarian diets does not interfere with adequate consumption of energy, protein, and other nutrients.[16,19]

Children

Except for those on severely restricted diets, most vegetarian children exhibit growth comparable to their omnivore peers.[92] The average calorie and protein intake generally meets or exceeds recommendations. Vegan children may have slightly higher protein needs than nonvegan children because of differences in plant-sourced protein bioavailability and quality, but protein requirements are usually met with an intake of a variety of plant foods. The importance of proper intake of calcium, zinc, and iron should be emphasized.[16,19]

Adolescents

Whether adolescents adopt a vegetarian diet at this age or have been vegetarians from infancy, nutritional imbalances in their diets may occur during this period of life. Vegetarianism may be adopted as a part of disordered eating attitudes and behaviors.[93,94] A vegetarian diet is practiced by some young women as a means of weight control.[95] Adolescent vegetarians were significantly more likely to exhibit bulimic behaviors in a Minnesota study.[96] Because adolescent vegetarians may be at increased risk for eating disorders, inquiry about current and former vegetarian status is prudent when assessing these patients.[97] Vegetarian males also appear more vulnerable to eating disorders.[98] In a Turkish study to evaluate the prevalence of eating disorders associated with vegetarianism, abnormal eating habits, low

Table 11.3.
Formulas for Gastrostomy Tube Feedings

Vegetarian		Vegan	
<1 y	>1 y	<1 y	>1 y
Alimentum	Kindercal	Isomil	Elecare
Enfamil	Next Step	Neocate	Isomil 2
Nutramigen	Nutren Jr/1.0/2.0	Prosobee	Neocate/Jr/One
Pregestamil	Pediasure	Carnation Soy	L-Emental
Similac	Peptamen/Jr	RCF (Ross)	Tolerex
Enfacare	Similac 2		Vivonex/Plus/Ten
Carnation	Ensure/Plus		Faa (Nestle)
	Jevity		Next Step Soy
	Isocal		
	Enfagrow Toddler Transitions		

self-esteem, high body image anxiety, and high trait anxiety were detected in Turkish vegetarian adolescents between 7 and 21 years of age.[99] Data from a study comparing fish-eating vegetarians with omnivores demonstrate that long-term adherence to a vegetarian diet is associated with maintained leanness and a lower body mass index (BMI).[100] Therefore, vegetarian practices may be a marker to help identify those adolescents or young adults with eating disorder tendencies or weight obsession, and adolescents who choose to become vegetarians may benefit significantly from dietary guidance (see Tables 11.2 and 11.4).

Athletes

With increasing interest in the potential health benefits of vegetarian diets, it is relevant to consider dietary practices that influence athletic performance. Athletes can meet their protein needs from a vegetarian diet.[5,101] Although long-term controlled studies are needed, a well-planned and appropriately supplemented vegetarian diet appears to effectively support the nutritional requirements of athletes.[5] Vegetarian female athletes should be informed of an increased risk of iron deficiency, which may limit endurance performance.[102] Vegetarian athletes have a lower mean muscle creatine concentration, and it has been suggested that they may experience greater performance increments after creatine loading in activities that rely on adenosine triphosphate/phosphocreatine systems,[103] although this requires substantiation. Trainers and coaches need to be made aware of the use of a

Table 11.4.

Modifications to the Vegetarian Food Guide (Fig 11.2 and 11.3) for Children, Adolescents, and Pregnant and Lactating Women

	Food Group[a]		
Stage	B$_{12}$-Rich Foods (Servings)	Beans/Nuts/ Seeds/Egg (Servings)	Calcium- Rich Foods (Servings)
Child, 4–8 y	2	5	6
Adolescent, 9–13 y	2	6	10
Adolescent, 14–18 y	3	6	10

[a]The number of servings in each group is the minimum amount needed. The minimum number of servings from other groups is not different from the vegetarian food guide (Fig 11.2 and 11.2). Additional foods can be chosen from any of the groups in the vegetarian food guide to meet energy needs.

Adapted from Messina et al.[47]

vegetarian diet as a form of weight control, and appropriate steps should be taken to determine that a balanced vegetarian diet is followed to ensure the good health of these athletes.

Developmentally and Neurologically Delayed Children

It is possible to provide oral and/or enteral feeding to pediatric patients with swallowing problems whose families elect to provide a vegetarian diet. A list of appropriate formulas for use by vegetarian and vegan diets at different ages is shown in Table 11.3.

Vegetarian Diets in Management of Metabolic Syndrome and Type 2 Diabetes Mellitus

Vegetarian diets present potential advantages for the management of type 2 diabetes mellitus.[104] Although most of the studies have been conducted in adults, the findings appear to be applicable to children and adolescents. The increased intake of soluble and insoluble fiber in a vegetarian diet improves glucose metabolism in both diabetic and normal subjects, along with a reduced intake of saturated fats and high-glycemic index foods.[105] Vegetarian diets have been shown to be efficacious, nutritionally complete under proper guidance, acceptable, and practical to follow.[106] The prevalence of type 2 diabetes mellitus in a large population of Adventists on different types of vegetarian diets was compared with that in omnivores using self-reported questionnaire.[106] Vegans had a significantly lower BMI than did nonvegetarians, even after adjustment for demographic and lifestyle factors, as well as a lower incidence of type 2 diabetes mellitus. This study provides further evidence of the advantage of a vegetarian lifestyle in protecting against obesity and reducing the risk of type 2 diabetes mellitus.

Vegetarian Diets and Obesity

Although there is an increased prevalence of childhood overweight and obesity globally, evidence from epidemiologic studies suggests that children and adults on vegetarian diets have a lower BMI and a decreased prevalence of obesity.[107,108] Because vegetarian diets may reduce the risk of overweight and obesity, they should be considered a possible preventive measure against obesity in at-risk pediatric patients, under supervision. The low energy density of vegetarian foods, along with increased consumption of complex carbohydrates, fiber, and water may increase satiety and metabolic rate. Vegetarian diets appeared to have significant benefits on weight reduction compared with nonvegetarian diets in a recent meta-analyses.[21,109] Both clinical trials and observational research indicate an advantage to adoption of plant-based diets for preventing overweight and obesity and promoting weight loss. In addition, these may also provide higher-quality diets than are observed with other therapeutic diet approaches, with similar levels of adherence and acceptability.[110] Additional long-term trials are needed to investigate the effects of vegetarian diets on body weight control, especially for the pediatric age group.

Conclusion

In general, vegetarian diets support growth and good health, despite concerns about their adequacy. A systematic review to evaluate studies on the dietary intake and the nutritional or health status of vegetarian infants, children, and adolescents in industrialized countries failed to provide any firm evidence of benefits versus risks because of heterogeneity of data from 16 studies.[111] The studies cited in this review are also from the 1980s-1990s. In the current Internet-savvy environment, many parents of vegetarian children proactively seek information about optimizing their diets. Thus, chances of extreme nutrient deficiencies are much less common today. Table 11.5 lists a few useful and "reliable" Web sites for use by consumers and pediatricians. Counseling families about the reliability of information available on the Internet on this topic is very important, because there is a significant amount of marketing and claims for vegetarian diets and foods that cannot be substantiated. Overall, vegetarian diets can meet the nutritional needs of children and adolescents if appropriately planned and

Table 11.5.

List of Useful Vegetarian Web Sites

https://www.nutrition.gov/smart-nutrition-101/healthy-eating/eating-vegetarian
https://www.healthlinkbc.ca/health-topics/zx3391
http://vegetariannutrition.net
http://kidshealth.org/en/parents/vegetarianism.html
http://www.heart.org/HEARTORG/GettingHealthy/NutritionCenter/Vegetarian-Diets_UCM_306032_Article.jsp
https://www.nal.usda.gov/fnic
http://www.theveganrd.com/
http://www.vrg.org
http://www.vegsoc.org/health

monitored by a health care professional or dietitian. The current evidence base of vegetarian studies convincingly indicates that plant-based diets have health benefits as well. In addition to maintaining awareness of various relevant nutritional issues, health care professionals should familiarize themselves with the wide range of vegetarian diets and the social, cultural, and ideological systems present among vegetarians in their practice. Those who are monitoring the nutritional status of children and adolescents who consume a vegetarian diet should bear in mind that despite advances, states of malnutrition can occur, even in higher-income families. Compliance with dietary counseling among vegetarians varies but has been reported to be better in those with a higher socioeconomic status.[112] Additional prospective long-term follow-up studies to assess the adequacy of the many and various diets included in the broad category of "vegetarian diets," with validated objective outcome markers and social gradient data, are urgently needed.

References

1. Melina V, Craig W, Levin S. Position of the Academy of Nutrition and Dietetics: Vegetarian diets. *J Acad Nutr Diet.* 2016;116(12):1970–1980
2. Kushi M, Jack A. *The Book of Macrobiotics: The Universal Way of Health, Happiness, and Peace.* Rev ed. Boston, MA: Japan Publications; 1987
3. Corliss R. Should we all be vegetarians? Would we be healthier? The risks and benefits of a meat free life. *Time.* 2002;160(3):48–56
4. Edmunds F. *An Introduction to Anthroposophy.* London, England: Rudolph Steiner Press; 2006
5. Fuhrman J, Ferreri DM. Fueling the vegetarian (vegan) athlete. *Curr Sports Med Rep.* 2010;9(4):233–241
6. Rosenfeld DL, Burrow AL. Vegetarian on purpose: understanding the motivations of plant-based dieters. *Appetite.* 2017;116:456–463
7. Fox N, Ward KJ. You are what you eat? Vegetarianism, health and identity. *Soc Sci Med.* 2008;66(12):2585–2595
8. Mathieu S, Dorard G. Vegetarianism and veganism lifestyle: Motivation and psychological dimensions associated with selective diet. *Presse Med.* 2016;45(9):726–733
9. Gale CR, Deary IJ, Schoon I, Batty GD. IQ in childhood and vegetarianism in adulthood: 1970 British cohort study. *BMJ.* 2007;334(7587):245–248
10. Group TVR. How many adults in the US are vegetarian or vegan? How many adults eat vegetarian and vegan meals when eating out? Available at: https://www.vrg.org/nutshell/Polls/2016_adults_veg.htm. Accessed April 14, 2017
11. The Vegetarian Resource Group. How many youth are vegetarian? February 24, 2010. Available at: https://www.vrg.org/press/youth_poll_2010.php. Accessed April 14, 2017

12. Quora.com. What is the percentage of vegetarians in world in 2015? Available at: https://www.quora.com/What-is-the-percentage-of-vegetarians-in-world-in-2015/. Accessed April 14, 2017

13. Melina V. Five decades: from challenge to acclaim. *Can J Diet Pract Res.* 2016;77(3):154–158

14. Amit M, Canadian Paediatric Society, Community Paediatrics Committee. Vegetarian diets in children and adolescents. *Paediatr Child Health.* 2010;15(5):303–314

15. Dharmapuri S, Hettich K, Goday PS. Contemporary Dietary Practices: FODMAPs and Beyond. *Adolesc Med.* 2016;27(1):109–124

16. Renda M, Fischer P. Pediatr Rev. *Vegetarian diets in children and adolescents.* 2009;30(1):e1–e8

17. Reid MA, Marsh KA, Zeuschner CL, Saunders AV, Baines SK. Meeting the nutrient reference values on a vegetarian diet. *Med J Aust.* 2013;199(4 Suppl): S33–S40

18. Craig WJ. Nutrition concerns and health effects of vegetarian diets. *Nutr Clin Pract.* 2010;25(6):613–620

19. McEvoy CT, Woodside JV. Vegetarian diets. *World Rev Nutr Diet.* 2015;113:134–138

20. Appleby PN, Key TJ. The long-term health of vegetarians and vegans. *75.* 2016;3(287–293)

21. Bennett WL, Appel LJ. Vegetarian Diets for Weight Loss: How Strong is the Evidence? *J Gen Intern Med.* 2016;31(1):9–10

22. Chiu YF, Hsu CC, Chiu THL, C.Y., et al. Cross-sectional and longitudinal comparisons of metabolic profiles between vegetarian and non-vegetarian subjects: a matched cohort study. *Br J Nutr.* 2015;114(8):1313–1320

23. Chuang SY, Chiu TH, Lee CY, et al. Vegetarian diet reduces the risk of hypertension independent of abdominal obesity and inflammation: a prospective study. *J Hypertens.* 2016;34(11):2164–2171

24. Dinu M, Abbate R, Gensini GF, Casini A, Sofi F. Vegetarian, vegan diets and multiple health outcomes: a systematic review with meta-analysis of observational studies. *Crit Rev Food Sci Nutr.* 2017;57(17):3640–3649

25. Le LT, Sabaté J. Beyond meatless, the health effects of vegan diets: findings from the Adventist cohorts. *Nutrients.* 2014;6(6):2131–2147

26. Printz C. Vegetarian diet associated with lower risk of colorectal cancer. *Cancer.* 2015;121(16):2667

27. Sabaté J, Wien M. A perspective on vegetarian dietary patterns and risk of metabolic syndrome. *Br J Nutr.* 2015;113(Suppl 2):S136–S143

28. Wise J. Vegetarians have lower risk of colorectal cancers, study finds. *BMJ.* 2015;350:h1313

29. Wong JM. Gut microbiota and cardiometabolic outcomes: influence of dietary patterns and their associated components. *Am J Clin Nutr.* 2014;100(Suppl 1): 369S–377S

30. Purschwitz K, Rassoul F, Reuter W, et al. Soluble leukocyte adhesion molecules in vegetarians of various ages. *Z Gerontol Geriatr.* 2001;34(6):476–479

31. Hare LG, Woodside JV, Young IS. Dietary salicylates: another benefit of fruit and vegetable consumption? (Editorial). *J Clin Pathol.* 2003;56(9):649–650

32. Blacklock CJ, Lawrence JR, Malcolm EA, Gibson IH, Kelly CJ, Paterson JR. Salicylic acid in the serum of subjects not taking aspirin. Comparison of salicylic acid concentrations in the serum of vegetarians, non-vegetarians, and patients taking low-dose aspirin. *J Clin Pathol.* 2001;54(7):553–555

33. Lawrence JR, Peter R, Baxter G, Robson J, Graham AB, Paterson JR. Urinary excretion of salicyluric and salicylic acids by non-vegetarians, vegetarians and patients taking low-dose aspirin. *J Clin Pathol.* 2003;56(9):651–653

34. Xu XM, Sansores-Garcia L, Chen XM, Matijevic-Aleksic N, Du M, Wu KK. Suppression of inducible cyclo-oxygenase 2 gene transcription by aspirin and sodium salicylate. *Proc Natl Acad Sci.* 1999;96(9):5292–5297

35. Leitzmann C. Vegetarian diets: what are the advantages? *Forum Nutr.* 2005;57:147–156

36. Pershagen G, Reinders C, Wreiber K, Scheynius A. An anthroposophic lifestyle and intestinal microflora in infancy. *Pediatr Allergy Immunol.* 2002;13(6):402–411

37. Kalliomaki M, Salminen S, Arvilommi H, Kero P, Koskinen P, Isolauri E. Probiotics in primary prevention of atopic disease: a randomized placebo controlled trial. *Lancet.* 2001;357(9262):1076–1079

38. Matsuzaki T, Yamazaki R, Hashimoto S, Yokokura T. The effect of oral feeding of *Lactobacilli casei* strain *Shirota* on immunoglobulin E production in mice. *J Dairy Sci.* 1998;81(1):48–53

39. Tanaka T, Kouda K, Kotani M, et al. Vegetarian diet ameliorates symptoms of atopic dermatitis through reduction of the number of peripheral eosinophils and of PGE2 synthesis by monocytes. *J Physiol Anthropol.* 2001;20(6):353–361

40. Gorczyca D, Pasciak M, Szponar B, Gamian A, Jankowski A. An impact of the diet on serum fatty acid and lipid profiles in Polish vegetarian children and children with allergy. *Eur J Clin Nutr.* 2011;65(2):191–195

41. Craig WJ. Health effects of vegan diets. *Am J Clin Nutr.* 2009;89(Suppl): 1627S–1633S

42. Ambroszkiewicz J, Laskowska-Klita T, Klemarczyk W. Low levels of osteocalcin and leptin in serum of vegetarian prepubertal children. *Med Wieku Rozwoj.* 2003;7(4 Pt 2):5870591

43. Colev M, Engel H, Mayers M, Markowitz M, Cahill L. Vegan diet and vitamin A deficiency. *Clin Pediatr (Phila).* 2004;43(1):107–109

44. Dunham L, Kollar LM. Vegetarian eating for children and adolescents. *J Pediatr Health Care.* 2006;20(1):27–34

45. Moilanen BC. Vegan diets in infants, children and adolescents. *Pediatr Rev.* 2004;25(5):174–176

46. Sanders TA, Purves R. An anthropometric and dietary assessment of the nutritional status of vegan preschool children. *J Hum Nutr.* 1981;35(5):349–357

47. Messina V, Melina V, Mangels AR. A new food guide for North American vegetarians. *J Am Diet Assoc.* 2003;103(6):771–775

48. Chiplonkar SA, Tupe R. Development of a diet quality index with special reference to micronutrient adequacy for adolescent girls consuming a lacto-vegetarian diet. *J Am Diet Assoc.* 2010;110(6):926–931

49. Segovia-Siapco G, Sabaté J. Using personal mobile phones to assess dietary intake in free-living adolescents: comparison of face-to-face versus telephone training. *JMIR Mhealth Uhealth.* 2016;4(3):e91

50. Bishnoi S, Khetarpaul N. Protein digestibility of vegetables and field peas (Pisum sativum). Varietal differences and effect of domestic processing and cooking methods. 46. 1994;1(71–76)

51. Platel K, Srinivasan K. Bioavailability of micronutrients from plant foods: an update. *Crit Rev Food Sci Nutr.* 2016;56(10):1608–1619

52. Institute of Medicine, Food and Nutrition Board. Dietary Reference Intakes for Energy, Carbohydrate, Fiber, Fat, Fatty Acids, Cholesterol, Protein and Amino Acids. Washington, DC: National Academies Press; 2005:386

53. Marsh KA, Munn EA, S.K. B. Protein and vegetarian diets. *Med J Aust.* 2013;199 (4 Suppl):S7–S10

54. Mathai JK, Liu Y, Stein HHBJNF-. Values for digestible indispensable amino acid scores (DIAAS) for some dairy and plant proteins may better describe protein quality than values calculated using the concept for protein digestibility-corrected amino acid scores (PDCAAS). *Br J Nutr.* 2017;117(4):490–499

55. Messina V, Mangels AR. Considerations in planning vegan diets: children. *J Am Diet Assoc.* 2001;101(6):661–669

56. Young VR, Fajardo L, Murray E, Rand WM, Scrimshaw NS. Protein requirements of man. Comparative nitrogen balance response within the submaintenance -to-maintenance range of intakes of wheat and beef proteins. *J Nutr.* 1975;105(5):534–542

57. Messina M, Messina V. The role of soy in vegetarian diets. *Nutrients.* 2010;2(8):855–888

58. Kumar P, Chatli MK, Mehta N. Meat analogues: health promising sustainable meat substitutes. *Crit Rev Food Sci Nutr.* 2017;57(5):923–932

59. Ensaff H, Homer M, Sahota P, Braybrook D, Coan S, McLeod H. Food choice architecture: an intervention in a secondary school and its impact on students' plant-based food choices. *Nutrients.* 2015;7(6):4426–4437

60. Lazor K, Chapman N, Levine E. Soy goes to school: acceptance of healthful, vegetarian options in Maryland middle school lunches. *J Sch Health.* 2010;80(4):200–206

61. Attwood CR. Low-fat diets for children: practicality and safety. *Am J Cardiol.* 1998;82(10B):77T–79T

62. World Health Organization, Food and Agriculture Organization of the United Nations. Diet, Nutrition and the Prevention of Chronic Diseases. Geneva, Switzerland: World Health Organization; 2003: Available at: http://whqlibdoc. who.int/trs/WHO_TRS_916.pdf. Accessed December 12, 2018

63. Kris-Etherton PM, Taylor DS, Yu-Poth S, et al. Polyunsaturated fatty acids in the food chain in the United States. *Am J Clin Nutr.* 2000;71(1 Suppl):179S–188S

64. Brenner RR, Peluffo RO. Regulation of unsaturated fatty acids biosynthesis. I. Effect of unsaturated fatty acid of 18 carbons of the microsomal desaturation of linoleic acid into gamma-linoleic acid. *Biochem Biophys Acta.* 1969;176(3):471–479

65. Conquer JA, Holub BJ. Supplementation with an algae source of docosahexanoic acid increases (n-3) fatty acid status and alters selected risk factors for heart disease in vegetarian subjects. *J Nutr.* 1996;126(12):3032–3039

66. Baker RD, Baker S. Infant and toddler nutrition. In: Wyllie R, Hyams J, eds. *Pediatric Gastrointestinal and Liver Disease.* 4th ed. Philadelphia, PA: Elsevier/ Saunders; 2010:935–945

67. Ribaya-Mercado JD. Influence of dietary fat on beta carotene absorption and bioconversion into vitamin A. *Nutr Rev.* 2002;60(4):104–110

68. Institute of Medicine. Dietary Reference Intakes for Thiamin, Riboflavin, Niacin, Vitamin B 6, Folate, Vitamin B12, Pantothenic Acid, Biotin, and Choline. Washington, DC: National Academies Press; 1998

69. Donaldson MS. Metabolic vitamin B12 status on a mostly raw vegan diet with follow up using tablets, nutritional yeast or probiotic supplements. *Ann Nutr Metab.* 2000;44(5–6):229–234

70. Pawlak R, Lester SE, Babatunde T. The prevalence of cobalamin deficiency among vegetarians assessed by serum vitamin B12: a review of literature. *Eur J Clin Nutr.* 2014;68(5):541–548

71. Dhananjaya S, Manjunatha N, Manjunatha R, Kumar SU. Dietary deficiency of cobalamin presented solely as schizoaffective disorder in a lacto-vegetarian adolescent. *Ind J Psychol Med.*37(3):339–341

72. Goraya JS, Kaur S, Mehra B. Neurology of nutritional vitamin B12 deficiency in infants: case series from India and literature review. *J Child Neurol.* 2015;30(13):1831–1837

73. Trang HM, Cole DE, Rubin LA, Pierratos A, Siu S, Vieth R. Evidence that vitamin D3 increases serum 25 hydroxyvitamin D more efficiently than does Vitamin D2. *Am J Clin Nutr.* 1998;68(4):854

74. Ambroszkiewicz J, Klemarczyk W, Gajewska J, Chelchowska M, Franek E, Laskowska-Klita T. The influence of vegan diet on bone mineral density and biochemical bone turnover markers. *Pediatr Endocrinol Diabetes Metab.* 2010;16(3):201–204

75. Institute of Medicine. *Dietary Reference Intakes for Vitamin A, Vitamin K, Arsenic, Boron, Chromium, Copper, Iodine, Iron, Manganese, Molybdenum, Nickel, Silicon, Vanadium, and Zinc.* Washington, DC: National Academies Press; 2001

76. Donovan UM, Gibson R. Iron and zinc status of young women aged 14 to 19 years consuming vegetarian and omnivorous diets. *J Am Coll Nutr.* 1995;14(5):463–472

77. Gibson RS, Heath AL, Szymlek-Gay EA. Is iron and zinc nutrition a concern for vegetarian infants and young children in industrialized countries? *Am J Clin Nutr.* 2014;100(Suppl 1):459S–468S

78. Haider LM, Schwingshackl L, Hoffmann G, Ekmekcioglu C. The effect of vegetarian diets on iron status in adults: a systematic review and meta-analysis. *Crit Rev Food Sci Nutr.* 2016;58(8):1359–1374

79. Hunt JR, Roughead ZK. Adaptation of iron absorption in men consuming diets with high or low iron bioavailability. *Am J Clin Nutr.* 2000;71(1):94–102

80. Foster M, Samman S. Vegetarian diets across the lifecycle: impact on zinc intake and status. *Adv Food Nutr Res.* 2015;74:93–131

81. Subar AF, Krebs-Smith SM, Cook A, Kahle LL. Dietary sources of nutrients among US adults, 1989 to 1991. *J Am Diet Assoc.* 1998;98(5):537–547

82. Harland BF, Oberleas D. Phytate in foods. *World Rev Nutr Diet.* 1987;52:235–259

83. Hunt JR, Matthys LA, Johnson LK. Zinc absorption, mineral balance and blood lipids in women consuming controlled lactoovovegetarian and omnivorous diets for 8 weeks. *Am J Clin Nutr.* 1998;67(3):421–430

84. Taylor A, Redworth EW, Morgan JB. Influence of diet on iron, copper and zinc status in children under 24 months of age. *Biol Trace Element Res.* 2004;94(3): 197–214

85. Heaney RP, Dowell MS, Rafferty K, Bierman J. Bioavailability of the calcium in fortified soy imitation milk, with some observations on method. *Am J Clin Nutr.* 2000;71(5):1166–1169

86. Weaver C, Proulx W, Heaney RP. Choices for achieving adequate dietary calcium with a vegetarian diet. *Am J Clin Nutr.* 1999;70(3 Suppl):543S–548S

87. Leung AM, Lamar A, He X, Braverman LE, Pearce EN. Iodine status and thyroid function of Boston-area vegetarians and vegans. *J Clin Endocrinol Metab.* 2011;96(8):E1303–E1307

88. Laidlaw SA, Shultz TD, Cecchino JT, Kopple JD. 47. 46. 1988;660–663

89. Lombard KA, Olson AL, Nelson SE, Rebouche CJ. Carnitine status of lacto-ovo vegetarians and strict vegetarian adults and children. *Am J Clin Nutr.* 1989;50(2):3010306

90. Mangels AR, Messina V. Considerations in planning vegan diets: infants. *J Am Diet Assoc.* 2001;101(6):670–677

91. Sanders TA. Vegetarian diets and children. *Pediatr Clin North Am.* 1995;42(4): 955–965

92. Hebbelinck M, Clarys P. Physical growth and development of vegetarian children and adolescents. In: Sabaté J, ed. *Vegetarian Nutrition.* Boca Raton, FL: CRC Press Inc; 2001:173–193

93. Freeland-Graves JH, Greninger SA, Graves GR, Young RK. Health practices, attitudes and beliefs of vegetarians and nonvegetarians. *J Am Diet Assoc.* 1986;86(7):913–918

94. Worsley A, Skrzypiec G. Teenage vegetarianism: prevalence, social and cognitive contexts. *Appetite.* 1998;30(2):151–170

95. Gillbody SM, Kirk SFL, Hill AJ. Vegetarianism in young women: another means of weight control? *Int J Eat Disord.* 1999;26(1):87–90

96. Neumark-Sztainer D, Story M, Resnick MD, Blum RW. Adolescent vegetarians. A behavioral profile of a school based population in Minnesota. *Arch Pediatr Adolesc Med.* 1997;151(8):833–838

97. Robinson-O'Brien R, Perry CL, Wall MM, Story M, Neumark-Sztainer D. Adolescent and young adult vegetarianism: better dietary intake and weight outcomes but increased risk of disordered eating behaviors. *J Am Diet Assoc.* 2009;109(4):648–655

98. Perry CL, Mcguire MT, Neumark-Sztainer D, Story M. Characteristics of vegetarian adolescents in a multi-ethnic urban population. *J Adolesc Health.* 2001;29(6):406–416

99. Bas M, Karabudak E, Kiziltan G. Vegetarianism and eating disorders: association between eating attitudes and other psychological factors among Turkish adolescents. *Appetite.* 2005;44(3):309–315

100. Phillips F, Hackett AF, Stratton G, Billington D. Effect of changing to a self-selected vegetarian diet on anthropometric measurements in UK adults. *J Hum Nutr Diet.* 2004;17(3):249–255

101. Nieman DC. Physical fitness and vegetarian diets. Is there a relation? . *Am J Clin Nutr.* 1999;70(3 Suppl):570S–575S

102. Snyder AC, Dvorak LL, Roepke JB. Influence of dietary iron source on measures of iron status among female runners. *Med Sci Sports Exerc.* 1989;21(1):7–10

103. Burke DG, Chilibeck PD, Parise G, Candow DG, Mahoney D, Tarnopolsky M. Effect of creatine and weight training on muscle creatine and performance in vegetarians. *Med Sci Sports Exerc.* 2003;35(11):1946–1955

104. Barnard ND, Katcher HI, Jenkins DJ, Cohen J, Turner-McGrievy G. Vegetarian and vegan diets in type 2 diabetes management. *Nutr Rev.* 2009;67(5):255–263

105. Turner-McGrievy GM, Barnard ND, Cohen J, Jenkins DJ, Gloede L, Green AA. Changes in nutrient intake and dietary quality among participants with type 2 diabetes following a low-fat vegan diet or a conventional diabetes diet for 22 weeks. *J Am Diet Assoc.* 2008;108(10):1636–1645

106. Tonstad S, Stewart K, Oda K, Batech M, Herring RP, Fraser GE. Vegetarian diets and incidence of diabetes in the Adventist Health Study–2. *Nutr Metab Cardiovasc Dis.* 2013;23(4):292–299

107. Galson SK. Childhood overweight and obesity prevention. *Public Health Rep.* 2008;123(3):258–259

108. Sabaté J, Wien M. Vegetarian diets and childhood obesity prevention. *Am J Clin Nutr.* 2010;91(5):1525S–1529S

109. Huang RY, Huang CC, Hu FB, Chavarro JE. Vegetarian diets and weight reduction: a meta-analysis of randomized controlled trials. *J Gen Intern Med.* 2016;31(1):109–116

110. Turner-McGrievy G, Mandes T, Crimarco A. A plant-based diet for overweight and obesity prevention and treatment. *J Geriatr Cardiol.* 2017;14(5):369–374

111. Schürmann S, Kersting M, Alexy U. Vegetarian diets in children: a systematic review. *Eur J Nutr.* 2017;56(5):1797–1817

112. Kersting M, Alexy U, Schurmann S. Critical Dietary Habits in early childhood: Principles and Practice. *World Rev Nutr Diet.* 2016;115:24–35

Chapter 12

Sports Nutrition

Introduction

The global sports nutrition market accounted for more than $28 billion in sales in 2016 and is expected to expand by over 8% annually through 2022.[1] This is a field in which marketing and hype are unencumbered by the need for peer-reviewed evidence, and the United States is by far the largest market, accounting for approximately 38% of sales in 2016.[1] This steady stream of new products can be quite alluring for young athletes and their families, especially when promoted by high-profile sports personalities and claims of performance enhancement spread rapidly through social media. It can be very difficult for families to sort truth from hyperbole and to determine what is most appropriate for their young athlete. Health care providers should be comfortable providing this guidance and steering families toward appropriate information resources.

Dietary patterns in young athletes may differ from their nonathlete peers. Male high school athletes place a larger emphasis on healthy diets as compared with nonathletes.[2] A review of studies on nutrition in adolescents found that those involved in youth sports ingested more fruits, vegetables, and milk as compared with their nonathletic peers.[3] However, athletes were also more likely to eat fast food and drink sugar-sweetened beverages. Although athletes are reported to have higher rates of disordered eating as compared with nonathletes, this is more of an issue in older and elite athletes than in the majority of athletes participating in scholastic and community sports.

It is important to emphasize that sports nutrition is not a "quick fix" in terms of fueling a particular workout or event, but rather considers how food and fluids support overall development in the young athlete over the longer term. Young athletes tend to think of sports nutrition as a strategy used primarily during periods of training and competition. However, there is increasing recognition of the critical role that "recovery nutrition" plays in optimizing athletic performance. This includes attention not only to the content of the athlete's diet, but the timing of ingestion as well.

Athlete Development

Questions about nutrition and performance-enhancing substances (PESs) are often raised by those seeking to improve strength, muscularity, and athletic achievement. The best guidance for patients and families places sports nutrition within the context of broader principles of athlete development. However, there is a general unawareness of the overall principles of athletic development in the young athlete. Athleticism is best built on a foundation of a variety of motor inputs and outputs, and any decision to specialize in a single sport should be delayed until later in adolescence.[4] When pediatricians are counseling patients and families on physical activity and sports, it is important to recognize that for the child younger than 8 or 9 years, diversity in physical activity is much more effective at enhancing motor development than is repetition.[4] This is the rationale behind the endorsement of "free play" for younger children and particularly for encouraging participation in a wide variety of sporting activities. Although varied activities and training remain important throughout an athletic career, as children move into early adolescence and beyond, repetition and practice become much more beneficial to refine specific motor movement patterns and enhance sports-specific skills. Nutrition and dietary supplements are not substitutes for the gains that come with development and appropriate training.

The United States Olympic Committee has adopted the "American Development Model" and is encouraging its use as a template for youth sports participation. This is outlined in Table 12.1. Further information

Table 12.1.

United States Olympic Committee American Development Model
(http://www.teamusa.org/About-the-USOC/Athlete-Development/
American-Development-Model)

Stage 1: Discover, learn, and play (ages 0–12)
- Learn core fundamental movements and enhance physical literacy
- Emphasize fun with unstructured play and sampling multiple sports
- Develop a passion for movement and physical activity

Stage 2: Develop and challenge (ages 10–16)
- Continued emphasis on fun and socialization
- Explore more organized training options within sport
- Development of physical, social, technical and tactical skills

Stage 3: Train and compete (ages 13–19)
- Train and compete in a program that matches goals and interests

Stage 4: Excel for high performance or participate and succeed (ages 15+)
- Higher-level sport-specific training

Stage 5: Mentor and thrive (Active for life)
- Maintenance of a healthy lifestyle

can be found at https://www.teamusa.org/About-the-USOC/Programs/
Coaching-Education/American-Development-Model and in a clinical report
from the American Academy of Pediatrics (AAP), "Sports Specialization and
Intensive Training in Young Athletes."[4]

Training Principles

Any discussion of sports nutrition needs to consider the volume and intensity of the athlete's training and ambition. Some athletes practice and play
several hours daily on a year-round basis. The problem with this becomes
evident with further consideration of some fundamental principles of
sports training. Exercise creates a training stimulus or stress that affects
not only musculoskeletal tissue but also multiple body systems. The body
adapts to this stimulus in such a way that builds exercise capacity. The most
successful training programs include:

1. Variety and periodicity in training:
   a. Throughout the course of a week, workouts should be of varying
      types and intensity (easier workouts should be interspersed be-
      tween those that are more difficult).
      i. Every workout should not be "hard."
      ii. Variety fosters muscle and motor adaptation and development.
   b. Throughout the course of a year, there should be at least one season
      of down time away from organized sport. Recreational activity with
      an emphasis on "fun" and enjoyment should be encouraged during
      this time.
   c. High-quality training sessions and athletic performance require
      appropriate dietary choices before and during activity.
2. Adequate recovery is essential for the increased strength and skill that
   comes from physical training and decreases risk of injury and burnout.
   a. High-intensity workouts require 24 to 72 hours for full recovery.
   b. Appropriate food and fluid choices during recovery optimize meta-
      bolic and soft tissue adaptations from training.

The goal of this chapter is to provide evidence-based information
regarding the role of nutrition in young athletes. As much as possible, this
information is based on results from studies performed in the pediatric
population. The key points that will be covered in this chapter include:

- The use of appropriate fluids and macronutrients to provide fuel for,
  and to enhance recovery from, exercise and physical exertion;
- The role of select vitamins and minerals in the young athlete's diet;

- Issues related to weight loss and weight gain in the athlete; and
- Information regarding nutritional supplements in common use in youth sports.

Fuels for Activity

Overview of Exercise Metabolism

One of the basic tenets of sports nutrition is to ensure adequate fuel and fluid to optimize athletic efforts. The preferred fuel for physical activity depends on the intensity and duration of the physical effort as well as the nutritional and training status of the athlete. A basic understanding of exercise metabolism (see Table 12.2) provides the foundation for dietary counseling as it pertains to physical activity.

Carbohydrates

Carbohydrate (CHO) requirements in athletes are dependent on volume and intensity of training and will, therefore, vary over the course of the athletic season. Although athletes may practice several hours per day, it is important to note that many young athletes are often relatively inactive for large parts of the time spent in practice or game situations. This varies widely by sport and position (ie, goaltenders often train very differently than offensive players). Therefore, it is "activity time" rather than "practice time" that determines these carbohydrate recommendations[5]:

Low-intensity/skill sessions: 3–5 g CHO/kg body weight/day
Moderate-intensity sessions (~1 h/day): 5–7 g CHO/kg body weight/day
High-intensity sessions (1–3 h/day): 6–10 g CHO/kg body weight/day

Despite the importance of carbohydrates in supporting optimal physical performance, young and adolescent athletes often consume significantly less than recommended amounts. Convincing athletes to increase carbohydrate intake to cover the caloric demand of their activity can be a "hard sell" for some athletes, who are often used to functioning on far less. When carbohydrate intake is inadequate, the metabolic response is to catabolize muscle to provide needed fuel. In these cases, it is often helpful to inform athletes that the muscle and strength they are working so hard to gain is being broken down and used as an expendable fuel source.

Carbohydrates should be ingested throughout the course of the day, but they are particularly important during the times surrounding athletic

Table 12.2.

Overview of Exercise Metabolism

1. Rest/low-intensity activity (ie, activities of daily living, walking)
   a. Fat stores are main fuel source.
   b. Smaller contribution from carbohydrates (CHOs [blood glucose and stored glycogen]).
2. Gradual increased intensity (ie, warmup before practice)
   a. Gradual shift from fat to carbohydrates as dominant energy source.
   PEDIATRIC PEARL: For a given level of exertion: children and adolescents remain more dependent on lipids than adults, which spares muscle glycogen. Endurance training increases this lipid reliance and allows the athlete to more readily tap into the vast amount of energy stored in body fat.
   b. As CHO metabolism increases: Stored glycogen is used initially, then blood glucose becomes more important with increasing duration of exercise.
   PEDIATRIC PEARL: As compared with adults, muscle glycogen stores may be 50%–60% lower in children and adolescents, and therefore, they are much more dependent on blood glucose and ingested carbohydrates for energy during moderate and intense activity.
3. Sudden initiation of high-intensity activity: (ie, short sprint)
   a. For activity lasting 10–30 seconds, the adenosine triphosphate (ATP)/phosphocreatine system is primary fuel substrate. As ATP is metabolized to adenosine diphosphate (ADP), stored phosphocreatine is used to regenerate ATP.
      i. This is the primary mechanism of action for creatine supplementation.
4. Continuation of high-intensity activity: (ie, competitive tennis match)
   a. CHOs become the dominant fuel source, with muscle glycogen providing energy via anaerobic pathway.
   PEDIATRIC PEARL: As compared with adults, decreased glycogen stores in children and adolescents increases the importance of glycogen replenishment after activity.
   b. Buildup of lactic acid prohibits sustained effort.

Table 12.3.

Carbohydrate Content of Sample Food and Products Commonly Ingested During Sports Activities

Food	Carbohydrate (g)
Apple, 1 medium	21
Banana, 1 medium	27
Clif Builders bar, 1 chocolate mint	30
Clif Kid Z bar, 1 chocolate brownie	23
Fig Newton, 2-oz single-serve packet	39
Fruit Roll Up, 1 strawberry roll	11
Kashi chewy granola bar, chocolate/peanut butter	21
Kind bar, 1 fruit and nut	17
Luna bar, 1 lemon zest	27
Nature Valley, 2 bars oats and honey	29
NutriGrain bar, 1 strawberry	24
Orange, ½ large	11
Power Bar Performance, 1 bar peanut butter	44
Pretzels, 1 oz (about 18 mini pretzels)	23
Raisins, 1.5-oz box	22
Trail mix ¼ cup (Planters tropical fruit and nut)	17

activity. Carbohydrate content of foods and products commonly consumed during this time period can be found in Table 12.3.

Before Exercise

Before working out, carbohydrates:

- Bolster muscle glycogen and blood glucose.
  - Optimal levels of muscle glycogen are best supported with a diet that is consistently high in carbohydrates throughout the athletic season. This can be particularly important in the days leading up to endurance events, or tournaments with multiple sustained efforts in a single day.

- Prevent muscle catabolism.
- Maintain fuel source for brain.

Current recommendations are for 1 to 4 g carbohydrate/kg body weight in the 1 to 4 hours preceding exercise sessions lasting for greater than 60 minutes.[5]

Some athletes may have difficulty with these pre-exercise feedings because of issues with gastric tolerance. Gastric emptying significantly slows with higher-intensity exercise, and some may complain of bloating, cramping, diarrhea, nausea, and/or vomiting. Athlete comfort should dictate the timing and content of any pre-exercise intake, but some trial and error often occurs when trying to determine the best fueling strategy for a given athlete. Successful fueling plans should be determined in advance of competitive events, and the following may be helpful for young athletes.

- Carbohydrates should form the foundation for pre-exercise meals and snacks.
  - Lunch typically occurs 3 to 4 hours before after-school training sessions, and examples of appropriate lunch selections can be found in Table 12.4.
- Dedicated effort can be made to "train the gut" using strategies that, over time, should enhance gastric emptying and carbohydrate absorption (Fig 12.1).[6]

Table 12.4.

Sample Lunch Choices for After-School Practice for a 50-kg (110-lb) Athlete

1–4 g of carbohydrate/kg of body weight = 50–200 g of carbohydrate (The higher range is for higher-intensity practice/competition)
2 turkey sandwiches[a] = 50 g
2 bananas = 54 g
2 cups chocolate milk = 52 r
2 oatmeal raisin cookies: 18 r
Total: 184 g of carbohydrates (in many cases this would be considered a "double lunch")

[a] Sandwich = 2 slices bread/4 oz turkey/1 tbsp mayo/lettuce/tomato.

Figure 12.1.

Summary of methods to "train the gut" to enhance gastric comfort for recommended fluid and food ingestion before and during physical activity

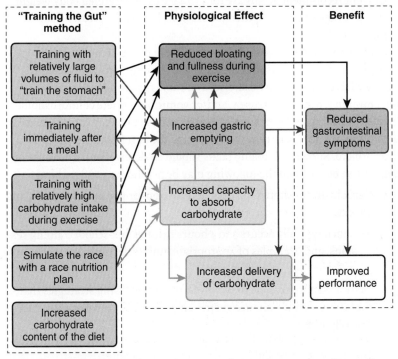

Reprinted under a Creative Commons license (http://creativecommons.org/licenses/by/4.0/) from Jeukendrup AE. Training the gut for athletes. *Sports Med.* 2017;47(Suppl 1):101–110.[6] Copyright © the authors; 2017.

- Gastric comfort for a given session is often enhanced with the following strategies for pre-exercise intake:
  - Smaller, more frequent snacks may be better tolerated than larger meals.
  - Choices should be relatively low in fat, protein, and/or fiber.
  - High-fructose intakes can cause gastrointestinal discomfort in some athletes.
    - Glucose and sucrose carbohydrate sources may be better tolerated.

Given the young athlete's reliance on blood glucose, some athletes may benefit from a small high-carbohydrate snack 30 to 60 minutes before beginning exercise.[7] It was previously reported that athletes benefited from ingesting foods with a low glycemic index before exercise. More recent data have shown that glycemic index of pre-exercise food choices does not seem to affect subsequent performance.[8] However, some athletes may experience a rebound hypoglycemia and subjective fatigue during the subsequent exercise session. In these cases, a trial of additional carbohydrate intake (~15 g) immediately before activity may mitigate the hypoglycemia and fatigue.

During Exercise

Intake of carbohydrates during activity appears to be beneficial as an ongoing fuel source and protects lean tissue from catabolism during and after exercise. This is best established for activity lasting longer than 1 hour but may also be true for shorter activity.[5] The following general principles apply:

- Athletes participating in sustained or "stop-and-start" activities lasting 60 to 150 minutes should consume 0.7 g of carbohydrate/kg/hour (up to 60 g of carbohydrate/hour for full-grown individuals), divided into 15- to 20-minute intervals.[5] Some authors recommend up to 90 g of CHO/hour for activities lasting >120 minutes.[6]

- The type and form of carbohydrate can be dictated by the athlete's preference and gastric tolerance. Hydration with recommended volumes of a 6% to 8% carbohydrate-containing sports drink during exercise also provides the recommended amount of carbohydrates (see Table 12.5 and fluid section later in this chapter).

- Exogenous carbohydrate utilization during exercise appears to be limited by intestinal transport. Ingesting different carbohydrates that utilize different transporters in the intestinal tract (ie, glucose and fructose) during exercise appears to increase available exogenous carbohydrate to fuel exercise in adults.[9] Intestinal transport appears to be of greater consequence with the higher CHO intakes recommended as above for longer activity. It is interesting to speculate how these differences in physiology may influence exercise performance in young athletes, who are already known to be more dependent on exogenous glucose, but no data are available to date.

- Strategies as listed above and in Fig 12.1 for enhancing gastric tolerance may help some athletes.

Current evidence seems to support use of a CHO mouth rinse (without subsequent ingestion) for high-intensity activities lasting less than 1 hour.[9]

Table 12.5.
Carbohydrate and Sodium Content of Several Common Sports Drinks and Comparison Fluids

Product	% Carbohydrate	Carbohydrate (g/8-oz serving)	Carbohydrate Type	Sodium mmol/L
Gatorade Original Thirst Quencher, Orange	6	14	Sucrose, dextrose	19
Gatorlytes (1 packet/20 oz fluid)				57 (in addition to any sodium in fluid)
Powerade ION4 Fruit Punch	6	15	High-fructose corn syrup	18
Propel Fitness Water	0	0	n/a	19
Apple juice	16	38	Fructose, sucrose, dextrose	1
Orange juice (from concentrate)	11	26	Sucrose, fructose, dextrose	<1
Cola (Pepsi)	12	28	High-fructose corn syrup, sucrose	2
Milk	6	14	Lactose	20
Milk, chocolate 2%	12	29	Lactose, added sugar source varies	26

Reward centers in the brain are activated by CHO receptors in the mouth, and this has been associated with a 2% to 3% performance improvement in efforts lasting about 1 hour. Specific protocols vary but generally include rinsing with a 6% to 10% CHO solution for +/− 10 seconds and repeating this 4 to 12 times during efforts lasting 30 to 60 minutes.[9] It is important to remember that mouth rinses do not contribute to the fuel and fluid requirements of exercise but may be of benefit to athletes who experience difficulty with gastrointestinal upset with recommended CHO intake.

Evidence is mounting that low CHO availability during exercise (eg, exercising after an overnight fast, participating in multiple training sessions/day, or following a low-CHO diet) appears to upregulate a number of factors that enhance muscle metabolism during exercise, especially oxidative capacity and lipid metabolism.[10] This is known as "training low" and should subsequently result in sparing of glycogen stores with activity and theoretically delay onset of fatigue. The trade-off for training with low CHO availability is that the quality of the associated workout tends to be low but is performed with the hope for building a better muscle metabolic profile and the potential for future enhanced performance. Although the metabolic effects of "training low" are well delineated, the performance effects on future training are not.[10] There is not enough evidence at this time to recommend this strategy for young athletes, but it is an area of very active study. Any athlete who attempts this approach needs to be aware of the effect on overall training quality and to discern those workouts that are for "physical training" as compared with those workouts that are for "metabolic training."

After Exercise

Many scholastic athletes train at least 5 days/week, with some preseason training involving multiple sessions per day. For athletes training at this frequency, postexercise carbohydrate intake becomes very important in replenishing diminished muscle glycogen, as this becomes an important fuel source for the next workout. It is currently recommended that athletes ingest 1 to 1.2 g of carbohydrates/kg/hour for 4 to 6 hours after exercise.[5] Athletes with limited time between training sessions or performances should start this as soon as possible after completion of activity, because glycogen resynthesis occurs at approximately 5% per hour.[5] In addition, carbohydrate ingestion once again protects muscle, as the postexercise meal appears to have an important role in sparing muscle from postexercise catabolism.

Fluids for the Workout

Adequate fluid volume during physical activity is important for the delivery of oxygen and nutrients to exercising muscle and assisting with heat dissipation in young athletes. Fluid requirements are highly variable across the spectrum of pediatric athletic participation and are affected by climate and acclimatization; conditioning; type, location, and intensity of activity; maturation; and intrinsic interindividual variability in sweat rate. Therefore, fluid recommendations need to be specific for the individual and the situation. This is particularly true for endurance, or aerobic, activities.

Unfortunately, young athletes and their parents are often uncertain about the appropriate types and quantities of fluid needed to maintain hydration before, during, and after physical activity. General hydration strategies can be found in Table 12.6, and a comparison of the carbohydrate and sodium content of various drinks is shown in Table 12.5.

One opportunity to educate patients and families about appropriate hydration is to check urine specific gravity. Although there is some evidence that a specific gravity of 1.010 indicates optimal hydration, the National Federation of High School Sports (NFHS) and the National Collegiate Athletic Association (NCAA) allow specific gravities of 1.025 and 1.020, respectively, when determining euhydration for preseason wrestling weigh-ins.[11]

Before Exercise

Young athletes should be fully hydrated before beginning any training session and ideally should maintain euhydration throughout the day. However, this can be challenging, particularly in cases in which training sessions occur on sequential days (especially in hot environments) or when multiple periods of activity occur in a single day (ie, tournament situations, or "two a day" practices in fall football). In these situations, it is easy for young athletes to experience cumulative fluid deficits from one session to the next. Practical prehydration guidance and strategies are found in Table 12.6.

During Exercise

Sweat rates are one of the chief determinants of fluid requirements during exercise. Sweat losses of 300 to 700 mL/hour have been reported in 9- to 12-year-olds who exercise in the heat.[12] Older or male athletes tend to have higher sweat rates than younger or female athletes, and can reach up 2.5 L/hour with strenuous activity in the heat. Although thirst is often recognized when dehydration approaches 3% to 5%, aerobic capacity, balance, and

Table 12.6.

Hydration Strategies for Young Athletes

Before exercise:
- Replenish any fluid losses from prior workouts
  - o Urine should be pale yellow
  - o Restoration of preexercise body weight
- Consider prehydration 2–4 hours before exercise with 5–10 mL fluid/kg body weight (~2–4 mL/lb)
  - o Allows sufficient time for gastric emptying and fluid absorption
  - o Sodium-containing fluids helps with absorption and retention
- Water or any nutritive beverage that is well-tolerated by the athlete is acceptable
  - o Sports drinks confer no added benefit over other fluid choices

During exercise:
- Fluid losses are highly variable and recommendations should be individualized to the athlete and training/competition situation
  - o A good starting point with strenuous activity:
    - – Young adolescents: 100–250 mL (3–8 oz) every 20 min
    - – Older adolescents: up to 350 mL (12 oz) every 20 min
  - o Both over- and underhydration should be avoided
- Fluid needs can be calculated by having athletes weigh themselves immediately before and immediately after workouts, after removal of any wet clothing
  - o 1 pound of weight change = 16 ounces of fluid
  - o Athletes then need to reconfigure their drinking strategy to avoid
    - – Fluid losses >2% of body mass
    - – Any weight gain
- In most cases, water is best choice for hydration during exercise
  - o When exercise is >60 minutes of sustained activity, 6–8% carbohydrate (CHO) solutions can provide both fluid and fuel
    - – In some athletes, low-CHO–containing fluids may be less likely to produce stomach upset than water
  - o 6–8% CHO concentration is found in many commercial sports drinks, or can be obtained by a 50:50 dilution of nonacidic fruit juice

After exercise:
- Replace fluid losses before next workout
  - o 16–20 oz of fluid replacement per 1 lb weight loss
- Fluid volume is of greater consequence than fluid type
  - o Young athletes will typically combine food and fluid during recovery
  - o Combination of CHOs, sodium, potassium, and protein in chocolate milk make it a good choice for recovery
  - o Sports drinks do not confer specific benefit over other fluid choices
    - – Do not contain enough CHOs for recovery on their own

mental/cognitive performance appear to fall off at approximately 2% dehydration.[13] Therefore, the goal for fluid intake during exercise is to keep fluid losses to less than 2% body weight.

Fluids with added sodium stimulate osmoreceptors and enhance additional intake. Many sports drinks contain 10 to 20 mmol of sodium/L, which appears sufficient to stimulate further drinking. However, contrary to common perception, this amount of sodium is not sufficient to significantly replace sweat-related sodium losses (sodium content in adolescent sweat is typically on the order of 40 to 70 mmol/L). Sweat sodium losses depend on genetics, acclimatization and training (decreases sodium content in sweat), and sweat rate (high sweat rate increases sodium content per volume).

Although sodium losses are usually not of clinical consequence for most young athletes, in some situations, these losses can be problematic. In most cases, sodium losses from a single training session are readily replaced with normal dietary intake. However, older adolescents participating in strenuous activity in heat may lose up to 2 to 5 g of sodium/hour and up to 20 g of sodium/day for those athletes involved in longer or multiple training/competition efforts per day.[12] Athletes with high sweat sodium losses may be identified by white salt crusting often noted on skin or clothes after training. These athletes are sometimes called "salty sweaters," and appear to be more prone to muscle cramping because of hyperexcitable neuromuscular junctions occurring with fluid contraction.[12] For individuals who sustain heavy salt losses, some products marketed for endurance activity contain higher sodium levels than traditional sport drink products (see Table 12.5). Another alternative is to add 1/8 to 1/4 teaspoon of table salt per serving of a standard sports beverage (1 tsp table salt = 2.3 g sodium).

Exercise-associated hyponatremia (EAH) is another clinical consequence of low sodium concentration. EAH appears to be attributable to overdrinking of hypotonic beverages in combination with arginine vasopressin (AVP)-induced impaired excretion of free water.[14] EAH was originally described in sustained endurance activities lasting >4 hours but has more recently been described in a much broader range of sporting activity. Although asymptomatic EAH may be more common than previously realized, the medical consequences of symptomatic EAH can be severe. From 2008–2014, 3 high school football players in the United States died as a result of EAH.[14]

Risk factors for EAH include:

- Overdrinking hypotonic fluids (including water and sports drinks)
  - Usually a result of overzealous attempts at avoiding dehydration

- High BMI/low BMI
- Long exercise duration (especially over 4 hours)
  - Especially in athletes performing at a slow pace
- Poor training and/or event inexperience

Case reports suggest that athletes with cystic fibrosis, anorexia, bulimia, and intrinsic kidney disease may be at elevated risk for EAH.[14,15] Athletes who actually gain weight over the course of a training session are overdrinking and need to have pre- and postexercise weight measured, as described in Table 12.6.

Similar to complaints often seen with food ingestion before or during exercise, athletes may report gastric discomfort or nausea when attempting to drink recommended volumes of fluid. Gastric emptying of fluids in individuals participating in high-intensity intermittent running (such as seen in practices and games of many team sports) is reduced by 50% to 70% as compared with lower-intensity activity and may contribute to issues with gastric tolerance for recommended volumes of fluid. For athletes complaining of stomach discomfort when attempting appropriate volume intake, the following may be helpful:

- Temperate fluids empty quicker from the stomach than do cold fluids and may be better tolerated by some.
- Smaller, more frequent sips are generally better tolerated than less frequent, higher-volume intakes (ie, "sips, not gulps").
- It may take some experimenting with different fluid types or combinations of fluid and food to find what works for individual athletes. "Training the gut," as outlined in Fig 12.1, provides strategies that may lead to improved tolerance for fluid volume.[6]

Young athletes often do not recognize the difference between energy drinks, which are formulated for performance enhancement, versus sports drinks, which are formulated for rehydration, but it is an important distinction. Although there is no formal definition for the term "energy drink," it is generally recognized as a flavored beverage containing relatively high amounts of caffeine, guarana, or other stimulants. Energy drinks are aggressively marketed to children and adolescents, and many companies are utilizing athletes in these marketing campaigns. The AAP states that energy drinks have no place in the diets of children and adolescents.[16] See Table 12.7 for comparison of caffeine amounts found in common energy drinks and other beverages.

Table 12.7.

Comparison of Caffeine Contained in Energy Drinks With Amounts Found in Other Common Sources of Dietary Caffeine

Product	Caffeine Content (mg/"usual" serving size)
Coffee (drip)	100 mg/8oz
Starbucks Grande Mocha	175 mg/16 oz
Mountain Dew	73 mg/16 oz
Coca Cola	48 mg/16 oz
Red Bull Energy Drink	80 mg/8 oz
Monster Energy Drink	140 mg/16 oz
No Fear Energy Drink	160 mg/16 oz
Energy "shots" (multiple brands)	200–350 mg/1–2 oz

After Exercise

Given the variation in sweat losses, postexercise fluid recommendations should start by encouraging athletes to determine their individual fluid status as outlined in Table 12.6. For postexercise hydration, the volume of beverage is more important than the type of beverage used. Water, milk, or other nutritive beverages are all appropriate choices. Most young athletes will be also be ingesting solid food during this time period, which will provide the carbohydrate and sodium that appear to enhance fluid retention during rehydration. If food is not available, studies performed with hypertonic solutions containing 10% carbohydrate and 25 mmol of sodium/L appear more effective at restoring hydration than do hypotonic solutions.[17] One way to achieve this content is to add ¼ teaspoon of table salt to 1 L of orange or other fruit juice.

Protein

There is a growing trend toward individualizing protein recommendations in athletes. Table 12.8 reviews the variables that contribute to protein needs for a given athlete. Protein recommendations in adult athletes are currently 1.2 to 2.0 g protein/kg/day.[5] Limited data suggest these ranges likely hold for adolescents as well. The higher range (or even slightly higher) may be appropriate for those training with a higher degree of intensity, initiating a new training regimen, trying to lose weight, or recovering from injury. (For

Table 12.8.

Determinants of Protein Requirements in Young Athletes

- Protein contains the building blocks that are needed for:
  - o Growth and development
  - o Synthesis and repair of muscle and other tissue:
    - – injury
    - – microtrauma associated with exercise
- Protein requirements in athletes are variable and depend on:
  - o Growth and development:
    - – protein requirements increase during periods of rapid growth
  - o Training status:
    - – protein requirements increase during periods of increased training volume and intensity
    - – protein requirements are higher in novice athletes
  - o Energy availability:
    - – protein requirements are higher during periods of decreased energy availability (ie, weight loss)
      - ■ Increased protein intake appears to minimize muscle catabolism

reference, the mean daily protein intake for 12- to 19-year-olds in the United States is 95 g for males and 62 g for females.[18])

When considering protein ingestion in athletes, much of the literature in this area is based on evaluation of muscle protein synthesis (MPS). MPS is needed for the repair and adaptation of muscle that produces strength improvements after training. A bout of high-intensity resistance exercise can stimulate MPS for at least 24 hours, and protein ingestion increases MPS by 30% to 100% for 1 to 4 hours.[19] These effects appear to be synergistic (as shown in Fig 12.2), and this is the rationale for the recent focus on "protein timing" as a factor in maximizing training gains with the following periods of particular significance:

- Before and during exercise: Metabolic studies show that ingestion of relatively small amounts of protein before or during exercise appears to increase MPS and protect against muscle breakdown during exercise.

- After exercise: MPS appears to be optimized with consumption of 0.3 to 0.5 g of protein/kg body weight shortly after exercise and at 3- to 5-hour intervals during the day in the 24 to 48 hours following exercise.[5] This appears to be a saturable process with optimal effect

Figure 12.2.

Enhanced protein synthesis after resistance exercise, which is augmented with protein ingestion during the postexercise period. Fed indicates fed (and no exercise); Ex-Fed, exercised and fed; Ex, exercise alone.

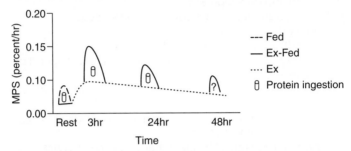

after ingestion of a total of 20 to 25 g of protein in young men. A recent study in children 9 to 13 years of age found maximal effect with a total of 5 to 10 g of protein when ingested at 15 minutes and again at 4 hours after an exercise session.[20] Adolescent needs would appear to lie between these two.

- Before sleep: MPS does occur during sleep, but overnight MPS is limited by amino acid availability. In adults, a protein serving before bed has been shown to enhance MPS, but this effect has not yet been studied in the pediatric population.

At this point it is not yet known whether the effects of these different "windows" of protein are additive. However, it is clear that the dominant factor determining MPS is the ingestion of appropriate amounts of protein periodically throughout the day.[5] If this is achieved, the issues of timing relative to exercise are likely less significant. See Table 12.9 for protein content of some common foods and supplements.

Table 12.9.

Protein Content of Some Common Foods and Supplements Used by Athletes

Food	Protein (g)
Meats/eggs	
Hamburger (3 oz, extra lean)	24
Chicken, roasted (3 oz)	21
Tuna (3 oz, water-packed)	20
Eggs (1 large)	6
Dairy	
Cottage cheese (1/2 cup, low-fat)	14
Yogurt (8 oz)	12
Milk (8 oz, whole or skim)	8
Nonfat dry milk (2 tablespoons)	3
Beans/legumes	
Tofu (1/2 cup)	10
Peanut butter (2 tablespoons)	10
Lentils (1/2 cup, cooked)	9
Black beans (1/2 cup)	8
Hummus (2 tablespoons)	3
Grains	
Pasta (1 cup, cooked)	7
Bread (whole wheat, 2 slices)	5
Other	
Protein supplements (per serving)	20–35
Promax bar	20
Clif bar (peanut butter flavor)	12
Carnation-brand instant breakfast (w/8 oz skim milk)	12
PowerBar	10
Ensure (8 oz)	9
Snickers bar	4
Nutri-Grain bar	2

Micronutrients

Minerals

IRON (SEE ALSO CHAPTER 19: IRON)

Iron status is a dynamic balance among iron stores, iron losses, and the rate of erythropoiesis. Pediatric athletes may tap into iron stores for:

1. Growth-related expansion of red cell mass;
2. Increased red cell mass to correct a dilutional "sports anemia" that occurs as plasma volume expands at onset of training (especially aerobic); and
3. Replacement of menstrual losses or exercise-related losses through feces, urine, and sweat, especially in endurance and ultra-endurance athletes.

Iron has an important role in oxygen delivery and energy generation in the young athlete, and there are iron-related stressors that are unique to athletes, increase their need for iron, and confound results for measurements of iron status biomarkers. These iron-related stressors include[5]:

- In endurance and ultra-endurance events: Some athletes will lose small amounts of iron via sweat or through the gastrointestinal or genitourinary tracts. These losses are typically compensated by enhanced dietary absorption and are likely not clinically significant in the majority of young athletes.
- In high-impact activity (especially running): Hemolysis can occur with the forces generated during footstrike. The body is generally very good at recovering iron after hemolysis, and athletes may have a macrocytosis resulting from increased reticulocyte formation.
- In weight controlled sports: Iron intake is often suboptimal in athletes who are restricting dietary intake.

There is a high degree of interest among athletes and coaches regarding iron intake and iron status, and athletes presenting with fatigue or poor performance are often first suspected to have iron deficiency.

It is important to recognize that supplies of iron in the human body appear to exist on a functional continuum. Athletes with fully replete iron stores are capable of completely supporting the increases in red cell mass that occur with aerobic training. Athletes with mild depletion may develop a "relative anemia" in which hemoglobin concentrations are below optimal for the individual but still within population norms. Athletes with more significant decreases in iron stores may develop a frank anemia.

Rates of iron-deficiency anemia are similar between athletes and nonathletes, and there is consensus that iron-deficiency anemia leads to significant decreases in athletic performance.[5] However, there is currently disagreement as to the definition and athletic impact of nonanemic iron-deficient states, and athletes do appear to be at greater risk of developing this condition.[21]

Ferritin is often used as a marker of iron stores, and there is disagreement over the lower concentration at which ferritin is still considered "normal." Many laboratories report the lower limit of normal ferritin concentrations at 12 ng/mL. However, iron absorption studies suggest that 35 ng/mL may be a more appropriate normal lower limit, and the upregulation of iron absorption that is seen in deficient states has been demonstrated in some studies with ferritin concentrations as high 60 ng/mL.[21] Given the difficulties with the definition of "iron deficiency," it is not surprising that methodology and results of studies looking at the effects of nonanemic low iron stores on athletic performance have been inconsistent. Some studies have shown significant changes in maximal oxygen uptake and exercise performance in the nonanemic athlete with low ferritin, but others have not.[5,21]

There should be a low threshold for checking hemoglobin, hematocrit, and ferritin in athletes presenting with fatigue (often reported as "dead legs" in running athletes) or decreases in performance. Although iron supplementation is common in young athletes, it is not without risk and should be reserved for those cases with documented iron deficiency in which symptoms, performance, and laboratory values are followed during treatment. Studies in nonanemic depleted athletes showed that doses of 50 mg of elemental iron/day have been sufficient at replenishing ferritin stores in an athletic population. A "relative anemia" can be detected by looking for a rebound in hemoglobin concentrations after supplementing for approximately 1 month.

CALCIUM (SEE ALSO CHAPTER 18: CALCIUM, PHOSPHORUS, AND MAGNESIUM)

Although calcium has multiple physiologic functions, its role in bone health is of particular interest in young athletes, and the relative importance of calcium intake on bone development has been evolving over the past decade. The highest rates of bone mass accrual in girls occurs between 10 and 14 years of age, whereas boys will continue to increase bone mass at higher rates up to 15 to 18 years.[22,23]

The AAP currently recommends 1300 mg of calcium/day in children and adolescents 9 to 18 years of age.[23,24] Overall, it appears that increasing calcium intake correlates with improvements in bone health, with this effect most pronounced in those with low baseline intakes.[25] However, the data supporting the role of calcium intake reducing fracture risk are less robust.[26] A recent prospective cohort study compared stress fracture risk in >6200 female adolescents between those with the highest quintile of calcium intake (average, 1891 mg/day) and those in the lowest quintile (average, 541 mg/day).[27] A curious finding was that among girls participating in high-impact activity, increasing calcium intakes was associated with a large (but statistically insignificant) trend toward increased fracture risk (hazard ratio [HR], 2.14 for those in the highest quintile as compared with those in the lowest quintile; P_{trend}, 0.11). This raises the question as to whether girls with the highest calcium intakes were trying to compensate for other fracture risk factors. Other reports have found that higher calcium intakes do appear to protect against fractures in adolescents,[25] and one review in younger adult female athletes found that calcium intakes greater than 1500 mg/day reduces the risk of stress fractures.[28]

Dietary calcium, and dairy sources in particular, appears to exert multiple influences on building bone, and calcium needs ideally should be met with dietary sources.[26] Calcium supplementation is only recommended for those who are unable to meet recommended intake.[24]

For a given level of calcium intake, most athletes, particularly those participating in high-impact activities, have higher bone density than their more sedentary peers. However, the athlete's demands for bone integrity are much greater than those of their peers, and athletes are at higher risk of developing stress fractures. This is particularly true for female athletes whose energy intake is too low to support their caloric requirements.[23] These girls often have suppressed estrogen production, possibly resulting in pubertal delay or oligomenorrhea or amenorrhea. This combination of low caloric intake and decreased estrogen production results in diminished bone formation. This condition is known as the "female athlete triad," and these young athletes typically have bone density below average for their age group and are at markedly higher risk of developing bony stress injuries. Further information on treatment of the female athlete triad can be found in the 2016 AAP clinical report "The Female Athlete Triad."[23]

Magnesium

Magnesium has a role in more than 300 metabolic reactions in the body, including calcium absorption/bone accretion; energy production; and cardiac, nerve, and skeletal muscle function. A 2012 study on swimmers found magnesium intake in adolescents to be an independent predictor of bone mineral density.[29] Low magnesium levels have been associated with proinflammatory states.[30]

Approximately half of the body's magnesium stores are found in bone, and the other half are found in soft tissues. Very little magnesium is in the circulation. Studies on adolescent athletes indicate that low magnesium intake is common in this population.[30] Sunflower and sesame seeds, almonds, and a variety of beans are good sources of magnesium.

Vitamin D (See Also Chapter 22.II, Fat-Soluble Vitamins)

The roles of vitamin D particularly pertinent to the athletic population include attainment of optimal bone mass and support of muscle function. Vitamin D and physical activity appear to exert separate but complementary roles on bone development.[31] A 2010 study in adolescents found that the positive correlation between exercise and bone density became stronger as vitamin D concentrations decreased, even as vitamin D concentrations decreased below 27.5 nmol/L.[31] This seems to indicate that exercise may provide increasing protection against bone loss as vitamin D levels fall.

A prospective cohort study from 2013 looked at the relationship between vitamin D intake and stress fracture risk in adolescent girls who participated in >1 hour of high-impact activity/day.[27] Girls in the highest quintile of vitamin D intake had a 52% reduced risk of stress fracture as compared with the lowest quintile (663 vs 107 IU/day).[27] It should be noted that average intake of the highest quintile was just above the 600 IU/day that is currently recommended by the AAP for children 1 year and older.[24]

Interaction between physical activity, calcium, vitamin D, and the more recent recognition of the role of vitamin D receptor polymorphisms may explain the variable findings in some of the literature that has evaluated the relationship between vitamin D and stress fracture development in athletes. A military study looking at stress fracture risk by quartile of vitamin D levels showed that female navy recruits with the lowest serum 25-hydroxyvitamin D (25-OH-D) concentrations (average, 20 ng/mL or approximately 50 nmol/L) were twice as likely to sustain stress fractures than those in the highest quartile (average, 50 ng/mL or approximately 125 nmol/L).[32] Studies in young adults appear to show that stress fractures are less frequent in subjects supplemented with calcium (2000 mg/day) and vitamin D (800 IU/day) compared with placebo as well as in athletes with higher dairy intakes.[33,34] On the basis of these findings, many practitioners ascribe a protective role for vitamin D in stress fracture development; however, there remains a paucity of rigorous studies on this topic and essentially no published prospective studies performed with adolescent athletes.

Vitamin D deficiency is also associated with poor muscle function. Although this has been well-studied in the elderly population, data are accumulating on vitamin D and muscle function in children and adolescents. Low vitamin D concentrations may produce fatty infiltration of muscle and atrophy of type 2 fibers (aka "fast twitch")[35] and in children are associated with reductions in strength and other measures of athletic performance.[36,37] A 2014 meta-analysis reported that vitamin D supplementation increased muscle strength, particularly in those with baseline vitamin D concentrations <30 nmol/mL or with vitamin D concentrations that increased by >25 nmol/mL over the course of the study.[38] Unfortunately, only one study looking at strength in the pediatric population was included in their analysis. A 2016 review on the topic concluded that vitamin D supplementation in deficient young adult athletes was ergogenic but was not beneficial if athletes were already replete.[39] Myopathy in children attributable to low vitamin D appears to readily reverse with supplementation.[35]

The current recommended Recommended Dietary Allowance for vitamin D was chosen to meet the daily needs of 97% of the population (and, therefore, to achieve a vitamin D concentration of 20 ng/mL).[24] However, some authors propose that young athletes benefit when serum 25-OH-D concentrations are >80 nmol/L and up to 125 nmol/L.[5] For those who pursue these higher concentrations, the daily upper limit of vitamin D_3 is 4000 IU/day for 9- to 18-year-olds.[24] Athletes at risk for low vitamin D concentrations include those who live at latitudes above the 35th parallel (north of Santa Barbara, CA, and north of the southern border of Tennessee); indoor athletes and dancers; those with dark complexion; those with high body fat content; and those who practice aggressive ultraviolet B ray blocking.[5]

Body Weight and Body Composition In Young Athletes

Appearance and performance are the main drivers for desired body shape and weight in young athletes. In modern culture, it has traditionally been held that boys seek muscularity and that girls strive for thinness. However, recent data in adolescents has shown that the majority of both males and females have made changes in diet and exercise for the specific goal of building muscle.[40] National media outlets reflect this trend in females with statements like "Muscle is the new skinny."[41] The balance between appearance and performance concerns will be different for each athlete, and young athletes are subject to the same (if not greater) appearance pressures that are ubiquitous in current society.

With regard to athletic performance, for a given athlete in a given sport, there is a range of body weights that support optimal performance. The specific weight range may change depending on choice of sport, developmental stage, body composition, and a variety of factors intrinsic to the individual. But this basic relationship holds: body weights at either extreme are associated with a decrease in athletic performance and increase the potential for injury.

Pediatric office visits typically include weight and body mass index (BMI) calculations. These measures are often used to help determine health risk and as a proxy for body composition (ie, high BMIs are associated with increased adiposity). However, these relationships do not necessarily apply to many athletes. High levels of muscularity may result in a relatively high BMI, yet low adiposity. On the other end of the spectrum, BMIs often underrepresent body fat content in individuals with eating disorders or others who have lost muscle content.[11] Any further pursuit of weight and body composition assessments beyond these office measures should be performed with caution and with an understanding of their rationale and implications.

Some sports (ie, wrestling and others with weight classifications) require calculations of body composition for weight class certification. This procedure is outlined in detail in the AAP clinical report "Promotion of Healthy Weight Control Practices in Young Athletes."[11] However, routine assessment of body composition in other athletes is not indicated and has the potential to be detrimental. Body composition issues have an emotional overlay for many young athletes, and inappropriate use may trigger disordered eating patterns. Sports performance measures (ie, speed, agility, jump height, etc) are far better gauges than body composition measures in determining optimal body weight for a given athlete.

Principles of Weight Gain in Young Athletes

Despite the continuing epidemic of obesity in youth, many adolescent males actively seek to gain weight and muscle mass. This is particularly true in American football, and pediatricians who provide care for young football players should understand size-related trends in that sport:

- A study looking at size trends in an NCAA Division III (ie, nonscholarship) football program found that over the past 60 years, most positions have seen marked increases in mean body weight of players: offensive lineman have increased in body weight by 14 lb/decade, defensive ends have increased in body weight by 11 lb/decade, and defensive lineman and tight ends have increased in body weight by 9 lb/decade.[42]

- A cross-sectional analysis of community football players in Michigan found that 11-year-olds had median heights and weights around the 75th percentile. In older cohorts (up to 14 years of age), median weights drifted upward toward the 90th percentile, while heights remained around the 75th percentile.[43]

- Between 2001 and 2009, average weights for college-recruited high school offensive linesmen and defensive tackles were approximately 130 kg (286 lb).[44]

There is currently debate about the roles fitness and physical activity may play in mitigating the cardiovascular risk associated with obesity in these athletes. Studies in current collegiate football players demonstrate that this is a group with higher rates of metabolic syndrome and other cardiovascular risk factors as compared with peers matched for activity level.[45] However, no published studies have been performed looking at size-matched controls. Any performance benefit to weight gain needs to be tempered by concerns that excessive weight gain during childhood and adolescence often leads to a lifetime of issues with overweight and obesity, and at present, athletic participation does not appear to protect these individuals from adverse health implications.

Table 12.10 offers practical recommendations for young athletes who are seeking to gain weight.

Table 12.10.

Strategies for Weight Gain in Young Athletes

GOAL: Maximize lean muscle gains and minimize fat gains
Potential rates of gains in lean muscle mass per week:
  • Girls and preadolescent males: 0.25–0.75 lb
  • Postadolescent males: 0.5–1.0 lb
 	
Training:
High-intensity resistance training is a key aspect of making gains in lean mass:
  • For muscle hypertrophy: 2–3 sets of 8–15 repetitions/set
  • For strength/power gain: multiple sets of 4–6 repetitions/set
Appropriate rest:
  • Strength training for a given body part should be done on nonconsecutive days to allow muscle recovery in between high-intensity workouts
  • Adequate sleep

Continued

Table 12.10. *Continued*

Nutrition:
Calories:
- Increase intake by 300–400 kcal/day over any increased expenditures

Carbohydrates:
- 1–4 g carbohydrates/kg body weight 1–4 hours before training provide fuel for high-intensity workout and minimizes muscle breakdown

Protein:
- Maintain 1.5–1.8 g/kg/day
  o 0.3 g/kg within 2 hours after exercise and every 3–5 hours throughout the day

Fat: consider increasing fat content of diet if:
- Difficulty gaining weight or ingesting adequate calories, after implementing above recommendations
- No contraindications/other risk factors for a higher-fat diet

Practical recommendations to attain above:
- Increase frequency of meals/snacks
- Do not skip breakfast
- Aim to eat 5–9 times/day
- Increase size of meals/portions
- Change dietary composition to include foods with higher caloric density

Examples of ways to enhance calorie/protein content of foods in diet:
- Enrich full-fat milk with nonfat dry milk, instant breakfast, other flavorings
- Reconstitute canned soup with evaporated milk instead of water
- Choose cranberry, grape, or pineapple juice instead of orange or grapefruit juice
- Add dried fruits and/or nuts to hot cereal, sandwich fillings, etc
- Create sandwiches with thick-sliced, dense bread instead of white

Weight gain supplements (ie, "weight gainers") are not necessary:
- Food and Drug Administration (FDA) regulation of supplements is much looser than for foods or drugs
  o High rates of contamination/impure product
- Many provide between 500–2000 kcal/serving
  o If used as directed, will often result in excessive fat gains
- For young athletes, liquid food products (eg, Ensure, Carnation-brand instant breakfast) are reasonable options
  o Regulated by Food and Drug Administration and widely available
  o 2 servings/day often provide appropriate calories and protein to support lean tissue growth

Principles of Weight Loss in Young Athletes

Pursuit of weight loss is ubiquitous in American culture for both health and aesthetic reasons. The 2015 Youth Risk Behavior Survey (YRBS) of high school students in the United States reported that 61% of high school females and 31% of males had tried to lose weight in the previous year.[46] This effort can be particularly problematic for some females (see earlier discussion of the female athlete triad). Weight issues in athletes are often compounded by the perception in some sports that competing at the lowest possible weight is advantageous. This may be attributable to appearance concerns (particularly in aesthetic sports, such as gymnastics or figure skating), increased strength-to-mass ratio, or the desire to compete in a lower weight class. Weight loss practices of athletes can be generally divided into those techniques that produce rapid loss of fluid weight (ie, dehydration, also known as "cutting weight") and those that result in more gradual reductions in lean tissue or fat mass.

Table 12.11 provides additional information that may assist athletes with healthy weight loss efforts, and greater detail can be found in the AAP clinical report "Promotion of Healthy Weight Control Practices in Young Athletes."[11] Once weight goals are met, weight maintenance should be emphasized. Cyclic fluctuations tend to produce significant decreases in metabolic rate and lean body mass over time and should be discouraged.

Vegetarian Athletes *(See Also Chapter 11: Nutritional Aspects of Vegetarian Diets)*

The pediatric prevalence of vegetarians, and the proportion of those who are vegans, have not been recently evaluated. However, older data from the 2007 National Health Interview Survey reported that 0.5% of children younger than 18 years follow a vegetarian diet.[47] Children and adolescents decide to become vegetarian for a variety of reasons: health, financial, social, or environmental concerns; animal compassion; or religious background. There are multiple benefits to a vegetarian diet in terms of decreased risk of obesity and chronic disease as well as increased fruit and vegetable intakes. However, any restrictive diet increases the risk for inadequate energy intake, and for some young athletes, a vegetarian diet may be a red flag for dietary restraint associated with disordered eating behaviors. Pediatric vegetarian athletes benefit from close attention to maintenance of appropriate growth trends and any indicators of inadequate energy availability or disordered eating patterns, as outlined earlier in this chapter.

Table 12.11.
Strategies for Weight Loss in Young Athletes

> **GOAL: Maintenance of lean muscle mass while decreasing fat**
> Recommended rates of weight loss:
> - Growing athletes: up to 1 lb/wk
> - Skeletally mature athletes: up to 2 lb/wk
>
> **Training:**
> - Monitor training quality and athletic performance during times of weight loss
> - Avoid detrimental effects of caloric/nutrient restriction
>
> **Nutrition:**
> Calories:
> - Decrease by 250–500kcal/day
>   - o Reduce portion sizes and energy density of food
>   - – Foods with low energy density: whole fruits/vegetables, whole grains, beans/legumes, low fat dairy, lean meats
> - Strategies:
>   - o Increase proportion of vegetables in mixed dishes
>   - o Use low fat dairy/leaner meats
>   - o Foods with high fiber and water content increase satiety
>   - o Eliminate sugar-sweetened beverages
> Carbohydrates:
> - Breakfast/morning meal replenishes glycogen and provides fuel for activity
> - After workout, replenishes glycogen and provides fuel for the next workout
> Protein:
> - High intake of up to 2 g of protein/kg of body weight can help minimize loss of muscle mass during weight reduction
> - Spread protein intake throughout the day
>   - o Particularly important at breakfast and after working out
>   - o Provides pool of amino acids for tissue maintenance and repair

The amount of planning required to meet nutritional recommendations may be difficult for many vegetarian children and adolescents. Adequate intakes of some nutrients can be more challenging in vegetarian diets, as outlined in Table 12.12. Many vegetarian athletes, particularly at higher performance levels, may benefit from consultation with a sports dietitian.

Performance Enhancing Substances

There is increasing recognition that athletes and nonathletes are using a variety of dietary supplements and drugs in attempts to improve not only athletic and/or academic performance but also appearance-related

Table 12.12.
Nutrients at Risk for Inadequate Intake in Vegetarian and Vegan Diets

Protein	Usually met with adequate energy intakes in a balanced vegetarian diet. Protein recommendations in vegans >6 y are 20% more than for nonvegans because of decreased protein digestibility. Legumes and soy products can help ensure ingestion of balance of essential amino acids.	Supports tissue recovery and muscle building.
Essential fatty acids	Intake of long-chain omega-3 fatty acids (eicosapentaenoic acid [EPA] and docosahexaenoic acid [DHA]) is low in vegetarian diets. These can be endogenously synthesized from alpha-linolenic acid (ALA). Good ALA sources include variety of seeds and oils: flax, chia, canola, hemp, and walnut.	Inadequate intake can decrease calcium absorption.
Iron	Supports red cell production. Nonheme iron less absorption than heme iron (ie, meat-based). However, vitamin C/ascorbic acid and low iron levels (as often seen in vegetarians) can markedly enhance absorption.	Iron-deficiency anemia decreases athletic performance. Controversial impact of nonanemic iron deficiency on athletic performance. Some recommend routine monitoring of athletes, especially during periods of rapid growth.

Vitamin D	Supplements often needed (especially for indoor athletes).	Bone health, skeletal muscle function
Zinc	Vegetarian diets generally lower than meat-based diets. Soaking and sprouting beans, grains and seeds can increase zinc bioavailability.	Impact of deficiency in athletes not known.
Calcium	Vegetable calcium sources are poorly absorbed. Tofu coagulated with calcium sulfate can be good source as well as fortified orange juice.	Bone health and muscle function.
Iodine	Variable amounts in dairy products. Sea vegetables and iodized salt are good sources.	Sweat losses can be significant. Role in athletic performance beyond impact on thyroid function is unknown.
Vitamin B_{12}	Not a component of plant-based foods. Milk and eggs contain vitamin B_{12}, but vegans need supplement or fortified foods.	Significant deficiency may cause anemia and decreased athletic performance. Mild deficiencies asymptomatic.

concerns. In particular, efforts to build muscularity seem to drive much use of these agents. An overview of the PESs most commonly used in the pediatric population can be found in Table 12.13.

Despite the prevalence of use, there is a paucity of data in children and adolescents on the safety and efficacy of many of the PESs in common use, and most PESs used in this population are sold as over-the-counter dietary supplements. The Dietary Supplement Health and Education Act of 1994 resulted in decreased oversight by the US Food and Drug Administration (FDA) for the manufacture and sale of supplements as compared with other food and drug products in the United States. Manufacturers do not have to prove safety or efficacy before bringing dietary supplements to market, and high rates of contamination have been found when PESs have been tested by independent laboratories.

- A 2010 evaluation of 15 popular protein supplements performed by Consumer Reports found that all tested products contained heavy metals, and 3 had levels exceeding maximum intake guidelines established by the United States Pharmacopeia (USP).[48]

- A 2014 study analyzed the content of dietary supplements after an FDA recall for adulteration with banned pharmaceuticals. The study found that 85% of recalled supplements sold for sports enhancement still contained the banned agent when purchased 6 months later.[49]

- In 2015, the New York attorney general sent cease-and-desist letters to 4 national retailers after an investigation revealed that only 5 of 20 herbal supplement products tested consistently contained active ingredients as listed.[50]

In young athletes, the most powerful factors that lead to improved athletic performance include adherence to nutrition fundamentals, appropriate coaching and practice, and the onset of puberty. An important point of emphasis is the role of puberty as the "ultimate performance enhancer," particularly when combined with appropriate nutrition and training. Although it is important to emphasize to athletes and their families that the vast majority of ergogenic claims by commercial products are unfounded, it is also important to acknowledge supplements that have been shown to be effective, such as caffeine and creatine. However, the small performance benefits associated with their use will not be detectable in the vast majority of adolescent athletes, and their use has not been shown to translate to improved "on-field" performance in the young athlete.

Text continued on page 360

Table 12.13.

Summary Table of PES Prevalence, Effects, and Safety Concerns in Children and Adolescents

PES	Available Prevalence Data	Usual Form of Intake	Purported Mechanism of Performance Effect	Data on Performance Effects	Potential Adverse Effects
Creatine	16.7% of 12th grade males and 1.4% of 12th grade females report use within the past year.[53]	Creatine monohydrate supplement. About 1 g/day found in omnivore diet.	Delays onset of muscle fatigue during high-intensity training by ATP production in high intensity activities that rely on phosphocreatine shuttle.	Performance benefit in most studies is small and primarily seen in short-duration, maximum-intensity resistance training. No benefit generally shown in aerobic activities or with "on field" athletic performance.	Short-term use at usual doses appears safe in normal adults. Most concern with impact on kidneys because of nephrotoxic metabolites (methylamine and formaldehyde), and specific recommendation against use for athletes at risk for kidney dysfunction.[54] May impair performance in endurance activities.

Continued

Table 12.13. *Continued*

Summary Table of PES Prevalence, Effects, and Safety Concerns in Children and Adolescents

PES	Available Prevalence Data	Usual Form of Intake	Purported Mechanism of Performance Effect	Data on Performance Effects	Potential Adverse Effects
Anabolic agents	The 2015 Youth Risk Behavior Survey: 4% of high school males and 2.7% of females have used nonprescribed anabolic steroids.[46]	Variety of testosterone derivatives. Schedule III drugs. Oral, injectable, buccal, and transdermal forms. Multiple forms often taken in "stacks" in 6-to 12-week cycles.	Enhances net protein synthesis by increasing transcription and decreasing catabolism.	Increased strength and lean muscle mass.	Possible long-term effects on brain remodeling with adolescent AAS exposure. Premature physeal closure with decreased final adult height. Acne. Gynecomastia (irreversible). Hair loss/male pattern baldness (irreversible). Hypogonadism/testicular atrophy. Dependence. Behavior change (hypomania, irritability, aggression). Cardiomyopathy. Increased low-density lipoproteins/decreased high-density lipoproteins. Cholestatic jaundice, liver tumors.

Prohormones	0.9% of high school seniors report use in past year.[53]	Variety of substances often taken in combination ("stacks") and in cyclical fashion. All except for DHEA are now scheduled drugs under the Anabolic Steroid Control Act of 2004 and Designer Anabolic Steroid Act of 2014.	Purported to enhance testosterone levels after ingestion, and potential direct anabolic effects as well.	Androstenedione and DHEA: repeated dosages do not appear to increase blood testosterone levels or increase muscle size or strength.[55]	Suppression of endogenous testosterone production, otherwise potentially same as for testosterone. Supplements contaminated with prohormones are common cause of doping violations in organized sports.[55]

Continued

Table 12.13. *Continued*

Summary Table of PES Prevalence, Effects, and Safety Concerns in Children and Adolescents

PES	Available Prevalence Data	Usual Form of Intake	Purported Mechanism of Performance Effect	Data on Performance Effects	Potential Adverse Effects
Caffeine/other stimulants	Diet pills: 71% of 12th grade girls have used diet pills in the past year.[53] 73% children consume caffeine on any given day.[56] Nonmedical use of amphetamines in 12th grade[57]: lifetime, 12.4 %; monthly, 4.4%.	Caffeine is ubiquitous in a variety of food and beverages, as well as OTC diet pills and "stay awake" medication. Amphetamines often diverted from prescription use.	Currently believed that performance benefit primarily due to CNS stimulation and enhanced muscle activation.	Most studies have examined caffeine doses of 3–6 mg/kg, but 1–3 mg/kg can be ergogenic, particularly in endurance activity. 4% improvements in strength of knee extensors (note: other muscle groups did not show strength improvements with caffeine).[58] 14% in muscular endurance and 10%–20% improvements in time to exhaustion studies.	Tolerance. Cardiac arrhythmias (PVCs), increased blood pressure. Headaches, irritability, sleep disruption, tremor. Gastric irritation. Increased core temperature with exertion, particularly in hot environments. Significant toxicity has been associated with ingestion of multiple energy drinks, leading to almost 1500 emergency room visits in 2011 in the 12- to 17-year age group.[59] FDA warning regarding increased availability of pure powdered caffeine is of particular concern and is responsible for at least two deaths in young people (1 tsp is equivalent to 25 cups of coffee).

Supplement	Prevalence of use	Form	Claimed benefit	Evidence	Adverse effects/risks
Protein supplements	Middle school girls: 25%. Middle school boys: 18%. High school girls: 30%. High school boys: 39%.[40]	Variety of powders/bars/Shakes.	Provides "building blocks" for muscle and lean tissue growth.	No performance benefit of protein supplement if diet provides adequate protein.	Risk of contaminated product: a 2010 report found that 100% of protein supplements had heavy metal contamination, with 20% of those levels exceeding USP recommendations.[48]
Amino acids and related compounds	N/A	Oral supplements. Individual amino acids or in combination. Diets with adequate amounts of complete proteins are replete with essential amino acids. Hydroxymethyl-butyrate (HMB) is a leucine metabolite.	Arginine and citrulline produce increases in nitric oxide (see below for further discussion). Beta-alanine and carnosine buffer H+ accumulation (see buffer discussion below). HMB is believed to enhance repair of damaged muscle tissue.	HMB: Meta-analysis of studies on young adults show untrained athletes with 6.6% gains in strength and only trivial strength impacts on trained athlete.[60]	Ingestion of single amino acids may result in imbalance of others. Short-term ingestion of HMB appears safe at 6 g/day.[61]
Human growth hormone (hGH)/insulin-like growth factor 1 (IGF-1)	11% high school students reported use.[62]	Injectable recombinant hGH or IGF-1	hGH acts primarily through IGF-1 resulting in increases in lean mass, decreases in fat mass.	Most recent reviews do not support performance benefit.	Elevated plasma glucose/insulin resistance, sodium retention and edema, benign intracranial hypertension, acromegaly, cardiovascular disease.

Continued

Table 12.13. *Continued*

Summary Table of PES Prevalence, Effects, and Safety Concerns in Children and Adolescents

PES	Available Prevalence Data	Usual Form of Intake	Purported Mechanism of Performance Effect	Data on Performance Effects	Potential Adverse Effects
Nitric oxide boosters (arginine, beetroot juice, citrulline,	N/A	Oral supplements and dietary forms.	Nitric oxide is a potent vasodilator. Synthesized from arginine. Citrulline is an arginine precursor.	Recent studies do not demonstrate significant improvement in trained athletes. Any potential benefit of arginine appears minimal in healthy young athletes who ingest sufficient protein.[63,64]	Supplementation with the amino acid arginine may create imbalance between other amino acids.

Buffers	N/A	Sodium bicarbonate or sodium citrate. Carnosine and beta-alanine.	Buffers the metabolic acidosis resulting from high-intensity physical activity. Beta-alanine is a precursor of carnosine.	Data are variable regarding endurance exercise. Studies in adolescent swimmers with sodium bicarbonate show some swimmers with >1 sec improvement in 200 meter efforts.[65]	Sodium bicarbonate with significant gastric upset in about 10%. Beta-alanine with paresthesias at higher doses.
Blood doping	N/A	Recombinant erythropoietin and synthetic analogues.	Increases oxygen delivery to exercising muscles.	Increases maximal oxygen uptake by 6%–12%.[66]	Hyperviscosity can lead to thrombogenic or embolic events. Increased cardiac afterload.

AAS, anabolic-androgenic steroid; ATP, adenosine triphosphate; CNS, central nervous system; DHEA, dehydroepiandrosterone; N/A, not applicable; OTC, over-the-counter; PVC, premature ventricular contraction.

Adapted with permission from: LaBotz M, Griesemer BA; American Academy of Pediatrics, Council on Sports Medicine and Fitness. Use of performance-enhancing substances. *Pediatrics.* 2016;138(1):e20161300.[52]

The changes in strength, speed, endurance, and athletic proficiency that come with maturation and practice dwarfs even the most optimistic results of performance enhancement with any dietary supplement. Youth resistance training programs 8 to 20 weeks in duration can produce strength gains of up to 30%,[51] and this is not likely to be noticeably enhanced by any nonanabolic agent in current use. Additional information can be found in the AAP clinical report "Use of Performance-Enhancing Substances."[52]

Resources

The evidence-based literature cannot maintain the pace of development and dissemination of information about sports nutrition, dietary supplements, and ergogenic aids. The Internet is a common source of nutritional information and misinformation for young athletes, and location of appropriate Internet resources can be very helpful for the health care professional as well as for the athlete and his or her family. Two high-quality sites include:

- www.healthychildren.org, an AAP Web site that provides basic information on a broad spectrum of sports- and nutrition-related topics.
- http://learn.truesport.org/topics/nutrition, is an educational Web site from the United States Anti-Doping Agency. This is an engaging site that provides a broad spectrum of articles and videos as well links for both parents and young athletes.

Where to Get Further Assistance

Some young athletes will benefit from dedicated and individualized guidance from a sports dietitian. However, many individuals and commercial enterprises purport to provide sports nutrition counseling and services.

- Sports nutritionist: There is no standard definition for a "nutritionist." This designation is often used by individuals with a particular interest in sports nutrition, but this term does not imply any specific level of training or credentials.
- Sports dietitian: Registered dietitians (RDs) have met education, experience, and testing standards as defined by the Academy of Nutrition and Dietetics, and young athletes should be steered toward an RD when seeking nutritional consultation. Additional licensure and certification requirements vary by state. Additional board certification as a Certified Specialist in Sports Dietetics (CSSD) requires

demonstration of clinical experience and knowledge specific to athletes and sports participation.

The Sports, Cardiovascular, and Wellness Nutrition practice group of the Academy of Nutrition and Dietetics can provide assistance for locating a credentialed dietician through its website at: https://www.scandpg.org/search-rd/.

References

1. Zion Market Research. Sports Nutrition Market (Sports Food, Sports Drink & Sports Supplements): Global Industry Perspective, Comprehensive Analysis and Forecast, 2016–2022. Available at: https://www.zionmarketresearch.com/report/sports-nutrition-market. Accessed July 1, 2017

2. Mikulan R, Piko BE. High school students' body weight control: differences between athletes and non-athletes. *Coll Antropol.* 2012;36(1):79–86

3. Manore MM, Patton-Lopez MY, Wong SS. Sport nutrition knowledge, behaviors and beliefs of high school soccer players. *Nutrients.* 2017;9(4):E350

4. Brenner JS, American Academy of Pediatrics, Council on Sports Medicine and Fitness. Clinical report: Sports specialization and intensive training in young athletes. *Pediatrics.* 2016;138(3):e20162148

5. Thomas DT, Erdman KA, Burke LM. American College of Sports Medicine Joint Position Statement. Nutrition and Athletic Performance. *Med Sci Sports Exerc.* 2016;48(3):543–568

6. Jeukendrup AE. Training the gut for athletes. *Sports Med.* 2017;47(Suppl 1):101–110

7. Kreider RB, Wilborn CD, Taylor Lea. ISSN exercise and sport nutrition review: research and recommendations. *J Int Soc Sports Nutr.* 2010;7:7

8. Baker LB, Rollo I, Stein KW, Jeukendrup AE. Acute effects of carbohydrate supplementation on intermittent sports performance. *Nutrients.* 2015;7:5733–5763

9. Burke LM, Hawley JA, Wong SH, Jeukendrup AE. Carbohydrates for training and competition. *J Sports Sci.* 2011;29(Suppl 1):S17–S27

10. Jeukendrup AE. Periodized nutrition for athletes. *Sports Med.* 2017;47(Suppl 1):51–63

11. Carl RL, Johnson MD, Martin TJ, American Academy of Pediatrics, Council on Sports Medicine and Fitness. Promotion of healthy weight control practices in young athletes *Pediatrics.* 2017;140(3):e20171871

12. Bergeron MF. Hydration in the pediatric athlete-how to guide your patients. *Curr Sports Med Rep.* 2015;14(4):288–293

13. Montain SJ. Hydration recommendations for sport 2008. *Curr Sports Med Rep.* 2008;7(4):187–192

14. Hew-Butler T, Rosner MH, Fowkes-Godek S, et al. Statement of the 3rd International Exercise-Associated Hyponatremia Consensus Development Conference, Carlsbad, California, 2015. *Br J Sports Med.* 2015;49:1432–1446

15. Ghoch ME, Calugi S, Grave RDCRiM, Article ID 8194160, 5 pages, 2016. doi:10.1155/2016/8194160. Management of severe rhabdomyolysis and exercise-associated hyponatremia in a female with anorexia nervosa and excessive compulsive exercising. *Case Rep Med.* 2016;2016:8194160

16. American Academy of Pediatrics, Committee on Nutrition, Council on Sports Medicine and Fitness. Clinical report: Sports drinks and energy drinks for children and adolescents: are they appropriate? *Pediatrics.* 2011;127(6):1182–1189

17. Evans GH, Shirreffs SM, Maughan RJ. Postexercise rehydration in man: the effects of osmolality and carbohydrate content of ingested drinks. *Nutrition.* 2009;25(9):905–913

18. US Department of Agriculture, Service AR. *Nutrient Intakes from Food and Beverages: Mean Amounts Consumed per Individual, by Gender and Age. What We Eat in America, NHANES 2013–2014.* Washington, DC: US Department of Agriculture; 2016

19. Phillips SM. A brief review of critical processes in exercise-induced muscular hypertrophy. *Sports Med.* 2014;44(Suppl 1):71–77

20. Volterman KA, Moore DR, Breithaupt P, et al. Timing and pattern of post-exercise protein ingestion affects whole body protein balance in healthy children: a randomized trial. *Appl Physio Nutr Met.* 2017;42(11):1142–1148

21. Rodenberg RE, Gustafson S. Iron as en ergogenic aid: ironclad evidence? *Curr Sports Med Rep.* 2007;6(4):258–264

22. Bonjour JP, Theintz G, Buchs B, Slosman D, Rizzoli R. Critical years and stages of puberty for spinal and femoral bone mass accumulation during adolescence. *J Clin Endocrinol Metab.* 1991;73(3):555–563

23. Weiss Kelly AK, Hecht S, American Academy of Pediatrics, Council on Sports Medicine and Fitness. The female athlete triad. *Pediatrics.* 2016;138(2):e20160922

24. Golden NH, Abrams SA, American Academy of Pediatrics, Committee on Nutrition. Optimizing bone health in children and adolescents. *Pediatrics.* 2014;134(4):e1229–e1243

25. Ackerman KE, Misra M. Bone Health in Adolescent Athletes with a Focus on Female Athlete Triad. *Phys Sportsmed.* 2011;39(1):131–141

26. Burckhardt P. Calcium revisited, part III: effect of dietary calcium on BMD and fracture risk. *Bonekey Rep.* 2015;4:708

27. Sonneville KR, Gordon CM, Kocher MS, Pierce LM, Ramappa A, Field AE. Vitamin D, Calcium, and Dairy Intakes and Stress Fractures Among Female Adolescents. *Arch Pediatr Adolesc Med.* 2012;166(7):595–600

28. Tenforde AS, Sayres LC, Sainani KL, Fredericson M. Evaluating the relationship of calcium and vitamin D in the prevention of stress fracture injuries in the young athlete: a review of the literature. *PM R.* 2010;2(10):945–949

29. Matias CN, Santos DA, Monteiro CP, et al. Magnesium intake mediates the association between bone mineral density and lean soft tissue in elite swimmers. *Magnes Res.* 2012;25(3):120–125

30. Volpe SL. Magnesium and the athlete. *Curr Sports Med Rep.* 2015;14(4):279–283

31. Constantini NW, Dubnov-Raz G, Chodick Gea, Rozen GS, Giladi A, Ish-Shalom S. Physical activity and bone mineral density in adolescents with vitamin D deficiency. *Med Sci Sports Exerc.* 2010;42(4):646–650

32. Burgi AA, Gorham ED, Garland CF, et al. High serum 25-hydroxyvitamin D is associated with low incidence of stress fractures. *J Bone Miner Res.* 2011;26(10):2371–2377

33. Lappe J, Cullen D, Haynatzki G, Recker R, Ahlf R, Thompson K. Calcium and vitamin d supplementation decreases incidence of stress fractures in female navy recruits. *J Bone Miner Res.* 2009;23(5):741–749

34. Nieves JW, Melsop K, Curtis M, et al. Nutritional factors that influence change in bone density and stress fracture risk among young female cross-country runners. *PM R.* 2010;2(8):740–750

35. Rosen CJ, Adams JS, Bikle DD. The nonskeletal effects of vitamin D: an Endocrine Society scientific statement. *Endocrinol Rev.* 2012;33(3):456–492

36. Bezrati I, Hammami R, Ben Fradj MK. Association of plasma 25-hydroxyvitamin D with physical performance in physically active children. *Appl Physio Nutr Met.* 2016;41(11):1124–1128

37. Carson EL, Pourshahidi LK, Hill TR. Vitamin D, muscle function, and cardiorespiratory fitness in adolescents from the Young Hearts Study. *J Clin Endocrinol Metab.* 2015;100(12):4621–4628

38. Beaudart C, Buckinx F, Gillain S. The effects of vitamin D on skeletal muscle strength, muscle mass, and muscle power: a systematic review and meta-analysis of randomized controlled trials. *J Clin Endocrinol Metab.* 2014;99(11): 4336–4345

39. Koundourakis NE, Avgoustinaki PD, Malliaraki N, Margioris AN. Muscular effects of vitamin D in young athletes and non-athletes and in the elderly. *Hormones.* 2016;15(4):471–488

40. Eisenberg ME, Wall M, Neumark-Sztainer D. Muscle–enhancing behaviors among adolescent girls and boys. *Pediatrics.* 2012;130(6):1019–1026

41. Muscle is the new skinny. *USA Today.* January 13, 2017. Available at: https://www.usatoday.com/videos/news/nation/2017/01/13/muscle-new-skinny/96566062/. Accessed March 6, 2019

42. Elliott KR, Harmatz JS, Zhao Y, Greenblatt DJ. Body size changes among National Collegiate Athletic Association New England Division III football players, 1956–22014: comparison with age-matched population controls. *J Athl Train.* 2016;51(5):373–381

43. Malina RM, Morano PJ, Barron M, Miller SJ, Cumming SP. Growth status and estimated growth rate of youth football players: a community-based study. *Clin J Sports Med.* 2005;15(3):125–132

44. Ghigiarelli JJ. Combine performance descriptors and predictors of recruit ranking for the top high school football recruits from 2001 to 2009: differences between position groups. *J Strength Cond Res*. 2011;25(5):1193–1203

45. Feairheller DL, Aichele KR, Oakman JE, et al. Vascular health in American football players: cardiovascular risk increased in Division III players. *Int J Vasc Med*. 2016;2016:6851256

46. Kann L, McManus T, Harris WA, et al. Youth Risk Behavior Surveillance – United States 2015. *MMWR Surveill Summ*. 2016;65(6):1–174

47. Barnes PM, Bloom B, Nahin RL. Complementary and alternative medicine use among adults and children: United States, 2007. *Natl Health Stat Rep*. 2008 (12):1–23

48. Health risks of protein drinks: You don't need the extra protein or heavy metals our tests found. *Consumer Reports*. July 2010. Available at: https://www.consumerreports.org/cro/2012/04/protein-drinks/index.htm. Accessed December 12, 2018

49. Cohen PA, Maller G, DeSouza R, Neal-Kababick J. Presence of Banned Drugs in Dietary Supplements Following FDA Recalls. *JAMA*. 2014;312(16):1691–1693

50. O'Connor A. New York Attorney General targets supplements at major retailers. *New York Times*. February 3, 2015. Available at: http://well.blogs.nytimes.com/2015/02/03/new-york-attorney-general-targets-supplements-at-major-retailers/. Accessed December 12, 2018

51. Faigenbaum AD, Kraemer WJ, Blimkie CJ, et al. Youth resistance training: updated position statement paper from the National Strength and Conditioning Association. *J Strength Cond Res*. 2009;23(5 Suppl):S60–S79

52. LaBotz M, Griesemer BA, American Academy of Pediatrics, Council on Sports Medicine and Fitness. Use of performance-enhancing substances. *Pediatrics*. 2016;138(1):e20161300

53. Miech RA, Johnston LD, O'Malley PM, Bachman JG, Schulenberg JE, Patrick ME. Monitoring the Future National Survey Results on Drug Use, 1975–2016: Volume I, Secondary School Students. Ann Arbor, MI: The University of Michigan; 2017: Available at: Available at: http://monitoringthefuture.org/pubs.html#monographs. Accessed December 12, 2018

54. Kim HJ, Kim CK, Carpentier A, Poortmans JR. Studies on the safety of creatine supplementation. *Amino Acids*. 2011;40(5):1409–1418

55. King DS, Baskerville R, Hellsten Y. A-Z of nutritional supplements: dietary supplements, sports nutrition foods and ergogenic aids for health and performance: part 34. *Br J Sports Med*. 2012;46(9):689–690

56. Branum AM, Rossen LM, Schoendorf KC. Trends in caffeine intake among U.S. children and adolescents. *Pediatrics*. 2014;133(3):386–393

57. Johnston LD, O'Malley PM, Bachman JG, Schulenberg JE, Miech RA. *Monitoring the Future: National Survey Results on Drug Use, 1975–2013, Vol. I: Secondary School Students*. Ann Arbor, MI: Institute for Social Research, The University of Michigan; 2014

58. Warren GL, Park ND, Maresca RD, McKibans KI, Millard-Stafford ML. Effect of caffeine ingestion on muscular strength and endurance: a meta-analysis. *Med Sci Sports Exerc.* 2010;42(7):1375–1387

59. Substance Abuse and Mental Health Services Administration, Center for Behavioral Health Statistics and Quality. *The DAWN Report: Update on Emergency Department Visits Involving Energy Drinks: A Continuing Public Health Concern.* Rockville, MD: Substance Abuse and Mental Health Services Administration; 2013

60. Rowlands DS, Thomson JS. Effects of beta-hydroxy-beta-methylbutyrate supplementation during resistance training on strength, body composition, and muscle damage in trained and untrained young men: a meta-analysis. *J Strength Cond Res.* 2009;23(3):836–846

61. Currell K, Derave W, Everaert I, et al. A-Z of nutritional supplements: dietary supplements, sports nutrition foods and ergogenic aids for health and performance: part 20. *Br J Sports Med.* 2011;45(6):530–532

62. Partnership for Drug-Free Kids. The 2013 Partnership Attitude Tracking Study. Available at: https://drugfree.org/research-reports/. Accessed July 31, 2017

63. Castell LM, Burke LM, Stear SJ. BJSM reviews: A-Z of supplements: dietary supplements, sports nutrition foods and ergogenic aids for health and performance Part 2. *Br J Sports Med.* 2009;2009(43):11

64. Sandbakk SB, Sandbakk O, Peacock O, et al. Effects of acute supplementation of L-arginine and nitrate on endurance and sprint performance in elite athletes. *Nitric Oxide.* 2015;48:10–15

65. Zajac A, Cholewa J, Poprzecki S, Waskiewicz Z, Langfort J. Effects of sodium bicarbonate ingestion on swim performance in youth athletes. *J Sports Sci Med.* 2009;8(1):45–50

66. Thomsen JJ, Rentsch RL, Robach P, et al. Prolonged administration of recombinant human erythropoietin increases submaximal performance more than maximal aerobic capacity. *Eur J Appl Physiol.* 2007;101(4):481–486

Chapter 13

Fast Foods, Organic Foods, Fad Diets, and Herbs, Herbals, and Botanicals

Fast Food

Most people have a mental image of what fast food is; however, there is no standard definition. If you ask a child in Vietnam, he is likely to point to a street vendor selling Pho; if you ask a child in Peru, she is likely to tell you it is anticuchos, a spicy bit of grilled beef heart sold on a skewer on the street. In the United States, however, fast food and fast food restaurants are associated with hamburgers, French fries, and sweetened beverages; hot dogs or other sandwiches; pizza; and fried chicken. Orders can be placed and picked up within a few minutes and be taken away or consumed on the premises. Generally, fast food is eaten without cutlery, and fast food restaurants have no wait staff. Failure to have a standardized definition of fast food makes it difficult to compare studies or to set standards.

The origin of the fast food restaurant is unclear, but some food historians believe the first fast food restaurants were the Harvey Houses along the Santa Fe Railroad beginning in 1879, where food was served and consumed quickly by travelers. The growth of the "fast food" industry in this country has been phenomenal. As of 2017, there were nearly 250 000 fast food restaurants in the United States.[1] Fast food outlets are ubiquitous and found in local communities, public schools, military bases, and even hospitals. However, similar to the problem with defining fast food itself, it has become more difficult to define a fast food restaurant. Fast-causal and "quick-service" restaurants often provide similar menu options, although the perception of the healthfulness of these options may vary.

In 2014, approximately $728 million dollars were spent on food at home and $731 million in total food expenditures outside the home; 34.7% of the monies spent outside the home were spent in "limited-service eating places."[2] These figures are well up from the 25% spent on food away from home in 1970.[2]

Characteristics of Fast Food Restaurants

Fast food restaurants have been defined as having "typical" meal costs of $5, minimal service, drive-through facilities, and advertising that "emphasizes convenience and affordability." This definition can be used to distinguish between fast food restaurants and fast-casual restaurants, which has been defined as having a "typical" meal cost of $9 to $13 dollars, with "limited service," and advertising "emphasizing flavor or freshness."[3] Categorizing fast food restaurants by the food served, such as hamburger, pizza, sandwich, Mexican, chicken, Asian, fish, and coffee shops, may allow more precise monitoring of intake by children.[4] However, these categories fail to clearly define some fast food restaurants; for example, a well-known sandwich food chain, which advertises some of their products as healthy and low fat, may not be perceived as being a fast food restaurant. It is more difficult to find a clear definition of "quick-service restaurants," which was a term used in some articles,[5] although most of these restaurants seem indistinguishable from fast food restaurants. These discrepancies make it difficult to compare studies. What We Eat in America (WWEIA),[6] the dietary component of the National Health and Nutrition Examination Survey (NHANES), included the source coded as: "Restaurant fast food/pizza," "Cafeteria NOT in a K-12 school," "Sport, recreation, or entertainment facility," or "Street vendor, vending truck" to distinguish among these restaurants. The question asked the participants in NHANES is "How many meals did you get from a fast-food or pizza place?"[7] Because of potential confusion about defining fast food or fast food restaurants, questions about consumption or place of consumption could be confusing to the participants, leading to misclassification of consumers and, thus, dietary intake.

With the exception of school meals, food consumed away from home is generally lower in some nutrients, including dietary fiber, calcium, and iron, and higher in energy, total and saturated fatty acids (SFAs), cholesterol, added sugars, and sodium than food consumed at home.[8] Fast food restaurants generally also promote meals low in fruits, vegetables, and dairy products.[9] One study showed that 99% of 1662 children's meal combinations from national chain restaurants were of poor nutritional quality.[10] However, nutrient quality varied considerably among fast food restaurants.[11]

Many fast food restaurants have made an effort to improve meals designed for children by including more fruit, salad, and dairy options. These changes are in part because of the National Restaurant Association's "Kids LiveWell program."[12] This program includes nearly 42 000 restaurant locations that, in connection with Healthy Dining,[13] help parents and children select healthy menu items when eating out. Participating restaurants must offer at least one "kids" menu (entrée, side, and beverage) that is ≤600 kilocalories (kcals); contains 2 or more servings of fruit, vegetables, whole grains, lean protein, or low-fat dairy; and limits sodium (≤770 mg), fat (≤35% total; ≤10% SFAs and <0.5 artificial trans-fats), and total sugars (≤35%). Restaurants participating must also offer at least one other individual menu item with ≤200 kcals with limits on fat (<35% total;

<10% SFAs and <0.5 artificial trans-fats), total sugars (<35%), and sodium (≤250 mg) and contains a serving of fruit, vegetables, whole grains, or lean protein or low-fat dairy. Finally, participating restaurants must also display or have available on request the nutrition information of the healthful menu options and promote those options. Although restaurants pay a nominal fee for participation, they receive promotional benefits.

Overall, fast food restaurants tend to provide large portions of foods, although this is changing, in large part in response to the movie "Super Size Me." Portion sizes are a critical issue for controlling energy intake. In infants, toddlers, and children up to 3 years of age, food intake is self-regulated.[14] By 4 years of age, however, larger portion sizes lead to increased consumption and energy intake.[14,15] Fisher et al[16] demonstrated that children consumed 25% more of an entree when a larger portion was presented on their plates, which negatively affected self-regulation of intake (see also Chapter 7: Feeding the Child). Portion size and energy density of food acted independently to increase intake.[17] Thus, having smaller-sized menu options available for children, like "kid's fries," may help children 5 years and older regulate intake.

The Effect That Fast Food Has on the Energy and Nutrient Intakes to the Diets of Children

The effect of fast food consumption by children and adolescents on dietary intake or eating patterns is unclear. The number of children consuming fast food depends on the study population, the age that defined children in the study, how fast food was defined, and some type of temporal element. Using nationally representative data from the NHANES, the number of children 4 to 19 years of age consuming fast food on a given day has dropped slightly from 38.8% (2003–2004) to 32.6% (2009–2010),[18] with this number increasing slightly to 34.3% of children 2 to 19 years of age in 2011–2012.[19]

Fast food consumption is associated with poor diet quality, with lower intake of fruit and vegetables and higher intake of sodium and SFAs, as compared with food consumed at home.[9,19–23] Food consumed away from home is also associated with higher energy intakes and compromised diet quality, as measured by the Healthy Eating Index (HEI), especially in adolescents 13 to 18 years of age. Sweetened beverages contributed to 35% of this increased energy intake and to approximately 20% of the decline in HEI scores. However, even after controlling for sweetened beverages, away-from-home meals contributed an extra 65 kcals to the diets of all children, 107 kcals to the diets of older children, and lowered diet quality by 4%.[8]

Data from What We Eat in America (2013–2014) appear to show gender and age differences in children eating at quick-service restaurants (there is no specific "fast food" restaurant category in this survey), although no statistical analyses were provided (Table 13.1). As children grow older, a higher percentage of their energy comes from quick-service restaurants, and as expected, intake of dietary fiber and selected nutrients also increase with age. The data suggest, however, that for the most part, children are not meeting recommended nutrient intakes. As discouraging as these data

Table 13.1.
Quick-Service Restaurants: Percent Reporting (41.1%; 1.1 [SE]), Mean Amounts (± SE) of Energy, Macronutrients, and Nutrients of Public Health Concern and Sodium, Foods Obtained from Quick-Service Restaurants, by Children, 2-19 Years of Age (n=3019) in the United States, 2013-2014

All individuals			
Gender and Age (y)	*Total Intake*	*Intake From Quick-Service Restaurants*	*Percentages From Quick-Service Restaurants*
Energy (kcals) (SE)			
Males 2-5	1571 (35.2)	147 (17.7)	9 (1.2)
Males 6-11	2036 (46.2)	261 (21.8)	13 (1.0)
Males 12-19	2376 (38.2)	478 (48.6)	20 (2.1)
Females 2-5	1395 (36.9)	161 (34.9)	12 (2.5)
Females 6-11	1786 (30.4)	274 (31.8)	15 (1.8)
Females 12-19	1689 (48.0)	313 (28.3)	19 (1.7)
Protein (g) (SE)			
Males 2-5	55.8 (2.36)	5.2 (0.57)	9 (1.1)
Males 6-11	72.9 (2.13)	9.2 (0.72)	13 (1.0)
Males 12-19	95.5 (3.51)	19.8 (2.43)	21 (2.3)
Females 2-5	50.3 (1.67)	5.3 (1.12)	10 (2.2)
Females 6-11	61.2 (1.14)	9.9 (1.23)	16 (2.0)
Females 12-19	61.9 (2.16)	12.2 (1.19)	20 (1.9)

Table 13.1. *Continued*

Gender and Age (y)		Total Intake	Intake From Quick-Service Restaurants	Percentages From Quick-Service Restaurants
Carbohydrates (g) (SE)				
Males	2–5	217 (5.2)	18 (3.0)	8 (1.4)
Males	6–11	270 (4.7)	31 (2.5)	12 (0.9)
Males	12–19	298 (7.9)	53 (5.8)	18 (2.1)
Females	2–5	186 (4.7)	20 (4.9)	11 (2.5)
Females	6–11	239 (5.9)	32 (3.6)	13 (1.6)
Females	12–19	220 (5.1)	36 (3.4)	16 (1.5)
Total Sugars (g) (SE)				
Males	2–5	104 (3.1)	5 (0.7)	4 (0.7)
Males	6–11	126 (2.8)	12 (1.4)	9 (1.0)
Males	12–19	139 (4.8)	20 (3.1)	15 (2.4)
Females	2–5	90 (3.2)	6 (1.3)	7 (1.4)
Females	6–11	107 (3.1)	11 (1.4)	10 (1.3)
Females	12–19	99 (2.5)	14 (1.6)	14 (1.6)
Dietary Fiber (g) (SE)				
Males	2–5	12.4 (0.48)	1.0 (0.10)	8 (0.9)
Males	6–11	15.0 (0.70)	1.7 (0.15)	11 (0.9)
Males	12–19	16.4 (0.43)	2.8 (0.23)	17 (1.5)
Females	2–5	10.8 (0.42)	1.1 (0.25)	10 (2.1)
Females	6–11	13.9 (0.51)	1.8 (0.22)	13 (1.7)
Females	12–19	12.5 (0.61)	1.9 (0.17)	15 (1.3)

Continued

Table 13.1. *Continued*

Gender and Age (y)		Total Intake	Intake From Quick-Service Restaurants	Percentages From Quick-Service Restaurants
Total Fat (g) (SE)				
Males	2–5	55.7 (1.27)	6.0 (0.59)	11 (1.1)
Males	6–11	76.2 (2.54)	11.2 (1.07)	15 (1.2)
Males	12–19	90.5 (1.59)	20.8 (1.94)	23 (2.0)
Females	2–5	51.9 (1.87)	6.6 (1.36)	13 (2.6)
Females	6–11	67.7 (1.22)	12.1 (1.43)	18 (2.0)
Females	12–19	64.2 (2.68)	13.6 (1.20)	21 (1.9)
Saturated Fatty Acids (g) (SE)				
Males	2–5	20.1 (0.57)	2.0 (0.21)	10 (0.9)
Males	6–11	28.5 (1.29)	4.1 (0.39)	14 (1.1)
Males	12–19	30.5 (0.82)	6.6 (0.53)	22 (1.6)
Females	2–5	18.8 (0.78)	2.3 (0.52)	12 (2.6)
Females	6–11	23.6 (0.52)	4.3 (0.58)	18 (2.3)
Females	12–19	21.3 (0.92)	4.6 (0.41)	22 (1.8)
Vitamin D (µg) (SE)				
Males	2–5	6.1 (0.52)	0.1 (0.02)	2 (0.4)
Males	6–11	6.1 (0.25)	0.2 (0.04)	2 (0.6)
Males	12–19	6.0 (0.30)	0.4 (0.05)	6 (0.9)
Females	2–5	5.6 (0.35)	0.2 (0.06)	4 (1.0)
Females	6–11	4.7 (0.10)	0.3 (0.07)	6 (1.4)
Females	12–19	3.7 (0.15)	0.3 (0.05)	8 (1.5)

Table 13.1. *Continued*

Gender and Age (y)		Total Intake	Intake From Quick-Service Restaurants	Percentages From Quick-Service Restaurants
Calcium (mg) (SE)				
Males	2–5	940 (33.6)	54 (6.0)	6 (0.6)
Males	6–11	1175 (41.5)	108 (7.9)	9 (0.5)
Males	12–19	1186 (35.4)	178 (14.7)	15 (1.2)
Females	2–5	926 (45.1)	72 (21.2)	8 (2.2)
Females	6–11	960 (28.1)	128 (22.2)	13 (2.1)
Females	12–19	842 (33.3)	138 (13.1)	16 (1.4)
Potassium (mg)				
Males	2–5	2019 (76.8)	129 (14.8)	6 (0.8)
Males	6–11	2332 (53.1)	235 (24.5)	10 (1.1)
Males	12–19	2665 (41.8)	450 (50.9)	17 (1.8)
Females	2–5	1811 (80.3)	146 (30.9)	8 (1.6)
Females	6–11	1962 (49.3)	250 (34.6)	13 (1.7)
Females	12–19	1873 (63.2)	296 (25.9)	15 (1.3)
Sodium (mg)				
Males	2–5	2396 (62.5)	280 (32.9)	12 (1.4)
Males	6–11	3185 (94.5)	445 (38.5)	14 (1.2)
Males	12–19	3960 (91.8)	894 (93.8)	23 (2.2)
Females	2–5	2110 (65.8)	272 (61.3)	13 (2.8)
Females	6–11	2767 (56.0)	492 (62.6)	18 (2.2)
Females	12–19	2844 (89.6)	556 (52.4)	20 (1.8)

Adapted from What we Eat in America, Table 49: Quick Service Restaurants: https://www.ars.usda.gov/ARSUserFiles/80400530/pdf/1314/Table_49_QSR_GEN_13.pdf. Accessed October 4, 2017. Data are from day 1 intake only.

are, Rehm and Drewnowski,[4] also using NHANES data, have shown temporal changes from 2003 to 2010 in fast food consumption by children 4 to 19 years of age. These data showed a significant decline in energy intake of 205 kcals/day, 109 kcals of which is attributed to a decline in consumption of foods from fast food restaurants. Also observed were decreases in solid fat and added sugar intakes, but there was no significant decrease in sodium intake.[4] Although these data are encouraging, intake of nutrients of public health concern (dietary fiber, vitamin D, calcium, and potassium) still fail to meet recommended dietary intakes.[4] Similarly, in a study of adolescents, consumption of fast foods has been associated with a lower likelihood of meeting dietary recommendations, with decreased intakes of vegetables, milk (boys), and fruits (girls) and increased intakes of total calories (girls), discretionary calories (boys and girls), and fat (girls).[24] This is consistent with findings from earlier studies.[21,25]

Accessibility of Nutrient Information on Food Consumed Away From Home

Americans are less likely to be aware of ingredients and nutrient content of foods prepared away from home compared with foods prepared in their own homes.[26] Menu labeling has been suggested as a way to make consumers more aware of foods that they consume away from home; and, in theory, improve their food choices. On March 23, 2010, the president signed into law the Patient Protection and Affordable Care Act (Pub L No. 111-148). Section 4205 of the Affordable Care Act amended section 403(q) of the Federal Food, Drug, and Cosmetic Act (FFDCA [21 USC 301]) to provide requirements for nutrition labeling for foods offered for sale at retail chains with 20 or more locations, regardless of ownership. On April 6, 2011, the US Food and Drug Administration (FDA) published the Food Labeling; Nutrition Labeling of Standard Menu Items in Restaurants and Similar Retail Food Establishments; Proposed Rule in the *Federal Register*.[27]

Restaurants covered by the ruling will need to provide energy information for standard menu items on menus and menu boards along with a succinct statement about suggested daily energy intake. Other nutrient information—total energy; energy from total-, saturated-, and trans-fat; cholesterol; sodium; total carbohydrates; dietary fiber; sugars; and protein must be available in writing on request. Although not yet mandatory, studies have looked at the theoretical and the actual impact on children and parents. A systematic review of the effect that menu labeling for "hypothetical food purchases in artificial environments" could be efficacious in reducing the total amount of food energy purchased for or by children and adolescents; however, "real-world" studies were less supportive.[28] Seven of the 11 available studies in that review were listed as "weak," and only one was deemed "strong," suggesting clearly the need for well-designed studies. A recent systematic review found that, in "real-life settings," qualitative symbols, such as traffic lights—green, yellow, and red may be more effective in helping individuals make better food choices[29]; however, this was not confirmed in a second review.[28]

For any nutrition labeling initiative to be successful, the public will need age-appropriately targeted nutrition education.[30] Intervention studies in the United States and South Korea showed that when provided with nutrition education and fast food menus with nutrition information, parents chose lower-energy meals for their children[31,32] but not for themselves.[32]

Association of Weight and Other Cardiovascular Risk Factors With Fast Food Consumption

The parallel rise of the fast food industry with the obesity epidemic has suggested to some that fast food consumption is a causative agent. This has been difficult to demonstrate conclusively because of a lack of consistent findings; a systematic review showed that only 1 in 5 studies in children demonstrated an association between body mass index (BMI) and the fast food environment.[33] A more recent review[34] suggested that consumption of "ultraprocessed foods," which included but was not limited to fast foods was associated with body fat in adolescents. This study, however, included "junk" (a nondefined term) and generic convenience foods, as well as individual foods including soft drinks/sweetened beverages, sweets, chocolate, and ready-to-eat cereals. A potential problem with this review is that some ultraprocessed foods, notably ready-to eat cereals, have consistently been shown to be associated with lower weights in children,[35] provide valuable nutrients,[36] and were associated with higher levels of milk and fruit consumption in children.[37] Some of the foods listed in the review, including sweetened beverages, have been positively associated with weight in some reviews, but not others.[20,38] Overall, however, a reduction in food consumed away from home has been associated with improved weight and body composition in children.[20]

There are studies linking fast food consumption with insulin resistance and other cardiovascular risk factors, including the metabolic syndrome in adolescents.[20,38–41] However, it is clear that all children who consume fast foods do not have these health issues. This may be related to how much and how often children eat energy-dense fast foods. Other notable variables include how much food was consumed from other sources and that consumers of fast foods may not have generally healthy eating habits.[42,43] Many fast food studies are cross-sectional in design and cannot be used to show a cause-and-effect relationship.[44] More longitudinal studies and randomized control trials are needed, particularly with larger samples of children from various ethnic groups and geographic locations, before any definitive conclusions can be made about the relationship of fast food consumption to childhood obesity. Despite the lack of a clear cause-and-effect relationship between consumption of fast food and overweight/obese status in children and adolescents, the American Academy of Pediatrics (AAP) recommends that eating at restaurants, particularly fast food restaurants, should be limited to help prevent pediatric obesity.[45]

Demographic and Other Factors Contributing to Fast Food Consumption

A number of studies have attempted to characterize who eats at fast food restaurants and why. Generally, those who are younger, employed, and living in large households are more likely to report eating fast food. Attempts to link gender, BMI, educational level, income, and race/ethnicity to fast food consumption have been inconclusive.[46]

A convenience sample of adolescents and adults[46] showed that overall, more than 50% of individuals (n=594) agreed or strongly agreed that they consumed fast food because it was quick (92.3%), it was easy to get (80.1%), they liked the taste (69.2%), they were too busy to cook (53.2%), or it was a "treat" (50.1%). Less than 50% of individuals agreed or strongly agreed that they consumed fast food because they did not like to prepare foods themselves (44.3%), their friends/family like fast food (41.8%), it was a way of socializing with friends and family (33.1%), they have many nutritious foods to offer (20.6%), and they were fun and entertaining (11.7%).

The family is a major influence on what young children and, to a lesser degree, what adolescents eat. Consumption of meals as a family has been associated with physical and psychosocial benefits to children.[47] The AAP recommends that families regularly eat meals together, without distractions such as television or the use of other "devices," as part of their childhood obesity prevention strategies.[48] The traditional pattern of the family eating at the kitchen table has changed over the years, with fewer families eating meals at home together. There has been an increase in the number of single-parent households and substantial growth in maternal employment over the past few decades. Households in which both parents work or in which there is a single parent have less time to prepare meals. Reliance on fast food is a convenient and relatively cheap alternative for these parents to feed their families. However, reliance on fast foods may undermine the benefits of a family meal.[47]

Media Influences and Product Branding and Fast Food Consumption

Public health experts have called for changes in the food environment to address the pediatric obesity epidemic and the overall poor diet in children and adolescents.[49] A principal concern is media marketing, especially of food-related products, to children. The volume of marketing for energy-dense, nutrient-poor foods targeted to children has been called one of the most "pernicious environmental influences on food consumption by youth,"[50] in part because most young children do not understand that the purpose of advertising is to sell them a product.[51,52] Foods advertised to children tend to be high in added sugars, SFAs, and sodium, which can contribute to obesity and other chronic diseases. Studies on children's choices have shown consistently that children exposed to advertising chose advertised food products at significantly higher rates than those not exposed.[53] As a corollary, children who watch more television tend to consume more energy than children who watch less.[54] Watching television may also influence food choice, with the foods selected being energy dense and nutrient poor.[55]

Children and adolescents live in a media-saturated environment. Television remains the principal vehicle for advertising.[56] Despite passage of the Children's Television Act of 1990 (Pub L No. 101-437), which places limits on advertising during children's TV programming hours, a 2007 survey reported that children are exposed to more than 40 000 television commercials/year,[57] of which approximately 5500 are food advertisements.[58]

There has been some improvement in television advertising food to children. The Children's Food and Beverage Advertising Initiative (CFBAI) is a voluntary, self-regulated program comprised of 18 of the nation's leading food and beverage companies and quick-service restaurants that works to shift the emphasis of foods advertised to children younger than 12 years to encourage healthier options.[59] The CFBAI lists of products and participating companies is available on its Web site.[59] The CFBAI has monitored food and beverage advertisements on the channel Nickelodeon, and from 2014 to 2016, the total number of televised ads decreased from 1274 to 1020, and the percentage of food ads of total ads decreased from 23% to 17%.[59] It should be noted, however, that although spending on television advertisements to children 2 to 17 years of age decreased by 19.5% from 2006 to 2009, food companies increased marketing efforts to children and adolescents in other media (eg, online, mobile phones) by 50%.

Advertising targeted to children and adolescents is not limited to television, and fast food companies are using newer forms of interactive media—for example, Facebook's social ad system and online videos.[60] A 2006 Institute of Medicine report[56] provided a comprehensive overview of the effect that media exposure can have on food preference, consumption, and obesity.

Environmental Influences on Fast Food Consumption

An obesogenic environment has been implicated in the dramatic increases in the prevalence of overweight in children of all racial and ethnic groups. As noted, children and adolescents have ready access to fast food restaurants. However, fast food restaurants are not the only source of available "fast foods"; neighborhood and convenience stores, gas stations, and even vending machines have similar foods for sale.[61]

Studies have suggested that fast food restaurants were more likely to be found in low-socioeconomic status (SES) areas than in middle- or upper-SES areas and in areas with higher concentrations of ethnic minority groups, including non-Hispanic black and Hispanic individuals, than in those with a higher population of non-Hispanic white individuals.[33] Locations of fast food restaurants have been implicated in the childhood obesity epidemic. In Chicago, IL, the median distance from any school to the nearest fast food restaurant was 0.52 km, and 78% of schools had at least 1 fast food restaurant within 800 m. There were 3 to 4 times as many fast food restaurants within 1.5 km from schools than would be expected if the restaurants were randomly distributed throughout the city.[62] Nearly all school children in New York City had high levels of access to fast food, and nearly 34% had a fast food restaurant within 400 m of the school. Low-income and Hispanic children had the highest level of access.[63] The effect that the proximity of fast food restaurants to schools may have on pediatric obesity is not clear, and it has been assumed that intake of these foods would be increased and that obesity would be more common[64] and that there would be higher levels of chronic disease, such as cardiac disease.[65] However, studies have failed to show these links to fast foods.[66-68] Burdette and Whitaker,[66] for example, showed that there was no relationship with the prevalence of overweight and the location of fast food restaurants.

However, their study was limited to preschool children, and further studies are needed to assess more fully the link between obesity in children and adolescents and the location of fast food outlets.

Virtually all schools in the United States participate in the National School Lunch Program (NSLP), and 92.2% of the schools participating in the NSLP participate in the National School Breakfast Program (see also Chapter 49). Schools participating in these programs are required to provide meals that meet strict dietary standards. Students participating in the NSLP have a higher intake of nutrient dense foods than students who do not[69]; however, many students do not meet dietary recommendations.[70] It is important to provide children with healthy food options at school rather than fast food options; and provide the nutrition education to help them make informed food choices (see also Chapter 9).

At any given time, approximately one third of all high school students are employed, at least part time. Although the majority of fast food workers are no longer teenagers, approximately 30% do still work in the industry.[71] These work sites may provide employee food discounts or free beverages during the work day; thus, many adolescents may eat meals on site during their shift, which may increase their intake fast foods.

Corporate Responsibility

As discussed earlier, some fast food restaurants have taken responsibility to improve the nutritional quality of their menu items, to modify advertising to children, and to make nutrition information about their foods easily available to the public. In addition, many fast food chains employ registered dietitians. Changes in their menu offerings include:

1) Offering water, milk, and juice as the beverage in kids meals on menu boards, in store, and in external advertising.
2) Offer customers a choice of side salad, fruit, or vegetable as a substitute for French fries in value meal bundles.
3) Packing innovations and designs that feature emphasis healthy choices that include fruit, vegetable, low-/reduced-fat dairy, whole grains, no added sugar, and decreased sodium content.

Other changes made by fast food restaurants to improve to improve dietary choices for children include making more product nutritional information available, using vegetable oil for all frying, offering grilled and broiled foods alongside their fried dishes, and reducing the sodium content of their products. However, an article appearing in the CDC's *Preventing Chronic Disease* that compared the CFBAI's 2014 lists of food and beverages approved to be advertised on children's television still found that 53% of the products did not meet the nutrition requirements and recommended that foods and beverages advertised to children continue to be monitored.[72]

Promotional items, especially toys, are often used to encourage children to choose fast food meals and encourage repeat business. Toys are often linked to television or movie characters or children's games[73] and are especially appealing to children.[74] On the positive side for toys, it has been shown in one study that when a toy was provided with a smaller-sized meal and no toy was provided with a larger sized meal, children opted for the toy and the smaller-sized meal.[75] If this study is confirmed, it is a potential strategy to encourage children to select smaller fast food meals containing healthier food items.

The CFBAI does not address child-targeted marketing through toys or other promotional items, and the National Restaurant Association Kids LiveWell program[12] does not include toys or other premiums as a part of its child-directed marketing policies. A list of participants in that program can be found on its Web site.[12] Table 13.2 provides information on where to find more about corporate efforts to improve the diets of children.

Table 13.2.
Where to Find More Information about Corporate Efforts to Improve the Diets of Children

Children's Food & Beverage Advertising Initiative (CFBAI) is a National Partner Program of the Better Business Bureau. There is a list of participants, along with the criteria that advertised foods must have. CFBAI updates it's Product Lists which lists foods and beverages that may be advertised to children under 12 years of age. Also available is a White Paper examining how these criteria were developed.
The National Academies of Sciences, Engineering, Medicine: Challenges and Opportunities for Change in Food Marketing to Children and Youth - Workshop Summary (2013) and **The National Academies of Sciences, Engineering, Medicine: Food Marketing and the Diets of Children and Youth** (2005) discuss a framework for marketing food and beverages to children.
Individual restaurants, restaurant chains, and food companies are also working to improved meals and foods served to children

Web sites accessed February 4, 2019.

Fast Food Summary—Going Forward

Fast food restaurants are an integral and pervasive part of our society. Three of 10 consumers state that meals away from home, including fast food meals, are essential to the way they live. Restrictive feeding practices in children have been associated with an increased preference for the forbidden foods[76] and have resulted in an increased intake when these foods were available.[77] Thus, it is important not to totally restrict fast food from the diets of children and adolescents if they wish to consume it occasionally. Parents, with the help of nutrition professionals, must teach children and adolescents to make the best choices at fast food restaurants by instruction and by modeling. Healthful choices for children at fast food restaurants include oatmeal or egg sandwich wraps and low-fat milk or 100% fruit juice for breakfast. For lunch and dinner, kids' meals with deli sandwiches, plain hamburgers, or grilled chicken with apple slices and 100% fruit juice or low-fat milk are healthful choices for young children. For older children and adolescents, healthful choices include plain hamburgers, grilled chicken, salads, chili, low-fat deli-style sandwiches, apple slices, 100% fruit juice, and low-fat milk. These foods should be associated with lower energy intake and improved diet quality and should not replace regular family meals at home.

Fast food restaurants and other outlets where these foods are sold must be sure that healthful foods and accurate nutrition information are available at the restaurant and on their Web sites. Responsible advertising to children must also be part of the corporate plan to improve the nation's health. Responsible advertising can be accomplished by advertising healthier menu options to children, emphasizing the importance of low-fat milk and other nutrient-dense foods in the diet. Sweden and Norway have an explicit ban on advertising targeted to children younger than 12 years; other countries also have limits on advertising to children. Although accessibility to global media through cable television and the Internet dilute the effect of this television advertising ban somewhat, it is still an important step. If marketing of fast foods to children cannot be stopped, then innovative advertising of healthful foods to children needs to occur.[78] Advertisement of healthful foods, like fruit and vegetables, may serve to increase awareness of these foods and increase consumption.

Organic Foods

What Are Organic Foods?

"Organic" is a production term and does not refer to characteristics of the foods themselves. Organic crop standards include that the land has had no prohibited substances applied to it for at least 3 years before the harvest of an organic crop. Use of genetic engineering, ionizing radiation, and sewage sludge is prohibited. Soil fertility and crop nutrients are managed through tillage and cultivation practices, crop rotations, and cover crops; soils can be supplemented with animal and crop waste materials and allowed synthetic materials. Crop pests, weeds, and diseases are controlled primarily through management practices including physical, mechanical, and biological controls. When these practices are not sufficient, a biological, botanical, or synthetic substance approved for use on the national list may be used.[79] Animals on organic farms eat organic feed, are not confined 100% of the time, and are raised without antibiotics or added hormones. Organic production is said to "promote and enhance biodiversity, biological cycles, and soil biological activity."[80]

In the United States, The Organic Foods Production Act of 1990 (OFPA) (Title XXI of the 1990 Farm Bill [Pub L No. 101-624])[81] originally mandated that the US Department of Agriculture (USDA): (1) establish national standards governing the marketing of certain agricultural products as organically produced products; (2) assure consumers that organically produced products meet a consistent standard; and (3) facilitate interstate commerce in fresh and processed food that is organically produced. Foods covered by this act are fruits, vegetables, mushrooms, grains, dairy products, eggs, livestock feed, meats, poultry, fish and other seafood, and honey.

The regulations have been modified several times, especially in Title 7, Part 205 of the Code of Federal Regulations. Regulations have been designed to respond to site-specific conditions by integrating cultural, biological, and mechanical practices that foster cycling of resources, promote ecological balance, and conserve biodiversity. If livestock are involved, the livestock must be reared with regular access to pasture and without the routine use of antibiotics or growth hormones; other regulations also apply.[81] Although the FDA does not define or regulate the term "organic" as it applies to cosmetics, body/personal care products, the USDA may regulate the term "organic through its National Organic Program regulation (7 CFR part 205).[82] Wines and textiles can also use organic labeling.

Labeling is strict for all organic products. Organic products must be "produced without exclusions according to the National List of Allowed and Prohibited Substances,[79] overseen by a USDA National Organic Program-authorized certifying agent, and follow all USDA organic regulations."[83] The accompanying wording of "100% organic" reflects a product that is 100% organic. Products with at least 95% organic ingredients (excluding added water and salt) can be called "organic." Note that for wine to be classified as "organic," it must not contain added sulfites. Products with at least 70% organic ingredients may say "made with organic ingredients;" and products with less than 70% of organic ingredients may list specific organically produced ingredients on the side panel of the product packaging but may not make any organic claims on the front panel. The name and address of the government-approved certifier must be on all products that contain at least 70% organic ingredients.

The USDA organic seal (Figure 13.1) is an official mark of the USDA Agricultural Marketing Service and is protected by federal regulation (7 CFR Part 205.311). There is a fine of up to $11 000 per violation for misuse. "The seal may not be used: 1) in any displays or on labels for products not certified organic according to the USDA organic regulations, 2) on broad display in stores or advertisements in a way that misrepresents non-organically produced products as organic, or by uncertified operations, or operations that have been suspended or revoked from organic certification."[84]

"Clear" Labeling Regulations May Lead to Consumer Confusion

Despite the clear labeling requirements for organic foods, consumers can be confused over a host of terms that imply that certain menus items are more healthful, free of additives, or "natural." This confusion has arisen because people are striving for healthier eating and because undefined terms are ill-defined in the media. If the consumer is aware and educated, foods labeled as organic have a clear definition. "Natural" is another confusing term, because all organic foods are natural, but not all natural foods are organic. Other terms, especially "clean," are not so clear, in part, because there is no standard definition.[85] The term clean has recently been used in food advertisements and is confusing and leaves the definition open to the consumer. For US consumers to be certain they are getting organic food, they need to look for the USDA Organic Seal.

Purchasing Trends for Organic Foods

Once sold only in premium markets or health food stores, organic foods are now widely available year-round in conventional supermarkets, and half

Figure 13.1.
The USDA Organic Seal. https://www.ams.usda.gov/rules-regulations/organic/organic-seal.

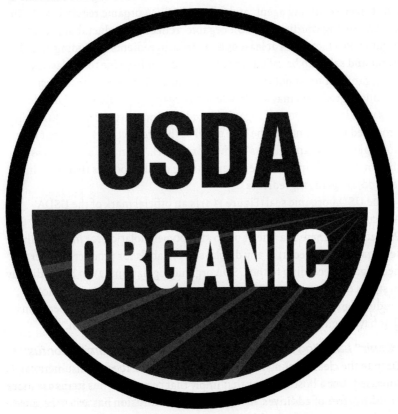

of all organic foods are purchased in supermarkets, club stores, or big-box stores.[86] Consumer demand for variety, convenience, and quality in fresh produce has boosted sales of organic foods and pressured farmers to expand acreage devoted to organic foods. The US organic food industry has grown substantially. Consumer demand for organic goods shows double-digit growth.[86]

Fresh fruits and vegetables have been the top selling category of organically grown food since the organic food industry started retailing products over 3 decades ago, and they are still outselling other food categories. Produce accounted for 43% of US organic food sales in 2012, followed by dairy (15%), packaged/prepared foods (11%), beverages (11%), bread/grains (9%), snack foods (55), meat/fish/poultry (3%), and condiments (3%).[86]

Organic produce is purchased at a premium price. The cost also varies with stores. For example, in a 2015 report, the percent difference between regular and organic apples per pound varied from +20% to +60%, ground beef per pound varied from +40% to +73%, and organic milk per half gallon varied from +20% to +67%.[87] Although prices have decreased somewhat over time, most are significantly more expensive than conventional meat, milk, and produce.[86]

Consumer Purchasing Behavior

In 2016, sales of organic foods were approximately $47 billion dollars; sales accounted for approximately 5% of total food sales and were 8.4% higher than in 2015.[88] On average, 82% of US households purchased organic products in 2016. Washington State had the highest percentage, with 92% of households making these purchases and Mississippi had the lowest with only 70% of households purchasing organic products.[88] Organic products are the fastest-growing section in the food industry. A survey of the shopping habits of more than 1800 families conducted by the Organic Trade Association showed that parents 18 to 34 years of age were the largest group of purchasers of organic foods in the United States.[89]

Consumer preferences for purchasing organic foods have been well reviewed[90] and include perceived benefits for environmental protection, supporting the local economy, animal welfare, food safety, perceived better taste, personal health or following an alternative lifestyle, and feelings of responsibility for one's family. Consumers are also willing to pay more money for organic foods because of their perceived health benefits. Perceived health benefits may apply more to some food groups than others; for example, chemicals in produce may engender more concern than chemicals in dairy products.[91]

Nutrients and Health Benefits of Organic Versus Conventional Foods

It is widely believed that organic foods are healthier and safer than conventional foods.[92,93] However, the effects of organic growing systems on nutrient bioavailability and nonnutrient components have received little attention, so this belief may not be evidence based. Many published studies comparing the nutrient content of organic to conventional produce have methodologic concerns. Natural products, including fruits and vegetables, vary in their nutrient content and nonnutrient substances. Moreover, it is difficult to compare studies performed over time, because regulations, recommendations, and analytical techniques vary.

The first systematic review of the literature that compared nutrient content between conventional and organic crops found that conventional crops had higher levels of nitrogen and organic crops had higher levels of phosphorus and higher titratable acidity. No other differences were found in the eight other nutrient categories examined (vitamin C, magnesium, potassium, calcium, zinc, copper, phenolic compounds, and total soluble solids). Differences observed were likely attributable to differences in fertilizers and ripeness at harvest rather than to any specific organic techniques used in production.[94] Some previous studies suggested higher levels of vitamin C were present in organically grown leafy green vegetables, peaches, tomatoes, and potatoes.[95] Overall, there is little convincing evidence that organic foods are more nutritious than conventional foods. Several recent meta-analyses have been published looking at compositional differences between organic and conventional meat.[96] Although for most nutrients, including minerals, antioxidants, and most individual fatty acids, the evidence base was too weak for meaningful analyses, concentrations of SFA and monounsaturated fatty acids were similar or slightly lower, respectively, in organic compared with conventional meat. Larger differences were detected for the increase in total polyunsaturated fatty acids (PUFAs) and omega-3 PUFAs in organic versus conventional milk. A similar analysis showed that organic milk had higher PUFAs, omega-3 PUFAs, conjugated linoleic acid, α-tocopherol, and iron but lower iodine and selenium concentrations than conventional milk.[97] Milk, however, is not a significant source of iron, iodine, or selenium.

No long-term studies have been conducted on the effects of consuming organic foods, and the Institute of Food Technologists,[98] the American Heart Association,[99] and the AAP[100] do not promulgate organically grown food as more healthful than conventional foods. Healthful foods, including fresh produce, whole grains, low-fat dairy, and antibiotic-free poultry may lead to health benefits, regardless of whether they are organic or not.

Nitrate Content of Organic Versus Conventional Foods

Nitrate is the main form of nitrogen fertilizer applied to crops. Nitrogenous fertilizers can, in turn, leech into the groundwater and contaminate well water and increase the nitrate content of food. Nitrate has low toxicity; however, nitrites and nitrosamines, conversion products of nitrates in foods, can cause adverse health effects. Nitrate-contaminated well water and vegetables high in nitrates have been shown to cause methemoglobinemia in infants, and this has been addressed by the AAP[101] (see also Chapter 52: Food Safety). The effects of the exposure to nitrates in drinking water on the incidence of birth defects, especially neural tube defects and cardiac anomalies, have also been reported[102]; however, the effect nitrate had in these studies was equivocal.

Nitrite and nitrate concentrations of organic and conventional vegetables from 5 metropolitan areas have been compared.[103] Although there were no differences in nitrite levels, there were differences in nitrate levels. Some differences were striking—for example, conventional broccoli from Raleigh, North Carolina, contained 553 mg/kg fresh weight (FW) of nitrate, compared with only 8 mg/kg in organic broccoli.[103] Other studies have also shown significantly lower levels of nitrates than in conventional crops.[104] However, levels of nitrates in plant foods are inconsistent and depend on the producer, crop, season in which the plants are grown, storage conditions, geographic location, and postharvest processing. Thus, it seems that the use of organic farming to reduce dietary nitrate intake is premature and not justified at this time.

Pesticides

A detailed look at the effects of pesticides on health is beyond the scope of this chapter (see also Chapter 52 for more information). However, some discussion is warranted as it relates specifically to organic foods. The 1993 National Research Council report "Pesticides in the Diets of Infants and Children" recognized that children have higher exposures and increased susceptibility to environmental toxicants, including pesticides.[105] Table 13.3 shows why children are more susceptible to environmental toxicants. Exposure to organophosphorus pesticides have been reported to have neurologic and neurodevelopmental effects in infants and children.[106,107] Data from the NHANES have suggested that children exposed to low levels of organophosphate pesticides, presumably through diet, were at higher risk of developing attention-deficit/hyperactivity disorder. The data also suggested that children received a continuous exposure to these pesticides.[108] Children tended to have diets high in foods that were potentially high in pesticide residues, including juices, fruits, and vegetables.[109]

The Food Quality Protection Act (FQPA) of 1996 (Pub L No. 104-170) amended the Federal Insecticide, Fungicide, and Rodenticide Act (FIFRA [Pub L No. 80-104]), and the US Federal Food, Drug, and Cosmetic Act (FFDCA) previously set high standards to protect infants and children from pesticide risks. Under the FIFRA, the Environmental Protection Agency (EPA) registers pesticides for use in the United States and prescribes labeling and other regulatory requirements to prevent unreasonable adverse effects on health or the environment. Under the FFDCA, the EPA establishes

Table 13.3.

Reasons Children Are at Increased Risk from Environmental Agents

Children have disproportionally higher exposures to many environmental agents.	Per unit weight, children drink more water, eat more food, and breathe more air than adults. Putting objects in their mouths and crawling or playing on the floor or ground also potentially contribute to higher exposures to pesticides.
A child's ability to metabolize, detoxify, or excrete environmental agents differs from adults.	Ironically, in some instances, children are protected against some agents, because they cannot make active metabolites required for toxicity.
Developmental processes are easily disrupted during rapid growth and development before and after birth.	
Children have more years of future life and this more time to develop diseases initiated by early exposures.	

Adapted with permission from Landrigan PJ, Kimmel CA, Correa A, Eskenazi B. Children's health and the environment: public health issues and challenges for risk assessment. *Environ Health Perspect.* 2004;112(2):257-265.

tolerances (maximum legally permissible levels) for pesticide residues in food. The Department of Health and Human Services/FDA enforces tolerances for most foods; the USDA Food Safety and Inspection Service enforce tolerances for meat, poultry, and some egg products. Conventional agricultural practices have changed over time, and consumer exposures to organophosphate pesticides and paradichlorobenzene are within EPA regulations and are consistent with safe food standards.

The FQPA explicitly requires the EPA to address risks to infants and children and to publish a specific safety finding before a tolerance can be established. It also provides for an additional safety factor (tenfold, unless reliable data show that a different factor will be safe) to ensure that tolerances are safe for infants and children and requires collection of better data on food consumption patterns, pesticide residue levels, and pesticide use.

The Organic Seal does not guarantee that the food products are free of pesticides. In the United States, for foods to be certified as organic, no synthetic pesticides can have been applied to the land for at least 3 years, and a "sufficient buffer zone" must also be in place to reduce the risk of contamination from conventional farming operations. However, unless products were grown under a cover, they could still become contaminated with pesticides. The persistence of pesticides in the environment was recently shown when organochlorine insecticides were shown to contaminate root crops and tomatoes[110] despite that these pesticides had been off the market for 20 years. Pesticide contamination of organic foods can occur from cultivation of previously contaminated soil, percolation of chemicals through soils, wind-drift, groundwater or irrigation water, or during transport, processing, or storage. Thus, contrary to popular belief, organic foods can be contaminated by pesticide residues; however, they are less likely to be contaminated than foods grown using conventional methods.[111,112] One report that compared results from 3 studies showed that organic crops were 10 times less likely to be contaminated with multiple pesticide residues.[111] However, it is important to recognize that measured levels of permitted pesticides are low and often undetectable in both organic and conventional foods.

Intuitively, it would seem that eating organic produce would reduce levels of pesticide residues in children; however, few data support this supposition. Several studies have used biological monitoring to examine dietary exposures to pesticides in children.[113,114] In a study of children 2 to 5 years of age (n=39), it was shown that those consuming primarily organic produce had levels of total dimethyl metabolites in their urine that were significantly lower than those who consumed conventional produce.[113] In a crossover study of 23 children 3 to 11 years of age, Lu et al[115] demonstrated that children consuming a conventional diet during phase 1 (days 1–3) and phase 3 (days 9–15) of the study had significantly higher organophosphorus pesticide levels than when they ate an organic diet during phase 2 of the study, days 4 through 8. A more recent study showed that long-term dietary exposure to organophosphate pesticides in the Multi-Ethnic Study of Atherosclerosis (n=4666) showed that lower levels of urinary dialkylphosphate were seen in more frequent consumers of organic foods.[116] These studies, although most of them are small, provide tantalizing information about the potential effects that consuming organic foods has on pesticide levels. What these studies do not show is a long-term health benefit to consuming organic foods or demonstrate any adverse health effects of consuming conventional foods.

Are There Adverse Health Concerns With Organic Foods?

The FDA has consumer information available explaining how to wash fresh produce to reduce the risk of foodborne illnesses http://www.fda.gov/downloads/Food/ResourcesForYou/Consumers/UCM174142.pdf

In theory, the small amounts of residual pesticides in both organic and conventional produce could pose a health threat for those consuming produce grown using either method. Ironically, the use of composted manure and the reduced use of fungicides and antibiotics in organic food production could lead to a higher level of contamination by microorganisms or microbial products. Whether organic foods are more susceptible to microbial contamination or whether they take up microbial contamination from organic manure is controversial. Organic foods, in common with conventionally produced foods, are not free from microbial contamination. In a study of vegetables sold in retail markets, the aerobic bacteria and coliform counts between organic and conventional produce were not significantly different; however, the occurrence of *Bacillus cereus*, which can cause gastrointestinal distress, was 40% higher in organic foods.[117] *Listeria monocytogenes*, which causes listeriosis, and *Escherichia coli*, another gut active pathogen, have been found on organically grown lettuce.[118] Organically grown chickens have not been shown to have less *Salmonella*[118,119] or *Campylobacter*[120] organisms than either conventional or free-range chickens. Although only a small sample, these studies suggest that foods bearing the Organic Seal must be treated, handled, and prepared in a manner consistent with reducing the risk of foodborne illness.

Organic Foods Summary and AAP Recommendations

Whether organic foods are safer or more nutritious or confer more health benefits than conventional foods is unclear, because studies are conflicting, but the preponderance of evidence suggests that organic foods are comparable in nutrient content and that both organic and conventionally grown foods have very low levels of approved pesticides. Organic foods are also subject to microbial contamination, like their conventionally grown counterparts, and must be treated, handled, and prepared in a manner consistent with practices that reduce the risk of foodborne illness. Because organic produce is not waxed, it may spoil more quickly—quick spoilage has been identified as a barrier to consumption of organic fruits and vegetables. However, the principal barrier to consuming organic foods is their higher cost.

> **AAP**
>
> "...organic diets have been convincingly demonstrated to expose consumers to fewer pesticides associated with human disease. Organic farming has been demonstrated to have less environmental impact than conventional approaches. However, current evidence does not support any meaningful nutritional benefits or deficits from eating organic compared with conventionally grown foods, and there are no well-powered human studies that directly demonstrate health benefits or disease protection as a result of consuming an organic diet. Studies also have not demonstrated any detrimental or disease-promoting effects from an organic diet. Although organic foods regularly command a significant price premium, well-designed farming studies demonstrate that costs can be competitive and yields comparable to those of conventional farming techniques. Pediatricians should incorporate this evidence when discussing the health and environmental impact of organic foods and organic farming while continuing to encourage all patients and their families to attain optimal nutrition and dietary variety consistent with the US Department of Agriculture's MyPlate recommendations."
>
> Forman J, Silverstein J; American Academy of Pediatrics, Committee on Nutrition, Council on Environmental Health. Clinical report: organic foods: health and environmental advantages and disadvantages.
>
> *Pediatrics.* 2012;130(5):e1406-e1415

At this time, there is no evidence-based information suggesting that organic foods have a nutrition or health advantage. The position of the AAP is clear on this issue:

In summary, it is important to consume a variety of foods to achieve nutrient adequacy and limit repeated exposure to a single contaminant, buy produce in season when possible, and use safe food–handling practices. Prepared products that use organic foods can also be high in fats and added sugars; thus, consumers need to read product labels to be able to make healthy selections.

Fad Diets

Fad Diet Overview

"Fads" refer to something that enjoys temporary popularity. Fad diets have been described variously as diets that make unrealistic claims, promise a "quick fix" and rapid weight loss, or eliminate foods or food groups, often stating these are toxic. One problem with these diets is that they are usually undertaken without medical advice or under medical supervision. This is of special concern for children and adolescents, because they may not disclose to parents or medical professionals that they are on a "diet" or they may be unaware of potential health risks. With the high prevalence of pediatric obesity, it is not surprising that children and adolescents may be driven to weight loss regimens including those that are untested or unsuitable for children or adolescents. There is a clear disparity between the number of children who are overweight, who perceive themselves as overweight, and those attempting to lose weight, suggesting that dieting practices to lose weight did not depend on actual overweight. These perceptions may lead to unhealthy weight loss practices, including fad diets (eg, the "military diet").

In 2011, a search on Amazon.com with the key words "weight loss" brought up 19 710 books. A 2017 search yielded 66 841 results. The overwhelming majority of these books describe what can be termed a "fad diet," and many are written by celebrities, rather than nutrition authorities. Table 13.4 describes how to determine whether a popular diet is actually a fad diet.

Table 13.4.
How to Determine Whether a Diet Is a Fad Diet

	Comment	*Example* = Sugar Busters
Step 1	Keep an open but informed mind. Many of the diets available on the market today are fad diets, but many are not. Do not automatically dismiss a popular diet as a fad diet.	*Sugar Busters* by H. Leighton Steward, Morrison C. Bethea, MD, Sam S. Andrews, MD, and Luis A. Balart, MD
Step 2	Look at the author(s) and their qualifications—are they trained in medicine or nutritional sciences or are they celebrity spokespeople?	3 medical doctors lend credence to this diet.
Step 3	Evaluate the overall tone of the writing—is it professional or is it biased?	The writing is casual, even for a popular press book— "How do I avoid getting arteriosclerosis? The answer is easy. Don't live long enough." And, "When the liver goes, 'Adios, Amigo'" are examples of this casual tone.

Table 13.4. *Continued*

	Comment	Example = Sugar Busters
Step 4	Understand the premise of the diet—is the diet low carbohydrate, low energy, low fat, or something else?	Is the effect of the diet biologically plausible? Yes and no. The diet is based on the glycemic index but makes comments like "insulin is toxic."
Step 5	Does the peer-reviewed literature support the effectiveness of the diet? Or do the authors rely on testimonials?	The authors of this book rely principally on testimonials; however, it should be noted that articles linking weight loss to eating low-glycemic index foods are beginning to appear in the peer reviewed literature. Long-term studies on the safety and effectiveness of these diets are lacking. There are other comments in the book that are of concern. For example, "Yet the standard diet recommended for patients with or at risk for coronary disease is to consume 80 to 85% of calories from carbohydrates with very low amounts of fat and protein!" This is clearly not consistent with recommendations from the National Cholesterol Education Program.
Step 6	Look at the claims the authors make. If it seems too good to be true…it probably is not.	There are no fantastic claims for this diet.
Step 7	Are any foods or supplements required for the diet? Are the authors of the diet selling their own foods or supplements? Are any health risks associated with the supplements?	There is a line of *Sugar Buster* products.

Continued

Table 13.4. *Continued*

	Comment	*Example* = Sugar Busters
Step 8	Are foods or food groups omitted?	Foods with high glycemic indices are omitted from this diet. Eliminating foods with simple sugars is an effective weight loss strategy; however, many wholesome foods like bananas, beets, and carrots are also eliminated.
Step 9	Is this diet potentially dangerous?	The diet is low in dairy and potentially low in fruits, vegetables, and fiber. The cumbersome schedule outlined for eating what fruits are allowed may limit intake.
Step 10	Are there any health warnings associated with the diet?	Yes, the authors do suggest that more carbohydrate foods may be needed for individuals with strenuous exercise schedules. There is no mention that insulin-dependent diabetics may need to adjust their insulin schedule. This diet should not be used by people with renal failure.
Step 11	Does the diet imply that weight loss and be maintained without physical activity and permanent lifestyle changes?	The diet encourages permanent lifestyle changes.
Step 12	Are there any good points associated with the diet?	Yes, there are many elements of this diet that can lead to weight loss. By omitting high-energy, simple carbohydrates, like cake and candy, as well as alcohol can eliminate many calories and lead to weight loss. *Sugar Busters* works principally because it is low energy.
Is this a fad diet? Yes, although elimination of foods high in simple sugars and the energy intake associated with this diet are likely to result in weight loss.		

Fad diets can be generally categorized in several ways: those that omit foods or entire food groups; those that require foods be consumed in a specific order or in a specific combination; those that are very low in carbohydrates and, hence, high in fat and protein; those with moderate carbohydrate content, which may incorporate principles of the glycemic index in carbohydrate selection; and those that are high in carbohydrates and, hence, low fat. Low-carbohydrate diets have emerged as perhaps the "most popular" of the fad diets, but it is not clear how many children and adolescents actually self-prescribe these diets.

Low-Carbohydrate Diets: The Classic "Fad Diet"

Dr. Atkins' New Diet Revolution, a very low-carbohydrate diet, is perhaps the most recognizable of the low-carbohydrate diets. Atkins diet books have sold more than 45 million copies. The proposed mechanism by which low-carbohydrate diets induce weight loss is that reduced carbohydrate intake lowers insulin levels, allows unrestrained lipolysis, increases lipid oxidation, and initiates ketone production, which in turn suppresses appetite. The Atkins diet is divided into 4 main phrases: induction, leading to rapid weight loss; ongoing weight loss when weight loss slows; premaintenance, with slow weight loss; and life-time maintenance. Energy levels are lowest during the induction phase and highest during maintenance, although all phases of the diet are low energy.[121] The carbohydrate content and the percent of energy from carbohydrates range from 15 g (3%) in the induction phase to 116 g (22%) of energy in the maintenance phase.

The rapid weight loss that is usually found at the outset of starting most low-carbohydrate diets results from diuresis as a result of mobilization of glycogen stores. It is not clear what actually causes the longer-term weight loss found in subjects on a low-carbohydrate diet. Authors of the diet books have suggested weight loss results because ketosis suppresses appetite or because the high protein levels suppress hunger and increase satiety. None of these factors has been confirmed, although other studies suggest that protein preloads significantly increased subjective ratings of satiety.[122] It has also been suggested that low-carbohydrate diets have less variety and are, therefore, less palatable, leading people to eat less. It is generally assumed, in the scientific community, that these diets are effective because they are low in energy and that diet duration is longer than other weight loss diets. Freedman et al[121] reported energy levels of 3 popular low-carbohydrate diets—the Atkins' induction diet (1152 kcals), the Carbohydrate Addict's Diet (1476 kcals), and Sugar Busters (1462 kcals). The majority of people will lose weight at these lower energy levels in the short term, regardless of the specific low-carbohydrate diet.

Other than ketogenic diets, used as a treatment for intractable epilepsy, none of the low-carbohydrate diets has been studied adequately or long-term in children and adolescents. A meta-analysis of 7 studies that looked at children 6 to 18 years of age (mean sample size of 71) treated in a hospital setting showed that only 3 of the studies reported an advantage of low-carbohydrate diets compared with low-fat diets. The effect of the low-carbohydrate diets on cardiovascular risk factors was also mixed.[123] An umbrella systematic review (n=16 systematic reviews) of treatments for pediatric obesity showed that low-carbohydrate diets had similar effects to low-fat diets in terms of BMI reduction (moderate quality of evidence).[124]

Health Concerns of Low-Carbohydrate Diets

Short-term effects of low-carbohydrate diets have been summarized by Freedman et al[121] and include bad taste, constipation, diarrhea, dizziness, headache, nausea, thirst, tiredness, weakness, and fatigue. It is unclear whether these are related to the low energy content of the diets or the composition of the diet. Ketoacidosis has also been reported.[125] There is also some evidence that in children, dietary restraint may be associated with decreased cognitive function.[126] Over a longer term, low-carbohydrate diets or other fad diets may not provide adequate energy for growth. This is a concern in the ketogenic diets used to treat some children with epilepsy (see Chapter 47: Ketogenic Diets) or, under medical supervision, some severely overweight children and adolescents. It is unclear whether lean body mass is spared in ketogenic diets.

Low-carbohydrate diets or other fad diets do not meet the dietary recommendations for children and adolescents[127] and are, therefore, not recommended for unsupervised use. Fruit and vegetable consumption in children is already low,[128] with some studies showing that when French fries are excluded, less than 20% of children ate the recommended number of fruits and vegetables a day.[129] If children or adolescents were to follow a low-carbohydrate diet, lack of fruits and vegetables could be exacerbated. Fruit and vegetable consumption has been associated with many health benefits; for example, fruit and salad consumption have been associated with lower diastolic blood pressure in adolescents.[130] It is important for children and adolescents to consume fruit and vegetables, because their dietary habits and health behaviors track into adulthood.[131] In adults, consumption of fruits or vegetables has been inversely related to the risk of chronic disease including some cancers,[132] coronary heart disease,[133] hypertension,[134] and type 2 diabetes mellitus.[135] Primary prevention through diet in childhood and adolescence may reduce the risk of these diseases in adulthood. Dairy foods, the major source of calcium in the diet, are also often omitted from low-carbohydrate diets. In the 2015 Dietary Guidelines for Americans,[136] calcium was identified as a nutrient of public health concern, because intake is low in many groups. Because low-carbohydrate diets are low in many wholesome foods, they also provide lower than recommended levels of vitamins A, E, and B$_6$; folate; thiamin; calcium; magnesium; iron; potassium; and dietary fiber.[121] For children older than 2 years, a diet containing fruits and vegetables, whole grains, low-fat and nonfat dairy products, beans, fish, and lean meats is needed to maintain health and support growth.[136]

The high-protein aspects of these diets, coupled with the lack of fruits and vegetables in the diet, pose concerns about bone health; however, the effect of dietary acid load in children and bone health is unclear.[137] There is also controversy whether high-protein diets in patients without renal disease damages the kidneys, although there is no evidence to substantiate this claim. Studies have not been performed in children or adolescents. It is clear that children with existing renal disease or diabetes with microalbuminuria or clinical albuminuria should not attempt a high-protein diet unless under medical supervision.

Medically Supervised Low-Carbohydrate Diets in Children: Lessons for Those on Fad Diets?

High-fat (90% of energy), low-carbohydrate (3% of energy) ketogenic diets are used to control seizures in children with epilepsy that are refractory to more traditional treatment (see also Chapter 47). Ketogenic diets have been reviewed recently.[138] In addition to the traditional ketogenic diet, a modified Atkins diet has also been used successfully to treat these children.[139] Children with higher levels of urinary ketones seem to have better seizure control than subjects reporting variable ketosis. Children on these diets may be deficient in calcium, magnesium, and iron. A major concern about these diets is that they adversely affect growth. It has also been shown[140] that the presence of urinary ketones adversely affects growth.

Early-onset adverse effects of ketogenic diets include hypertriglyceridemia, transient hyperuricemia, hypercholesterolemia, various infectious diseases, symptomatic hypoglycemia, hypoproteinemia, hypomagnesemia, repetitive hyponatremia, low concentrations of high-density lipoprotein, aspiration pneumonia, hepatitis, acute pancreatitis, and persistent metabolic acidosis. Late-onset adverse effects include growth abnormalities, osteopenia, renal stones, cardiomyopathy, secondary hypocarnitinemia, and iron-deficiency anemia.[141] These findings suggest that diets, including low-carbohydrate diets, that induce ketosis have the potential to cause potentially severe adverse reactions in children and should not be undertaken lightly or without medical supervision. These diets should not be undertaken unless under the guidance of a medical team. Children and adolescents, who self-select similar diets, should be counseled against this choice.

Gluten-Free Diets

A gluten-free diet has become the new popular fad diet of choice. A gluten-free diet, which is a diet that does not include wheat, barley, and rye, is the only effective treatment for celiac disease, nonceliac gluten sensitivity, and wheat (or barley or rye) allergy. Celiac disease is a genetic gluten-induced immune-mediated enteropathy. Although many symptoms are intestinal, celiac disease is a systemic disease with extraintestinal symptoms. Nonceliac gluten sensitivity has been diagnosed in individuals without celiac disease or wheat allergy but who have intestinal symptoms, extraintestinal symptoms, or both, related to ingestion of gluten-containing grains, with symptomatic improvement on their withdrawal.[142] Celiac disease is relatively uncommon, but the prevalence varies by country and has been reported to be as high as 1 in 37 and as low as 1 in 658. In the United States, the prevalence is approximately 1 in 100. There are 2 peaks of onset; one between 1 and 2 years of age and the other at approximately 30 years of age.[143]

If a gluten-free diet is so important in treating the symptoms of celiac disease, including diarrhea, vomiting, malabsorption, anemia, and failure to thrive in infants and very young children, and reducing long-term health risks, including osteoporosis, why is it included under the "fad diet" section of this chapter? In a Google Trend plot of search histories, interest in "celiac disease" as a search term has been consistent at approximately 10% of the search histories over the past 10 years; whereas, the popularity of the term "gluten free" has increased from 10% to nearly 100% in that time frame. Marketing research has suggested gluten-free diets have reached fad diet status, as by 2015, 25% of individuals reported consuming gluten free foods and estimated sales were $11.6 billion. These figures do not reflect the number of individuals with celiac disease or other diseases treated by this diet.[144]

Although virtually nothing is known about why children without celiac disease or nonceliac sensitivity consume gluten-free diets, some information is available on why adults choose to follow a gluten-free diet. The choice of an adult to eat gluten free may influence the diet of the entire household, including the children. In a 2015 survey of 1500 American adults, 35% gave no reason for "jumping on board the gluten-free fad" and an additional 26% thought it was a healthier option. In that survey, only 8% stated they had a gluten sensitivity and 10% said they had a family member with a gluten sensitivity.[145] Television and online advertisements, especially of ready-to-eat cereals, have also advertised gluten-free products heavily, especially to the parents of young children.

If gluten-free diets were benign, it would not be a problem if individuals preferred to eat this way for themselves or their children, but they are not. Gluten-free diets are very difficult and inconvenient to follow, even for those with celiac disease or nonceliac sensitivity; gluten-free foods are also more expensive than traditional grain foods. A social stigma has also been listed as a disadvantage, although with the burgeoning popularity of this diet, this has become less of a concern. There are a number of risks associated with this diet, including micronutrient deficiencies such as vitamins B_{12} and D, folate, iron, zinc, magnesium, and calcium as well as protein and dietary fiber.[146] Gluten-free foods are also higher in fat and carbohydrates.[146] Besides causing an actual nutrient deficiency, gluten-free diets can lead to health problems including constipation, weight gain, and a lower quality of life. However, the most important point is that following a gluten-free diet without the advice of a physician could lead to a missed diagnosis of celiac disease.[142] Parents who suspect their child has celiac disease, nonceliac gluten sensitivity, or a wheat allergy should consult their physician for a definitive diagnosis.

Other Types of Fad Diets

Table 13.5 reviews other types of fad diets, most of which are for weight loss, but some also promise improved quality of life or feeling of well-being. There is a paucity of evidence in children about the types of diets they may follow or of the effects of these diets, but the diets are available on the Internet and through books, and older children may elect to follow these diets.

Table 13.5.

Sample Fad Diets With the Basic Premise of the Diet[a] and Where to Find More Information About Them

Diet	Basic Premise of the Diet	Web Site[b,c]
Beverly Hills Diet—updated as the New Beverly Hills Diet	A diet in which food groups (carbohydrates, proteins, fruit, and fasts) must be consumed in a certain order with a waiting period between consumption of the next food group: fruit is consumed first, then carbohydrates, and then proteins. Milk is a protein food, so consumption is limited. Wine is categorized as a fruit (except champagne which is neutral).	https://www.diet.com/g/beverly-hills-diet https://www.webmd.com/diet/a-z/new-beverly-hills-diet
Blood Type Diet	This diet is based on consuming foods "compatible" with the participants' blood type. For example, individuals with type A blood should consume vegetarian meals; type B individuals should consume no chicken, but game meats, green vegetables, eggs, and low fat dairy; and type O individuals should focus on lean, organic meats, vegetables and fruit, and avoid wheat and dairy. Those with type AB should focus on tofu, seafood, dairy and green vegetables for weight loss, and avoid all smoked or cured meats. One problem here is that there are other blood groups, in addition to the ABO group; for example Rhesus.	https://dadamo.com/txt/index.pl?0000
Cabbage Soup Diet	A low-energy diet that is heavily based on consumption of low-energy cabbage soup.	https://www.cabbage-soup-diet.com

Cookie Diets: The Hollywood Cookie Diet and the Smart for Life Cookie Diet	Specially made cookies are consumed for breakfast, lunch, dinner, and snacks with a "sensible" dinner. The "Hollywood Cookie Diet has a free diet advice hotline."	https://www.webmd.com/diet/a-z/cookie-diet
Detox Diets	Although not necessarily for weight loss, detox diets purport to "cleanse" the body of endotoxins such as waste products from the gut or exotoxins, such as environmental toxins, pesticides, or phthalates. "Most detoxification programs recommend removing processed foods and foods to which some people are sensitive, such as dairy, gluten, eggs, peanuts and red meat, and eating mostly organically grown vegetables, fruit, whole nonglutinous grains, nuts, seeds, and lean protein. Other programs recommend fasting, a potentially risky practice for some people [especially for children], which may actually suppress detoxification pathways in the body."	http://www.eatright.org/resource/health/weight-loss/fad-diets/whats-the-deal-with-detox-diets
Grapefruit Diet (also known as Hollywood Diet)	This is a low-energy, protein-rich diet plan that focuses on consuming grapefruit or grapefruit juice at every meal. Most versions of the diet are approximately 1000 kcal. This diet can be harmful for those taking medications that interact with grapefruit or grapefruit juice.	https://www.healthline.com/health/grapefruit-diet#2

Continued

[a] None of these diets are nutritionally balanced and in compliance with the Dietary Guidelines for Americans.
[b] These are mostly commercial Web sites that may not be evidence based.
[c] All Web sites accessed January 21, 2019.

Table 13.5. *Continued*

Sample Fad Diets With the Basic Premise of the Diet[a] and Where to Find More Information About Them

Diet	Basic Premise of the Diet	Web Site[b,c]
HMR Diet[d,e]	This is a for-cost meal plan called *Healthy Solutions at Home* and uses a 3+2+5 structure with 3 HMR Shakes, 2 HMR Entrees, and 5 servings of fruit and vegetables. It also gives the option to eat more if hungry. A 3-week quick start kit is $201.65 and a Healthy Shakes 2-week starter kit is $111.15.	https://www.hmrprogram.com/learn-more-zip-code
Israeli Army Diet	An 8-day, rapid weight loss diet with very limited foods allowed: days 1 and 2 = apples; days 3 and 4 = cheese; days 5 and 6 = chicken; and days 7 and 8 = salad. Coffee and tea are allowed daily. Note: this is not followed by the Israel Defense Forces.	https://www.dietsinreview.com/diets/isreali-army-diet
Junk Food Diet	This diet is largely made up of foods considered to be unhealthy, such as high-fat or processed foods. A daily multivitamin, whole milk, and a small serving of vegetables can be added.	https://health.usnews.com/health-news/diet-fitness/diet/articles/2010/09/29/junk-food-the-new-weight-loss-diet

Diet	Description	Web site
Military Diet	The Military Diet is a 1500-kcal diet split into 2 parts over a week—3 days on and 4 days off. The diet is Spartan—grains, protein, fruit, and vegetables, but has 1 cup of vanilla ice cream with each dinner.	http://themilitarydiet.com http://themilitarydiet.com/military-diet-plan
Paleo Diet	The Paleo Diet eschews grains, legumes (including peanuts), refined sugars, dairy, potatoes, processed foods, salt, and refined vegetable oils.	http://thepaleodiet.com
Simple Seven = The Green Smoothies Diet	Consumption of one daily green smoothie purports to overcome cravings for coffee and ice cream and help with weight loss. A cookbook is available to help individuals prepare a variety of green smoothies.	https://www.simplegreensmoothies.com/simple7

a None of these diets are nutritionally balanced and in compliance with the Dietary Guidelines for Americans.

b These are mostly commercial Web sites that may not be evidence based.

c All Web sites accessed January 21, 2019.

d The HMR diet was chosen as the best diet for weight loss and the best diet for fast weight loss in 2017 by US News and World Report.

e Meal plans such as HMR are similar in structure to Nutrisystem (https://www.nutrisystem.com/jsps_hmr/home/index.jsp) and Jenny Craig (http://www.jennycraig.com), in which food is delivered to the home, but may be supplemented with fresh fruit and vegetables.

Recommendations Concerning Weight Loss in Children (See Chapter 33: Pediatric Obesity)

No unsupervised weight loss program should be undertaken by children or adolescents. Overweight or obese children would be better served with medically supervised programs that rely on behavior modification techniques to improve diet and lifestyle. Because of the potential link to dieting, notably severe dieting and eating disorders, education programs in the schools should be established to alert children, adolescents, and their parents to potential dangers of fad diets or unsupervised attempts at weight loss. It is also important that physicians and registered dietitians discuss healthy weight and healthful dietary patterns with children, adolescents, and their parents. The Evidence Analysis Library of the Academy of Nutrition and Dietetics recommends a multicomponent weight management intervention for overweight or obese children with diet therapy, physical activity, and behavior modification.[147]

Use of Botanicals By Children and Adolescents

Background

Complementary and alternative medicine (CAM) or complementary and integrative medicine and health care practices are defined simply as those that are not presently part of conventional medicine. Included in CAM is phytotherapy, or using plant-derived substances to treat or prevent disease. Technically, plant parts, including leaves, stems, flowers, berries, rhizomes, or roots, are called botanicals. They are valued for their therapeutic qualities, flavor, or scent. The terms "herb" and "herbals" are often used interchangeably with botanicals; however, by definition, herbs are nonwoody, seed-producing plants that die to the ground at the end of the growing season. For the purposes of this review, the terms "herbals" and "botanicals" are used interchangeably.

The Dietary Supplement Health and Education Act (DSHEA) of 1994 (Pub L No. 103-417) created a new framework for supplements by defining a dietary supplement as "a product taken by mouth that contains a 'dietary ingredient' intended to supplement the diet. The 'dietary ingredients' in these products may include: vitamins, minerals, herbs or other botanicals, amino acids, and substances such as enzymes, organ tissues, glandulars, and metabolites. Dietary supplements can also be extracts or concentrates, and may be found in many forms such as tablets, capsules, softgels, gelcaps, liquids, or powders. They can also be in other forms, such as a bar, but if they are, information on their label must not represent the product as a conventional food or a sole item of a meal or diet. Whatever their form may be, DSHEA places dietary supplements in a special category under the general umbrella of 'foods,' not drugs, and requires that every supplement be labeled a dietary supplement. A 'new dietary ingredient' is one that meets the above definition for a 'dietary ingredient' and was not sold in the U.S. in a dietary supplement before October 15, 1994."[148]

Manufacturers are responsible for determining that the dietary supplements they produce or distribute are safe and that any representations or claims made about them are substantiated by adequate evidence to show that they are not false or misleading. Dietary supplements do not need approval from the FDA before they are marketed. Except in the case of a new dietary ingredient, for which premarket review for safety data and other information is required by law, manufacturers of dietary supplements do not have to provide the FDA with the evidence they relied on to substantiate safety or effectiveness before or after they market their products. Manufacturers also need to register pursuant to the Bioterrorism Act with the FDA before producing or selling supplements. In June, 2007, the FDA published comprehensive regulations for Current Good Manufacturing Practices for those who manufacture, package, or hold dietary supplement products.[149] These regulations focus on practices that ensure the identity, purity, quality, strength, and composition of dietary supplements, including vitamins, minerals, and herbal preparations.

Information that must be included on a dietary supplement label includes: a descriptive name of the product stating that it is a "supplement"; the name and place of business of the manufacturer, packer, or distributor; a complete list of ingredients; and the net contents of the product. In addition, each dietary supplement must have nutrition labeling in the form of a "Supplement Facts" panel, which must identify each dietary ingredient contained in the product. Because only drugs can make such claims, dietary supplements must bear on the label that "This statement has not been evaluated by the Food and Drug Administration. This product is not intended to diagnose, treat, cure, or prevent disease."[148]

Much of the information available about an herb or herbal supplement is available online; and it is important that parents and older children and adolescents can evaluate this information. The Office of Dietary Supplements of the National Institutes of Health[150] provides information on how to assess information on the Internet and has a downloadable app to make the material more available. The site also explains how to spot a health fraud.

Herbal Medicines

Herbal medicines are widely available in drugstores, in supermarkets, and over the Internet, and their sales are increasing. In 2015, sales of herbal dietary supplements were estimated at almost $7 billion,[151] compared with $5.2 billion in 2010.[152] It is not clear what percentage of these sales were made to children and adolescents; however, in a 2012 survey of complementary health approaches among children 4 to 17 years of age (n=10 218), 11.6% of children used some type of alternative medicine. The study showed that 5.2% of males and 4.6% of females used nonvitamin, nonmineral dietary supplements. Garlic supplements, combination herb pills, ginseng, cranberry, and glucosamine or chondroitin were used by approximately 0.1% of children.[153] CAM use among children could be higher than reported, especially among adolescents, because some children and adolescents may neglect to tell their parents they are using CAM.[154] Children are more than 5 times more likely to use CAM, including herbals, if their parents use them.

Herbal medicines are available in several forms. Children may consume teas, which are made by pouring boiling water over herbal parts, such as the leaves or flowers, and allowing them to steep. Decoctions are similar; they are made by boiling parts of the herb, usually woody parts like roots or bark, in water and then straining and drinking the extract. Tinctures are hydroalcoholic or glycerol solutions that usually contain 1 to 2 g of active ingredient(s)/mL of solution. Fluid extracts contain a ratio of 1 part solvent to 1 part herb; these are more concentrated than tinctures. Powdered herbs can be pressed into tablets or made into capsules. Salves, ointments, shampoos, and poultices can also be used for external use. Aromatherapy uses inhalation of volatile oils from herbs to treat illnesses or reduce stress.

Aside from their classification as dietary supplements, herbal medicines differ from conventional medicines in other ways. In common with other plant extracts, herbals are not limited to a single agent, and the actual therapeutic component(s) and mechanism of action may not be known. Herbs can be grown, harvested, processed, and sold by anyone. The concentration of active ingredients is influenced by growing conditions, time of harvest, and storage and processing. The species used may be in question if herbs are harvested locally using common names. Finally, herbal medicines have not been subjected to the rigorous clinical trials that traditional medicines have. Previously, "caveat emptor" (or buyer beware) was the advice that consumers needed to heed when purchasing herbals as studies showed that the assayed species content was inconsistent with the content on the label.[155,156] As regulatory controls such as the FDA's comprehensive regulations for Current

Good Manufacturing Practices have been implemented and improved analytical techniques to assess bioactive constituents of herbal preparations have been applied, the standardization of herbal preparations appears to have improved.

Specific Uses of Botanicals by Children and Adolescents

Seventy percent of the world's sick or injured children are treated, often by physicians, using CAM; these treatments include use of traditional herbal medicines. In the United States, use of botanicals is self-selected, and most dietary supplements marketed to children and adolescents are vitamin and mineral preparations, not herbals. However, there are some mixtures of herbal preparations marketed specifically to children, including: honeysuckle flower, European elder berry, lemon balm leaf, chamomile flower, catnip aerial parts, *Echinacea purpurea* root and leaf, cassia twig, and licorice root. Another that is marketed as an "immune protect" contains astragalus root, baizhu atractylodes rhizome, and siler root. Another product with extracts of ginger root, fennel seed, and chamomile flowers is marketed for teething infants, including those as young as 0 to 1 month of age.

Botanicals are used by children and adolescents because of dissatisfaction with conventional medicine, fear of adverse effects of conventional medicine, perceived benefits, and the belief that herbals are "more natural" and, therefore, safer than conventional medications. In 2012, the most commonly used nonvitamin, nonmineral, natural products used by children for health reasons in the past 30 days were *Echinacea* (0.8%), fish oil (0.7%), and combination herb pill (0.5%). In children, natural products were used for back or neck pain, head or chest colds, anxiety or stress, and other musculoskeletal problems.[153]

In children, use of nontraditional and potentially toxic products, such as turpentine, pine needles, and cow chip tea, has also been reported.[157] Other studies have reported aloe vera, chamomile, garlic, peppermint, lavender, cranberry, ginger, *Echinacea*, lemon balm/grass, licorice, goldenseal, St. John wort, gingko, sweet oil, and milk thistle as common botanicals taken by children (and their caregivers).[157–159] Table 13.6 reviews some of the natural products commonly used in pediatric populations.

Fewer than 50% of children, adolescents, or their parents informed their primary health care professional about herbal use, because they did not believe botanicals would have adverse effects or that they could interact with conventional medications. Many patients who did try to discuss use of botanicals with health care professionals were not given information to

Table 13.6.
Natural Products That Are Commonly Used by Pediatric Populations

Natural Products	Use	Comments
Aloe (*Aloe ferox*)	Internal: purgative External: burns and other skin conditions	Internal use is contraindicated in children younger than 12 y because of potential for diarrhea, dehydration, and electrolyte loss.
Chamomile (*Anthemis nobilis*)	Internal uses: gastrointestinal distress—indigestion, colic, heartburn, anorexia, diarrhea External: swelling, inflammation	Allergic reactions. Inhibits cytochromes, potentially leading to drug interactions or toxicities. May be effective in treatment of infantile colic.
Combination herb pill	These are made up of different herbs	Some herbs may have side effects and may interact with other dietary supplements or medications. Parents should know that their children are taking these and what the specific combination is; they should also be aware that these pills may not have been tested for safety or efficacy in children.
Cranberry (*Vaccinium macrocarpon*)	Primarily used for urinary tract infections, also used for *Helicobacter* infections	Appears safe, but excess amounts can lead to stomach upset and diarrhea.
Echinacea (*Echinacea angustifolio*; *Echinacea purpurea*)	Colds, flu, coughs, bronchitis, fever, immune stimulant	Not recommended for individuals with autoimmune disorders. Allergic reactions may occur in some individuals. No benefit for upper respiratory infection has been shown for children from 2 to 11 y.
Fish oil/Omega-3 fatty acids	Fish oil contains omega-3 fatty acids (specifically docosahexaenoic acid [DHA] and eicosapentaenoic acid [EPA]) that may be important for children's brain and eye development	DHA and EPA are found in most seafoods, with the highest amounts in "oily" or "fatty" fish like tuna, salmon, mackerel, herring, and sardines. Dietary sources are a better source of these nutrients than supplements. Fish oil supplements can cause adverse effects including belching, bad breath, heartburn, nausea, and loose stools.

Herb	Uses	Notes
Garlic (*Allium sativum*)	Internal: colds, bronchitis, fever, hypertension, dyslipidemia. External: antibacterial, antifungal	Not well studied in children. Possible adverse effects include: allergic reaction, stomach disorders, odor of skin or breath, diarrhea, and rash. Dysrhythmias have also been reported.
Ginger (*Zingiber officinale*)	Anti-nausea, motion sickness, indigestion, anti-inflammatory, headache	Has been used in children undergoing cancer chemotherapy. Allergic reactions are seen, as is heartburn, if taken in excess. Ginger may interfere with blood clotting although there are no reports of interactions with blood-thinning medications; there is a report of a ginger and drug bezoar small bowel obstruction.
Ginkgo (*Ginkgo biloba*)	Asthma, bronchitis, tinnitus, multiple sclerosis, memory improvement	Adverse effects include headache, nausea, gastrointestinal upset, diarrhea, dizziness, and allergic skin reactions. There is an increased risk of bleeding, and ginkgo is contraindicated in patients taking anticoagulants.
Ginseng Asian ginseng (*Panax ginseng*) American ginseng *Panax quinquefolius*	Asian ginseng has been studied for lowering blood sugar levels and improving immune function. American ginseng: stress, immune system "boost," stimulant, infections, and gastrointestinal upset	*Panax ginseng* should not be given to children because of possible side effects, including insomnia and gynecomastia (in boys).
Melatonin	Sleep disorders	Better solutions to sleep disorders in children may be a set bedtime routine, avoiding caffeine, and limiting screen time.

Principally taken from: Black LI, Clarke TC, Barnes PM, Stussman BJ, Nahin RL. Use of complementary health approaches among children aged 4-17 years in the United States: National Health Interview Survey, 2007-2012. *Natl Health Stat Rep.* 2015;(78):1-19 help them make an informed decision about use and instead got information from friends or relatives. Most pediatricians surveyed believe their patients use CAM, but few ask about use. Physicians with a higher comfort level discussing CAM therapies with patients were more likely to discuss it with patients; however, fewer than 5% of physicians surveyed felt very knowledgeable about CAM and its use, and most believe that they need more education.[160] Because use of botanicals can pose health risks, especially in children, it is important that physicians are knowledgeable about botanicals and their effects, possible toxicities, and potential interactions with conventional medication. It is also important that they ask parents and children about their use. Parents and older children should disclose the use of any herbals children are taking—along with conventional medications.

Botanical Use and Potential Risks and Benefits in Children With Surgery or Chronic Health Problems

Use of CAM by children, especially those scheduled for surgery or with chronic conditions, is increasing. The percentage of children or adolescents using herbals that were surgical patients varies greatly, ranging from as few as 3.5% or 4%[161] to as many as 12.8%.[162]

Echinacea was the most commonly reported herbal used by children presenting for elective surgery. Up to 42% of these children were also using conventional medications. The recommended preoperative discontinuation times of botanical vary, but in general, it is recommended that any herbal medication be discontinued 2 weeks in advance of elective surgery. CAM use, including the use of botanicals, is up to 3 times more common in children with chronic disease, including asthma, inflammatory bowel disease and other gastrointestinal diseases, and cancer or recurrent diseases. It is especially important to assess potential benefits and risks of botanical use in these children.

Up to 29% of children with asthma use botanicals. Although they were perceived as being safe, use of botanicals has been associated with persistent asthma, use of high-dose inhaled or oral steroids, poor or very poor control of symptoms, more frequent doctor visits, and increased risk of hospitalization.[163-167] Some clinical trials have supported the use of an herbal preparation called Food Allergy Herbal Formula-2 (FAHF-2) for food-allergic reactions in children.[168,169] Meta-analyses, however, have suggested that there were insufficient data supporting the safety and efficacy of herbal preparations for the treatment of asthma, and what data were available were suggestive of only subjective improvement and were usually not supported by objective findings.[170] It should also be noted that although some treatments, like quail eggs, are benign, others, like lobelia, possibly pennyroyal mint, and tree tea oil, are potentially toxic.

A study in Australia suggested that as many as 72% of children with inflammatory bowel disease used CAM[171]; however, each child used an average of 2.4 therapies. Probiotics (78%) and fish oil (56%) were the most commonly used products; however, (unidentified) herbal therapies were used by 8% of children. Only a minority of patients believed the treatments were efficacious.[172] Other studies have shown the prevalence of children with inflammatory bowel disease using CAM treatments is below that of generally healthy children. A wide variety of CAM therapies are used by children with cancer. One study showed that 35% of pediatric cancer patients used herbals.[173] In most surveys, these therapies are used as adjunct therapies rather than primary ones. Ginger, an antiemetic, may benefit children undergoing highly emetogenic cancer chemotherapy treatments.[174]

However, herbals also have the potential to interact with traditional pharmaceuticals.[175] Herbs with the highest likelihood of this include those that modulate the activity of drug-metabolizing enzymes, especially cytochrome p450 isoenzymes and the drug transporter P-glycoprotein.[176] Thus, it is critical for parents to discuss with health care professionals any herbal medications their children are taking.

Herbal medicines also have more novel uses for children. A sugar-free lollipop containing Glycyrrhiza A from licorice roots was developed to reduce the risk of cariogenic bacteria[177] and, with twice-a-day use, was shown to work in children at high risk of dental caries. Ginkgolide B complex may be useful as a prophylaxis for migraine symptoms in children.[178]

Safety of Botanicals in Children

A wide variety of drug-herbal or food-herbal adverse effects and toxicities has been reported; however, very little is known about this in children and adolescents. Randomized controlled trials are lacking; the few that have been performed are difficult to interpret, because the herbals were not always characterized, making it difficult to understand fully any therapeutic effects or any adverse effects.

Of major concern is that in the United States, herbals are self-prescribed, usually without an understanding of their potential toxicity or adverse effects. Moreover, dosages for children are unknown and may differ from those appropriate for adults. Infants and children differ from adults in the absorption, distribution, metabolism, and excretion of drugs, including herbals. Few studies have been conducted in children.

The developing central nervous system and immune system of young children may make them more susceptible to adverse effects of herbals. Paradoxically, young children may be more efficient in detoxifying these substances, but the growing number of reports of hepatotoxicity of herbals is of concern.[179] Laxatives, such as aloe and senna, and diuretics, including fennel and licorice, have the potential to cause dehydration and electrolyte imbalances in infants and young children. Children are also at high risk of developing allergic reactions to commonly used herbs, such as *Echinacea* and chamomile, both members of the family *Compositae*.

The effect of long-term exposures of herbals on the fetus and breast-feeding infants is unknown. Woolf[180] reviewed a case of a newborn infant whose mother drank senecionine-containing herbal tea daily during her pregnancy. The infant was born with hepatic vaso-occlusive disease; senecionine is one of the pyrrolizidine alkaloids associated with hepatic venous injury. Comfrey is an example of an herb containing pyrrolizidine; although oral comfrey preparations have been banned from the US and European markets, topical preparations are still available.

German Commission E[151] listed aloe, buckthorn, camphor, Cajeput oil, cascara sagrada bark, eucalyptus leaf and oil, fennel oil, horseradish, mint oils (external), nasturtium, rhubarb root, senna, and watercress as contraindicated in children. More research is clearly needed to establish the safety and efficacy of botanicals in children.

Resources and Recommendations

Herbals have been used for centuries and are still used by the majority of the world's children. As use in the United States continues to grow, it is critical that reliable information be available to parents, adolescents, and physicians. Rigorous scientific studies should be conducted to determine the safety and efficacy of phytotherapy in children and adolescents.

Practitioners should be familiar with the Natural Medicines Comprehensive Database, which provides information on product specific efficacy and safety data.[181] The National Center for Complementary and Integrative Health[182] provides information on herbs, including uses and adverse effects; evidence-based medicine, continuing education, and clinical practice guidelines; and how to find practitioners. The Dietary Supplement Label Database provides information on herbals, randomized controlled trials, adverse effects, and manufacturers.[183] The Office of Dietary Supplements also provides dietary supplement fact sheets, definition of terms, and health professional fact sheets.[150] Courses on CAM, including phytotherapy, should be offered as part of the education of pediatricians and pharmacists, and health care professionals should be prepared to discuss CAM therapies with their patients.

Parents or caregivers may not tell pediatricians or other health care professionals that their child is receiving CAM. It is important, however, that parents or caregivers speak with their child's health care professional about any CAM therapy being used or considered. Full disclosure will help manage their child's health and will help ensure coordinated and safe care. The National Center for Complementary and Integrative Health provides online and printed information describing how patients can talk to their health care professional about CAM.[181] Points to consider for parent/health care professional discussions on CAM, taken from the National Center for Complementary and Integrative Medicine Web site, are shown in Table 13.7. Other sources of reliable information about herbals are presented in Table 13.8. All health care professionals should ask pediatric surgical and medical patients about use of CAM, especially herbals.

Table 13.7.
Points to Consider When Considering Complementary and Integrative Medicine Use for Children

Selecting a Complementary Health Practitioner
If you are looking for a complementary health practitioner for your child, be as careful and thorough in your search as you are when looking for conventional care. Be sure to ask about the practitioner's:
- Experience in coordinating care with conventional health care providers.
- Experience in delivering care to children.
- Education, training, and license. For more information on credentialing, see the NCCIH Web site.

Additional points to consider:
- Make sure that your child has received an accurate diagnosis from a licensed health care provider.
- Educate yourself about the potential risks and benefits of complementary health approaches.
- Ask your child's health care provider about the effectiveness and possible risks of approaches you're considering or already using for your child.
- Remind your teenagers to talk to their health care providers about any complementary approaches they may use.
- Do not replace or delay conventional care or prescribed medications with any health product or practice that hasn't been proven safe and effective.
- If a health care provider suggests a complementary approach, do not increase the dose or duration of the treatment beyond what is recommended (more isn't necessarily better).
- If you have any concerns about the effects of a complementary approach, contact your child's health care provider.
- As with all medications and other potentially harmful products, store dietary supplements out of the sight and reach of children.
- The NCCIH Web site offers safety tips on dietary supplements and mind and body practices for children and teens.
- Tell all your child's health care providers about any complementary or integrative health approaches your child uses. Give them a full picture of what you do to manage your child's health. This will help ensure coordinated and safe care.

From: National Institutes of Health. National Center for Complementary and Integrative Medicine. Children and the Use of Complementary Health Approaches. Available at: https://nccih.nih.gov/health/children#consider. Accessed January 21, 2019.

Table 13.8.
Where To Get Reliable Information About Herbs

Books
Awang DVC. *Tyler's Herbs of Choice: The Therapeutic Use of Phytochemicals.* 3rd ed. Boca Raton, FL: CRC Press; 2009. ISBN:13-978-0-7890-2809-9 Foster S, Tyler VE. *Tyler's Honest Herbal: A Sensible Guide to the Use of Herbs and Related Remedies.* 4th ed. New York, NY, and London, England: Routledge; 1999. ISBN-13: 978-0789008756 Herr SM. *Herb-Drug Interaction Handbook.* 3rd ed. New York, NY: Church Street Books; 2005. ISBN: 0-9678773-2-6 *PDR for Herbal Medicine.* 4th ed. Montvale, NJ: PDR Network; 2004. ISBN-13: 978-1563635120
Online Databases Agricola: http://agricola.nal.usda.gov Amazon Plants Tropical Plant Database: http://www.rain-tree.com/plants.htm American Indian Ethnobotany Database: http://naeb.brit.org Botanical Dermatology Database: http://bodd.cf.ac.uk Dr. Duke's Phytochemical and Ethnobotanical Databases: https://phytochem.nal.usda.gov/phytochem/search FDA Poisonous Plant Database: https://www.accessdata.fda.gov/scripts/plantox Garden Gate: Roots of Botanical Names: http://www1.biologie.uni-hamburg.de/b-online/library/glossary/botrts0.htm Medical Herbalism: Poisonous Plant Database: http://medherb.com/POISON.HTM NAPRALERT: https://www.napralert.org Natural Standard: http://www.naturalstandard.com Plants Database: https://plants.usda.gov/java Plants for a Future Database Search: http://www.pfaf.org/user/plantsearch.aspx Poisonous Plant Database (PLANTOX): https://www.accessdata.fda.gov/scripts/plantox. PubMed: https://www.ncbi.nlm.nih.gov/pubmed
Reliable Information About Botanicals on the Internet The American Herbalist Guild: http://www.americanherbalistsguild.com American Herbal Products Association: http://www.ahpa.org American Botanical Council: http://www.herbalgram.org Herb Research Foundation: http://www.herbs.org Food and Drug Administration: http://www.fda.gov MedLine Plus Health Information Drugs and Supplements: http://www.nlm.nih.gov/medlineplus/druginformation.html National Center for Complementary and Integrative Medicine: https://nccih.nih.gov Office of Dietary Supplements, National Institutes of Health: http://dietary-supplements.info.nih.gov World Health Organization: http://www.who.int/en

All Web sites accessed January 21, 2019.

References

1. Statista. Number of establishments in the United States fast food industry from 2004 to 2018. Available at: https://www.statista.com/statistics/196619/total-number-of-fast-food-restaurants-in-the-us-since-2002. Accessed June 23, 2017

2. US Department of Agriculture, Economic Research Service. Food Expenditures Overview. Available at: http://www.ers.usda.gov/data-products/food-expenditures.aspx. Accessed June 23, 2017

3. Schoffman DE, Davidson CR, Hales SB, Crimarco AE, Dahl AA, Turner-McGrievy GM. The fast-casual conundrum: fast-casual restaurant entrées are higher in calories than fast food. *J Acad Nutr Diet.* 2016;116(10):1606–1612

4. Rehm CD, Drewnowski A. Trends in consumption of solid fats, added sugars, sodium, sugar-sweetened beverages, and fruit from fast food restaurants and by fast food restaurant type among US children, 2003–2010. *Nutrients.* 2016;8(12):E804

5. Cohen JF, Roberts SB, Anzman-Frasca S, et al. A pilot and feasibility study to assess children's consumption in quick-service restaurants using plate waste methodology. *BMC Public Health.* 2017;17(1):259

6. US Department of Agriculture, Agricultural Research Service. What we Eat in America 2013–2014. Available at: https://www.ars.usda.gov/northeast-area/beltsville-md/beltsville-human-nutrition-research-center/food-surveys-research-group/docs/wweia-data-tables. Accessed June 23, 2017

7. US Department of Agriculture. National Health and Nutrition Examination Survey. 2013–2014 Data Documentation, Codebook, and Frequencies. Diet Behavior & Nutrition (DBQ_H). Available at: https://wwwn.cdc.gov/nchs/nhanes/2013–2014/dbq_h.htm#DBD900. Accessed July 6, 2017

8. Mancino L, Todd JE, Guthrie J, Lin B-H. *How Food Away From Home Affects Children's Diet Quality. Economic Research Report No. ERR-104.* Washington, DC: US Department of Agriculture, Economic Research Service; October 2010

9. French SA, Story M, Neumark-Sztainer D, Fulkerson JA, Hannan P. Fast food restaurant use among adolescents: associations with nutrient intake, food choices and behavioral and psychosocial variables. *Int J Obes.* 2001;25(12): 1823–2833

10. Batada A, Bruening M, Marchlewicz EH, Story M, Wootan MG. Poor nutrition on the menu: children's meals at America's top chain restaurants. *Child Obes.* 2012;8(3):251–254

11. Hobin E, White C, Li Y, Chiu M, O'Brien MF, Hammond D. Nutritional quality of food items on fast-food 'kids' menus': comparisons across countries and companies. *Public Health Nutr.* 2014;17(10):2263–2269

12. The National Restaurant Association. Kids LiveWell Program. Available at: http://www.restaurant.org/Industry-Impact/Food-Healthy-Living/Kids-LiveWell/About. Accessed July 6, 2017

13. The National Restaurant Association. Healthy Dining. Available at: http://www.restaurant.org/Industry-Impact/Food-Healthy-Living/Healthy-Dining. Accessed July 6, 2017

14. Rolls BJ, Engell D, Birch LL. Serving portion size influences 5-year-old but not 3-year-old child's food intakes. *J Am Diet Assoc.* 2000;100(2):232–234

15. Diliberti N, Bordi PL, Conklin MT, Roe LS, Rolls BJ. Increased portion size leads to increased energy intake in a restaurant meal. *Obes Res.* 2004;12(3):562–568

16. Fisher JO, Rolls BJ, Birch LL. Children's bite size and intake of an entrée are greater with large portions than with age-appropriate or self-selected portions. *Am J Clin Nutr.* 203;77(5):1164–1170

17. Fisher JO, Liu Y, Birch LL, Rolls BJ. Effects of portion size and energy density on young children's intake at a meal. *Am J Clin Nutr.* 2007;86(1):174–179

18. Rehm CD, Drewnowski A. Trends in Energy Intakes by Type of Fast Food Restaurant Among US Children From 2003 to 2010. *JAMA Pediatr.* 2015;169(5): 502–504

19. Centers for Disease Prevention and Control, National Center for Health Statistics. Caloric Intake From Fast Food Among Children and Adolescents in the United States, 2011–2012. Available at: https://www.cdc.gov/nchs/data/databriefs/db213.htm. Accessed June 23, 2017

20. Altman M, Cahill Holland J, Lundeen D, et al. Reduction in food away from home is associated with improved child relative weight and body composition outcomes and this relation is mediated by changes in diet quality. *J Acad Nutr Diet.* 2015;115(9):1400–1407

21. Bowman SA, Gortmaker SL, Ebbeling CB, Pereira MA, Ludwig DS. Effects of fast-food consumption on energy intake and diet quality among children in a national household survey. *Pediatrics.* 2004;113(1 Pt 1):112–118

22. Lipsky LM, Nansel TR, Haynie DL, et al. Diet quality of US adolescents during the transition to adulthood: changes and predictors. *Am J Clin Nutr.* 2017;105(6): 1424–1432

23. Powell LM, Nguyen BT. Fast-food and full-service restaurant consumption among children and adolescents: effect on energy, beverage, and nutrient intake. *JAMA Pediatr.* 2013;167(1):14–20

24. Sebastian RS, Wilkinson Enns C, Goldman JD. US adolescents and MyPyramid: associations between fast-food consumption and lower likelihood of meeting recommendations. *J Am Diet Assoc.* 2009;109(2):226–235

25. Paeratakul S, Ferdinand DP, Champagne CM, Ryan DH, Bray GA. Fast-food consumption among US adults and children: dietary and nutrient intake profile. *J Am Diet Assoc.* 2003;103(10):1332–1338

26. Variyam JN. *Nutrition Labeling in the Food-Away-From-Home Sector: An Economic Assessment.* Washington, DC: US Department of Agriculture, Economic Research Service; 2005

27. Food Labeling; Nutrition Labeling of Standard Menu Items in Restaurants and Similar Retail Food Establishments; Proposed Rule. *Fed Regist.* 2011;76(66): 19191–19236

28. Sacco J, Lillico HG, Chen E, Hobin E. The influence of menu labelling on food choices among children and adolescents: a systematic review of the literature. *Perspect Public Health.* 2017;137(3):173–181

29. Fernandes AC, Oliveira RC, Proença RP, Curioni CC, Rodrigues VM, Fiates GM. Influence of menu labeling on food choices in real-life settings: a systematic review. *Nutr Rev.* 2016;74(8):534–548

30. Krukowski RA, Harvey-Berino J, Kolodinsky J, Narsana RT, Desisto TP. Consumers may not use or understand calorie labeling in restaurants. *J Am Diet Assoc.* 2006;106(6):917–920

31. Ahn JY, Park HR, Lee K, et al. The effect of providing nutritional information about fast-food restaurant menus on parents' meal choices for their children. *Nutr Res Pract.* 2015;9(6):667–672

32. Tandon PS, Wright J, Zhou C, Rogers CB, Christakis DA. Nutrition menu labeling may lead to lower-calorie restaurant meal choices for children. *Pediatrics.* 2010;125(2):244–248

33. Fleischhacker SE, Evenson KR, Rodriguez DA, Ammerman AS. A systematic review of fast food access studies. *Obes Res.* 2011;12(5):e460–e471

34. Costa CS, Del-Ponte B, Assunção MCF, Santos IS. Consumption of ultra-processed foods and body fat during childhood and adolescence: a systematic review. *Public Health Nutr.* 2018;21(1):148–159

35. Williams PG. The benefits of breakfast cereal consumption: a systematic review of the evidence base. *Adv Nutr.* 2014;5(5):636S–673S

36. Fulgoni VL, Buckley RB. The contribution of fortified ready-to-eat cereal to vitamin and mineral intake in the U.S. population, NHANES 2007–2010. *Nutrients.* 2015;7(6):3949–3958

37. Michels N, De Henauw S, Beghin L, et al. Ready-to-eat cereals improve nutrient, milk and fruit intake at breakfast in European adolescents. *Eur J Nutr.* 2016;55(2):771–779

38. Asghari G, Yuzbashian E, Mirmiran P, Mahmoodi B, Azizi F. Fast food intake increases the incidence of metabolic syndrome in children and adolescents: Tehran Lipid and Glucose Study. *PLoS One.* 2015;10(10):e0139641

39. Fulkerson JA, Farbakhsh K, Lytle L, Hearst MO, Dengel DR, Pasch KEea. Away-from-home family dinner sources and associations with weight status, body composition, and related biomarkers of chronic disease among adolescents and their parents. *J Am Diet Assoc.* 2011;111(12):1892–1897

40. Hsieh S, Klassen AC, Curriero FC, et al. Fast-food restaurants, park access, and insulin resistance among Hispanic youth. *Am J Prev Med.* 2014;46(4):378–387

41. Tavares LF, Fonseca SC, Garcia Rosa ML, Yokoo EM. Relationship between ultra-processed foods and metabolic syndrome in adolescents from a Brazilian Family Doctor Program. *Public Health Nutr.* 2012;15(1):82–87

42. Mancino L, Todd J, Lin BH. Separating what we eat from where: measuring the effect of food away from home on diet quality. *Food Policy.* 2009;34:557–562

43. Poti JM, Duffey KJ, Popkin BM. The association of fast food consumption with poor dietary outcomes and obesity among children: is it the fast food or the remainder of the diet? *Am J Clin Nutr.* 2014;99(1):162–171

44. Kant AK, Whitley MI, Graubard BI. Away from home meals: associations with biomarkers of chronic disease and dietary intake in American adults, NHANES 2005–2010. *J Obes (Lond)*. 2015;39(5):820–827

45. Barlow SE, Expert Committee. Expert committee recommendations regarding the prevention, assessment, and treatment of child and adolescent overweight and obesity: summary report. *Pediatrics*. 2007;120(Suppl 4):S164–S192

46. Rydell SA, Harnack LJ, Oakes JM, Story M, Jeffery RW, French SA. Why eat at fast-food restaurants: reported reasons among frequent consumers. *J Am Diet Assoc*. 2008;108(12):2066–2070

47. Martin-Biggers J, Spaccarotella K, Berhaupt-Glickstein A, Hongu N, Worobey J, Byrd-Bredbenner C. Come and Get It! A Discussion of Family Mealtime Literature and Factors Affecting Obesity Risk. *Adv Nutr*. 2014;5(3):235–247

48. Daniels SR, Sandra G, Hassink SG, American Academy of Pediatrics, Committee on Nutrition. The role of the pediatrician in primary prevention of obesity. *Pediatrics*. 2015;136(1):e275–e292

49. Frieden TR, Dietz W, Collins J. Reducing childhood obesity through policy change: acting now to prevent obesity. *Health Aff (Millwood)*. 2010;29(3):357–363

50. Andreyeva T, Kelly IR, Harris JL. Exposure to food advertising on television: associations with children's fast food and soft drink consumption and obesity. *Econ Hum Biol*. 2011;9(3):221–233

51. Carter OB, Patterson LJ, Donovan RJ, Ewing MT, Roberts CM. Children's understanding of the selling versus persuasive intent of junk food advertising: implications for regulation. *Soc Sci Med*. 2011;72(6):962–968

52. Oates C, Blades M, Gunter B, Don J. Children's understanding of television advertising: a qualitative approach. *J Marketing Commun*. 2003;9:59–71

53. Coon KA, Tucker KL. Television and children's consumption patterns. A review of the literature. *Minerva Pediatr*. 2002;54(5):423–436

54. Wiecha JL, Peterson KE, Ludwig DS, Kim J, Sobol A, Gortmaker SL. When children eat what they watch. Impact of television viewing on dietary intake in youth. *Arch Pediatr Adolesc Med*. 2006;160(4):436–442

55. Marquis M, Filion YP, Dagenais F. Does eating while watching television influence children's food-related behaviours? . *Can J Diet Pract Res*. 2005;66(1): 12–19

56. Institute of Medicine, Committee on Food Marketing and the Diets of Children and Youth. *Food Marketing to Children and Youth: Threat or Opportunity?* Washington, DC: National Academies Press; 2006

57. American Academy of Pediatrics, Committee on Communications. Policy statement: Children, adolescents, and advertising. *Pediatrics*. 2006;118(6): 2563–2569

58. Holt DJ, Ippolito PM, Desrochers DM, Kelley CR. *Children's Exposure to TV Advertising in 1977 and 2004: Information for the Obesity Debate*. Washington, DC: Federal Trade Commission; 2007

59. Children's Food & Beverage Advertising Initiative. Available at: https://www. bbb.org/council/the-national-partner-program/national-advertising-review-services/childrens-food-and-beverage-advertising-initiative. Accessed August 10, 2017

60. Freeman B, Kelly B, Baur L, et al. Digital junk: food and beverage marketing on Facebook. *Am J Public Health*. 2014;104(12):e56–e64

61. Sharkey JR, Johnson CM, Dean WR, Horel SA. Focusing on fast food restaurants alone underestimates the relationship between neighborhood deprivation and exposure to fast food in a large rural area. *Nutr J*. 2011;10:10

62. Austin SB, Melly SJ, Sanchez BN, Patel A, Buka S, Gortmaker SL. Clustering of fast-food restaurants around schools: a novel application of spatial statistics to the study of food environments. *Am J Public Health*. 2005;95(9):1575–1581

63. Neckerman KM, Bader MD, Richards CAea. Disparities in the food environments of New York City public schools. *Am J Prev Med*. 2010;39(3): 195–202

64. Block JP, Scribner RA, DeSalvo KB. Fast food, race/ethnicity, and income: a geographic analysis. *Am J Prev Med*. 2004;27(3):211–217

65. Alter DA, Eny K. The relationship between the supply of fast-food chains and cardiovascular outcomes. *Can J Public Health*. 2005;96(3):173–177

66. Burdette HL, Whitaker RC. Neighborhood playgrounds, fast food restaurants, and crime: relationships to overweight in low-income preschool children. *Prev Med*. 2004;38(1):57–63

67. Jeffery RW, Baxter J, McGuire M, Linde J. Are fast food restaurants an environmental risk factor for obesity? *Int J Behav Nutr Phys Act*. 2006;3:2

68. Sturm R, Datar A. Body mass index in elementary school children, metropolitan area food prices and food outlet density. *Public Health*. 2005;119(12):1059–1068

69. Vernarelli JA, O'Brien B. A vote for school lunches: school lunches provide superior nutrient quality than lunches obtained from other sources in a nationally representative sample of US children. *Nutrients*. 2017;9(9):e924

70. Mansfield JL, Savaiano DA. Effect of school wellness policies and the Healthy, Hunger-Free Kids Act on food-consumption behaviors of students, 2006–2016: a systematic review. *Nutr Rev*. 2017;75(7):533–552

71. Schmitt J, Jones J. *Slow Progress for Fast-Food Workers. Issue Brief*. Washington, DC: Center for Economic Policy and Research; August 2013

72. Schermbeck RM, Powell LM. *Nutrition Recommendations and the Children's Food and Beverage Advertising Initiative's 2014 Approved Food and Beverage Product List*. Atlanta, GA: Centers for Disease Control and Prevention; 2015

73. Federal Trade Commission. A review of food marketing to children and adolescents: Follow up report. 2012

74. Jenkin G, Madhvani N, Signal L, Bowers S. A systematic review of persuasive marketing techniques to promote food to children on television. *Obes Res*. 2014;15(4):281–293

75. Reimann M, Lane K. Can a toy encourage lower calorie meal bundle selection in children? A field experiment on the reinforcing effects of toys on food choice. *PLoS One.* 2017;12(1):e0169638

76. Birch LL, Zimmerman S, Hind H. The influence of social-affective context on preschool children's food preferences. *Child Dev.* 1980;51:856–861

77. Fisher JO, Birch LL. Restricting access to palatable foods affects children's behavioral response, food selection, and intake. *69.* Am J Clin Nutr;6(1264–1272)

78. Nicklas TA, Goh ET, Goodell LS, et al. Impact of commercials on food preferences of low-income, minority preschoolers. *J Nutr Educ Behav.* 2011;43(1): 35–41

79. Steinbrenner H, Al-Quraishy S, Dkhil MA, Wunderlich F, Sies H. Dietary selenium in adjuvant therapy of viral and bacterial infections. *Adv Nutr.* 2015;6(1):73–82

80. Winter CK, Davis SF. Organic foods. *J Food Sci.* 2006;71(9):R117–R124

81. US Department of Agriculture. Agricultural Marketing Service. Organic Standards. Available at: https://www.ams.usda.gov/grades-standards/organic-standards. Accessed August 11, 2017

82. US Department of Agriculture, Agricultural Marketing Service. National Organic Program. Available at: https://www.ams.usda.gov/sites/default/files/media/OrganicCosmeticsFactSheet.pdf. Accessed August 11, 2017

83. US Department of Agriculture. Labeling Organic Products. Available at: https://www.ams.usda.gov/sites/default/files/media/Labeling%20Organic%20Products%20Fact%20Sheet.pdf. Accessed August 11, 2017

84. US Department of Agriculture. Using the USDA Organic Seal: Media, Marketing & Educational Materials. Available at: https://www.ams.usda.gov/sites/default/files/media/Using%20the%20Organic%20Seal%20Factsheet.pdf. Accessed August 11, 2017

85. Asioli D, Aschemann-Witzel J, Caputo V, et al. Making sense of the "clean label" trends: A review of consumer food choice behavior and discussion of industry implications. *Food Res Int.* 2017;99(Pt 1):58–71

86. Dimitri C, Oberholtzer L. *Marketing U.S. Organic Foods: Recent Trends From Farms to Consumers. Economic Information Bulletin No. 58.* Washington, DC: US Department of Agriculture, Economic Research Service; 2009

87. Oberholtzer L, Dimitri C, Greene C. Washington, DC: US Department of Agriculture, Economic Research Service; 2005

88. Organic Trade Association. Organic Market Analysis. Available at: https://www.ota.com/resources/market-analysis. Accessed August 14, 2017

89. Organic Trade Association. Consumer Attitudes and Beliefs Study

90. Baudry J, Péneau S, Allès B, et al. Food choice motives when purchasing in organic and conventional consumer clusters: focus on sustainable concerns (The NutriNet-Santé Cohort Study). *Nutrients.* 2017;9(2):E88

91. Foster C, Padel S. Exploring the gap between attitudes and behaviour: Understanding why consumers buy or do not buy organic food. *Br Food J.* 2005;107:606–625

92. Magnusson MK, Arvola A, Hursti UK, Aberg L, Sjoden PO. Choice of organic foods is related to perceived consequences for human health and to environmentally friendly behaviour. *Appetite.* 2003;40(2):109–117

93. Shepherd R, Magnusson M, Sjoden PO. Determinants of consumer behavior related to organic foods. *Ambio.* 2005;34(4-5):352–359

94. Dangour AD, Dodhia SK, Hayter A, Allen E, Lock K, Uauy R. Nutritional quality of organic foods: a systematic review. *Am J Clin Nutr.* 2009;90(3):680–685

95. Magkos F, Arvaniti F, Zampelas A. Organic food: buying more safety or just piece of mind? A critical review of the literature. *Crit Rev Food Sci Nutr.* 2006;46(1): 23–56

96. Średnicka-Tober D, Barański M, Seal C, et al. Composition differences between organic and conventional meat: a systematic literature review and meta-analysis. *Br J Nutr.* 2016;115(6):994–1011

97. Średnicka-Tober D, Barański M, Seal CJ, et al. Higher PUFA and n-3 PUFA, conjugated linoleic acid, α-tocopherol and iron, but lower iodine and selenium concentrations in organic milk: a systematic literature review and meta- and redundancy analyses. *Br J Nutr.* 2016;115(6):1043–1060

98. Winter CK. Institute of Food Technologists. Organic Foods. Available at: http://www.ift.org/Knowledge-Center/Read-IFT-Publications/Science-Reports/Scientific-Status-Summaries/Editorial/~/media/Knowledge%20Center/Science%20Reports/Scientific%20Status%20Summaries/Editorial/editorial_1106_organicfoods.pdf. Accessed August 14, 2017

99. American Heart Association. Organic Food: Fact vs Perception. Available at: http://www.heart.org/HEARTORG/HealthyLiving/HealthyEating/Nutrition/Organic-Food-Fact-vs-Perception_UCM_425671_Article.jsp#.WZHWXzeYacw. Accessed August 14, 2017

100. American Academy of Pediatrics. American Academy of Pediatrics Weighs in for the First Time on Organic Foods for Children. Available at: https://www.aap.org/en-us/about-the-aap/aap-press-room/pages/american-academy-of-pediatrics-weighs-in-for-the-first-time-on-organic-foods-for-children.aspx. Accessed August 14, 2017

101. Sanchez-Echaniz J, Benito-Fernandez J, Mintegui-Raso S. Methemoglobinemia and consumption of vegetables in infants. *Pediatrics.* 2001;107(5):1021–1028

102. Croen LA, Todoroff K, Shaw GM. Maternal exposure to nitrate from drinking water and diet and risk for neural tube defects. *Am J Epidemiol.* 2001;153(4): 325–331

103. Nuñez de González MT, Osburn WN, Hardin MD, et al. A survey of nitrate and nitrite concentrations in conventional and organic-labeled raw vegetables at retail. *J Food Sci.* 2015;80(5):C942–C949

104. Worthington V. Nutritional quality of organic versus conventional fruits, vegetables, and grains. *J Altern Complement Med.* 2001;7(2):161–173

105. National Research Council. *Pesticides in the Diets of Infants and Children.* Washington, DC: National Academies Press; 1993

106. Eskenazi B, Bradman A, Castorina R. Exposures of children to organophosphate pesticides and their potential adverse health effects. *Environ Health Perspect.* 1999;107(Suppl 3):409–419

107. Eskenazi B, Marks AR, Bradman A, et al. Organophosphate pesticide exposure and neurodevelopment in young Mexican-American children. *Environ Health Perspect.* 2007;115(5):792–798

108. Bouchard MF, Bellinger DC, Wright RO, Weisskopf MG. Attention-deficit/hyperactivity disorder and urinary metabolites of organophosphate pesticides. *Pediatrics.* 2010;125(6):e1270–e1277

109. Benbrook CM. Organochlorine residues pose surprisingly high dietary risks. *J Epidemiol Community Health.* 2002;56(11):822–823

110. Gonzales M, Miglioranza KS, Aizpun de Moreno JE, Moreno VJ. Occurrence and distribution of organochlorine pesticides (OCPs) in tomato (Lycopersicon esculentum) crops from organic production. *J Agric Food Chem.* 2003;51(5):1353–1359

111. Baker BP, Benbrook CM, Groth E, Benbrook L. Pesticide residues in conventional, integrated pest management (IPM)-grown and organic foods: insights from three US data sets. *Food Addit Contam.* 2002;19(5):427–446

112. Crinnion WJ. Organic foods contain higher levels of certain nutrients, lower levels of pesticides, and may provide health benefits for the consumer. *Altern Med Rev.* 2010;15(1):4–12

113. Curl CL, Fenske RA, Elgethun K. Organophosphorus pesticide exposure of urban and suburban preschool children with organic and conventional diets. *Environ Health Perspect.* 2003;111(3):377–382

114. MacIntosh DL, Kabiru C, Echols SL, Ryan PB. Dietary exposure to chlorpyrifos and levels of 3,5,6 trichloro-2-pyridinol in urine. *J Expo Anal Environ Epidemiol.* 2001;11(4):279–285

115. Lu C, Toepel K, Irish R, Fenske RA, Barr DB, Bravo R. Organic diets significantly lower children's dietary exposure to organophosphorus pesticides. *Environ Health Perspect.* 2006;114(2):260–263

116. Curl CL, Beresford SA, Fenske RA, et al. Estimating pesticide exposure from dietary intake and organic food choices: the Multi-Ethnic Study of Atherosclerosis (MESA). *Environ Health Perspect.* 2015;123(5):475–483

117. Kim YJ, Kim HS, Kim KY, Chon JW, Kim DH, Seo KH. High occurrence rate and contamination level of *Bacillus cereus* in organic vegetables on sale in retail markets. *Foodborne Pathog Dis.* 2016;13(12):656–660

118. Loncarevic S, Johannessen GS, Rorvik LM. Bacteriological quality of organically grown leaf lettuce in Norway. *Lett Appl Microbiol.* 2005;41(2):186–189

119. Bailey JS, Cosby DE. *Salmonella* prevalence in free-range and certified organic chickens. *J Food Prot.* 2005;68(11):2451–2453

120. Cui S, Ge B, Zheng J, Meng J. Prevalence and antimicrobial resistance of *Campylobacter* spp. and *Salmonella* serovars in organic chickens from Maryland retail stores. *Appl Environ Microbiol.* 2005;71(7):4108–4111

121. Freedman MR, King J, Kennedy E. Popular diets: a scientific review. *Obes Res.* 2001;9(Suppl 1):1S–40S

122. Halton TL, Hu FB. The effects of high protein diets on thermogenesis, satiety, and weight loss: a critical review. *J Am Coll Nutr.* 2004;23(5):373–385

123. Gow ML, Ho M, Burrows TL, et al. Impact of dietary macronutrient distribution on BMI and cardiometabolic outcomes in overweight and obese children and adolescents: a systematic review. *Nutr Rev.* 2014;72(7):453–470

124. Rajjo T, Mohammed K, Alsawas M, et al. Treatment of pediatric obesity: an umbrella systematic review. *J Clin Endocrinol Metab.* 2017;102(3):763–775

125. Shah P, Isley WL. Ketoacidosis during a low-carbohydrate diet. *N Engl J Med.* 2006;354(1):97–98

126. Brunstrom JM, Davison CJ, Mitchell GL. Dietary restraint and cognitive performance in children. *Appetite.* 2005;45(3):235–241

127. Giddling SS, Dennison BA, Birch LL, et al. American Heart Association. Dietary recommendations for children and adolescents: a guide for practitioners. *Pediatrics.* 2006;117(2):544–559

128. Kimmons J, Gillespie C, Seymour J, Serdula M, Blanck HM. Fruit and vegetable intake among adolescents and adults in the United States: percentage meeting individualized recommendations. *Medscape J Med.* 2009;11(1):26

129. Dennison BA, Rockwell HL, Baker SL. Fruit and vegetable intake in young children. *J Am Coll Nutr.* 1998;17(4):371–378

130. McNaughton SA, Ball K, Mishra GD, Crawford DA. Dietary patterns of adolescents and risk of obesity and hypertension. *J Nutr.* 2008;138(2):364–370

131. Tercyak KP, Tyc VL. Opportunities and challenges in the prevention and control of cancer and other chronic diseases: children's diet and nutrition and weight and physical activity. *J Pediatr Psychol.* 2006;31(8):750–763

132. World Cancer Research Fund/American Institute for Cancer Research. *Food, Nutrition, Physical Activity, and the Prevention of Cancer: A Global Perspective.* Washington, DC: American Institute for Cancer Research; 2007

133. Mente A, de Koning L, Shannon HS, Anand SS. A systematic review of the evidence supporting a causal link between dietary factors and coronary heart disease. *Arch Intern Med.* 2009;169(7):659–669

134. Dauchet L, Amouyel P, Dallongeville J. Fruits, vegetables and coronary heart disease. *Nat Rev Cardiol.* 2009;6(9):599–608

135. Esposito K, Kastorini CM, Panagiotakos DB, Giugliano D. Prevention of type 2 diabetes by dietary patterns: a systematic review of prospective studies and meta-analysis. *Metab Syndr Relat Disord.* 2010;8(6):471–476

136. US Department of Agriculture. Dietary Guidelines for Americans 2015–2020. Available at: https://health.gov/dietaryguidelines. Accessed August 17, 2017

137. Garcia AH, Franco OH, Voortman T, et al. Dietary acid load in early life and bone health in childhood: the Generation R Study. *Am J Clin Nutr.* 2015;102(6): 1595–1603

138. Cai QY, Zhou ZJ, Luo R, et al. Safety and tolerability of the ketogenic diet used for the treatment of refractory childhood epilepsy: a systematic review of published prospective studies. *World J Pediatr.* 2017;13(6):528–536

139. Sharma S, Jain P. The modified Atkins diet in refractory epilepsy. *Epilepsy Res Treat.* 2014;2014(404202)

140. Groleau V, Schall JI, Stallings VA, Bergqvist CA. Long-term impact of the ketogenic diet on growth and resting energy expenditure in children with intractable epilepsy. *Dev Med Child Neurol.* 2014;56(9):898–904

141. Willi SM, Oexmann MJ, Wright NM, Collop NA, Key Jr LL. The effects of a high-protein, low-fat, ketogenic diet on adolescents with morbid obesity: Body composition, blood chemistries, and sleep abnormalities. *Pediatrics.* 1998;101 (1 Pt 1):61–67

142. Leonard MM, Sapone A, Catassi C, Fasano A. Celiac disease and nonceliac gluten sensitivity: a review. *JAMA.* 2017;381(7):647–656

143. Garnier-Lengliné H, Cerf-Bensussan N, Ruemmele FM. Celiac disease in children. *Clin Res Hepatol Gastroenterol.* 2015;39(5):544–551

144. Reilly NR. The gluten-free diet: recognizing fact, fiction, and fad. *J Pediatr.* 2016;175:206–210

145. The Hartman Group. The Hartman Group's Health & Wellness 2015 and Organic & Natural 2014 reports. Available at: http://www.hartman-group.com/ acumenPdfs/gluten-free-2015-09-03.pdf. Accessed August 17, 2017

146. Vici G, Belli L, Biondi M, Polzonetti V. Gluten free diet and nutrient deficiencies: A review. *Clin Nutr.* 2016;35(6):1236–1241

147. Academy of Nutrition and Dietetics. Evidence Analysis Library. Pediatric Weight Management. Available at: https://www.andeal.org/topic.cfm?menu=5296. Accessed September 12, 2017

148. US Food and Drug Administration. Overview of Dietary Supplements. Available at: http://www.fda.gov/food/dietarysupplements/default.htm. Accessed September 12, 2017

149. US Food and Drug Administration. Current Good Manufacturing Practices (CGMPs). Dietary Supplements. Available at: https://www.fda.gov/food/ guidanceregulation/cgmp/ucm079496.htm. Accessed September 12, 2007

150. National Institutes of Health. Office of Dietary Supplements. Available at: https://ods.od.nih.gov. Accessed September 12, 2007

151. American Botanical Council. The Complete German Commission E Monographs Therapeutic Guide to Herbal Medicines. 1999. Available at: http://cms. herbalgram.org/commissione/intro/comm_e_int.html. Accessed September 13, 2017

152. Blumenthal M, Lindstrom A, Lynch ME, Rea P. Herb sales continue growth – Up 3.3% in 2010. *HerbalGram.* 2011;90:64–67

153. Black LI, Clarke TC, Barnes PM, Stussman BJ, Nahin R. Use of Complementary Health Approaches Among Children Aged 4–17 Years in the United States: National Health Interview Survey, 2007–2012. *Natl Health Stat Rep.* 2015(78):1–19

154. Barnes PM, Bloom B, Nahin RL. Complementary and alternative medicine use among adults and children: United States, 2007. *Natl Health Stat Rep.* 2008;10(12):1–23

155. Garrard J, Harms S, Eberly LE, Matiak A. Variations in product choices of frequently purchased herbs: caveat emptor. *Arch Intern Med.* 2003;163(19): 2290–2295

156. Gilroy CM, Steiner JF, Byers T, Shapiro H, Georgian W. Echinacea and truth in labeling. *Arch Intern Med.* 2003;163:699–704

157. Lanski SL, Greenwald M, Perkins A, Simon HK. Herbal therapy use in a pediatric emergency department population: expect the unexpected. *Pediatrics.* 2003;111(5 Pt 1):981–985

158. Lohse B, Stotts JL, Priebe JR. Survey of herbal use by Kansas and Wisconsin WIC participants reveals moderate, appropriate use and identifies herbal education needs. *J Am Diet Assoc.* 2006;106(2):227–337

159. Wilson KM, Klein JD, Sesselberg TS, et al. Use of complementary medicine and dietary supplements among U.S. adolescents. *J Adolesc Health.* 2006;38:385–394

160. Ottolini MC, Hamburger EK, Loprieato JO, et al. Complementary and alternative medicine use among children in the Washington DC area. *Ambul Pediatr.* 2001;1(2):122–125

161. Noonan K, Arensman RM, Hoover JD. Herbal medication use in the pediatric surgical patient. *J Pediatr Surg.* 2004;39(3):500–503

162. Lin YC, Bioteau AB, Ferrair LR, Berde CB. The use of herbs and complementary and alternative medicine in pediatric preoperative patients. *J Clin Anesth.* 2004;16(1):4–6

163. Anheyer D, Frawley J, Koch AK, et al. Herbal Medicines for Gastrointestinal Disorders in Children and Adolescents: A Systematic Review. *Pediatrics.* 2017;139(6):e20170062

164. Clark CE, Arnold E, Lasserson TJ, Wu T. Herbal interventions for chronic asthma in adults and children: a systematic review and meta-analysis. *Prim Care Respir J.* 2010;19(4):307–314

165. Mazur LJ, De Ybarrondo L, Miller J, Colasurdo G. Use of alternative and complementary therapies for pediatric asthma. *Tex Med.* 2001;97:64–68

166. Nunes MA, Rodrigues F, Alves RC, Oliveira MBPP. Herbal products containing *Hibiscus sabdariffa L.*, *Crataegus* spp., and *Panax* spp.: labeling and safety concerns. *Food Res Int.* 2017;100(Pt 1):529–540

167. Shenfield G, Lim E, Allen H. Survey of the use of complementary medicines and therapies in children with asthma. *J Paediatr Child Health.* 2002;38(3):252–257

168. Nowak-Węgrzyn A, Sampson HA. Future therapies for food allergies. *J Allergy Clin Immunol.* 2011;127:558–573

169. Wang J, Jones SM, Pongracic JA, et al. Safety, clinical, and immunologic efficacy of a Chinese herbal medicine (Food Allergy Herbal Formula-2) for food allergy. *J Allergy Clin Immunol*. 2015;136(4):962–970

170. Kohn CM, Paudyal P. A systematic review and meta-analysis of complementary and alternative medicine in asthma. *Eur Respir Rev*. 2017;56(143):160092

171. Day AS, Whitten KE, Bohane TD. Use of complementary and alternative medicines by children and adolescents with inflammatory bowel disease. *J Paediatr Child Health*. 2004;40(12):681–684

172. Neuhouser ML, Patterson RE, Schwartz SM, Hedderson MM, Bowen DJ, Standish LJ. Use of alternative medicine by children with cancer in Washington state. *Prev Med*. 2001;33(5):347–354

173. Haidar C, Jeha S. Drug interactions in childhood cancer. *Lancet Oncol*. 2011;12(1): 92–99

174. Pillai AK, Sharma KK, Gupta YK, Bakhshi S. Anti-emetic effect of ginger powder versus placebo as an add-on therapy in children and young adults receiving high emetogenic chemotherapy. *Pediatr Blood Cancer*. 2011;56(2):234–238

175. Sparreboom A, Cox MC, Acharya MR, Figg WD. Herbal remedies in the United States: potential adverse interactions with anticancer agents. *J Clin Oncol*. 2004;22(12):2489–2503

176. Ondieki G, Nyagblordzro M, Kikete S, Liang R, Wang L, He X. Cytochrome P450 and P-glycoprotein-mediated interactions involving African herbs indicated for common noncommunicable diseases. *Evid Based Complement Altern Med*. 2017;2017:2582463

177. Peters MC, Tallman JA, Braun TM, Jacobson JJ. Clinical reduction of S. mutans in pre-school children using a novel liquorice root extract lollipop: a pilot study. *Eur Arch Paediatr Dent*. 2010;11(6):274–278

178. Usai S, Grazzi L, Bussone G. Gingkolide B as migraine preventive treatment in young age: results at 1-year follow-up. *Neurol Sci*. 2011;32(Suppl 1):197–199

179. Teschke R, Eickhoff A. Herbal hepatotoxicity in traditional and modern medicine: actual key issues and new encouraging steps. *Front Pharmacol*. 2015;6:72

180. Woolf AD. Herbal remedies and children: Do they work? Are they harmful? *Pediatrics*. 2003;112:240–246

181. The Natural Medicines Comprehensive Database. Available at: http://naturaldatabase.therapeuticresearch.com/home.aspx?cs=&s=ND. Accessed September 14, 2017

182. National Institutes of Health, National Center for Complementary and Integrative Health. Available at: https://nccih.nih.gov. Accessed September 14, 2017

183. National Institutes of Health. Dietary Supplement Label Database. Available at: https://ods.od.nih.gov/Research/Dietary_Supplement_Label_Database.aspx. Accessed September 14, 2017

Micronutrients and Macronutrients

Chapter 14

Energy

Introduction

Energy flow through living systems encompasses cellular respiration and metabolic processes that lead to production and utilization of energy in forms such as adenosine triphosphate (ATP). Chemical energy in food is transformed and made available for biosynthesis, anabolic process, and mechanical work. Energy is required for all the biochemical and physiologic functions that sustain life: respiration, circulation, maintenance of electrochemical gradients across cell membranes, and maintenance of body temperature as well as for growth and physical activity.[1,2] Energy provided in the diet by protein, carbohydrate, and fat is expressed as a unit of heat, the calorie. A calorie is defined as the amount of heat required to raise the temperature of 1 g of water by 1°C from 15°C to 16°C. The scientific international unit of energy is the joule (J), defined as the energy expended when 1 kg is moved 1 m by a force of 1 newton. In the field of nutrition, a kilocalorie (kcal), which is 1000 times the energy of a calorie (cal), is commonly used. Hence, 1 kcal = 4.184 kJ, and 1 kJ = 0.239 kcal.

Energy Balance

Energy balance is the accounting for energy consumption; excretion in feces, urine, and combustible gases; expenditure; and retention of organic compounds (ie, protein and fat accretion).[3] Implicit in the definition of energy balance is that energy is conserved. Energy balance may be expressed as:

Energy Intake − Energy Excretion − Energy Expenditure = Energy Retention

Digestible energy is the dietary energy absorbed by the gastrointestinal tract after accounting for loss in feces.[4] Metabolizable energy is energy available after accounting for losses in feces, urine, and combustible gases. The Atwater factors of 4, 9, and 4 kcal of metabolizable energy per g of protein, fat, and carbohydrate, respectively, are widely used to express the energy content of foods in food composition tables.[5] Atwater factors are applied to the protein estimated from its nitrogen content, fat determined by extraction, and carbohydrates determined by difference after taking into account the protein, fat, water, and ash in the food.

Although food intake is the result of complex interactions among central nervous system regulating regions (mainly hypothalamic) and peripheral neural (eg, vagal) and humoral (eg, gut peptides and insulin) signals and environmental factors, energy balance at all ages is regulated with a fair degree of precision. This is reflected in the observation that most infants and children grow in regular fashion, and many adults maintain stable body weight for long periods. Infants appear to eat to satisfy energy needs and will compensate for low food energy density and poor digestibility by increasing food intake.[6] Observations of young children fed ad libitum while recovering from malnutrition showed that their voracious appetites abated as they approached normal weight for height.[7] Despite the innate balancing of energy intake against energy expenditure and energy needs for growth, obesity (see also Chapter 33: Obesity), a consequence of long-term energy intake in excess of energy requirements, has become alarmingly prevalent among children in the United States.[8]

Most clinical problems involving energy balance can be approached by systematic evaluation of the terms in the energy balance equation, although specific macronutrient effects on metabolism may need to be considered in certain clinical settings.[6,9] Inadequate energy intake may be a consequence of insufficient provision of appropriate food by the child's caregivers or may be attributable to problems inherent to the child (eg, neurologic, behavioral, or certain gastrointestinal tract disorders). Fecal excretion of fat usually accounts for most of the energy excretion, although in some instances, carbohydrate and nitrogenous losses also may be clinically important. Clinically significant increased energy excretion most commonly is secondary to intestinal, pancreatic, or hepatobiliary disorders that result in macronutrient maldigestion and/or malabsorption. In some situations (eg, diabetes mellitus, ketosis), energy losses in urine may be significant.

Components of Energy Expenditure

Energy expenditure includes energy expended for basal metabolic processes, the thermic effect of food ingestion, energy expended for thermoregulation, and energy expended for physical activity.[1-3]

Basal Metabolism

Basal metabolic rate (BMR) is energy expenditure under standard conditions—for example, after a 12- to 18-hour fast, awake, but quietly lying down (in early morning after awakening), in a thermoneutral environment (eg, an environmental temperature at which the metabolic rate and, therefore, oxygen consumption are at a minimum), bodily and mentally at rest. BMR reflects energy required for vital body processes during physical, emotional, and digestive rest.[1] Important factors that affect energy expenditure at rest include age, body size and composition, and presence of disease (eg, infection, fever, or trauma). If the experimental conditions required for the measurement of BMR are not practical, resting metabolic rate is often measured instead. Resting metabolic rate, the energy expended by a person at rest in a thermoneutral environment, is 10% to 20% higher than the BMR because of recent food intake or physical activity. In the case of infants, sleeping metabolic rate is often measured to avoid uncontrollable body movement.

Because of the dominant contribution of the brain (60%-70%), weight-adjusted BMR (kcal·kg⁻¹·day⁻¹) is highest during the first years of life.[10] BMR of term infants ranges from 43 to 60 kcal·kg⁻¹·day⁻¹ or 2 to 3 times greater than that in adults.[11] Absolute BMR (kcal/day) is influenced by age (greater in older than in younger children), gender (greater in males than in females), and feeding mode (less in breastfed than in formula-fed infants).[12] BMR of healthy children younger than 3 years may be predicted by the following equations derived by Schofield et al[11]:

Boys: BMR (kcal/day) = 0.1673 weight (kg) + 1517 length (m) − 618

Girls: BMR (kcal/day) = 16.25 weight (kg) + 1023 length (m) − 413

Similarly, the BMR for older children and adolescents may be estimated from the Schofield equations. These equations may not apply to sick children, in whom metabolism and/or body composition may be altered. For children 3 to 10 years of age:

Boys: BMR (kcal/day) = 19.60 weight (kg) + 130.26 length (m) + 414.90

Girls: BMR (kcal/day) = 16.97 weight (kg) + 161.80 length (m) + 371.17

For children 10 to 18 years of age:

Boys: BMR (kcal/day) = 16.25 weight (kg) + 137.19 length (m) + 515.52

Girls: BMR (kcal/day) = 8.365 weight (kg) + 465.57 length (m) + 200.04

Thermic Effect of Food

The thermic effect of feeding (TEF) or specific dynamic action is the increase in energy expenditure resulting from ingestion of food.[3] The TEF is mainly attributable to the obligatory metabolic costs of processing a meal, which include nutrient digestion, absorption, transport, and storage. The remaining facultative TEF reflects heat production that does not result in net synthesis or mechanical work and likely involves uncoupling of oxidative phosphorylation (ie, substrates are oxidized but heat is produced instead of ATP). The TEF is computed as the increment in energy expenditure above BMR, divided by the energy content of the food consumed; TEF varies from 5% to 10% for carbohydrate, 0% to 5% for fat, and 20% to 30% for protein. A mixed meal elicits an increase in energy expenditure equivalent to approximately 10% of the calories consumed.

Thermoregulation

Humans, like all homeotherms, maintain an almost constant body temperature over a wide range of environmental temperatures.[3] Energy required to maintain body temperature depends on environmental temperature. When ambient temperatures are below or above the zone of thermoneutrality, energy expenditure will increase. A narrower range of higher temperatures is needed to maintain thermoneutrality in neonates, particularly for those born preterm. However, beyond infancy, little additional energy is needed between environmental temperatures of 20°C and 30°C. Outside these limits, an additional 5% to 10% of total energy may be necessary to maintain body temperature.

Facultative thermogenesis is defined as heat production in response to cold (shivering and nonshivering thermogenesis), diet, or exercise, and involves the transformation of chemical energy into heat at the expense of ATP production.[13–15] Facultative thermogenesis occurs mainly in brown adipose tissue (BAT) and skeletal muscle and is mediated by acetylcholine, norepinephrine, and thyroid hormones. BAT possesses the ability to transfer energy from food into heat using uncoupling protein 1 (UCP1).

Until recently, BAT was thought to be present and active in humans only during infancy. However, during fluorodeoxyglucose (^{18}F) positron emission tomography (FDG PET) used to image tumors, BAT was visualized unexpectedly in several anatomical areas initially in adults [16] and later in children.[17] Presence of metabolically active BAT is markedly higher in pediatric than adult populations.[18] The functional role of BAT in children has yet to be thoroughly investigated.

Physical Activity

Marked variability exists in the energy requirements of children and adolescents because of variable physical activity levels.[1,2] The amount of time children spend in recreational activities and domestic and productive work varies across societies. The energy costs of discrete physical activities have been measured using indirect calorimetry and are usually expressed in terms of metabolic equivalents (METs) or physical activity ratios.[19] The energetic efficiency for physical work is remarkably constant for non–weight-bearing activities.[20] Under optimal conditions, the net efficiency (external work/internal energy conversion rate necessary to accomplish the work) of the body is approximately 25%. However, this does not imply that the energy cost of activities is constant among individuals. Energy cost (kcal/min) of activities among individuals varies because of differences in age, weight, and skill. For weight-bearing physical activities, the cost is roughly proportional to body weight.

Ainsworth and colleagues provided comprehensive MET tables to estimate the energy expended in discrete physical activities for adults.[21] However, adult MET values are not applicable to children.[22–24] Children have higher basal metabolism per unit of body mass than adults, and it declines with age because of sex-specific developmental changes in organ weights, organ-specific metabolic rates, muscle mass, and adiposity.[25,26]

A Youth Compendium of Physical Activities has recently been published based on empirical energy expenditure measurements in children.[27] The Youth Compendium consists of METy (or MET for youth) values for 196 specific activities classified into 16 major categories for 4 age groups: 6 through 9 years, 10 through 12 years, 13 through 15 years, and 16 through 18 years. The methods used in formulating the Youth Compendium addressed the unique developmental challenges in determining the energy costs of physical activities in children. First, all METy values were measured or derived from pediatric data only. METy was defined as the measured energy cost of the activity divided by the BMR predicted using the age-, sex-, and mass-specific Schofield equations.[11] Second, missing METy data were predicted using an imputation mixed model for each major activity category. Third, METy values for each activity were provided for the 4 age groups to address the age dependency of METy values.[28] Selected METy values are presented in Table 14.1, and complete downloadable METy tables are available at nccor.org/youthcompendium.

Table 14.1.
Youth MET$_y$ Values for Selected Activities

Activity Category	Specific Activity	MET$_y$			
		Ages 6–9	Ages 10–12	Ages 13–15	Ages 16–18
Active play	Free play (basketball, rope, hoop, climb)	**5.0**	**5.8**	5.8	5.9
Active play	Playing tag – moderate	**5.9**	**6.1**	6.5	6.5
Active video games (full body)	Active video games (compilation)	**4.5**	**5.4**	**6.0**	5.9
Active video games (upper body)	Active video games – Wii (compilation of games)	**2.5**	**2.6**	**2.8**	**2.4**
Bike/scooter riding	Riding a bike – self paced	4.4	**5.4**	5.3	7.0
Bike/scooter riding	Riding scooter	**5.0**	**5.9**	6.1	6.6
Calisthenics/gymnastics	Gymnastics	2.7	2.9	**2.4**	2.7
Calisthenics/gymnastics	Jumping jacks	**4.8**	4.8	4.7	4.7
Computer/video games (sitting)	Computer games (compilation)	**1.6**	**1.5**	**1.4**	**1.3**
Dance/aerobics/steps	Aerobic dance/dance	**3.6**	**4.0**	**4.8**	**4.0**
Housekeeping/work	Housework	**4.0**	**4.3**	**4.4**	**2.9**
Lying	Quietly lying	**1.3**	**1.2**	**1.1**	**1.1**
Lying	Watching TV/DVD – lying	**1.3**	**1.0**	1.1	1.1

Quiet play/schoolwork/TV (sitting)	Schoolwork	**1.5**	**1.8**	**1.4**	1.5
Quiet play/schoolwork/TV (sitting)	Watching TV/DVD – sitting	**1.3**	**1.3**	**1.2**	**1.2**
Running	Run 4.0 mph	**6.5**	**6.6**	**7.4**	8.2
Running	Run 6.0 mph	**8.4**	**8.8**	**10.3**	**10.6**
Running	Run 8.0 mph	10.9	11.6	**13.1**	**12.7**
Sports/games	Basketball – game	**6.2**	**7.8**	**7.3**	**6.2**
Sports/games	Soccer – game	**8.5**	**8.5**	**9.0**	8.3
Sports/games	Volleyball	5.0	**4.4**	5.0	5.8
Standing	Standing	1.7	1.6	**1.6**	1.2
Swimming	Swimming – front crawl 1.0 m/sec	9.9	**9.6**	8.5	9.8
Walking	Walk 2.0 mph	**2.7**	**3.1**	**3.1**	**3.3**
Walking	Walk 3.0 mph	**3.7**	**4.4**	**4.0**	**4.7**
Walking	Walk 4.0 mph	**4.9**	**5.3**	**5.3**	**6.2**
Weight lifting	Hand weight exercises	**3.0**	**3.3**	3.2	3.2

Metabolic equivalent for youth (MET_y) defined as the measured energy cost of the activity divided by the BMR predicted using the age-, sex- and mass-specific Schofield equations.[11] Bolded MET_y values are observed values from the literature; other values are imputed.

Measurement of Energy Expenditure

Energy expenditure can be measured by direct calorimetry, indirect calorimetry, and noncalorimetric methods.[29] For practical reasons, the most commonly used method is indirect calorimetry, in which energy expenditure is computed from oxygen consumption (Vo_2), carbon dioxide production (Vco_2), and the respiratory quotient (RQ), which is equal to the ratio of Vco_2 to Vo_2. Substrate utilization can be determined from rates of Vo_2, Vco_2, and urinary nitrogen excretion.[30] The complete oxidation of glucose results in an RQ equal to 1.0. The complete oxidation of fat and protein results in an RQ averaging about 0.7 and 0.85, respectively, depending on the chemical structure of the foodstuff. The RQ for lipogenesis (conversion of carbohydrate to stored fat) is greater than 1. The ingestion or administration of a high percentage of calories as carbohydrate may cause difficulties for children with respiratory insufficiency, because excess carbon dioxide is produced. This is especially true if the energy intake from carbohydrate exceeds the energy expenditure.

The Weir equation[31] is the most widely used equation for the calculation of energy expenditure (EE):

$$EE \text{ (kcal)} = 3.941 \times Vo_2 \text{ (L)} + 1.106\, Vco_2 \text{ (L)} - (2.17 \times UrN \text{ (g))} \text{ or}$$

$$EE \text{ (kcal)} = 3.941 \times Vo_2 \text{ (L)} + 1\, Vco_2 \text{ (L)}/(1 + 0.082\, p)$$

where UrN is urinary nitrogen and p is the fraction of calories resulting from protein. Weir demonstrated that the error in neglecting the effect of protein metabolism on the caloric equivalent of oxygen is 1% for each 12.3% of the total calories that arise from protein. Under usual conditions, approximately 12.5% of total calories will arise from protein; therefore, the foregoing equation can be reduced to the following:

$$EE \text{ (kcal)} = 3.9 \times Vo_2 \text{ (L)} + 1.1\, Vco_2 \text{ (L)}.$$

The doubly labeled water method, which provides an indirect measure of Vco_2, has been used to estimate total EE in a number of different research settings.[32,33] Doubly labeled water is a stable (nonradioactive) isotope method that provides an estimate of total EE in free-living individuals. Two stable isotopic forms of water ($H_2{}^{18}O$ and ^2H_2O) are administered to the individual, and their ^{18}O and ^2H disappearance rates from the body are monitored for 7 to 21 days. The disappearance rate of ^2H_2O reflects water flux, whereas that of $H_2{}^{18}O$ reflects water flux plus Vco_2, and the difference between the 2 disappearance rates is used to calculate Vco_2. Applying a value for RQ based on food intake, V_{O_2} is calculated ($V_{O_2} = V_{CO_2}/$ RQ); hence, total EE is calculated using the Weir equation. The doubly labeled water method may be used to assess energy requirements in weight-stable individuals.

Energy Cost of Growth

The energy cost of growth also is a component of total energy requirements.[1] The energy needed for growth represents approximately 35% of total energy requirements at 1 month of age, decreases to approximately 3% at 12 months of age because of slower growth, and remains almost negligible until the onset of puberty. The energy cost of growth is estimated from the individual costs of protein and fat deposition and ranges from 2.4 to 6.0 kcal/g, depending on the composition of the tissues deposited.[34,35] For the US Dietary Reference Intakes, the energy cost of growth was estimated to be 175 kcal/day for the age interval 0 through 3 months, 60 kcal/day for 4 through 6 months, and 20 kcal/day for 7 through 35 months.[1] Although the composition of newly synthesized tissues varies in childhood and adolescence, these variations have a minor effect on total energy requirements, because approximately 20 to 25 kcal/day only are required for growth.

Energy Requirements of Infants, Children, and Adolescents

Energy requirements of infants, children, and adolescents are defined as the amount of food energy needed to balance total energy expenditure at a desirable level of physical activity and to support optimal growth and development consistent with long-term health.[1,2] In 2002, the Institute of Medicine (now the National Academy of Medicine) published estimated energy requirements (EERs) for infants and children based on total energy expenditure measured by the doubly labeled water method.[1] EER equations for estimation of energy requirements for sedentary, low active, active, and very active categories of physical activity are provided in Table 14.2. The sedentary level reflects BMR, TEF, and the minimal activity required for daily living. Incorporating approximately 120, 230, and 400 minutes/day walking at 2.5 miles per hour or equivalent activity corresponds to the low active, active, and very active categories, respectively. Clearly, children in the active and very active categories are participating in moderate and vigorous activities, in addition to walking. Even though energy requirements also are

Table 14.2.
Estimated Energy Requirements

Estimated Energy Requirements (EERs)[a]	
0–3 mo	(89 × weight [kg] − 100) + 175 kcal
4–6 mo	(89 × weight [kg] − 100) + 56 kcal
7–12 mo	(89 × weight [kg] − 100) + 22 kcal
13–36 mo	(89 × weight [kg] − 100) + 20 kcal
3–8 y (boys)	88.5 − (61.9 × age [y]) + PA × (26.7 × weight [kg] + 903 × height [m]) + 20 kcal
3–8 y (girls)	135.3 − (30.8 × age [y]) + PA × (10.0 × weight [kg] + 934 × height [m]) + 20 kcal
9–18 y (boys)	88.5 − (61.9 × age [y]) + PA × (26.7 × weight [kg] + 903 × height [m]) + 25 kcal
9–18 y (girls)	135.3 − (30.8 × age [y]) + PA × (10.0 × weight [kg] + 934 × height [m]) + 25 kcal

Adapted from Institute of Medicine.[1]

[a] EER = total energy expenditure + energy deposition.

Where PA is the physical activity coefficient:
For boys 3 through 18 years:
      PA = 1.00 (sedentary, estimated PAL ≥1.0<1.4)
      PA = 1.13 (low active, estimated PAL ≥1.4<1.6)
      PA = 1.26 (active, estimated PAL ≥1.6<1.9)
      PA = 1.42 (very active, estimated PAL ≥1.9<2.5)
For girls 3 through 18 years:
      PA = 1.00 (sedentary, estimated PAL ≥1.0<1.4)
      PA = 1.16 (low active, estimated PAL ≥1.4<1.6)
      PA = 1.31 (active, estimated PAL ≥1.6<1.9)
      PA = 1.56 (very active, estimated PAL ≥1.9<2.5)

presented for varying levels of physical activity, moderately active lifestyles are strongly encouraged to maintain fitness and health and to reduce the risk of developing obesity and its comorbidities.

At the time of the formulation of the 2002 Dietary Reference Intakes, the doubly labeled water database was limited in the 3- to 5-year-old range, resulting in EER equations that overestimate energy requirements of preschool-aged children.[36] The erroneous predictions stemmed from the fact that physical activity (PAL) categories used were developmentally inappropriate for this young age group. Observed PAL values gradually

Table 14.3.

Revised Estimated Energy Requirements for Preschool-Aged Children

Estimated Energy Requirements[a]	
3–5 y (boys)	358 + PA × (16 × weight [kg] + 356 × height [m]) + 20 kcal
3–5 y (girls)	352 + PA × (11.6 × weight [kg] + 347 × height [m]) + 20 kcal

Adapted from Butte.[36]

[a] EER = total energy expenditure + energy deposition.

Where PA is the physical activity coefficient:
For boys 3 through 5 years:
PA = 1.00 (sedentary, estimated PAL ≥1.0<1.2)
PA = 1.20 (low active, estimated PAL ≥1.2<1.35)
PA = 1.37 (active, estimated PAL ≥1.35<1.5)
PA = 1.64 (very active, estimated PAL ≥1.5)

For girls 3 through 18 years:
PA = 1.00 (sedentary, estimated PAL ≥1.0<1.2)
PA = 1.25 (low active, estimated PAL ≥1.2<1.35)
PA = 1.46 (active, estimated PAL ≥1.35<1.5)
PA = 1.62 (very active, estimated PAL ≥1.5)

increase from infancy to early childhood because of declining BMR and developmental maturation. New total energy expenditure (TEE) prediction equations based on doubly labeled water and developmentally appropriate PAL categories are presented for preschool-aged children in Table 14.3.[36]

Macronutrient Distribution Ranges

Acceptable macronutrient distribution ranges, as a percent of total energy intake, for fat are slightly higher in children than adults (30%–40% for children 1–3 years of age and 25%–35% for children 4–18 years of age vs 20%–35% in adults) and for protein are lower (5%–20% for children 1–3 years of age and 10%–30% for children 4–18 years of age vs 10%–35% in adults).[1] The acceptable macronutrient distribution ranges for carbohydrates are the same for all ages—45% to 65% of energy intake from carbohydrates, with added sugars constituting no more than 25% of total energy intake. The average diet of individuals in the United States supplies 12% to 15% of calories from protein and the remainder from carbohydrates and fat. An appropriate balance of total calories and protein is required for adequate growth, especially in response to malnutrition. The more rapid the weight gain, the higher the dietary protein-to-energy (P:E) ratio required. Growth rates of

10, 30, and 50 g/day required P:E ratios of 5.6%, 6.9%, and 8.1%, respectively, in infants recovering from malnutrition.[7] Standard infant formulas and human milk have P:E ratios of approximately 12% and 8%, respectively.

Altered Energy Requirements

Many common pathologic conditions may alter energy requirements, interfere with nutrient availability, affect substrate utilization, or impair physical activity. Provision of adequate energy may be especially important in certain clinical situations, particularly if a patient's ability to regulate intake is impaired. Energy deficit in children leads to growth retardation; loss of fat and muscle; delayed motor, cognitive, and behavioral development; diminished immunocompetence; and increased morbidity and mortality.[2] Excess energy intake can lead to obesity and its comorbidities, including type 2 diabetes mellitus, hyperlipidemia, hypertension, hyperandrogenism in girls, sleep disorders, respiratory difficulties, nonalcoholic fatty liver disease, gall bladder disease, orthopedic problems, and idiopathic intracranial hypertension.[37] During infancy, childhood, and adolescence, growth rate may serve as a good "bioassay" for dietary adequacy in terms of meeting energy requirements. Careful consideration of the factors affecting energy balance (eg, energy intake, energy excretion, energy expenditure, and energy retention) can often clarify seemingly complex clinical problems.

Infection and Trauma

A characteristic response to infection and trauma is an increase in core body temperature and resting energy expenditure. Oxygen consumption was measured in adult patients with several febrile illnesses (eg, tuberculosis, typhoid fever, malaria, bacterial pneumonia, and rheumatic fever).[38] These studies indicated that for each degree centigrade increase in body temperature, the metabolic rate increased up to 13%.

During infection, fatty acids continue to be the major fuel source, but utilization of ketone bodies is decreased.[38] Uptake and utilization of branched-chain amino acids are accelerated in skeletal muscles to fuel gluconeogenesis in the liver and kidney.

When the energy cost of measles was estimated in Kenyan children 28 months of age, a 75% decrease was seen in energy intake and a slight decrease in absorption during the acute illness.[39] BMR was similar during measles and after recovery. The energy density of the diet tolerated during illness decreased from 0.9 kcal/g to 0.6 kcal/g. Inadequate intake, not elevated expenditure, was responsible for the energy deficit with this infectious disease.

The degree of hypermetabolism with trauma varies with the extent of the injury, the most extensive being in burn patients.[40] A 50% total body surface burn may double the metabolic rate. If the burn patient's body temperature is regulated at a high set point, the patient must be kept warm and heat losses must be minimized during the febrile state. If heat production exceeds thermoregulatory needs, physical and pharmacologic measures should be used to lower body temperature. In either case, energy requirements should be determined and met with vigorous nutritional support. In 91 children 3 to 18 years of age with severe burns, the Schofield equation underestimated measured resting energy expenditure by 635 ± 526 kcal/day.[41] Another study of 15 children with burns showed that measured basal energy expenditure was 1.16 ± 0.10 times predicted BEE and TEE was 1.33 ± 0.27 times predicted basal energy expenditure.[42]

Critically Ill Children

The American Society of Parenteral and Enteral Nutrition (ASPEN) and the Society of Critical Care Medicine (SCCM) presented best practices in nutrition therapy in critically ill pediatric patients hospitalized for greater than 2 or 3 days in a pediatric intensive care unit admitting medical, surgical, and cardiac patients[43] (see also Chapter 37: Nutrition of Children Who Are Critically Ill). Because of the diversity of this clinical population, energy expenditure should be measured by indirect calorimetry and used to estimate energy requirements. If indirect calorimetry is not feasible, the Schofield weight-height or weight equations[11] may be used cautiously to estimate energy expenditure, with subsequent weight monitoring.

Energy balance studies were performed in 46 mechanically ventilated and spontaneously breathing children admitted with sepsis or following surgery or trauma.[44] Measured energy expenditure did not differ from predicted values. Patients receiving parenteral nutrition achieved adequate energy intake and were more likely to be overfed. Enterally fed patients were frequently underfed mainly because of prescription and administration of energy amounts less than measured values.

Other Diseases

Bronchopulmonary dysplasia typically is associated with slow growth. The impaired growth rate has been attributed to decreased intake during acute illness and increased work of respiration. Oxygen consumption was 25%

higher in infants with bronchopulmonary dysplasia than that in controls.[45] Indirect calorimetry studies have shown an increase of 15 to 25 kcal/kg/day in infants with bronchopulmonary dysplasia compared with controls.[46] Doubly labeled water studies confirm higher rates of total energy expenditure in this patient population.[47] The increased energy requirements should be supported with aggressive nutritional therapy (see also Chapter 5: Nutritional Needs of the Preterm Infant).

Energy imbalance in children with congenital heart disease (CHD) is common and is influenced by age, cardiac diagnoses, preoperative nutritional status, the surgery itself, and postoperative care[48] (see also Chapter 44: Cardiac Disease). Because predictive equations have been shown to be inaccurate in estimating energy requirements, indirect calorimetry should be used to assess energy requirements throughout the hospitalization. The metabolic rates of infants with congestive heart failure were elevated in proportion to their degree of growth retardation and heart failure. The oxygen consumption of infants with congestive heart failure was 9.4 mL/kg/min, compared with 6.5 mL/kg/min in infants with CHD but not in failure.[49] Infants with severe CHD who were markedly undergrown had abnormally high rates of oxygen consumption, whereas those with CHD whose growth was normal consumed oxygen at normal rates.[50] Higher rates of total energy expenditure by doubly labeled water, resting energy expenditure by indirect calorimetry, and energy intake were demonstrated in infants with cyanotic congenital heart disease compared with healthy control infants.[51]

In children with Prader-Willi syndrome, total energy expenditure, resting energy expenditure, sleep energy expenditure, activity energy expenditure, and diet-induced thermogenesis were demonstrated to be lower compared with age-, sex-, and body mass index-matched controls.[52] Lower lean body mass, endocrine dysfunction, and lower fat oxidation, sympathetic activity, and spontaneous physical activity all contribute to the reduction in energy expenditure in Prader-Willi syndrome.

References

1. Institute of Medicine. *Dietary Reference Intakes for Energy, Carbohydrate, Fiber, Fat, Fatty Acids, Cholesterol, Protein, and Amino Acids.* 5 ed. Washington DC: National Academy of Science; 2002

2. FAO/WHO/UNU Expert Consultation. *Human energy requirements.* Rome: World Health Organization; 2004

3. Blaxter K. *Energy metabolism in animals and man.* 1 ed. Cambridge: Cambridge University Press; 1989

4. Consolazio CF, Johnson RE, Pecora LJ. The computation of metabolic balances. *Physiological Measurements of Metabolic Functions in Man.* New York: McGraw-Hill Book Company, Inc.; 1963. p. 313–325

5. Watt BK, Merrill AL. *Composition of foods.* ARS Handbook No. 8 ed. Washington DC: US Government Printing Office; 1963

6. Krieger JW, Sitren HS, Daniels MJ, Langkamp-Henken B. Effects of variation in protein and carbohydrate intake on body mass and composition during energy restriction: a meta-regression 1. *Am J Clin Nutr* 2006 February;83(2):260–274

7. Ashworth A, Millward DJ. Catch-up growth in children. *Nutr Rev* 1986;44:157–163

8. Ogden CL, Carroll MD, Lawman HG et al. Trends in Obesity Prevalence Among Children and Adolescents in the United States, 1988–1994 Through 2013–2014. *JAMA* 2016 June 7;315(21):2292–2299

9. Feinman RD, Fine EJ. "A calorie is a calorie" violates the second law of thermodynamics. *Nutr J* 2004 July 28;3:9

10. Holliday M, Potter D, Jarrah A, Bearg S. Relation of metabolic rate to body weight and organ size. *Pediatr Res* 1967;1:185–195

11. Schofield WN, Schofield C, James WPT. Basal metabolic rate-review and prediction, together with annotated bibliography of source material. *Hum Nutr: Clin Nutr* 1985;39C:1–96

12. Butte NF, Wong WW, Hopkinson JM, Heinz CJ, Mehta NR, Smith EO. Energy requirements derived from total energy expenditure and energy deposition during the first 2 years of life. *Am J Clin Nutr* 2000;72:1558–1569

13. Cannon B, Nedergaard J. Nonshivering thermogenesis and its adequate measurement in metabolic studies. *J Exp Biol* 2011 January 15;214(Pt 2):242–253

14. van Marken Lichtenbelt WD, Schrauwen P. Implications of nonshivering thermogenesis for energy balance regulation in humans. *Am J Physiol Regul Integr Comp Physiol* 2011 August;301(2):R285–R296

15. Muller MJ, Bosy-Westphal A. Adaptive thermogenesis with weight loss in humans. *Obesity (Silver Spring)* 2013 February;21(2):218–228

16. Nedergaard J, Bengtsson T, Cannon B. Unexpected evidence for active brown adipose tissue in adult humans. *Am J Physiol Endocrinol Metab* 2007 August;293(2): E444–E452

17. Hu HH, Yin L, Aggabao PC, Perkins TG, Chia JM, Gilsanz V. Comparison of brown and white adipose tissues in infants and children with chemical-shift-encoded water-fat MRI. *J Magn Reson Imaging* 2013 February 25

18. Ponrartana S, Hu HH, Gilsanz V. On the relevance of brown adipose tissue in children. *Ann N Y Acad Sci* 2013 October;1302:24–29

19. Brooks GA, Fahey TD, Baldwin KM. *Exercise Physiology: Human Bioenergetics and its Applications.* 4th ed. New York: McGraw-Hill; 2004

20. McArdle WD, Katch FI, Katch VL. *Exercise Physiology, Energy Nutrition, and Human Performance.* 5th ed. 2001

21. Ainsworth BE, Haskell WL, Whitt MC et al. Compendium of physical activities: an update of activity codes and MET intensities. *Med Sci Sports Exerc* 2000 September;32(9 Suppl):S498–S504

22. Torun B. Energy cost of various physical activities in healthy children. In: Schürch B, Scrimshaw NS, editors. *Activity, energy expenditure and energy requirements of infants and children.* Lausanne: International Dietary Energy Consultancy Group; 1990. p. 139–183

23. McMurray RG, Butte NF, Crouter SE et al. Exploring Metrics to Express Energy Expenditure of Physical Activity in Youth. *PLoS One* 2015;10(6):e0130869

24. Rowland TW. Children's Exercise Physiology. 2nd ed. Champaign IL: Human Kinetics; 2005. p. 80–84

25. Gallagher D, Belmonte D, Deurenberg P et al. Organ-tissue mass measurement allows modeling of REE and metabolically active tissue mass. *Am J Physiol* 1998 August;275(2 Pt 1):E249–E258

26. Muller MJ, Bosy-Westphal A, Kutzner D, Heller M. Metabolically active components of fat-free mass and resting energy expenditure in humans: recent lessons from imaging technologies. *Obes Rev* 2002 May;3(2):113–122

27. Butte NF, Watson KB, Ridley K et al. A Youth Compendium of Physical Activities: Activity Codes and Metabolic Intensities. *Med Sci Sports Exerc* 2018 February;50(2):246–256

28. Pfeiffer KA, Watson KB, McMurray RG et al. Energy cost expression for a Youth Compendium of Physical Activities: Rationale for using age groups. Pediatric Exercise Science. 2017

29. Jequier E, Acheson K, Schutz Y. Assessment of energy expenditure and fuel utilization in man. *Ann Rev Nutr* 1987;7:187–208

30. Livesey G, Elia M. Estimation of energy expenditure, net carbohydrate utilization, and net fat oxidation and synthesis by indirect calorimetry: evaluation of errors with special reference to the detailed composition of fuels. *Am J Clin Nutr* 1988;47:608–628

31. Weir JB. New methods for calculating metabolic rate with special reference to protein metabolism. *J Physiol* 1949;109:1–9

32. Schoeller DA, Van Santen E. Measurement of energy expenditure in humans by doubly labeled water method. *J Appl Physiol* 1982;53:955–959

33. Schoeller DA. Measurement of energy expenditure in free-living humans by using doubly labeled water. *J Nutr* 1988 November;118(11):1278–1289

34. Butte NF, Wong WW, Garza C. Energy cost of growth during infancy. *Proc Nutr Soc* 1989;48:303–312

35. Roberts SB, Young VR. Energy costs of fat and protein deposition in the human infant. *Am J Clin Nutr* 1988;48:951–955

36. Butte NF, Wong WW, Wilson TA, Adolph AL, Puyau MR, Zakeri IF. Revision of Dietary Reference Intakes for energy in preschool-age children. *Am J Clin Nutr* 2014 July;100(1):161–167

37. Barlow SE. Expert committee recommendations regarding the prevention, assessment, and treatment of child and adolescent overweight and obesity: summary report. *Pediatrics* 2007 December;120 Suppl 4:S164–S192

38. Beisel WR, Wannemacher RW, Neufeld HA. Relation of fever to energy expenditure. *Assessment of Energy Metabolism in Health and Disease.* Columbus: Ross Laboratories; 1980. p. 144–150

39. Duggan MB, Milner RDG. Energy cost of measles infection. *Arch Dis Child* 1986;61:436–439

40. Aulick LH. Studies in heat transport and heat loss in thermally injured patients. *Assessment of Energy Metabolism in health and Disease.* Columbus: Ross Laboratories; 1980. p. 141–144

41. Suman OE, Mlcak RP, Chinkes DL, Herndon DN. Resting energy expenditure in severely burned children: analysis of agreement between indirect calorimetry and prediction equations using the Bland-Altman method. *Burns* 2006 May;32(3):335–342

42. Goran MI, Peters EJ, Herndon DN, Wolfe RR. Total energy expenditure in burned children using the doubly labeled water technique. *Am J Physiol* 1990 October;259(4 Pt 1):E576–E585

43. Mehta NM, Skillman HE, Irving SY et al. Guidelines for the Provision and Assessment of Nutrition Support Therapy in the Pediatric Critically Ill Patient: Society of Critical Care Medicine and American Society for Parenteral and Enteral Nutrition. *JPEN J Parenter Enteral Nutr* 2017 July;41(5):706–742

44. Oosterveld MJ, Van Der KM, De MK, De Greef HJ, Gemke RJ. Energy expenditure and balance following pediatric intensive care unit admission: a longitudinal study of critically ill children. *Pediatr Crit Care Med* 2006 March;7(2):147–153

45. Weinstein MR, Oh W. Oxygen consumption in infants with bronchopulmonary dysplasia. *J Pediatr* 1981;99:958–993

46. Wilson DC, McClure G. Energy requirements in sick preterm babies. *Acta Paediatr Suppl* 1994 December;405:60–64

47. Denne SC. Energy expenditure in infants with pulmonary insufficiency: is there evidence for increased energy needs? *J Nutr* 2001 March;131(3):935S–937S

48. Wong JJ, Cheifetz IM, Ong C, Nakao M, Lee JH. Nutrition Support for Children Undergoing Congenital Heart Surgeries: A Narrative Review. *World J Pediatr Congenit Heart Surg* 2015 July;6(3):443–454

49. Krauss AN, Auld PAM. Metabolic rate of neonates with congenital heart disease. *Arch Dis Child* 1975;50:539–541

IV

50. Lees MH, Bristow JD, Griswold HE, Olmsted RW. Relative hypermetabolism in infants with congenital heart disease and undernutrition. *Pediatrics* 1965;36: 183–191

51. Leitch CA, Karn CA, Peppard RJ et al. Increased energy expenditure in infants with cyanotic congenital heart disease. *J Pediatr* 1998 December;133(6):755–760

52. Alsaif M, Elliot SA, MacKenzie ML, Prado CM, Field CJ, Haqq AM. Energy Metabolism Profile in Individuals with Prader-Willi Syndrome and Implications for Clinical Management: A Systematic Review. *Adv Nutr* 2017 November;8(6):905–915

Chapter 15

Protein

Introduction

Proteins are the major structural and functional components of all cells in the body. They are macromolecules comprising 1 or more chains of amino acids that vary in their sequence and length and are folded into specific 3-dimensional structures. The sizes and conformations of proteins, therefore, are infinitely diverse and complex, and this enables them to serve an extensive variety of functions in the cell. Dietary protein provides the amino acids required for both the synthesis of body proteins and the production of other nitrogenous compounds with important functional roles, such as glutathione, creatine, polyamines, phosphatidyl choline, heme, nucleotides, hormones, nitric oxide, carnitine, bile acids, and some neurotransmitters. Amino acids are also critical contributors to one-carbon metabolism that is responsible for the generation of methyl groups. In this nonnitrogenous role, they can affect a large number of cellular processes, including DNA and histone methylation, to modulate gene expression. Amino acids can exist as various stereoisomers in nature. Only the L-amino acids are biologically active and can be incorporated into proteins. Body proteins also can be catabolized and serve as an energy source when energy intake, in particular carbohydrate intake, is inadequate.

From the dietary perspective, it is the amino acid composition of a protein that is its most relevant property, although for some, the structure can dictate digestibility—for example, keratin, an insoluble protein that makes up hair, skin, and nails. Protein digestion begins in the stomach through the activity of pepsin in the presence of hydrochloric acid. Pepsin activity and hydrochloric acid have been identified in the stomachs of fetuses by 20 weeks of gestation, and preterm infants as young as 24 weeks of gestation can reduce their gastric pH soon after birth. However, the frequent milk ingestion in newborn infants buffers the acidity and delays gastric proteolysis; nonetheless, the stomach is believed to present no limitations to the digestibility of proteins even at the youngest ages. Similar pepsin levels have been observed in infants, children, and adults. Protein digestion continues in the presence of pancreatic enzymes in the duodenum and the enzymes in the brush border of the jejunum and proximal ileum. Pancreatic proteases (trypsin and chymotrypsin) are present from about 20 weeks of gestation and increase progressively attaining adult levels during infancy. However, enterokinase, required for the activation of trypsin, is not detected until 26 weeks of gestation and is only at 20%

of adult levels by term.[1] This low enterokinase activity may limit luminal
protein digestion, enabling increased passage of larger proteins, such as
immunoglobulin G (IgG) into the intestine, where they can be digested or
absorbed. Peptidases on the intestinal brush border continue the hydrolysis of proteins to oligopeptides and amino acids, and these are absorbed
primarily in the jejunum via a large area of amino acid transporters in the
brush-border membrane. Oligopeptides are hydrolyzed to amino acids by
enzymes in the cells of the intestinal epithelium, but some can be absorbed
also as di- and tripeptides. The peptidases and amino acid transporters
are present and active before 24 weeks of gestation and are not limiting for
protein digestion in neonates.[2] Generally, more than 90% of the amino acids
ingested as dietary protein are absorbed by the small intestine. The protein
that escapes digestion in the small intestine, together with secreted proteins, mucins, and sloughed off intestinal cells, are metabolized by bacterial
proteases and peptidases secreted by the microbiota in the large intestine.
With the possible exception of the neonate, however, the amino acids generated cannot be absorbed by the large intestine. Amino acids that are not
incorporated into microbial proteins are metabolized by the gut microbiota
into a wide assortment of metabolites, including short-chain fatty acids,
polyamines, neuroactive molecules, sulfur-containing and aromatic compounds, and ammonia.[3] The nitrogenous products of bacterial fermentation
can be absorbed by the intestine, where they can directly influence intestinal
cell physiology, or they are transported to the liver, where they are detoxified
or further metabolized. The ammonia provides nitrogen for the synthesis
of amino acids. The products of bacterial fermentation of amino acids and,
thus, the systemic effects they incur, are a function of the specific microbiota present in the gut, which in turn, is influenced by the individual's age,
metabolic phenotype, and diet.[3] The human infant microbiome is present
starting at birth and undergoes profound diversification until approximately
3 years of age.[4] The infant's diet and environmental exposures dictate the
compositional development of the microbiota. Thus, although it is likely that
these changes affect nitrogen metabolism of the microbiome, the effect on
the infant's protein metabolism is uncertain and is an area of active research.

Amino acids absorbed from the small intestine are first transported to
the liver, where they are metabolized or enter the general amino acid pool of
the body in the plasma and exchange with tissue pools. Some amino acids
are used directly by the intestine itself, as an energy source, to synthesize
gut proteins, or in the production of other nitrogen-containing biological

molecules. Indeed, the gut derives most of its energy from the metabolism of glutamate, glutamine, and aspartate. The gut's high capacity to metabolize glutamate serves to prevent excessive increases in plasma glutamate and the potential development of neurotoxicity, from a high dietary intake of glutamate, such as when foods supplemented with monosodium glutamate are consumed.[5] In the growing organism, an influx of amino acids to the tissues from the diet rapidly stimulates protein synthesis.[6-8] This response is dampened as the organism matures, and in adults, protein consumption primarily reduces protein breakdown with only a moderate response in protein synthesis.[9,10] Dietary amino acids consumed in excess of the body's needs cannot be stored. The nitrogen component of amino acids is converted to urea, and the remaining keto-acids are used directly for energy production or converted to glucose and fat for storage when energy intake is adequate. Therefore, blood urea nitrogen is a good indicator of recent protein intake when hydration and renal function are normal. The stimulation of protein synthesis by the influx of amino acids from the diet, together with the body's inability to store excess dietary amino acids, are primary reasons for the recommendation that in infants and children the daily protein requirement should be consumed as meals at regular intervals throughout the day.

Body proteins and other nitrogenous compounds are continuously degraded and resynthesized. Several times more endogenous protein is turned over every day than is usually consumed. The rate of turnover can be rapid, as in bone marrow and in gastrointestinal mucosa, or it can be slow, as in muscle and collagen. Protein turnover also changes with age; it is highest during early life when tissues are maturing and their growth rates are at their highest.[10] The amino acids released from the breakdown of endogenous proteins are recycled, but this process is not completely efficient. Amino acids that are not reused are catabolized or lost in urine, feces, sweat, desquamated skin, hair, and nails. These losses create an obligatory requirement for dietary amino acids, in addition to any requirement for the net accretion of body protein. This obligatory fraction constitutes the maintenance or basal needs of the organism, and once growth has ceased, this fraction represents an individual's entire protein requirement. The magnitude of these basal losses is dictated by the individual's total lean mass and basal metabolic rate.

Amino acids are usually categorized into 3 groups: indispensable, dispensable, and conditionally indispensable. Amino acids with carbon skeletons that cannot be synthesized de novo in adults are regarded as indispensable (essential) amino acids and must be provided by the diet; they include leucine, isoleucine, valine, threonine, methionine, phenylalanine, tryptophan, lysine, and histidine. To sustain normal growth and the maintenance of the body's protein mass after the requirements for indispensable amino acids have been met, the additional dietary nitrogen required must be provided as dispensable (nonessential) amino acids. Dispensable amino acids are those that can be synthesized in the body from other amino acids or nitrogen containing molecules. These are usually divided into 2 categories: the truly dispensable amino acids and the conditionally indispensable amino acids. Conditionally indispensable amino acids are those that ordinarily can be synthesized, but an exogenous source is required under certain circumstances. The designation varies according to the age of the individual and the presence of genetic or acquired disease conditions. For all humans, alanine, aspartic acid, asparagine, serine, and glutamic acid can be classified as dispensable. Arginine, glutamine, proline, glycine, cysteine, and tyrosine are in the conditionally indispensable category. Cysteine, tyrosine, and arginine must be provided to the preterm infant because of the immaturity of the enzyme activities necessary for their synthesis from precursors. Recent studies suggest that by term, the necessary enzyme activities to generate these amino acids from their precursors is present and they are no longer indispensable.[11] Glycine is required for the synthesis of creatine, porphyrins, glutathione, nucleotides, and bile salts and is present in relatively high amount in collagen; therefore, the requirement for this amino acid during times of rapid growth is relatively high.[12] Glycine is present in relatively small amounts in milk and may be a conditionally indispensable amino acid for the preterm infant and neonate. Various disease conditions can also interfere with the synthesis of amino acids that can normally be synthesized from other amino acids. Arginine is essential in patients with defects of the urea cycle. Arginine is also important for immune function and is the precursor for nitric oxide, which is a pivotal intracellular signaling molecule. During critical illness, there is an accelerated loss of arginine, which diminishes its availability to support immune function and is believed to contribute to an increased risk of infection in critically ill patients.[13] Therefore, its supplementation in these conditions has been investigated but has yielded controversial outcomes, and thus, it is not recommended in the pediatric population.[14] In addition to the preterm infant, cysteine may be essential in patients with hepatic disease or homocystinuria. Tyrosine is essential for people with phenylketonuria and may be required for patients with hepatic disease. Glutamine is the preferred fuel for rapidly dividing cells, such as enterocytes and lymphocytes; it is also a precursor for glutathione, citrulline, and arginine synthesis. Thus, during times of critical stress, such as after surgical procedures, nonsurgical trauma, or sepsis, or in patients with gastrointestinal mucosal injury, large amounts of glutamine are synthesized by the skeletal muscle from the amino acids of skeletal muscle proteins. Numerous clinical studies have assessed the benefits of glutamine supplementation in critically ill patients. Although little benefit has been demonstrated in neonates and critically ill children, its use may be indicated in adult patients in the intensive care unit without multiple organ failure.[15] Taurine and carnitine are amino acids that serve important and specific functions in the cell but are not incorporated into proteins. They can be synthesized by the body from cysteine and lysine, respectively, and are present in a mixed diet containing proteins of animal origin. The rates of synthesis in infants fed by total parenteral nutrition or receiving synthetic formulas devoid of taurine and carnitine may be insufficient to meet all of their needs and necessitate dietary supplementation.[16,17] Nearly all infant formulas today contain added taurine and carnitine.

Recommended Dietary Intake for Protein and Amino Acids

The appropriate amount of protein that should be consumed is expressed in a number of different ways according to the information it is meant to convey, how the values are derived, and the purpose for which the information will be used. The Recommended Dietary Allowance (RDA) for protein is the average daily intake of protein that meets the nutrient needs of most healthy individuals of a particular life stage and sex (see Appendix E).[18,19] The RDA is derived from:

1. *The Estimated Average Requirement (EAR) for protein.* The EAR is the daily protein intake that meets the protein needs of 50% of all healthy individuals of a specific age and sex. The physiologic requirement is defined as the lowest level of protein intake needed to replace losses from the body when energy intake is in balance (maintenance requirement). In growing individuals and pregnant and lactating women, the protein requirement also includes the protein required for tissue accretion and milk production at a level associated with good health. The need for growth decreases from approximately 55% of total intake over the first

3 months of life to 10% or less by 8 years of age and accounts largely for the reduction with age in protein requirements (Table 15.1). These intakes assume that the protein source is of high quality on the basis of its amino acid composition.

2. *The variability in protein needs for specific population groups.* The RDA defines the protein need of 97.5% of individuals in a particular age group. Thus, the RDA must be increased above the EAR to account for the variability in the requirements among groups of similar individuals. This includes the variation in maintenance needs, the variation in protein accretion rate (if relevant), and the variation in the efficiency with which dietary protein is accumulated. It is important to note that because of this adjustment, the RDA exceeds the protein needs of most individuals within a specified group.

For some nutrients and/or certain populations, the scientific data (either average intakes or their variability) for estimating an EAR are not sufficiently robust to make a definitive recommendation. In these cases, a level defined as an Adequate Intake (AI) is used. This value is based on the average protein intake of a group of individuals who appear to be healthy and in a good nutritional state. The recommendation for daily protein and amino acid intake of infants from birth to 6 months falls in this category and is based on the average daily protein intake of infants fed principally with human milk.

Table 15.1.
Contribution of Maintenance and Growth to Protein Needs of Infants and Children[a]

| Age | Protein Gain[b] | Intake | |
| | | Growth | Maintenance |
	(g/(kg/d))	(% of total)	
0.5–3 mo	0.49	55	45
3–6 mo	0.30	43	57
6–12 mo	0.18	31	69
1–3 y	0.10	20	80
4–8 y	0.046	10	90

[a] Sources: Institute of Medicine,[18] Butte et al,[24] and Ellis et al.[25]

[b] Average for boys and girls.

The Dietary Reference Intake guidelines[18] define 2 additional parameters that should be taken into consideration in the evaluation of diets and in making dietary recommendations: the Tolerable Upper Intake Level (UL) and the Acceptable Macronutrient Distribution Range (AMDR). No ULs have been set for protein or amino acid intakes because of the absence of sufficient data on which to base recommendations. This does not imply that high levels are not harmful; some of the current concerns regarding less beneficial effects of high protein intakes will be discussed later. The AMDRs were developed because of the increasing evidence that the dietary sources from which individuals obtain their energy may play a role in the development of chronic diseases.[20] Protein, fats, and carbohydrates can substitute for each other as sources of dietary energy; thus, for a given energy intake, if the proportion of one varies, so must the others. The AMDR for protein is the proportion of the total energy intake that is protein and that is associated with a reduced risk for chronic disease. The AMDR for protein is 5% to 20% of total energy intake in 1- to 3-year-old children and 10% to 30% of total energy intake for 4- to 18-year-old children and adolescents.

For the 9 indispensable amino acids, EARs and RDAs have been developed for individuals from 7 months to 18 years of age, and AIs have been determined for infants from birth through 6 months. The requirement for methionine is frequently given as a composite value for total sulfur-containing amino acids (ie, methionine and cysteine, the latter being a metabolic product of methionine catabolism). Thus, the requirement for cysteine is dependent on there being sufficient methionine in the diet to meet the needs for synthesis of both amino acids, although it is clear that in some circumstances, such as in preterm infants, the metabolism of methionine to cysteine may not be sufficient to meet the entire cysteine requirement. Similarly, the requirements for phenylalanine and tyrosine, the aromatic amino acids, are pooled because tyrosine can be formed from the metabolism of phenylalanine.

Methods for Determining Protein and Amino Acid Requirements

Protein

Protein requirements and balance data are frequently measured and expressed on the basis of nitrogen content. On average, nitrogen constitutes 16% of the weight of a protein, although the exact value varies from protein to protein. The recommendations for protein intakes have used a factor of 6.25 to convert g of nitrogen to g of protein.

Protein needs have been estimated using various approaches.[18,19,21–23] During the first 6 months of life, human milk is the optimal source of protein for infants and, when freely fed, is sufficient to sustain good health and optimal growth. Thus, the average intake of healthy breastfed infants has been used to define an AI for this age group. The intake of the infants was determined from the volume of milk consumed (measured by weighing infants before and after a feed) and the average protein content of human milk. However, because the protein content and composition of milk changes both within individual feeds and over time as lactation proceeds from birth, this leaves some uncertainty on the absolute requirement for protein.

Recommendations for dietary protein intakes of infants older than 6 months (once supplementation with weaning foods begins) have been estimated using the factorial method. The factorial method provides an estimate of protein needs for maintenance and growth and adjusts for the efficiency with which dietary protein is used according to age, size, and gender.

Maintenance protein requirements are derived from nitrogen balance studies.[23] This method involves determination of the difference between the intake and excretion of nitrogen in urine, feces, sweat, and minor losses via other routes for 1 to 3 weeks or longer. Several different levels of a quality protein source, such as milk or egg, legume and cereal mixes, or mixed vegetable and animal sources, are tested at a constant and adequate energy intake. From the relationship between intake and balance (intake minus excretion), the amount of nitrogen required for maintenance (zero balance) is extrapolated.

To the maintenance requirements, additional amounts of protein that would be sufficient to support appropriate body protein gains have been added. The mean rate of protein gain during growth has been estimated from the body composition data of infants from 9 months through 3 years of age[24] and children from 4 to 18 years of age.[25] In both studies, body composition was measured using a combination of total body water by deuterium dilution, total body potassium, and dual-energy x-ray absorptiometry. The conversion of dietary protein to body proteins, however, is not 100% efficient. In growing individuals, the slope of the relationship between balance and intake provides a measure of the efficiency with which dietary protein is used for growth (58% from 0.5 through 13 years of age; 43% from

14 to 18 years[18]). Thus, the amount of dietary protein needed for growth must be adjusted to account for this inefficiency.

Amino Acids

Estimation of the requirements of amino acids can be determined by a number of approaches. The general approach involves measuring the relationship between the intake of the amino acid and a relevant indicator of nutritional adequacy in the context of an otherwise adequate diet. The indicator can be a measure of protein metabolism, such as nitrogen balance or whole body protein turnover, or it can be a measure of the metabolism of the amino acid of interest (eg, from the effect of graded intakes of individual amino acids on their plasma concentration, or various assessments of the rate of amino acid oxidation using stable-isotope labeled amino acids as tracers). The various methods have advantages and disadvantages and do not all result in the same values. Because of this uncertainty, together with the paucity of direct measurements of amino acid metabolism in the pediatric population, a factorial approach was used to estimate individual amino acid EARs from 6 months to 18 years of age. For infants through 6 months of age, AIs have been defined based on data from human milk fed infants.[18,19,21,22] These were calculated from the average volume of milk consumed and the amino acid composition of human milk proteins of normally growing, healthy infants.

To define the growth component of the requirement for individual amino acids, the factorial approach uses data for tissue protein accretion, and the amino acid composition of body tissues, corrected for the inefficiency of dietary utilization. Because the maintenance protein requirement does not vary with age in children, and the values are very similar to adult values (expressed per unit of body weight), the values for the maintenance component of the amino acid requirements are based on adult maintenance values. The adult values are derived from direct measurements of amino acid kinetics and yield a different amino acid pattern from that of body proteins. Hence, as the total amount of amino acid deposited decreases with age, the composition of amino acids required changes (reflected in Table 15.2): the indispensable amino acids comprise approximately 42% of the tissue amino acid pattern but only 23% of the maintenance pattern.[22] The RDA for amino acids adds an amount to the EAR to include an allowance for variability in the population in growth and maintenance requirements.

Table 15.2.

Amino Acid Scoring Patterns Based on the Estimated Average Requirements for Protein and Indispensable Amino Acids[a,b]

Amino Acid	Infants	Children (1–3 y)	Adults (18+ y)
	(mg/g protein)		
Histidine	23	18	17
Isoleucine	57	25	23
Leucine	101	55	52
Lysine	69	51	47
Methionine + Cysteine	38	25	23
Phenylalanine + Tyrosine	87	47	41
Threonine	47	27	24
Tryptophan	18	7	6
Valine	56	32	29
Total indispensable amino acids	495	287	262

[a] Indispensable amino acid EAR/EAR for protein for an individual age group.

[b] Source: Institute of Medicine.[18]

Protein Quality

In many respects, the ultimate test of the protein quality of a particular food must take into consideration not only its ability to support body function, such as appropriate growth, immunity, and mental development of the individual consuming that food protein, but also its bioavailability. When human milk is no longer the only source of protein, the quality and digestibility of food protein becomes important. Because of the wide variation in amino acid composition and digestibility, proteins differ in their ability to provide the nitrogen and amino acids required for growth and maintenance. The amino acid composition of the food consumed is important, because if the content of a single indispensable amino acid is insufficient to meet an individual's need for that amino acid, it will limit the ability of the body to utilize the remaining amino acids in the diet, even if the total amount of protein consumed would appear to be adequate. The recommendations for protein intake assume that the sources of protein are highly digestible (greater than 95%) and that the indispensable amino acid composition closely meets human needs. These properties apply to animal proteins, such as those from egg, milk, meat, and fish. Vegetable proteins often have a lower digestibility (70%–80%), and they often provide inadequate amounts of individual amino acids. For example, cereals are relatively deficient in lysine, whereas the sulfur-containing amino acids are low in legumes (for examples, see Table 15.3).[18,19,26] Although plant proteins are generally of a lower quality than proteins of animal origin, equivalent

Table 15.3.

Mean Values for Digestibility and Amino Acid Scores of Various Protein Sources

Protein Source	True Digestibility[a]	Amino Acid Score[b]	
	(%)	6 mo to 1 y	School-Aged Child
Whole egg (hen)	97	0.74 (trp)	1.36 (his)
Cow milk	95	0.52 (thr)	0.90 (thr)
Beef (cooked)	94	0.54 (trp)	1.39 (trp)
Corn, whole	85	0.41 (lys)	0.55 (lys)
Rice, white, cooked	88	0.59 (lys)	0.80 (lys)
Wheat, flour, whole	86	0.40 (lys)	0.54 (lys)
Wheat, flour, refined	96	0.37 (lys)	0.50 (lys)
Peanut butter	95	0.40 (lys)	0.55 (lys)
Beans, navy cooked	78	0.60 (S)	0.91 (S)
Soy protein isolate	95	0.75 (S)	1.14 (S)
Rice + beans	78	0.70 (trp)	1.02 (lys)

[a] True digestibility in man (%) =

$$\frac{\text{Nitrogen intake - (Fecal N on test protein - Fecal N on nonprotein diet)} \times 100}{\text{Nitrogen intake}}$$

A factor of 6.25 is used to convert nitrogen to protein. Data from Institute of Medicine[18] and Food and Agriculture Organization, World Health Organization.[26]

[b] The amino acid score for various protein sources was derived using the amino acid requirement pattern shown in Table 15.2. The amino acid of the protein sources was obtained from the USDA Nutrient Database for Standard Reference, Release 19, 2006. The abbreviation shown in parenthesis is for the most limiting amino acid; Trp, tryptophan; lys, lysine; S, cysteine + methionine; thr, threonine; his, histidine. Values more than 1 indicate that the protein source contains relatively more of that amino acid than the ideal reference protein.

amino acid patterns can be achieved by mixing plant proteins from different sources such as legumes and cereals.[23] Processing of foods, including cooking, can also increase or decrease the digestibility of dietary proteins. An important example is the chemical modification to lysine with cooking, which renders it unavailable. Thus, to apply the recommendations for protein intake to mixed diets containing protein sources other than animal-based foods, it is necessary to adjust for the protein digestibility and correct for the adequacy of the amino acid composition of the food.

For the purpose of evaluating the adequacy of the amino acid content of food proteins, an amino acid scoring pattern provided by a dietary protein can be derived by dividing the indispensable amino acid EAR by the EAR for protein for an individual age group (Table 15.2).[18] Thus, an ideal protein is one containing all the indispensable amino acids in amounts sufficient to meet requirements without any excess. For infants to 1 year of age, the amino acid pattern of human milk proteins is considered the ideal, and provided the protein requirement is met with human milk, the amino acid intake will be appropriate. The scoring pattern for toddlers older than 1 year is significantly different from that for infants because of the smaller and different requirement pattern for growth. Thus, as maintenance requirements come to dominate, the requirement for indispensable amino acids diminishes. Because the scoring pattern is similar for young children and adults, the most recent recommendations propose that the scoring pattern for children from 1 to 3 years of age also be used in the assessment of the diets of adolescents and adults.[18]

The effectiveness with which the food source of an absorbed dietary protein can meet the indispensable amino acid requirement is determined by the protein's amino acid score (Table 15.3). This is determined by the amount of the amino acid in the food source that least meets the individual's amino acid requirements. To determine the amino acid score, the amount of an amino acid in 1 g of the protein of the food source is divided by the amount in 1 g of the reference protein for the relevant population (Table 15.2). The amino acid that has the lowest score is the limiting amino acid, and its value represents the amino acid score of that specific protein.

$$\text{amino acid score} = \frac{\text{mg of limiting amino acid in 1 g of food protein}}{\text{mg of amino acid in 1 g of reference pattern}}$$

The amino acid score corrected for the digestibility of the protein is termed the protein digestibility corrected amino acid score (PDCAAS)[18,19,26]:

$$PDCAAS (\%) = \text{true digestibility} \times \text{amino acid score} \times 100$$

Of the indispensable amino acids, only four are likely to affect the quality of a food protein: lysine, the sulfur-containing amino acids (methionine + cysteine), threonine, and tryptophan. Examples of the amino acid score for various protein sources if they were the only protein source in the diet of a young child are shown in Table 15.3. In the formulation of special purpose diets in clinical practice, it is essential that the scoring pattern for all indispensable amino acids is considered.

The PDCAAS, therefore, takes into account both the biological value of the protein and its bioavailability. However, this measure of the protein quality of a food has a number of inherent shortcomings and is believed to overestimate the true availability of amino acids in some foods.[27] The inaccuracies arise for a variety of reasons including: (1) it makes no allowance for additional nutritional value when high biological value proteins are consumed; (2) it does not consider the presence of antinutritional factors; (3) it does not take into account the bioavailability of amino acids; and (4) it overestimates protein foods of lower digestibility when these are supplemented with limiting amino acids. An alternative metric aimed to address these shortcomings, the Digestible Indispensable Amino Acid Score (DIAAS), has been proposed and is currently under development.[27,28]

Protein Requirements

Because of the differences in the quality of proteins available in the diet and other factors such as age, sex, activity levels, and methodological limitations, confidence in the recommendations for protein and amino acid intakes for individuals or populations is somewhat tenuous. Nonetheless, recommendations are needed to guide the design of diets and for planning specific intervention programs. The recommendations for protein intake are categorized by life stage and sex, because among healthy individuals these are the 2 primary parameters that are responsible for variations in the body's need for protein. The pediatric stage of life has been subdivided into 6 groupings: infancy, approximately 0 to 6 months, and 7 to 12 months; toddlers, approximately 1 through 3 years of age; early

IV

childhood, approximately 4 through 8 years of age; puberty, approximately 9 through 13 years of age; and adolescence, approximately 14 to 18 years of age. Differences between boys and girls are only defined for the adolescent group.[18] Preterm infants have higher protein requirements per kilogram of weight, and are not discussed here (see Chapter 5: Nutritional Needs of the Preterm Infant).

Infants

The optimal food for full-term infants is human milk, and it is recommended that this be the sole source of nutrition for infants for approximately the first 6 months of life. Current recommendations are based on the average value determined from a number of different studies of exclusively breastfed infants. These results indicate that, on average, infants to 6 months of age consume 0.78 L of milk per day (reviewed by the Institute of Medicine and Dewey et al[18,21]). The protein content of human milk is the lowest of any species, with values decreasing from approximately 15 g/L of true protein after the first few days through 2 weeks postpartum to approximately 9 g/L with the establishment of lactation (Appendix A). An average value of 11.7 g/L was used to calculate the AI for protein during this period. Human milk also contains significant amounts of nonprotein nitrogenous compounds, such as free amino acids, including carnitine, taurine, and glutamine (the most abundant), polyamines, nucleotides, urea, and creatine. Together, they constitute 17% to 23% of the total nitrogen content, or 0.5 to 0.4 g/L (Appendix A). Variability in the nitrogen components of human milk can be attributed in part to maternal nutrition.[29] The proportion of the nonprotein nitrogen that is bioavailable and spares the utilization of milk protein amino acids is uncertain; estimates from 46–61% have been proposed.[21] The protein composition of human milk, in which the whey proteins rather than the caseins are the dominant protein constituents, is unique among mammals because of its high cysteine content and high cysteine/methionine ratio.[30] The nonprotein nitrogen component of human milk also contains substantial quantities of taurine, which is present in much lower amounts in cow milk[31] and is added to commercially prepared infant formulas. It is important to note, however, because the nitrogenous components of human milk change as lactation advances, the precise protein requirement needed to support the optimal growth and health of infants to 6 months of age is uncertain.

Although the protein content of human milk is less than that of commercial infant formulas, the human milk proteins have a high nutritional quality and are digested and absorbed more efficiently than bovine milk proteins. Thus, a 6-kg infant ingesting 780 mL/day of human milk receives approximately 9.1 g protein, which is about 1.52 g/kg/day of high-quality protein, the AI (using 11.7 g/L) for infants up to 6 months of age. Because of the uncertainty of its availability, the contribution of nonprotein nitrogen is **not included.** On the other hand, data from infants freely fed commercial formulas consume more on the order of 2 g/kg/day.[21,22] The consensus from a number of studies seems to be that although the total weight and lean mass gain of infants fed formula is higher than for exclusively human milk-fed infants after 3 months of age, this difference likely is attributable not only to the higher protein content of formulas but also their higher nutrient intake in general. Thus, after adjusting for differences in energy intake, differences in growth rate attributable to milk source are no longer evident.[18,21] There is no indication that the lower protein intake of breastfed infants has adverse effects.[22] Their protein intake appears to satisfy the infant requirements for maintenance and growth without an amino acid or solute excess.

Commercial infant formulas for term infants in the United States contain a protein equivalent of 14 to 16 g/L or 2.0 to 2.5 g/100 kcal (see also Chapter 4: Formula Feeding of Term Infants). This concentration is higher than for human milk and provides a margin of safety for the lower digestibility of cow milk proteins. In Europe, the recommended range is 1.8 to 2.5 g/100 kcal. Most cow milk-based commercial infant formulas are supplemented with bovine whey to create a whey protein-to-casein ratio similar to that of mature term human milk. Although the specific proteins of bovine whey differ considerably from those of human whey, the amino acid composition (especially for cysteine and methionine) of these "humanized" formulas is closer to that of human milk proteins than are formulas with the lower whey protein-to-casein ratio of bovine milk. Some formulas are also supplemented with nonnutritive proteins, such as lactalbumin and lactoferrin, that have antimicrobial and prebiotic activities and also improve mineral absorption. For soy-based formulas, in which the digestibility of proteins is lower and the indispensable amino acid composition not ideal, the protein content is a minimum of 2.25 g/100 kcal.[32]

For 7- to 12-month-old infants, nitrogen balance and body composition data are available from which average requirements can be derived. Maintenance requirements for children from 9 months to 14 years of age were determined to be similar, and thus a constant value equivalent to 0.688 g/(kg/d) is suggested for all ages. The growth requirement over this

6-month age range (corrected for the efficiency of utilization of dietary protein for growth, ie, 58%) yielded a value of 0.312 g/ (kg/d), so that the EAR for the older infant was estimated at 1 g/(kg/d), and the RDA is 1.2 g/(kg/d). This is lower than the measured AI of healthy 7- to 12-old infants with an average weight of 9 kg (1.52 g/[kg/d]) fed human milk supplemented with weaning foods.[18]

Children

During the preschool and school-age years, there is a continuing decline in protein needs relative to body weight. This reflects the decreasing contribution of the growth requirement relative to the constant maintenance requirement (Table 15.1). Current protein allowances have been derived from estimates of the average requirements by the factorial method and by assuming that the variability of protein needs among individual children is the same as that of other age groups. On the other hand, a 2011 study of 7 healthy school-aged children using the indicator amino acid oxidation method estimated requirements that were almost twice the DRI,[33] suggesting that the current recommendations are inaccurate. Although extensive concerns have been expressed regarding the applicability of these limited data to the population at large, it does emphasize the uncertainty in our understanding of protein metabolism and the current recommended intakes for this age group.

There are few data on the amino acid requirements of children and adolescents and, thus, current recommendations also have been derived using the factorial approach. The requirement for growth (calculated from body composition measurements) contributes only a small proportion of total needs after the first few years of life (Table 15.1). As maintenance protein requirements have been demonstrated to change little with age, the amino acid requirement for maintenance has been based on the EAR for adults determined by direct amino acid oxidation measurements, which are generally believed to be more accurate than those derived from measuring obligatory losses or based on maintenance protein requirements at nitrogen equilibrium.

The amino acid requirement values for the 1- to 3-year-old child are only slightly higher than for adults and, thus, the scoring pattern for dietary proteins will also be very similar. Therefore, the recommendation has been made that the reference amino acid pattern for preschool children should be used for assessing the protein components of foods for all individuals older than 1 year.[18] Food consumption surveys in the United States have established that the amino acid patterns and digestibility of proteins in foods commonly consumed is uniform from 1 year of age onward and that no adjustment to the RDA is required for individuals consuming a typical US diet.[18] However, appropriate corrections must be made if a diet of lower-quality protein than any acceptable reference protein, is customarily consumed.[19]

In children, there has been cross-validation of the recommendations for some amino acids based on the factorial method, with estimates derived using the indicator amino acid oxidation approach. These give similar values for lysine and the total sulfur amino acids (methionine and cysteine), but for the branched chain amino acids (leucine, isoleucine and valine), values using the indicator amino acid oxidation approach were almost 50% higher.[34]

Adolescents

Few data are available on the protein requirements of adolescents specifically. Values have been estimated using the factorial approach, using the adult value for maintenance needs (0.66 g/(kg/day)), estimated from nitrogen balance studies. The growth component is derived from body composition studies corrected for the efficiency of utilization derived from the nitrogen balance studies (47%). Although the growth spurt is small relative to body size, the values are slightly higher for boys than girls; thus, the calculated EAR for 14- to 18-year-old boys is 0.73 g/(kg/day) compared with 0.71 g/(kg/day) for 14- to 18-year-old girls. However, the RDA for adolescent boys and girls have both been set at 0.85 g/(kg/day). There have been no further developments in identifying any specific amino acid needs for adolescents, and the recommendations are the same as for children.

Factors Affecting Dietary Protein Requirements

The RDAs proposed are derived for healthy individuals on the basis of age and sex. However, dietary requirements for protein are affected by a variety of factors including pregnancy, lactation, illness, the adequacy of other nutrients in the diet, and possibly, genetic variation. These factors influence in various ways the bioavailability of all nutrients, the maintenance needs of the organism, and the efficiency with which amino acids can be used for body functions, including growth. Examples of some of the factors that can modify this basic requirement are described below.

Energy Intake

Following removal of the amino group, the carbon skeleton of amino acids can be channeled to oxidative metabolism and contribute to the body's energy supply. When energy intake does not meet the body's energy needs because intake is low and/or expenditure is elevated, protein (dietary and body tissues) catabolism and amino acid oxidation are upregulated and can make a considerable contribution to the body's energy needs. Similarly, up to a certain point, when protein intake is low, increasing energy intake can improve the efficiency of dietary protein for protein deposition. Indeed, the attainment of protein balance depends on both protein and energy intake, and recommendations regarding the physiologic requirement for protein are based on the assumption that the individual is in energy equilibrium. Thus, when energy needs are not met protein requirements are effectively increased. This is an important consideration mainly for individuals in negative energy balance due to high activity levels or illness, and when protein intakes are marginally adequate.[35]

Pregnancy and Lactation

Protein requirements for pregnancy are increased to meet the need for maternal and fetal tissue deposition.[18,19] During the first trimester there are changes in maternal protein metabolism but relatively insignificant amounts of tissue growth, and requirements are the same as for nonpregnant females. During the second and third trimesters of pregnancy, higher protein intakes are required for both maternal and fetal tissue deposition and the maintenance needs of the deposited, metabolically active tissue. The demand for amino acids to support gluconeogenesis and the provision of glucose to the growing fetus also increases as pregnancy progresses. These increased anabolic needs are met in part by adaptations in maternal protein and amino acid metabolism to reduce amino acid oxidation and increase protein synthesis, but also require an increased dietary intake. The EAR to meet these needs is 0.88 g/(kg/day), or 33% higher than for adult women, and the RDA for pregnancy is 1.1 g/(kg/day). Pregnant adolescents, although still growing, are able to undergo the same adaptive changes in protein and amino acid metabolism as pregnant adults, provided they are in well-nourished and receive adequate prenatal care.[36] In these circumstances, their protein and amino acid needs are likely to be met by the standard recommendations for adult pregnancy. However, in pregnant adolescents with marginal nutrition status or in younger adolescents, these adaptive responses are blunted, and they may be less capable of meeting some of their dispensable amino acid needs when food intake is limited and, thereby, put their fetus at risk for impaired growth. In support of this possibility, studies of undernourished adolescent girls demonstrated improved birth outcomes, especially the number of preterm and low birth weight infants, when they received food supplements to increase their protein and energy intake during the latter half of pregnancy.[37]

Additional dietary protein also is required for lactation to supply amino acids for the production of milk proteins and nonprotein nitrogen. These values are adjusted for the efficiency of dietary protein utilization. The published recommendations specify the increase in the protein intake over the nonlactating value for adolescent girls and women that are necessary at different stages of lactation. Again, similar values (EAR, 1.05 [kg/day]; RDA, 1.3 [kg/day]) have been proposed for lactating adolescent and adult females, even though the requirements for the nonpregnant adolescent are slightly higher than the adult.

There are no data on the amino acid requirements of pregnancy and lactation specifically, so it is generally assumed that the indispensable amino acid needs are increased in the same proportions as the increased protein needs.

Disease and Injury

Conditions that increase protein catabolism, reduce bioavailability, increase insensible losses, or need to support tissue accretion will increase individual protein and energy requirements. Trauma in general, but especially severe burn injury, results in hypermetabolism, and both protein and energy maintenance needs are increased because of increased rates of protein and amino acid catabolism and increased losses. These responses are often compounded by a loss of appetite and reduced food intake. With burn injuries, the hypermetabolism persists for an extensive period after the burn, leading to severe loss of lean body mass. In pediatric patients, protein intakes of 2.5 g/(kg/day) are recommended during the rehabilitative phase from burn injury, and during the acute phase, up to 4 times the requirement has demonstrated beneficial effects. These protein intakes must be accompanied by higher energy intakes to ensure appropriate utilization of the amino acids.[38]

Infections also result in a state of hypermetabolism with increased nitrogen losses frequently compounded by reduced food intake and impaired nutrient absorption. When these are persistent and/or the disease burden is high, such as with repeated respiratory and/or gastrointestinal disturbances, linear growth and lean body mass are compromised if the

IV

increased demand for protein is not met. This compromise is exacerbated if energy needs are also insufficiently met. Despite the clear-cut evidence for a greater protein need during periods of infection and stress, specific recommendations are not available. On the basis of some studies, a reasonable estimate is a 20% to 30% increase in total protein with an infection (30% to 50% in the case of diarrhea) and during the recovery period, which is 2 to 3 times longer than the duration of the illness.[19] In patients with symptom-free HIV, intakes 50% higher than normal maybe required. These estimates, however, are based on the assumption that energy needs are met and that the protein is of high quality and digestibility. In resource-limited countries where diet quality is poor or with a diet containing predominantly plant source proteins, these intakes need to take into account the lower quality of the protein.[39]

Activity

Although exercise and heavy physical work increase energy needs, whether the need for protein is also increased once the energy needs are met is hotly debated[40] (see also Chapter 12: Sports Nutrition). An important distinction that must be made when considering this issue is that optimal protein needs for an athlete and the needs for exercising nonathletes are dictated by different outcomes; whereas in exercising nonathletes, optimal health and body composition are the usual desired goal, for the athlete, performance is paramount. Because the protein needs associated with different training regimens and competition vary among sports, for athletes general recommendations must be made on an individual basis. Both endurance and resistance exercise result in increased amino acid oxidation, which, in theory, increases protein and amino acid needs. With low- to moderate-intensity endurance exercise, an acute absolute increase in lysine and leucine acid oxidation have been measured, but with training, in the resting state, a decrease has been observed and overall nitrogen balance is maintained when the RDA for protein is consumed, provided that energy intake is sufficient.[40,41] For endurance competition, additional protein does not appear to enhance athletic performance.[42] Resistance exercise, in contrast, promotes muscle hypertrophy, which is essential for power and strength-based sports. Current recommendations by sports nutrition organizations for individuals wanting to increase muscle mass and improve body composition are for intakes of 1.4 to 2.0 g/(kg/day) with a resistance training program.[42] Increased protein intake in itself will not increase skeletal muscle protein deposition. However, the extent to which protein intakes above recommended levels improve muscle strength in nonathletes is variable.[42] There is good evidence that the timing of the feed in relation to the exercise, the amino acid composition of the protein, and the digestibility of the protein all interact to determine the degree of muscle anabolism.[40,42] Specifically, studies have shown that in the period following a bout of resistance exercise, skeletal muscle is more responsive to protein and amino acids, especially the branched-chain amino acids. Thus, the provision of a protein supplement preferably enriched in indispensable or branched chain amino acids over this time can promote muscle anabolism. Chronic, well-controlled studies in which the effects of these dietary variables on muscle accretion have been performed in nonathletes, but not athletes. Nonetheless, it is important to note that with a few exceptions, protein intakes are unlikely to be of practical concern,[40] because, provided individuals consume a well-balanced diet (in which approximately 15% to 20% of the total energy content is made up of proteins), the increased food consumption that usually accompanies the increased energy needs of physical activity ensures that protein intake also is increased. Thus, any increased needs will be met without the need for specific supplements or a change in the composition of the diet. Exceptions to this may occur with individuals consuming proteins of low biological value or in those attempting to lose weight while attempting to maintain their lean mass and performance standards. Most of our understanding of the effects of activity on protein requirements is based on studies of adults. Few studies have evaluated the consequences of physical activity for protein metabolism in the pediatric population. Thus, there are no specific recommendations targeted to this demographic.

Catch-up Growth

Protein requirements are increased in infants and children undergoing catch-up growth following a period of restricted growth.[19,43] The additional amount of protein that must be supplied depends on the desired rate and composition of weight gain. With intensive supplementation, rates of weight gain up to 20 g/(kg/day) can be achieved in infants with severe wasting. The protein needs for a gain of 1g body weight/(kg/day) can be calculated using the factorial method, and assumptions about the composition of the tissue gain and the efficiency of utilization of dietary proteins.[43] Assuming a composition of 14% protein and that the efficiency of conversion of dietary protein to body protein is 70% during catch-up growth, 0.2g/(kg/day) of protein above the maintenance protein requirement will be needed. Along with the additional protein, energy must also be supplemented to support catch-up growth. The level of energy supplementation that is needed varies depending on numerous considerations, including whether the child has wasting or not and underlying morbidities.[43] Weight gain in a child with wasting will have a larger proportion of fat, which carries a greater energy cost than an equivalent weight of lean body mass. Thus, when refeeding malnourished children, careful consideration must be given to the overall protein-to-energy ratio of the diet, because this will influence the composition of the weight gain.[19] Because children who have severe wasting are often stunted, feedings with high protein-to-energy ratios to minimize the likelihood of excessive fat deposition are preferable. In practice, rates of fat and lean vary during recovery, so weight gain on a given intake may be faster than expected initially because of higher lean tissue deposition and slower subsequently as a greater proportion of fat deposition occurs as the child's catch-up growth trajectory declines. Catch-up growth also increases the requirements for micronutrients, such as zinc, magnesium, iron, and copper. Thus, the intake of these nutrients must be increased to maximize the efficiency of dietary protein utilization.[43]

Assessment of Protein Nutritional Status *(see also Chapter 24: Assessment of Nutritional Status)*

Both insufficient or excessive protein intake can have deleterious consequences and contribute to various morbidities, especially in the pediatric population. Thus, in the clinical assessment of patients, an evaluation of nutritional status is often warranted. The assessment of protein status usually entails a measure of the size of protein stores (ie, lean mass and/or skeletal muscle) and a measure of protein and/or amino acid metabolism. These measures are best obtained using a combination of anthropometric, clinical, and biochemical data. Ideally, interpretation of these results requires consideration of the patient's diet to assess the extent to which any emerging issue can be attributed primarily to a poor diet (primary deficiency) or to increased needs because of potential underlying disease (secondary deficiency).

In the pediatric population, assessment of growth status (weight and height) and body composition provide an index of the protein stores. Although deviations from the norm are frequently indicative of a relatively chronic condition, the same is not necessarily true for monitoring the

improvement in nutritional status, when rapid changes can occur following the implementation of therapeutic measures to combat the underlying
disease condition.[43] The value of these measurements is critically dependent
on the availability of appropriate norms for the specific parameter that
is being evaluated and the technique used to make the measurement. In
general, lean mass reflects the protein mass of the body. In childhood, the
primary determinants of lean mass are the height/length of the child, tissue
hydration, and skeletal muscle mass.[44] Although assessment protocols and
standards for height/length for all ages are widely available, body composition standards are less inclusive. Sex- but not race-specific reference
standards for lean mass measured by dual energy X-ray absorptiometry
(DXA) based on data collected from 1999 to 2004 in the National Health and
Nutrition Examination Survey (NHANES) for 8- to 20-year-olds are now
available.[45,46] Although some reference data for younger infants and children are available, their use could be limiting because of the methodologies
used and the populations for which they were derived (reviewed by Wells[47]).
For routine clinical practice and public health settings, these whole-body
measurements are not practical, and anthropometric measures indicative of
lean mass can be used. Mid-upper arm muscle area derived from measurements of upper arm skinfolds and circumference has been used extensively
and is readily applicable in all settings, and reference norms are available
for comparison.[48] Although bioelectrical impedance analysis (BIA) provides
values for whole-body lean mass and can be readily used in nonspecialized
settings, its predictive accuracy, especially in the pediatric patient, often
precludes its usefulness at the individual level.[47,49]

A number of biochemical tests, predominantly of blood and urine, can
provide objective and quantitative measures of the underlying state of an
individual's protein and amino acid metabolism.[50] The concentrations of
serum proteins, primarily albumin, transferrin, transthyretin, and retinol-
binding protein, are often used to assess protein nutritional status, because
their synthesis in the liver is responsive to protein intake. These proteins
differ in their rates of turnover (approximately 18, 8, 2, and 0.5 days,
respectively) and, therefore, can provide a measure of severity and duration
of the deficit. There are important limitations in the use of these measures,
however, because they are affected by a variety of factors independently of
protein status—for example, liver disease, infections, enteropathies, renal
disease, and other nutrient deficiencies (eg, vitamin A and iron). Although
plasma amino acid levels also respond to changes in protein intake, their

concentrations reflect the product of all the mechanisms that release amino acids into the extracellular compartment and those that remove them. Thus, with the possible exception of patients in whom a disorder of amino acid metabolism is suspected, their use for a routine assessment of protein nutritional status is not warranted. Urinary creatinine and 3-methylhistidine are derived primarily from the turnover of skeletal muscle proteins and, under specific conditions, can provide a measure of skeletal muscle mass.[50] However, there are several factors that can confound the interpretation of these measurements, and together with the practical limitations of their measurement, their usefulness is limited to clinical studies rather than for routine nutritional assessment. The urinary output of the major end-products of nitrogen catabolism (urea, ammonia), in theory, is indicative of protein status. However, in additions to the practical limitations in conducting and interpreting the measurements, the information it yields is influenced by the immediate status of the individual's protein metabolism, which is not necessarily the status of their protein stores. As described previously, measures of amino acid flux and protein turnover at the whole-body and individual organ levels can provide specific, objective, and quantitative measures of protein and amino acid status. The procedures and analyses required, however, are not readily implemented, and thus, their use is limited to experimental protocols.

Effects of Insufficient and Excessive Protein Intake

The consequences of inadequate protein intake vary according to the severity of the deficiency relative to the need of the individual, the duration of the insult, and the adequacy of the intake of other macro- and micronutrients. Thus, younger individuals with higher requirements are often at the greatest risk, especially once human milk is insufficient to meet their nutrient needs, necessitating the introduction of complementary foods; these frequently are cereal-based with a lower protein density than milk and suboptimal amino acid composition. Indeed, a recent analysis of protein intakes in low-income communities identified the highest prevalence of insufficient protein intake in 6- to 8-month-old infants.[51] These marginal protein intakes, especially if accompanied by conditions that reduce absorption and produce hypermetabolism (such as enteric dysfunction and infections), impair growth and chronically contribute to stunting and reduced lean mass. Additionally, immune function becomes compromised and neurologic development is delayed, although the extent to which this can be attributed to insufficient dietary protein per se is uncertain. The relationship between the severity of the inadequacy in protein intake and the degree to which various functions are compromised is uncertain. This requires longitudinal randomized controlled trials in which protein intakes of a large number of infants is controlled or monitored and the population is well-characterized.

More severe childhood protein-energy malnutrition encompasses a wide spectrum of conditions, the main clinical syndromes being kwashiorkor, characterized by the presence of edema, low plasma protein concentrations, skin lesions, compromised antioxidant status, and hepatic steatosis; marasmus, in which the child has severe wasting; and marasmic kwashiorkor. Especially in kwashiorkor, the condition is often precipitated by the development of conditions that increase the child's protein needs, such as an infection or diarrhea. Both whole-body protein kinetics and the metabolism of individual amino acids differ in children with infections and edematous malnutrition compared with nonedematous malnutrition.[52,53] These differences in protein and amino acid metabolism among clinical syndromes characterized by malnutrition contribute to their different pathophysiology and also have consequences for the development of refeeding strategies appropriate for the different conditions. Although protein-energy malnutrition is observed even in industrialized countries, such as the United States, the cause is usually associated with the presence of clinical conditions that decrease food intake or impair the digestion or absorption of food.

The effects of dietary protein intakes above the RDA have not been studied extensively, and the findings are equivocal (summarized by the Institute of Medicine[18]). The suggestion has been made that a high protein intake during the first 2 years life promotes more rapid growth and increases the risk for the development of obesity in later life.[54,55] The proposal is based on the comparison between the long-term growth of infants fed human milk or infant formula in early postnatal life as well as studies in older infants that relate protein intake and protein source to weight gain in later life. Although the findings are suggestive, they are by no means conclusive, and before changes in infant feeding practices are considered, a number of issues require greater evaluation. These include a clearer understanding of the relationships between appetite control, food composition, and energy intake[56]; accurate measurements of body composition to demonstrate increased adiposity rather than just greater BMI values; assessment of the contribution of differences in socioeconomic factors

IV

that frequently confound the comparison between formula and breastfed infants; and, importantly, whether there are critical windows during which a metabolic phenotype is influenced by protein intakes. Although data showing that growth rate is higher in healthy infants fed higher protein intakes (often associated with the consumption of formula rather than just breast-feeding) are convincing, higher weight gains have been associated with greater length and lean body mass gains during the first year of life and not necessarily greater adiposity.[57–59] Longitudinal randomized trials rather than observational studies that examine the long-term consequences will be needed to determine whether these effects carry a long-term risk. The protein source is also an important variable to consider, with a high protein intake from animal sources, especially dairy, but not vegetable or cereal protein sources, being associated with the development of greater adiposity.[60] However, animal protein sources are also associated with higher intakes of micronutrients, such as iron and zinc, which could provide additional benefits. Thus, it is not possible to discern whether it is the protein intake per se or the composite nature of the protein-containing food that might be responsible for the observed associations between early protein intake and the risk of developing obesity in later life.

Urinary calcium excretion increases linearly at protein intakes above the RDA, with a doubling of protein intake leading to a 50% increase in urinary calcium in adults in the absence of any change in other nutrients. This increased protein intake was believed to promote bone demineralization and to increase the risk for kidney stone formation. The increased bone demineralization was attributed to the increased acid load produced from the metabolism of the sulfur-containing amino acids, methionine and cysteine, when high-protein diets were consumed. Subsequently, it has been demonstrated that the increased excretion of urinary calcium with high-protein diets is attributable in part to increased intestinal calcium absorption. Thus, the net effect of dietary protein intake on bone appears to be a balance between the catabolic effects of a high acid load and an otherwise general anabolic effect of protein on bone formation.[61] Several studies have demonstrated that the beneficial effects of protein on bone are evident only in the presence of an adequate calcium intake.[61] The presence of adequate fruit and vegetables that serve to "alkalinize" the diet can further modulate the effects of dietary protein and calcium intake on bone mineralization.

There is little evidence for other adverse effects of high protein intakes on healthy individuals. As protein intake increases, plasma amino acids and urea concentrations increase, which might present difficulties for individuals in whom the mechanisms to eliminate nitrogenous metabolites are compromised, but not otherwise. High intakes of protein, especially casein, by small infants can result in acidosis, aminoacidemia, and cylinduria. For many years, the concern for the development of metabolic derangements limited the amount of amino acids that would be administered to preterm infants. However, this practice is being abandoned as it is clear that the provision of protein intakes as high as 4 g/(kg/day) can be tolerated and improve short- and long-term outcomes.[62] Although some studies in adults have shown a correlation between protein intake and the prevalence of atherosclerosis or the risk for cancer, these findings have not been consistent. The positive associations seem to be more prevalent when meat is the source of dietary protein; thus, a causative role for protein itself is uncertain. Given the paucity of data and the inconsistent nature of the conclusions derived from them, the only safe recommendation that can be made regarding high protein intakes is that the maximal levels of protein intake should be dictated by the overall macronutrient composition of the diet and should fall within the AMDR.[18]

References

1. McClean P, Weaver LT. Ontogeny of human pancreatic exocrine function. *Arch Dis Child.* 1993;68(1 Spec No):62–65

2. Neu J. Gastrointestinal maturation and implications for infant feeding. *Early Hum Dev.* 2007;83(12):767–775

3. Portune KJ, Beaumont M, Davila A-M, Tome D, Blachier F, Sanz Y. Gut microbiota role in dietary protein metabolism and health-related outcomes: the two sides of the coin. *Trends Food Sci Technol.* 2016;57:213–232

4. Yatsunenko T, Rey FE, Manary MJ, Trehan I, Dominguez-Bello MG, Contreras MM, M. Human gut microbiome viewed across age and geography. *Nature.* 2012;486(7402):222–227

5. Burrin DG, Stoll B. Metabolic fate and function of dietary glutamate in the gut. *Am J Clin Nutr.* 2009;90(3):850S–856S

6. Davis TA, Fiorotto ML. Regulation of muscle growth in neonates. *Curr Opin Clin Nutr Metab Care.* 2009;12(1):78–85

7. Denne SC, Kalhan SC. Leucine metabolism in human newborns. *Am J Physiol.* 1987;253(6 Pt 1):E608–E615

8. Denne SC, Rossi EM, Kalhan SC. Leucine kinetics during feeding in normal newborns. *Pediatr Res.* 1991;30(1):23–27

9. Matthews DE. Observations of branched-chain amino acid administration in humans. *J Nutr.* 2005;135(6 Suppl):1580S–1584S

10. Waterlow JC, Jackson AA. Nutrition and protein turnover in man. *Br Med Bull.* 1981;37(1):5–10

11. Kalhan SC, Bier DM. Protein and amino acid metabolism in the human newborn. *Annu Rev Nutr.* 2008;28:389–410

12. Jackson AA. The glycine story. *Eur J Clin Nutr.* 1991;45(2):59–65

13. Rosenthal MD, Carrott PW, Patel J, Kiraly L, Martindale RG. Parenteral or enteral arginine supplementation safety and efficacy. *J Nutr.* 2016;146(12): 2594S–2600S

14. Mehta NM, Skillman HE, Irving SY, et al. Guidelines for the provision and assessment of nutrition support therapy in the pediatric critically ill patient: Society of Critical Care Medicine and American Society for Parenteral and Enteral Nutrition. *JPEN J Parenter Enteral Nutr.* 2017;41(5):706–742

15. Ginguay A, De Bandt JP, Cynober L. Indications and contraindications for infusing specific amino acids (leucine, glutamine, arginine, citrulline, and taurine) in critical illness. *Curr Opin Clin Nutr Metab Care.* 2016;19(2):161–169

16. Crill CM HR. The use of carnitine in pediatric nutrition. *Nutr Clin Pract.* 2007;22(2):204–213

17. Verner A, Craig S, McGuire W. Effect of taurine supplementation on growth and development in preterm or low birth weight infants. *Cochrane Database Syst Rev.* 2007(4):CD006072

18. Institute of Medicine, Food and Nutrition Board. Protein and amino acids. *Dietary Reference Intakes for Energy, Carbohydrates, Fiber, Fat, Fatty Acids, Cholesterol, Protein, and Amino Acids.* Washington, DC: National Academies Press; 2005: 589–768

19. World Health Organization, Food and Agriculture Organization of the United Nations, United Nations University. *Protein and amino acid requirements in human nutrition: report of a joint WHO/FAO/UNU Expert Consultation.* Geneva, Switzerland: World Health Organization;2007

20. Institute of Medicine, Food and Nutrition Board. Macronutrients and healthful diets. *Dietary Reference Intakes for Energy, Carbohydrates, Fiber, Fat, Fatty Acids, Cholesterol, Protein, and Amino Acids.* Washington, DC: National Academies Press; 2005:769–879

21. Dewey KG, Beaton G, Fjeld C, Lonnerdal B, Reeds P. Protein requirements of infants and children. *Eur J Clin Nutr.* 1996;50(Suppl 1):S119–S147

22. Nestle' Nutrition Workshop Series Pediatric Program. *Protein and Energy Requirements in Infancy and Childhood.* Basel, Switzerland: Karger; 2006

23. Viteri FE. INCAP studies of energy, amino acids, and protein. *Food Nutr Bull.* 2010;31(1):42–53

24. Butte NF, Hopkinson JM, Wong WW, Smith EO, Ellis KJ. Body composition during the first 2 years of life: an updated reference. *Pediatr Res.* 2000;47(5): 578–585

25. Ellis KJ, Shypailo RJ, Abrams SA, Wong WW. The reference child and adolescent models of body composition. A contemporary comparison. *Ann N Y Acad Sci.* 2000;904:374–382

26. Food and Agriculture Organization of the United Nations, World Health Organization. *Protein Quality Evaluation.* Rome, Italy: Food and Agriculture Organization of the United Nations; 1991

27. Food and Agriculture Organization of the United Nations. *Dietary protein quality evaluation in human nutrition. FAO food and nutrition paper 92.* Rome, Italy: Food and Agriculture Organization of the United Nations;2013

28. Lee WT, Weisell R, Albert J, Tome D, Kurpad AV, Uauy R. Research approaches and methods for evaluating the protein quality of human foods proposed by an FAO Expert Working Group in 2014. *J Nutr.* 2016;146(5):929–932

29. Picciano MF. Nutrient composition of human milk. *Pediatr Clin North Am.* 2001;48(1):53–67

30. Davis TA, Nguyen HV, Garcia-Bravo R, et al. Amino acid composition of human milk is not unique. *J Nutr.* 1994;124(7):1126–1132

31. Sarwar G, Botting HG, Davis TA, Darling P, Pencharz PB. Free amino acids in milks of human subjects, other primates and non-primates. *Br J Nutr.* 1998;79(2):129–131

32. Turck D. Soy protein for infant feeding: what do we know? *Curr Opin Clin Nutr Metab Care.* 2007;10(3):360–365

33. Elango R, Humayun MA, Ball RO, Pencharz PB. Protein requirement of healthy school-age children determined by the indicator amino acid oxidation method. *Am J Clin Nutr.* 2011;94(6):1545–1552

34. Pillai RR, Kurpad AV. Amino acid requirements in children and the elderly population. *Br J Nutr.* 2012;108(Suppl 2):S44–S49

35. Pellett PL, Young VR. The effects of different levels of energy intake on protein metabolism and of different levels of protein intake on energy metabolism: a statistical evaluation from the published literature. In: Scrimshaw NS, Schurch B, eds. *Protein Energy Interactions.* Lausanne, Switzerland: International Dietary Energy Consultancy Group Switzerland; 1992:81–136

36. Thame MM, Hsu JW, Gibson R, et al. Adaptation of in vivo amino acid kinetics facilitates increased amino acid availability for fetal growth in adolescent and adult pregnancies alike. *Br J Nutr.* 2014;112(11):1779–1786

37. Dubois S, Coulombe C, Pencharz P, Pinsonneault O, Duquette MP. Ability of the Higgins Nutrition Intervention Program to improve adolescent pregnancy outcome. *J Am Diet Assoc.* 1997;97(8):871–878

38. Prelack K, Yu YM, Sheridan RL. Nutrition and metabolism in the rehabilitative phase of recovery in burn children: a review of clinical and research findings in a speciality pediatric burn hospital. *Burns Trauma.* 2015;3:7

39. Ghosh S, Suri D, Uauy R. Assessment of protein adequacy in developing countries: quality matters. *Br J Nutr.* 2012;108(Suppl 2):S77–S87

IV

40. Tipton KD, Witard OC. Protein requirements and recommendations for athletes: relevance of ivory tower arguments for practical recommendations. *Clin Sports Med.* 2007;16(1):17–36

41. Gaine PC, Viesselman CT, Pikosky MA, Martin WF, Armstrong LE, Pescatello LS. Aerobic exercise training decreases leucine oxidation at rest in healthy adults. *J Nutr.* 2005;135(5):1088–1092

42. Jager R, Kerksick CM, Campbell BI, et al. International Society of Sports Nutrition Position Stand: protein and exercise. *J Int Soc Sports Nutr.* 2017;14:20

43. Golden MH. Proposed recommended nutrient densities for moderately malnourished children. *Food Nutr Bull.* 2009;30(3 Suppl):S267–S342

44. Forbes GB. *Human Body Composition: Growth, Aging, Nutrition and Activity.* New York, NY: Springer-Verlag; 1987

45. Fan B, Shepherd JA, Levine MA, et al. National Health and Nutrition Examination Survey whole-body dual-energy X-ray absorptiometry reference data for GE Lunar systems. *J Clin Densitom.* 2014;17(3):344–377

46. Weber DR, Moore RH, Leonard MB, Zemel BS. Fat and lean BMI reference curves in children and adolescents and their utility in identifying excess adiposity compared with BMI and percentage body fat. *Am J Clin Nutr.* 2013;98(1):49–56

47. Wells JC. Toward body composition reference data for infants, children, and adolescents. *Adv Nutr.* 2014;5(3):320S–329S

48. Addo OY, Himes JH, Zemel BS. Reference ranges for midupper arm circumference, upper arm muscle area, and upper arm fat area in US children and adolescents aged 1-20 y. *Am J Clin Nutr.* 2017;105(1):111–120

49. Brantlov S, Ward LC, Jodal L, Rittig S, Lange A. Critical factors and their impact on bioelectrical impedance analysis in children: a review. *J Med Eng Technol.* 2017;41(1):22–35

50. Young VR, Marchini JS, Cortiella J. Assessment of protein nutritional status. *J Nutr.* 1990;120(Suppl 11):1496–1502

51. Arsenault JE, Brown KH. Dietary protein intake in young children in selected low-income countries is generally adequate in relation to estimated requirements for healthy children, except when complementary food intake is low. *J Nutr.* 2017;147:932–030

52. Jahoor F. Effects of decreased availability of sulfur amino acids in severe childhood undernutrition. *Nutr Rev.* 2012;70(3):176–187

53. Jahoor F, Badaloo A, Reid M, Forrester T. Protein kinetic differences between children with edematous and nonedematous severe childhood undernutrition in the fed and postabsorptive states. *Am J Clin Nutr.* 2005;82(4):792–800

54. Grote V, von Kries R, Closa-Monasterolo R, et al. Protein intake and growth in the first 24 months of life. European Childhood Obesity Trial Study Group. *J Pediatr Gastroenterol Nutr.* 2010;51(Suppl 3):S117–S118

55. Patro-Golab B, Zalewski BM, Kouwenhoven SM, et al. Protein concentration in milk formula, growth, and later risk of obesity: a systematic review. *J Nutr.* 2016;146:551–564

56. Kalhan SC. Optimal protein intake in healthy infants. *Am J Clin Nutr.* 2009;89(6): 1719–1720

57. Bell KA, Wagner CL, Feldman HA, Shypailo RJ, Belfort MB. Associations of infant feeding with trajectories of body composition and growth. *Am J Clin Nutr.* 2017;106(2):491–498

58. Putet G, Labaune JM, Mace K, et al. Effect of dietary protein on plasma insulin-like growth factor-1, growth, and body composition in healthy term infants: a randomised, double-blind, controlled trial (Early Protein and Obesity in Childhood (EPOCH) study). *Br J Nutr.* 2016;115(2):271–284

59. Tang M, Krebs NF. High protein intake from meat as complementary food increases growth but not adiposity in breastfed infants: a randomized trial. *Am J Clin Nutr.* 2014;100(5):1322–1328

60. Gunther AL, Remer T, Kroke A, Buyken AE. Early protein intake and later obesity risk: which protein sources at which time points throughout infancy and childhood are important for body mass index and body fat percentage at 7 y of age? *Am J Clin Nutr.* 2007;86(6):1765–1772

61. Jesudason D, Clifton P. The interaction between dietary protein and bone health. *J Bone Miner Metab.* 2011;29(1):1–14

62. Ziegler EE. Meeting the nutritional needs of the low-birth-weight infant. *Ann Nutr Metab.* 2011;58(Suppl 1):8–18

IV

Chapter 16

Carbohydrate and Dietary Fiber

Overview

Carbohydrates provide 50% to 60% of the calories consumed by the average American. Although relatively little carbohydrate is needed in the diet, carbohydrate spares protein and fat from being metabolized for calories. The principal dietary carbohydrates are sugars and starches. In addition to providing energy, carbohydrates have numerous other potential effects, such as lowering cholesterol, increasing calcium absorption, acting as a source of short-chain fatty acids in the colon, and increasing fecal bulk (Table 16.1).

By convention, dietary carbohydrates can be classified by several components of their chemical nature, including degree of polymerization (number of sugar molecules), the type of linkage between sugar molecules, and the character of individual monomers (Table 16.2).[1] This classification system results in the division of dietary carbohydrates into 3 main categories: sugars, oligosaccharides, and polysaccharides. Sugars include monosaccharides, disaccharides, and polyols. The monosaccharides include glucose, galactose, and fructose, and disaccharides include lactose, sucrose, maltose, and trehalose. Lactose is derived from milk, whereas fructose, glucose, and sucrose are contained in the cells of fruits and vegetables. Sucrose for example is generally purified from cane or beet sources for common uses. Processed foods may contain a significant amount of fructose and corn syrup; the latter also contains oligosaccharides and polysaccharides because it is derived from cornstarch. Maltose can be found in sprouted wheat and barley. Fructose is the sweetest of the dietary carbohydrates. Trehalose is often used as a substitute for sucrose in the food industry as a less sweet option and is found in nature in yeast, fungi, and honey and may be used in small amounts in bread. Besides being used as sweeteners, sugars also confer functional characteristics to foods (eg, viscosity, texture, control of moisture to prevent drying out).[1] The polyols (eg, sorbitol) are alcohols of sugars commonly found as sweeteners in commercial food products. They are found naturally in some fruits but also can be manufactured from monosaccharides or polysaccharides.[2] Polyols often are used as a replacement for sucrose in the diet of people with diabetes mellitus.[1] Foods labeled as sugar free contain polyols and no additional added sugar.[2]

Oligosaccharides contain between 3 and 9 sugars (3–9 degrees of polymerization or DP3-9; Table 16.2). Food oligosaccharides fall into 2 groups, maltodextrins (glucose-based) and oligosaccharides not composed solely of glucose molecules. Maltodextrins are mostly derived from starch and

Table 16.1.

Principal Physiological Properties of Dietary Carbohydrates

	Provide Energy	Increase Satiety	Glycemic	Cholesterol Lowering	Increase Calcium Absorption	Source of Short-Chain Fatty Acids	Prebiotic	Increase Stool Output	Immuno-modulatory
Monosaccharides	✓		✓						
Disaccharides	✓		✓		✓				
Polyols	✓		✓			✓[a]		✓	
Maltodextrins	✓		✓						
Oligosaccharides (Non-α-glucan)	✓				✓	✓	✓		✓
Starch	✓		✓			✓[b]		✓[b]	
Nonstarch polysaccharides	✓	✓		✓[c]		✓		✓	

Adapted from Cummings and Stephen.[1]

[a] Except erythritol.

[b] Resistant starch.

[c] Some forms of nonstarch polysaccharides only.

Table 16.2.
Major Dietary Carbohydrates

Class (Degree of Polymerization)	Subgroup	Principal Components
Sugars (1-2)	Monosaccharides	Glucose, fructose, galactose
	Disaccharides	Sucrose, lactose, maltose, trehalose
	Polyols (sugar alcohols)	Xylitol, erythritol, isomalt, maltitol
Oligosaccharides (3-9)	Malto-oligosaccharides (a-glucans)	Maltodextrins
	Non-α-glucan oligosaccharides	Raffinose, stachyose, fructo- and galacto-oligosaccharides, polydextrose, inulin
Polysaccharides (≥10)	Starch (α-glucans)	Amylose, amylopectin, modified starches
	Nonstarch polysaccharides	Cellulose, hemicellulose, pectin, arabinoxylans, β-glucan, glucomannans, plant gums and mucilages, hydrocolloids

Adapted from Cummings and Stephen.[1]

include maltotriose and α-limit dextrins, which contain both α-1,4 and α-1,6 linkages (bonds) with an average DP8. They are used by the food industry as sweeteners, fat substitutes, and texture modifiers.[1] Oligosaccharides (composed of glucose and fructose molecules linked to varying numbers of galactose molecules) include raffinose, stachyose, and verbascose and are found in a variety of plant seeds (eg, peas, beans, lentils).[1] Included in this group are inulin and fructo-oligosaccharides. These oligosaccharides fall under the category of fructans and do not contain any α-1,4 or α-1,6 bonds and are, thus, not susceptible to pancreatic enzyme or brush-border enzyme hydrolysis.[1,3] This property makes these oligosaccharides useful as prebiotics. Oligosaccharides in human milk, which are predominantly galactose based, also are prebiotics.

Polysaccharides are ≥10 sugars in length and consist of starches and nonstarch polysaccharides (Table 16.2). Starches are the storage carbohydrates of plants and consist of sugars (eg, glucose) linked together. Starches exist as either amylose (nonbranched with α-1-4 bonds) or amylopectin (branched with α-1-4 and α-1-6 bonds) (see section on Starches).

Historically, dietary fiber has been divided into 2 primary groups based on water solubility and viscosity. This categorization changed in 2005 when the National Academy of Sciences proposed a new definition of dietary fiber based on the concept that the classification should determine the analytical methods needed to measure it rather than have the method determine what qualified as fiber or not.[4] The definition proposes that total fiber equals dietary fiber plus functional fiber. Dietary fiber consists of nondigestible carbohydrates and lignins, which are intrinsic and intact in plants (eg, gums, cellulose, oat, and wheat bran). Functional fiber consists of isolated, nondigestible carbohydrates that have beneficial physiological effects in humans and may be derived from plants (eg, resistant starches from bananas or potatoes) or animals (eg, chitin and chitosan from crab and lobster shells).

Digestion of Disaccharides and Starches

Lactose and sucrose are hydrolyzed to monosaccharides via lactase and sucrase, respectively (Fig 16.1). These enzymes are located in the brush border of the small intestine and are responsible for hydrolyzing lactose into glucose and galactose and sucrose into fructose and glucose. Lactase activity increases primarily during the third trimester, whereas sucrase activity is already at levels found at birth by the onset of the last trimester.[5,6]

Figure 16.1.

Absorption of carbohydrate. Carbohydrates in the form of glycogen begins to be digested within the intestinal lumen through the action of α-amylase into α-limit dextrins and oligosaccharides. They are further digested into glucose hexoses through the action of disaccharidases and oligosaccharidases. Sucrose, and lactose are broken down into their respective hexoses: glucose (G), galactose (Ga), and fructose (F). Glucose is subsequently absorbed via active transport through a carrier-mediated Na+ glucose cotransporter. Fructose is absorbed via facilitated diffusion.

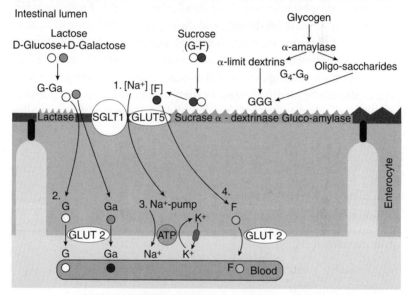

Adapted under a Creative Commons License from Paulev PE, Zubieta-Calleja G. *New Human Physiology. Textbook in Medical Physiology and Pathophysiology: Essentials and Clinical Problems.* 2nd ed. Copenhagen, Denmark; 2004. Available at: http://www.zuniv.net/physiology/book/

Throughout the fetal and neonatal period, disaccharidase activity remains highest in the proximal jejunum, as is found in adults.[7]

Starch digestion is more complex. The production of pancreatic amylase, the enzyme primarily responsible for the digestion of starches, increases to mature levels during the first year of life.[8-13] Salivary, and more likely, mucosal enzymes (glucoamylase, sucrase, and isomaltase) are responsible for starch digestion in young infants.[9,14,15] Pancreatic and salivary amylase hydrolyze the interior α-1,4 bonds (Fig 16.1). Glucoamylase sequentially cleaves α-1,4 bonds from the nonreducing end of the molecule (Fig 16.1).[16-18]

It is most active against starches between 5 and 9 glucose residues in length.[16] [17,18] Deficiencies in this enzyme have been described as a cause of chronic diarrhea and malabsorption in the pediatric population.[19] Isomaltase (a-dextrinase) and sucrase also have some activity in starch digestion. Isomaltase is primarily responsible for cleaving the α-1,6 bonds. At the brush border, starch polymers are further broken down by disaccharidases and oligosaccharidases into glucose (Fig 16.1).

The digestibility of starches can vary depending on the chemical nature of the starch, the physical form of the starch, the presence of possible inhibitors (eg, alpha amylase inhibitors), and the physical distribution of starch in relation to fiber components.[20] In general, starches can be divided into 3 categories according to digestibility: poorly digested starches, intermediate digested starches, and highly digested starches (Table 16.3). The property of starches also can be modified using a variety of chemical treatments including oxidation, substitution, and cross-bonding.[20] These modifications allow

Table 16.3.
Digestibility of Unmodified Starches

Digestibility	Examples
Least digestible	Potato Canna Plantain fruit Arrowroot Sago palm Lily Chestnuts Buffalo gourd Banana
Intermediate digestible	Sweet potato Tree fern Legumes
Most digestible	Wheat Maize Barley Rice Mung bean Cassava Taro

Adapted from Dreher.[20]

for changes in the natural consistency and shelf life of these starches and will naturally affect the digestibility of the starch depending on the specific modification.[20]

Absorption of Monosaccharides

The end products of disaccharide and starch digestion are monosaccharides, which are absorbed in the small intestine (Fig 16.1). Access into enterocytes occurs via 2 main families of transporters. The GLUT family of transporters allow for the passive transport of glucose and fructose (see below) across the cell membrane. In comparison, glucose and galactose are actively transported via the sodium-glucose–linked transporter (SGLT1).[21,22] In this system, glucose and galactose entry is coupled to the entry of sodium along its electrochemical gradient.[21,22] The electrochemical gradient is maintained via sodium-potassium-adenosine triphosphatase (Na^+-K^+ ATPase) located at the basolateral surface. SGLT1 has binding sites for both glucose and sodium.[21] Two sodium molecules are absorbed for every glucose molecule.[21] Once both sites are occupied, the transporter translocates across the brush-border membrane and releases the glucose and sodium into the enterocyte.[21] The sodium-linked transport of glucose provides the basis for adding glucose or starches to oral rehydration solutions.[21]

Fructose transport across the brush border membrane can occur passively down its concentration gradient via facilitated diffusion via GLUT5, a mechanism that is not sodium dependent.[23,24] This facilitated transport system limits the ability of fructose to be absorbed when it is consumed in large amounts or high concentrations.[24] However, in reality, coingestion of fructose with glucose (as the monosaccharide or the disaccharide sucrose) significantly raises the threshold for fructose malabsorption.[24] The mechanism whereby glucose facilitates the absorption of fructose is unclear.[24]

Classically, GLUT2, a sodium independent transporter, is thought to be responsible for the passive movement of glucose, fructose, and galactose across the basolateral surface of the enterocyte and into the circulation.[21–23,25] There remains much debate regarding the potential role of GLUT2 in the transport of glucose and fructose across the brush border of the enterocyte.[21,22,24–26] Conflicts in the data may relate to errors in experimental design and/or differences in methodology, fasting versus nonfasting responses, and/or animal models.[21,22,24–26] A number of other GLUT transporters (GLUT9, GLUT12, GLUT 7) have been identified in the small intestine, but their physiologic roles remain unclear.[23,27]

That said, ingestion of carbohydrates in combinations that use different apical transport systems will increase the overall rate of carbohydrate
absorption.[28] This concept plays an important role in exercise physiology
because the ingestion of multiple types of sugars can increase the total
delivery of carbohydrates into circulation and increase oxidation by muscle
in excess of the previously accepted maximum rate of 1 g/minute (Fig 16.2).[28]
This effect is observed most dramatically in prolonged periods of exercise
(2.5 hours or longer).[28] An additional metabolic effect to improve exercise
tolerance may relate to the oxidation of fructose to lactate, which is used as
an energy source in muscle.[28]

Figure 16.2.

**When multiple carbohydrates are ingested (squares), the total
carbohydrate oxidation rate is increased compared with the ingestion
of a single carbohydrate (circles). This is related, in part, to faster and
more efficient intestinal absorption. Ingestion of multiple (eg, glucose
and fructose) as opposed to single carbohydrates (eg, glucose) improves
exercise performance.**

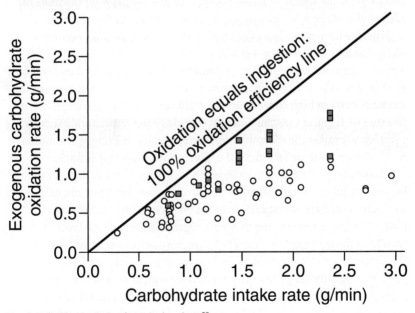

Reprinted with permission from Jeukendrup.[28]

Carbohydrates not absorbed in the small intestine are fermented by colonic bacteria and converted to short chain fatty acids, which are, in turn, absorbed by the colon.[29,30] When the ability of the fermentative rate is exceeded, the remaining mono-, di-, and oligosaccharides create an osmotic gradient that drives water into the lumen and results in an osmotic diarrhea.[17]

Metabolism of Glucose

Dietary carbohydrates are converted to glucose in the liver. Glucose is the most abundant carbohydrate and the majority of it is metabolized for energy.[31] Quantitatively, the brain is the largest utilizer of glucose as an energy source.[31] Amino acids and glycerol from lipids also can be converted to glucose. However, in the case of amino acids, this potentially shunts substrate away from protein synthesis. Additionally, glucose synthesis from both amino acids and glycerol is not very metabolically efficient. There are few data that allow the limits of carbohydrate intake to be defined.[31] Estimates of minimum glucose requirements based on cerebral glucose utilization are shown in Table 16.4. The upper limits of glucose requirements should be defined by the amount that defines a minimal need for fat and protein and maximum glucose oxidation rates (Table 16.5).[31] In contrast, the minimal glucose requirement for children is defined as the amount

IV

Table 16.4.

Estimates of Glucose Consumption by the Brain

	Body Weight	Brain Weight	Glucose Consumption		
	(kg)	(g)	$(mg \cdot kg^{-1} \cdot min^{-1})$	$(g \cdot kg^{-1} \cdot d^{-1})$	(g/d)
Newborn	3.2	399	6.0	11.5	37
1 y	10.0	997	7.0	10.1	101
5 y	19.0	1266	4.7	6.8	129
Adolescent	50.0	1360	1.9	2.7	135
Adult	70.0	1400	1.0	1.4	98

Adapted from Kalhan and Kilic.[31]

Table 16.5.
Upper Limit of Carbohydrate Intake for Infants and Children[a]

Age	Total Energy Expenditure[b] (kcal · kg^{-1} · d^{-1})	Carbohydrate Equivalent[c] (g·kg^{-1} · d^{-1})
Newborn	73	19
1–3 y	85	22
4–6 y	68	18
12–13 y	55	14
18–19 y	44	12
Adult	35	9

Adapted from Kalhan and Kilic.[31]

[a] Upper limit should be determined by the minimal need for protein and fat obtained. Therefore, the described upper limits here are theoretical maximal to meet all the energy needs.

[b] Average of data for boys and girls. Estimate based on double-labeled water method.

[c] Carbohydrate equivalent = total energy expenditure/3.8, assuming each g of carbohydrate yields 3.8 kcal.

required to meet the energy needs of the brain and other glucose dependent organs while minimizing gluconeogenesis and preventing ketosis.[31] These are theoretical limits, because they presume the minimal intake of protein and fat with glucose providing essentially all energy needs. However, doing so can be associated with adverse effects, such as hyperglycemia.

Current data suggest that in the human newborn infant, gluconeogenesis appears soon after birth and contributes to 30% of glucose produced in the term infant and 20% to 40% in the preterm infant.[32] Gluconeogenesis allows for the production of glucose and glycogen from nonglucose precursors.[31,32] As noted previously, the majority of glucose is used by the central nervous system. Glucose that is not immediately oxidized can be polymerized to form glycogen. Storage and mobilization of glycogen are under the hormonal control of insulin and glucagon (see Chapter 30: Nutrition Therapy for Children and Adolescents With Type 1 and Type 2 Diabetes Mellitus, and Chapter 31: Hypoglycemia in Infants and Children). During periods of fasting, the liver and kidney can mobilize glucose from glycogen. If fasting is prolonged, hepatic glycogen stores will be drained in a few hours and gluconeogenesis from lactate, alanine, glycerol, and glutamine must be stimulated to maintain euglycemia.[33] The newborn infant has approximately 34 g of glycogen, only 6 g of which is in the liver and is accumulated during the last weeks of fetal life. Hepatic glycogen is totally depleted during the first few days postnatally and then reaccumulates.[34] Carbohydrate-free diets lead to ketosis, as does fasting. Ketosis occurs when carbohydrate intake drops below about 10% of total calories. It occurs more readily in children than in adults during fasting or when extremely low-carbohydrate diets are consumed.[35] Low-carbohydrate diets and low-carbohydrate, high-fat diets (the ketogenic diet; see Chapter 13) have been used in the treatment of epilepsy and as a diagnostic test for ketotic hypoglycemia.

In addition to glycogen stores in the liver and skeletal muscle, the body contains carbohydrate in many different forms. These include mucopolysaccharides (structural carbohydrates that are important constituents of connective and collagenous tissues) and components of nucleic acids, glycoproteins, glycolipids, and various hormones and enzymes.

Abnormalities in these structural carbohydrates have been associated with specific symptoms or disorders. Genetic defects in glycoprotein metabolism usually result in neurologic symptoms. However, defects in glycoprotein biosynthesis known as congenital disorders of glycosylation (formerly known as the carbohydrate-deficient glycoprotein syndromes) also present with hypoglycemia, protein-losing enteropathy, and hepatic pathology.[36] In these conditions, the N-glycosylation pathway is affected, resulting in alterations in the number or structure of sugar chains on the proteins. The diagnosis often can be made via isoelectric focusing of transferrin.[36]

Glycemic Index

The Glycemic Index (GI) is a numerical scale first introduced by Jenkins et al in 1981 to determine how rapidly affected and elevated blood glucose will be after consuming a particular food.[37,38] The index is calculated by first measuring the area under the 2-hour blood glucose response curve after ingestion of a fixed amount of carbohydrate (usually 50 g).[37] This area is then divided by the area under the curve of a standard, based on ingestion of an equal amount of carbohydrate (commonly glucose). This value is then multiplied by 100 to determine the index value.[37] Per equal gram of carbohydrate, a high-GI food will elevate blood glucose concentration higher than a low-GI food.[39] Disaccharides have a high GI, whereas fiber generally has a low GI. Evidence suggests that long-term consumption of a diet with a high GI may predict the risk of developing type 2 diabetes mellitus and cardiovascular disease.[39] Thus, many groups recommend a diet rich in foods with a low GI.[39] However, there are limitations to the GI. For example, the GI of a particular food can vary significantly depending on the variety of a specific food, storage conditions, cooking methods, other foods consumed at the same time, and differences in testing techniques.[39]

Lactose

Lactose is present in almost all mammalian milks and is the major carbohydrate consumed by young infants.[40] Lactase, an enzyme on the brush border of the enterocyte in the small intestine, hydrolyzes the disaccharide lactose into the monosaccharides glucose and galactose (Fig 16.1).

Although a congenital form of lactase deficiency exists (also termed primary lactase deficiency), it is extremely rare. It manifests at birth with diarrhea, gaseous distention, and malnutrition in the presence of a lactose-containing diet.[41] Lactase activity is normally at detectable levels by 12 weeks' gestation. Lactase activity increases most rapidly during the last trimester of gestation.[5] By 34 weeks' gestation, however, lactase activity is only at 30% of that of a term infant. Thus, in preterm infants (born at <34 weeks' gestation), developmental lactase deficiency is a temporary form of lactase deficiency that may be clinically significant.[42] Likely because of the later increase in lactase activity compared with the mucosal enzyme responsible for the digestion of short-chain glucose polymers (maltase-glucoamylase),[9,43] preterm infants do not digest lactose as well as glucose polymers.[44] Several studies suggest that the feeding of formula containing lactose as the sole carbohydrate to very preterm infants may be associated with an increased risk of feeding intolerance and that the risk of feeding intolerance is inversely related to lactase activity.[45,46] The one randomized controlled trial evaluating the effectiveness of adding lactase to the feedings of preterm infants found benefit for weight gain but not feeding intolerance; however, the treatment was not started until the infants had reached 75% of their goal feeding.[47] One study in preterm infants reported increased lactase activity in breastfed infants when compared with formula-fed infants.[42] Thus, lactose from human milk may be less problematic than that from formula. Developmental lactase deficiency improves as the intestinal mucosa matures.[42]

Most commonly, lactase activity begins to decline in a genetically programmed (autosomal recessive) fashion so that by adulthood lactase activity is low in approximately 65% of the world's population.[48] The prevalence of lactase deficiency varies depending on whether the diagnosis is made phenotypically (eg, with lactose breath testing), genetically, or in combination.[49] On the basis of phenotypic diagnosis, the US prevalence of lactase deficiency is approximately 6% to 22% in white people and 80% to 100% in American Indian/Alaska Native populations.[50] Recent genetic studies have shown that the prevalence of lactase deficiency can vary widely even in populations traditionally thought to be lactase deficient.[49] For example, the prevalence of lactase deficiency is approximately 100% in black African people, but in parts of Sudan it is 55%; it is approximately 100% in Asian people, but in parts of Northern India it is only 45%; and in the Middle East it can range from 100% to as low as 27%.[49] Persistence of lactase activity is predicted by the presence of polymorphisms in the lactase gene and potentially, epigenetic modifications affecting expression.[48] On the basis of phenotypic data, the decline in lactase activity usually begins to occur around 3 to 7 years of age; ethnic groups with a higher prevalence of lactase deficiency typically have an earlier decline.[40] People with low lactase activity often do not manifest symptoms of lactose intolerance, such as flatulence, bloating, abdominal pain, and nausea and diarrhea (also see Chapter 27: Chronic Diarrheal Disease).[40,50] In fact, most people with low lactase activity can tolerate some lactose intake, particularly when it is part of a meal.[40,50]

Symptoms of lactase intolerance are caused by lactose that escapes digestion in the small intestine and passes into the colon, where it is fermented by enteric bacteria into organic acids, hydrogen, methane, and other gases.[29,30] These gases can cause bloating and pain; the unabsorbed sugar and acids cause an increase in osmotic pressure, resulting in osmotic diarrhea. However, the likelihood of developing symptoms depends on the amount of residual lactase activity, the amount of lactose ingested, the composition of the meal, and the presence or absence of visceral hypersensitivity.[40,51]

Lactase activity also can be diminished secondary to mucosal injury in the small intestine (secondary lactase deficiency). This is observed most commonly in infants with viral gastroenteritis and is a consequence of damage to the intestinal villi that resolves with resolution of the illness. In an otherwise healthy infant, the lactase deficiency may not be clinically significant. For example, most infants with rotavirus are not lactose intolerant.[52] However, infants with inadequate weight gain or prolonged diarrhea may have clinical lactose intolerance until the illness resolves; using a lactose-free formula until the infant recovers from diarrhea may be beneficial.[40] The intolerance usually lasts 1 to 2 weeks, except in severe cases. Secondary lactase deficiency also can be seen in other diseases associated with damage to the small bowel, including inflammatory bowel disease and celiac disease.

Currently, there are several different methods of diagnosing lactase deficiency. The hydrogen breath test is considered by many to be the best tool for the diagnosis of lactose malabsorption (presumably attributable to lactase deficiency) because of its ease of use and inexpensive nature.[40,48,53] Lactose malabsorption is detected by an increase in expired breath hydrogen after lactose ingestion.[50] Conditions that cause small intestinal damage can result in secondary lactase deficiency and a positive breath test (see above).[53] Although false-negative results are believed to occur as a result of individuals whose gut microbiota are incapable of producing hydrogen, there is evidence that all individuals are hydrogen producers if the breath test is conducted long enough.[54] That said, studies in children and adults show strong correlation between the results of breath testing and genetic testing (see below).[38,55]

Specific evaluation for lactose intolerance (presumably caused by lactase deficiency) can be achieved relatively easily by dietary elimination and challenge.[40] However, the lactose content of foods can vary because of its use as an ingredient in processed foods or as a bulking agent in pharmaceuticals, facts that need to be considered when using a lactose-free diet as a diagnostic aid.[56]

Genetic testing also is available that can detect polymorphisms associated with lactase (non)persistence. Genetic testing results strongly correlate with those from measurement of lactase activity.[57] The number of alleles associated with lactase persistence continues to expand.[48]

Lactase deficiency can be diagnosed invasively via enzymatic testing performed on mucosal biopsies, but there is disagreement regarding the correlation between activity and clinical symptoms, which is understandable, given that lactase activity will depend on the site of the biopsy and the number of biopsies taken.[58,59] In practice, mucosal biopsy is rarely necessary to diagnose lactase deficiency. Other testing modalities are currently being explored, including the lactose quick test, which uses a colorimetric assay on duodenal biopsy samples.[59]

Clinically significant carbohydrate malabsorption (including that from lactose) can also be detected by testing the pH of the stool by using nitrazine paper (pH <5.5 indicates carbohydrate fermentation attributable to malabsorption) and testing for glucose (based on copper reduction) using the same products used to test for glucose in the urine.[40] The glucose derives from the breakdown of lactose by the colonic microbiota. It is important to test the watery part of the stool, because the formed part of the stool is likely to give a false-negative result. This test can be used to detect the presence of other sugars, such as sucrose and starches, because bacteria will degrade some proportion of these sugars to glucose. Detectable carbohydrate malabsorption should be treated to reduce fluid losses attributable to osmotic diarrhea with the consequent risks of dehydration and acidosis.

Special Carbohydrate Diets and Supplements

Lactose and fructose, along with fructans, galactans, and polyols, constitute a group of carbohydrates termed fermentable oligosaccharide, disaccharide, monosaccharide, and polyol (FODMAP) carbohydrates[60] (Table 16.6). These carbohydrates are poorly (or not at all) digested in the small intestine but can be rapidly fermented by colonic bacteria resulting in colonic distension, flatus, bloating, and/or watery diarrhea. FODMAP carbohydrates have been implicated to play a role in adult and childhood abdominal pain-related functional gastrointestinal disorders, and studies have suggested a low

Table 16.6.

Carbohydrates included in FODMAP Group

Carbohydrate	*Common Foods*
Oligosaccharides	
Fructans	Wheat, onions, rye
Galactans	Beans, legumes, asparagus
Disaccharides	
Lactose	Cow milk, cheese
Monosaccharides	
Fructose	Apples, pears, honey; juices
Polyols	
Sorbitol	Certain fruits and vegetables: apricots, cherries, pears

Adapted from Barrett and Gibson.[95]

FODMAP diet may be beneficial in the treatment of such disorders.[61,62] A typical treatment course with a low-FODMAP diet involves an initial elimination period of approximately 4 to 6 weeks, during which time foods high in FODMAPS are excluded from the patient's diet. When symptomatic relief is achieved, gradual reintroduction of FODMAPs helps to determine which of the carbohydrates are responsible for symptoms and the amount of FODMAPs that might be tolerated. Although the results have thus far been promising, further studies are necessary to delineate the true short- and long-term efficacy of FODMAP elimination, which patients are most likely to respond, the optimal method for reintroduction into the diet, and which other disorders (eg, inflammatory bowel disease) may respond to the treatment.[63,64]

Prebiotics consist of nondigestible supplements or foods, usually oligosaccharides, which provide a benefit to the host by stimulating the growth or activity of one or more indigenous probiotic bacteria. These oligosaccharides often are composed of multiple chains of fructose with a terminal glucose. Although indigestible by humans, they allow for the proliferation of bacteria such as those of the *Bifidobacteria* species, which are thought to be beneficial to health. Fructo-oligosaccharides (FOSs), inulin, and galacto-oligosaccharides (GOSs) are just a few examples of prebiotic oligosaccharides. Human milk is a natural source of high levels of prebiotics, containing up to 14g/L of oligosaccharides.[65] Prebiotics also are often added as supplements to a variety of foods, drinks, and infant formula. Currently, no definitive statement can be made as to their efficacy in the treatment or prevention of childhood diseases such as atopic dermatitis and other allergic disorders or growth or clinical outcomes in term infants.[66–68] Some evidence suggests that prebiotics may reduce the number of infectious episodes requiring antibiotic therapy in infants and children 0 to 24 months of age.[69] That said, overall, to date, there is insufficient evidence to clearly support or refute the use of prebiotics in the pediatric diet.

Starches

As noted previously, starches are the storage carbohydrate of plants consisting of amylose (a linear α-1,4 polysaccharide of glucose molecules) and amylopectin (an α-1,4 polysaccharide of glucose molecules with α-1,6 branch points). Chains between DP3 and DP9 and those $\geq$DP10 are termed oligosaccharides and polysaccharides, respectively (Table 16.2). The larger the starch, the less osmotically active it is.

Corn syrup is a generic term for products derived from cornstarch by hydrolysis with acid or enzymes. These products are classified according to their chemical-reducing power relative to glucose, which has a dextrose equivalent (DE) of 100%. The DE of corn syrups ranges from less than 20% to more than 95%. A low-DE corn syrup is somewhat hydrolyzed and is, therefore, more like starch than a high-DE corn syrup. Glucose polymer (or maltodextrin) is another term for corn syrup that has been hydrolyzed to (usually) a high DE carbohydrate. They often are added to formulas to provide additional calories without greatly increasing the osmolality of the feeding. Approximately 20% to 25% of infants in the United States are fed lactose-free soy isolate formulas containing sucrose or corn syrup solids or a combination of both as the carbohydrate source(s).

Modified food starches possess certain technical properties, such as altered viscosity and "mouth feel," freeze-thaw stability, gel clarity, and stability in acid products. In animal models, caloric availability of modified food starches is similar to unmodified starches. Modified food starches have been used for many years in infant foods and are "generally recognized as safe" (GRAS) by the US Food and Drug Administration. Many powdered special formulas and strained foods contain modified corn or tapioca starches. Special formulas may provide approximately 15% of the total calories in the form of modified starch, which is used to facilitate suspension of insoluble nutrients during feeding. The amount of modified starch in a few commercial infant desserts may amount to as much as 45% of the total content of the solids. Modified food starches may have modest effects on increasing or decreasing the availability of minerals depending on the type of starch used.[70–72]

Fiber

The term fiber has multiple definitions in the nutrition world, but fiber generally refers to intrinsic plant cell polysaccharides, which are derived from the cellular walls and are poorly digestible.[1] Fiber is also called bulk or roughage and is composed predominantly of nonstarch polysaccharides and nonpolysaccharides (mainly lignins). Nonstarch polysaccharides are the most diverse of all the carbohydrate groups and include cellulose (β-1-4 linkages) and noncellulosic polysaccharides (eg, hemicelluloses, pectins, gums, and mucilages), which contain a mixture of hexose and pentose sugars. Pectin often is used to improve the gel consistency of jams. Gums also are used as thickeners. Mucilages are used as thickeners in mayonnaise, soups,

498   Chapter 16

and toothpaste. Carrageenan, derived from algae, is used in dairy products and chocolate. The definition of nonstarch polysaccharides excludes other substances in the plant materials, such as phytates, cutins, saponins, lectins, proteins, waxes, silicon, and other organic constituents.

Crude fiber refers to the residue left after strong acid and base hydrolysis of plant material. This process dissolves pectin, gums, mucilages, and most of the hemicellulose. Thus, crude fiber is mainly a measure of cellulose and lignin and tends to underestimate the total amount of fiber in the food. Most food composition tables provide only crude fiber values. Appendix I lists the fiber content of common foods. It has been estimated in adults that 5% to 10% of dietary starch (20–40 g in a Western diet) is "resistant starch," which is not digested in the small intestine and, therefore, reaches the colon in its intact form.[16,33] Table 16.7 lists the effects of various nonstarch polysaccharides on stool output.[30]

Historically, fiber was classified as soluble (some hemicelluloses, pectins, gums, and mucilages found in beans, fruits, psyllium, and oat products) or insoluble (most hemicelluloses, celluloses, and lignins found in whole-grain

Table 16.7.

Effects of Various Nonstarch Polysaccharides on Bowel Habit

Source	No. of Subjects	Increase in Stool Weight (mean g/g 'fiber' fed)	Median	Range
Raw bran	82	7.2	6.5	3–14.4
Fruit and vegetables	175	6.0	3.7	1.4–19.6
Cooked bran	338	4.4	4.9	2–12.3
Psyllium/ispaghula	119	4.0	4.3	0.9–6.6
Oats	53	3.4	4.8	1–5.5
Other gums and mucilages	66	3.1	1.9	0.3–10.2
Corn	32	2.9	2.9	2.8–3.0
Soya and other legumes	98	1.5	1.5	0.3–3.1
Pectin	95	1.3	1.0	0–3.6

Modified from Elia and Cummings.[1]

products and vegetables). This original classification appeared useful in understanding the properties of dietary fibers implying a division into those that primarily had effects on glucose and lipid absorption in the small intestine (soluble) and those that were slowly and incompletely fermented and had greater effects on facilitating defecation (insoluble).[1] However, the distinction between soluble and insoluble fibers is primarily dependent on pH, weakening the physiological link. For example, psyllium, which is considered a soluble fiber, is actually poorly fermented.[73]

The National Academy of Sciences has proposed the terms dietary fiber and functional fiber.[74] Dietary fiber consists of nondigestible carbohydrates and lignin that are intrinsic and intact in plants. Functional fiber consists of isolated, nondigestible carbohydrates that have beneficial physiological effects in humans. Total fiber is the sum of dietary fiber and functional fiber.

The definition of fiber has important nutritional implications. The health benefits of fiber (see below) depend on the type of fiber, with those from fruits and vegetables generally being regarded as contributing most to health.[75] A working definition (Table 16.8) to resolve this potential dilemma of how best to define fiber has been put forth by the World Health Organization/Food and Agriculture Organization of the United Nations 30th Session of the Codex Alimentarius Commission (http://www.fao.org/fao-who-codexalimentarius/en).[75]

Table 16.8.
Definition of Fiber

Dietary fiber means carbohydrate polymers with 10 or more monomeric units, which are not hydrolyzed by the endogenous enzymes in the small intestine of humans and belong to the following categories:
• Edible carbohydrate polymers naturally occurring in the food as consumed
• Carbohydrate polymers, which have been obtained from food raw material by physical, enzymatic or chemical means and which have been shown to have a physiological effect of benefit to health as demonstrated by generally accepted scientific evidence to competent authorities
• Synthetic carbohydrate polymers which have been shown to have a physiological effect of benefit to health as demonstrated by generally accepted scientific evidence to competent authorities

Adapted from the World Health Organization/Food and Agriculture Organization of the United Nations 30th Session of the Codex Alimentarius Commission (http://www.fao.org/fao-who-codexalimentarius/en).[75]

Potential Benefits of Fiber Intake

The current interest in fiber was stimulated in part by the suggestion that fiber could help prevent and/or treat certain diseases common in the United States, such as cancer of the colon, irritable bowel syndrome, constipation, obesity, and coronary heart disease. Epidemiologic studies noted that African people in rural areas where fiber intake was high rarely developed these diseases. However, as urban migration has increased, the adoption of Western habits and dietary patterns has coincided with the increased incidence of Western diseases. According to the National Health and Nutrition Examination Survey (NHANES) 2009–2010 report, the average fiber intake of all individuals 2 years and older in the United States was 16 g/day with the majority coming from fruit and vegetable sources.[76] This falls far below the recommended daily intake from multiple expert groups.

Increased dietary fiber has been found to have numerous positive health benefits. In adults, there is strong evidence that mortality from cardiovascular disease, coronary artery disease, and all cancers is reduced (9%, 11%, 6%, respectively) related to dietary fiber intake when the highest versus lowest intakes are compared or as a dose response (10 g/day increment in intake).[74,77] Fiber from cereal and legumes were beneficial for cardiovascular disease mortality, but vegetable and fruit were not.[77–79] Evidence supports the ability of dietary fiber to reduce both total and low-density lipoprotein cholesterol concentrations and, perhaps, serum triglycerides.[74] Similarly, studies support additional benefit in reducing the risk of type II diabetes.[74,78] Whether these benefits relate to reductions in inflammatory pathways remains controversial.[79]

Much fewer data are available regarding potential health benefits of dietary fiber in children.[80] Epidemiologic studies are split as to whether dietary fiber intake affects glucose regulation and/or metabolic syndrome prevalence in children, likely related to differences in study design, study populations, and the type of dietary fiber investigated.[80] Studies examining the effect of psyllium fiber on blood lipids in children suggest modest but significant benefit in most,[81–83] but not all, double-blind randomized controlled trials.[84]

Given the high prevalence of constipation in children, there have been a number of studies examining the role of increased dietary fiber in its treatment and/or prevention. As noted previously, the effect of fiber on stooling pattern depends on the type of dietary fiber. Thus, it is not surprising that the benefit of increased dietary fiber in the treatment and prevention of constipation in children is unclear given the variation in types and dose of fibers used (eg, general increase in dietary fiber versus use of a fiber supplement).[80,85] A recent report by the North American Society for Pediatric Gastroenterology, Hepatology and Nutrition did not recommend fiber supplements in the treatment of constipation.[86]

Given the increasing prevalence of childhood obesity in the United States, there is interest in the role of fiber in reducing the risk of obesity. However, there is a paucity of randomized controlled trials. Observational studies are plagued by differences in study populations, study design, and types of dietary fiber evaluated, leading to lack of clarity.[80]

Potential Adverse Effects of Fiber Intake

Although there have been numerous proposed health benefits to a high-fiber diet, some concerns have been raised, primarily related to possible adverse effects on the absorption of minerals.[87] Both soluble and insoluble fibers have mineral binding properties dependent on the specific type of fiber and pH.[88,89] Although this may inhibit, to some degree, absorption in the small intestine, if the fiber is fermented in the colon, the minerals are liberated and can be absorbed.[88] Some fibers actually enhance the absorption of minerals but these effects are very specific (eg, low-molecular weight pectins do, but high-molecular weight pectins do not).[88] In situations of adequate nutrition, mineral binding by fiber is unlikely to be of importance.[74,88] However, it may be of relevance in situations in which mineral intake is low.[87,89]

Another potential issue relates to decreased energy absorption in the face of high fiber intake.[87,89] As in the case of interference with mineral absorption, this concern appears potentially to be more relevant in populations with either poor baseline energy intake and/or who are already undernourished.[87,89] In a study in 1-month-old healthy infants, the addition of rice cereal in relatively large amounts to infant formula (4 g/30 mL) did not lead to decreased energy or nitrogen absorption.[90]

Current Dietary Recommendations

Over the years, the amount of recommended dietary fiber has been increasing. Previous recommendations suggested that between 6 and 12 months of age, fruits and vegetables be introduced gradually, increasing to 5 g/day by the first year.[91] The American Health Foundation had set forth a guideline suggesting that children older than 2 years consume an amount of fiber approximately equivalent to the child's age plus 5 g/day.[92] This "age plus 5" guideline results in a gradual increase of fiber intake over time, with older teenagers achieving the recommended intake for adults. The amount recommended for an older adolescent was also within the range endorsed by a conference that was held on dietary fiber in childhood in 1995.[93]

The most recent recommendations come from The National Academy of Medicine and the United States Department of Agriculture. The National Academy of Medicine report on Dietary Reference Intakes in 2005 established the Allowable Intake for fiber for children (Table 16.9).[74,94] The recommendations are fairly aligned, except for 4- to 8-year-old-children, for whom the US Department of Agriculture recommendations run lower than those from the National Academy of Medicine. Refined flour commonly found in breads, rolls, buns, and pizza crust contribute substantially to dietary fiber consumption, even though they are not the best sources of dietary fiber. The reports recommend that one should increase the consumption of beans and peas, other vegetables, fruits, whole grains, and other foods with naturally occurring fiber as opposed to refined fibers or by fiber supplementation with over-the-counter supplements.

Table 16.9.
Daily Recommended Intake of Fiber

Gender/Age (y)	Fiber (g)[a]	Fiber (g)[b]
0–1	ND	ND
≥1–3	19	14
4–8 Female Male	 25 25	 16.8 19.6
9–13 Female Male	 26 31	 22.4 25.2
14–18 Female Male	 26 38	 25.2 30.8

[a] Institute of Medicine.[74]

[b] USDA Dietary Guidelines.[94]

ND indicates not determinable.

References

1. Cummings JH, Stephen AM. Carbohydrate terminology and classification. *Eur.J Clin.Nutr.* 2007;61 Suppl 1:S5–18

2. Fitch C, Keim KS, Academy of N, Dietetics. Position of the Academy of Nutrition and Dietetics: use of nutritive and nonnutritive sweeteners. *J Acad Nutr Diet.* May 2012;112(5):739–758

3. Cummings JH, Macfarlane GT, Englyst HN. Prebiotic digestion and fermentation. *Am J Clin Nutr.* Feb 2001;73(2 Suppl):415S–420S

4. Trumbo P, Schlicker S, Yates AA, Poos M. Dietary reference intakes for energy, carbohydrate, fiber, fat, fatty acids, cholesterol, protein and amino acids. *J Am. Diet.Assoc.* 2002;102(11):1621–1630

5. Antonowicz I, Chang SK, Grand RJ. Development and distribution of lysosomal enzymes and disaccharidases in human fetal intestine. *Gastroenterology.* Jul 1974;67(1):51–58

6. Koldovsky O. Development of human gastrointestinal functions: interaction of changes in diet composition, hormonal maturation, and fetal genetic programming. *J Am Coll Nutr.* 1984;3(2):131–138

7. Mobassaleh M, Montgomery RK, Biller JA, Grand RJ. Development of carbohydrate absorption in the fetus and neonate. *Pediatrics.* Jan 1985;75(1 Pt 2): 160–166

8. Christian M, Edwards C, Weaver LT. Starch digestion in infancy. *J Pediatr Gastroenterol Nutr.* Aug 1999;29(2):116–124

9. Raul F, Lacroix B, Aprahamian M. Longitudinal distribution of brush border hydrolases and morphological maturation in the intestine of the preterm infant. *Early human development.* Apr 1986;13(2):225–234

10. Hadorn B, Zoppi G, Shmerling DH, Prader A, McIntyre I, Anderson CM. Quantitative assessment of exocrine pancreatic function in infants and children. *J Pediatr.* Jul 1968;73(1):39–50

11. Lebenthal E, Lee PC. Development of functional responses in human exocrine pancreas. *Pediatrics.* Oct 1980;66(4):556–560

12. Kamaryt J, Fintajslova O. [Development of salivary and pancreatic amylase in children during the 1st year of life]. *Z Klin Chem Klin Biochem.* Nov 1970;8(6): 564–566

13. Klumpp TGN, A.V. The gastric and duodenal contents of normal infants and children. *Am J Dis Child.* 1930;40:1215–1229

14. Shulman RJ, Kerzner B, Sloan HR, et al. Absorption and oxidation of glucose polymers of different lengths in young infants. *Pediatr Res.* 1986;20(8):740–743

15. Shulman RJ, Feste A, Ou C. Absorption of lactose, glucose polymers, or combination in premature infants. *J Pediatr.* Oct 1995;127(4):626–631

16. Eggermont E. The hydrolysis of the naturally occurring alpha-glucosides by the human intestinal mucosa. *European journal of biochemistry / FEBS.* Jul 1969;9(4):483–487

17. Nichols BL, Eldering J, Avery S, Hahn D, Quaroni A, Sterchi E. Human small intestinal maltase-glucoamylase cDNA cloning. Homology to sucrase-isomaltase. *J Biol Chem.* Jan 30 1998;273(5):3076–3081

18. Kelly JJ, Alpers DH. Properties of human intestinal glucoamylase. *Biochim Biophys Acta.* Jul 05 1973;315(1):113–122

19. Lebenthal E, Khin MU, Zheng BY, Lu RB, Lerner A. Small intestinal glucoamylase deficiency and starch malabsorption: a newly recognized alpha-glucosidase deficiency in children. *J Pediatr.* 1994;124(4):541–546

20. Dreher ML, Dreher CJ, Berry JW. Starch digestibility of foods: a nutritional perspective. *Crit Rev Food Sci Nutr.* 1984;20(1):47–71

21. Wright EM, Loo DD, Hirayama BA. Biology of human sodium glucose transporters. *Physiological reviews.* Apr 2011;91(2):733–794

22. Roder PV, Geillinger KE, Zietek TS, Thorens B, Koepsell H, Daniel H. The role of SGLT1 and GLUT2 in intestinal glucose transport and sensing. *PloS one.* 2014;9(2):e89977

23. Augustin R. The protein family of glucose transport facilitators: It's not only about glucose after all. *IUBMB.Life.* 2010;62(5):315–333

24. Jones HF, Butler RN, Brooks DA. Intestinal fructose transport and malabsorption in humans. *Am.J Physiol Gastrointest.Liver Physiol.* 2011;300(2): G202–G206

25. Schmitt CC, Aranias T, Viel T, et al. Intestinal invalidation of the glucose transporter GLUT2 delays tissue distribution of glucose and reveals an unexpected role in gut homeostasis. *Mol Metab.* Jan 2017;6(1):61–72

26. Kellett GL, Brot-Laroche E. Apical GLUT2: a major pathway of intestinal sugar absorption. *Diabetes.* 2005;54(10):3056–3062

27. Ebert K, Ludwig M, Geillinger KE, et al. Reassessment of GLUT7 and GLUT9 as Putative Fructose and Glucose Transporters. *J Membr Biol.* Jan 12 2017

28. Jeukendrup AE. Carbohydrate and exercise performance: the role of multiple transportable carbohydrates. *Curr.Opin.Clin.Nutr.Metab Care.* 2010;13(4):452–457

29. Cummings JH, Macfarlane GT. Role of intestinal bacteria in nutrient metabolism. *JPEN J Parenter.Enteral Nutr.* 1997;21(6):357–365

30. Elia M, Cummings JH. Physiological aspects of energy metabolism and gastrointestinal effects of carbohydrates. *Eur J Clin Nutr.* Dec 2007;61 Suppl 1: S40–74

31. Kalhan SC, Kilic I. Carbohydrate as nutrient in the infant and child: range of acceptable intake. *Eur.J Clin.Nutr.* 1999;53 Suppl 1:S94–100

32. Kalhan SC, Parimi P, Van Beek R, et al. Estimation of gluconeogenesis in newborn infants. *Am J Physiol Endocrinol Metab.* Nov 2001;281(5):E991–997

33. Halliday D, Bodamer OA. Measurement of glucose turnover—implications for the study of inborn errors of metabolism. *Eur J Pediatr.* Aug 1997;156 Suppl 1: S35–38

34. Devi BG, Habeebullah CM, Gupta PD. Glycogen metabolism during human liver development. *Biochem Int.* Oct 1992;28(2):229–237

35. Lieberman MM, A.D. *Marks' Basic Medical Biochemistry: A Clinical Approach.* 4th ed. Philadelphia, P.A.: Lippincott Williams & Wilkins; 2013

36. Scott K, Gadomski T, Kozicz T, Morava E. Congenital disorders of glycosylation: new defects and still counting. *J Inherit Metab Dis.* Jul 2014;37(4):609–617

37. Jenkins DJ, Wolever TM, Taylor RH, et al. Glycemic index of foods: a physiological basis for carbohydrate exchange. *Am J Clin Nutr.* Mar 1981;34(3): 362–366

38. Alliende F, Vial C, Espinoza K, et al. Accuracy of a Genetic Test for the Diagnosis of Hypolactasia in Chilean Children: Comparison With the Breath Test. *J Pediatr Gastroenterol Nutr.* Jul 2016;63(1):e10–13

39. Foster-Powell K, Holt SH, Brand-Miller JC. International table of glycemic index and glycemic load values: 2002. *Am.J Clin.Nutr.* 2002;76(1):5–56

40. Heyman MB, Committee on N. Lactose intolerance in infants, children, and adolescents. *Pediatrics.* Sep 2006;118(3):1279–1286

41. Diekmann L, Pfeiffer K, Naim HY. Congenital lactose intolerance is triggered by severe mutations on both alleles of the lactase gene. *BMC Gastroenterol.* Mar 21 2015;15:36

42. Shulman RJ, Schanler RJ, Lau C, Heitkemper M, Ou CN, Smith EO. Early feeding, feeding tolerance, and lactase activity in preterm infants. *J Pediatr.* Nov 1998;133(5):645–649

43. Lebenthal E, Lee PC. Glucoamylase and disaccharidase activities in normal subjects and in patients with mucosal injury of the small intestine. *J.Pediatr.* 1980;97(3):389–393

44. Stathos TH, Shulman RJ, Schanler RJ, Abrams SA. Effect of carbohydrates on calcium absorption in premature infants. *Pediatr Res.* Apr 1996;39(4 Pt 1):666–670

45. Griffin MP, Hansen JW. Can the elimination of lactose from formula improve feeding tolerance in premature infants? *J Pediatr.* Nov 1999;135(5):587–592

46. Shulman RJ, Ou CN, Smith EO. Evaluation of potential factors predicting attainment of full gavage feedings in preterm infants. *Neonatology.* 2011;99(1): 38–44

47. Erasmus HD, Ludwig-Auser HM, Paterson PG, Sun D, Sankaran K. Enhanced weight gain in preterm infants receiving lactase-treated feeds: a randomized, double-blind, controlled trial. *J Pediatr.* Oct 2002;141(4):532–537

48. Ingram CJ, Mulcare CA, Itan Y, Thomas MG, Swallow DM. Lactose digestion and the evolutionary genetics of lactase persistence. *Hum Genet.* Jan 2009;124(6): 579–591

49. Itan Y, Jones BL, Ingram CJ, Swallow DM, Thomas MG. A worldwide correlation of lactase persistence phenotype and genotypes. *BMC Evol Biol.* Feb 09 2010;10:36

50. Harrington LK, Mayberry JF. A re-appraisal of lactose intolerance. *Int J Clin Pract.* Oct 2008;62(10):1541–1546

51. Zhu Y, Zheng X, Cong Y, et al. Bloating and distention in irritable bowel syndrome: the role of gas production and visceral sensation after lactose ingestion in a population with lactase deficiency. *Am J Gastroenterol.* Sep 2013;108(9):1516–1525

IV

52. Brown KH, Peerson JM, Fontaine O. Use of nonhuman milks in the dietary management of young children with acute diarrhea: a meta-analysis of clinical trials. *Pediatrics.* Jan 1994;93(1):17–27

53. Gasbarrini A, Corazza GR, Gasbarrini G, et al. Methodology and indications of H2-breath testing in gastrointestinal diseases: the Rome Consensus Conference. *Alimentary pharmacology & therapeutics.* Mar 30 2009;29 Suppl 1:1–49

54. Strocchi A, Corazza G, Ellis CJ, Gasbarrini G, Levitt MD. Detection of malabsorption of low doses of carbohydrate: accuracy of various breath H2 criteria. *Gastroenterology.* 1993;105(5):1404–1410

55. Marton A, Xue X, Szilagyi A. Meta-analysis: the diagnostic accuracy of lactose breath hydrogen or lactose tolerance tests for predicting the North European lactase polymorphism C/T-13910. *Alimentary pharmacology & therapeutics.* Feb 2012;35(4):429–440

56. Lomer MC, Parkes GC, Sanderson JD. Review article: lactose intolerance in clinical practice—myths and realities. *Alimentary pharmacology & therapeutics.* Jan 15 2008;27(2):93–103

57. Baffour-Awuah NY, Fleet S, Montgomery RK, et al. Functional significance of single nucleotide polymorphisms in the lactase gene in diverse US patients and evidence for a novel lactase persistence allele at -13909 in those of European ancestry. *J Pediatr Gastroenterol Nutr.* Feb 2015;60(2):182–191

58. Gupta SK, Chong SK, Fitzgerald JF. Disaccharidase activities in children: normal values and comparison based on symptoms and histologic changes. *J Pediatr Gastroenterol Nutr.* Mar 1999;28(3):246–251

59. Furnari M, Bonfanti D, Parodi A, et al. A comparison between lactose breath test and quick test on duodenal biopsies for diagnosing lactase deficiency in patients with self-reported lactose intolerance. *J Clin Gastroenterol.* Feb 2013;47(2):148–152

60. Barrett JSG, P.R. Clinical ramifications of malabsorption of fructose and other short-chain carbohydrates. *Pract Gastroenterol.* 2007(August):51–65

61. Halmos EP, Power VA, Shepherd SJ, Gibson PR, Muir JG. A diet low in FODMAPs reduces symptoms of irritable bowel syndrome. *Gastroenterology.* Jan 2014;146(1):67–75 e65

62. Chumpitazi BP, Cope JL, Hollister EB, et al. Randomised clinical trial: gut microbiome biomarkers are associated with clinical response to a low FODMAP diet in children with the irritable bowel syndrome. *Alimentary pharmacology & therapeutics.* Aug 2015;42(4):418–427

63. Krogsgaard LR, Lyngesen M, Bytzer P. Systematic review: quality of trials on the symptomatic effects of the low FODMAP diet for irritable bowel syndrome. *Alimentary pharmacology & therapeutics.* Apr 25 2017

64. Gibson PR. Use of the low-FODMAP diet in inflammatory bowel disease. *J Gastroenterol Hepatol.* Mar 2017;32 Suppl 1:40–42

65. Boehm G, Stahl B. Oligosaccharides from milk. *J Nutr.* Mar 2007;137(3 Suppl 2): 847S–849S

66. van der Aa LB, Heymans HS, van Aalderen WM, Sprikkelman AB. Probiotics and prebiotics in atopic dermatitis: review of the theoretical background and clinical evidence. *Pediatr Allergy Immunol.* Mar 2010;21(2 Pt 2):e355–367

67. Cuello-Garcia CA, Fiocchi A, Pawankar R, et al. World Allergy Organization-McMaster University Guidelines for Allergic Disease Prevention (GLAD-P): Prebiotics. *World Allergy Organ J.* 2016;9:10

68. Mugambi MN, Musekiwa A, Lombard M, Young T, Blaauw R. Synbiotics, probiotics or prebiotics in infant formula for full term infants: a systematic review. *Nutr J.* Oct 04 2012;11:81

69. Lohner S, Kullenberg D, Antes G, Decsi T, Meerpohl JJ. Prebiotics in healthy infants and children for prevention of acute infectious diseases: a systematic review and meta-analysis. *Nutr Rev.* Aug 2014;72(8):523–531

70. Gonzalez-Bermudez CA, Frontela-Saseta C, Lopez-Nicolas R, Ros-Berruezo G, Martinez-Gracia C. Effect of adding different thickening agents on the viscosity properties and in vitro mineral availability of infant formula. *Food Chem.* Sep 15 2014;159:5–11

71. Bosscher D, Van Caillie-Bertrand M, Van Cauwenbergh R, Deelstra H. Availabilities of calcium, iron, and zinc from dairy infant formulas is affected by soluble dietary fibers and modified starch fractions. *Nutrition.* Jul-Aug 2003;19 (7-8):641–645

72. Wurzburg OB. Modified Starches. In: Stephen AM, ed. *Food Polysaccharides and Their Applications.* New York: Marcel Dekker; 1995:67

73. Marlett JA, Fischer MH. The active fraction of psyllium seed husk. *The Proceedings of the Nutrition Society.* Feb 2003;62(1):207–209

74. Board IoMFaN. *Dietary Reference Intakes for Energy, Carbohydrate, Fiber, Fat, Fatty Acids, Cholesterol, Protein, and Amino Acids.* Washington, DC: National Academy Press; 2005

75. Mann JI, Cummings JH. Possible implications for health of the different definitions of dietary fibre. *Nutr Metab Cardiovasc Dis.* Mar 2009;19(3):226–229

76. Hoy MKG, J.D. Fiber Intake of the US Population. 2014; https://www.ars.usda.gov/ARSUserFiles/80400530/pdf/DBrief/12_fiber_intake_0910.pdf, 2017

77. Kim Y, Je Y. Dietary fibre intake and mortality from cardiovascular disease and all cancers: A meta-analysis of prospective cohort studies. *Arch Cardiovasc Dis.* Jan 2016;109(1):39–54

78. Seal CJ, Brownlee IA. Whole-grain foods and chronic disease: evidence from epidemiological and intervention studies. *The Proceedings of the Nutrition Society.* Aug 2015;74(3):313–319

79. Kaczmarczyk MM, Miller MJ, Freund GG. The health benefits of dietary fiber: beyond the usual suspects of type 2 diabetes mellitus, cardiovascular disease and colon cancer. *Metabolism.* Aug 2012;61(8):1058–1066

80. Kranz S, Brauchla M, Slavin JL, Miller KB. What do we know about dietary fiber intake in children and health? The effects of fiber intake on constipation, obesity, and diabetes in children. *Adv Nutr.* Jan 2012;3(1):47–53

IV

81. Ribas SA, Cunha DB, Sichieri R, Santana da Silva LC. Effects of psyllium on LDL-cholesterol concentrations in Brazilian children and adolescents: a randomised, placebo-controlled, parallel clinical trial. *Br J Nutr.* Jan 14 2015;113(1):134–141

82. Davidson MH, Dugan LD, Burns JH, Sugimoto D, Story K, Drennan K. A psyllium-enriched cereal for the treatment of hypercholesterolemia in children: a controlled, double-blind, crossover study. *Am J Clin Nutr.* Jan 1996;63(1):96–102

83. Williams CL, Bollella M, Spark A, Puder D. Soluble fiber enhances the hypocholesterolemic effect of the step I diet in childhood. *J Am.Coll.Nutr.* 1995;14(3):251–257

84. Dennison BA, Levine DM. Randomized, double-blind, placebo-controlled, two-period crossover clinical trial of psyllium fiber in children with hypercholesterolemia. *J Pediatr.* Jul 1993;123(1):24–29

85. Stewart ML, Schroeder NM. Dietary treatments for childhood constipation: efficacy of dietary fiber and whole grains. *Nutr Rev.* Feb 2013;71(2):98–109

86. Tabbers MM, DiLorenzo C, Berger MY, et al. Evaluation and treatment of functional constipation in infants and children: evidence-based recommendations from ESPGHAN and NASPGHAN. *J Pediatr Gastroenterol Nutr.* Feb 2014;58(2):258–274

87. Williams CL. Dietary fiber in childhood. *J Pediatr.* 2006;149(5):S121–S130

88. Baye K, Guyot JP, Mouquet-Rivier C. The unresolved role of dietary fibers on mineral absorption. *Crit Rev Food Sci Nutr.* Mar 24 2017;57(5):949–957

89. Aggett PJ, Agostoni C, Axelsson I, et al. Nondigestible carbohydrates in the diets of infants and young children: a commentary by the ESPGHAN Committee on Nutrition. *J Pediatr Gastroenterol.Nutr.* 2003;36(3):329–337

90. Shulman RJ, Boutton TW, Klein PD. Impact of dietary cereal on nutrient absorption and fecal nitrogen loss in formula-fed infants. *J Pediatr.* Jan 1991;118(1):39–43

91. Agostoni C, Riva E, Giovannini M. Dietary fiber in weaning foods of young children. *Pediatrics.* Nov 1995;96(5 Pt 2):1002–1005

92. Williams CL, Bollella M, Wynder EL. A new recommendation for dietary fiber in childhood. *Pediatrics.* 1995;96:985–988

93. A summary of conference recommendations on dietary fiber in childhood. Conference on Dietary Fiber in Childhood, New York, May 24, 1994. *Pediatrics.* 1995;96:1023–1028

94. Dietary Guidelines for Americans 2015–2020. In: Agriculture USDo, ed. Eighth ed2015

95. Barrett JS, Gibson PR. Fermentable oligosaccharides, disaccharides, monosaccharides and polyols (FODMAPs) and nonallergic food intolerance: FODMAPs or food chemicals? *Therapeutic advances in gastroenterology.* Jul 2012;5(4):261–268

Chapter 17

Fats and Fatty Acids

General Considerations

The absolute fat requirement of the human species is the amount of essential fatty acids needed to maintain optimal fatty acid composition of all tissues and normal eicosanoid and docosanoid synthesis. At most, this requirement is no more than approximately 5% of an adequate energy intake. However, fat accounts for approximately 50% of the nonprotein energy content of both human milk and currently available infant formulas. This fat content is believed to be necessary to ensure that total energy intake is adequate to support growth and optimal utilization of dietary protein. In theory, the energy supplied by fat could be supplied by carbohydrate, from which all fatty acids except the essential ones can be synthesized. In practice, however, it is difficult to ensure an adequate energy intake without a fat intake considerably in excess of the requirement for essential fatty acids. In part, this is difficult because the osmolality of such a diet containing simple carbohydrates (eg, monosaccharides and disaccharides) will be sufficiently high to result in diarrhea and because such a diet containing more complex carbohydrates may not be fully digestible, particularly during early infancy. Moreover, because approximately 25% of the energy content of carbohydrate that is converted to fatty acids is consumed in the process of lipogenesis, metabolic efficiency is greater if nonprotein energy is provided as a mixture of fat and carbohydrate rather than predominately carbohydrate. Fat also facilitates the absorption, transport, and delivery of fat-soluble vitamins and is an important satiety factor.

Dietary Fats

Triglycerides account for the largest proportion of dietary fat. Structurally, these have 3 fatty acid molecules esterified to a single molecule of glycerol. They usually contain at least 2, often 3, different fatty acids. Other dietary fats include phospholipids, free fatty acids, monoglycerides and diglycerides, and small amounts of sterols and other nonsaponifiable compounds.

Naturally occurring fatty acids contain 4 to 26 carbon atoms. Some of these are saturated (ie, no double bonds in the carbon chain), some are monounsaturated (ie, 1 double bond), and some are polyunsaturated (ie, 2 or more double bonds). All have common names but, by convention, are identified by their number of carbon atoms, their number of double bonds, and the site of the first double bond from the terminal methyl group of the

Table 17.1.

Common Names and Numerical Nomenclature of Selected Fatty Acids

Common Name	Numerical Nomenclature
Caprylic acid	8:0
Capric acid	10:0
Lauric acid	12:0
Myristic acid	14:0
Palmitic acid	16:0
Stearic acid	18:0
Oleic acid	18:1ω-9[a]
Linoleic acid	18:2ω-6[a]
Arachidonic acid	20:4ω-6[a]
Linolenic acid[b]	18:3ω-3[a]
Eicosapentaenoic acid	20:5ω-3[a]
Docosahexaenoic acid	22:6ω-3[a]

[a] ω-9, ω-6, and ω-3 are used interchangeably with n-9, n-6, and n-3.
[b] Usually designated α-linolenic acid to distinguish it from 18:3ω-6 or γ-linolenic acid.

molecule. For example, palmitic acid, a saturated, 16-carbon fatty acid, is designated 16:0, and oleic acid, an 18-carbon, monounsaturated fatty acid with the single double bond located between the ninth and tenth carbon from the methyl terminal, is designated 18:1ω-9. Linoleic acid, 18:2ω-6, is an 18-carbon fatty acid with 2 double bonds, the first between the sixth and seventh carbon from the methyl terminal. The common names as well as the shorthand numerical designations of a number of common fatty acids are shown in Table 17.1.

Unsaturated fatty acids are folded at the site of each double bond; in this configuration, they are said to be in the cis form. During processing, the molecules may become unfolded, transforming them to trans fatty acids, which have been implicated in development of atherosclerosis. In general, the amount of trans fatty acids in infant formulas and foods is low; however, some processed fats (eg, margarines) may have a higher content. The trans fatty acid content of human milk also is reasonably low unless the mother's diet is high in trans fatty acids.

Fat Digestion, Absorption, Transport, and Metabolism

At birth, the infant must adjust from using carbohydrate as the major energy source to using a mixture of carbohydrate and fat. Hence, some aspects of fat digestion and metabolism are not fully developed, even at term. However, most term infants have sufficient fat digestive capacity to adjust satisfactorily. The limitations of fat digestion are somewhat more serious in the preterm infant, but there is little evidence that these infants have significant limitations beyond the first few weeks of life.

Fat digestion begins in the stomach, where lingual lipase hydrolyzes short- and medium-chain fatty acids from triglycerides and gastric lipase hydrolyzes long- as well as medium- and short-chain fatty acids.[1] The intragastric release of fatty acids with formation of monoglycerides delays gastric emptying and facilitates emulsification of fat in the intestine. Further, some of the released short- and medium-chain fatty acids can be absorbed directly from the stomach.[2] When they enter into the duodenum, the monoglycerides and free fatty acids stimulate release of a number of enteric hormones; among these is cholecystokinin, which stimulates contraction of the gall bladder and secretion of pancreatic enzymes.[3] Lingual and gastric lipases are largely inactivated in the duodenum, and fat digestion continues through the action of pancreatic lipase and colipase, which may be somewhat limited during the first few weeks of life. Like lingual and gastric lipase, pancreatic lipase hydrolyzes triglycerides into free fatty acids and a monoglyceride.

Human milk contains 2 additional lipases, lipoprotein lipase and bile salt-stimulated lipase. The former is essential for formation of milk lipid in the mammary gland but plays little role in intestinal fat digestion. The latter is present in much larger amounts. It is stable at a pH as low as 3.5 if bile salts are present and it is not affected by intestinal proteolytic enzymes.[4] However, it is heat labile and, hence, is inactivated by pasteurization, which is believed to be a major factor in the poor fat absorption of infants fed pasteurized human milk.[5]

Bile salt-stimulated lipase hydrolyzes triglyceride molecules into free fatty acids and glycerol rather than into free fatty acids and a monoglyceride. In theory, the bile salt-stimulated lipase of human milk can substitute for limited pancreatic lipase[4]; however, this does not appear to be of great importance for fat digestion of most infants. On the other hand, because bile salt-stimulated lipase is much more effective than pancreatic lipase in hydrolyzing esters of vitamin A, the primary form of this vitamin in human milk and many other foods, it may be important for optimal vitamin A absorption.

The bile acids released by contraction of the gall bladder help emulsify the intestinal contents, thereby facilitating triglyceride hydrolysis and fat absorption. They are released primarily as salts of taurine or glycine and, hence, have both a water-soluble and a lipid soluble portion. Alone, bile salts are poor emulsifiers, but in combination with monoglycerides, fatty acids, and phospholipids, they are quite effective. Thus, the fat hydrolysis that occurs in the stomach is an important adjunct to intestinal fat digestion.

The rate of synthesis of bile salts by newborn infants is less than that of adults, and the bile salt pool of newborn infants is only about one quarter that of adults.[6] However, an intraduodenal concentration of bile salts below 2 to 5 mM, the critical concentration required for the formation of micelles, is unusual.[6] Bile salts are actively reabsorbed in the distal ilium, transported back to the liver, and eventually reappear in bile.[7] This enterohepatic circulation occurs approximately 6 times daily, with loss of only approximately 5% of the bile salts with each circulation, although the enterohepatic circulation of bile salts is likely to be less mature in preterm infants.[8]

The monoglycerides and diglycerides and long-chain fatty acids resulting from lipolysis as well as phospholipids, cholesterol, and fat-soluble vitamins are insoluble in water but are solubilized by physicochemical combination with bile salts to form micelles.[8] Because of their amphiphilic nature, bile salts aggregate with their hydrophobic region to the interior, or core, of the micelle and their hydrophilic region to the exterior. The components of the micelle are transferred into the enteric mucosal cell, where long-chain fatty acids and monoglycerides are re-esterified into triglycerides and subsequently combined with protein, phospholipid, and cholesterol to form chylomicrons or very low-density lipoproteins. In this form, they enter the intestinal lymphatics, then the thoracic duct, and finally, the peripheral circulation.

Medium-chain triglycerides can be absorbed into the enteric cells without being hydrolyzed.[8] However, they also are rapidly hydrolyzed in the duodenum, and because the released medium-chain fatty acids are relatively soluble in the aqueous phase of the intestinal lumen, they can be absorbed without being incorporated into micelles, making them particularly useful in treatment of infants and children with a variety of pancreatic, hepatic, biliary, and/or intestinal disorders, as well as with preterm infants.

In general, long-chain unsaturated fatty acids are absorbed more readily than long-chain saturated fatty acids. Apart from the degree of unsaturation, to position of the fatty acid on the triglyceride molecule also influences absorption.[9] For the most common dietary saturated fatty acids, palmitic acid (16:0), the 2-monoglyceride of palmitic acid, is well absorbed, but free palmitic acid released from the terminal positions of the triglyceride molecule is not. The palmitic acid content of human milk is esterified primarily to the 2-position of glycerol, and this is believed to account for the better absorption of palmitic acid from human milk than from formulas containing butterfat. Synthetic fats that contain palmitic acid, primarily in the 2 position, are available[10,11] and are increasingly being used in infant formula.

In the circulation, chylomicrons acquire a specialized apoprotein from high-density lipoproteins.[8] This enables the triglycerides of the chylomicron to be hydrolyzed by lipoprotein lipase, the major enzyme responsible for intravascular hydrolysis of chylomicrons and very low-density lipoproteins.[12] Lipoprotein lipase is synthesized in most tissues, and the flow of fatty acids to tissues reflects its activity in the tissue's capillary bed. Levels of lipoprotein lipase are somewhat low in preterm and small-for-gestational-age infants, but this does not appear to impose major difficulties except, perhaps, in tolerance of intravenously administered lipid emulsions.[13]

The phospholipid and most of the apoproteins remaining after hydrolysis of chylomicron triglyceride are transferred to high-density lipoprotein, and the remainder of the apoproteins is transferred to other lipoprotein particles. This reduces the chylomicron to a fraction of its original mass, resulting in a chylomicron remnant that is removed from the circulation by specialized hepatic receptors.

Essential Fatty Acids

Fatty acids with double bonds in the ω-6 and ω-3 positions cannot be synthesized endogenously by the human species.[14] Therefore, specific ω-6 and ω-3 fatty acids or their precursors with double bonds at these positions—that is, linoleic acid (LA [18:2ω-6]) and α-linolenic acid (ALA [18:3ω-3])—must be provided in the diet. The precursor fatty acids are metabolized by the same series of desaturases and elongases to longer-chain, more unsaturated fatty acids,[14] referred to collectively as long-chain polyunsaturated fatty acids (LC-PUFAs). This pathway is outlined in Fig 17.1. Important metabolites of 18:2ω-6 and 18:3ω-3 include 18:3ω-6 (gamma linolenic acid [GLA]), 20:3ω-6 (dihomogamma linolenic acid [DHLA]), 20:4ω-6 (arachidonic acid [ARA]), 20:5ω-3 (eicosapentaenoic acid [EPA]), and 22:6ω-3 (docosahexaenoic acid [DHA]).

Figure 17.1.
Metabolism of omega-6 and omega-3 fatty acids

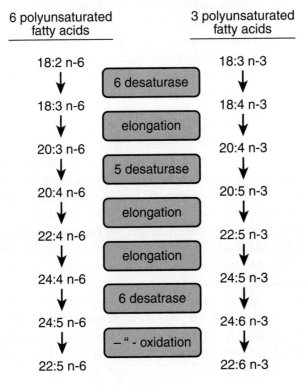

Metabolism of 6 and 3 Fatty Acids

6 polyunsaturated fatty acids		3 polyunsaturated fatty acids
18:2 n-6		18:3 n-3
↓	6 desaturase	↓
18:3 n-6		18:4 n-3
↓	elongation	↓
20:3 n-6		20:4 n-3
↓	5 desaturase	↓
20:4 n-6		20:5 n-3
↓	elongation	↓
22:4 n-6		22:5 n-3
↓	elongation	↓
24:4 n-6		24:5 n-3
↓	6 desatrase	↓
24:5 n-6		24:6 n-3
↓	– " - oxidation	↓
22:5 n-6		22:6 n-3

LA (18:2ω-6) and ALA (18:3ω-3) are present in many vegetable oils (see Table 17.2). In vivo, they are found in storage lipids, cell membrane phospholipids, intracellular cholesterol esters, and plasma lipids. The longer-chain, more unsaturated fatty acids synthesized from these precursors, in contrast, are found primarily in specific cell membrane phospholipids. DHLA, ARA, and EPA are immediate precursors of eicosanoids,[14,15] and DHA is the precursor of the docosanoids,[16] each being converted to a different series with different biological activities and/or functions.

The same series of desaturases and elongases that catalyze desaturation and elongation of ω-6 and ω-3 fatty acids also catalyze desaturation and elongation of ω-9 fatty acids. The substrate preference of these enzymes is

Table 17.2.

Fatty Acid Composition of Common Vegetable Oils[a]

Fatty Acid	Canola	Corn	Coconut	Palm Olein	Safflower[b]	Soy	High-Oleic Sunflower
6:0–12:0	–	0.1	62.1	0.2	–	–	–
14.0	–	0.1	18.1	1.0	0.1	0.1	–
16:0	4.0	12.1	8.9	39.8	6.8	11.2	3.7
18:0	2.0	2.4	2.7	4.4	2.4	0.4	5.4
18:1ω-9	55.0	32.1	6.4	42.5	76.8	22.0	81.3
18:2ω-6	26.0	50.9	1.6	11.2	12.5	53.8	9.0
18:3ω-3	10.0	0.9	–	0.2	0.1	7.5	–
Other	2.0	1.0	–	<1.6	<1.0	<1.0	<1.0

[a] Percent of total fatty acids (g/100 g).

[b] High-oleic safflower oil: approximately 77% 18:1ω-9 and 12.5% 18:2ω-6.

ω-3, ω-6, and finally, ω-9.[14] Thus, competition between the ω-9 fatty acids and either the ω-6 or ω-3 fatty acids is not an issue unless LA and/or ALA concentrations are very low, as occurs in deficiency states. In this case, oleic acid (18:1ω-9) is readily desaturated and elongated to eicosatrienoic acid (20:3ω-9). The ratio of this fatty acid to 20:4ω-6, called the triene-to-tetraene ratio, has been used as a diagnostic index of ω-6 fatty acid deficiency. This ratio usually is <0.1. A ratio of >0.4 is usually cited as indicative of deficiency,[17] but most believe that an even lower value (eg, >0.2) might be more reasonable. In the few documented cases of isolated 18:3ω-3 deficiency in which the triene-to-tetraene ratio was measured (see later discussion), it was not elevated.

LA (18:2ω-6) has been recognized as an essential nutrient for the human species for more than 85 years.[18,19] The most common symptoms of deficiency are poor growth and scaly skin lesions. These symptoms are usually preceded by an increase in the triene-to-tetraene ratio of plasma lipids. It is now clear that ALA (18:3ω-3) also is an essential nutrient. In animals, deficiency of this fatty acid results in visual and neurologic abnormalities.[20–23] Neurologic abnormalities also were observed in a human infant who had been maintained for several weeks on a parenteral nutrition regimen lacking ALA[24] and in elderly nursing home residents who were receiving intragastric feedings of an elemental formula with no ALA.[25]

Although symptoms related to deficiency of the 2 series of fatty acids seem to differ, many studies on which the description of ω-6 fatty acid deficiency are based used a fat-free or very low-fat diet rather than a diet deficient in only 18:2ω-6. Thus, there may be some overlap in the symptoms of LA and ALA deficiency. The clinical symptoms of ω-6 fatty acid deficiency can be corrected by LA or ARA; those related to ALA deficiency can be corrected by ALA, EPA, or DHA. Thus, it is not clear whether LA and ALA serve specific functions other than as precursors of LC-PUFAs.

LA usually represents between 8% and 20% of the total fatty acid content of human milk, and ALA usually represents between 0.5% and 1%.[26] Human milk also contains small amounts of a number of longer-chain, more unsaturated metabolites of both fatty acids, primarily AA (20:4ω-6) and DHA (22:6ω-3). Maternal diet has a marked effect on the concentration of most fatty acids in human milk. The concentration of DHA in the milk of women consuming a typical North American diet is generally in the range of 0.1% to 0.3% of total fatty acids, and the level of ARA ranges from 0.4% to 0.6%.[26] The milk of vegetarian women contains less DHA,[27] and that of women whose dietary fish consumption is high or who take DHA supplements is higher.[28,29] The ARA content of human milk is less variable and appears to be less dependent on maternal ARA intake, perhaps reflecting the relatively high LA intake of most populations.

Corn, coconut, safflower, and soy oils as well as high-oleic safflower and sunflower oils and palm olein oil are commonly used in the manufacture of infant formulas (see Table 18.2). All except coconut oil contain adequate amounts of LA, but only soybean oil contains an appreciable amount of ALA (6% to 9% of total fatty acids). Canola oil, a component of many formulas available outside the United States, contains somewhat less LA and more ALA. Until the 1990s, little emphasis was placed on the ALA content of infant formulas, and many with virtually no ALA were available (see also Chapter 4: Formula Feeding, and Appendix B). Current recommendations specify minimal intakes of LA ranging from 2.7% to 8% of total fat and maximum intakes ranging from 21% to 35% of total fatty acids.[30,31] The most recent recommendations for the minimum and maximum contents of ALA in term infant formulas are 1.75% and 4% of total fatty acids, respectively.[30,31] Some recommendations aim to maintain a reasonable balance between LA and ALA and recommend that the LA-to-ALA ratio be between 5 and 15,[30] and others suggest that a ratio is unnecessary.[31] Term and preterm infant formulas currently available in the United States contain approximately 20% of total fatty acids as LA and approximately 2% as ALA; hence, their LA-to-ALA ratios are approximately 10.

Long-Chain Polyunsaturated Fatty Acids

LC-PUFAs are fatty acids with a chain length of more than 18 carbons and 2 or more double bonds. Those of primary interest for infant nutrition are ARA ($20:4\omega$-6) and DHA ($22:6\omega$-3), the plasma and erythrocyte lipid contents of which are higher in breastfed than formula-fed infants.[32,33] Because human milk contains these fatty acids but, until 2002, formulas did not, the lower content of these fatty acids in plasma lipids of formula-fed infants were interpreted as indicating that the infant cannot synthesize enough of these fatty acids to meet ongoing needs. Prior and concurrent observations of better cognitive function of breastfed versus formula-fed infants[34-37] focused attention on the possibility that the lower cognitive function of formula-fed infants might be related, in part, to inadequate LC-PUFA intake.

The possibility that cognitive function is related to LC-PUFA intake is supported by the facts that ARA and DHA are the major ω-6 and ω-3 fatty acids of neural tissues[38–40] and that DHA is a major component of retinal photoreceptor membranes.[40] Further, the major supply of these fatty acids to the fetus during development is from maternal plasma.[41] Thus, the need for these fatty acids by the infant born before or during the third trimester of pregnancy and, hence, receiving a limited supply of LC-PUFA prior to birth is thought to be greater than that of the term infant. However, the daily rates of accumulation of these fatty acids in the developing central nervous system change minimally between mid-gestation and 1 year of age.[40]

On the basis of postmortem studies,[42,43] the cerebral content of DHA, but not ARA, is minimally but significantly lower in formula-fed term infants. However, the DHA content of the retina does not differ between breastfed and formula-fed infants,[43] perhaps because the content of this fatty acid in retina reaches adult levels at approximately term, whereas adult levels in the cerebrum are not reached until much later. In piglets, the cerebral DHA content of formula-fed infants reflected the ALA content of the formula received before death.[44] In this study, ALA intakes less than 0.7% of total energy resulted in low brain levels of DHA.[44] Further, studies in infants have shown a positive relationship between ALA intake and rates of DHA synthesis.[45]

Both term and preterm infants can convert LA to ARA and ALA to DHA.[46–50] This has been established by studies in which the precursor fatty acids labeled with stable isotopes of either carbon (^{13}C) or hydrogen (^{2}H) were administered to the infant and blood concentrations of the labeled fatty acids as well as labeled metabolites of each were measured by gas chromatography/mass spectroscopy (see Fig 17.1). The studies of Sauerwald et al[45,49] and Uauy et al[50] suggested that the overall ability of preterm infants to convert LA and ALA to LC-PUFAs is at least as good as that of term infants. On the other hand, there is considerable variability in conversion among both preterm and term infants fed the same formula. Moreover, because measurements of enrichment have been limited to plasma, which represents only a small fraction of the body pool of precursor as well as product fatty acids and may not be representative of fatty acid pools of other tissues, including the central nervous system, the amount of LC-PUFAs that either preterm or term infants can synthesize is not known.

The higher DHA content of plasma and erythrocyte lipids of breastfed infants and infants fed formulas supplemented with LC-PUFAs versus infants fed unsupplemented formulas, including those with a relatively high

ALA content,[51–53] suggests that the amounts of LC-PUFAs formed endogenously are less than the amounts provided by human milk or supplemented formulas. However, the extent to which the concentration of individual LC-PUFAs in plasma reflects the content of these fatty acids in tissues, particularly the brain, is not known.

In this regard, animal studies have demonstrated that the content of LC-PUFAs in plasma is much less highly correlated with the content of these fatty acids in brain than with the content in erythrocytes and liver.[54] In contrast, postmortem studies in human infants have demonstrated a weak but statistically significant, correlation between erythrocyte and brain contents of DHA.[43] Correlation between the content of this fatty acid in erythrocyte membranes and the contents of other tissues was not reported. Studies in isolated cell systems suggest that precursors of DHA are transferred from plasma to astrocytes where they are converted to DHA, which is subsequently transferred to neurons.[55] This pathway for direct synthesis of DHA within the central nervous system appears to occur in vivo in some animal species,[56] but the extent to which it occurs in humans is not known.

Importance of LC-PUFAs in Development

The findings discussed previously, although far from definitive, are compatible with the possibility that failure to provide preformed LC-PUFAs during early infancy, perhaps longer, may compromise development of tissues/organs with a high content of these fatty acids, particularly 22:6ω-3. However, the specific roles of LC-PUFAs in normal development are not clear.[57] These fatty acids affect gene transcription and may produce post-translational modifications. Moreover, many are precursors of eicosanoids and docosanoids that, in turn, modify several processes. These fatty acids also have effects on signal transduction, and the amount of these fatty acids in cell membranes can modify membrane fluidity, membrane thickness, and the microenvironment of the membrane as well as interactions between the fatty acid and membrane proteins. Such changes, in turn, can affect receptor function, and the fatty acids also may exert direct effects on receptor function. Although the degree of unsaturation of membrane fatty acids affects fluidity, this effect is most marked by substituting a monounsaturated or polyunsaturated fatty acid for a saturated fatty acid. In 22:6ω-3 deficiency, 22:5ω-6 replaces 22:6ω-3 with little effect on fluidity.

Despite the lack of a clear mechanism of the role of LC-PUFAs in development, numerous studies over the past 2 decades have focused on differences in visual acuity and neurodevelopmental indices between breastfed and formula-fed infants. Because human milk contains several factors other than LC-PUFAs that might affect visual acuity and/or neurodevelopmental indices, studies comparing breastfed versus formula-fed infants cannot help resolve the specific role of LC-PUFAs in infant development. Rather, intervention studies comparing infants fed LC-PUFA-supplemented and unsupplemented formulas and studies comparing different LC-PUFA intakes of breastfed infants secondary to maternal supplementation can provide important insights into cause-and-effect relationships between LC-PUFA intake and early childhood outcomes.

LC-PUFA Intake and Visual Function

Early studies in rodents established the importance of ω-3 fatty acids for normal retinal function,[20,23] and subsequent studies established this in primates.[21,22] These studies showed that abnormal retinal/visual function of ω-3 fatty acid-deficient animals clearly resulted from an inadequate intake of 18:3ω-3 and were partially reversed by adding this fatty acid or DHA. It is with this rationale that many human studies of assessed the effects of DHA (22:6ω-3) intake on retinal and/or visual function in babies. The early randomized controlled trials of LC-PUFA interventions were designed to assess whether infant formulas required supplementation with ω-3 (and often ω-6 LCPUFA) as formulas were devoid of all LCPUFA and contained only the precursor essential fatty acid ALA (18:3ω-3) in small amounts and much larger quantities of the ω-6 EFA and LA (18:2 ω-6).

Because infants in these studies were preverbal, visual acuity was most often assessed behaviorally or electrophysiologically. The most common behavioral assessment of visual acuity is the Teller Acuity Card procedure and is based on the innate tendency to look toward a discernible pattern rather than a blank field.[58] The infant is shown a series of cards with stripes (gratings) of different widths on one side and a blank field on the other, and his or her looking behavior is observed through a peephole in the center of the card.[59] Cards with wider stripes are shown initially followed by cards with progressively decreasing stripe widths. The infant's visual acuity is the finest grating toward which he or she clearly looks preferentially (ie, the finest grating that he or she is able to resolve).

The electrophysiologically based tests use visual evoked potentials (VEPs) that measure the activation of the visual cortex in response to visual information that is processed by the retina and transmitted to the visual cortex.[60,61] The presence of a reliable evoked response indicates that the stimulus information was resolved up to the visual cortex, where the response is processed. Use of VEPs to assess visual acuity requires measuring the electrical potentials of the visual cortex in response to patterns of contrast reversal with vertical square wave gratings or checkerboards. The frequency of the gratings or checkerboards is decreased from low (large) to high (small), and the visual acuity threshold is estimated by linear regression of the VEP amplitudes versus the frequency, or size, of the grating or checkerboard stimulus.[60,61] A rapid VEP method (sweep VEP) has been developed for use in infant populations.[62]

Electroretinography, unlike the aforementioned procedures that measure the response of the entire visual system, measures only the activity of the retina.[63–65] However, this methodology is somewhat more invasive and time consuming than the other methods and has been used to assess effects of LC-PUFAs in only a few studies. The primary components of the electroretinogram generated in response to a flash of light are the a-wave, which is produced by hyperpolarization of the photoreceptor, and the b-wave, which reflects the subsequent activation of retinal neurons. Performance is quantified by parameters such as the threshold (the minimal intensity of light necessary to elicit a small amplitude), the implicit time or peak latency (the time from the presentation of a brief flash of light to the response peak), the maximal amplitude, and the sensitivity (the intensity of light that elicits a response of half the maximal amplitude).

To date, there have been 9 trials assessing the effect of LC-PUFA supplementation of infant formulas for term infants that have included a measure of visual acuity. VEP acuity was assessed in 6 trials, the behavioral method of Teller Acuity Cards was used in 2 studies, and another trial used both electrophysiological and behavioral methods. These have recently been summarized in a Cochrane systematic review.[66] Four of the 9 included studies reported a beneficial effect of supplementation on visual acuity, and the 5 remaining studies reported no effect of supplementation. All of the included studies have compared a low to modest dose of DHA supplementation (up to approximately 0.3% of total fatty acids) with no supplementation. The results of the meta-analyses were inconsistent, although all meta-analyses assessing visual acuity using Teller Acuity Cards at different ages consistently showed no effect of supplementation. Because the electrophysiological protocols for assessing visual acuity were different between trials, it is not possible to ascertain whether the inconsistent results are attributable to methodologic differences, random error, or some other factor.

IV

Some have suggested that dietary DHA dose may be an important factor and that at least 0.3% of total fatty acids as DHA is required in the infant diet to document a beneficial effect of supplementation on visual acuity.[52,53] This view has recently been supported in a dose-response trial involving 4 different doses of DHA. This was a 2-site trial in which formula-fed infants were randomly allocated to equivalent formulas containing either 0%, 0.32%, 0.64%, or 0.96% DHA as total fatty acids.[67] All formulas also contained 0.64% total fatty acids as AA. Infants fed the control formula (0% DHA) had poorer visual evoked potential acuity compared with DHA-supplemented infants. There were no differences in the visual acuity between the groups fed the 3 different doses of DHA at any time point.[67] Although the overall data from this trial are suggestive that a dose of at least 0.3% DHA may be needed to maximize visual acuity development, a significant study site by formula group interaction suggested that the visual acuity response to the formulas varied by enrolling site, with differences between control and DHA-supplementation being most marked in only one of the study sites. Interestingly, a dose-response trial conducted in breastfed infants some 13 years earlier reported that supplementation of lactating women to increase the average DHA concentration of their human milk from a mean of approximately 0.2% total fatty acids as DHA to either 0.35%, 0.46%, 0.86%, or 1.13% DHA as total fatty acids resulted in no differences in infant visual evoked potential acuity or latency between groups.[68] Unfortunately, the visual acuity estimates from the 2 trials do not appear to be directly comparable because of methodologic differences.

Maternal supplementation with DHA during pregnancy has been investigated in 4 randomized controlled trials, including 467 infants, with visual outcomes in term infants.[69-72] Three of the 4 studies reported no differences in VEP latency[71,72] and no difference in visual acuity measured either using VEPs[72] or the card procedure.[69] Only 1 study with a small sample size suggested improvement with Teller acuity card acuity at 4 but not 6 months of age.[70]

Infants born preterm are at greatest risk of dietary LC-PUFA insufficiency, because they miss the large and active accumulation of LC-PUFAs that occurs during the last trimester of pregnancy, they are born with few fat reserves, and their feeding regimens often contain minimal LC-PUFA. Therefore, it follows that any beneficial effects of LC-PUFAs will be more obvious in preterm infants rather than their counterparts who are born at term. However, this hypothesis has not been consistently supported by studies investigating the effects on LC-PUFA supplementation of preterm infant formulas and visual outcomes. The relevant trials have been summarized in a recent Cochrane systematic review.[73] Eight randomized trials were included; 3 tested the addition of only ω-3 LC-PUFAs to infant formulas, 4 tested the addition of ω-3 LC-PUFAs and AA, and another had 2 intervention groups – 1 with ω-3 LC-PUFAs only and 1 with ω-3 LC-PUFAs and AA. Seven trials have visual acuity outcomes, and 4 of these studies reported beneficial effects of supplementation during early infancy,[63,74–76] although in 2 cases this was confined to specific subgroups.[75,76] It is important to note that the methodologies of assessing acuity differed, the sample sizes were generally small, and some of the randomization processes were not adequately reported. Similar issues were apparent in the 2 trials that assessed electroretinographic responses, with 1 study reporting a positive effect of supplementation and the other reporting no effect.[53,77]

Most recently, the dose of DHA in milks fed to preterm infants has been assessed in a randomized trial based on realistic feeding practices in which infants are fed a combination of expressed human milk and infant formula.[78] This trial tested a high dose of DHA (1% total fatty acid) against a standard dose of DHA (0.3% total fatty acids), with the ARA concentration being held constant in both groups at about 0.4% of total fatty acids, and found that infants fed the high-DHA diet had better visual acuity at 4 months' corrected age compared with control infants. No differences were noted at 2 months' corrected age.[78]

LC-PUFAs and Cognitive, Behavioral, and Other Neurodevelopmental Outcomes

Most studies addressing the cognitive or behavioral development of infants fed LC-PUFA-supplemented versus unsupplemented formulas have used the Bayley Scales of Infant and Toddler Development, which are considered the "gold standard" for assessing global abilities of infants from birth to about 42 months of age. They provide standardized indices of both mental/cognitive and motor development. However, they are intended to distinguish between "normal" and "abnormal," not degrees of either. Thus, unless cognitive and/or psychomotor function as assessed by the Bayley Scales early in life is abnormal, the relationship between these early scores and later function is relatively poor.[79]

Other nonstandardized or more experimental approaches have also been used to assess specific developmental domains. Tests have included novelty preference, auditory evoked potentials, problem-solving ability, measures of attention, measures of general movements, and most recently, assessment of brain structure using magnetic resonance imaging. Although it has been argued that the standardized tests assessing global developmental measures (such as the Bayley Scales) are less sensitive than some of the more targeted experimental approaches, the data gained from both standardized and experimental approaches in studies of LC-PUFA supplementation have been variable. Some of the studies utilizing these tests have shown advantages of LC-PUFA supplementation with both approaches, some with one but not the other, and still others with neither approach. Available studies in term infants were initially critically reviewed in 1998 by an expert panel appointed by the Life Sciences Research Organization to assess the nutrient requirements for term infant formulas.[30] These studies were criticized by consultants to the panel for including too few infants, failing to control adequately for confounding factors, failing to assess function at more than one age, failing to examine individual differences in development, and failing to follow the infants for a sufficiently long period (eg, none of the studies available at that time included data beyond 1 year of age). Partially on the basis of these criticisms, the panel did not recommend addition of LC-PUFAs to term infant formulas but suggested that the issue be reevaluated.

The randomized trials involving term infants published since 1998[30,80-84] have not resolved many of these criticisms, although infant formula with LC-PUFAs became widely available since the early 2000s. The trials have differed with respect to the source of LC-PUFA supplementation, the duration of supplementation, the amounts of 22:6ω-3 and 20:4ω-6 supplementation, and the ratio of 22:6ω-3 to 20:4ω-6. There also were differences in the 18:2ω-6 and 18:3ω-3 contents of the control and experimental formulas. The variance in Bayley mental and motor scores also varied among studies, being smallest in the one study that showed an advantage of 22:6ω-3 and 20:4ω-6 supplementation for the first 4 months of life on the Bayley mental development score at 18 months of age.[81]

Relevant data from LC-PUFA intervention trials involving term formula-fed infants have most recently in a Cochrane systematic review,[66] including 11 trials with neurodevelopmental outcomes. This systematic review[66] as well as an earlier review[85] both reported no effect of LC-PUFA supplementation of infant formula for term infants on Bayley mental or motor scores.

Two recent systematic reviews and meta-analyses are also available summarizing the randomized controlled trials assessing LC-PUFA–supplemented versus –unsupplemented formulas for preterm infants.[73,86] Both reviews included the same 7 trials with Bayley outcomes, and both reported no overall effect of LC-PUFA supplementation on Bayley mental or psychomotor scores, although these trials are subject to many of the same criticisms levied against the studies in term infants.[73,86] Indeed, some sensitivity analyses have suggested that the heterogeneity between trials may be related to the administration of different versions of the Bayley Scales, the sample population studied, the way the intervention was applied, or trial methodology.[86] Interestingly, the subgroup of 5 of the 7 studies using the second version of the Bayley Scales and including the majority of infants tested (n=879) demonstrated that supplementation of preterm formula with LC-PUFAs resulted in an increase in mental development scores by 3.4 points (95% confidence interval [CI], 0.6–6.3) compared with controls.[86] Further high-quality trials are clearly needed to substantiate these findings but are probably unlikely to occur, because most infant formulas for preterm infants are now supplemented with LC-PUFAs.

Of more current clinical relevance are 2 recent trials in which DHA doses reflective of the estimated in utero accretion rate were used.[87–89] These trials also included infants fed human milk. Both trials reported no differences in mental development scores at 18 to 20 months of age.[88,89] However, the larger and more robust of the 2 trials demonstrated that girls had a 4.5 point (approximately 0.3 standard deviations [SDs]) improvement in mental development scores (95% CI, 0.5–8.5), and significant mental delay (mental development scores <70) was reduced from 10.5% in the control group to 5% in the higher DHA group (relative risk, 0.50; 95% CI, 0.26–0.93).[88] Although there was some suggestion of benefit with DHA supplementation at 18 months of age, there was no benefit of DHA supplementation at 7 years of age.[90]

The effects of maternal supplementation with ω-3 LC-PUFAs, either in pregnancy or during lactation, on childhood developmental outcomes has also been investigated in randomized controlled trials, and some of these trial have been large and rigorous and followed children until 7 years of age. These studies[91–93] as well as the available systematic reviews[94,95] indicate no consistent benefit of ω-3 LC-PUFA supplementation on childhood developmental outcomes.

Effects of LC-PUFAs on Pregnancy Outcomes and Childhood Allergies

Outside the sphere of neurologic development, interest has focused on the anti-inflammatory and immune-modulating effects of ω-3 LC-PUFAs. Increased ω-3 LC-PUFAs, particularly EPA, antagonize the actions of ARA and can lead to a range of biochemical and immunologic changes that limit inflammatory responses, which has been an important aspect of the rationale to explain the effects of dietary LC-PUFAs on childhood allergies and pregnancy duration.

With regard to childhood allergic disease, some postnatal dietary intervention studies designed to increase ω-3 LC-PUFA status through a combination of DHA-rich tuna oil supplementation and a reduction in dietary LA intake have suggested that dietary intervention lowers the prevalence of early asthma symptoms, such as cough and wheeze, but follow-up studies have generally failed to detect an effect.[96,97]

Randomized trials that have commenced intervention with ω-3 LC-PUFA, mainly as fish oil, during pregnancy have produced some interesting results and are summarized in a Cochrane systematic review.[98] There is some supportive evidence from the Cochrane systematic review that suggests that at least 1 g of ω-3 LC-PUFA supplementation during pregnancy results in a reduction in atopic eczema in the first 3 years of life and a reduction in sensitization during the first year of life in children who have a higher-than-normal risk of allergic disease.[98] The review showed no clear effects on asthma or wheeze outcomes.[98] However, the 2 largest and highest-quality trials show contrasting results, with the most recent trial being published after the Cochrane review. The newest trial by Bisgaard et al[99] showed a 25% reduction in persistent wheeze/asthma at 3 to 5 years with no effects on eczema or sensitization, whereas Palmer et al[100] demonstrated reductions in sensitization and atopic eczema at 1 year that were no longer evident at 3 or 6 years.[101,102] There were no effects of ω-3 LC-PUFA supplementation during on wheeze or asthma at 3 and 6 years.[101,102] This inconsistency is perplexing and may relate to the different interventions (about 1 g of ω-3 LC-PUFA, largely as DHA, vs 3 g of ω-3 LC-PUFA, largely as EPA), the different populations studied, or the definitions used to diagnose asthma. Asthma can be difficult to accurately diagnose in early childhood, and not all persistent wheeze is asthma.[103] Further work is needed, using standardized assessments, to understand the responsiveness of fetus and child based on maternal and family allergic history and if dose or class of ω-3 LC-PUFA are important in determining outcome.

Supplementation studies with ω-3 LC-PUFA during pregnancy, regardless of the longer-term infant or childhood outcome, have generally all collected basic information relating to birth outcomes and this has provided the most solid evidence base for the effects of ω-3 LC-PUFA on pregnancy outcomes. More than 50 trials with data from more than 15 000 women have been included in the most recent systematic review.[104] This review shows that ω-3 LC-PUFA supplementation during pregnancy is clearly associated with an increase in the mean length of gestation, resulting in a 39% reduction in early preterm birth at <34 weeks' gestation and an 8% reduction in preterm births at <37 weeks' gestation.[104] However, the results also indicate that ω-3 LC-PUFA supplementation also results in a 57% increase in the risk of prolonged gestation (>42 weeks' gestation).[104] Modern obstetric practice generally will not allow women to progress their pregnancies beyond the middle of their 41st week of gestation, and indeed, the largest and one of the most recent trials also demonstrates that ω-3 LC-PUFA supplementation during pregnancy also resulted in need for obstetric intervention (induction or elective caesarian section) because of post-term gestations.[91] The reductions observed in the rate of early preterm birth also had the expected consequences of reducing the number of low birth weight infants and the frequency of admission to the neonatal intensive care unit.[91] However, these promising data have not resulted in widespread implementation into clinical practice, because it is not yet fully understood how to identify the group of pregnant women who are most likely to benefit from ω-3 LC-PUFA supplementation and avoid supplementation of women who may not benefit or may even be exposed to increased risks.

Effects of LC-PUFAs on Postnatal Growth

The observation in the early 1990s that preterm infants assigned to a formula supplemented with fish oil (0.3% of total fatty acids as 20:5ω-3 and 0.2% as 22:6ω-3) versus an unsupplemented formula had lower normalized weight and lower normalized length at various times during the first year of life[105] generated considerable concern. In this study, weight at 12 months' corrected age was correlated with plasma phospholipid 20:4ω-6 content at various times during the first year of life.[106] This led to the assumption that the lower rate of weight gain was related in some way to the 20:5ω-3 content of the fish oil. Two additional studies in preterm infants[75,107] demonstrated an adverse effect of ω-3 LC-PUFAs on growth, whereas another trial suggested a positive effect,[108] and yet others demonstrated no effects.[52] These confusing data may be the result of random error and/or the small sample sizes in most trials. It is difficult to think of a biologic mechanism by which ω-3 fatty acids may inhibit growth. Possibilities that have been suggested include inhibition of desaturation and elongation of 18:2ω-6 to 20:4ω-6 by the ω-3 fatty acids, inhibition of eicosanoid synthesis from 20:4ω-6 by the intake of preformed 20:5ω-3 or endogenous synthesis of 20:5ω-3 from a moderately high intake of 18:3ω-3, and effects of ω-3 and ω-6 fatty acids on transcription of genes controlling lipolysis and lipogenesis.[109]

Trials of infant formula feeding for preterm infants including a combination of ω-3 LC-PUFAs with ARA have generally been of higher quality than the earlier trials of formula feeding that have included only ω-3 LC-PUFAs, and these trials most consistently have demonstrated no effect of LC-PUFA supplementation on the growth of preterm infants, as summarized in the most recent Cochrane systematic review.[73] Interestingly, the only growth effects noted are higher weights and higher lengths in infants at 2 months post-term, and the meta-analysis included a combination of trials that supplemented infants with ω-3 LC-PUFAs alone or in combination with ARA.[73]

The single largest trial of LC-PUFA supplementation to assess growth, involving more than 650 infants born at <33 weeks' gestation, compared supplementation with DHA of approximately 1% total fatty acids and supplementation with DHA of approximately 0.3% total fatty acids, supplied through human milk, infant formula, or a combination of both to mimic typical feeding practices in neonatal intensive care units.[110] All milks contained approximately 0.5% total fatty acids. There was no effect of higher dietary DHA on weight or head circumference at any age, but infants given more DHA were 0.7 cm (95% CI, 0.1–1.4 cm; $P = .02$) longer at 18 months' corrected age. There was an interaction effect between treatment and birth weight strata for weight and length. Higher DHA supplementation resulted in increased length in infants born weighing ≥1250 g at 4 months' corrected age and in both weight and length at 12 and 18 months' corrected age.[110] Although complex, these data indicate that DHA up to 1% total dietary fatty acids does not adversely affect growth.

The data regarding LC-PUFA supplementation and growth of term infants are more straightforward. A meta-analysis of growth data from 14 (from a total of 21 known trials) generally high-quality trials that involved LC-PUFA supplementation of infant formula fed to term infants found no evidence that such supplementation influences the growth of term infants in either a negative or a positive way.[111] Subgroup analyses showed that neither supplementation with only ω-3 LC-PUFAs nor source of LC-PUFA supplementation affected infant growth. This analysis of data from 1846 infants has put to rest the question of growth inhibition by ω-3 LC-PUFAs.

Possible Adverse Effects of LC-PUFAs

In addition to the original concerns about adverse effects of ω-3 fatty acids on growth, a number of theoretical concerns related to the known biologic effects of ω-6 and ω-3 LC-PUFAs should be considered. Among these is the possibility that supplementation with highly unsaturated oils will increase the likelihood of oxidant damage. This is because peroxidation occurs at the site of double bonds, making membranes with unsaturated fatty acids more vulnerable to oxidant damage. Thus, it is possible that LC-PUFA supplementation will increase the incidence of conditions thought to be related to oxidant damage (eg, necrotizing enterocolitis, bronchopulmonary dysplasia, retrolental fibroplasia). There has also been concern that unbalanced supplementation with ω-3 and/or ω-6 LC-PUFAs will result in altered eicosanoid and docosanoid metabolism with potential effects on a variety of physiological mechanisms (eg, blood clotting, infection). There are few data to support these theoretical concerns with respect to the small amounts of LC-PUFAs that are added to infant formulas.

Many of the randomized controlled trials comparing the outcomes of preterm infants receiving supplemented formulas with either DHA or both DHA and ARA from a variety of sources (single-cell oils, fish oil, egg yolk triglyceride, egg yolk phospholipids) with infants receiving unsupplemented formula have reported a range of clinical outcomes, including necrotizing enterocolitis, sepsis, retinopathy of prematurity, intraventricular hemorrhage, and bronchopulmonary dysplasia (BPD). The relevant trials have been summarized in a systematic review and meta-analysis specifically designed to consider the effects of LC-PUFA supplementation of infant formula on the typical diseases of prematurity.[86] The clinical signs and symptoms used to diagnose a disease may differ between neonatal units and may change with improvements in clinical practice over time. Thus, the reported meta-analyses included all outcomes according to any definition as well as sensitivity analyses including trials only using internationally accepted definitions or trials with a low risk of bias on the basis of reporting adequate concealment of randomization and analysis according to the intention-to-treat principle. In meta-analyses of data from approximately 1500 preterm infants, the risk of necrotizing enterocolitis and sepsis did not differ between infants fed LC-PUFA–supplemented or control formula when all available data were included, when necrotizing enterocolitis or sepsis were confirmed, or in sensitivity analysis.[86] There were also no clear differences in rates of retinopathy of prematurity, intraventricular hemorrhage, or bronchopulmonary dysplasia between preterm infants fed LC-PUFA–supplemented or control formula in overall analyses or when trials reported diseases according to the prespecified definitions or in sensitivity analysis.[86] However, in many cases, the small numbers of infants and low disease rates limited these analyses. Collectively, these data together with those from LC-PUFA supplementation of infant formulas have not resulted in a greater incidence of adverse conditions and suggest that the amounts and the sources of LC-PUFAs used in these studies are safe. Furthermore, supplementation with DHA at higher doses (up to 1% of total fatty acids) has had no effect on the incidence of sepsis, necrotizing enterocolitis, or intraventricular hemorrhage.[88,112] However, a trial published in 2017 with 1273 infants born at <29 weeks' gestation showed that a high-dose enteral DHA emulsion (providing a total of 60 mg DHA/kg/day, about 1% total dietary fatty acids) compared with a soy oil emulsion (without DHA) may increase the risk of BPD.[112] In this study,[112] all infants in the control group received DHA according to standard feeding practice, which provided about 20 mg/kg/day. Further work is needed to understand the relationship of DHA dose with BPD and whether there is any interplay with oxidant damage or the balance of bioactive lipid mediators, such as the eicosanoids and docosanoids.

Sources for LC-PUFA Supplementation
Available sources for LC-PUFA supplementation include egg yolk lipid, phospholipid, and triglyceride, all of which contain ω-6 as well as ω-3 LC-PUFAs; fish oils; and oils produced by single-cell organisms (ie, microalgal and fungal oils). Few untoward effects of the available supplements have been noted at the relatively modest doses that are commonly used for infants. In vitro and animal studies of toxicity also have revealed little toxicity of any of these sources. In fact, the US Food and Drug Administration has accepted the conclusion of a manufacturer of a combination of algal and fungal oils as well as that of a manufacturer of a combination of low-EPA tuna and a fungal oil that their products are generally regarded as safe sources of DHA and ARA for addition to formulas intended for normal infants.

Supplementation of Infant Formulas With LC-PUFAs
The American Academy of Pediatrics has no official position on supplementation of term or preterm infant formulas with LC-PUFAs. The Life Sciences Research Organization Expert Panel on Nutrient Composition of Term

Infant Formulas recommended neither a minimum nor maximum content of either AA or DHA.[30] The Life Sciences Research Organization Expert Panel on Nutrient Composition of Preterm Formulas specified a maximum amount of ARA and DHA for preterm infant formulas but did not specify a minimum amount of either fatty acid.[113] In contrast, regulatory and advisory groups from other countries recommend that infant formulas, particularly those intended for preterm infants, be supplemented with these 2 fatty acids,[31] although a more recent option has suggested that term infants only require additional DHA. [31] Formulas with both DHA and ARA are available in most countries, including the United States. It has been estimated that approximately 75% of the term formulas and 100% of the preterm formulas sold in the United States are supplemented with DHA and ARA.

The evidence for efficacy of supplementing term infant formulas with these fatty acids is only modestly different from that available to the Life Sciences Research Organization term formula panel in 1998, but the evidence for efficacy of modest supplementation of preterm formulas is more convincing, with a few studies suggesting that there may be advantages to early childhood development. Moreover, most of the safety concerns expressed earlier have been resolved.

Finally, considering the marked variability among infants of apparent conversion of ALA to DHA and LA to ARA, it is conceivable that some infants will benefit from supplementation, whereas others will not. Such a scenario certainly would help explain the marked variability in outcomes documented by virtually every study. It also is likely that any beneficial effects of LC-PUFA supplementation will be subtle and possibly not detectable with all methodologies.

References

1. Hamosh M. A review. Fat digestion in the newborn: role of lingual lipase and preduodenal digestion. *Pediatr Res.* May 1979;13(5 Pt 1):615–622

2. Faber J, Goldstein R, Blondheim O, et al. Absorption of medium chain triglycerides in the stomach of the human infant. *J Pediatr Gastroenterol Nutr.* Mar-Apr 1988;7(2):189–195

3. Linscheer WG, Vergroesen AJ. Lipids. In: ME S, VR Y, eds. *Modern Nutrition in Health and Disease.* 7th ed. Philadelphia, PA: Lea & Febiger; 1988:72–1007

4. Hernell O, Blackberg L, Fredrikzon B, al. e. Bile salt stimulated lipase in human milk and lipid digestion during the neonatal period. In: Lebenthal E, ed. *Textbook of Gastroenterology and Nutrition in Infancy.* New York, NY: Raven Press; 1987:465–471

5. Williamson S, Finucane E, Ellis H, Gamsu HR. Effect of heat treatment of human milk on absorption of nitrogen, fat, sodium, calcium, and phosphorus by preterm infants. *Arch Dis Child.* Jul 1978;53(7):555–563

6. Watkins JB. Lipid digestion and absorption. *Pediatrics.* Jan 1985;75(1 Pt 2):151–156

7. Hofmann AF, Roda A. Physicochemical properties of bile acids and their relationship to biological properties: an overview of the problem. *J Lipid Res.* Dec 15 1984;25(13):1477–1489

8. Gray GM. Mechanisms of digestion and absorption of food. In: Sleisenger MH, Fordtran JS, eds. *Gastrointestinal Disease. Pathophysiology, Diagnosis, Management.* 3rd ed. Philadelphia, PA: W.B. Saunders; 1983:844–858

9. Filer LJ, Jr., Mattson FH, Fomon SJ. Triglyceride configuration and fat absorption by the human infant. *J Nutr.* Nov 1969;99(3):293–298

10. Carnielli VP, Luijendijk IH, van Goudoever JB, et al. Structural position and amount of palmitic acid in infant formulas: effects on fat, fatty acid, and mineral balance. 1996/12// 1996;23(5):553–560

11. Kennedy K, Fewtrell MS, Morley R, et al. Double-blind, randomized trial of a synthetic triacylglycerol in formula-fed term infants: effects on stool biochemistry, stool characteristics, and bone mineralization. *Am J Clin Nutr.* Nov 1999;70(5):920–927

12. Bensadoun A. Lipoprotein lipase. *Annu Rev Nutr.* 1991;11:217–237

13. Griffin EA, Bryan MH, Angel A. Variations in intralipid tolerance in newborn infants. *Pediatr Res.* Jun 1983;17(6):478–481

14. Innis SM. Essential fatty acids in growth and development. *Prog.Lipid Res.* 1991;30:39–103

15. Oliw E, Gramstrom E, Anggard E. The Prostaglandins and Related Substances. In: Pace-Asciak C, Gramstron E, eds. *Prostaglandins and Related Substances.* Amsterdam, The Netherlands: Elsevier; 1983:1–19

16. Calder PC. Immunomodulation by omega-3 fatty acids. *Prostaglandins Leukot Essent Fatty Acids.* Nov-Dec 2007;77(5-6):327–335

17. Holman RT. The ratio of trienoic: tetraenoic acids in tissue lipids as a measure of essential fatty acid requirement. *J Nutr.* Mar 1960;70:405–410

18. Burr GO, Burr MM. A new deficiency disease produced by the rigid exclusion of fat from the diet. *J.Biol.Chem.* 1929;82:345–367

19. Hansen AE, Stewart RA, Hughes G, Soderhjelm L. The relation of linoleic acid to infant feeding. *Acta Paediatr Suppl.* 1962;137:1–41

20. Benolken RM, Anderson RE, Wheeler TG. Membrane fatty acids associated with the electrical response in visual excitation. *Science.* 1973;182:1253–1254

21. Neuringer M, Connor WE, Lin DS, Barstad L, Luck S. Biochemical and functional effects of prenatal and postnatal omega-3 fatty acid deficiency on retina and brain in rhesus monkeys. *Proc.Natl.Acad.Sci.USA.* 1986;83:4021–4025

22. Neuringer M, Connor WE, Van Petten C, Barstad L. Dietary omega-3 fatty acid deficiency and visual loss in infant rhesus monkeys. *J.Clin.Invest.* 1984;73: 272–276

23. Wheeler TG, Benolken RM, Anderson RE. Visual membranes: specificity of fatty acid precursors for the electrical response to illumination. *Science*. 1975;188: 1312–1314

24. Holman RT, Johnson SB, Hatch TF. A case of human linolenic acid deficiency involving neurological abnormalities. *Am J Clin Nutr*. 1982;35:617–623

25. Bjerve KS, Fischer S, Alme K. Alpha-linolenic acid deficiency in man: effect of ethyl linolenate on plasma and erythrocyte fatty acid composition and biosynthesis of prostanoids. *Am J Clin Nutr*. 1987;46:570–576

26. Jensen RG. Lipids in human milk. *Lipids*. Dec 1999;34(12):1243–1271

27. Sanders TAB, Reddy S. The influence of a vegetarian diet on the fatty acid composition of human milk and the essential fatty acid status of the infant. *J.Pediatr*. 1992;120:S71–S77

28. Jensen CL, Maude M, Anderson RE, Heird WC. Effect of docosahexaenoic acid supplementation of lactating women on the fatty acid composition of breast milk lipids and maternal and infant plasma phospholipids. *Am J Clin Nutr*. Jan 2000;71(1 Suppl):292S–299S

29. Makrides M, Neumann MA, Gibson RA. Effect of maternal docosahexaenoic acid (DHA) supplementation on breast milk composition. *European Journal of Clinical Nutrition*. 1996;50(6):352–357

30. Raiten DJ, Talbot JM, Waters JH. Assessment of nutrient requirements for infant formulas. *The Journal of Nutrition*. 1998;128(11S):S2110–S2130

31. EFSA Panel on Dietetic Products Nutrition and Allergies. Scientific Opinion on the essential composition of infant and follow-on formulae. *EFSA Journal*. 2014;12(7):3760–n/a

32. Carlson SE, Rhodes PG, Ferguson MG. Docosahexaenoic acid status of preterm infants at birth and following feeding with human milk or formula. *Am J Clin Nutr*. 1986;44:798–804

33. Innis SM, Akrabawi SS, Diersen-Schade DA, Dobson MV, Guy DG. Visual acuity and blood lipids in term infants fed human milk or formulae. *Lipids*. Jan 1997;32(1):63–72

34. Lucas A, Morley R, Cole TJ. Randomised trial of early diet in preterm babies and later intelligence quotient. *Br.Med.J. J1 - BMJ*. 1998;317(7171):1481–1487

35. Lucas A, Morley R, Cole TJ, et al. Early diet in preterm babies and developmental status at 18 months. *Lancet*. 1990;335:1477–1481

36. Morrow Tlucak M, Haude RH, Ernhart CB. Breastfeeding and cognitive development in the first 2 years of life. *Social Sci.Med*. 1988;26(6):635–639

37. Rogan WJ, Gladen BC. Breast-feeding and cognitive development. *Early Hum. Dev*. 1993;31(1993):181–193

38. Clandinin MT, Chappell JE, Leong S, Heim T, Swyer PR, Chance GW. Intrauterine fatty acid accretion rates in human brain: implications for fatty acid requirements. *Early Hum.Dev*. 1980;4:121–129

IV

39. Clandinin MT, Chappell JE, Leong S, Heim T, Swyer PR, Chance GW. Extrauterine fatty acid accretion in infant brain: implications for fatty acid requirements. *Early Hum.Dev.* 1980;4:131–138

40. Martinez M. Tissue levels of polyunsaturated fatty acids during early human development. *J.Pediatr.* 1992;120:S129–S138

41. Dutta-Roy AK. Transport mechanisms for long-chain polyunsaturated fatty acids in the human placenta. 2000/01// 2000;71(1 Suppl):315S–322S

42. Farquharson J, Cockburn F, Patrick WA, Jamieson EC, Logan RW. Infant cerebral cortex phospholipid fatty-acid composition and diet. *Lancet.* 1992;340:810–813

43. Makrides M, Neumann MA, Byard RW, Simmer K, Gibson RA. Fatty acid composition of brain, retina, and erythrocytes in breast- and formula-fed infants. *Am J Clin Nutr.* 1994;60:189–194

44. Arbuckle LD, MacKinnon MJ, Innis SM. Formula 18:2(n-6) and 18:3(n-3) content and ratio influence long-chain polyunsaturated fatty acids in the developing piglet liver and central nervous system. *J.Nutr.* 1994;124:289–298

45. Sauerwald TU, Hachey DL, Jensen CL, Chen H, Anderson RE, Heird WC. Effect of dietary alpha-linolenic acid intake on incorporation of docosahexaenoic and arachidonic acids into plasma phospholipids of term infants. *Lipids.* 1996/03// 1996;31 Suppl:S131–S135

46. Carnielli VP, Wattimena DJL, Luijendijk IHT, Boerlage A, Degenhart HJ, Sauer PJJ. The very low birth weight premature infant is capable of synthesizing arachidonic and docosahexaenoic acids from linoleic and linolenic acids. *Pediatr. Res.* Jul 1996;40(1):169–174

47. Demmelmair H, v.Schenck U, Behrendt E, Sauerwald T, Koletzko B. Estimation of arachidonic acid synthesis in fullterm neonates using natural variation of 13C-abundance. *J.Pediatr.Gastroenterol.Nutr.* 1995;21:31–36

48. Salem N, Jr., Wegher B, Mena P, Uauy R. Arachidonic and docosahexaenoic acids are biosynthesized from their 18-carbon precursors in human infants. *Proc.Natl. Acad.Sci.USA.* Jan 9 1996;93(1):49–54

49. Sauerwald TU, Hachey DL, Jensen CL, Chen HM, Anderson RE, Heird WC. Intermediates in endogenous synthesis of C22:6 omega 3 and C20: 4 omega 6 by term and preterm infants. *Pediatr.Res.* Feb 1997;41(2):183–187

50. Uauy R, Mena P, Wegher B, Nieto S, Salem N, Jr. Long chain polyunsaturated fatty acid formation in neonates: effect of gestational age and intrauterine growth. *Pediatr Res.* Jan 2000;47(1):127–135

51. Carlson SE, Cooke RJ, Rhodes PG, Peeples JM, Werkman SH, Tolley EA. Long-term feeding of formulas high in linolenic acid and marine oil to very low birth weight infants: phospholipid fatty acids. *Pediatr Res.* Nov 1991;30(5):404–412

52. Uauy R, Hoffman DR, Birch EE, Birch DG, Jameson DM, Tyson J. Safety and efficacy of omega-3 fatty acids in the nutrition of very low birth weight infants: Soy oil and marine oil supplementation of formula. *J.Pediatr.* 1994;124:612–620

53. Uauy RD, Birch DG, Birch EE, Tyson JE, Hoffman DR. Effect of dietary omega-3 fatty acids on retinal function of very-low-birth-weight neonates. *Pediatr.Res.* 1990;28:485–492

54. Rioux FM, Innis SM, Dyer R, MacKinnon M. Diet-induced changes in liver and bile but not brain fatty acids can be predicted from differences in plasma phospholipid fatty acids in formula- and milk-fed piglets. *J Nutr.* Feb 1997;127(2): 370–377

55. Moore SA. Cerebral endothelium and astrocytes cooperate in supplying docosahexaenoic acid to neurons. *Adv Exp Med Biol.* 1993;331:229–233

56. Pawlosky RJ, Denkins Y, Ward G, Salem N, Jr. Retinal and brain accretion of long-chain polyunsaturated fatty acids in developing felines: The effects of corn oil-based maternal diets. Feb 1997;65(2):465–472

57. Heird WC, Lapillonne A. The role of essential fatty acids in development. *Annu Rev Nutr.* 2005;25:549–571

58. Dobson V. Clinical applications of preferential looking measures of visual acuity. *Behav Brain Res.* Oct 1983;10(1):25–38

59. McDonald MA, Dobson V, Sebris SL, Baitch L, Varner D, Teller DY. The acuity card procedure: a rapid test of infant acuity. *Invest.Ophthalmol.Vis.Sci.* 1985;26:1158–1162

60. Sokol S, Hansen VC, Moskowitz A, Greenfield P, Towle VL. Evoked potential and preferential looking estimates of visual acuity in pediatric patients. *Ophthalmology.* 1983;90(5):552–562

61. Uauy R, Birch E, Birch D, Peirano P. Visual and brain function measurements in studies of n-3 fatty acid requirements of infants [published erratum appears in J Pediatr 1992 Aug;121(2):329]. *J.Pediatr.* 1992;120(4 Pt 2):S168–180

62. Norcia AM, Tyler CW. Spatial frequency sweep VEP: visual acuity during the first year of life. *Vision Res.* 1985;25:1399–1408

63. Birch DG, Birch EE, Hoffman DR, Uauy RD. Retinal development in very-low-birth-weight infants fed diets differing in omega-3 fatty acids. *Invest.Ophthalmol. Vis.Sci.* 1992;33:2365–2376

64. Hood DC, Birch DG. The A-wave of the human electroretinogram and rod receptor function. *Invest.Ophthalmol.Vis.Sci.* 1990;31(10):2070–2081

65. Naka KI, Rushton WA. S-potentials from colour units in the retina of fish (Cyprinidae). 1966;185(3):536–555

66. Jasani B, Simmer K, Patole SK, Rao SC. Long chain polyunsaturated fatty acid supplementation in infants born at term. *Cochrane Database Syst Rev.* Mar 10 2017;3:CD000376

67. Birch EE, Carlson SE, Hoffman DR, et al. The DIAMOND (DHA Intake And Measurement Of Neural Development) Study: a double-masked, randomized controlled clinical trial of the maturation of infant visual acuity as a function of the dietary level of docosahexaenoic acid. *Am J Clin Nutr.* Apr 2010;91(4):848–859

68. Gibson RA, Neumann MA, Makrides M. Effect of increasing breast milk docosahexanoic acid on plasma and erythrocyte phospholipid fatty acids and neural indices of exclusively breast fed infants. *European Journal of Clinical Nutrition.* 1997;51:578–584

69. Innis SM, Friesen RW. Essential n-3 fatty acids in pregnant women and early visual acuity maturation in term infants. *Am.J.Clin.Nutr.* 2008;87(3):548–557

70. Judge MP, Harel O, Lammi-Keefe CJ. A docosahexaenoic acid-functional food during pregnancy benefits infant visual acuity at four but not six months of age. *Lipids.* 2007;42(2):117–122

71. Malcolm CA, McCulloch DL, Montgomery C, Shepherd A, Weaver LT. Maternal docosahexaenoic acid supplementation during pregnancy and visual evoked potential development in term infants: a double blind, prospective, randomised trial. *Arch Dis Child Fetal Neonatal Ed.* Sep 2003;88(5):F383–390

72. Smithers LG, Gibson RA, Makrides M. Maternal supplementation with docosahexaenoic acid during pregnancy does not affect early visual development in the infant: a randomized controlled trial. *Am J Clin Nutr.* Apr 13 2011;93:1293–1299

73. Moon K, Rao SC, Schulzke SM, Patole SK, Simmer K. Longchain polyunsaturated fatty acid supplementation in preterm infants. *Cochrane Database of Systematic Reviews.* 2016(12)

74. Carlson SE, Werkman SH, Rhodes PG, Tolley EA. Visual-acuity development in healthy preterm infants: effect of marine-oil supplementation. *Am J Clin Nutr.* 1993;58:35–42

75. Carlson SE, Werkman SH, Tolley EA. Effect of long-chain n-3 fatty acid supplementation on visual acuity and growth of preterm infants with and without bronchopulmonary dysplasia. *Am J Clin Nutr.* May 1996;63(5):687–697

76. O'Connor DL, Hall R, Adamkin D, et al. Growth and development in preterm infants fed long-chain polyunsaturated fatty acids: a prospective, randomized controlled trial. *Pediatrics.* 2001/08// 2001;108(2):359–371

77. Faldella G, Govoni M, Alessandroni R, et al. Visual evoked potentials and dietary long chain polyunsaturated fatty acids in preterm infants. *Arch.Dis.Child.Fetal Neonatal.* Sep 1996;75(2):F108–F112

78. Smithers LG, Gibson RA, McPhee A, Makrides M. Higher dose of docosahexaenoic acid in the neonatal period improves visual acuity of preterm infants: results of a randomized controlled trial. *Am J Clin Nutr.* Oct 2008;88(4):1049–1056

79. McCall RB, Mash CW, Dobbing J. Long-chain polyunsaturated fatty acids and the measurement and prediction of intelligence (IQ). *Developing Brain and Behaviour: the role of lipids in infant formula.* Vol 1st. London: Academic Press; 1997:295–338

80. Auestad N, Halter R, Hall RT, et al. Growth and development in term infants fed long-chain polyunsaturated fatty acids: a double-masked, randomized, parallel, prospective, multivariate study. *Pediatrics.* 2001/08// 2001;108(2):372–381

81. Birch EE, Garfield S, Hoffman DR, Uauy R, Birch DG. A randomized controlled trial of early dietary supply of long-chain polyunsaturated fatty acids and mental development in term infants. *Dev.Med.Child Neurol.* 2000/03// 2000; 42(3):174–181

82. Bouwstra H, Dijck-Brouwer DA, Wildeman JA, et al. Long-chain polyunsaturated fatty acids have a positive effect on the quality of general movements of healthy term infants. *Am J Clin Nutr.* Aug 2003;78(2):313–318

83. Lucas A, Stafford M, Morley R, et al. Efficacy and safety of long-chain polyunsaturated fatty acid supplementation of infant-formula milk: a randomised trial. *Lancet.* Dec 4 1999;354(9194):1948–1954

84. Makrides M, Neumann MA, Simmer K, Gibson RA. A critical appraisal of the role of dietary long-chain polyunsaturated fatty acids on neural indices of term infants: A randomized, controlled trial. *Pediatrics.* 2000/01// 2000;105 (1 Pt 1):32–38

85. Makrides M, Smithers LG, Gibson RA. Role of long-chain polyunsaturated fatty acids in neurodevelopment and growth. Nestle Nutr Workshop Ser Pediatr Program; 2010

86. Smithers LG, Gibson RA, McPhee AJ, M M. Effect of LCPUFA supplementation of preterm infants on disease risk and neurodevelopment: a systematic review of randomised controlled trials. *Am J Clin Nutr* 2008;87(4):912–920

87. Henriksen C, Haugholt K, Lindgren M, et al. Improved cognitive development among preterm infants attributable to early supplementation of human milk with docosahexaenoic acid and arachidonic acid. *Pediatrics.* 2008;121(6): 1137–1145

88. Makrides M, Gibson RA, McPhee AJ, et al. Neurodevelopmental outcomes of preterm infants fed high-dose docosahexaenoic acid: a randomized controlled trial. *Journal of the American Medical Association.* Jan 14 2009;301(2):175–182

89. Westerberg AC, Schei R, Henriksen C, et al. Attention among very low birth weight infants following early supplementation with docosahexaenoic and arachidonic acid. *Acta Paediatr.* Jan 2011;100(1):47–52

90. Collins CT, Gibson RA, Anderson PJ, et al. Neurodevelopmental outcomes at 7 years' corrected age in preterm infants who were fed high-dose docosahexaenoic acid to term equivalent: a follow-up of a randomised controlled trial. *BMJ Open.* Mar 18 2015;5(3):e007314

91. Makrides M, Gibson RA, McPhee AJ, et al. Effect of DHA supplementation during pregnancy on maternal depression and neurodevelopment of young children: a randomized controlled trial. *JAMA.* Oct 20 2010;304(15):1675–1683

92. Makrides M, Gould JF, Gawlik NR, et al. Four-year follow-up of children born to women in a randomized trial of prenatal DHA supplementation. *JAMA.* May 07 2014;311(17):1802–1804

93. Gould JF, Treyvaud K, Yelland LN, et al. Seven-Year Follow-up of Children Born to Women in a Randomized Trial of Prenatal DHA Supplementation. *JAMA.* Mar 21 2017;317(11):1173–1175

94. Dziechciarz P, Horvath A, Szajewska H. Effects of n-3 long-chain polyunsaturated fatty acid supplementation during pregnancy and/or lactation on neurodevelopment and visual function in children: a systematic review of randomized controlled trials. *J Am Coll Nutr.* Oct 2010;29(5):443–454

95. Gould JF, Smithers LG, Makrides M. The effect of maternal omega-3 (n-3) LCPUFA supplementation during pregnancy on early childhood cognitive and visual development: a systematic review and meta-analysis of randomized controlled trials. *Am J Clin Nutr.* Mar 2013;97(3):531–544

96. Marks GB, Mihrshahi S, Kemp AS, et al. Prevention of asthma during the first 5 years of life: a randomized controlled trial. *Journal of Allergy and Clinical Immunology*. 2006;118(1):53–61

97. Peat JK, Mihrshahi S, Kemp AS, et al. Three-year outcomes of dietary fatty acid modification and house dust mite reduction in the Childhood Asthma Prevention Study. *Journal of Allergy and Clinical Immunology*. 2004;114(4):807–813

98. Gunaratne AW, Makrides M, Collins CT. Maternal prenatal and/or postnatal n-3 long chain polyunsaturated fatty acids (LCPUFA) supplementation for preventing allergies in early childhood. *Cochrane Database Syst Rev.* Jul 22 2015;(7):CD010085

99. Bisgaard H, Stokholm J, Chawes BL, et al. Fish Oil-Derived Fatty Acids in Pregnancy and Wheeze and Asthma in Offspring. *N Engl J Med.* Dec 29 2016;375(26):2530–2539

100. Palmer DJ, Sullivan T, Gold MS, et al. Effect of n-3 long chain polyunsaturated fatty acid supplementation in pregnancy on infants' allergies in first year of life: randomised controlled trial. *BMJ.* 2012;344:e184

101. Palmer DJ, Sullivan T, Gold MS, et al. Randomized controlled trial of fish oil supplementation in pregnancy on childhood allergies. *Allergy.* Nov 2013;68(11):1370–1376

102. Best KP, Sullivan T, Palmer D, et al. Prenatal Fish Oil Supplementation and Allergy: 6-Year Follow-up of a Randomized Controlled Trial. *Pediatrics.* Jun 2016;137(6)

103. Bush A, Fleming L. Diagnosis and management of asthma in children. *BMJ.* Mar 05 2015;350:h996

104. Middleton P, Gould J, Shepherd E, Makrides M. Omega-3 supplementation during pregnancy: an updated Cochrane review. *Journal of Paediatrics and Child Health.* 2017;53:68–69

105. Carlson SE, Cooke RJ, Werkman SH, Tolley EA. First year growth of preterm infants fed standard compared to marine oil n-3 supplemented formula. *Lipids.* 1992;27:901–907

106. Carlson SE, Werkman SH, Peeples JM, Cooke RJ, Tolley EA. Arachidonic acid status correlates with first year growth in preterm infants. *Proc.Natl.Acad.Sci. USA.* 1993;90:1073–1077

107. Ryan AS, Montalto MB, Groh-Wargo S, et al. Effect of DHA-containing formula on growth of preterm infants to 59 weeks postmenstrual age. *American Journal of Human Biolog.* 1999;11:457–467

108. Fewtrell MS, Abbott RA, Kennedy K, et al. Randomized, double-blind trial of long-chain polyunsaturated fatty acid supplementation with fish oil and borage oil in preterm infants. *J.Pediatr.* 2004;144(4):471–479

109. Lapillonne A, Clarke SD, Heird WC. Plausible mechanisms for effects of long-chain polyunsaturated fatty acids on growth. *J Pediatr.* Oct 2003;143 (4 Suppl):S9-16

110. Collins CT, Makrides M, Gibson RA, et al. Pre- and post-term growth in pre-term infants supplemented with higher-dose DHA: a randomised controlled trial. *Br J Nutr.* Mar 29 2011:1635–1643

111. Makrides M, Gibson RA, Udell T, Ried K, Invesitgators atIL. Supplementation of infant formula with long-chain polyunsaturated fatty acids does not influence the growth of term infants. *Am J Clin Nutr.* May 2005;81509(5):1094–1101

112. Collins CT, Makrides M, McPhee AJ, et al. Docosahexaenoic Acid and Bronchopulmonary Dysplasia in Preterm Infants. *N Engl J Med.* Mar 30 2017;376(13):1245–1255

113. Klein CJ. Nutrient requirements for preterm infant formulas. *J. Nutr.* 2002;132(6 Suppl 1):1395S–1577S

IV

Chapter 18

Calcium, Phosphorus, and Magnesium

Basic Physiology/Homeostasis

The minerals calcium, magnesium, and phosphorus participate in many of the body's most important functions. These elements play prominent roles in energy processes and transport of metabolites in a host of molecular biochemical reactions. In addition, calcium and phosphorus constitute the principal components of the skeleton in the form of hydroxyapatite, $Ca_{10}(PO_4)_6(OH)_2$. Magnesium, which is mainly an intracellular cation, is a cofactor in a wide variety of enzymatic reactions. Thus, these minerals are essential nutrients for life processes and for forming the mineral skeleton.[1-3]

Naturally occurring calcium sources include milk and other dairy products, animal bones, and in lesser amounts, a number of vegetables (Appendix J). In addition, calcium is widely found in fortified food products, such as breakfast cereals and fruit juices, especially orange juice. Phosphorus is abundantly available from virtually all animal and vegetable sources and is most abundant in dairy products, seafood, meat, soy, whole grains, lentils, and nuts. Magnesium, like phosphorus, is abundant in animal and plant cells and is commonly found in legumes, nuts, seeds, and seafood. Together, these 3 elements constitute 98% of body minerals by weight. Bone accounts for 99% of the calcium, 80% of the phosphorus, and 60% of the magnesium in the body.

Both calcium and phosphorus appear in the serum and extracellular fluid in low concentrations. Total serum calcium concentration is closely maintained in a narrow range of 2.13 to 2.63 mmol/L (8.5–10.5 mg/dL). Approximately half of the calcium in the serum is bound to albumin at normal levels of the latter; most of the remainder is ionized. The ionized fraction is the physiologically active portion, and in health, the concentration is constant. If hypoalbuminemia should occur, the total calcium concentration decreases, but the ionized portion remains undisturbed. The phosphorus concentration varies and is age and diet dependent. The normal range is 1.6 to 2.4 mmol/L (5.0–7.5 mg/dL) in infants, 1.3 to 1.78 mmol/L (4–5.5 mg/dL) in older children and 0.8 to 1.6 mmol/L (2.5–4.5 mg/dL) in adolescents and adults.[4]

Calcium is regulated by various hormones (parathyroid hormone, calcitonin, 1,25-dihydroxyvitamin D [1,25-$(OH)_2$-D]) and a number of organs (skin, small intestine, kidney, and bone). The gastrointestinal tract regulates calcium absorption; a portion of the calcium is absorbed by passive diffusion, and a portion of it is actively transported. Parathyroid hormone enhances serum calcium primarily by releasing calcium from bone. The concentration of ionized calcium in the fluid perfusing the parathyroid gland is a major determinant of the rate of synthesis and release of this hormone. Calcitonin, a hormone elaborated by the parafollicular cells of the thyroid, inhibits bone reabsorption.[4-6] The kidney is an important site of action of parathyroid hormone and is also the site of synthesis of the active hormonal form of vitamin D, 1,25-$(OH)_2$-D.

Vitamin D facilitates transcellular calcium intestinal absorption. To achieve this effect, it must undergo sequential hydroxylation in the liver to calcidiol and in the kidney to the final product, 1,25-$(OH)_2$-D also known as calcitriol.[7,8] Calcidiol (25-hydroxyvitamin D [25-OH-D]) represents the primary circulatory and storage form of vitamin D. Anticonvulsant drugs, such as phenobarbital and phenytoin, can interfere with vitamin D hydroxylation and metabolism, increasing the daily requirement. The large reservoir of calcium in bone is important in maintaining calcium homeostasis, because a portion of bone calcium exchanges readily with the calcium of extracellular fluid.

Factors other than calcium and vitamin D that are important in maintaining bone health are genetic factors; hormonal factors, especially levels of growth hormone and estrogen; and physical activity. In children, evidence suggests that a combination of adequate mineral intake and weight-bearing physical activity are optimal for bone formation and mineralization.[9-12] Disuse osteoporosis, as may occur in children with chronic illnesses, also leads to marked bone loss. Although only partially understood, bone formation and calcium metabolism are also regulated via genetic factors. Recent data implicate specific vitamin D receptor genes as affecting calcium absorption in children.[13] Other data indicate that race and gender also affect calcium absorption.[14-17]

AAP

AAP Statement on Optimizing Bone Health in Children and Adolescents

- Higher recommended dietary allowances for vitamin D as advised by the Institute of Medicine are endorsed
- Supports testing for vitamin D deficiency in children and adolescents with conditions associated with increased bone fragility
- Insufficient evidence to support universal screening for vitamin D deficiency among healthy children or children with dark skin or obesity

Pediatrics. 2014;134(4):e1229-e1243

Less is known about the regulation of phosphorus. Phosphorus is absorbed efficiently in the small intestine, and its absorption is inhibited by aluminum-containing antacids. It is filtered and reabsorbed in the kidney, and parathyroid hormone inhibits its renal reabsorption. A significant aspect of phosphorus regulation is by renal excretion, such that renal insufficiency leads to decreased renal phosphate excretion and hyperphosphatemia.[7]

Only a small fraction of total body magnesium is present in serum. The normal serum total magnesium concentration is 1.6 to 2.5 mg/dL. Approximately half of this magnesium is protein bound, principally to albumin. Magnesium homeostasis is maintained partly by control of intestinal absorption but also by control of renal excretion. Magnesium appears to be absorbed principally in the ileum by 3 mechanisms: passive diffusion, "solvent drag," and active transport.[7] Absorption of magnesium is inversely related to intake and is minimally affected by vitamin D.

Parathyroid hormone decreases renal reabsorption of filtered magnesium. Release of parathyroid hormone is modestly suppressed by increased concentrations of magnesium in extracellular fluid, an action that may be mediated by an increase in calcium in the cytosol of parathyroid cells. Conversely, acute (but not chronic) hypomagnesemia stimulates the release of parathyroid hormone.[7,18–21]

Transient neonatal hypomagnesemia has been observed in association with both hypocalcemia and hyperphosphatemia. Transient neonatal hypomagnesemia is more common in infants with intrauterine growth restriction and infants of mothers with diabetes, hypophosphatemia, or hyperparathyroidism. Magnesium supplementation or even intravenous magnesium may be required for these infants. Rarely, severe hypomagnesemia associated with convulsions occurs in early infancy as a result of a genetically determined disorder of magnesium metabolism. This disorder probably results from a defective intestinal absorption of magnesium. Long-term magnesium supplementation is necessary.[18]

Calcium Requirements

The specific requirements for calcium intake by full-term infants, children, and adolescents have been extensively reviewed in recent years.[22,23] Dietary Reference Intakes (DRIs) for calcium and vitamin D were established in 1997 relied on bone health as the indicator in setting reference values for adequacy.[7] That report established an Adequate Intake (AI) for all life stage groups for calcium in lieu of an Estimated Average Requirement (EAR) and Recommended Dietary Allowance (RDA) as a result of uncertainties associated with balance studies, lack of concordance between observational and experimental data, and lack of longitudinal data to verify the relationship among calcium intake, calcium retention, and bone loss. The EAR is a DRI term that represents the intake level for a nutrient at which the needs of 50% of the population will be met, and the RDA is the average daily level of intake sufficient to meet the nutrient needs of nearly all (97%-98%, or EAR plus 2 standard deviations) healthy individuals. In 2011, the Institute of Medicine (IOM; now the National Academy of Medicine) released a new DRI report in which an EAR and RDA for calcium were set for children 1 year and older and adults on the basis of newer evidence on skeletal health that emerged from a combination of large-scale randomized trials and calcium balance studies.[23] The AI for children 1 to 3 years of age was revised from 500 mg to an EAR of 500 mg and RDA of 700 mg. The AI for children 4 to 8 years of age was revised from 800 mg to an EAR of 800 mg and RDA of 1000 mg.[7,23] These updated DRIs, as well as the Tolerable Upper Intake Level (ULs), are shown in Table 18.1. It is important to understand the goal of nutritional policy is not to ensure that virtually all members of a population are above the RDA, as this will lead to intakes in most members of the population above their requirements.[24,25]

Multiple approaches are used to assess the requirements for calcium in older children. They include the following: (1) measurement of calcium balance in people with various levels of calcium intake; (2) measurement of bone mineral content, by dual-energy x-ray absorptiometry (DXA) or other techniques, in groups of children before and after calcium supplementation; and (3) epidemiologic studies relating bone mass or fracture risk in adults with childhood calcium intake.[20] However, even the use of multiple techniques is inadequate to identify a single optimal daily calcium "requirement" for all children.[24]

The calcium balance technique consists of measuring the effects of any given calcium intake on the net retention of calcium by the body. This approach is commonly used to estimate the minimal requirement. Its usefulness is based on the principle that all retained calcium is used, and that unused calcium is excreted and, thus, unnecessary. In children, optimizing calcium retention from the diet should lead to the highest degree of skeletal mineralization and, thus, decrease the relative risk of osteoporosis in adults.[26,27]

Table 18.1.

Calcium Intake From the Diet and All Sources Compared With DRI Recommendations Among Children in the United States, 2003–2006

	Age Group, y	n	EAR	RDA	UL	CALCIUM Total Intake, mg/d	% Below EAR cut-point
Males	1–3	758	500	700	2500	1008 ± 28.3	5%
	4–8	807	800	1000	2500	1087 ± 31.0	19%
	9–13	1009	1100	1300	3000	1093 ± 32.9	54%
	14–18	1351	1100	1300	3000	1296 ± 41.1	41%
Females	1–3	745	500	700	2500	977 ± 28.1	4%
	4–8	869	800	1000	2500	974 ± 27.1	32%
	9–13	1039	1100	1300	3000	988 ± 47.1	65%
	14–18	1249	1100	1300	3000	918 ± 29.7	75%

Adapted from Bailey RL, Dodd KW, Goldman JA, et al. *J Nutr*, 2010 and Table H-2 NHANES 2003–2006 (https://www.ncbi.nlm.nih.gov/books/NBK56051/table/appendixes.app8.t2/?report=objectonly)

EAR, Estimated Average Requirement; RDA, = Recommended Dietary Allowance; UL, Upper Limit. All values are mg/d.

The substantial limitations involved in obtaining and interpreting data about calcium balance are well known. These include substantial technical problems with measuring calcium excretion and the difficulty obtaining dietary intake control in children. These problems have been partly overcome by the development of stable isotopic methods to assess calcium absorption and excretion.[27] Because the majority of these data are from studies in infants and adolescent girls, more data are needed to establish the "optimal" level of calcium retention at different ages. Recent data have clarified that very low calcium intakes, such as those <600 mg/day, lead to much lower levels of total calcium absorption and retention than recommended intake levels.[28]

A major advance in the field during the last 25 years has been improved methods of measuring total body and regional bone mineral content by various radiologic techniques. Currently, the technique used in the majority of studies is DXA.[29] This technique can rapidly measure the bone mineral content and bone mineral density of the entire skeleton or of regional sites with a minimal level of radiation exposure. Furthermore, enhancements in the precision of the technique have made it suitable for assessing the short- and long-term effects of calcium supplementation on bone mass in children of all ages.[30-33] Nonetheless, substantial limitations in current DXA technology has led to increased interest in the use of newer techniques, including quantitative computed tomography and bone ultrasonography.[34]

Preterm Infants

Calcium and phosphorus accretion rates increase exponentially during the third trimester in utero. Decreased calcium intake is common in preterm infants and may be less than the postconceptional requirement. This decrease places preterm infants at risk of osteopenia and rickets. It is a common problem in infants with birth weight less than 1000 g who have relatively low intakes of calcium and phosphorus that do not meet the needs for bone growth and mineralization. The frequency of osteopenia is also increased in preterm infants who require long-term parenteral nutrition or who require medications, such as diuretics and steroids, which may adversely affect mineral metabolism.[35] In small preterm infants fed parenterally, the danger of calcium-phosphorus precipitation in the solution limits the amount of these minerals that can be administered intravenously. As a result, prenatal retention rates of calcium and phosphorus are not achieved in preterm infants, although if optimized in intravenous solutions, should be adequate to prevent severe osteopenia or rickets. In situations in which fluids are being restricted, this may be more difficult to achieve.[36,37]

The presence of osteopenia can be assessed by direct radiologic evaluation.[38] Increased lucency of the cortical bone with or without epiphyseal changes is characteristic of significant osteopenia. Frank rickets is identified using standard criteria for older infants and children including cupping and fraying at the epiphyses. Although the presence of a fracture can be the presenting sign of osteopenia or rickets, most infants with decreased bone mineralization, including some with severe rickets, do not have fractures. Fractures can occur in preterm infants, however, as part of caregiving by family or medical staff even without the presence of obvious osteopenia or rickets.

Human milk is relatively low in calcium and phosphorus relative to the in utero accretion rates of these minerals. Although minerals are well absorbed from human milk (60%–70%), the net retention of calcium and phosphorus are far below the rates in utero, which leads to the development of undermineralized bones. Supplementary calcium and phosphorus are needed to sustain optimal calcium balance in preterm infants. Currently, human milk fortifiers (for human milk-fed infants) and special formulas with added minerals are marketed in the United States and many other countries for feeding preterm infants (see Appendix D). Use of these products has led to net calcium retention comparable to that achieved in utero.[39] After preterm infants with birth weight <1500 g are discharged from the hospital, there may be benefits to providing a higher mineral intake than is available from human milk or from routine cow milk-based formulas.[23,40–42] This is particularly true for infants who require oxygen or fluid restriction after hospital discharge. Multiple strategies are in clinical use for this situation without clear identification of an optimal approach (see also Chapter 5: Nutritional Needs of the Preterm Infant). One recent randomized control study has shown the benefit of continuing human milk fortifier in preterm infants after hospital discharge.[43]

Full-Term Infants and Children

The optimal primary nutritional source during the first year of life for healthy full-term infants is human milk. No available evidence shows that exceeding the amount of calcium retained by the exclusively breastfed full-term infant during the first 6 months of life or the amount retained by

> **AAP**
>
> ## AAP Recommendations for
> ## Calcium Requirements of Preterm Infants[38]
>
> - Preterm infants, especially those born at <27 weeks' gestation or with birth weight <1000 g with complex medical conditions are at high risk of rickets.
> - Infants <1500 g birth weight should have routine evaluation of bone mineral status via biochemical testing, starting 4 to 5 weeks after birth.
> - Serum alkaline phosphatase >800 to 1000 IU/L or evidence of fractures should be followed up with radiographic evaluation of rickets.
> - Preterm infants with birth weight <1800 to 2000 g should be fed human milk fortified with minerals or formulas designed for preterm infants.
> - At discharge, very low birth weight infants may often receive higher intakes of minerals with the use of transitional formulas for preterm infants, than are typically provided by human milk or formulas for term infants. If exclusively breastfed, obtain a serum alkaline phosphatase at 2 to 4 weeks after discharge.
>
> *Pediatrics.* 2013;131(5):e1676–e1683

the human milk-fed infant given complementary foods during the second 6 months of life is beneficial to achieving long-term increases in bone mineralization. Cow milk-based formulas contain more calcium than does human milk. Relatively greater calcium concentrations are found in specialized formulas, such as soy formulas and casein hydrolysates, to account for the potential lower bioavailability of the calcium from these formulas relative to cow milk-based formula.[18] Of note is the fact that the fractional absorption of calcium from some formulas is similar to that of human milk.[44,45] Thus, the much higher calcium content in such formulas may lead to greater net calcium retention in the formula-fed infant than in the breastfed infant.[46,47]

Some variations exist in the amount of calcium absorbed from different formulas and the bone mineral mass accumulated during infancy.[48,49] Studies comparing the bone mineral content of full-term infants during the first year of life have generally found a slightly greater value for those fed infant formulas than those fed human milk, likely because of the usual greater net calcium retention, as noted previously.[46,47,50] However, there are no data suggesting that such a difference is maintained through adolescence, and there is no evidence at present that these differences lead to clinically significant differences in bone mass.[51] Longer-term studies are needed to evaluate these issues, but at the present time, the bone mass of the breastfed infant remains the reference standard for appropriate bone mineral mass accumulation in infancy.

One should be cautious about using the AI guidelines of the IOM (now the National Academy of Medicine) in infants to determine the appropriate intake of calcium for formula-fed infants. The AI guidelines are specific to breastfed infants, and the AI value for calcium does not hold for infants who are not breastfed. The concentration of calcium (and phosphorus and the calcium-to-phosphorous ratio) in infant formulas is set by the Infant Formula Act, and there is no specific science-based rationale for specific AIs of calcium for formula-fed infants.[52] The IOM did not make any specific recommendations in this regard in its 2011 guidelines.[23]

Few data are available about the calcium requirements of children before puberty.[22] Calcium retention is relatively low in toddlers and slowly increases as puberty approaches. The benefits of calcium intakes above the RDA are uncertain. High levels of calcium intake may negatively affect other minerals, especially iron, although adaptation to this effect occurs and the intake of calcium containing beverages such as dairy should not be restricted solely for this reason.[53] Because these minerals are important for growth and development and may be marginal in toddlers and preschool-aged children, more data regarding the risks and benefits of a calcium intake above the RDA are needed before it can be recommended prior to puberty.

In 2011, the IOM differed from its previous calcium recommendations. Instead of using an AI for calcium intakes, the IOM determined there was sufficient evidence for an EAR and RDA for calcium. Shown in Table 18.1 are the proportion of infants and children below the EAR, which defines the deficient proportion of the population. The prevalence of inadequate dietary intakes is determined by the EAR cut-point method. This represents the proportion of the population with intakes below the median requirement (EAR). In the case of calcium, data from the National Health and Nutrition Examination Survey (NHANES) 2003–2006 reveal that children 1 to 3 years of age at the 50th percentile for calcium intake consume approximately 955 mg/day and that about 5% of that population has an intake below the EAR of 500 mg/day that would be considered inadequate.[23]

Perhaps of most importance in young children is the development of eating patterns that will be associated with adequate calcium intake later in life. As such, it is important that families learn to identify the calcium content of foods (see Appendix J) based on the food label and incorporate this information into their food-buying habits. The most readily available food source of calcium (70%–80% of calcium content in US diets) is from dairy products, and the current Dietary Guidelines for Americans recommend 3 to 4 servings a day.[54] The food label currently provides the amount of calcium as a proportion of the Daily Value, which is 1000 mg; thus, a 20% Daily Value on the food label equates to 200 mg per serving. The US Food and Drug Administration has recently required that the new revised food labels for older children and adults also include the actual amounts of calcium per serving (see also Chapter 50.II: Food Labeling).

Preadolescents and Adolescents

The majority of research in children about calcium requirements has been directed toward 9- to 18-year-old females. The efficiency of calcium absorption is increased during puberty, and the majority of bone formation occurs during this period. Data from balance studies suggest that for most healthy children in this age range, an intake of 1300 mg/day will support optimal bone growth.[23,55]

Numerous controlled trials have found an increase in the bone mineral content in children in this age group who have received calcium supplementation.[7,37,56–59] However, the available data suggest that if calcium intake is augmented only for relatively short periods (ie, 1 to 2 years), there may be minimal or no long-term benefits to establishing and maintaining a maximum peak bone mass.[37,60,61] Even longer-term increased intake of calcium may only lead to relatively small benefits in bone mass,[58] although calcium supplementation may be more beneficial in some subgroups of children, such as those with early puberty or those of greater height.[58,62,63] The implications of such findings for dietary guidance are unclear. In general, the available data emphasize the importance of a well-balanced diet in achieving adequate calcium intake and in establishing dietary patterns with a calcium intake at or near recommended levels throughout childhood and adolescence.[22]

In addition to calcium intake, exercise is an important aspect of achieving maximal peak bone mass. There is evidence that childhood and adolescence may represent an important period for achieving long-lasting skeletal benefits from regular exercise.[56] Low bone mass may be a contributing factor to some fractures in children.[64]

Although virtually all data regarding the importance of calcium intake has focused on the bone health benefits, emerging evidence, both in adults and in some studies performed in children, suggest that calcium intake may be important in both blood pressure and weight regulation. However, some but not all evidence supports the conclusion that children who have an adequate intake of calcium are more likely to have an optimal weight for age.[59,65–70]

It is recommended that pediatricians actively discuss issues of bone health with families during routine visits. Recommended ages for such discussions are 2 to 3 years of age, 8 to 9 years of age, and then later during adolescence. The 1997 AI for children 9 to 13 years old was revised in 2011 from 1300 mg to an EAR of 1100 mg and RDA of 1300 mg.[7,23] An emphasis should be placed on preventing inadequate calcium intake, encouraging weight-bearing exercise, and ensuring adequate vitamin D status.[22]

Adolescent Pregnancy and Lactation

At birth, the fetus contains approximately 30 g of calcium. This represents approximately 2.5% of typical maternal body calcium stores.[18] Evidence suggests that, in adult women, much of this 30 g comes from increases in dietary calcium absorption during pregnancy.[71] A similar increase in calcium absorption during pregnancy occurs in adolescents.[72]

During lactation, a period of 6 months of exclusive breastfeeding would lead to an additional 45 g of calcium secreted by the mother. Although some of this is accounted for by decreased urinary calcium excretion during lactation, there is extensive evidence demonstrating a loss of maternal bone calcium during lactation.[73–75] In adult women, however, bone remineralization occurs after weaning, and neither pregnancy nor lactation is associated with persistent bone loss. Because of data demonstrating that calcium supplementation is not effective in preventing lactation-associated bone loss or enhancing postweaning bone mass recovery,[75] dietary recommendations do not suggest increases in calcium for healthy adult women who are pregnant or lactating above the 1000 mg/day RDA for nonlactating adult women.[23]

The situation for pregnant and lactating adolescents is less clear. Current guidelines do not recommend an increased intake above the age-appropriate maximum for adolescents (1300 mg/day) who are either pregnant or lactating.[7] Shorter femur length in fetuses of pregnant African American adolescents with low dairy intake compared with those with higher intakes has been observed.[76] This is consistent with earlier similar data demonstrating a lower neonatal bone mineral density associated with low calcium intake during pregnancy in adults.[77]

At the present time, the available evidence supports the recommendation that the benefits of breastfeeding greatly outweigh any demonstrated risks to adolescents in terms of achieving either optimal growth or peak bone mass.[72,78] No available data suggest that calcium intakes above the recommended amounts are beneficial to pregnant or lactating adolescents. However, it should be noted that these recommended intake levels are far above those typical of the diet of even most nonpregnant adolescents.

Phosphorous Requirements

As with calcium, the recommended AI for phosphorus for infants was based on usual dietary intakes of breastfed infants. These values are 100 mg/day from ages 0 through 6 months and 275 mg/day from ages 7 through 12 months. The higher value in older infants reflects the considerable contribution of solid foods to usual phosphorus intakes of these infants. There are few data on which to base estimates of phosphorus requirements for older children. The DRIs used a factorial approach based on limited estimates of phosphorus absorption, excretion, and accretion to determine average requirements.[7] An allotment of an additional 20% was provided to calculate the RDA. Using this method, values for the RDA of 460 mg/day for children 1 through 3 years of age and 500 mg/day for children 4 through 8 years of age were derived. These values are well below typical intakes for children of these ages, suggesting that deficient phosphorus intake is an uncommon problem in small children. Dietary requirements for phosphorus were not considered by the recent RDA committee evaluating calcium and vitamin D requirements.[23] Thus, the recommendations from 1997 were not changed (see Appendix E).

For adolescents, both the factorial method and estimates of intake needed to maintain typical serum phosphorus were used to determine RDAs. An RDA of 1250 mg/day was calculated for boys and girls ages 9 through 18 years.[7] This value is much closer to typical intake values for adolescents and reflects the rapid bone and muscle growth during this time period. No increase was added for pregnant or lactating adolescents (see Appendix E).

Magnesium Requirements

Current dietary guidelines for magnesium for infants are based on the intakes of human milk-fed infants. The recommended AI is 30 mg/day for infants in the first 6 months of life and 75 mg/day from 7 through 12 months of age (see Appendix E). Commercial cow-milk based infant formulas are generally higher in magnesium concentration (40–50 mg/L) than is human milk (34 mg/L). Soy-based formulas may have even higher levels of magnesium (50–80 mg/L).[7,13] In a large series of studies, Fomon and Nelson reported approximately 40% absorption of magnesium in infants fed soy- or cow milk-based formulas (based on total intake of 53–59 mg/day) with a net retention of 9 to 10 mg/day.[7,18]

Few metabolic balance studies have been performed for magnesium in children, especially those 1 through 8 years of age. On the basis of limited available data, it appears that a magnesium intake of 5 mg/kg/day should lead to positive magnesium balances in most children. Using average weight-for-age data, this intake leads to an RDA of 80 mg/day for ages 1 through 3 years, 130 mg/day for ages 4 through 8 years, and 240 mg/day for 9 through 13 years. For adolescents ages 14 through 18 years, slightly greater average intakes are needed (5.3 mg/kg/day) to account for increased pubertal magnesium needs. Differences in average weights of boys and girls were used to calculate RDAs of 410 mg/day for boys and 360 mg/day for girls (see Appendix E).[7]

Because of efficient homeostatic mechanisms, especially renal conservation of magnesium, low dietary magnesium alone does not usually cause clinically apparent magnesium deficiency. Magnesium deficiency is, however, quite common in young children with protein-energy malnutrition, especially when accompanied by gastroenteritis. Muscle magnesium is depressed, but serum magnesium may be normal. Hypomagnesemia sometimes occurs in malabsorption syndromes, and magnesium depletion may develop in subjects with severe diarrhea. Convulsions are the most clearly documented feature of hypomagnesemia with or without total body magnesium deficiency in infants and young children.[79] Neuropsychiatric disorders are well documented in magnesium-depleted adults. Hypocalcemia associated with magnesium deficiency may be the result of defective synthesis or release of parathyroid hormone. Hypokalemia also occurs secondarily to magnesium deficiency.[80]

Numerous conditions may be related to subacute magnesium deficiency, however. For example, evidence has also linked magnesium deficiency with insulin resistance and worsening diabetic regulation. Increased blood pressure, migraines, and inadequate bone mineralization may also be linked to habitually low magnesium intake, although data for these relationships continues to be incomplete.[7]

IV

Dietary Sources: Calcium

Knowledge of dietary calcium sources is a first step toward increasing the intake of calcium-rich foods.[81] The largest source of dietary calcium for most people is milk and other dairy products. Most vegetables contain calcium, although at low density, making it difficult to achieve required intakes from vegetables without additional calcium sources. Therefore, relatively large servings are needed to equal the total intake achieved with typical servings of dairy products. The bioavailability of calcium from vegetables is generally high. An exception is spinach, which is high in oxalate, making the calcium virtually nonbioavailable. Several products have been introduced that are fortified with calcium. These products, most notably orange juice, are fortified to achieve a calcium concentration similar to that of milk. Breakfast cereals also are frequently fortified with minerals, including calcium. The gap between the recommended calcium intakes and the typical intakes of children and adolescents is substantial. A list of foods relatively high in calcium is given in Appendix J. Most adolescents, especially females, have calcium intakes below the recommended levels (see Table 18.1).[82] Preoccupation with being thin is common in this age group, especially among females, as is the misconception that all dairy foods are fattening. Many children and adolescents are unaware that low-fat milk contains at least as much calcium as whole milk.[22]

For children with lactose intolerance, several alternatives exist. Lactose intolerance is more common in African American, Mexican American, and Asian/Pacific Islander individuals than in white individuals. Many children with lactose intolerance can drink small amounts of milk without discomfort. Other alternatives include the use of other dairy products, such as solid cheeses and yogurt, which may be better tolerated than milk. Lactose-free and low-lactose milks are widely available as are nondairy "milks" fortified with calcium such as soy milk.

In general, dietary sources of calcium, including fortified foods, are preferred to calcium supplementation via pill or similar nondietary supplements because of the range of nutrients and the establishment of good dietary habits that are enhanced by the use of food sources of calcium. Furthermore, nutrient interactions may be decreased and tolerance may be greater for minerals provided from food sources.

Dietary Sources: Magnesium

Quantities of magnesium in infant formulas range from 40 to 70 mg/L (3.3–5.8 mEq/L). Whole grains, beans, and legumes are good sources of magnesium. Because magnesium is a component of chlorophyll, green leafy vegetables are high in magnesium. Other dietary sources include milk, eggs, and meat. Depending on its "hardness," water may also significantly contribute to dietary magnesium intake.

References

1. Cohn SH, Vaswani A, Zanzi I, Aloia JF, Roginsky MS, Ellis KJ. Changes in body chemical composition with age measured by total-body neutron activation. *Metabolism.* 1976;25(1):85–95

2. Widdowson EM, McCance RA, Spray CM. The chemical composition of the human body. *Clin Sci.* 1951;10(1):113–125

3. Widdowson EM, Spray CM. Chemical development in utero. *Arch Dis Child.* 1951;26(127):205–214

4. Broadus AE. Physiological functions of calcium, magnesium, and phosphorus and mineral ion balance. In: Favus MJ, ed. *Primer on the Metabolic Bone Diseases and Disorders of Mineral Metabolism.* New York, NY: Raven Press; 2003:105–111

5. Bronner F, Pansu D. Nutritional aspects of calcium absorption. *J Nutr.* 1999;129(1):9–12

6. Salle BL, Delvin EE, Lapillonne A, Bishop NJ, Glorieux FH. Perinatal metabolism of vitamin D. *Am J Clin Nutr.* 2000;71(5 Suppl):1317S-1324S

7. Institute of Medicine, Food and Nutrition Board. *Dietary Reference Intakes for Calcium, Phosphorus, Magnesium, Vitamin D, and Fluoride.* Washington, DC: National Academies Press; 1997

8. Kim Y, Linkswiler HM. Effect of level of protein intake on calcium metabolism and on parathyroid and renal function in the adult human male. *J Nutr.* 1979;109(8):1399–1404

9. Baptista F, Barrigas C, Vieiera F, et al. The role of lean body mass and physical activity in bone health in children. *J Bone Miner Res.* 2012;30(1):100–108

10. Pitukcheewanont P, Punyasavatsut N, Feuille M. Physical activity and bone health in children and adolescents. *Pediatr Endocrinol Rev.* 2010;7(3):275–282

11. Tan VP, Macdonald HM, Kim S, et al. Influence of physical activity on bone strength in children and adolescents: a systematic review and narrative synthesis. *J Bone Miner Res.* 2014;29(10):2161–2181

12. Hind K, Burrows M. Weight-bearing exercise and bone mineral accrual in children and adolescents: a review of controlled trials. *Bone.* 2007;40(1):14–27

13. Abrams SA, Griffin IJ, Hawthorne KM, et al. Vitamin D receptor Fok1 polymorphisms affect calcium absorption, kinetics and bone mineralization rates during puberty. *J Bone Miner Res.* 2005;20(6):945–953

14. Abrams SA, O'Brien KO, Liang LK, Stuff JE. Differences in calcium absorption and kinetics between black and white girls age 5-16 years. *J Bone Miner Res.* 1995;10(5):829–833

IV

15. Koay MA, Tobias JH, Leary SD, Steer CD, Villarino-Guell C, Brown MA. The effect of LRP5 polymorphisms on bone mineral density is apparent in childhood. *Calcif Tissue Int.* 2007;81(1):1-9

16. Utriainen P, Jaaskelainen J, Saarinen A, Vanninen E, Makitie O, Voutilainen R. Body composition and bone mineral density in children with premature adrenarche and the association of LRP5 gene polymorphisms with bone mineral density. *J Clin Endocrinol Metab.* 2009;94(11):4144–4151

17. Wigertz K, Palacios C, Jackman LA, et al. Racial differences in calcium retention in response to dietary salt in adolescent girls. *Am J Clin Nutr.* 2005;81(4):845–850

18. Fomon SJ, Nelson SE. Calcium, phosphorus, magnesium, and sulfur. In: Fomon SJ, ed. *Nutrition of Normal Infants.* St Louis, MO: Mosby-Year Book Inc; 1993: 192–218

19. Hardwick LL, Jones MR, Brautbar N, Lee DB. Magnesium absorption: mechanisms and the influence of vitamin D, calcium, and phosphate. *J Nutr.* 1991;121(1):13–23

20. Shils ME. Magnesium in health and disease. *Annu Rev Nutr.* 1988;8:429–460

21. Yamamoto T, Kabata H, Yagi R, Takashima M, Itokawa Y. Primary hypomagnesemia with secondary hypocalcemia: report of a case and review of the world literature. *Magnesium.* 1985;4(2-3):153–164

22. Greer FR, Krebs NF, American Academy of Pediatrics, Committee on Nutrition. Clinical report: Optimizing bone health and calcium intakes of infants, children, and adolescents. *Pediatrics.* 2006;117(2):578–585

23. Institute of Medicine, Food and Nutrition Board. *Dietary Reference Intakes for Calcium and Vitamin D.* Washington, DC: National Academies Press; 2011

24. Abrams SA. What does it mean to target specific serum 25-hydroxyvitamin D concentrations in children and adolescents? *Am J Clin Nutr.* 2016;104(5):1193–1194

25. Manson JE, P.M. B, C.J. R, Taylor CL. Vitamin D deficiency - is there really a pandemic? *N Engl J Med.* 2016;375(19):1817–1820

26. Abrams SA, Grusak MA, Stuff J, O'Brien KO. Calcium and magnesium balance in 9-14-y-old children. *Am J Clin Nutr.* 1997;66(5):1172–1177

27. Jackman LA, Millane SS, Martin BR, et al. Calcium retention in relation to calcium intake and postmenarcheal age in adolescent females. *Am J Clin Nutr.* 1997;66(2):327–333

28. Abrams SA, Griffin IJ, Hicks PD, Gunn SK. Pubertal girls only partially adapt to low dietary calcium intakes. *J Bone Miner Res.* 2004;19(5):759–763

29. Kalkwarf HJ, Abrams SA, DiMeglio LA, Koo WWK, Specker BL, Weiler H. Bone densitometry in infants and young children: the 2013 ISCD pediatric official positions. *J Clin Densitom.* 2014;17(2):243–257

30. Adams JE. Bone densitometry in children. *Semin Musculoskeletal Radiol.* 2016;20(3):254–268

31. Christiansen C, Rodbro P, Nielsen CT. Bone mineral content and estimated total body calcium in normal children and adolescents. *Scand J Clin Lab Invest.* 1975;35(6):507–510

32. Ellis KJ, Abrams SA, Wong WW. Body composition of a young, multiethnic female population. *Am J Clin Nutr.* 1997;65(3):724–731

33. Wren TA, Gilsanz V. Assessing bone mass in children and adolescents. *Curr Osteoporos Rep.* 2006;4(4):153–158

34. Wren TA, Liu X, Pitukcheewanont P, Gilsanz V. Bone densitometry in pediatric populations: discrepancies in the diagnosis of osteoporosis by DXA and CT. *J Pediatr.* 2005;146(6):776–779

35. Atkinson SA. Human milk feeding of the micropremie. *Clin Perinatol.* 2000;27(1): 235–247

36. Prestridge LL, Schanler RJ, Shulman RJ, Burns PA, Laine LL. Effect of parenteral calcium and phosphorus therapy on mineral retention and bone mineral content in very low birth weight infants. *J Pediatr.* 1993;122(5 Pt 1):761–768

37. Wizenberg TM, Shaw K, Fryer J, Jones G. Calcium supplementation for improving bone mineral density in children. *Cochrane Database Syst Rev.* 2006;19(2):CD005119

38. Abrams SA, American Academy of Pediatrics, Committee on Nutrition. Calcium and vitamin D requirements of enterally fed preterm infants. *Pediatrics.* 2013;131(5):e1676–e1683

39. Schanler RJ, Abrams SA. Postnatal attainment of intrauterine macromineral accretion rates in low birth weight infants fed fortified human milk? *J Pediatr.* 1995;126(3):441–447

40. Carver JD, Wu PY, Hall RTea. Growth of preterm infants fed nutrient-enriched or term formula after hospital discharge. *Pediatrics.* 2001;107(4):683–689

41. Hawthorne KM, Griffin IJ, Abrams SA. Nutritional approaches to the care of preterm infants. *Minerva Pediatr.* 2004;56(4):359–372

42. Lapillonne A, Salle BL, Glorieux FH, Claris O. Bone mineralization and growth are enhanced in preterm infants fed an isocaloric, nutrient-enriched preterm formula through term. *Am J Clin Nutr.* 2004;80(6):1595–1603

43. Almone A, Rovet J, Ward W, et al. Growth and body composition of human milk-fed premature infants provided with extra energy and nutrients early after hospital discharge:1-year follow-up. *J Pediatr Gastroenterol Nutr.* 2009;49(4): 456–466

44. Abrams SA. Calcium absorption in infants and small children: Methods of determination and recent findings. *Nutrients.* 2010;2(4):474–480

45. Hicks PD, Hawthorne KM, Berseth CL, Marunycz JD, Heubi JE, Abrams SA. Total calcium absorption is similar from infant formulas with and without prebiotics and exceeds that in human milk-fed infants. *BMC Pediatr.* 2012;12:118

46. Abrams SA, Griffin IJ, Davila PM. Calcium and zinc absorption from lactose-containing and lactose-free infant formulas. *Am J Clin Nutr.* 2002;76(2):442–446

47. Abrams SA, Wen J, Stuff JE. Absorption of calcium, zinc and iron from breast milk by 5- to 7-month-old infants. *Pediatr Res.* 1997;41(3):384–390

IV

48. Koo WW, Hammami M, Margeson DP, Nwaesei C, Montalto MB, Lasekan JB. Reduced bone mineralization in infants fed palm olein-containing formula: a randomized, double-blinded, prospective trial. *Pediatrics.* 2003;111(5 Pt 1): 1017–1023

49. Nelson SE, Frantz JA, Ziegler EE. Absorption of fat and calcium by infants fed a milk-based formula containing palm-olein. *J Am Coll Nutr.* 1998;17(4):327–333

50. Specker BL, Beck A, Kalkwarf H, Ho M. Randomized trial of varying mineral intake on total body bone mineral accretion during the first year of life. *Pediatrics.* 1997;99(6):e12

51. Young RJ, Antonson DL, Ferguson PW, Murray ND, Merkel K, Moore TE. Neonatal and infant feeding: effect on bone density at 4 years. *J Pediatr Gastroenterol Nutr.* 2005;41(1):88–93

52. Abrams SA. What are the risks and benefits to increasing dietary bone minerals and vitamin D intake in infants and small children? *Annu Rev Nutr.* 2011;31: 285–297

53. Ames SK, Gorham BM, Abrams SA. Effects of high vs low calcium intake on calcium absorption and red blood cell iron incorporation by small children. *Am J Clin Nutr.* 1999;70(1):44–48

54. US Department of Health and Human Services, US Department of Agriculture. *2015–2020 Dietary Guidelines for Americans.* 8th ed. Washington, DC: US Department of Health and Human Services, US Department of Agriculture; December 2015

55. Vatanparast H, Bailey DA, Baxter-Jones AD, Whiting SJ. Calcium requirements for bone growth in Canadian boys and girls during adolescence. *Br J Nutr.* 2010;103(4):575–580

56. Lloyd T, Petit MA, Lin HM, Beck TJ. Lifestyle factors and the development of bone mass and bone strength in young women. *J Pediatr.* 2004;144(6):776–782

57. Matkovic V, Goel PK, Badenhop-Stevens NE, et al. Calcium supplementation and bone mineral density in females from childhood to young adulthood: a randomized controlled trial. *Am J Clin Nutr.* 2005;81(1):175–188

58. Matkovic V, Landoll JD, Badenhop-Stevens NE, et al. Nutrition influences skeletal development from childhood to adulthood: a study of hip, spine, and forearm in adolescent females. *J Nutr.* 2004;134(3):701S-705S

59. Merrilees MJ, Smart EJ, Gilchrist NL, et al. Effects of diary food supplements on bone mineral density in teenage girls. *Eur J Nutr.* 2000;39(6):256–262

60. Lanou AJ, Berkow SE, Barnard ND. Calcium, dairy products, and bone health in children and young adults: a reevaluation of the evidence. *Pediatrics.* 2005;115(3):736–743

61. Abrams SA. Calcium supplementation during childhood: long-term benefits on bone mineralization. *Nutr Rev.* 2005;63(7):251–255

62. Abrams SA, Griffin IJ, Hawthorne KM, Liang L. Height and height Z-score are related to calcium absorption in 5 to 15 yr-old girls. *J Clin Endocrinol Metab.* 2005;90(9):5077–5081

63. Ferrari SL, Chevalley T, Bonjour JP, Rizzoli R. Childhood fractures are associated with decreased bone mass gain during puberty: an early marker of persistent bone fragility? *J Bone Miner Res.* 2006;21(4):501–507

64. Goulding A, Cannan R, Williams SM, Gold EJ, Taylor RW, Lewis-Barned NJ. Bone mineral density in girls with forearm fractures. *J Bone Miner Res.* 1998;13(1): 143–148

65. Dixon LB, Pellizzon MA, Jawad AF, Tershakovec AM. Calcium and dairy intake and measures of obesity in hyper- and normocholesterolemic children. *Obes Res.* 2005;13(10):1727–1738

66. Huang TT, McCrory MA. Dairy intake, obesity, and metabolic health in children and adolescents: knowledge and gaps. *Nutr Rev.* 2005;63(3):71–80

67. Lorenzen JK, Molgaard C, Michaelsen KF, Astrup A. Calcium supplementation for 1 y does not reduce body weight or fat mass in young girls. *Am J Clin Nutr.* 2006;83(1):18–23

68. Murphy MM, Douglass JS, Johnson RK, Spence LA. Drinking flavored or plain milk is positively associated with nutrient intake and is not associated with adverse effects on weight status in US children and adolescents. *J Am Diet Assoc.* 2008;108(4):631–639

69. Samadi M, Sadrzadeh-Yeganeh H, Azadbakht L, Jafarian K, Sotoudeh G. Dietary calcium intake and risk of obesity in school girls aged 8-10 years. *J Res Med Sci.* 2012;17(2):1102–1107

70. Zheng M, Rangan A, Olsen NJ, et al. Substituting sugar-sweetened beverages with water or milk is inversely associated with body fatness development from childhood to adolescence. *Nutrition.* 2015;31(1):38–44

71. Heaney RP, Skillman TG. Calcium metabolism in normal human pregnancy. *J Clin Endocrinol Metab.* 1971;33(4):661–670

72. O'Brien KO, Nathanson MS, Mancini J, Witter FR. Calcium absorption is significantly higher in adolescents during pregnancy than in the early postpartum period. *Am J Clin Nutr.* 2003;78(6):1188–1193

73. Hopkinson JM, Butte NF, Ellis K, Smith EO. Lactation delays postpartum bone mineral accretion and temporarily alters its regional distribution in women. *J Nutr.* 2000;130(4):777–783

74. Kalkwarf HJ, Specker BL. Bone mineral loss during lactation and recovery after weaning. *Obstet Gynecol.* 1995;86(1):26–32

75. Kalkwarf HJ, Specker BL, Bianchi DC, Ranz J, Ho M. The effect of calcium supplements on bone density during lactation and after weaning. *N Engl J Med.* 1997;337(8):523–528

76. Chang SC, O'Brien KO, Nathanson MS, Caulfield LE, Mancini J, Witter FR. Fetal femur length is influenced by maternal diary intake in pregnant African American adolescents. *Am J Clin Nutr.* 2003;77(5):1248–1254

77. Koo WW, Walters JC, Esterlitz J, Levine RJ, Bush AJ, Sibai B. Maternal calcium supplementation and fetal bone mineralization. *Obstet Gynecol.* 1999;94(4): 577–584

78. Bezerra FF, Mendonca LM, Lobato EC, O'Brien KO, Donangelo CM. Bone mass is recovered from lactation to postweaning in adolescent mothers with low calcium intakes. *Am J Clin Nutr.* 2004;80(5):1322–1326

79. Capalleri AM, Tardini G, Mazzoni MBM, Belli M, Milani GP, Fossali EF. Neonatal focal seizures and hypomagnesemia: a case report. *Eur J Pediatr Neurol.* 2016;20(1):176–178

80. Rude RK. Magnesium deficiency: a cause of heterogeneous disease in humans. *J Bone Miner Res.* 1998;13(4):749–758

81. Golden NH, Abrams SA, American Academy of Pediatrics, Committee on Nutrition. Clinical report: Optimizing bone health in children and adolescents. *Pediatrics.* 2014;134(4):e1229–e1243

82. Hamner HC, Perrine CG, Scanlon KS. Usual intakes of key minerals among children in the second year of life, NHANES 2003–2012. *Nutrients.* 2016;8(8):E468

Chapter 19

Iron

Introduction

Iron deficiency has recently been defined by a group of international experts as: "a health-related condition in which iron availability is insufficient to meet the body's needs which can be present with or without anemia."[1] Iron is critical for the generation and functioning of numerous proteins as well as cells with high energy demand, such as cardiac and skeletal myocytes. Also vulnerable to iron depletion are cells with a high mitogenic potential, including hematopoietic, epithelial, and immune cells.[2]

Iron deficiency (ID) and iron deficiency anemia (IDA) continue to be of worldwide concern. Among children in the developing world, iron is the most common single-nutrient deficiency.[3] Even in industrialized countries, despite a demonstrable decline in prevalence, it is still a more prevalent problem in medically underserved populations.[4] ID remains a common cause of anemia in young children, and according to the National Health and Examination Survey (NHANES) 2003–2010, IDA occurs in up to 3% of children age 1 to 2 years of age[5] and 2.4% of adolescent girls in the United States.[6] ID is more common and occurs in 13.5% of 1- to 2-year-olds, 3.7% of 3- to 5-year-olds, and up to 16% of adolescent girls. ID is twice as likely in overweight adolescents than those with normal weight. ID in early life, with or without anemia, is associated with long-term neurodevelopment and behavior impairment, which may persist into adulthood.[7-9] In adolescents with ID, iron fortification has demonstrated improved verbal learning, concentration, and memory.[8] Iron supplementation has also improved aerobic capacity,[10] decreased fatigue scores,[11] and decreased restless leg syndrome (RLS)[12] among nonanemic but iron-deficient girls. In 2010, the American Academy of Pediatrics (AAP) published a clinical report with recommendations on the prevention and diagnosis of IDA in infants and young children (see AAP text box).[4] An updated AAP clinical report focused on the treatment of children with IDA across the pediatric lifespan is currently under development.

Iron Metabolism

Iron is highly regulated, primarily at the site of dietary absorption in the apical surface of duodenal enterocytes. Heme iron is efficiently transported into the enterocyte via heme carrier protein 1 (HCP1),[13] explaining why iron in red meat is well absorbed. Nonheme iron is less readily absorbed.

In exclusively breastfed or formula-fed infants, nonheme iron (iron 3+ or ferric iron) is the primary source. Iron 3+ is reduced to iron 2+ (ferrous iron) at the duodenal brush border via the enzyme ferric reductase associated with the divalent metal transporter 1 (DMT-1) that internalizes iron 2+ within an endosome.[14] Within the enterocyte, iron can be either stored as ferritin for later mitochondrial use or sloughed with enterocyte senescence into the lumen. If signaled to do so, nonheme iron is exported across the enterocyte basolateral membrane after oxidation via the exporter, ferroportin, into the villus capillaries bound to transferrin. Once in circulation, transferrin-bound iron is transported to the site of either use or storage. Erythrocyte precursors express high densities of transferrin receptor 1 (TfR1) and, thus, have preferred access to circulating iron. If not needed for bone marrow erythrocytes or tissues, iron is taken up through membrane TfR1 on hepatocytes and macrophages. Throughout life, but especially in early infancy, iron from senescent erythrocytes is recycled via the reticuloendothelial system and stored in the liver to support growth. Storage iron is exported from hepatocytes via ferroportin, the same iron exporter found on enterocytes.

The communication needed to traffic iron between transport, storage, and cells utilizing iron is mediated by hepcidin, an antimicrobial peptide synthesized in hepatocytes that serves as the negative feedback regulator of iron homeostasis.[15] When iron is not needed for erythrocyte precursors or other tissues, hepcidin induces internalization and degradation of ferroportin, which then limits iron export from enterocytes, hepatocytes, or liver macrophages. Chronic inflammatory conditions lead to elevated levels of hepcidin which also decreases the availability of iron for cellular functions.[16] Conversely, low levels of hepcidin activate ferroportin, increasing export of iron from intestinal enterocytes, hepatocytes, and macrophages.

Hepcidin is also the master iron regulator during human development. Maternal hepcidin levels normally decrease in pregnancy to meet the sixfold higher needs for the woman's iron absorption[17] and facilitate placental syncytiotrophoblast transfer through the apical TfR1 importer and basal ferroportin exporter.[18] During normal third trimester growth, decreasing fetal hepcidin levels also signal for increased placental iron delivery. However, during intrauterine inflammation, fetal liver hepcidin can increase and downregulate placental iron delivery. Inflammation in obesity or maternal diabetes can also inhibit the normal fall in maternal hepcidin during pregnancy.[19] Thus transfer of placental iron can be limited, despite the lower levels of iron that normally signal decreased hepcidin levels.[20] Placental dysfunction sufficiently severe to cause intrauterine growth restriction may also limit placental iron transfer, despite already low fetal iron levels.[21] Under normal conditions, fetal iron acquisition supplies half of the iron needed for postnatal infant growth. However, with placental dysfunction and/or preterm birth, infants are born with an inadequate iron endowment unable to meet their needs for postnatal growth, especially with breastfeeding.

The human body can prioritize available iron both between and within organs. As iron is prioritized to erythrocytes, its role in oxygen transport is its most critical function. ID with inadequate oxygen transport in the fetus or young infant causes hepatic stores to be depleted first, followed by other lower-priority tissues, such as skeletal muscle and intestine. With worsening ID, cardiac iron is compromised, followed by brain iron, and lastly erythrocyte iron. Thus, IDA represents a severe form of ID, and the prioritization of iron for erythrocytes even over the brain accounts for the adverse neurodevelopmental effects seen even in ID without anemia,[22] as is observed in infants after 4 to 6 months of age not receiving supplemental iron.

Iron plays a key role in neurotransmission and brain development and maturation. Animal data have shown that iron is necessary for synthesis and packaging of neurotransmitters, especially dopamine. Iron is also an essential factor in myelination.[2] Intraorgan prioritization also occurs, and this has been demonstrated in the developing rat brain. The selective hippocampal and cortical vulnerability to perinatal ID results in an early critical loss of recognition memory.[23]

Numerous neurobehavorial studies on the effect of iron therapy on in young children have been conducted. The majority of these studies have looked at the effect of IDA rather than ID, and thus, the impact of ID in the absence IDA on cognition is not clear cut.[24] A series of systematic reviews of randomized controlled trials in which infants[25-27] and older children[25,28-30] with various stages of ID and who did or did not receive oral iron therapy showed mixed results.

Nutritional Requirements for Iron

Iron requirements of healthy children have been established by the Institute of Medicine (IOM; now the National Academy of Medicine [NAM]) and published in the Dietary Reference Intakes (DRIs).[31] These values are given in Table 19.1. The source of the recommendations is listed in the first column.

Table 19.1.
Daily Recommended Intake of Dietary Iron

Strength of Recommendation	Age	Gender	Elemental Iron (mg/day)
Adequate Intake	0–6 mo	All	0.27
Recommended Dietary Allowance	7–12 mo	All	11
	1–3 y	All	7
	4–8 y	All	10
	9–13 y	All	8
	14–18 y	Female Male	15 11
ESPGHAN	Preterm <2 kg infants 1–6 mo	All	2–3 mg/kg up to 15 mg/day
ESPGHAN	LBW 2–2.5 kg 1–6 mo	All	1–2 mg/kg

Source: Institute of Medicine, Food and Nutrition Board. *Dietary Reference Intakes for Vitamin A, Vitamin K, Arsenic, Boron, Chromium, Copper, Iodine, Iron, Manganese, Molybdenum, Nickel, Silicon, Vanadium, and Zinc.* Washington, DC: National Academies Press; 2003.

When the recommendation is based on sound and adequate scientific evidence, a Recommended Dietary Allowance (RDA) is given. If sufficient scientific evidence is lacking, the best estimate based on the available information is listed as Adequate Intake (AI). Both the RDA and the AI should supply adequate amounts of the nutrient to cover the needs of almost all (97%–98%) healthy individuals. Levels of iron intake are given in milligrams (mg) of elemental iron per day.

Full-Term Infants
Most healthy infants born at term have sufficient iron stores to last until 4 to 6 months of age, largely because of their high hemoglobin (Hb) concentration and blood volume relative to body weight. Both decline during the first months of life with the preservation of the Hb iron, which diminishes the requirement for iron and likely accounts for human milk iron content evolving to be relatively low—on average, 0.35 mg/L. The iron concentration of human milk is also variable between days and between individuals. The IOM used the average iron content of human milk and an average intake of

human milk (0.78 L/day) to determine the AI of 0.27 mg/day for full-term healthy breastfed infants through 6 months of age (Table 19.1).[31] The IOM recommendations, however, do not take into account at-risk infants born with a lower-than-usual iron endowment (Table 19.2).[4,32,33] It is important to identify low fetal iron status, because infants born with low iron endowment and breastfed exclusively until 4 months of age were at much higher risk for developing ID before 6 months.[34]

In addition to other benefits, the Neonatal Resuscitation Program of the AAP and American Heart Association, in addition to the American College of Obstetricians and Gynecologists,[35] recommend delayed cord clamping or placental transfusion at nearly all births to improve erythrocyte iron endowment and, thus, both short- and long-term iron status in infancy.[36] Delaying cord clamping may also improve neurocognitive development at school age.[37] A number of studies have shown that exclusively breastfed infants supplemented with iron before 6 months of age exhibit higher Hb concentrations compared with unsupplemented infants at 6 months of age.[38,39] Iron supplementation also resulted in improved visual acuity and higher Bayley psychomotor developmental indices by 13 months of age.[38] Infant iron supplementation between 6 and 9 months improved 9-month motor scores more than maternal iron supplementation during pregnancy alone.[40] Such findings support the AAP recommendation that all exclusively breastfed term infants receive iron supplementation of 1 mg/kg/day elemental iron starting at 4 months of age using either iron drops or iron-containing multivitamin drops that also provide vitamin D.[4] Such supplementation should continue until appropriate iron-containing complementary foods are introduced.[4] For partially breastfed infants, the proportion of human milk versus formula is uncertain. Therefore, the AAP recommends that infants receiving more than half of their daily feedings as human milk and who are not receiving iron-containing complementary foods should also receive 1 mg/kg/day of supplemental iron beginning at 4 months of age to help prevent breastfeeding infants from developing ID (see AAP text box).[4]

For infants 7 to 12 months of age, the RDA for iron is 11 mg/day[31] (Table 19.1), as determined by a factorial approach that calculated iron losses, iron requirements for growth (increased blood volume, tissue mass), and storage iron. The disjuncture that occurs when contrasting to 0.27 mg/day to 11 mg/day by 6 months of age results from the very different methods of determining these values (see Table 19.1). Other recommendations in resource-rich countries ranged from 6.9 to 11 mg/day on the basis of different levels of iron

Table 19.2.
Risk Factors and Presentation of ID

Age Group	Medical Risk Factors	Dietary Risk Factors	Clinical Presentations
Newborns and infants up to 12 mo	Prematurity, IUGR, SGA, LGA, twin, maternal diabetes, maternal obesity, immediate cord clamping, milk protein allergy, ethnic minority (especially Mexican American), low socioeconomic status, PPI or H2 acid blockers, lead exposure	Exclusive breastfeeding for 4 months, early cow milk	Sleep disturbance, irritability, breath holding spells, febrile seizures
Toddlers 1 through 3 y	Rapid growth, lead exposure, cows milk protein allergy, PPI or H2 acid blockers	Excessive cow milk, autism or developmental delay with restrictive diet	Sleep disturbance, RLS/PLMD, pica, irritability, decreased energy, pallor
4 through 8 y	Family history, PPI or H2 acid blockers, renal failure	Obesity, vegetarian or restricted diet (especially in autism/developmental delay)	RLS/PLMD, pica, fatigue, dizziness, irritability, poor concentration, cold hands/feet, headache

Age	Medical risk factors	Dietary risk factors	Symptoms
9 through 13 y	Gastrointestinal risk factors (inflammatory bowel disease, *Helicobacter pylori* infection, PPI or H2 acid blockers), menstrual blood loss (early menarche, heavy menstrual bleeding and/or abnormal uterine bleeding), family history, renal failure	Obesity, vegetarian or restricted diet (especially in autism/developmental delay or in menstruating girls)	Pica, fatigue, dizziness, palpitations, poor exercise tolerance, headache, poor concentration, cold hands/feet, RLS
14 through 18 y	Menstrual blood loss (heavy menstrual bleeding and/or abnormal uterine bleeding), gastrointestinal risk factors (inflammatory bowel disease, *H pylori* infection, PPI or H2 acid blockers), high endurance athletes (long-distance runners, athlete's anemia), renal failure, family history, blood donors, bariatric surgery	Obesity, vegetarian or restricted diet (especially in autism/developmental delay, eating disorder or in menstruating girls)	Pica, fatigue, dizziness, syncope, palpitations or tachycardia, poor exercise tolerance, headache, poor concentration, cold hands/feet, RLS

H2 indicates histamine 2 acid blockers; IUGR, intrauterine growth restriction; LGA, large for gestational age; PPI, proton pump inhibitor; RLS, restless leg syndrome; SGA, small for gestational age.

AAP

AAP Recommendations for Diagnosis and Prevention of Iron Deficiency and Iron-Deficiency Anemia in Infants and Young Children (0-3 Years of Age)

1. Full-term, healthy infants have sufficient iron for at least the first 4 months of life. Human milk contains very little iron. Exclusively breastfed infants are at increasing risk of ID after 4 completed months of age. Therefore, at 4 months of age, breastfed infants should be supplemented with 1 mg/kg/day of oral iron beginning at 4 months of age until appropriate iron-containing complementary foods (including iron-fortified cereals) are introduced in the diet (see Table 19.1). For partially breastfed infants, the proportion of human milk versus formula is uncertain; therefore, beginning at 4 months of age, partially breastfed infants (more than half of their daily feedings as human milk) who are not receiving iron-containing complementary foods should also receive 1 mg/kg/day of supplemental iron.

2. For formula-fed infants, the iron needs for the first 12 months of life can be met by a standard infant formula (iron content, 10-12 mg/dL) and the introduction of iron-containing complementary foods after 4 to 6 months of age, including iron-fortified cereals (Appendix K). Whole milk should not be used before 12 completed months of age.

3. The iron intake between 6 and 12 months of age should be 11 mg/day. When infants are given complementary foods, red meat and vegetables with higher iron content should be introduced early (Appendix K). To augment the iron supply, liquid iron supplements are appropriate if iron needs are not being met by the intake of formula and complementary foods.

4. Toddlers 1 through 3 years of age should have an intake of iron intake of 7 mg/day. This would be best delivered by eating red meats, cereals fortified with iron, vegetables that contain iron, and fruits with vitamin C, which augments the absorption of iron (Appendix K). For toddlers not receiving this iron intake, liquid supplements are suitable for children 12 through 36 months of age, and chewable multivitamins can be used for children 3 years and older.

5. All preterm infants should have an intake of iron of at least 2 mg/kg/day through 12 months of age, which is the amount of iron supplied by iron-fortified formulas. Preterm infants fed human milk should receive an iron supplement of 2 mg/kg/day by 1 month of age, and this should be continued until the infant is weaned to iron-fortified formula or begins eating complementary foods that supply the 2 mg/kg of iron. An exception to this practice would include infants who have received an iron load from multiple transfusions of packed red blood cells during their hospitalization.

AAP

6. Universal screening for anemia should be performed at approximately 12 months of age with determination of Hb concentration and an assessment of risk factors associated with ID/IDA. These risk factors would include low socioeconomic status (especially children of Mexican American descent [Table 19.2]), a history of prematurity or low birth weight, exposure to lead, exclusive breastfeeding beyond 4 months of age without supplemental iron, and weaning to whole milk or complementary foods that do not include iron-fortified cereals or foods naturally rich in iron (Appendix K). Additional at-risk factors are feeding problems, poor growth, and inadequate nutrition, typically seen in infants with special health care needs. For infants and toddlers (1 through 3 years of age), additional screening can be performed at any time if there is a risk of ID/IDA, including inadequate dietary iron intake.

7. If Hb concentration is less than 11.0 mg/dL at 12 months of age, then further evaluation for IDA is required to rule this out as a cause of anemia (See Table 19.4). If there is a high risk of dietary iron deficiency as described in recommendation 6, then further testing for ID should be performed, given the potential adverse effects on neurodevelopmental outcomes. Additional screening tests for ID or IDA should include:
   - SF and CRP; or
   - CHr

8. If a child has mild anemia (Hb 10-11 mg/dL) and can be closely monitored, an alternative method of diagnosis would be to document a 1 g/dL increase in plasma Hb concentration after 1 month of appropriate iron replacement therapy, especially if the history indicates that the diet is likely to be iron deficient.

9. Use of the TfR1 assay as screening for ID is promising, and the AAP supports the development of TfR1 standards for use of this assay in infants and children.

10. If IDA (or any anemia) or ID has been confirmed by history and laboratory evidence, a means of carefully tracking and following infants and toddlers with a diagnosis of ID/IDA should be implemented. Electronic health records could be used not only to generate reminder messages to screen for IDA and ID at 12 months of age but also to document that IDA and ID have been adequately treated once diagnosed.

Pediatrics. 2010;126(5):1040-1050

bioavailability.[41] Infants in the second 6 months of life do not need iron supplementation if receiving adequate amounts of iron from iron-containing formula, iron-fortified cereals, or appropriate amounts of iron-rich complementary foods (see Appendix K, and AAP text box).[4] Meats containing heme iron should be encouraged, given its better bioavailability and improved enteral absorption (20% to 35%) than iron in fruits and vegetables.

Healthy full-term, formula-fed infants do not need additional iron. For the last 20 years, standard infant formulas in the United States have contained 12 mg of iron/L, higher than in other countries. This amount was calculated to supply all of the exogenous iron requirements of a normal formula-fed full-term infant for the first year of life. Because a normal infant has iron sources other than formula (especially cereal and meats), the 12 mg/L iron formula appears to supply more iron than is necessary.[5] Concerns have been expressed that this amount of iron may have associated risks; however, the AAP has concluded that infant formula containing 12 mg of elemental iron/L is safe for its intended use.[4] Although some concerns are expressed about linear growth in iron-replete infants receiving additional iron, no published studies have convincingly documented decreased linear growth in iron-replete infants receiving formulas containing high amounts of iron.[42] Evidence is also insufficient to associate formulas containing 12 mg of iron/L with gastrointestinal tract symptoms. At least 4 studies found no adverse effects.[43-46]

Reports have conflicted on whether excess iron fortification is associated with increased risk of infection in higher-income, temperate climates. Decreased incidence, increased incidence, and no change in number of infections have all been reported.[45,47] A systematic review concluded that "iron supplementation has no apparent harmful effect on the overall incidence of infectious illnesses in children," although risk of developing diarrhea increases slightly.[48] On the other hand, observations studies in children have shown that iron-deficient individuals have defective immune function, particularly T-lymphocyte immunity.[49-52] These observations in children are supported by animal studies showing lower T-lymphocyte numbers and reduced proportion of mature T-lymphocytes, with inhibition of cytokine secretion.[2] Thus, the relationship between iron and the immune system is complicated.

After 12 months of age, children can begin consuming cow milk, but intake should be limited to 16 ounces or less per day and preferably given in a cup in lieu of a bottle. Intake of iron-fortified infant cereals substantially improves daily iron intake above those not normally consuming cereal.[53]

Iron contained in wet-packed cereals with fruit was equally well absorbed as medicinal iron in infants.[54]

Preterm Infants

Accretion of iron occurs predominantly in the last 3 months of intrauterine life; therefore, preterm infants lack sufficient iron. This iron deficit increases with decreasing gestational age. Late preterm or low birth weight infants also do not have the full fetal iron endowment. Delaying umbilical cord clamping or placental transfusion is highly recommended when possible in these infants.[55] In addition to preterm birth, factors that further impede iron endowment at birth include intrauterine growth restriction, maternal anemia, hypertension, obesity, and diabetes, common diagnoses in mothers' of preterm infants. Postnatal events can also affect an infant's iron status, including frequent blood sampling, which can further deplete body iron. The use of erythropoietin or erythrocyte-stimulating agents to avoid transfusions can also dramatically increase the need for exogenous iron. On the other hand, sick preterm infants frequently receive multiple blood transfusions, an excellent source of iron. Delaying umbilical cord clamping in preterm infants may improve neonatal physiology and iron status, in addition to decreasing the numbers of postnatal transfusions in the neonatal intensive care unit (see AAP text box).[56,57] Identifying which preterm infants are at risk for ID and how much and how the iron should be supplied is challenging because of the individual variations in iron requirements of preterm infants, which makes establishing recommendations difficult. The AAP and European Society for Pediatric Gastroenterology, Hepatology and Nutrition have recommended that all preterm infants be provided an intake of iron of at least 2 mg/kg/day through 12 months of age, which is the amount of iron supplied by iron-fortified formulas.[4,58] Early iron supplementation in preterm infants resulted in improved iron indices and did not impact linear growth.[59] Although neurocognitive sequelae of ID is of concern, a meta-analysis of 15 studies in low birth weight infants included only 2 reporting neurocognitive outcomes, and no difference in these outcomes was found.[59] Despite feeding iron-containing formulas, 14% of preterm infants still develop ID between 4 and 8 months of age.[60] Preterm infants fed human milk should receive an iron supplement of 2 mg/kg/day by 1 month of age, and this should be continued until infants are weaned to iron-fortified formula or consume complementary foods that supply 2 mg/kg/day of iron. A potential exception may be those iron loaded from multiple transfusions during their hospitalization.[4] Because of this, preterm infants may benefit from a personalized approach, monitoring serum ferritin and other iron indices at 1 and 6 months, especially when fed human milk.

Toddlers 1 Through 3 Years of Age

Toddlers 1 through 3 years of age should have an iron intake of 7 mg/day (Table 19.1).[31] Toddlers go through many dietary changes that affect their iron status. In their transition from "infant food" to more adult-like food, they leave behind iron-fortified formula and cereal, but they potentially gain a variety of iron-containing foods, such as meats and some vegetables, which should be encouraged (see Appendix K). Fruits containing vitamin C, which augments iron absorption, should also be encouraged. Many toddlers are picky eaters and their food choices may select against iron-rich foods. Given the diet variability within this age group, the iron status of toddlers is often difficult to predict. Historical, medical, and dietary risk factors, as well as certain clinical presentations should be considered in decisions to evaluate (Table 19.2).[4] For example, pica, an intense craving to eat, lick, or chew nonfood items (ie, dirt, rocks, paper, baby wipes, or cardboard), is highly associated with ID. Because of such diet variability, the AAP recommends universal screening of toddlers for ID at approximately 12 months of age, with repeat screening at 18 months of age or older in the presence of dietary risk factors, such as excessive cow milk intake.[4] All children treated should be followed closely until resolution of ID or IDA (see AAP text box).

ID and lead poisoning are associated morbidities in this age group (Table 19.2). Children with IDA have enhanced lead absorption, because lead substitutes for iron in the duodenal divalent metal transporter and because of poorer physiological lead chelation in the gut. Correction of ID limits lead absorption and restores the response to chelation. Thus, primary ID prevention could reduce the risk of lead intoxication and neurotoxicity as well.[61] For toddlers not receiving the recommended 7 mg/day of iron or who are at increased risk of ID, liquid iron supplements or multivitamins with iron are suitable for children 12 to 36 months of age, and chewable vitamins can be used for children 3 years and older (Table 19.3).[4] It is important to note, however, that many gummy or jelly vitamins do not contain iron, making it important to read labels. In gummy or jelly multivitamins containing iron, however, risk for accidental iron overdose is high, and care should be taken to ensure child-safe storage.

School-Aged Children: 4 Through 8 Years of Age

In young school-aged children, iron-containing foods (Appendix K), as part of a well-balanced diet, should be promoted by providers and caregivers

Table 19.3.

Oral Iron Preparations for Children

Compound	Trade Name	Formulation	Compound Quantity	Elemental Iron (mg)	Other Ingredients
	Fer-in-sol	Drops	75 mg/1 mL	15 mg/1 mL	0.2% alcohol, sugar, sorbitol
	Ferrous Sulfate (generic)	Drops	15 mg/1 mL	15 mg/1 mL	0.2% alcohol, sorbitol
	Ferrous Sulfate (generic)	Elixir	220 mg/5 mL	44 mg/5 mL	5% alcohol
	MyKidz Iron 10	Drop	75 mg/1.5 mL	15 mg/1.5 mL	No alcohol, dye, or sugar
Ferrous Sulfate	Feosol	Tablet	324 mg	65 mg	
	Slow-Fe	Slow-release tablet	142 mg	45 mg	
Ferrous Gluconate	Fergon	Tablet	240 mg	27 mg	
	Nature's Way Iron	Tablet	160 mg	18 mg	
	Whole Foods Chelated Iron (Ferrous Bisglycinate)	Liquid	10 mg/5 mL	10 mg/5 mL	Herbs, but alcohol free
Ferrous Fumarate	Ircon	Tablet	200 mg	66 mg	
	Ferretts	Tablet	325 mg	106 mg	
	Ferrocite	Tablet	324 mg	106 mg	

Continued

IV

Table 19.3. *Continued*
Oral Iron Preparations for Children

Compound	Trade Name	Formulation	Compound Quantity	Elemental Iron (mg)	Other Ingredients
Iron Complex Polysaccharide	NovaFerrum	Drop	50 mg/mL	15 mg/1 mL	Both products free of alcohol, sugar, dye, and gluten; Kosher and vegan verified
	NovaFerrum 125	Elixir		125 mg/5 mL	
	NovaFerrum	Capsule		50 mg	Kosher
	Nu-Iron 150	Capsule	219 mg	150 mg	
	Ferrex Forte	Capsule	219 mg	150 mg	Folic acid, vitamin B_{12}
Chelated Iron		Liquid			
Upspring Bab Iron+Immunity		Liquid			
Carbonyl Iron	Feosol Carbonyl	Drop	50 mg/mL	15 mg/1 mL	
	NutriPure Chewable Iron with Vitamin C	Tablet melt	18 mg for children 4+ years	18 mg for children 4+ years	Stevia leaf extract, xylitol, mannitol
	Enfamil Poly-Vi-Sol with iron (Ferrous Sulfate)	Drop	15 mg/mL	15 mg/1 mL	Vitamins A, D, and E, and B vitamins
	Upspring Baby Iron+Immunity (Ferric Glycinate)	Liquid	10 mg/5 mL	15 mg/ 5 mL	Vitamins A, C, D, and E; B vitamins; zinc

Multivitamin + Iron					
	Zarbees Naturals Multivitamin +Fe (Ferrous Gluconate)	Liquid			Vitamins A, C, D, and E, and B vitamins Contains xylitol
	NovaFerum Pediatric Multivitamin with Iron (Iron Polysaccharide)	Liquid	10 mg/mL	10 mg/mL	Vitamins A, D, and E and B vitamins Free of alcohol, sugar, dye, and gluten; Kosher and vegan verified
	Flintstone's Chewable Multivitamin with Iron (Ferrous Fumarate)	½ tablet for children 2 and 3 years old, 1 tablet for 4+ years	18 mg	9 mg for children 2 and 3 years old or 18 mg for 4+ years	Vitamins A, D, and E, and B vitamins Contains fructose, sorbitol, artificial flavors
	Rite Aid Chewable (Ferrous Fumarate)	½ tablet for children 2 and 3 years old, 1 tablet for 4+ years	18 mg	9 mg for children 2 and 3 years old or 18 mg for 4+ years	Vitamins A, D, and E, and B vitamins Contains orbitol, mannitol, monoglycerides and diglycerides
	Nature's Plus Iron +C +Herbs Chewable (amino acid chelate complex)	1/2 tablet	27 mg	13.5 mg for children (1/2 tablet)	Vitamin C Contains fructose, rose hips, beet, raspberry

Continued

IV

Table 19.3. *Continued*

Oral Iron Preparations for Children

Compound	Trade Name	Formulation	Compound Quantity	Elemental Iron (mg)	Other Ingredients
	BellyBar Prenatal Vitamin (Iron reduced from Pentacarbonyl)	1 chewable tablet	13.5 mg/tablet	1 tablet for children, 2 tablets for pregnant women	Vitamins A, C, D, and E, and B vitamins, calcium, zinc
Multivitamin + Iron *Continued*	Vitamin Friends Vegetarian gummies (Ferrous fumarate)	1 gummy	15 mg	15 mg	Vitamin C and B vitamins, zinc Sugar cane, glucose, citrus pectin, black carrot; risk for accidental overdose with candy-like quality
	Navitco NutriBear Iron Vegetarian Jellies (Ferrous fumarate)	1 bear	5 mg	5 mg	Vitamin C, folate, vitamin B_{12} Sucrose, glucose, citrus pectin, natural flavors: risk for accidental overdose with candy-like quality

with the goal of achieving an iron intake of 10 mg per day.[17] Prevalence of ID and IDA is significantly less in this age group compared with young children but is more common in combination with certain historical, medical, or dietary risk factors (Table 19.2). Therefore, children in this age group who develop ID or IDA warrant not only a full dietary review but also assessment of overall growth, illnesses, and potential gastrointestinal blood loss. If anemia or ID is suspected, screening for both ID and IDA should be performed (see "Screening for ID and IDA" below). In addition to addressing the underlying etiology (diet versus blood loss), ID should be treated with therapeutic iron supplementation and followed closely until resolution.

School-Aged Children: 9 Through 13 Years of Age

Older school-aged children and adolescents have increasing discretion in food selection and may consume more than half of their food outside of the home (ie, snacks/meals at school or extracurricular activities as well as meals on the go). These factors result in decreased supervision of meal content and quality, thereby increasing the risk of restricted diets and poorer nutritional choices (see also Chapter 8: Adolescent Nutrition). Iron needs in this group are heterogeneous because of variability in growth spurts, which result in increased Hb and muscle mass, as well as menstrual blood loss in girls with the onset of menarche. In general, children 9 through 13 years of age should receive approximately 8 mg/day of iron (Table 19.1), and foods with high iron content should be encouraged (Appendix K).

Increased iron demands may exceed dietary iron availability and deplete iron stores. Therefore, any adolescent with poor diet, restricted dietary behaviors (ie, vegetarian, vegan), or pica (ie, paper, starch, ice), as well as girls with early menarche, especially those who are obese, should be screened for ID. Age-specific historical, medical, and dietary risks should be considered (Table 19.2). Dietary modifications should be initiated, in addition to oral iron therapy. Girls with excessive menstrual blood loss resulting in ID or IDA should have hormonal therapy recommended to minimize future blood loss until successful iron replacement therapy. All children should be followed until resolution of IDA, including normalization of iron stores.

Adolescents: 14 Through 18 Years of Age

As in preadolescence, iron needs in older adolescents must account for basal losses, increased Hb and muscle mass, and menstrual blood loss in girls. Lifestyle and variations in food preferences, including alternative diets or missed meals, may also occur (see Chapter 8: Adolescent Nutrition).

Recommended iron intake for this age group is 11 mg for males and 15 mg for females (Table 19.1). Nutritious diets with regular meals including iron-rich foods should be encouraged (Appendix K). Any adolescent with a restricted diet, inconsistent eating patterns, or symptoms of pica should be screened for ID and IDA. Young women with heavy menstrual bleeding or abnormal uterine bleeding, particularly within the first 2 years after menarche, and those who are obese should also be considered for screening. Age-specific historical, medical, and dietary risks should be considered (Table 19.2). Once identified, the underlying etiology for the IDA should be addressed and iron replacement therapy should be initiated and followed until resolution. In addition to poor concentration and fatigue, several other neurologic and sleep conditions have been associated with ID, particularly in the adolescent age group. Pediatric RLS, a disorder that results in the urge to move the legs, typically accompanied by uncomfortable and unpleasant sensations, has been strongly associated with ID.[12,62] Likewise, periodic limb movement disorder (PLMD), which is characterized by repetitive, stereotyped movements involving the lower limbs resulting in sleep disturbance, is associated with ID. Patients with both RLS and PLMD receiving iron therapy have reported subsequent improved symptom management.[63,64] Both RLS and PLMD can have a strong family predominance, and as such, genome-wide association studies found a total of 4 single nucleotide polymorphisms that conferred increased risk for RLS or PLMD, 1 of which on chromosome 6 that also confers greater risk for developing ID. At least 1 study has found that children with neurally mediated syncope (ie, simple faint), the most common type of syncope in pediatrics, had a higher prevalence of ID compared with children with other forms of syncope.[65] Adolescents with postural tachycardia syndrome, an autonomic disorder of orthostatic tolerance, also have higher prevalence of ID and anemia compared with the typical US pediatric population and may have symptomatic improvement with iron therapy.[66]

Screening for ID and IDA

ID progresses through 3 phases: iron depletion, iron restricted-erythropoiesis, and finally, frank IDA. Severe anemia resulting from long-standing ID may require emergency medical care. However, even mild ID without anemia warrants identification and appropriate treatment given the potential neurocognitive impact. Although no single laboratory test can definitively diagnose ID or IDA, many laboratory tests are available and can confirm the diagnosis when assessed in combination and within the context of a child's clinical presentation and history (Table 19.4). From a complete blood cell (CBC) count, a microcytic anemia demonstrated by a low Hb and mean corpuscular volume (MCV) in combination with an elevated red cell distribution width (RDW) is most consistent with IDA. In the absence of anemia, the reticulocyte Hb content (CHr) obtained with many automated hematology analyzers, is the first peripheral blood marker that becomes abnormal in ID by identifying iron deficient reticulocytes. Serum ferritin is the most commonly used iron measure to determine overall body iron stores.

Ideally, initial screening should be performed with a full CBC. If an isolated point-of-care Hb is used to identify anemia, a full CBC and/or serum ferritin should then be obtained to confirm the presence of a microcytic

Table 19.4.

Measurement of Iron Status

Parameter	Iron Overload	Depleted Iron Stores (Stage I)	ID Without Anemia (Stage II)	IDA (Stage III)	Anemia of Inflammation
SF	↑	↓	↓	↓↓	↑↑
Transferrin saturation	↑↑	Normal	↓	↓	↓
TfR1	↓	↑	↑↑	↑↑↑	↑↑↑
CHr	Normal	Normal	↓	↓	↓
Hemoglobin	Normal	Normal	Normal	↓	↓
MCV	Normal	Normal	Normal	↓	↓
ZnPP/H	Normal	Normal	↓	↓	↓
Plasma Hepcidin[a]	↑	Normal	↓	↓	↑

Modified from Tussing-Humphreys, 2012.

CHr, reticulocyte hemoglobin content; MCV, mean corpuscular volume; SF, serum ferritin; ZnPP/H, Zinc protoporhyrin/heme.

[a] Clinical availability limited in US to 1 reference laboratory, but potentially available soon.

anemia and low stores, which confirms the diagnosis of IDA. Serum ferritin is an acute-phase reactant and may be elevated in patients with anemia associated with inflammation or in obesity (Table 19.4). Thus, in patients with an acute or chronic inflammation, assessment of concomitant C-reactive protein can be considered to determine whether inflammation is contributing to the anemia. Other specific tests for measuring iron status include: transferrin saturation (calculated value of serum iron over total iron binding capacity), the serum or soluble transferrin receptor 1 (sTfR1) concentration, zinc protoporphyrin/heme ratio, and plasma hepcidin (Table 19.4).

Historical recommendations established cutoff values for iron screening in children as Hb of 11.0 g/dL and serum ferritin of 10 to 12 µg/L.[4] However, recent data in 1257 children at 6 to 36 months of age show that the inflection point for Hb plotted against serum ferritin was at Hb of 12.1 g/dL and serum ferritin of 17.9 µg/L.[67] A Hb level of 11.0 g/dL was associated with extremely low serum ferritin (2.4-4.6 µg/L) in these young children.[67] Recent work also shows that capillary Hb values measured by point-of-care instrument readings in toddlers were numerically higher and suboptimal in assessing anemia compared with venous blood collected simultaneously and assay by standard instrumentation.[68] Capillary samples and point-of-care machines are not well studied in older children. Specific newer data about how to screen for ID in older children are limited, but using other measures of erythrocyte iron (erythrocyte protoporphyrin, zinc protoporphyrin/heme ratio, or reticulocyte Hb content) may be more effective than Hb and traditional erythrocyte indices in this population, even in anemia of chronic disease.[69-72] Development of age-based reference intervals for these newer biomarkers is needed.[73]

Iron Therapy

Oral Iron Therapy

In children in whom ID or IDA has been identified, therapeutic iron replacement should be initiated. Although ideal for supplementation and prevention, multivitamins containing iron (Table 19.3) **should not** be used for the treatment of ID and IDA. Many formulations of therapeutic oral iron are available (Table 19.3). At least 1 randomized clinical trial in 80 young children demonstrated that ferrous sulfate was more effective in improving the Hb concentration over 12 weeks compared with iron polysaccharide complex, although both groups demonstrated improvement.[74] The recommended dosing range varies widely from 3 to 6 mg/kg/day, yet low-dose iron (3 mg/kg elemental iron administered once daily) has demonstrated efficacy even in patients with moderate to severe IDA.[75,76] Several studies in adults also suggest that low-dose therapy is effective therapy while minimizing adverse effects and improving adherence.[77–79] Thus, 60 to 120 mg/day of elemental iron (1 to 2 tablets), administered once daily, in older children should be effective.[4]

Treatment Response

Follow-up should occur *in all* patients to ensure appropriate response (see AAP text box). In children with mild anemia, the Hb should increase by at least 1 g/dL within 4 weeks, or approximately 1 month, of beginning therapy. In contrast, for children with moderate to severe anemia (Hb <9 g/dL), an increase of 1 g/dL should occur within the first 2 weeks. After ensuring an appropriate initial response, all patients should be reassessed at approximately 3 months after initiating therapy. Providers may consider assessing a serum ferritin in addition to a CBC to ensure that iron is replenished in addition to resolution of anemia. If oral iron is discontinued prior to normalizing iron stores, the patient is at risk of recurrent IDA.

The most common reason for oral iron failure is nonadherence to therapy or intolerance because of adverse effects.[80] Such effects are primarily gastrointestinal and may include nausea, vomiting, abdominal pain, diarrhea, and/or constipation. However, a randomized controlled trial of oral iron versus placebo in young children with IDA found no difference in reported adverse effects,[81,82] and a systematic analysis of gastrointestinal adverse effects in infants receiving iron-fortified formula found no significant difference between groups.[43] Regardless, some reports suggest that adverse gastrointestinal effects may be lessened by treatment with low dose oral iron therapy, as recommended above. Another reason for failure is insufficient dosage, using supplemental amounts instead of treatment dosing.[80]

Alternative and Herbal Oral Iron Supplements

Many newer iron supplements on the market advertise less preservatives and colorings, are Kosher, and use natural flavorings (Table 19.3). These may be more acceptable to families who wish to avoid artificial ingredients. Alternative strategies, although not well studied in pregnancy and childhood, include multiherbal preparations containing stinging nettle and beet juice because they have high iron content.[83] However, iron content in these plants varies based on soil iron content and processing, and the iron is poorly bioavailable. If estimated dosages of these remedies are sufficiently high to meet iron needs, then concerns for developing toxicity from other herbal components are high. Iron ingots shaped like fish (Lucky Iron Fish) used in cooking water have been studied in women from Southeast Asia and have been effective[84] and are without heavy metal contamination.[85] However, these have not been studied in children. Beef liver heme concentrates have also been used as nutritional supplements, but these remedies contain large amounts of vitamin B_{12} that are potentially toxic.

Intravenous Iron Therapy

Initial formulations of intravenous iron in the mid-20th century resulted in high rates of serious adverse effects, including anaphylaxis, which limited its use. Iron formulations developed since 2000 have improved safety profiles and also allow for greater doses of iron to be administered over shorter infusions. Thus, in children who have failed oral iron therapy, intravenous iron therapy is an alternative treatment option. Children with complex medical conditions, significant dietary restrictions, dependence on total parental nutrition, inflammatory bowel disease, short gut syndrome, other chronic inflammatory conditions, or recurrent blood loss may also benefit from intravenous iron therapy in lieu of oral iron.[86] Although adult literature on the safety and efficacy of intravenous iron is extensive, data in children are limited. Yet, several published studies have demonstrated efficacy of various intravenous iron formulations (iron sucrose, low-molecular weight iron dextran, and ferric carboxymaltose) in diverse groups of children and adolescents with ID and IDA.[87–90] Table 19.5 lists the current intravenous iron formulations available in the United States. Although the risk of serious adverse effects is very low with intravenous iron therapy, administration should be performed at a center with experience in its administration, often a pediatric hematology center, and staff to provide appropriate care in the event of an adverse event, including early recognition and management of anaphylaxis.[91]

Summary

Despite a decline in prevalence, IDA remains the most common hematologic condition in the world.[2] Because of the effects of ID on neurodevelopment in young children as well as concentration and learning in adolescents, it is imperative that providers carefully assess all patients for ID risk factors. Routine iron supplementation or fortification for infants

Table 19.5.
Intravenous Iron Preparations Approved in the United States

Generic Name	Trade Name	FDA Indication (Adult)	FDA Approved (Pediatrics)	Pediatric Dosing per Infusion (Max Dose)	Infusion Time	Test Dose Required	Black Box Warning	Iron Concentration
Ferric gluconate	Ferrlecit	Patients with chronic kidney disease on dialysis + erythropoiesis-stimulating agents	Yes, >6 y		60 minutes	No	No	12.5 mg/mL
Iron sucrose	Venofer	Patients with chronic kidney disease	Yes, >2 y		2-5 minutes	No	No	20 mg/mL
Low-molecular weight iron dextran	INFeD	Patients in whom oral iron administration is unsatisfactory or impossible	Yes, >4 mo		60 minutes	Yes	Yes	50 mg/mL
Ferumxytol	Feraheme	Patients with chronic kidney disease	No		15-60 minutes	No	Yes	30 mg/mL
Ferric Carboxy-maltose	Injectafer	Patients with intolerance or unsatisfactory response to oral iron; nondialysis-dependent chronic kidney disease	No	15 mg/kg (750 mg)	60 minutes	No	No	50 mg/mL

IV

until 12 months of age is recommended. Cow milk should not be introduced before 12 months. Children beyond 12 months of age should have limited cow milk intake and appropriate iron-rich foods incorporated within the diet. School-aged children and adolescents have increased iron requirements during rapid periods of growth. They are also at risk for ID because of inconsistent dietary habits. In adolescent girls, the potential for excessive blood loss should also result in a low threshold for screening. Point-of-care Hb testing has limited value in initial screening. Initial screening, ideally with a CBC with erythrocyte indices and serum ferritin, should be followed with appropriate identification of the underlying etiology and initiation of iron replacement therapy at therapeutic dosing. Low-dose iron therapy (3 mg/kg once daily) minimizes adverse effects and may improve adherence. All patients receiving iron therapy should be followed until resolution, which typically requires a minimum of 3 months of therapy. Finally, newer intravenous iron preparations can be considered in patients who fail or are intolerant to oral iron therapy but should be administered under the supervision of a treatment center with expertise in the use of intravenous iron for the treatment of IDA.

References

1. Cappellini MD, Comin-Colet J, de Francisco A, et al. Iron deficiency across chronic inflammatory conditions: International expert opinion on definition, diagnosis, and management. *Am J Hematol.* Oct 2017;92(10):1068–1078

2. Musallam KM, Taher AT. Iron deficiency beyond erythropoiesis: should we be concerned? *Curr Med Res Opin.* Jan 2018;34(1):81–93

3. WHO. WHO Micronutrient Deficiencies: IDA. 2017. Accessed July 13, 2017

4. Baker RD, Greer FR. Diagnosis and prevention of iron deficiency and iron-deficiency anemia in infants and young children (0-3 years of age). *Pediatrics.* Nov 2010;126(5):1040–1050

5. Gupta PM, Perrine CG, Mei Z, Scanlon KS. Iron, Anemia, and Iron Deficiency Anemia among Young Children in the United States. *Nutrients.* May 30 2016;8(6)

6. Sekhar DL, Kunselman AR, Chuang CH, Paul IM. Optimizing hemoglobin thresholds for detection of iron deficiency among reproductive-age women in the United States. *Transl Res.* Feb 2017;180:68–76

7. Lozoff B, Beard J, Connor J, Felt BT, Georgieff M, Challert T. Long-lasting neural and behavioral effects of iron deficiency in infancy. *Nutr Rev.* 2006;64:S34–S43

8. Bruner AB, Joffe A, Duggan AK, Casella JF, Brandt J. Randomised study of cognitive effects of iron supplementation in non-anaemic iron-deficient adolescent girls. *Lancet.* Oct 12 1996;348(9033):992–996

9. McCann JC, Ames BN. An overview of evidence for a causal relation between iron deficiency during development and deficits in cognitive or behavioral function. *Am J Clin Nutr.* Apr 2007;85(4):931–945

10. Zhu YI, Haas JD. Iron depletion without anemia and physical performance in young women. *Am J Clin Nutr.* Aug 1997;66(2):334–341

11. Sharma R, Stanek JR, Koch TL, Grooms L, O'Brien SH. Intravenous iron therapy in non-anemic iron-deficient menstruating adolescent females with fatigue. *Am J Hematol.* Oct 2016;91(10):973–977

12. Dosman C, Witmans M, Zwaigenbaum L. Iron's role in paediatric restless legs syndrome - a review. *Paediatr Child Health.* Apr 2012;17(4):193–197

13. Sharp P, Srai SK. Molecular mechanisms involved in intestinal iron absorption. *World J Gastroenterol.* Sep 21 2007;13(35):4716–4724

14. Andrews NC. Forging a field: the golden age of iron biology. *Blood.* Jul 15 2008;112(2):219–230

15. Ganz T, Nemeth E. Iron metabolism: interactions with normal and disordered erythropoiesis. *Cold Spring Harb Perspect Med.* May 2012;2(5):a011668

16. Wang J, Pantopoulos K. Regulation of cellular iron metabolism. *Biochem J.* Mar 15 2011;434(3):365–381

17. O'Brien KO, Zavaleta N, Abrams SA, Caulfield LE. Maternal iron status influences iron transfer to the fetus during the third trimester of pregnancy. *Am J Clin Nutr.* Apr 2003;77(4):924–930

18. Rehu M, Punnonen K, Ostland V, et al. Maternal serum hepcidin is low at term and independent of cord blood iron status. *European journal of haematology.* Oct 2010;85(4):345–352

19. Dao MC, Sen S, Iyer C, Klebenov D, Meydani SN. Obesity during pregnancy and fetal iron status: is Hepcidin the link? *J Perinatol.* Mar 2013;33(3):177–181

20. Dosch NC, Guslits EF, Weber MB, et al. Maternal Obesity Affects Inflammatory and Iron Indices in Umbilical Cord Blood. *J Pediatr.* Mar 9 2016

21. Briana DD, Boutsikou T, Baka S, et al. Perinatal role of hepcidin and iron homeostasis in full-term intrauterine growth-restricted infants. *European journal of haematology.* Jan 2013;90(1):37–44

22. East P, Delker E, Lozoff B, Delva J, Castillo M, Gahagan S. Associations among infant iron deficiency, childhood emotion and attention regulation, and adolescent problem behaviors. *Child Dev in press.* 2017

23. Siddappa AJM, Rao RB, Wobken JD, et al. Iron deficiency alters iron regulatory protein and iron transport protein expression in perinatal rat brain. *Pediatr Res.* 2003;53:800–807

24. Georgieff MK. Long-term brain and behavioral consequences of early iron deficiency. *Nutr Rev.* Nov 2011;69 Suppl 1:S43–48

25. Falkingham M, Abdelhamid A, Curtis P, Fairweather-Tait S, Dye L, Hooper L. The effects of oral iron supplementation on cognition in older children and adults: a systematic review and meta-analysis. *Nutr J.* Jan 25 2010;9:4

IV

26. Pasricha SR, Hayes E, Kalumba K, Biggs BA. Effect of daily iron supplementation on health in children aged 4-23 months: a systematic review and meta-analysis of randomised controlled trials. *Lancet Glob Health.* Aug 2013;1(2):e77–e86

27. Wang B, Zhan S, Gong T, Lee L. Iron therapy for improving psychomotor development and cognitive function in children under the age of three with iron deficiency anaemia. *Cochrane Database Syst Rev.* Jun 06 2013(6):CD001444

28. Guo XM, Liu H, Qian J. Daily iron supplementation on cognitive performance in primary-school-aged children with and without anemia: a meta-analysis. *Int J Clin Exp Med.* 2015;8(9):16107–16111

29. Hermoso M, Vucic V, Vollhardt C, et al. The effect of iron on cognitive development and function in infants, children and adolescents: a systematic review. *Ann Nutr Metab.* 2011;59(2-4):154–165

30. Low M, Farrell A, Biggs BA, Pasricha SR. Effects of daily iron supplementation in primary-school-aged children: systematic review and meta-analysis of randomized controlled trials. *CMAJ.* Nov 19 2013;185(17):E791–802

31. IOM. Dietary Reference Intakes. 2017. Accessed July 13, 2017

32. Lozoff B, Kaciroti N, Walter T. Iron deficiency in infancy: applying a physiologic framework for prediction. *Am J Clin Nutr.* Dec 2006;84(6):1412–1421

33. Ru Y, Pressman EK, Cooper EM, et al. Iron deficiency and anemia are prevalent in women with multiple gestations. *Am J Clin Nutr.* Oct 2016;104(4):1052–1060

34. Ziegler EE, Nelson SE, Jeter JM. Iron stores of breastfed infants during the first year of life. *Nutrients.* May 21 2014;6(5):2023–2034

35. Committee Opinion No. 684 Summary: Delayed Umbilical Cord Clamping After Birth. *Obstet Gynecol.* Jan 2017;129(1):232–233

36. Andersson O, Hellstrom-Westas L, Andersson D, Domellof M. Effect of delayed versus early umbilical cord clamping on neonatal outcomes and iron status at 4 months: a randomised controlled trial. *BMJ.* Nov 15 2011;343:d7157

37. Andersson O, Lindquist B, Lindgren M, Stjernqvist K, Domellof M, Hellstrom-Westas L. Effect of Delayed Cord Clamping on Neurodevelopment at 4 Years of Age: A Randomized Clinical Trial. *JAMA Pediatr.* Jul 2015;169(7):631–638

38. Friel JK, Aziz K, Andrews WL, Harding SV, Courage ML, Adams RJ. A double-masked, randomized control trial of iron supplementation in early infantcy in healthy term breast-fed infants. *J Pediatr.* 2003;143:582–586

39. Dewey KG, Domellof M, Cohen RJ, Landa Rivera L, Hernell O, Lonnerdahl B. Iron supplementation affects growth and morbidity of breast-fed infants: Results of a randomized trial in Sweden and Honduras. *J Nutr.* 2002;132:3249–3255

40. Angulo-Barroso RM, Li M, Santos DC, et al. Iron Supplementation in Pregnancy or Infancy and Motor Development: A Randomized Controlled Trial. *Pediatrics.* Apr 2016;137(4)

41. Hernell O, Fewtrell MS, Georgieff MK, Krebs NF, Lonnerdal B. Summary of Current Recommendations on Iron Provision and Monitoring of Iron Status for Breastfed and Formula-Fed Infants in Resource-Rich and Resource-Constrained Countries. *J Pediatr.* Oct 2015;167(4 Suppl):S40–47

42. Iannotti LL, Tielsch JM, Black MM, Black RE. Iron supplementation in early childhood: health benefits and risks. *Am J Clin Nutr.* Dec 2006;84(6):1261–1276

43. Hyams JS, Treem WR, Etienne NL, et al. Effect of infant formula on stool characteristics of young infants. *Pediatrics.* Jan 1995;95(1):50–54

44. Bradley CK, Hillman L, Sherman AR, Leedy D, Cordano A. Evaluation of two iron-fortified, milk-based formulas during infancy. *Pediatrics.* May 1993;91(5): 908–914

45. Baqui AH, Zaman K, Persson LA, et al. Simultaneous weekly supplementation of iron and zinc is associated with lower morbidity due to diarrhea and acute lower respiratory infection in Bangladeshi infants. *J Nutr.* Dec 2003;133(12):4150–4157

46. Nelson SE, Ziegler EE, M CA, Edwards BB, Fomon SJ. Lack of adverse reactions to iron-fortified formula. *Pediatrics.* 1988;81:360–364

47. Murray MJ, Murray A, B, Murray NJ, Murray MB. The effect of iron status on Nigerien mothers on that of their infants at birth and 6 months, and on the concentration of Fe in breast milk. *Br J Nutr.* 1978;39:627–630

48. Gera T, Sachdev HS, Boy E. Effect of iron-fortified foods on hematologic and biological outcomes: systematic review of randomized controlled trials. *Am J Clin Nutr.* Aug 2012;96(2):309–324

49. Das I, Saha K, Mukhopadhyay D, et al. Impact of iron deficiency anemia on cell-mediated and humoral immunity in children: A case control study. *Journal of natural science, biology, and medicine.* Jan 2014;5(1):158–163

50. Hassan TH, Badr MA, Karam NA, et al. Impact of iron deficiency anemia on the function of the immune system in children. *Medicine (Baltimore).* Nov 2016;95(47):e5395

51. Galan P, Thibault H, Preziosi P, Hercberg S. Interleukin 2 production in iron-deficient children. *Biol Trace Elem Res.* Jan-Mar 1992;32:421–426

52. Drakesmith H, Prentice AM. Hepcidin and the iron-infection axis. *Science.* Nov 9 2012;338(6108):768–772

53. Finn K, Callen C, Bhatia J, Reidy K, Bechard LJ, Carvalho R. Importance of Dietary Sources of Iron in Infants and Toddlers: Lessons from the FITS Study. *Nutrients.* Jul 11 2017;9(7)

54. Ziegler EE, Nelson SE, Jeter JM. Iron status of breastfed infants is improved equally by medicinal iron and iron-fortified cereal. *The American journal of clinical nutrition.* Jul 2009;90(1):76–87

55. McDonald SJ, Middleton P, Dowswell T, Morris PS. Effect of timing of umbilical cord clamping of term infants on maternal and neonatal outcomes. *Cochrane Database Syst Rev.* Jul 11 2013(7):CD004074

56. Backes CH, Rivera BK, Haque U, et al. Placental transfusion strategies in very preterm neonates: a systematic review and meta-analysis. *Obstet Gynecol.* Jul 2014;124(1):47–56

57. Mercer JS, Erickson-Owens DA. Rethinking placental transfusion and cord clamping issues. *J Perinat Neonatal Nurs.* Jul-Sep 2012;26(3):202–217; quiz 218–209

58. Domellof M, Braegger C, Campoy C, et al. Iron requirements of infants and toddlers. *J Pediatr Gastroenterol Nutr.* Jan 2014;58(1):119–129

59. Long H, Yi JM, Hu PL, et al. Benefits of iron supplementation for low birth weight infants: a systematic review. *BMC Pediatr.* 2012;12:99

60. Griffin IJ, Cooke RJ, Reid MM, McCormick KP, Smith JS. Iron nutritional status in preterm infants fed formulas fortified with iron. *Arch Dis Child Fetal Neonatal Ed.* Jul 1999;81(1):F45–49

61. Canfield RL, Henderson CR, Jr., Cory-Slechta DA, Cox C, Jusko TA, Lanphear BP. Intellectual impairment in children with blood lead concentrations below 10 microg per deciliter. *N Engl J Med.* Apr 17 2003;348(16):1517–1526

62. Tilma J, Tilma K, Norregaard O, Ostergaard JR. Early childhood-onset restless legs syndrome: symptoms and effect of oral iron treatment. *Acta Paediatr.* May 2013;102(5):e221–226

63. Dye TJ, Jain SV, Simakajornboon N. Outcomes of long-term iron supplementation in pediatric restless legs syndrome/periodic limb movement disorder (RLS/PLMD). *Sleep Med.* Apr 2017;32:213–219

64. Grim K, Lee B, Sung AY, Kotagal S. Treatment of childhood-onset restless legs syndrome and periodic limb movement disorder using intravenous iron sucrose. *Sleep Med.* Nov 2013;14(11):1100–1104

65. Jarjour IT, Jarjour LK. Low iron storage in children and adolescents with neurally mediated syncope. *J Pediatr.* Jul 2008;153(1):40–44

66. Jarjour IT, Jarjour LK. Low iron storage and mild anemia in postural tachycardia syndrome in adolescents. *Clin Auton Res.* Aug 2013;23(4):175–179

67. Abdullah K, Birken CS, Maguire JL, et al. Re-Evaluation of Serum Ferritin Cut-Off Values for the Diagnosis of Iron Deficiency in Children Aged 12–36 Months. *J Pediatr.* Sep 2017;188:287–290

68. Boghani S, Mei Z, Perry GS, Brittenham GM, Cogswell ME. Accuracy of Capillary Hemoglobin Measurements for the Detection of Anemia among U.S. Low-Income Toddlers and Pregnant Women. *Nutrients.* Mar 9 2017;9(3)

69. Uijterschout L, Domellof M, Vloemans J, et al. The value of Ret-Hb and sTfR in the diagnosis of iron depletion in healthy, young children. *Eur J Clin Nutr.* Aug 2014;68(8):882–886

70. Davidkova S, Prestidge TD, Reed PW, Kara T, Wong W, Prestidge C. Comparison of reticulocyte hemoglobin equivalent with traditional markers of iron and erythropoiesis in pediatric dialysis. *Pediatr Nephrol.* May 2016;31(5):819–826

71. Mei Z, Flores-Ayala RC, Grummer-Strawn LM, Brittenham GM. Is Erythrocyte Protoporphyrin a Better Single Screening Test for Iron Deficiency Compared to Hemoglobin or Mean Cell Volume in Children and Women? *Nutrients.* May 31 2017;9(6)

72. Rettmer RL, Carlson TH, Origenes ML, Jack RM, Labb RF. Zinc protoporphyrin/heme ratio for diagnosis of preanemic iron deficiency. *Pediatrics.* Sep 1999;104(3):e37

73. Lopez-Ruzafa E, Vazquez-Lopez MA, Lendinez-Molinos F, et al. Reference Values of Reticulocyte Hemoglobin Content and Their Relation With Other Indicators of Iron Status in Healthy Children. *J Pediatr Hematol Oncol.* Oct 2016;38(7):e207–212

74. Powers JM, Buchanan GR, Adix L, Zhang S, Gao A, McCavit TL. Effect of Low-Dose Ferrous Sulfate vs Iron Polysaccharide Complex on Hemoglobin Concentration in Young Children With Nutritional Iron-Deficiency Anemia: A Randomized Clinical Trial. *JAMA.* Jun 13 2017;317(22):2297–2304

75. Zlotkin S, Arthur P, Antwi KY, Yeung G. Randomized, controlled trial of single versus 3-times-daily ferrous sulfate drops for treatment of anemia. *Pediatrics.* Sep 2001;108(3):613–616

76. Oski FA. Iron deficiency in infancy and childhood. *New Engl J Med.* 1993;329: 190–193

77. Moretti D, Goede JS, Zeder C, et al. Oral iron supplements increase hepcidin and decrease iron absorption from daily or twice-daily doses in iron-depleted young women. *Blood.* Oct 22 2015;126(17):1981–1989

78. Schrier SL. So you know how to treat iron deficiency anemia. *Blood.* Oct 22 2015;126(17):1971

79. Rimon E, Kagansky N, Kagansky M, et al. Are we giving too much iron? Low-dose iron therapy is effective in octogenarians. *Am J Med.* Oct 2005;118(10): 1142–1147

80. Powers JM, Daniel CL, McCavit TL, Buchanan GR. Deficiencies in the Management of Iron Deficiency Anemia During Childhood. *Pediatr Blood Cancer.* Apr 2016;63(4):743–745

81. Yip R, Reeves JD, Lonnerdal B, Keen CL, Dallman PR. Does iron supplementation compromise zinc nutrition in healthy infants? *Am J Clin Nutr.* Oct 1985;42(4):683–687

82. Reeves JD, Yip R. Lack of adverse side effects of oral ferrous sulfate therapy in 1-year-old infants. *Pediatrics.* Feb 1985;75(2):352–355

83. Holst L, Nordeng H, Haavik S. Use of herbal drugs during early pregnancy in relation to maternal characteristics and pregnancy outcome. *Pharmacoepidemiol Drug Saf.* Feb 2008;17(2):151–159

84. Charles CV, Dewey CE, Hall A, Channary S, Summerlee AJ. A randomized control trial using a fish-shaped iron ingot for the amelioration of iron deficiency anemia in rural Camboidian Women. *Trop Med Surg.* 2015;3(3): 1000195

85. Armstrong GR, Dewey CE, Summerlee AJ. Iron release from the Lucky Iron Fish(R): safety considerations. *Asia Pac J Clin Nutr.* Jan 2017;26(1):148–155

86. Laass MW, Straub S, Chainey S, Virgin G, Cushway T. Effectiveness and safety of ferric carboxymaltose treatment in children and adolescents with inflammatory bowel disease and other gastrointestinal diseases. *BMC Gastroenterol.* Oct 17 2014;14:184

87. Crary SE, Hall K, Buchanan GR. Intravenous iron sucrose for children with iron deficiency failing to respond to oral iron therapy. *Pediatr Blood Cancer.* Apr 2011;56(4):615–619

88. Plummer ES, Crary SE, McCavit TL, Buchanan GR. Intravenous low molecular weight iron dextran in children with iron deficiency anemia unresponsive to oral iron. *Pediatr Blood Cancer.* Nov 2013;60(11):1747–1752

89. Powers JM, Shamoun M, McCavit TL, Adix L, Buchanan GR. Intravenous Ferric Carboxymaltose in Children with Iron Deficiency Anemia Who Respond Poorly to Oral Iron. *J Pediatr.* Jan 2017;180:212–216

90. Mantadakis E, Tsouvala E, Xanthopoulou V, Chatzimichael A. Intravenous iron sucrose for children with iron deficiency anemia: a single institution study. *World J Pediatr.* Feb 2016;12(1):109–113

91. Auerbach M, Macdougall IC. Safety of intravenous iron formulations: facts and folklore. *Blood Transfus.* Jul 2014;12(3):296–300

Chapter 20

Trace Elements

Introduction

A trace element can be arbitrarily defined as a mineral that constitutes less than 0.01% of total body weight or one for which requirements in adults are in the mg/day range (1–100 mg/day). Some trace elements are clearly essential for human health, such as iron, zinc, copper, manganese, molybdenum, chromium, iodine, selenium, and vanadium. Others are not essential but are beneficial for human health (fluoride), of uncertain importance (arsenic, boron, cobalt, silicon, manganese, and nickel), or important mostly in terms of their potential toxicity (aluminum, manganese). Iron and fluoride are discussed in Chapters 19 and 48, respectively; the rest are discussed in this chapter.

The Food and Nutrition Board of the Institute of Medicine (now the National Academy of Medicine) has established Dietary Reference Intakes (DRIs) for humans for iron, zinc, copper, manganese, chromium, iodine, molybdenum, and selenium using a framework containing 4 sets of dietary intake levels: Estimated Average Requirements (EARs), Recommended Dietary Allowances (RDAs), Adequate Intakes (AIs), and Tolerable Upper Intake Levels (Upper Levels or ULs).[1] The EAR is the intake expected to be adequate for 50% of a population, and the RDA is the nutrient intake that is sufficient to meet the needs for nearly all individuals (approximately 97%) in an age and gender group. If insufficient data are available to determine the EAR and RDA, an AI is determined—the intake expected to meet the needs of the vast majority of people within a population. The RDAs or the AIs of the major trace minerals discussed in this chapter are shown in Table 20.1 (see also Appendix E). Table 20.1 also summarizes normal serum values, biochemical actions, effects of deficiency, effects of excess, and food sources of the trace elements.

Zinc

Basic Science/Background

Zinc is an essential cofactor for several hundred enzymes with a multitude of functions.[2] These enzymes are involved in nucleic acid and protein metabolism, histone stability, apoptosis, cell division, and energy metabolism. Zinc is also important for the maintenance of protein stability and is a component of several transcription factors (in so-called zinc fingers). Considering these varied effects, it is not surprising that in many species,

Table 20.1.

Trace Elements

Name/Normal Serum Values	Biochemical Action	Effects of Deficiency	Effects of Excess	RDA or AI	Food Sources
Zinc (Zn)/ 0.75–1.20 mg/L or 11.5–18.5 µmol/L	Components of many enzymes and transcription factors	Anorexia, hypogeusia, retarded growth, delayed sexual maturation, impaired wound healing, skin lesions	Few toxic effects; may aggravate marginal copper deficiency	Infants, 0–6 mo: 2 mg/d[a] 7–12 mo: 3 mg/d[a] Children, 1–3 y: 3 mg/d 4–8 y: 5 mg/d Males, 9–13 y: 8 mg/d 14–18 y: 11 mg/d Females, 9–13 y: 8 mg/d 14–18 y: 9 mg/d	Oysters, liver, meat, cheese, legumes, whole grains
Copper (Cu)/ 1.10–1.45 mg/L or 11–22 µmol/L	Constituent of ceruloplasmin; component of key metalloenzymes; role in connective tissue biosynthesis	Sideroblastic anemia, retarded growth, osteoporosis, neutropenia, decreased pigmentation	Few toxic effects; Wilson disease, liver dysfunction	Infants, 0–6 mo: 0.20 mg/d[a] 7–12 mo: 0.22 mg/d[a] Children, 1–3 y: 0.34 mg/d 4–8 y: 0.44 mg/d Adolescents, 9–13 y: 0.70 mg/d 14–18 y: 0.89 mg/d	Shellfish, meat, legumes, nuts, cheese

Manganese (Mn)[b]/ 4–12 µg/L or 73–210 µmol/L	Activator of metal-enzyme complexes important for synthesis of polysaccharides and glycoproteins; constituent of pyruvate carboxylase and Mn-superoxide dismutase	Human, not documented; animals, growth retardation, ataxia of newborn, bone abnormalities, reduced fertility	Few toxic effects; neurologic manifestations from industrial contamination and in long-term total parenteral nutrition	Infants, 0–6 mo: 0.003 mg/d[a] 7–12 mo: 0.6 mg/d[a] Children, 1–3 y: 1.2 mg/d 4–8 y: 1.5 mg/d Males, 9–13 y: 1.9 mg/d 14–18 y: 2.2 mg/d Females, 9–13 y: 1.6 mg/d 14–18 y: 1.6 mg/d	Nuts, whole grains, tea
Selenium (Se)/ 30–75 µg/L or 0.35–1.00 µmol/L	Component of enzymes: glutathione peroxidase and deiodinase	Humans, cardiomyopathy; animals, hepatic necrosis, muscular dystrophy, exudative diathesis, pancreatic fibrosis	Irritation of mucous membranes (nose, eyes, upper respiratory tract), pallor, irritability, indigestion	Infants, 0–6 mo: 15 µg/d[a] 7–12 mo: 20 µg/d[a] Children, 1–3 y: 20 µg/d 4–8 y: 30 µg/d Adolescents, 9–13 y: 40 µg/d 14–18 y: 55 µg/d	Seafood, meat, whole grains

[a] For healthy breastfed infants, the AI is the mean intake.
[b] Whole blood.

Continued

Table 20.1. *Continued*
Trace Elements

Name/Normal Serum Values	Biochemical Action	Effects of Deficiency	Effects of Excess	RDA or AI	Food Sources
Chromium (Cr)	Required for maintenance of normal glucose metabolism; potentiates the action of insulin	Humans, impairment of glucose utilization; animals, impaired growth, disturbances of carbohydrate, protein, and lipid metabolism	Few toxic effects; humans, not well documented; animals, growth retardation, hepatic and kidney damage	Infants, 0–6 mo: 0.2 μg/d[a] 7–12 mo: 5.5 μg/d[a] Children, 1–3 y: 11 μg/d 4–8 y: 15 μg/d Males, 9–13 y: 25 μg/d 14–18 y: 35 μg/d Females, 9–13 y: 21 μg/d 14–18 y: 24 μg/d	Meat, cheese, whole grains, brewer's yeast
Cobalt (Co)	Component of vitamin B_{12}	Humans, unknown; animals, anemia, growth retardation	Few toxic effects; polycythemia, myocardial degeneration	Not established	Green leafy vegetables

Pediatric Nutrition, 8th Edition

| Molybdenum (Mo) | Component of enzymes involved in production of uric acid (xanthine oxidase) and in oxidation of aldehydes and sulfides | Humans, unknown; animals: growth retardation, anorexia | Humans, gout-like syndrome, antagonist of copper | Infants, 0–6 mo: 2 µg/d[a] 7–12 mo: 3 µg/d[a] Children, 1–3 y: 17 µg/d 4–8 y: 22 µg/d Adolescents, 9–13 y: 34 µg/d 14–18 y: 43 µg/d | Meats, grains, legumes |
| Iodine (I) | Component of thyroid hormones (T_3, T_4), enzymes involved in production of | Goiter, impaired mental function, delayed development | "Toxic goiter" | Infants, 0–6 mo: 110 µg/d[a] 7–12 mo: 130 µg/d[a] Children, 1–3 y: 90 µg/d 4–8 y: 90 µg/d Adolescents, 9–13 y: 120 µg/d 14–18 y: 150 µg/d | Iodized salt, dairy products, saltwater fish, seafood |

[a] For healthy breastfed infants, the AI is the mean intake.
[b] Whole blood.

including humans, zinc deficiency limits growth prenatally as well as in infants and children. Nor is it unexpected that rapidly turning over tissues are affected relatively early in zinc deficiency, with the immune system, the intestinal mucosa, and the skin being particularly susceptible. Zinc is essential for proper immune function.[3] It is important for barrier function in the skin and mucosa as well as humoral and cellular immunity.

Zinc is known to reduce the mortality and morbidity from acute and chronic diarrhea in high-risk populations, both as a treatment of established diarrhea and as a preventive public health measure.[4-6] It may have beneficial effects on other diseases, such as lower respiratory tract infections.[7-9] Furthermore, zinc has also been shown to have a positive effect on physical activity of preschool children[10] and on cognition and neurodevelopment.[11-13]

Zinc is absorbed in the small intestine by active transport, is resecreted into the gastrointestinal tract, and is excreted in the urine. Biliary and pancreatic secretions contain large amounts of zinc, most of which is reabsorbed more distally in the gastrointestinal tract. There is homeostatic regulation of absorption, both by uptake and endogenous secretion.[14] Reductions in urinary zinc excretion appear to be an extremely late sign of deficiency. Small amounts of zinc are also lost in sweat and in desquamated skin cells.

Two large families of zinc transporters have been described. The ZIP family appears to be responsible for zinc influx into cells and intracellular compartments, and the ZnT family regulates zinc efflux across the plasma membrane and out of intracellular organelles.[15-17] The regulation of these transporters by hormonal and dietary modifiers is complex, and there appears to be a large degree of duplication and redundancy in the system. The mechanisms by which these systems regulate zinc homeostasis continues to be an active area of research.[18] Zinc is transported in serum bound to serum albumin and α_2-macroglobulin, and further homeostasis of zinc metabolism occurs in the liver, where zinc may be stored as metallothionein.

Zinc Deficiency

For many years, it was believed that free-living humans consuming self-selected diets would not be zinc deficient, because zinc was so widely spread throughout the environment and in the food supply. Therefore, the first reports of zinc deficiency from Egypt and Iran were surprising.[19] Although uncommon in children, severe zinc deficiency is well characterized. Its clinical features include acro-orificial skin lesions, diarrhea, increased susceptibility to infection, immune dysfunction, delayed pubertal development, short stature, and slow growth.[20] These features are found in the autosomal-recessive genetic disorder of zinc metabolism, acrodermatitis enteropathica (AE), which causes severe zinc deficiency by decreased cellular retention of zinc. AE is caused by a mutation in ZIP4, a key zinc transporter in the brush-border membrane, regulating zinc uptake into the enterocyte.[21] People with AE require daily zinc supplements for alleviation of all symptoms. In children, the proper daily dose may be difficult to determine, particularly during periods of rapid growth, and there is a risk of excessive doses causing copper deficiency.[22] A dose of 20 to 30 mg/day of elemental zinc should usually be adequate to meet the zinc requirements of AE infants and children. Recovery from zinc deficiency is rapid after introduction of oral zinc, and the dermatitis often completely resolves within 4 to 5 days of adequate treatment. Severe zinc deficiency may also be observed in infants, particularly those with mothers with a defect in mammary gland zinc secretion[23] (see "Zinc Requirements") and in preterm infants with excessive losses—for example, those with proximal ileostomies because of necrotizing enterocolitis or intestinal resections. In the latter case, the loss of bilious fluid from an ostomy should caution that zinc is probably also being lost, and zinc intake should be increased by between 2 and 3 times the maintenance requirements.

Since Prasad's first description of severe human zinc deficiency,[19] severe zinc deficiency is now well recognized. What remains problematic is diagnosing and understanding the true incidence and importance of milder forms of zinc deficiency, largely because of the lack of reliable measures of zinc status in individuals. Although the incidence of stunting and plasma zinc measurements are useful for assessing the zinc status of populations, they perform poorly as measures of the zinc status of an individual.[24,25]

Mild zinc deficiency in infants was first described by Walravens and Hambidge, who found slower-than-normal growth in male formula-fed infants[26] and lower plasma zinc concentrations[27] than in breastfed infants. Fortification of formula to a zinc content of 5.8 mg/L led to normal growth. Several recent studies have shown a positive effect of zinc supplements on the growth of infants and children,[28–30] but others have failed to show an effect.[31] Zinc status at baseline, the dose of zinc given, growth rate, infections, compliance, and other factors may affect the outcome.[32] Whether growth impairment in children with suboptimal zinc status is attributable to effects on hormonal mediators of growth, reduced appetite, and food intake or more frequent infections is not yet known. Preterm infants are born with lower stores of zinc, and 2 small studies on such infants demonstrated beneficial effects of zinc supplementation on their growth rate.[33,34]

In recent years, an acrodermatitis-like syndrome has been reported in human milk feed infants. This syndrome is now known to be caused by loss of function mutation in the maternal ZnT2 transporter.[35] The transporter is required for efflux of zinc into maternal milk; in its absence, zinc content of milk is very low and transient neonatal zinc deficiency may result.[36] This condition can be distinguished from true AE by its rapid response to oral zinc supplementation or the addition of zinc-containing foods into the diet.

During the last several decades, the significance of zinc deficiency in childhood growth, morbidity, and mortality has been recognized by a number of large-scale, randomized, controlled supplementation trials in developing countries, and zinc deficiency has been identified as a leading cause of preventable deaths in children worldwide.[37] Systematic reviews have shown that in children with stunting, zinc supplementation was associated with significantly increased height and weight.[31] Similar reviews in young children evaluating the effect of daily or weekly zinc supplementation on infectious disease have reported a robust decrease (approximately 40%) in treatment failure and death secondary to diarrhea and pneumonia.[4,7,38] The consistent positive effects on diarrhea prompted the inclusion of zinc into oral rehydration solution (ORS),[39] which showed beneficial effects on stool output and diarrhea duration.[40] Although successful implementation has proved difficult,[41] it appears to be both efficacious and cost-effective.[42] Zinc supplements may have benefits in other infectious diseases, but data are insufficient to draw meaningful conclusions for either malaria or tuberculosis at the current time.[19] Zinc fortification of food staples may also increase the zinc status of high-risk populations but seems less effective if other micronutrients are added to the food staple in addition to zinc.[43]

Zinc has also been studied as a treatment for the common cold. Most recent analysis suggest that zinc may shorten the duration of the common cold. A recent Cochrane review found that despite heterogeneous evidence, zinc lozenges providing at least 75 mg/day of zinc seemed to shorted the duration of the common cold if started within 24 hours of symptom onset.[44]

Mild to moderate zinc deficiency can be difficult to diagnose because of the lack of specific features. Slow growth, frequent infections, minor rashes, lack of appetite, and compromised immune function may be suggestive of zinc deficiency. Zinc status is often evaluated by measurement of the plasma or serum zinc concentration. However, neither is a sensitive indicator, and infection, stress, growth rate, and other factors can affect these values.[45] Hair zinc concentration is sometimes used, but it is difficult to analyze and may be affected by factors other than zinc status.[46] When zinc deficiency is suspected, a zinc supplementation trial (usually 1 mg/kg per day) may provide a measurable response.[47] The supplement can be administered as an oral solution of zinc acetate (30 mg of zinc acetate in 5 mL of water). For term infants receiving total parenteral nutrition, intravenous requirements have been estimated to 100 µg/kg/day, and in preterm infants, up to 300 µg/kg/day has been recommended to prevent zinc deficiency.[48] Infants with cystic fibrosis have been shown to have low plasma zinc and abnormal zinc homeostasis[49] and may, therefore, have a higher requirement for zinc, as may those with Crohn disease or sickle cell disease.[50,51]

IV

Zinc Requirements

Zinc intake from human milk averages 0.5 to 1.0 mg/day but decreases over time as the human milk zinc content decreases with increasing duration of lactation. Infant formulas are fortified with zinc to a level higher than that of human milk (to compensate for lower bioavailability). Thus, intake is usually around 3 to 5 mg/day (or 1 mg/kg per day). Lower zinc intakes may be adequate for healthy term infants, because human milk zinc concentrations as low as 1.1 mg/L do not result in zinc deficiency.[52] However, overt zinc deficiency can occur in some infants receiving human milk with a lower-than-normal level of zinc.[53] This is of particular concern in preterm infants, because their rapid growth increases their zinc requirement. In preterm infants, deficiency because of low human milk content of zinc can occur quickly. Maternal zinc supplementation does not increase the content of zinc in the milk. Some women with abnormally low milk zinc have a genetic defect in ZnT2, one of the transporters regulating mammary zinc metabolism.[54] It is not yet known how common this specific mutation is among afflicted mothers, but these infants may present with features of AE that respond to relatively low levels of zinc supplementation or to the introduction of other sources of zinc into the diet (eg, complementary foods or infant formula). Unlike children with AE, zinc supplements are not required lifelong but for only as long as they rely on human milk as a source of dietary zinc. The disorder, if appropriately recognized and treated, is self-limiting. However, as the cause is the deficiency of the maternal transporter, the recurrence rate in subsequent pregnancies would be expected to be 100%.

If a sibling has had transient neonatal zinc deficiency, subsequent infants should still be breastfed, but they should receive an oral zinc supplement.

The RDA for zinc for older (7–12 months of age) infants and toddlers (1–3 years of age) is 3 mg/day. Exclusively breastfed infants ingest only 0.4 to 0.6 mg of zinc per day at 6 months of age without signs of overt zinc deficiency.[55] Little is known about the infant's capacity to homeostatically regulate zinc metabolism, but several of the zinc transporters described previously are affected by zinc intake and zinc status. Stable isotope studies in infants have suggested that zinc absorption is increased and fecal losses are decreased when zinc intake is low.[14] For several age groups, the margin between the EAR and the UL is relatively narrow. Among preschool-aged children in the United States, zinc intakes are relatively high compared with recommended intakes and are more likely to exceed the UL than to be below the EAR.[56] For example, data from the Feeding Infants and Toddlers Study reveal that zinc intakes below the EAR are observed in 6% of 5- through 11-month-old US children but <1% of 12- through 47-month-old children.[57] Conversely, the number of children consuming diets containing more than the UL for zinc varies between 47% (12- to 23-month-olds) and 74% (24- to 47-month-olds). Although the incidence of low zinc intakes is more common in adolescents,[58,59] the absence of obvious adverse effects in young children from this nominally "excessive" zinc intakes does raise questions about the UL for zinc for young children. The UL was set on the basis of concerns that zinc may impair copper absorption, and this interaction is exploited clinically in the early management of Wilson disease (see "Zinc Toxicity").

Dietary Sources/Bioavailability

Zinc absorption from human milk has been shown to be high compared with that from cow milk-based formula or cow milk.[60] Zinc from human milk may have higher bioavailability because zinc is loosely bound to citrate and serum albumin in human milk[61] rather than tightly bound to casein as in cow milk and cow milk-based formula. Citrate-bound zinc is readily absorbed, and the limited digestive capacity of neonates may be sufficient to release zinc from serum albumin but possibly inadequate for complete digestion of casein, resulting in unabsorbed zinc.[62] Zinc absorption from soy formula and infant cereals is even lower than from cow milk-based formula, most likely because of the high phytate content of these diets.[63] Phytic acid contains several negative charges and can bind divalent cations like zinc, iron, and calcium. Because humans cannot digest phytate to any significant degree, fecal zinc losses increase. Because removal of phytate increases zinc absorption considerably,[64] efforts are being made to reduce the phytate content of staple foods (corn, rice, barley) by fermentation, precipitation, phytase treatment, or genetic selection.[65] However, such products are not yet commercially available, and phytate reduction of food crops is problematic, because it may have adverse effects on crop yields. High intake of phytate-containing foods (cereals, legumes) and the low intake of zinc-rich foods such as meat (see Appendix L) are the most important reasons for the high prevalence of low zinc status in resource-limited countries.

When oral supplements are given, iron may partially inhibit zinc absorption,[66] and combined supplements of iron and zinc have been shown to be less effective in preventing low zinc status in infants than zinc supplementation alone.[67]

During the second 6 months of life, zinc requirements remain relatively high, and the amount of zinc provided from human milk may be inadequate. The concentration of zinc in human milk is approximately 2 to 3 mg/L during early lactation, but by 6 months postpartum, the concentration usually is only approximately 0.5 mg/L.[68] The quantity of zinc provided from human milk may be too low to meet the requirement; however, another likely reason for the beneficial effect of zinc supplements on growth of these infants may be that phytate-containing weaning foods reduce the bioavailability of zinc from human milk. It is apparent that zinc intake is a limiting factor during recovery from malnutrition and during rapid catch-up growth after stunting.[69] This was considered when new recommendations for complementary foods were issued by the World Health Organization (WHO)/United Nations Children's Fund.[70]

Zinc Toxicity

Acute zinc toxicity is rare but may occur from ingestion of pharmacologic preparations of zinc. Symptoms are usually diarrhea and vomiting. The Institute of Medicine used data on zinc intake and copper status to determine UL for zinc, and high amounts of oral zinc do reduce copper absorption. This may lead to desirable effects, such as when oral zinc is used as a treatment for Wilson disease (a disorder of inappropriate copper absorption and hyperaccumulation; see "Copper"), and undesirable effects, such as the case report of copper deficiency in an adolescent boy given excessive amounts of zinc for the treatment of AE.[22]

Copper

Basic Science/Background

Copper is essential in several physiologically important enzymes, such as lysyl oxidase, elastase, monoamine oxidases, cytochrome oxidase, ceruloplasmin, and copper-zinc-superoxide dismutase.[71] Lysyl oxidase and elastase are involved in connective tissue synthesis and collagen cross-linking, cytochrome oxidase is involved in the electron transport system as well as energy metabolism, ceruloplasmin (ferroxidase) is involved in iron metabolism, and superoxide dismutase is an antioxidant and scavenger of free radicals. The signs of copper deficiency can all be related to impaired activities of these enzymes.[71,72] Our knowledge regarding copper absorption and homeostasis is limited, but recently, several novel copper transporters (ATP7A, ATP7B, Ctr1) have been discovered,[71] in part because of their role in genetic disorders of copper metabolism.

Copper Deficiency

An x-linked recessive genetic disorder of copper metabolism, Menkes syndrome, usually manifests early in life and is characterized by depigmentation, anemia, steely hair, and a progressive degeneration of the brain.[73] Patients become copper deficient at a very young age, and aggressive treatment with copper should be used, but the long-term outcome for these patients is poor.[73,74] The gene involved has now been identified by work on mouse models of Menkes disease.[75] The defective protein is a P-type ATPase, ATP7A, which is involved in cellular copper metabolism, particularly the export of copper out of the cell.[76] Thus, copper is enters the enterocyte, but insufficient copper is transported out of the enterocyte and into the systemic circulation, resulting in severe copper systemic deficiency.

Risk factors for copper deficiency include low hepatic stores and rapid growth, malabsorption syndromes, and increased copper losses, but deficiency is usually not precipitated unless the dietary intake of copper is also low.[71,77]

Preterm infants have substantially lower hepatic stores of copper (which mainly accumulate during the third trimester); these prenatal stores are normally used during neonatal life by copper being incorporated into ceruloplasmin and exported into the bloodstream, causing an early increase in serum copper and ceruloplasmin.[78] Thus, many of the first descriptions of copper deficiency were from preterm infants who had been fed low-copper diets for prolonged periods. Iatrogenic copper deficiency continues to be seen in preterm infants, particularly those with short gut syndrome and parenteral nutrition-associated liver disease or parenteral nutrition-associated cholestasis (PNALD/PNAC, aka "TPN cholestasis"), in whom copper is often removed from or severely reduced in the parenteral nutrition. Copper deficiency has also been found in malnourished infants and children.[71] Signs of copper deficiency include neutropenia, hypochromic anemia (which does not respond to iron supplementation), bone abnormalities (osteoporosis, metaphyseal cupping), skin disorders, and depigmentation of skin and hair.[71,72] The immune system is also affected, reflected by decreased phagocytic capacity of neutrophils and impaired cellular immunity.[79] The anemia is caused by the low levels of ceruloplasmin, which is needed in several steps leading to the incorporation of iron into hemoglobin. Patients with aceruloplasminemia (a genetic defect in ceruloplasmin production) have normal copper status but pronounced iron deficiency anemia[80] resulting from decreased incorporation of iron into developing erythrocytes. Anemia attributable to copper deficiency may be mistaken for iron deficiency anemia, although it will not respond to iron supplementation.

Patients with copper deficiency usually respond rapidly to adequate treatment. Clinical parameters that are used to assess copper status include serum copper and ceruloplasmin, hair copper, and erythrocyte superoxide dismutase.[72] In infants older than 1 or 2 months, serum copper concentrations lower than 0.5 µg/mL or ceruloplasmin concentrations lower than 15 µg/100 mL should be considered abnormally low. However, serum copper and ceruloplasmin are not very responsive to marginal copper deficiency and are affected by other conditions, such as infection, which may raise concentrations. The level of hair copper also has limited value, because it may be affected by external factors.[46] The erythrocyte level of superoxide dismutase has been suggested as a good indicator of long-term copper status,[72] but the measurement has not reached routine clinical use.

Copper Requirement

The copper intake of infants is usually low, because human milk contains only 0.2 to 0.4 mg copper/L, and infant formulas are usually fortified to a similar level (0.4–0.6 mg/L).[77] This level of copper intake appears adequate in healthy term infants, because copper deficiency is rare.[19] In fact, even formula that had not been fortified with copper and only contained 0.08 mg/L resulted in adequate copper status in term infants.[81] The WHO has set the minimum recommended intake for infants at 60 µg/kg per day, and the current RDA for copper is 200 µg/day.[1]

After weaning, cereals and other foods provide more copper than does milk, and copper intake increases rapidly. Studies with older infants and children[82] indicate that copper intake at this age meets the requirements for growth and maintenance. Although there has been some concern that drinking water may be excessively high in copper in some areas, either because of the environment (eg, copper-mining areas) or copper pipes, infants fed formula at the current maximum copper content according to the WHO (2 mg/L) exhibited no signs of copper excess after 6 months of exposure.[83]

Dietary Sources/Bioavailability

Copper absorption in infants is high, approximately 80%, and does not appear to be dependent on age.[84] Increasing the copper intake of infants did not affect copper absorption, suggesting no or limited homeostatic regulation at a young age.[84] Stable isotope studies in preterm infants,[85] balance studies in term infants,[86] and radioisotope studies in experimental animals[87] demonstrated higher bioavailability of copper from human milk than from cow milk-based formula and cow milk. Copper bioavailability from soy formula and infant cereals appears to be even lower than that of cow milk, although phytate present in these products does not seem to have the same strong inhibitory effect on the absorption of copper as found for zinc absorption.[88] Dietary factors known to decrease copper absorption include high levels of ascorbic acid, zinc, iron, and cysteine. However, levels of these nutrients used in infant diets are moderate and usually exert no pronounced effects on copper absorption.[89] Some types of heat processing of infant formula, however, may have a negative effect on copper absorption,[90] possibly by formation of unabsorbable complexes.

Copper Toxicity

Acute copper toxicity is rare and is usually attributable to the consumption of contaminated foods or beverages or accidental or deliberate ingestion of large quantities of copper salts.[91] Symptoms include nausea, vomiting, and diarrhea. Chronic toxicity is also rare but appears to appear in geographic clusters. Indian childhood cirrhosis has been reported in families consuming milk boiled or stored in brass or copper containers,[92] and the Institute of Medicine selected changes in liver enzymes as a measure of excessive copper intake.[1] In the Austrian Tyrol, infants and children were reported to have died from liver cirrhosis resulting from high chronic copper intake.[93,94] In these cases, inheritance followed the typical pattern of a Mendelian recessive trait, suggesting that these individuals were particularly sensitive to copper exposure. This was supported by the observation that many children who had similar copper exposure were determined to have no liver damage. Sporadic cases have been reported in other areas, and some of these cases have occurred in consanguineous marriages.[93] Cases were much more frequent in boys, and a genetic origin is possible.

Wilson disease is an autosomal-recessive genetic disorder of copper metabolism that results in copper hyperaccumulation. Excessive amounts of copper are accumulated in the body, particularly in the liver and brain, and lead to liver cirrhosis, eye lesions (Kayser-Fleisher ring), renal impairment, and neurologic problems.[95] Despite very high levels of copper in the liver, serum copper and ceruloplasmin are low. Treatment includes a variety of chelating agents and large doses of oral zinc to reduce copper absorption.[96] In advanced cases, hepatic transplantation may be required. This disorder of copper metabolism has also been shown to be attributable to a defective transporter, in this case ATP7B,[97] which is responsible for copper trafficking and excretion of excess copper into the biliary canalicular system. Several different mutations of ATP7B have been described, and the severity of the disease varies with the type of mutation.[98] Genotyping of presymptomatic infants and children is, therefore, important for early and appropriate medical intervention. Copper absorption does not appear to be dysregulated in these patients; rather, tissue copper metabolism, particularly in the liver, is affected, causing excessive cellular accumulation of copper.[95] The outcome for these patients under treatment is usually good, but continuous monitoring of copper, zinc, and iron status is needed.

Manganese

Basic Science/Background

The essentiality of manganese in humans has not been fully established, although it has been determined for most other species. Manganese is a cofactor for enzymes including arginase, glutamate-ammonia ligase, manganese superoxide dismutase, and pyruvate carboxylase. In many cases, magnesium ions can replace manganese with continued enzyme activity.[99] Only one potential case of human manganese deficiency has been described.[100] It is possible that manganese deficiency does not occur in infants and children and that, instead, concern should be directed toward toxic effects of manganese excess.

Manganese Requirements

Requirements for manganese of infants and children are likely very small, and the current AI for 0- to 6-month-old infants is 3 µg/day.[1] However, for 9- to 13-year-old children, the AI is 1.6 to 1.9 mg/day, and this considerably higher level reflects the fact that manganese at this age is retained by the body to a very limited extent.

Assessment of Status

Manganese status is difficult to assess because of the very low concentrations of manganese in biological tissues and fluids; blood concentrations are only 10 µg/L, and serum concentrations are approximately 1 µg/L,[101] making analysis impossible for most laboratories. Because few of the manganese-dependent enzymes are found in blood, they are not helpful in the evaluation of manganese status. The identification of manganese transporters in mice, may lead to a better understanding of manganese homeostasis.[102]

Dietary Sources/Bioavailability

The concentration of manganese in human milk is very low, only 4 to 8 µg/L,[103] and most is bound to lactoferrin.[104] Cow milk and cow milk-based formula are about 10 times higher in manganese concentration (30 to 60 µg/L), and soy formula is about 50 to 75 times higher in manganese than is human milk.[105] Although in the past, some formulas were fortified with manganese,[106] the present levels of manganese in cow's milk formula and soy formula reflect the natural levels of manganese in the protein sources used. Of potential concern is the increasing use of soy and rice beverages ("milks") for feeding infants. These beverages contain 2 to 17 times the manganese content of soy formula and exceed the UL for 1- to 3-year-old children (there is no established UL for infants).[107]

Drinking water can contain significant concentrations of manganese.[107,108] In a recent US Geological Survey of glacial aquifers, manganese was the metal most commonly seen at levels above "benchmark," with 18.5% of samples containing >300 µg/L of manganese.[108] This source needs to be taken into account when estimating the manganese intake of children and also of infants fed powdered infant formula diluted in such water.

Manganese Toxicity

Although the bioavailability of manganese from human milk appears high relative to that from cow milk-based formula and soy formula,[109] there appears to be little regulation of manganese absorption at young ages, and it is strongly correlated with dietary intake.[110] Thus, the body burden of absorbed and retained manganese will be much larger in infants fed cow milk-based formula or, in particular, soy formula than in breastfed infants.[104] This is reflected in higher whole blood manganese concentrations in formula-fed infants.[111]

Toxic effects of manganese in human adults are manifested by central nervous system dysfunction, such as lack of coordination and balance, mental confusion, and muscle cramps.[112] The major site for the toxic effects of manganese is the extrapyramidal tracts. Although most reports on manganese toxicity in humans are on workers exposed to manganese by inhalation, there are cases of manganese toxicity in children who have ingested high doses of manganese.[113,114] In such cases, lack of attention, poor memory test results, and an epileptic syndrome were described. It has been shown in young animals that the brain may be particularly sensitive to manganese. Ingestion of modest amounts of manganese during early life caused a dose-dependent depletion of striatum dopamine and adverse effects on motor development and behavior in rats.[115] A negative correlation between blood manganese and cord blood monoamine metabolites was has been reported in healthy women.[116] It was also shown that cord blood manganese was negatively correlated to nonverbal psychomotor scores in 3-year-old children of these women. Behavioral studies in infant rhesus monkeys exposed to high levels of manganese in soy formula demonstrated that these infant monkeys engaged in less play behavior and more affiliative clinging and had shorter wake cycles and shorter daytime inactivity than controls,[117] suggesting signs of attention-deficit/hyperactivity disorder. Higher levels of manganese in drinking water have been shown to be associated with poor developmental scores in children.[107,118]

In North America, drinking water may be sufficient to meet the manganese requirements of formula-fed infants.[119] Indeed, in the United States, some household wells have water manganese levels exceeding 300 µg/L, the current lifetime health advisory level set by the US Environmental Protection Agency. It should be noted that soy formulas usually contain manganese at amounts exceeding this level.

Children receiving long-term parenteral nutrition may be at risk of excessive manganese exposure, because parenteral nutrition solutions frequently are high in manganese.[120] In such patients, cholestatic disease and nervous system disorders have been associated with high blood concentrations of manganese. The normal homeostatic mechanisms of the liver and gut are bypassed in these patients, leading to hypermanganesemia, and a reduction in the manganese concentration of parenteral nutrition solutions has been advocated.[121] Manganese is excreted via bile, so elevated plasma manganese concentrations are seen in children with biliary obstruction.[122] Given the questionable need for parenteral manganese and the risk of manganese toxicity, there is a good case for arguing that manganese should not be added to parenteral nutrition.[123]

Balance studies in infants show that breastfed infants accumulate little manganese, but formula-fed infants are in positive balance.[86] Little is known about the threshold for development of toxic effects of manganese, but because manganese absorption is high at young ages,[110] the possibility should be considered. This high absorption of manganese may be accentuated, because manganese absorption increases substantially during iron deficiency,[105] which is not uncommon in children.

Selenium

Basic Science/Background

Selenium is required in a limited number of proteins, including selenium-dependent glutathione peroxidase, selenoprotein P in serum, and iodothyronine-5'-deiodinase. In these proteins, selenium is incorporated into the proteins as selenocysteine via a unique transfer-RNA.[124] Thus, the number of selenocysteine residues in each protein is tightly regulated. Selenium can also be incorporated nonspecifically into methionine. A typical US diet consists of organic selenium (largely selenomethionine) and inorganic selenium in the form of selenite and selenate. Knowledge is limited about the metabolism of these different forms of selenium in humans, but they appear to be metabolized quite differently.[125,126] Glutathione peroxidase participates in the antioxidant defense and helps to scavenge free radicals that may cause tissue damage. Selenium is an integral part of cellular glutathione peroxidase, serum glutathione peroxidase, and a membrane-bound form of glutathione peroxidase, but there are also selenium-independent glutathione peroxidases.[124] Type I iodothyronine-5'-deiodinase catalyzes the conversion of thyroxine (T_4) to triiodothyronine (T_3) in liver and other tissues[127] and is, therefore, involved in thyroid function.

Selenium Deficiency

The essentiality of selenium in human nutrition was discovered recently, although selenium deficiency in animals had been known for some time. In Keshan province of China, a cardiomyopathy of unknown etiology was known to lead to high mortality in children.[128] Because of similarities between the pathologic changes of Keshan disease and selenium deficiency in cattle and the fact that the local soil was found to be low in selenium, deficiency of selenium was suspected as a cause. A large study evaluating the effects of selenium fortification of salt was begun, and mortality decreased significantly; selenium fortification has since been used routinely. However, other factors may have contributed to the cause of Keshan disease, because Keshan disease is not evident in other areas with similarly low intakes of selenium, and there is evidence to support a viral etiology.[129] It has been suggested that the low-selenium environment puts evolutionary pressure on normally harmless viruses (such as Coxsackie virus), causing them to mutate, which makes them pathogenic.[130] Evidence for such mutations in Coxsackie virus that can cause cardiomyopathy has been obtained at the molecular level.[129] Selenium deficiency has also been found in children receiving long-term total parenteral nutrition solutions that were not supplemented with selenium.[131] Signs of deficiency include macrocytosis and loss of skin and hair pigmentation. In severe pediatric cases, cardiomyopathy is also observed.[132] Selenium supplementation of parenteral solutions is, therefore, recommended at 2 µg/kg/day.

Low levels of erythrocyte glutathione peroxidase activity and serum and hair selenium concentrations have been found in low birth weight infants,[133] but the clinical significance of these observations is questionable. Low selenium status in pediatric patients with HIV infection has been shown to be a predictor of more rapid disease progression and mortality,[134] and selenium supplementation of such patients may, therefore, be beneficial.

Selenium Requirements

Tissue selenium and plasma selenium concentrations are lower in preterm infants than in term infants.[135] A selenium intake of at least 1 µg/kg/day is recommended to achieve intrauterine tissue accretion. However, evaluation of the selenium status of preterm infants is difficult. When preterm infants were fed human milk (containing 24 µg/L selenium) or infant formula with or without selenium fortification (34.8 and 7.8 µg/L selenium, respectively), no differences were found in plasma selenium, erythrocyte selenium, or glutathione peroxidase concentrations.[135] However, all of these infants may have had suboptimal selenium status, and selenium may have been quickly removed from the circulation and incorporated into newly synthesized tissue. Selenium fortification of infant formula improves selenium status of preterm infants,[136] and selenium supplementation may reduce the risk of sepsis.[137]

There is also limited evidence that low maternal selenium concentrations in the first trimester may increase the risk of preterm birth and maternal pregnancy-induced hypertension[138] and that selenium supplementation may reduce the risk of pregnancy-induced hypertension.[139]

Dietary Sources/Bioavailability

Selenium in the diet is strongly affected by local conditions; soil and water selenium levels affect plant selenium levels and the levels in grazing animals and their milk.[125] Similarly, selenium in human milk is affected by maternal selenium intake.[140] Thus, the selenium intake of infants and children is affected by geographic location. Some areas of the United States have high levels of selenium, and other areas have considerably lower levels. The raw materials used for infant formulas, such as skim milk powder, whey protein, and soy protein isolate, strongly affect the selenium content of the formulas.

The selenium concentration of human milk has been shown to be as low as 3 µg/L in some areas of China, while levels in other low-selenium areas, such as Finland and New Zealand, are around 10 µg/L.[125] Selenium levels in human milk from women in the United States vary but are usually approximately 15 µg/L.[141] A lower level of selenium was shown in formula-fed infants than in breastfed infants in several studies.[141,142] Infant formulas that are not fortified with selenium often contain considerably lower selenium levels (2 to 6 µg/L) than the level in human milk. Furthermore, the bioavailability of selenium in human milk, which is mostly in protein-bound form,[143] seems higher than that of selenium-fortified formula. A study in which the selenium status of formula-fed infants was lower than that in breastfed infants, even though the formula was fortified with selenium to a level higher than that of human milk, supports this.[142] At least part of the difference in selenium bioavailability may be related to the form of selenium in the diet; selenite or selenate (ie, inorganic selenium) is used in infant formula, whereas most selenium in human milk is protein bound (organic selenium). A difference in utilization of selenium given in different forms was shown in a study in which lactating women were given selenium supplements. Yeast selenium (ie, organic selenium) resulted in higher selenium levels in human milk than when selenite was given.[140] These differences were also manifested in the selenium status of the breastfed infants of mothers in the study.

Soy formula often provides even less selenium than does cow milk-based formula. Again, this depends on the soy protein source used, but several commercial soy formulas have been reported to contain only 2 to

6 µg selenium/L.[144,145] Selenium fortification of soy formula has, therefore, recently been implemented. Both selenite[144] and selenate[145] have been studied; stable isotope studies in infants show that the latter form is better absorbed, but selenium retention is similar from both forms.[146] The level of fortification has been chosen to provide the infant with an amount equal to the RDA of 15 to 20 µg/kg per day for infants from birth to 6 months of age. Another factor to consider is the selenium status of infants at birth. Markedly different concentrations of plasma selenium in infants in Finland and the United States may explain why increases after birth were seen in one study[142] but not in another.[147]

Selenium Toxicity

Acute selenium toxicity is very rare in humans, and cases are usually caused by ingestion of selenium supplements. Signs include diarrhea and garlic-smelling breath. Chronic selenium toxicity also appears rare, with signs such as brittle nails, hair loss, and fatigue.

Iodine

Basic Science/Background

The primary biological role of iodine is in the synthesis of thyroid hormones, particularly T_4. Iodine deficiency is a particular concern in pregnant women and in children, because it may lead to irreversible growth impairment and developmental delays.[148] Iodine is readily absorbed and then is rapidly taken up by the thyroid gland, as well as other tissues. Excess iodine is excreted via the urine, and urinary iodine is often used as an indicator of iodine status.[149]

Iodine Deficiency

Although iodine deficiency is one of the most common nutrient deficiencies worldwide, it is very uncommon among infants and children in the United States. Children in the United States will get an ample supply of iodine from iodination of table salt, dairy products, and baked goods,[149,150] although concerns have been raised about the increased use of noniodized salt in the fast food industry in the United States.[151] There are also concerns about the possible reemergence of childhood iodine deficiency in other industrialized countries.[152]

Children with goiter and iron-deficiency anemia do not respond to iodine supplementation,[153] suggesting that iron may be important for some vital step in iodine metabolism. Oral iron supplementation of such children led to a significantly improved response to iodine supplementation.[154]

Adequate selenium status is also vital for normal iodine metabolism, because the enzyme converting T_4 to T_3 (deiodinase) is selenium dependent (see "Selenium"). It may, therefore, be prudent to evaluate T_4 and T_3 status of infants and children with suspected selenium deficiency. Human milk, infant formulas, and parenteral nutrition solutions appear to contain insufficient iodine to meet the requirement of the preterm infant.[155] A Cochrane review found only 1 randomized controlled trial on iodine supplementation of preterm infants and morbidity and neurodevelopment and found insufficient data to make any conclusions.[156]

Iodine Requirement

The RDA of iodine for infants up to 6 months of age is 110 µg/day and for those 6 to 12 months of age, 130 µg/day. The concentration of iodine in human milk depends on maternal intake and, therefore, varies, but values of <100 µg/L were found in a multicenter international study.[157] The iodine concentration in human milk of women in the United States appears to be higher, with a mean value up to 155 µg/L.[158] Cow milk is a rich source of iodine, and cow milk-based infant formula is, therefore, a good source of iodine. Soy formula usually contains approximately 70 to 100 µg/L. Thus, it is evident that formula-fed and breastfed infants will receive adequate quantities of iodine. Children in the United States will get an ample supply of iodine from table salt, dairy products, and baked goods. For areas that are not reached by iodine fortification, low-dose oral iodized oil has been developed for children.[159]

Iodine Toxicity

Although goiter attributable to iodine deficiency is rare in the United States, there is an increasing risk of goiter attributable to excessive iodine intake. Several sources contribute to the iodine intake of children, and it is possible that iodination of salt is no longer needed.[159]

Other Trace Elements

Chromium functions as a cofactor for insulin. In experimental animals, chromium deficiency is characterized by impaired growth and longevity and by impaired glucose, lipid, and protein metabolism. However, chromium deficiency in infants is rare and has only been reported associated with protein-calorie malnutrition. The only reliable indicator of chromium deficiency is the demonstration of a beneficial effect of chromium supplementation. There appears to be no role for chromium supplementation in people with diabetes mellitus.[160]

Cobalt is considered essential for humans only because it is a component of the vitamin B_{12} molecule. Cobalt deficiency has never been demonstrated in humans or laboratory animals, and the requirement for cobalt is considered minute.

Molybdenum's biochemical functions are in the synthesis and function of xanthine oxidase, aldehyde oxidase, and sulfite oxidase. Molybdenum deficiency has not been reported under any natural conditions in humans, but it has recently been suggested that low birth weight infants may not meet their molybdenum requirement, particularly when receiving parenteral nutrition.[161]

Arsenic, nickel, silicon, and vanadium are probably not nutritionally important. Human deficiency states have not been demonstrated, and dietary requirements have not been set because of insufficient evidence.

There is no human requirement for aluminum. However, the American Academy of Pediatrics has recently reviewed the concerns for aluminum exposure and aluminum toxicity in infants and children.[162] Aluminum, although poorly absorbed, can accumulate in patients with renal insufficiency, and this accumulation has been associated with osteomalacia and encephalopathy. Care should be taken when administering aluminum-containing antacids to children with renal insufficiency (who may be less able to excrete aluminum).

Although many commercial infant formulas contain relatively high levels of aluminum,[163] particularly soy formulas,[164] the functional effects (if any) of this are unclear, and presently there are no associated negative effects.[164,165] The greatest concern is for preterm infants exposed to high amounts of aluminum with micronutrient delivery in parenteral nutrition solutions.[162,166,167] Of concern is a study in preterm infants that has shown that higher aluminum intakes are associated with both poorer neurodevelopmental outcome at 18 months[166] and lower bone mineral density at 15 years.[168] There are several approaches to limiting the exposure of preterm infants to aluminum in parenteral nutrition solutions,[169] but using the presently available solutions, aluminum exposure is still too high in preterm infants.[162]

References

1. Institute of Medicine, Food and Nutrition Board. *Dietary Reference Intakes for Vitamin A, Vitamin K, Arsenic, Boron, Chromium, Copper, Iodine, Iron, Manganese, Molybdenum, Nickel, Silicon, Vanadium, and Zinc.* Washington, DC: National Academies Press; 2001

2. Prasad AS. Clinical and biochemical spectrum of zinc deficiency in human subjects. In: Prasad AS, ed. *Clinical, Biochemical, and Nutritional Aspects of Trace Elements.* New York, NY: Alan R Liss Inc; 1982:3–62

3. Shankar AH, Prasad AS. Zinc and immune function: the biological basis of altered resistance to infection. *Am J Clin Nutr.* 1998;68(2 Suppl):447S–463S

4. Bhutta ZA, Bird SM, Black RE, et al. Zinc Investigators Collaborative Group. Therapeutic effects of oral zinc in acute and persistent diarrhea in children in developing countries: pooled analysis of randomized controlled trials. *Am J Clin Nutr.* 2000;72(6):1516–1522

5. Ruel MT, Rivera JA, Santizo MC, Lonnerdal B, Brown KH. Impact of zinc supplementation on morbidity from diarrhea and respiratory infections among rural Guatemalan children. *Pediatrics.* 1997;99(6):808–813

6. Sazawal S, Black RE, Bhan MK, Jalla S, Sinha A, Bhandari N. Efficacy of zinc supplementation in reducing the incidence and prevalence of acute diarrhea—a community based, double blind, controlled trial. *Am J Clin Nutr.* 1997;66(2):413–418

7. Bhutta ZA, Black RE, Brown KH, et al. Prevention of diarrhea and pneumonia by zinc supplementation in children in developing countries: pooled analysis of randomized controlled trials. Zinc Investigators Collaborative Group. *J Pediatr.* 1999;135(6):689–697

8. Black RE. Therapeutic and preventive effects of zinc on serious childhood infectious diseases in developing countries. *Am J Clin Nutr.* 1998;68(2 Suppl):476S–479S

9. Sazawal S, Black RE, Jalla S, Mazumdar S, Sinha A, Bhan MK. Zinc supplementation reduces the incidence of acute lower respiratory infections in infants and preschool children: a double blind, controlled trial. *Pediatrics.* 1998;102(1 Pt 1):1–5

10. Sazawal S, Bentley M, Black RE, Dhingra P, George S, Bhan MK. Effect of zinc supplementation on observed activity in low socioeconomic Indian preschool children. *Pediatrics.* 1996;98(6 Pt 1):1132–1137

11. Castillo-Duran C, Perales CG, Hertrampf ED, Marín VB, Rivera FA, Icaza G. Effect of zinc supplementation on development and growth of Chilean infants. *J Pediatr.* 2001;138(2):229–235

12. Frederickson CJ, Suh SW, Silva D, Frederickson CJ, Thompson RB. Importance of zinc in the central nervous system: the zinc containing neuron. *J Nutr.* 2000;130(5 Suppl):S1471–S1483

13. Sandstead HH, Penland JG, Alcock NW, et al. Effects of repletion with zinc and other micronutrients repletion on neuropsychological performance and growth of Chinese children. *Am J Clin Nutr.* 1997;16(2 Suppl):268–272

14. Hambidge KM, Krebs NF, Westcott JE, Miller LV. Changes in zinc absorption during development. *J Pediatr.* 2006;149(5 Suppl):S64–S68

15. Eide DJ. Zinc transporters and the cellular trafficking of zinc. *Biochim Biophys Acta.* 2006;1763(7):711–722

16. Gaither LA, Eide DJ. The human ZIP1 transporter mediates zinc uptake in human K562 erythroleukemia cells. *J Biol Chem.* 2001;276(25):22258–22264

17. McMahon RJ, Cousins RJ. Mammalian zinc transporters. *J Nutr.* 1998;128(4): 667–670

18. Hara T, Takeda TA, Takagishi T, Fukue K, Kambe T, Fukada T. Physiological roles of zinc transporters: molecular and genetic importance in zinc homeostasis. *J Physiol Sci.* 2017;67(2):283–301

19. Prasad AS. Impact of the discovery of human zinc deficiency on health. *J Am Coll Nutr.* 2009;28(3):257–265

20. Walravens PA. Nutritional importance of copper and zinc in neonates and infants. *Clin Chem.* 1980;26(2):185–189

21. Wang K, Zhou B, Kuo YM, Zemansky J, Gitschier J. A novel member of a zinc transporter family is defective in acrodermatitis enteropathica. *Am J Hum Genet.* 2002;71(1):66–73

22. Sandström B, Cederblad Å, Lindblad BS, Lönnerdal B. Acrodermatitis enteropathica, zinc metabolism, copper status and immune function. *Arch Pediatr Adolesc Med.* 1994;148(9):980–985

23. Zimmerman AW, Hambidge KM, Lepow MI, Greenberg RD, Stover ML, Casey CE. Acrodermatitis in breast-fed premature infants: evidence for a defect of mammary zinc secretion. *Pediatrics.* 1982;69(2):176–183

24. de Benoist B, Darnton-Hill I, Davidsson L, Fontaine O, Hotz C. Conclusions of the Joint WHO/UNICEF/IAEA/IZiNCG Interagency Meeting on Zinc Status Indicators. *Food Nutr Bull.* 2007;28(3 Suppl):S480–S484

25. Gibson RS, Hess SY, Hotz C, Brown KH. Indicators of zinc status at the population level: a review of the evidence. *Br J Nutr.* 2008;99(Suppl 3):S14–S23

26. Walravens PA, Hambidge KM. Growth of infants fed a zinc supplemented formula. *Am J Clin Nutr.* 1976;29(10):1114–1121

27. Hambidge KM, Walravens PA, Casey CE, Brown RM, Bender C. Plasma zinc concentrations of breast-fed infants. *J Pediatr.* 1979;94(4):607–608

28. Rivera JA, Ruel MT, Santizo MC, Lönnerdal B, Brown KH. Zinc supplementation improves the growth of stunted rural Guatemalan infants. *J Nutr.* 1998;128(3): 556–562

29. Ruz M, Castillo Duran C, Lara X, Codoceo J, Rebolledo A, Atalah E. A 14 mo zinc supplementation trial in apparently healthy Chilean preschool children. *Pediatrics.* 1997;66(6):1406–1413

30. Umeta M, West CE, Haidar J, Deurenberg P, Hautvast JG. Zinc supplementation and stunted infants in Ethiopia: a randomized controlled trial. *Lancet.* 2000;355(9220):2021–2026

IV

31. Brown KH, Peerson JM, Rivera J, Allen LH. Effect of supplemental zinc on the growth and serum zinc concentrations of prepubertal children: a meta-analysis of randomized controlled trials. *Am J Clin Nutr.* 2002;75(6):1062–1071

32. Brown KH. Commentary: zinc and child growth. *Int J Epidemiol.* 2003;32(6): 1103–1104

33. Diaz-Gomez NM, Domenech E, Barroso F, Castells S, Cortabarria C, Jiménez A. The effect of zinc supplementation on linear growth, body composition, and growth factors in preterm infants. *Pediatrics.* 2003;115(5 Pt 1):1002–1009

34. Islam MN, Chowdhury MA, Siddika M, et al. Effect of oral zinc supplementation on the growth of preterm infants. *Indian Pediatr.* 2010;47(10):845–849

35. Golan Y, Kambe T, Assaraf YG. The role of the zinc transporter SLC30A2/ZnT2 in transient neonatal zinc deficiency. *Metallomics.* 2017;9(10):1352–1366

36. Kambe T, Fukue K, Ishida R, Miyazaki SJNSVTSS-. Overview of inherited zinc deficiency in infants and children. *J Nutr Sci Vitaminol (Tokyo).* 2015;61(Suppl): S44–S46

37. Jones G, Steketee RW, Black RE, Bhutta ZA, Morris SS, Bellagio Child Survival Study Group. How many child deaths can we prevent this year? *Lancet.* 2003;362(9377):65–71

38. Brooks WA, Santosham M, Naheed A, et al. Effect of weekly zinc supplements on incidence of pneumonia and diarrhea in children younger than 2 years in an urban, low-income population in Bangladesh: randomised controlled trial. *Lancet.* 2005;366(9490):999–1004

39. Robberstad B, Strand T, Black RE, Sommerfelt H. Cost-effectiveness of zinc as adjunct therapy for acute childhood diarrhea in developing countries. *Bull World Health Organ.* 2004;82(7):523–531

40. Bhatnagar S, Bahl R, Sharma PKea. Zinc with oral rehydration therapy reduces stool output and duration of diarrhea in hospitalized children: a randomized controlled trial. *J Pediatr Gastroenterol Nutr.* 2004;38(1):34–40

41. Fischer Walker CL, Fontaine O, Young MW, Black RE. Zinc and low osmolarity oral rehydration salts for diarrhoea: a renewed call to action. *Bull World Health Organ.* 2009;87(10):780–786

42. Shillcutt SD, LeFevre AE, Fischer-Walker CL, Taneja S, Black RE, Maxumder S. Cost-effectivess, analysis of the diarrhea alleviation through zinc and oral rehydration therapy (DAZT) program in rural Gujarat India; an application of the net-benefit regression framework. *Cost Effect Resource Alloc.* 2017;15:9

43. Hemilä H. Zinc lozenges and the common cold: a meta-analysis comparing zinc acetate and zinc gluconate, and the role of zinc dosage. *JRSM Open.* 2017;8(5):2054270417694291

44. Shah D, Sachdev HS, Gera T, De-Regil LM, Peña-Rosas JP. Fortification of staple foods with zinc for improving zinc status and other health outcomes in the general population. *Cochrane Database Syst Rev.* 2016(6):CD010697

45. Brown KH. Effect of infections on plasma zinc concentration and implications for zinc status in low income populations. *Am J Clin Nutr.* 1998;68(2 Suppl): S425–S429

46. Hambidge KM. Hair analyses: worthless for vitamins, limited for minerals. *Am J Clin Nutr.* 1982;36(5):943–949

47. Hotz C, Brown KH. Identifying populations at risk of zinc deficiency: the use of supplementation trials. *Nutr Rev.* 2001;59(3 Pt 1):80–84

48. Greene HL, Hambidge KM, Schanler R, Tsang R. Guidelines for the use of vitamins, trace elements, calcium, magnesium, and phosphorus in infants and children receiving total parenteral nutrition. Report of Subcommittee. Committee on Clinical Practice Issues of the ASCN. *Am J Clin Nutr.* 1988;48(5): 1324–1342

49. Krebs NF, Westcott JE, Arnold TD, et al. Abnormalities in zinc homeostasis in young infants with cystic fibrosis. *Pediatr Res.* 2000;48(2):256–261

50. Solomons NW, Rosenberg IH, Sandstead HH, Vo-Khactu KP. Zinc deficiency in Crohn's disease. *Digestion.* 1977;16(1-2):87–95

51. Zemel BS, Kawchak DA, Fung EB, Ohene-Frempong K, Stallings VA. Effect of zinc supplementation on growth and body composition in children with sickle cell disease. *Am J Clin Nutr.* 2002;75(2):300–307

52. Krebs NF, Reidinger CJ, Robertson AD, Hambidge KM. Growth and intakes of energy and zinc in infants fed human milk. *J Pediatr.* 1994;124(1):32–39

53. Atkinson SA, Whelan D, Whyte RK, Lönnerdal B. Abnormal zinc content in human milk. *Am J Dis Child.* 1989;143(5):608–611

54. Chowanadisai W, Lonnerdal B, Kelleher SL. Identification of a mutation in SLC30A2 (ZnT-2) in women with low milk zinc concentration that results in transient neonatal zinc deficiency. *J Biol Chem.* 2006;281(51):39699–36707

55. Krebs NF, Hambidge KM. Zinc requirements and zinc intakes of breast fed infants. *Am J Clin Nutr.* 1986;43(2):288–292

56. Arsenault JE, Brown KH. Zinc intake of US preschool children exceeds new dietary reference intakes. *Am J Clin Nutr.* 2003;78(5):1011–1017

57. Butte NF, Fox MK, Briefel RR, et al. Nutrient intakes of US infants, toddlers, and preschoolers meet or exceed dietary reference intakes. *J Am Diet Assoc.* 2010;110(12 Suppl):S27–S37

58. Affenito SG, Thompson DR, Franko DL, et al. Longitudinal assessment of micronutrient intake among African American and White girls: The National Heart, Lung, and Blood Institute Growth and Health Study. *J Am Diet Assoc.* 2007;107(7):1113–1123

59. Schenkel TC, Stockman NKA, Brown JN, Duncan AM. Evaluation of energy, nutrient and dietary fiber intakes in adolescents males. *J Am Coll Nutr.* 2007;26(3):264–271

60. Sandstrom B, Cederblad A, Lonnerdal B. Zinc absorption from human milk, cow's milk, and infant formulas. *Am J Dis Child.* 1983;137(8):726–729

61. Lönnerdal B, Hoffman B, Hurley LS. Zinc and copper binding proteins in human milk. *Am J Clin Nutr.* 1982;36(6):1170–1176

62. Lönnerdal B. Dietary factors influencing zinc absorption. *J Nutr.* 2000;130(6): 1378S–1383S

IV

63. Lönnerdal B, Cederblad A, Davidsson L, Sandstrom B. The effect of individual components of soy formula and cow's milk formula on zinc bioavailability. *Am J Clin Nutr.* 1984;40(6):1064–1070

64. Lönnerdal B, Bell JG, Hendrickx AG, Burns RA, Keen CL. Effect of phytate removal on zinc absorption from soy formula. *Am J Clin Nutr.* 1988;48(5): 1301–1306

65. Gibson RS, Yeudall F, Drost N, Mtitimuni B, Cullinan T. Dietary interventions to prevent zinc deficiency. *Am J Clin Nutr.* 1998;68(2 Suppl):484S–487S

66. Sandström B, Davidsson L, Cederblad Å, Lönnerdal B. Oral iron, dietary ligands and zinc absorption. *J Nutr.* 1985;115(3):411–414

67. Lind T, Lönnerdal B, Stenlund H, et al. A community-based randomized controlled trial of iron and zinc supplementation in Indonesian infants: interactions between iron and zinc. *Am J Clin Nutr.* 2003;77(3):883–890

68. Krebs NF, Reidinger CJ, Hartley S, Robertson AD, Hambidge KM. Zinc supplementation during lactation: effects on maternal status and milk zinc concentrations. *Am J Clin Nutr.* 1995;61(5):1030–1036

69. Castillo Duran C, Heresi G, Fisberg M, Uauy R. Controlled trial of zinc supplementation during recovery from malnutrition: effects on growth and immune function. *Am J Clin Nutr.* 1987;45(3):602–608

70. Brown KH. WHO/UNICEF review on complementary feeding and suggestions for future research: WHO/UNICEF guidelines on complementary feeding. *Pediatrics.* 2000;106(5):1290

71. Olivares M, Araya M, Uauy R. Copper homeostasis in infant nutrition: deficit and excess. *J Pediatr Gastroenterol Nutr.* 2000;31(2):102–111

72. Milne DB. Copper intake and assessment of copper status. *Am J Clin Nutr.* 1998;67(5 Suppl):1041S–1045S

73. Kaler SG. Diagnosis and therapy of Menkes syndrome, a genetic form of copper deficiency. *Am J Clin Nutr.* 1998;67(5 Suppl):1029S–1034S

74. Sheela SR, Latha M, Liu P, Lem K, Kaler SG. Copper-replacement treatment for symptomatic Menkes disease: ethical considerations. *Clin Genet.* 2005;68(3): 278–283

75. Mercer JF, Livingston J, Hall B, et al. Isolation of a partial candidate gene for Menkes disease by positional cloning. *Nat Genet.* 1993;3(1):20–25

76. Camakaris J, Petris MJ, Bailey L, et al. Gene amplification of the Menkes (MNK; ATP7A) P type ATPase gene of CHO cells is associated with copper resistance and enhanced copper efflux. *Hum Mol Genet.* 1995;4(11):2117–2123

77. Lönnerdal B. Copper nutrition during infancy and childhood. *Am J Clin Nutr.* 1998;67(5 Suppl):1046S–1053S

78. Salmenperä L, Perheentupa J, Pakarinen P, Siimes MA. Cu nutrition in infants during prolonged exclusive breast feeding: low intake but rising serum concentrations of Cu and ceruloplasmin. *Am J Clin Nutr.* 1986;43(2):251–257

79. Percival SS. Copper and immunity. *Am J Clin Nutr.* 1998;67(5 Suppl):1064S–1068S

80. Harris ZL, Takahashi Y, Miyajima H, Serizawa M, MacGillivray RT, Gitlin JD. Aceruloplasminemia: molecular characterization of this disorder of iron metabolism. *Proc Natl Acad Sci U S A.* 1995;92(7):2539–2543

81. Salmenperä L, Siimes MA, Näntö V, Perheentupa J. Copper supplementation: failure to increase plasma copper and ceruloplasmin concentrations in healthy infants. *Am J Clin Nutr.* 1989;50(4):843–847

82. Sorenson AW, Butrum RR. Zinc and copper in infant diets. *J Am Diet Assoc.* 1983;83(3):291–297

83. Olivares M, Pizarro F, Speisky H, Lönnerdal B, Uauy R. Copper in infant nutrition: safety of World Health Organization provisional guideline value for copper content of drinking water. *J Pediatr Gastroenterol Nutr.* 1998;26(3):251–257

84. Olivares M, Lönnerdal B, Abrams SA, Pizarro F, Uauy R. Age and copper intake do not affect copper absorption, measured with the use of stable isotopes. 76. 2002;3(641–645)

85. Ehrenkranz RA, Gettner PA, Nelli CM. Zinc and copper nutritional studies in very low birth weight infants: comparison of stable isotopic extrinsic tag and chemical balance methods. 26. 1989;4(298–307)

86. Dörner K, Dziadzka S, Hohn A, et al. Longitudinal manganese and copper balances in young infants and preterm infants fed on breast milk and adapted cow's milk formulas. *Br J Nutr.* 1989;61(3):559–572

87. Lönnerdal B, Bell JG, Keen CL. Copper absorption from human milk, cow's milk and infant formulas using a suckling rat model. *Am J Clin Nutr.* 1985;42(5): 836–844

88. Lönnerdal B, Jayawickrama L, Lien EL. Effect of reducing the phytate content and of partially hydrolyzing the protein in soy formula on zinc and copper absorption and status in infant rhesus monkeys and rat pups. *Am J Clin Nutr.* 1999;69(3):490–496

89. Stack T, Aggett PJ, Aitken E, Lloyd DJ. Routine L ascorbic acid supplementation does not alter iron, copper, and zinc balance in low birthweight infants fed a cow's milk formula. *J Pediatr Gastroenterol Nutr.* 1990;10(3):351–356

90. Lönnerdal B, Kelleher SL, Lien EL. Extent of thermal processing of infant formula affects copper status in infant rhesus monkeys. *Am J Clin Nutr.* 2001;73(5):914–919

91. Pizarro F, Olivares M, Uauy R, Contreras P, Rebelo A, Gidi V. Acute gastrointestinal effects of graded levels of copper in drinking water. *Environ Health Perspect.* 1999;107(2):117–121

92. Tanner MS, Kantarjian AH, Bhave SA, Pandit AN. Early introduction of copper contaminated animal milk feeds as a possible cause of Indian childhood cirrhosis. *Lancet.* 1983;2(8357):992–995

93. Müller Höcker J, Meyer U, Wiebecke B, et al. Copper storage disease of the liver and chronic dietary copper intoxication in two further German infants mimicking Indian childhood cirrhosis. *Pathol Res Pract.* 1998;183(1):39–45

IV

94. Müller T, Feichtinger H, Berger H, Müller W. Endemic Tyrolean infantile cirrhosis: an ecogenetic disorder. *Lancet*. 1996;347(9005):877–880

95. Danks DM. Disorders of copper transport. In: Scriver CL, Beaudet AL, Sly WS, Valle D, eds. *The Metabolic and Molecular Bases of Inherited Disease*. New York, NY: McGraw Hill; 1995:2211–2235

96. Brewer GJ, Hill GM, Prasad AS, Cossack ZT, Rabbani P. Oral zinc therapy for Wilson's disease. *Ann Intern Med*. 1983;99(3):314–319

97. Petrukhin K, Lutsenko S, Chernov I, Ross BM, Kaplan JH, Gilliam TC. Characterization of the Wilson disease gene encoding a P type copper transporting ATPase: genomic organization, alternative splicing, and structure/function predictions. *Hum Mol Genet*. 1994;3(9):1647–1656

98. Panagiotataki E, Tzetis M, Manolaki N, et al. Genotype-phenotype correlations for a wide spectrum of mutations in the Wilson disease gene (ATP7B). *Am J Med Genet*. 2004;131(1):168–173

99. Tian G, Kane LS, Holmes WD, Davis ST. Modulation of cyclin-dependent kinase 4 by binding of magnesium (II) and manganese (II). *Biophys Chem*. 2002;95(1):79–90

100. Doisy EA. Effects of deficiency in manganese upon plasma levels of clotting proteins and cholesterol in man and chick. In: Hoekstra WG, Suttie JW, Ganther HE, Mertz W, eds. *Trace Elements in Man and Animals: 2*. Baltimore, MD: University Park Press; 1974:668–670

101. Stastny D, Vogel RS, Picciano MF. Manganese intake and serum manganese concentration of human milk fed and formula fed infants. *Am J Clin Nutr*. 1984;39(6):872–878

102. Xin Y, Gao H, Wang J, et al. Manganese transporter Slc39a14 deficiency revealed its key role in maintaining manganese homeostasis in mice. *Cell Discov*. 2017;3(17025)

103. Vuori E. A longitudinal study of manganese in human milk. *Acta Paediatr Scand*. 1979;68:571–573

104. Lönnerdal B, Keen C, Hurley LS. Manganese binding proteins in human and cow's milk. *Am J Clin Nutr*. 1985;41(3):550–559

105. Lönnerdal B. Manganese nutrition of infants. In: Klimis Tavantzis DJ, ed. *Manganese in Health and Disease*. Boca Raton, FL: CRC Press Inc; 1994:175–191

106. Cockell KA, Bonacci G, Belonje B. Manganese content of soy or rice beverages is high in comparison to infant formulas. *J Am Coll Nutr*. 2004;23(2):124–130

107. Wasserman GA, Liu X, Parvez F, et al. Water manganese exposure and children's intellectual function in Araihazar, Bangladesh. *Environ Health Perspect*. 2006;114(1):124–129

108. Groschen GE, Arnold TL, Morrow WS, Warner KL. *Occurrence and distribution of iron, manganese, and selected trace elements in ground water in the glacial aquifer system of the Northern United States. US Geological Survey Scientific Investigations Report 2009–5006*. Washington, DC: US Department of the Interior; 2008

109. Davidsson L, Cederblad Å, Lönnerdal B, Sandström B. Manganese absorption from human milk, cow's milk and infant formulas in humans. *Am J Dis Child.* 1989;143(7):823–827

110. Keen CL, Bell JG, Lönnerdal B. The effect of age on manganese uptake and retention from milk and infant formulas in rats. *J Nutr.* 1986;116(3):395–402

111. Hatano S, Aihara K, Nishi Y, Usui T. Trace elements (copper, zinc, manganese, and selenium) in plasma and erythrocytes in relation to dietary intake during infancy. *J Pediatr Gastroenterol Nutr.* 1985;4(1):87–92

112. Mena I. Manganese. In: Bronner F, Coburn JW, eds. *Disorders of Mineral Metabolism.* Orlando, FL: Academic Press Inc; 1981:233–270

113. Herrero Hernandez E, Discalzi G, Dassi P, Jarre L, Pira E. Manganese intoxication: the cause of an inexplicable epileptic syndrome in a 3 year old child. *NeuroToxicology.* 2003;24(4-5):633–639

114. Woolf A, Wright R, Amarasiriwardena C, Bellinger D. A child with chronic manganese exposure from drinking water. *Environ Health Perspect.* 2002;110(6): 613–616

115. Tran TT, Chowanadisai W, Crinella FM, Chicz-DeMet A, Lönnerdal B. Effect of high dietary manganese intake of neonatal rats on tissue mineral accumulation, striatal dopamine levels, and neurodevelopmental status. *NeuroToxicology.* 2002;23(4-5):635–643

116. Takser L, Mergler D, Hellier G, Sahuquillo J, Huel G. Manganese, monoamine metabolite levels at birth, and child psychomotor development. *NeuroToxicology.* 2003;24(4-5):667–674

117. Golub MS, Hogrefe CE, Germann SL, et al. Neurobehavioral evaluation of rhesus monkeys fed cow's milk formula, soy formula, or soy formula with added manganese. *Neurotoxicol Teratol.* 2005;27(4):615–627

118. Deveau M. Contribution of drinking water to dietary requirements of essential metals. *J Toxicol Environ Health A.* 2010;73(2):235–241

119. Bouchard MF, Sauvé S, Barbeau B, et al. Intellectual impairment in school-age children exposed to manganese from drinking water. *Environ Health Perspect.* 2011;119(1):138–143

120. Dickerson RN. Manganese intoxication and parenteral nutrition. *Nutrition.* 2001;17(7-8):689–693

121. Fell JM, Reynolds AP, Meadows N, et al. Manganese toxicity in children receiving long term parenteral nutrition. *Lancet.* 1996;347(9010):1218–1221

122. Bayliss EA, Hambidge KM, Sokol RJ, Stewart B, Lilly JR. Hepatic concentrations of zinc, copper and manganese in infants with extrahepatic biliary atresia. *J Trace Elem Med Biol.* 1995;9(1):40–43

123. Hardy IJ, Gillanders L, Hardy G. Is manganese an essential supplement for parenteral nutrition? . *Curr Opin Clin Nutr Metab Care.* 2008;11(3):289–296

124. Sunde RA. Molecular biology of selenoproteins. *Annu Rev Nutr.* 1990;10:451–474

125. Litov RE, Combs Jr GF. Selenium in pediatric nutrition. *Pediatrics.* 1991;87(3): 339–351

IV

126. Thomson CD, Robinson MF. Urinary and fecal excretion and absorption of a large supplement of selenium: superiority of selenate over selenite. *Am J Clin Nutr.* 1986;44(5):659–663

127. Berry MJ, Banu L, Larsen PR. Type I iodothyronine deiodinase is a selenocysteine-containing enzyme. *Nature.* 1991;349(6308):438–440

128. Observations on effect of sodium selenite in prevention of Keshan disease. *China Med J (Engl).* 1979;92(7):471–476

129. Peng T, Li Y, Yang Y, et al. Characterization of enterovirus isolates from patients with heart muscle disease in a selenium-deficient area of China. *J Clin Microbiol.* 2000;38(10):3538–3543

130. Nelson HK, Shi Q, Van Dael P, et al. Host nutritional status as a driving force for influenza virus. *FASEB J.* 2001;15(10):U488–U499

131. Vinton NE, Dahlström KA, Strobel CT, Ament ME. Macrocytosis and pseudoalbinism: manifestations of selenium deficiency. *J Pediatr.* 1987;111(5): 711–717

132. Lockitch G, Taylor GP, Wong LT, et al. Cardiomyopathy associated with nonendemic selenium deficiency in a Caucasian adolescent. *Am J Clin Nutr.* 1990;52(3):572–577

133. Lockitch G, Jacobson B, Quigley G, Dison P, Pendray M. Selenium deficiency in low birth weight neonates: an unrecognized problem. *J Pediatr.* 1989;114(5): 865–870

134. Campa A, Shor-Posner G, Indacochea F, et al. Mortality risk in selenium-deficient HIV-positive children. *J Acquire Immune Defic Syndr Hum Retrovirol.* 1999;20(5):508–513

135. Smith AM, Chan GM, Moyer Mileur LJ, Johnson CE, Gardner BR. Selenium status of preterm infants fed human milk, preterm formula, or selenium supplemented preterm formula. *J Pediatr.* 1991;119(3):429–433

136. Tyrala EE, Borschel MW, Jacobs JR. Selenate fortification of infant formulas improves the selenium status of preterm infants. *Am J Clin Nutr.* 1996;64(6): 860–865

137. Darlow BA, Austin NC. Selenium supplementation to prevent short-term morbidity in preterm neonates. *Cochrane Database Syst Rev.* 2003;(4):CD003312

138. Rayman MP, Wijnen H, Vader H, Kooistra L, V. P. Maternal selenium status during early gestation and risk for preterm birth. *CMAJ.* 2011;183(5):549–555

139. Tara F, Maamouri G, Rayman MP, et al. Selenium supplementation and the incidence of preeclampsia in pregnant Iranian women: a randomized, double-blind, placebo-controlled pilot trial. *Taiwan J Obstet Gynecol.* 2010;49(2):181–187

140. Kumpulainen J, Salmenperä L, Siimes MA, Koivistoinen P, Perheentupa J. Selenium status of exclusively breast fed infants as influenced by maternal organic or inorganic selenium supplementation. *Am J Clin Nutr.* 1985;42:829–835

141. Smith AM, Picciano MF, Milner JA. Selenium intakes and status of human milk and formula fed infants. *Am J Clin Nutr.* 1982;35(3):521–526

142. Kumpulainen J, Salmenperä L, Siimes MA, Koivistoinen P, Lehto J, Perheentupa J. Formula feeding results in lower selenium status than breast feeding or selenium supplemented formula feeding: a longitudinal study. *Am J Clin Nutr.* 1987;45:49–53

143. Milner JA, Sherman L, Picciano MF. Distribution of selenium in human milk. *Am J Clin Nutr.* 1987;45(3):617–624

144. Johnson CE, Smith AM, Chan GM, Moyer Mileur LJ. Selenium status of term infants fed human milk or selenite supplemented soy formula. *J Pediatr.* 1993;122(5 Pt 1):739–741

145. Smith AM, Chen LW, Thomas MR. Selenate fortification improves selenium status of term infants fed soy formula. *Am J Clin Nutr.* 1995;61(1):44–47

146. Ehrenkranz RA, Gettner PA, Nelli CM, et al. Selenium absorption and retention by very low birth weight infants: studies with the extrinsic stable isotope tag 74Se. *J Pediatr Gastroenterol Nutr.* 1991;13(2):125–133

147. Litov RE, Sickles VS, Chan GM, Hargett IR, Cordano A. Selenium status in term infants fed human milk or infant formula with or without added selenium. *Nutr Res.* 1989;9(6):585–596

148. Zimmermann MB. The adverse effects of mild-to-moderate iodine deficiency during pregnancy and childhood: a review. *Thyroid.* 2007;17(9):829–835

149. Caldwell KL, Miller GA, Wang RY, Jain RB, Jones RL. Iodine status of the US population, National health and Nutrition Examination Survey 2003–2004. *Thyroid.* 2008;18(11):1207–1214

150. Zimmermann MB. The impact of iodised salt or iodine supplements on iodine status during pregnancy, lactation and infancy. *Public Health Nutr.* 2007;10(12A):1584–1595

151. Lee SY, Leung AM, He X, Braverman LE, Pearce EN. Iodine content in fast foods: Comparison between two fast food chains in the United States. *Endocr Pract.* 2010;16(6):1071–1072

152. Vanderpump MP, Lazarus JH, Smyth PP, et al. British Thyroid Association UK Iodine Survey Group. Iodine status of UK schoolgirls: a cross-sectional survey. *Lancet.* 2011;377(9782):2007–2012

153. Zimmermann M, Adou P, Torresani T, Zeder C, Hurrell R. Low dose oral iodized oil for control of iodine deficiency in children. *Br J Nutr.* 2000;84(2):139–141

154. Zimmermann M, Adou P, Torresani T, Zeder C, Hurrell R. Persistence of goiter despite oral iodine supplementation in goitrous children with iron deficiency anemia in Cote d'Ivoire. 71. 2000;1(88–93)

155. Ares S, Quero J, Morreale de Escobar G. Neonatal iodine deficiency: clinical aspects. *J Pediatr Endocrinol Metab.* 2005;18(Suppl 1):1257–1264

156. Ibrahim M, Sinn J, McGuire W. Iodine supplementation for the prevention of mortality and adverse neurodevelopmental outcomes in preterm infants. *Cochrane Database Syst Rev.* 2006(2):CD005253

157. Azizi F, Smyth PP. Breastfeeding and maternal and infant iodine concentration. *Clin Endocrinol.* 2009;70(5):803–809

IV

158. Pearce EN, Leung AM, Blount BC, et al. Breast milk iodine and perchlorate concentrations in lactating Boston-area women. *J Clin Endocrinol Metab.* 2007;92(5):1673–1677

159. Zimmermann MB, Adou P, Torresani T, Zeder C, Hurrell RF. Effect of oral iodized oil on thyroid size and thyroid hormone metabolism in children with concurrent selenium and iodine deficiency. *Eur J Clin Nutr.* 2000;54(3):209–213

160. Landman GW, Bilo HJ, Houweling ST, Kleefstra N. Chromium does not belong in the diabetes treatment arsenal: current evidence and future perspectives. *World J Diabetes.* 2014;5(2):160–164

161. Friel JK, MacDonald AC, Mercer CN, et al. Molybdenum requirements in low birth weight infants receiving parenteral and enteral nutrition. *JPEN J Parenter Enteral Nutr.* 1999;23(3):155–159

162. Corkins MR, American Academy of Pediatrics, Committee on Nutrition. Technical report: Aluminum toxicity in infants and children. *Pediatrics.* 2019;in press

163. Burrell SA, Exley C. There is (still) too much aluminum in infant formulas. *BMC Pediatr.* 2010;10:63

164. Agostoni C, Axelsson I, Goulet O, et al. Soy protein infant formulae and follow-on formulae: a commentary by the ESPGHAN Committee on Nutrition. *J Pediatr Gastroenterol Nutr.* 2006;42(4):352–361

165. Litov RE, Sickles VS, Chan GM, Springer MA, Cordano A. Plasma aluminum measurements in term infants fed human milk or a soy based infant formula. *Pediatrics.* 1989;84(6):1105–1107

166. Bishop NJ, Morley R, Day JP, Lucas A. Aluminum neurotoxicity in preterm infants receiving intravenous-feeding solutions. *N Engl J Med.* 1997;336(22):1557–1561

167. Bohrer D, Oliveira SM, Garcia SC, Nascimento PC, Carvalho LM. Aluminum loading in preterm neonates revisited. *J Pediatr Gastroenterol Nutr.* 2010;51(2):237–241

168. Fewtrell MS, Bishop NJ, Edmonds CJ, Isaacs EB, Lucas A. Aluminum exposure from parenteral nutrition in preterm infants: bone health at 15-year follow-up. *Pediatrics.* 2009;124(5):1372–1379

169. Fanni D, Ambu R, Gerosa C, et al. Aluminum exposure and toxicity in neonates: a practical guide to halt aluminum overload in the prenatal and perinatal periods. *World J Pediatr.* 2014;10(2):101–107

Chapter 21

Vitamins

Table 21.1.

Vitamin Deficiency States, Recommended Intake, Deficiency Symptoms, Deficiency Risk Factors, Diagnostic Tests, and Therapeutic Dosages

Nutrient	Recommended Intake	Deficiency Name	Deficiency Symptoms	Deficiency Risk Factors	Diagnostic Tests	Food Sources	Recommended Therapeutic Dosage
Vitamin A AI infants	0–6 mo 1320 IU/d 7–12 mo 1650 IU/d		Night blindness, Infection (measles), keratomalacia	Fat malabsorption	Serum retinol Serum retinol-binding protein	Liver, eggs, dairy, vegetables	100 000–200 000 IU, orally
RDA 1–18 y	1–3 y 1000 IU/d 4–8 y 1430 IU/d 9–13 y 2000 IU/d 14–18 y 2310–3000 IU/d						
Vitamin D AI infants	Infants 400 IU/d Preterm infants: <1000 g 200–400 IU/d >1500 g 400 IU/d >1 y 600 IU/d	Rickets	Rickets, hypocalcemia, tetany, osteomalacia, hypophosphatemia	Fat malabsorption, lack of sunshine	X-ray, serum 25-OH-D	Fatty fish egg yolk	2000–5000 IU day (see text)
RDA 1–18y							
Vitamin E RDA all ages	0–6 mo 4 mg/d 7–12 mo 5 mg/d 1–3 y 6 mg/d 4–8 y 7 mg/d 9–13 y 11 mg/d 14–18 y 15 mg/d		Neuropathy, ataxia	Fat malabsorption	Serum alpha-tocopherol	Grain and vegetable oils	25 IU/kg/day for fat malabsorption

Vitamin K AI all ages 0–6 mo 2 µg/d 7–12 mo 2.5 µg/d 1–3 y 30 µg/d 4–8 y 55 µg/d 9–18 y 60–75 µg/d	Newborn deficiency bleeding	Bleeding	Fat malabsorption, breastfeeding	PT, PIVKA, clotting factors	Green vegetables, soy oil, seeds, fruits	1 mg, intramuscularly, in newborn infants
Thiamine (B$_1$) AI infants 0–6 mo 0.2 mg/d 7–12 mo 0.3 mg/d RDA 1–18y 1–3 y 0.5 mg/d 4–8 y 0.6 mg/d 9–13 y 0.9 mg/d 14–18 y 1–1.2 mg/d	Beriberi or Wernicke encephalopathy	Beriberi: symmetrical, peripheral neuropathy, edema; Wernicke; ophthalmoplegia, nystagmus, ataxia	HIV, alcohol abuse, dialysis, gastrointestinal tract disease, total parenteral nutrition, anorexia, furosemide, food faddism; inflammation in pediatric intensive care unit	Whole blood/RBC transketolase activation test, baseline and after thiamine pyrophosphate (TPP); or TPP level, urinary total thiamine	Unrefined grain, liver, pork, vegetables, dairy, peanuts, legumes, fruits, eggs	Severe infantile: 50–100 mg parenteral X1; children: 10–25 mg/day parenteral X 2 wk, followed by 5–10 mg/day, orally, X 1 mo. Mild: 10 mg/day, orally, until resolution
Riboflavin (B$_2$) AI infants 0–6 mo 0.3 mg/d 7–12 mo 0.4 mg/d RDA 1–18y 1–3 y 0.5 mg/d 4–8 y 0.6 mg/d 9–13 y 0.9 mg/d 14–18 y 1–1.3 mg/d		Pharyngitis, cheilosis, angular stomatitis, glossitis, seborrheic dermatitis	Weaning from breastfeeding, breastfed from deficient mother, alcoholism, phototherapy, cystic fibrosis, malnutrition, thyroid insufficiency, adrenal insufficiency	RBC or 24-h urine riboflavin level or RBC glutathione reductase (but of limited value in glutathione reductase deficiency, G6PD deficiency, or beta-thalassemia)	Milk, cheese, eggs, liver, lean meats, green vegetables	Infants: 0.5 mg, orally, twice/wk. Children: 1 mg, orally, dose 3 X/day until resolution

Continued

Table 211. *Continued*

Vitamin Deficiency States, Recommended Intake, Deficiency Symptoms, Deficiency Risk Factors, Diagnostic Tests, and Therapeutic Dosages

Nutrient	Recommended Intake	Deficiency Name	Deficiency Symptoms	Deficiency Risk Factors	Diagnostic Tests	Food Sources	Recommended Therapeutic Dosage
Niacin (B₃) AI infants RDA 1-18y	0-6 mo 2 mg/d 7-12 mo 4 mg/d 1-3 y 6 mg/d 4-8 y 8 mg/d 9-13 y 12 mg/d 14-18 y 14-16 mg/d	Pellagra	Diarrhea, dermatitis, dementia, glossitis, angular stomatitis, sun-exposed	Crohn disease; anorexia nervosa; Hartnup disease; Carcinoid syndrome; immigrant from area with nonfortified grains; medications isoniazid, anticonvulsants, antidepressants, 5-fluorouracil, 6-mercaptopurine, chloramphenicol, sulfas	24-h niacin and N-methylnicotinamide; or RBC NAD/NADP niacin number	Beef, liver, fish, pork, wheat flour, eggs	50-100 mg/dose, orally, 3 X/day for several wk

Pantothenic acid (B₅) AI all ages	0–6 mo 1.7 mg/d 7–12 mo 1.8 mg/d 1–3 y 2 mg/d 4–8 y 3 mg/d 9–13 y 4 mg/d 14–18 y 5 mg/d		Not characterized		24-h pantothenic acid	Chicken, beef, potatoes, oats, tomatoes, liver, kidney, yeast, egg yolk, broccoli	
Pyridoxine (B₆) AI infants RDA 1–18 y	0–6 mo 0.1 mg/d 7–12 mo 0.3 mg/d 1–3 y 0.5 mg/d 4–8 y 0.6 mg/d 9–13 y 1 mg/d 14–18 y 1.2–1.3 mg/d	Glossitis, cheilosis, angular stomatitis, depression, confusion	Chronic renal failure, leukemia; pyridoxine-dependent seizure; alcoholism; Medications isoniazid, hydralazine, penicillamine, theophylline	Plasma pyridoxal 5'-phosphate; 24-h urine 4-pyridoxic acid	Meat, liver, kidneys	Without neuropathy: 5–25 mg orally/day X 3 wk, with neuropathy: 10–50 mg/day, orally X 3 wk; then followed by 1.5–2.5 mg/day, orally. Seizures: 50–100 mg, intravenously or intramuscularly
Biotin (B₇) AI all ages	0–6 mo 5 µg/d 7–12 mo 6 µg/d 1–3 y 8 µg/d 4–8 y 12 µg/d 9–13 y 20 µg/d 14–18 y 25 µg/d	Hypotonia, exfoliative dermatitis	Infants with TPN without biotin, eating large amounts of undercooked eggs, holocarboxylase synthase deficiency, biotinidase deficiency, biotin transport defect, anticonvulsants	Urinary biotin or urinary 3-hyroxyi-sovaleric acid; lymphocyte propionyl-CoA carboxylase concentration, or leukocyte LSC19A3 transporter	Chard, tomatoes, romaine lettuce, carrots	Acquired deficiency: 150 µg/d

Continued

Table 21.1. *Continued*

Vitamin Deficiency States, Recommended Intake, Deficiency Symptoms, Deficiency Risk Factors, Diagnostic Tests, and Therapeutic Dosages

Nutrient	Recommended Intake	Deficiency Name	Deficiency Symptoms	Deficiency Risk Factors	Diagnostic Tests	Food Sources	Recommended Therapeutic Dosage
Folate (B₉) AI infants RDA 1–18y	0–6 mo 65 µg/d 7–12 mo 80 µg/d 1–3 y 150 µg/d 4–8 y 200 µg/d 9–13 y 300 µg/d 14–18 y 400 µg/d		Megaloblastic anemia, neural tube defect, cleft lip/palate	Poor intakes relatively common at 12 mo; consuming carbonated beverages; Crohn disease; fruit and carb; diarrhea; HIV, familial; medications methotrexate, trimethoprim, oral contraceptives, pyrimethamine, phenobarbital, phenytoin	Plasma or serum folate (acute); RBC folate (chronic deficiency); 5-methyltetrahy-drofolate; or urinary total folate	Cauliflower, green vegetables, yeast, liver, kidney	Infants: 15 µg/kg/day, orally or intramuscularly. Children 1–13: 1 mg/day, followed by 0.1–0.5 mg/d; Children >13: 1 mg/day.
Cobalamin (B₁₂) AI infants RDA 1–18y	0–6 mo 0.4 µg/d 7–12 mo 0.5 µg/d 1–3 y 0.9 µg/d 4–8 y 1.2 µg/d 9–13 y 1.8 µg/d 14–18 y 2.4 µg/d		Megaloblastic anemia, ataxia, muscle weakness, spasticity, incontinence, hypotension, vision problems,	Breastfed children of strict vegans; post bariatric surgery or stomach or ileal resection; pernicious anemia; bacterial	Serum cobalamin concentration, plasma homo-cysteine or serum methyl-malonic acid in PKU patient	Fish, eggs, cheese	Children: 30–50 µg/day, intramuscularly, X 2 wk, followed by 100 µg, intramuscularly, every mo, or 1 mg orally/day

	dementia, psychosis, mood disturbance, neural tube defect	overgrowth of gut; phenylketonuria; Whipple disease; Zollinger-Ellison syndrome; celiac disease; medications H_2 blockers					
Vitamin C AI infants RDA 1-18y 0-6 mo 40 mg/d 7-12 mo 50 mg/d 1-3 y 15 mg/d 4-8 y 25 mg/d 9-13 y 45 mg/d 14-18 y 65-75 mg/d	Scurvy	Osmotic diarrhea, bleeding gums, arthropathy, perifollicular hemorrhage	Overcooked foods, with minimal fruits and vegetables, anorexia nervosa, autism, ulcerative colitis, Whipple disease, dialysis, alcoholics, tobacco, total parenteral nutrition without vitamin C	White blood cell ascorbate concentration, urinary ascorbate, capillary fragility, widening of zone of provisional calcification bone ends on x-rays	Citrus fruits	Children: 25-100 mg, orally, intramuscularly, or intravenously, 3X/day X 1 wk, followed by 100 mg orally/day

IV

References for the table:

1. Institute of Medicine, Food and Nutrition Board. *Dietary Reference Intakes for Thiamin, Riboflavin, Nicacin, Vitamin B6, Folate, Vitamin B12, Pantothenic Acid, Biotin, and Choline.* Washington, DC: National Academies Press; 1998

2. Institute of Medicine, Food and Nutrition Board. *Dietary Reference Intakes for Vitamin C, Vitamin E, Selenium, and Carotenoids.* Washington, DC: National Academies Press; 2000

3. Institute of Medicine, Food and Nutrition Board. *Dietary Reference Intakes for Calcium and Vitamin D.* Washington, DC: National Academies Press; 2011

4. Institute of Medicine, Food and Nutrition Board. *Dietary Reference Intakes for Vitamin A,Vitamin K, Arsenic, Boron, Chromium, Copper, Iodine, Manganese, Molybdenum, Nickel, Silicon, Vanadium, and Zinc.* Washington, DC: National Academies Press; 2001

5. Setharaman U. Vitamins. *Pediatr Rev.* 2006;27(2):44-55

Table 21.2.
Vitamin Tolerable Upper Limits, Adverse Effects/Overdose Symptoms, Overdose Risk Factors, and Drug Interactions

Nutrient	Tolerable Upper Limits	Adverse Effects/Overdose Symptoms	Drug Interactions (Ref 5)
Vitamin A	2000 to 10 000 IU dependent on age in children	Anorexia, increased intracranial pressure, painful bone lesions, hepatotoxicity	Iron, retinoids, hepatotoxic drugs, tetracycline, warfarin
Vitamin D	1000 to 4000 IU dependent on age in children	Hypercalcemia	Aluminum, calcipotriene, digoxin, magnesium, thiazides, verapamil
Vitamin E	0–12 mo not established 1–3 y 200 mg/d 4–8 y 300 mg/d 9–13 600 mg/d 14–18 800 mg/d	Toxicity is rare—see text	Aspirin, chemotherapy, ibuprofen, iron, naproxen, warfarin
Vitamin K	Not established	Toxicity is rare—see text	Warfarin
Thiamine (B₁)	Not established, but symptoms can occur with parenteral dosing	Parenteral may cause dermatitis, hypersensitivity, tenderness, tingling, pruritus, pain, weakness, sweating, nausea, gastrointestinal tract distress, restlessness, respiratory distress, pulmonary edema, vascular collapse, death; >10 mg/d X 2 mo, with pantothenic A, eosinophilic pleuropericardial effusion	High dose >10 mg/d X 2 mo with pantothenic A; chemotherapy agents

		Diarrhea, polyuria, orange urine	Sulfamethoxazole
Riboflavin (B₂)	Not established but >400 mg/d suggested		
Niacin (B₃)	0-12 mo unknown 1-3 y unknown 4-8 y 15 mg/d 9-13 y 20 mg/d 14-18 y 30 mg/d	Flushing (niacin flush), pruritus, nausea, headache, vomiting, bloating, diarrhea, anorexia, peptic ulcer, impaired glucose control, impaired uric acid excretion, rare hepatotoxicity	Ibuprofen, insulin, oral diabetes drugs, nonsteroidal anti-inflammatory drugs, aspirin, carbamazepine, primidone, valproic acid, clobazam, clonidine, statins, warfarin
Pantothenic Acid (B₅)	Not established	Diarrhea, peripheral sensory neuropathy with paresthesia, high dose with riboflavin, eosinophilic pleuropericardial effusion	High dose >10 mg/d X 2 mo with riboflavin, statins, nicotinic acid
Pyridoxine (B₆)	0-12 mo unknown 1-3 y 30 mg/d 4-8 y 40 mg/d 9-13 y 60 mg/d 14-18 y 80 mg/d	Peripheral sensory neuropathy, nausea, vomiting, somnolence, allergic reactions, breast soreness and enlargement, increased ulcerative colitis; high dose combined with B₁₂, rosacea fulminans	High dose combined with B₁₂, corticosteroids, phenobarbital, phenytoin, levodopa
Biotin (B₇)	Not established	High dose combined with pantothenic A, eosinophilic pleuropericardial effusion	High dose combined with pantothenic A

Continued

Table 21.2. *Continued*

Vitamin Tolerable Upper Limits, Adverse Effects/Overdose Symptoms, Overdose Risk Factors, and Drug Interactions

Nutrient	Tolerable Upper Limits	Adverse Effects/Overdose Symptoms	Drug Interactions (Ref 5)
Folate (B_9)	1–3 y 300 mg/d 4–8 y 400 mg/d 9–13 y 600 mg/d 14–18 y 800 mg/d	Abdominal cramps, diarrhea, rash, high doses altered sleep patterns, irritability, confusion, exacerbation of seizures, nausea, flatulence, worsening B_{12} deficiency, increased risk of adverse coronary events	Corticosteroids, nonsteroidal anti-inflammatory drugs, aspirin, methotrexate, phenobarbital, phenytoin, primidone, pyrimethamine, alcohol, oral contraceptives, trimethoprim
Cobalamin (B_{12})	Not established	Diarrhea, peripheral vascular thrombosis, itching, urticaria, anaphylaxis; 20 µg/d, combined with 80 mg/d pyridoxine, may cause rosacea fulminans with nodules, papules, pustules; skin cream with avocado oil may cause itching	20 µg/d, combined with 80 mg/d pyridoxine; corticosteroids; ibuprofen; antiretroviral drugs; H_2 blockers; proton pump inhibitors

Vitamin C	Children not established Adults 2 g/d	Nausea, vomiting, esophagitis, heartburn, abdominal cramps, gastrointestinal tract obstruction, fatigue, flushing, headache, insomnia, sleepiness, diarrhea, urinary tract stones, increased coronary events	Acetaminophen, aspirin, warfarin, aluminum hydroxide, beta blockers, chemotherapy, estrogens, fluphenazine, protease inhibitors, antiviral drugs, iron

References for the table:

1. Institute of Medicine, Food and Nutrition Board. *Dietary Reference Intakes for Thiamin, Riboflavin, Niacin, Vitamin B6, Folate, Vitamin B12, Pantothenic Acid, Biotin, and Choline.* Washington, DC: National Academies Press; 1998

2. Institute of Medicine, Food and Nutrition Board. *Dietary Reference Intakes for Vitamin C, Vitamin E, Selenium, and Carotenoids.* Washington, DC: National Academies Press; 2000

3. Institute of Medicine, Food and Nutrition Board. *Dietary Reference Intakes for Calcium and Vitamin D.* Washington, DC: National Academies Press; 2011

4. Institute of Medicine, Food and Nutrition Board. *Dietary Reference Intakes for Vitamin A, Vitamin K, Arsenic, Boron, Chromium, Copper, Iodine, Manganese, Molybdenum, Nickel, Silicon, Vanadium, and Zinc.* Washington, DC: National Academies Press; 2001

5. Rogovik AL, Vohra S, Goldman RD. Safety considerations and potential interactions of vitamins: should vitamins be considered drugs? *Ann Pharmacother.* 2010;44(2):311-324

6. Setharaman U. Vitamins. *Pediatr Rev.* 2006;27(2):44-55

Table 21.3.
Multivitamin Preparations for Children

Formulation	Content Given Per	A (IU)	C (IU)	D (IU)	E (mg)	B₁ (mg)	B₂ (mg)	B₃ (mg)	B₆ (mg)	Folate (μg)	B₁₂ (μg)	Elemental Fe (mg)	Sweetener	Other
Drops														
Poly-Vi-Sol	1 mL	1500	35	400	5	0.5	0.6	8	0.4		2		Glycerin	
Poly-Vi-Sol w/ Iron	1 mL	1500	35	400	5	0.5	0.6	8	0.4			10	Glycerin	
Tri-Vi-Sol	1 mL	1500	35	400									Glycerin	
Tri-Vi-Sol w/ Iron	1 mL	1500	35	400								10	Glycerin	
AquADEK Pediatric Liquid	1 mL	5751	45	400	50	0.6	0.6	6	0.6				Corn starch, mannitol	Biotin 15 μg, pantothenic acid, Zn, Se, vit K 400 μg, CoQ10
TwinLab Infant Care w/ DHA	1 mL	1500	35	400	5	0.5	0.6	8	0.4		2		Glycerin	DHA 20.0 mg Pantothenic acid 3.0 mg
Tablets														
Flintstones Complete	1 tab	3000	60	400	30	1.5	1.7	15	2	400	6	18	Sorbitol, sucrose, xylitol, aspartame	Biotin 40 μg, pantothenic acid, Ca, P, I, Zn, Mg, Cu, Na, choline

	Serving												Other ingredients	Additional nutrients
Centrum Kids	1 tab	3500	60	400	30	1.5	1.7	20	2	400	6	18	Sucrose, dextrose, lactose, mannitol, aspartame	Vit K 10 µg, Biotin 45 µg, pantothenic acid, Zn, Ca, Mg, Mn, P, I, Cu, Cr, Mo
Windmill Bite-A-Mins	1 tab	2500	60	400	15	1.05	1.2	13.5	1.05	300	4.5		Sucrose, mannitol	
AquADEK Chewable Tablets	2 tabs	18167	70	800	100	1.5	1.7	10	1.9		12		Sorbitol, fructose, corn starch, sucrose 15 calories	Vit K 700 µg, biotin 100 µg, pantothenic acid, Zn, Se, CoQ10
Gummies														
Flintstones Complete	2 gummies	2000	30	400	18				1	200	3		Glucose syrup, sucrose 15 calories	Biotin 75 µg, pantothenic acid, I, Zn, Choline
L'il Critters Gummy Vites	2 gummies	2100	20	400	16.5				2	260	6		Glucose syrup, sucrose 10 calories	Biotin 60 µg, pantothenic acid, I, Zn, Choline, Inositol
Disney Gummies	2 gummies	1500	15	400	15				0.5	200	3		Sugar, corn syrup 15 calories	Biotin 45 µg, pantothenic acid, I, Mg, Zn, inositol, DHA 100 µg

Fat-Soluble Vitamins

Introduction

Intestinal absorption of the fat-soluble vitamins (A, D, E, and K) is strongly dependent on adequate secretion of pancreatic enzymes and of bile acids from the liver into the intestinal lumen. In addition, vitamin A and vitamin E esters require hydrolysis before intestinal absorption by an intestinal esterase that is bile acid dependent. Therefore, each of these vitamins may be poorly absorbed if any phase of fat digestion, absorption, or transport is interrupted. Therefore, deficiency in people with conditions associated with fat malabsorption, such as cystic fibrosis, celiac disease, and cholestatic liver diseases, is common.[1] Deficiency of these vitamins is also associated with inadequate intake in specific clinical situations. A detailed description of each fat-soluble vitamin is provided in this chapter.

IV

Vitamin A

The term vitamin A refers to retinol and derivatives that have the same β-ionone ring and qualitatively similar biologic activities. The principal vitamin A compounds—retinol, retinal (retinaldehyde), retinoic acid, and retinyl esters—differ in the terminal C-15 group at the end of the side chain. The functions of vitamin A are maintenance of proper vision, epithelial cell integrity, and regulation of glycoprotein synthesis and cell differentiation.

Vitamin A is present in the diet as retinyl esters derived almost exclusively from animal sources (liver and fish liver oils, dairy products, kidney, and eggs) and as provitamin A carotenoids (mainly beta-carotene) that are distributed widely in green, yellow, orange, and red fruits and vegetables. A report by the Institute of Medicine suggested that carotene-rich fruits and vegetables (carrots, sweet potatoes, broccoli) provide the body with half as much vitamin A as previously thought.[2] Vitamin A activity is expressed as retinol activity equivalents (RAEs; 1 RAE = 3.3 IU of vitamin A activity). The recommended intakes for vitamin A (Adequate Intake [AI] for infants 0–12 months of age and Recommended Dietary Allowance [RDA] for children 1–18 years) vary with age and are given in Table 21.I.1 in international units. (To convert to RAEs, divide IU by 3.3.) Human milk, cow milk (full fat or fortified reduced fat), and commercial infant formulas are excellent sources of vitamin A.

Table 21.I.1.

Vitamin A Adequate Intake by Age (See Also Appendix J, Table J-1)

Age	Vitamin A Dose (RAE)	Vitamin A Dose
0–6 mo	400 µg	1320 IU
7–12 mo	500 µg	1650 IU
1–3 y	300 µg	990 IU
4–8 y	400 µg	1320 IU
>8 y and adults	600–900 µg	1980–2970 IU

RAE indicates retinal activity equivalent: 1 RAE = 3.3 IU vitamin A.

Source: Institute of Medicine. *Dietary Reference Intakes for Vitamin A, Vitamin K, Arsenic, Boron, Chromium, Copper, Iodine, Iron, Manganese, Molybdenum, Nickel, Silicon, Vanadium and Zinc.* Washington, DC: National Academies Press; 2000

Deficiency

Vitamin A deficiency may occur in children receiving less than the AI and in those with fat malabsorption. Deficiency may lead to xerophthalmia, keratomalacia, and irreversible damage to the cornea as well as night blindness and pigmentary retinopathy. Deficiency may also increase morbidity and mortality from various infections, such as measles. Administration of the vitamin may be lifesaving in children with chronic deficiency and malnutrition.[3] Additionally, routine supplementation with vitamin A during early childhood has decreased visual complications of malnutrition and measles as well as childhood mortality from measles in resource-limited countries.[4]

The role of supplementation in infectious diseases other than measles is less clear. In several studies and a Cochrane review, vitamin A supplementation made no difference in clinical symptoms in infections other than measles (pneumonia, respiratory syncytial virus infection, infectious diarrhea)[5-8] and, in several instances, worsened clinical symptoms.[9-11]

Assessment

Vitamin A status is monitored by serum retinol and retinol-binding protein (RBP) concentrations. In children with chronic liver disease, a modified relative dose response test may be a more specific means of assessing deficiency,[12] although this approach should be validated in prospective studies. In resource-limited countries, screening has been performed using conjunctival impression cytology.[13,14]

Prevention and Treatment

The AI for infants is approximately 1320 to 1650 IU/day. The RDA for older children varies with age and peaks at 3000 IU/day (Table 21.1).[2] Children with conditions associated with fat malabsorption (cystic fibrosis, cholestatic liver disease) may require supplemental oral doses (2000–5000 IU/day) of a water miscible preparation to prevent deficiency. Treatment of frank vitamin A deficiency depends on the clinical manifestations. Significant eye findings, such as the presence of Bitot spots, xerophthalmia, and/or keratomalacia, should be treated with 50 000 to 100 000 IU of vitamin A administered parenterally. In patients without deficiency, supplementation with 1500 to 3000 μg (4950–9900 IU) of vitamin A during acute measles infection has been shown to be associated with lower morbidity and mortality.[15] Additionally, the World Health Organization (WHO) recommends administration of an oral dose of vitamin A (100 000 IU in infants and 200 000 IU in children older than 1 year) each day for 2 consecutive days to children with measles if they live in areas where vitamin A deficiency is common. A Cochrane review revealed that this approach was associated with a decrease in mortality in children younger than 2 years with measles.[16]

Toxicity

Claims that extremely high doses of vitamin A (24 750–49 500 IU/day) improve visual acuity in those who work in bright or dim light are unsubstantiated. As little as 19 800 IU (6000 μg RAE) daily can produce serious toxic effects in children, and the Tolerable Upper Intake Level (UL) in children is 2000 to 10 000 IU depending on age (Table 21.2). Vitamin A toxicity is manifested by anorexia, increased intracranial pressure (vomiting and headaches), painful bone lesions, precocious bone growth, desquamating dermatitis, and hepatotoxicity.[17–19] More than 75 years ago, Caffey warned that the hazards of vitamin A poisoning from the routine prophylactic use of concentrates of vitamins A in well-fed healthy infants and children in the United States are considerably greater than the hazards of vitamin A deficiency in healthy infants and children not fed vitamin concentrates.[20] Toxic effects of vitamin A were found in young children who were fed large amounts of chicken liver, which contains 300 IU (90 μg RAE) of vitamin A per gram, for 1 month or longer.[21] Vitamin A excess, including vitamin A derivatives, such as retinoic acid, are teratogenic; teenagers who may become pregnant should be informed of the dangers of vitamin A or derivatives used in the treatment of acne.[22]

Assessment

To monitor for vitamin A toxicity during high-dose vitamin A therapy, serum retinyl esters, normally not present, should be monitored. Plasma concentrations of retinol and RBP are not always reliable means of detecting vitamin A toxicity.[18,23]

Vitamin D

Vitamin D (calciferol) refers to 2 secosteroids, vitamin D_2 (ergocalciferol) and vitamin D_3 (cholecalciferol). Vitamin D_2 is derived from plants and fungi, and its use as a food or dietary supplement has largely been replaced by vitamin D_3. Vitamin D_3 is synthesized in the skin from 7-dehydrocholesterol on exposure to sunlight and is present in nature primarily in the fat of ocean-dwelling fish. Vitamins D_2 and D_3 are considered prohormones and subsequently undergo 25-hydroxylation in the liver to form 25-hydroxyvitamin D (25-OH-D, calcidiol), which is the major circulating form of vitamin D. From the liver, 25-OH-D is transported to the kidney for hydroxylation to form the biologically active hormone 1,25-dihydroxyvitamin D (1,25-OH_2-D, calcitriol).[24] Calcitriol is the biologically active form of vitamin D, which stimulates intestinal absorption of calcium and phosphorous, renal reabsorption of filtered calcium, and the mobilization of calcium and phosphorous from bone. Vitamin D is, therefore, essential for bone formation and mineral homeostasis. Although some recent evidence suggests that vitamin D may have other nonskeletal actions and health benefits, such as modulating the risk of heart disease, cancer, multiple sclerosis, and diabetes, a report from the Institute of Medicine (IOM) stated that the evidence was inconclusive and that no true cause-and-effect relationship could be proven.[24]

Vitamin D is synthesized in the skin by the action of ultraviolet light on a cholesterol precursor (the most effective wavelengths are in the range of 290–315 nm); therefore, the requirement for dietary vitamin D depends exposure to sunlight, taking into account the effects of the environment. The actual requirement for vitamin D in the absence of sunlight is unknown. The heightened awareness of the hazards of ultraviolet radiation exposure, highlighted in the policy statement from the American Academy of Pediatrics (AAP) on the subject, has resulted in revised recommendations for sunlight exposure as a means of maintaining adequate vitamin D stores.[25] Therefore, exposure to sunlight should not be used as a method to ensure adequate vitamin D status. Accordingly, ensuring adequate vitamin

D status while promoting sun-protection strategies requires attention to the use of dietary supplementation of vitamin D.[26]

Deficiency

The primary manifestations of vitamin D deficiency are related to the effects on calcium metabolism. Hypocalcemia, hypophosphatemia, tetany, osteomalacia, and rickets are the most common clinical features. Children at higher risk of deficiency include preterm infants, exclusively breastfed infants, children with dark skin pigmentation, and children with dietary fat malabsorption such as those with cholestatic liver disease, cystic fibrosis, and Crohn disease. More recently, obese children have also been identified as being at risk of vitamin D deficiency.[24,27]

Preterm infants, especially extremely low birth weight infants (<1000 g), are at high risk for radiographically defined rickets.[28] Risk factors, in addition to birth weight, include gestational age at birth <27 weeks, long-term need for total parental nutrition (TPN) and an inability to tolerate high-mineral content formulas or human milk fortifiers, severe broncho-pulmonary dysplasia (BPD) with the use of diuretics and fluid restriction, exposure to long-term steroids, and history of necrotizing enterocolitis.[29]

Assessment

The best indicator of vitamin D status is serum 25-OH-D concentration, which reflects absorption from the diet and synthesis by the skin. Other potentially useful tests include serum calcium, phosphorous, alkaline phosphatase, and parathyroid hormone concentrations. The AAP, the IOM, and the Pediatric Endocrine Society recommend a target for serum 25-OH-D concentration of ≥50 nmol/L (20 ng/mL).[24,30,31] However, it is recognized that there exists controversy over a true diagnosis of vitamin D deficiency versus biochemical deficiency that can be further complicated by variations in analytical measurements.[32,33] The diagnosis of rickets is made on the basis of a history of inadequate intake and clinical findings (craniotabes, enlargement of the costochondral junctions, beading of the ribs) and is confirmed by biochemical indices and radiographic findings. Parathyroid hormone generally is elevated in rickets associated with vitamin D deficiency.

Prevention and Treatment

In 2011 the IOM increased the recommended intake of vitamin D, establishing an AI of 400 IU/day for infants up to 1 year of age and an RDA of 600 IU/day for children 1 to 18 years of age.[24] This was endorsed by the AAP.[26] This new RDA for children older than 1 year of 600 IU/day is higher

AAP

AAP Statement on Calcium and Vitamin D Requirements of Enterally Fed Preterm Infants

1. Preterm infants, especially those <27 weeks' gestation or with birth weight <1000 g with a history of multiple medical problems, are at high risk of rickets.
2. Routine evaluation of bone mineral status by using biochemical testing is indicated for infants with birth weight <1500 g but not those with birth weight >1500 g. Biochemical testing should usually be started 4 to 5 week after birth.
3. Serum APA >800 to 1000 IU/L or clinical evidence of fractures should lead to a radiographic evaluation for rickets and management focusing on maximizing calcium and phosphorus intake and minimizing factors leading to bone mineral loss.
4. A persistent serum phosphorus concentration less than ~4.0 mg/dL should be followed, and consideration should be given for phosphorus supplementation.
5. Routine management of preterm infants, especially those with birth weight <1800 to 2000 g, should include human milk fortified with minerals or formulas designed for preterm infants.
6. At the time of discharge from the hospital, VLBW infants will often be provided higher intakes of minerals than are provided by human milk or formulas intended for term infants through the use of transitional formulas. If exclusively breastfed, a follow-up serum APA at 2 to 4 weeks after discharge from the hospital may be considered.
7. When infants reach a body weight of 1500 g and tolerate full enteral feeds, vitamin D intake should generally be ~400 IU/day, up to a maximum of 1000 IU/day.

Pediatrics. 2013;131(5):e1676-1683

than the amount provided by food fortification and above typical dietary intakes for most children; however, the vitamin D content of human milk is low (22 IU/L), and most infant formulas contain 1.5 μg (62 IU) of vitamin D/100kcal or 10 μg/L (400 IU/L), as do cow milk and evaporated milks. Consequently, vitamin D supplementation will be required for many children, in addition to exclusively breastfed infants. At the present time, the AAP recommends vitamin D supplementation at 400 IU/day for all breastfed infants and all nonbreastfed infants and older children ingesting <1000 mL/day of vitamin D-fortified formula or milk.

Patients with diseases associated with fat malabsorption (cholestatic liver disease, cystic fibrosis [see Chapter 43: Liver Disease, and Chapter 46: Nutrition in Cystic Fibrosis]) may become vitamin D deficient despite an intake of 400 IU/day. Higher doses of vitamin D supplementation may be necessary to achieve normal vitamin D status in these children. Vitamin D deficiency can be treated with oral vitamin D supplementation (ergocalciferol [Drisdol], 50 000 IU/capsule [800 U/mL]), at a dose range of 600 to 2000 IU/day. If a vitamin supplement is prescribed, 25-OH-D concentrations should be measured at 3-month intervals until normal concentrations have been achieved.[31]

Despite limited data, in 2013 the AAP developed recommendations for preventing vitamin D deficiency in preterm infants. When able to be enterally fed, 200 to 400 IU of vitamin D is recommended for ELBW infants <1000 g.[29] Once infants reach ~1500 to 2000 g and are taking full enteral feeds, supplementation should be increased to 400 IU as often intake remains <1 L of transitional preterm formula.[29] Preterm infants with rickets may require an increase in vitamin D supplementation (up to the established upper tolerable intake of 1000 IU/day) as well as addition of calcium and phosphorus supplementation.

Several approaches have been used for the treatment of nutritional or vitamin D-deficient rickets, including daily oral administration of 2000 to 5000 IU of ergocalciferol in children with normal gastrointestinal tract function or oral administration of 10 000 to 25 000 IU/day in children with malabsorption for 2 to 4 weeks. Vitamin D supplementation recommendations for children with liver and renal failure are provided in Chapters 43 and 40, respectively.

Toxicity
The principal manifestations of vitamin D intoxication are hypercalcemia, leading to depression of the central nervous system and ectopic calcification, and hypercalciuria, leading to nephrocalcinosis and nephrolithiasis. The UL, or the highest daily intake that is likely to pose no risk, was revised by the IOM to 1000 IU/day for infants 0 to 6 months of age, 1500 IU/day for infants 6 to 12 months of age, 2500 IU/day for children 1 through 3 years of age, 3000 IU for children 4 through 8 years of age, and 4000 IU/day for children 9 years and older[24] (Table 21.2).

Vitamin E
There are 4 major forms (alpha, beta, delta, and gamma) of tocopherol and tocotrienols, the 2 main forms of vitamin E. Alpha tocopherol has the highest biological activity and is the predominant form in foodstuffs, with the exception of soy oil, which contains high levels of gamma tocopherol. The major function of vitamin E is its role as an antioxidant, protecting cell

AAP

AAP Recommendations on Prevention of Rickets and Vitamin D Deficiency

To prevent rickets and vitamin D deficiency in healthy infants, children, and adolescents, a vitamin D intake of at least 400 IU/day is recommended. To meet this intake requirement, we make the following suggestions:

1. Breastfed and partially breastfed infants should be supplemented with 400 IU/day of vitamin D beginning in the first few days of life. Supplementation should be continued unless the infant is weaned to at least 1 L/day or 1 qt/day of vitamin D–fortified formula or whole milk. Whole milk should not be used until after 12 months of age. In those children between 12 months and 2 years of age for whom over-weight or obesity is a concern or who have a family history of obesity, dyslipidemia, or cardiovascular disease, the use of reduced-fat milk would be appropriate.

2. All nonbreastfed infants, as well as older children who are ingesting <1000 mL/day of vitamin D–fortified formula or milk, should receive a vitamin D supplement of 400 IU/day. Other dietary sources of vitamin D, such as fortified foods, may be included in the daily intake of each child.

3. Adolescents who do not obtain 400 IU of vitamin D per day through vitamin D–fortified milk (100 IU per 8-oz serving) and vitamin D–fortified foods (such as fortified cereals and eggs [yolks]) should receive a vitamin D supplement of 400 IU/day.

4. On the basis of the available evidence, serum 25-OH-D concentrations in infants and children should be ≥50 nmol/L (20 ng/mL).

5. Children with increased risk of vitamin D deficiency, such as those with chronic fat malabsorption and those chronically taking antisei-zure medications, may continue to be vitamin D deficient despite an intake of 400 IU/day. Higher doses of vitamin D supplementation may be necessary to achieve normal vitamin D status in these children, and this status should be determined with laboratory tests (eg, for serum 25-OH-D and PTH concentrations and measures of bone min-eral status). If a vitamin D supplement is prescribed, 25-OH-D levels should be repeated at 3-month intervals until normal levels have been achieved. PTH and bone-mineral status should be monitored every 6 months until they have normalized.

6. Pediatricians and other health care professionals should strive to make vitamin D supplements readily available to all children within their community, especially for those children most at risk.

Pediatrics 2008;122(5):1142–1152

membrane polyunsaturated fatty acids, thiol-rich proteins, and nucleic acids from oxidant damage initiated by free radical reactions. Vitamin E is essential for the maintenance of structure and function of the human nervous system, retina, and skeletal muscle. The common dietary sources of vitamin E are the oil-containing grains, plants, and vegetables. Vitamin E supplementation prevents severe neuropathy in infants with biliary atresia and other forms of chronic cholestatic liver disease, and it prevents muscle weakness in children with cystic fibrosis.[34] Little or no basis exists for the claims that high dietary intakes of vitamin E prolong life, increase sexual potency, prevent cancer, or improve cognitive function in Alzheimer's disease. Although it was suggested that vitamin E supplementation may play a role in prevention of cardiovascular disease,[35] recent large-scale prospective studies have not shown any beneficial effect.[36,37] In contrast, recent evidence suggests that treatment with vitamin E may be of benefit in patients with obesity-related non-alcoholic fatty liver disease and improves steatohepatitis in children[38] and serum alanine aminotransferase levels and liver histology in adults[39] (see Chapter 33: Pediatric Obesity).

Deficiency

The wide distribution of vitamin E in vegetable oils and cereal grains makes deficiency in people from industrialized countries unlikely. Vitamin E supplements are necessary for those with malabsorption (eg, pancreatic insufficiency or cystic fibrosis), biliary atresia and other biliary tract disorders, cirrhosis, and lipid transport disorders. Uncorrected vitamin E deficiency during childhood leads to a progressive neurologic disorder, including truncal and limb ataxia, hyporeflexia, depressed vibratory and position sensation, impairment in balance and coordination, peripheral neuropathy, proximal muscle weakness, ophthalmoplegia, and retinal dysfunction.[34] Significant cognitive and behavioral abnormalities have been described in association with prolonged vitamin E deficiency. The neurologic lesions may be irreversible to a substantial degree if vitamin E deficiency remains untreated. Congenital deficiency of the hepatic tocopherol transport protein also results in vitamin E deficiency and ataxia, despite normal absorption of vitamin E.[40]

Assessment

Vitamin E status is monitored by serum α-tocopherol concentrations and serum a-tocopherol-to-total lipid ratios.

Prevention and Treatment

The AI for α-tocopherol is 4 mg/day for infants 0 through 6 months of age and 5 mg/day for infants 7 to 12 months of age. The RDA for α-tocopherol is 6 mg/day for children 1 through 3 years of age, 7 mg/day for children 4 through 8 years of age, and 11 to 15 mg/day for children 9 through 18 years of age[41] (see Table 21.1).

For children with conditions associated with fat malabsorption (cystic fibrosis, cholestatic liver disease), supplemental doses (25 IU/kg/day) of vitamin E are required to prevent deficiency. The water miscible form of vitamin E, α-tocopherol polyethylene glycol succinate (TPGS) is the preferable form for oral supplementation during cholestasis and may even improve the absorption of other fat-soluble vitamins or drugs when given concurrently.[42,43]

Toxicity

Vitamin E toxicity is rare, and there have been no reports in children. Normal adults appear to tolerate oral doses of 100 to 800 mg/day without clinical signs or biochemical evidence of toxicity.[41] The IOM has set the UL in children at 200 to 800 mg/day depending on age, although no limit has been established for the first 12 months of life (Table 21.2).[41]

Vitamin K

Vitamin K belongs to the family of 2 methyl-1,4 naphthoquinones and exists naturally in 2 forms.[44] Phylloquinone (vitamin K_1) is obtained from leafy vegetables, soybean oil, fruits, seeds, and cow milk. Menaquinone (vitamin K_2), which has 60% of the activity of vitamin K_1 is synthesized by intestinal bacteria. Vitamin K is necessary for the post-translational carboxylation of glutamic acid residues of the vitamin K-dependent coagulation proteins (factors II, VII, IX, and X, protein C, and protein S). Carboxylation allows these proteins to bind calcium, thus, leading to activation of the clotting factors.[44,45] Other proteins undergoing this carboxylation of glutamic acid residues include osteocalcin, which is involved in bone mineralization.

Deficiency

Vitamin K deficiency leads to hypoprothrombinemia and hemorrhagic disorders. Newborn infants are especially at risk of newborn deficiency bleeding secondary to the inherently poor placental transport of vitamin K and the low concentration of vitamin K in human milk (20 IU/L compared with 60 IU/L in cow milk).[45] Common locations of bleeding include the gastrointestinal tract, the umbilicus, or the site of circumcision. In older children and adults, hypoprothrombinemia associated with vitamin K deficiency is usually secondary to disorders of fat malabsorption or chronic liver disease.[46] Vitamin K deficiency may also be seen in children on highly restricted diets or following bariatric surgery. Several studies have suggested an association between low vitamin K concentrations and abnormal bone mineral density, bone turnover, and even osteoarthritis, although a causal relationship has not been definitively established.[47,48]

Assessment

Vitamin K status is monitored by prothrombin time, the measurement of vitamin K-dependent factors (factors II, VII, IX, and X), plasma phylloquinone (vitamin K_1), or the analysis of proteins-induced-in-vitamin K absence (PIVKA).[2]

Prevention and Treatment

The newborn infant usually receives vitamin K soon after birth for prophylaxis against hemorrhagic disease of the newborn. Vitamin K should be administered as a single intramuscular dose of 1 mg (0.3–0.5 mg/kg for preterm infants with birth weights <1000 g). If this is not possible, then an oral dose of 2 mg should be administered at birth, 1 to 2 weeks of age, and 4 weeks of age.[45,49] Following the prophylactic dose of vitamin K at birth, most infants receive adequate vitamin K from cow milk-based formulas, and the formula-fed infant ordinarily does not need additional vitamin K. The AI for infants is 2 μg/day of phylloquinone or menaquinone for the first 6 months and 2.5 μg/day for the second 6 months of life. The AI for older children is 30 μg/day for children 1 through 3 years of age, 55 μg/day for children 4 through 8 years of age, and 60 to 75 μg/day for older children and adolescents[2] (Table 21.1).

In conditions associated with fat malabsorption (cystic fibrosis, cholestatic liver disease), supplemental doses of 2.5 to 5 mg, 2 to 7 times/week, may be required to prevent deficiency. Hypoprothrombinemia associated with chronic liver disease may be corrected by the administration of 5 to 10 mg of vitamin K given intramuscularly. Failure of the prothrombin time to improve following adequate administration of vitamin K suggests severe liver synthetic dysfunction. There have not been any prospective studies of vitamin K treatment for gastrointestinal tract bleeding in patients with liver disease, as highlighted by a Cochrane database review.[50] Vitamin K does not appear to be an effective treatment for the reversal of excessive anticoagulation secondary to oral anticoagulants.[51]

AAP

AAP Recommendations Concerning the Administration of Vitamin K to Newborn Infants

Because parenteral vitamin K has been shown to prevent vitamin K deficiency bleeding (VKDB) of the newborn and young infant and the risks of cancer have been unproven, the American Academy of Pediatrics recommends the following:

1. Vitamin K_1 should be given to all newborns as a single, intramuscular dose of 0.5 to 1 mg.
2. Additional research should be conducted on the efficacy, safety, and bioavailability of oral formulations and optimal dosing regimens of vitamin K to prevent late VKDB.
3. Health care professionals should promote awareness among families of the risks of late VKDB associated with inadequate vitamin K prophylaxis from current oral dosage regimens, particularly for newborns who are breastfed exclusively.

Pediatrics. 2003;112(1):191-192

Toxicity

Vitamin K toxicity is rare. In newborn infants, intravenous administration of water-soluble synthetic vitamin K (vitamin K_3) has been associated with hemolytic anemia, hyperbilirubinemia, and kernicterus.[45] No toxicity states have been associated with administration of the natural forms of vitamin K (K_1 and K_2).[2]

A Note on Vitamin K and Cancer Risk

In 1990, Golding et al reported on a study of a 1970 birth cohort in Great Britain that noted an unexpected association between childhood cancer and pethidine administered during labor and the neonatal administration of vitamin K.[52] Subsequently, they reported in a retrospective, case-controlled study a significant association between intramuscular vitamin K and cancer when compared with no vitamin K or oral vitamin K.[53] Draper and Stiller have questioned this study on the basis of other data from Great Britain and have called for large cohort studies.[54] The AAP formed a Vitamin K Ad Hoc Task Force to study this area in greater detail. The task force found no convincing links between vitamin K administration and childhood cancer.[49] On the basis of these observations, the committee continues to recommend the routine administration of vitamin K to newborn infants (see text box).

References

1. Sokol RJ. Fat-soluble vitamins and their importance in patients with cholestatic liver diseases. *Gastroenterol Clin North Am.* 1994;23(4):673–705

2. Institute of Medicine, Food and Nutrition Board. *Dietary Reference Intakes for Vitamin A,Vitamin K, Arsenic, Boron, Chromium, Copper, Iodine, Manganese, Molybdenum, Nickel, Silicon, Vanadium, and Zinc.* Washington, DC: National Academies Press; 2001

3. Rahmathullah L, Underwood BA, Thulasiraj RD, et al. Reduced mortality among children in southern India receiving a small weekly dose of vitamin A. *N Engl J Med.* 1990;323(14):929–935

4. Underwood BA, Arthur P. The contribution of vitamin A to public health. *FASEB J.* 1996;10(9):1040–1048

5. Bresee JS, Fischer M, Dowell SF, et al. Vitamin A therapy for children with respiratory syncytial virus infection: a multicenter trial in the United States. *Pediatr Infect Dis J.* 1996;15(9):777–782

6. Henning B, Stewart K, Zaman K, Alam AN, Brown KH, Black RE. Lack of therapeutic efficacy of vitamin A for non-cholera, watery diarrhoea in Bangladeshi children. *Eur J Clin Nutr.* 1992;46(6):437–443

7. Kjolhede CL, Chew FJ, Gadomski AM, Marroquin DP. Clinical trial of vitamin A as adjuvant treatment for lower respiratory tract infections. *J Pediatr.* 1995;126 (5 Pt 1):807–812

8. Ni J, Wei J, Wu T. Vitamin A for non-measles pneumonia in children. *Cochrane Database Syst Rev.* 2005(3):CD003700

9. Fawzi WW, Mbise RL, Fataki MR, et al. Vitamin A supplementation and severity of pneumonia in children admitted to the hospital in Dar es Salaam, Tanzania. *Am J Clin Nutr.* 1998;68(1):187–192

10. Long KZ, Montoya Y, Hertzmark E, Santos JI, Rosado JL. A double-blind, randomized, clinical trial of the effect of vitamin A and zinc supplementation on diarrheal disease and respiratory tract infections in children in Mexico City, Mexico. *Am J Clin Nutr.* 2006;83(3):693–700

11. Stephensen CB, Franchi LM, Hernandez H, Campos M, Gilman RH, Alvarez JO. Adverse effects of high-dose vitamin A supplements in children hospitalized with pneumonia. *Pediatrics.* 1998;101(5):e3

12. Feranchak AP, Gralla J, King R, et al. Comparison of indices of vitamin A status in children with chronic liver disease. *Hepatology.* 2005;42(4):782–792

13. Amedee-Manesme O, Luzeau R, Wittepen JR, Hanck A, Sommer A. Impression cytology detects subclinical vitamin A deficiency. *Am J Clin Nutr.* 1988;47(5): 875–878

14. Tseng SC. Staging of conjunctival squamous metaplasia by impression cytology. *Ophthalmology.* 1985;92(6):728–733

15. Hussey GD, Klein M. A randomized, controlled trial of vitamin A in children with severe measles. *N Engl J Med.* 1990;323(3):160–164

16. Huiming Y, Chaomin W, Meng M. Vitamin A for treating measles in children. *Cochrane Database Syst Rev.* 2005(4):CD001479

17. Lippe B, Hensen L, Mendoza G, Finerman M, Welch M. Chronic vitamin A intoxication. A multisystem disease that could reach epidemic proportions. *Am J Dis Child.* 1981;135(7):634–636

18. Mobarhan S, Russell RM, Underwood BA, Wallingford J, Mathieson RD, Al-Midani H. Evaluation of the relative dose response test for vitamin A nutriture in cirrhotics. *Am J Clin Nutr.* 1981;34(10):2264–2270

19. Rubin E, Florman AL, Degnan T, Diaz J. Hepatic injury in chronic hypervitaminosis A. *Am J Dis Child.* 1970;119(2):132–138

20. Caffey J. Chronic poisoning due to excess of vitamin A; description of the clinical and roentgen manifestations in seven infants and young children. *Pediatrics.* 1950;5(4):672–688

21. Mahoney CP, Margolis MT, Knauss TA, Labbe RF. Chronic vitamin A intoxication in infants fed chicken liver. *Pediatrics.* 1980;65(5):893–897

22. Lammer EJ, Chen DT, Hoar RM, et al. Retinoic acid embryopathy. *N Engl J Med.* 1985;313(14):837–841

23. Smith FR, Goodman DS. Vitamin A transport in human vitamin A toxicity. *N Engl J Med.* 1976;294(15):805–808

24. Institute of Medicine, Food and Nutrition Board. *Dietary Reference Intakes for Calcium and Vitamin D.* Washington, DC: National Academies Press; 2011

25. Balk SJ. Ultraviolet radiation: a hazard to children and adolescents. *Pediatrics.* 2011;127(3):e791–e817

26. Abrams SA. Dietary guidelines for calcium and vitamin D: a new era. *Pediatrics.* 2011;127(3):566–568

27. Moore CE, Liu Y. Low serum 25-hydroxyvitamin D concentrations are associated with total adiposity of children in the United States: National Health and Examination Survey 2005 to 2006. *Nutr Res.* 2016;36(1):72–79

28. Mitchell SM, Rogers SP, Hicks PD, Hawthorne KM, Parker BR, Abrams SA. High frequencies of elevated alkaline phosphatase activity and rickets exist in extremely low birth weight infants despite current nutritional support. *BMC Pediatr.* 2009;9:47

29. Abrams SA, American Academy of Pediatrics, Committee on Nutrition. Calcium and Vitamin D requirements of enterally fed preterm infants. *Pediatrics.* 2013;131(5):e1676–e1683

30. Misra M, Pacaud D, Petryk A, Collett-Solberg PF, Kappy M. Vitamin D deficiency in children and its management: review of current knowledge and recommendations. *Pediatrics.* 2008;122(2):398–417

31. Wagner CL, Greer FR. Prevention of rickets and vitamin D deficiency in infants, children, and adolescents. *Pediatrics.* 2008;122(5):1142–1152

32. Black LJ, Anderson D, Clarke MW, Ponsonby AL, Lucas RM, Ausimmune Investigator Group. Analytical bias in the measurement of serum 25-hydroxyvitamin D concentrations impairs assessment of vitamin D status in clinical and research settings. *PLoS One.* 2015;10(8):e0135478

33. Shah D, Gupta P. Vitamin D deficiency: Is the pandemic for real? *Indian J Community Med.* 2015;40(4):215–217

34. Sokol RJ. Vitamin E and neurologic deficits. *Adv Pediatr.* 1990;37:119–148

35. Pryor WA. Vitamin E and heart disease: basic science to clinical intervention trials. *Free Radic Biol Med.* 2000;28(1):141–164

36. Hercberg S, Galan P, Preziosi P, et al. The SU.VI.MAX Study: a randomized, placebo-controlled trial of the health effects of antioxidant vitamins and minerals. *Arch Intern Med.* 2004;164(21):2335–2342

37. Tornwall ME, Virtamo J, Korhonen PA, et al. Effect of alpha-tocopherol and beta-carotene supplementation on coronary heart disease during the 6-year post-trial follow-up in the ATBC study. *Eur Heart J.* 2004;25(13):1171–1178

38. Lavine JE, Schwimmer JB, Van Natta ML, et al. Effect of vitamin E or metformin for treatment of nonalcoholic fatty liver disease in children and adolescents: the TONIC randomized controlled trial. *JAMA.* 2011;305(16):1659–1668

39. Hoofnagle JH, Van Natta ML, Kleiner DE, et al. Vitamin E and changes in serum alanine aminotransferase levels in patients with non-alcoholic steatohepatitis. *Aliment Pharmacol Ther.* 2013;38(2):134–143

40. Traber MG, Sokol RJ, Burton GW, et al. Impaired ability of patients with familial isolated vitamin E deficiency to incorporate alpha-tocopherol into lipoproteins secreted by the liver. *J Clin Invest.* 1990;85(2):397–407

41. Institute of Medicine, Food and Nutrition Board. *Dietary Reference Intakes for Vitamin C, Vitamin E, Selenium, and Carotenoids.* Washington, DC: National Academies Press; 2000

42. Sokol RJ, Butler-Simon N, Conner C, et al. Multicenter trial of d-alpha-tocopheryl polyethylene glycol 1000 succinate for treatment of vitamin E deficiency in children with chronic cholestasis. *Gastroenterology.* 1993;104(6):1727–1735

43. Sokol RJ, Johnson KE, Karrer FM, Narkewicz MR, Smith D, Kam I. Improvement of cyclosporin absorption in children after liver transplantation by means of water-soluble vitamin E. *Lancet.* 1991;338(8761):212–214

44. Shearer MJ, Newman P. Metabolism and cell biology of vitamin K. *Thromb Haemost.* 2008;100(4):530–547

45. Greer FR. Vitamin K the basics—what's new? *Early Hum Dev.* 2010;86(Suppl 1):S43–S47

46. Mager DR, McGee PL, Furuya KN, Roberts EA. Prevalence of vitamin K deficiency in children with mild to moderate chronic liver disease. *J Pediatr Gastroenterol Nutr.* 2006;42(1):71–76

IV

47. Conway SP, Wolfe SP, Brownlee KG, et al. Vitamin K status among children with cystic fibrosis and its relationship to bone mineral density and bone turnover. *Pediatrics.* 2005;115(5):1325–1331

48. Neogi T, Booth SL, Zhang YQ, et al. Low vitamin K status is associated with osteoarthritis in the hand and knee. *Arthritis Rheum.* 2006;54(4):1255–1261

49. American Academy of Pediatrics, Committee on Fetus and Newborn. Policy statement: Controversies concerning vitamin K and the newborn. *Pediatrics.* 2003;112(1):191–192

50. Marti-Carvajal AJ, Marti-Pena AJ. Vitamin K for upper gastrointestinal bleeding in patients with liver diseases. *Cochrane Database Syst Rev.* 2005(3):CD004792

51. DeZee KJ, Shimeall WT, Douglas KM, Shumway NM, O'Malley PG. Treatment of excessive anticoagulation with phytonadione (vitamin K): a meta-analysis. *Arch Intern Med.* 2006;166(4):391–397

52. Golding J, Paterson M, Kinlen LJ. Factors associated with childhood cancer in a national cohort study. *Br J Cancer.* 1990;62(2):304–308

53. Golding J, Greenwood R, Birmingham K, Mott M. Childhood cancer, intramuscular vitamin K, and pethidine given during labour. *BMJ.* 1992;305(6849):341–346

54. Draper GJ, Stiller CA. Intramuscular vitamin K and childhood cancer. *BMJ.* 1992;305(6855):709

Water-Soluble Vitamins

Introduction

Deficiencies of the water-soluble vitamins (WSVs) are rare. Most children and adolescents who eat a diet consisting of fruits, vegetables, animal protein (meat, dairy, and egg), cereals, and breads consume sufficient WSVs to meet daily allowances. This includes formula-fed infants and breastfed infants of mothers consuming a diverse and healthy diet. Appreciating who might be at risk for deficiency of WSVs, however, is important because of limited total body stores and lack of endogenous synthesis of most WSVs. However, not all WSV deficiency states in infancy and childhood are due to dietary deficiency, because diseases caused by WSV deficiency can result from inborn errors of metabolism with genetic and epigenetic aleterations in the human genome. Additionally, medical conditions that may predispose someone to WSV deficiency include malabsorption secondary to celiac disease, Crohn disease, cystic fibrosis, food refusal, anorexia nervosa, HIV/AIDS, and bariatric surgery. Adolescent athletes, especially females with disorded eating habits or vegetarians, may suffer from poorer WSV status because of the twofold increased need for B-complex vitamins.[1] Children with autism may also suffer from restrictive diets.[2] Table 21.1 shows a list of WSVs, recommended intake, deficiency symptoms, deficiency risk factors, diagnostic tests, and therapeutic dosages.

Health and dietary fads may influence WSV status even in the pediatric population. The increasing utilization of complementary and alternative medicine (CAM) in the United States and abroad highlights this notion.[3,4] Children and adolescents have been reported to account for one third of visits to homeopathic and naturopathic providers,[5] and 68% of adolescents use CAM.[4] Nearly one third of children with autism are treated with multivitamin therapy,[6] the most common form of CAM product prescribed for children and adults by a naturopathic provider.[4,5] Single fat-soluble or WSV preparations are also commonly prescribed.[4,7,8] Energy drinks (including "shot" sized) and vitamin water products contain variable amounts of WSVs but may contain extremely high amounts. For example, the label of a 2-ounce energy "shot" product (5-Hour Energy) reports 2000% of the recommended intake of vitamin B_6 and more than 8000% of vitamin B_{12}.[9] Use of these energy drinks in adolescents is known to be associated with alcohol and substance use, risky behavior, sensation seeking, depression, and/or anxiety.[10] Energy drink consumption is inversely associated with sleep duration.[10] A widely-held belief is that WSVs are safe if given in excess; however,

Section IV: Micronutrients and Macronutrients **655**

they have the potential for serious toxicity if consumed in excessive quantities, in combinations with other medications, or over a prolonged period of time.[4] Table 21.2 shows tolerable upper limits, adverse effects/overdose symptoms, risk factors for symptoms, and drug interactions for WSVs.

The increasing population of overweight children and adolescents in the United States is also affecting WSV intakes.[11,12] Analysis of data from the National Health and Nutrition Examination Survey III reveals that foods with low nutrient density contribute more than 30% of the daily energy to the diets of children and adolescents. Studies show that the mean intake of vitamins A, C, and B_6, folate, and riboflavin decreased as foods low in nutrient density or high in fat increased.[13,14] Conversely, research in Scandinavian children showed that diets low in fat positively correlated with increased intake of several WSVs.[15] In US adolescents, a low-fat and high-fiber diet was associated with a greater likelihood of adequate B_6, B_{12}, C, niacin, thiamin, riboflavin, and folate intakes.[16] Not surprisingly, children and adolescents who regularly eat dinner with their family ingested higher amounts of vitamins B_6, B_{12}, C, and folate. Taken together, these studies demonstrate that diets high in fat or with a preponderance of foods with low nutrient density will place children and adolescents at risk for WSV deficiency.

Thiamine (Vitamin B_1)

Thiamine is an essential coenzyme involved in carbohydrate metabolism. Thiamine pyrophosphate (TPP) is the primary active form, as TPP and nicotinamide adenine dinucleotide (NAD) are coenzymes to pyruvate dehydrogenase in the oxidative decarboxylation of pyruvate to acetyl conenzyme A (CoA). Thiamine also plays an integral role with transketolase in the pentose phosphate pathway, which provides substrates for nucleic acid and fatty acid synthesis. In addition to being a coenzyme, thiamine also plays a key a role in nerve impulse conduction and voluntary muscle action.[17] Several mutations in thiamine transporter (THTR1) genes may potentially be responsive to thiamine, including TPK1 mutations causing episodic encephalopathy and Rogers syndrome (SLC19A2 mutation) with megaloblastic anemia, diabetes mellitus, and deafness.[18,19] THTR2 deficiency (SLC19A3 mutation) presents in childhood with basal ganglia disease, including encephalopathy, speech and swallowing difficulties, dystonia and rigidity, as well as other symptoms that can be responsive to biotin and thiamine.[19,20] Others include the mitrochondrial TPP transporter, Amish lethal microencephalopathy (SLC25A19 gene).[19] Additionally, clinical or biochemical responses to pharmacologic doses of thiamine have been reported in a small number of patients with pyruvate dehydrogenase deficiency or maple syrup urine disease.[19]

Foods rich in thiamine include yeast, legumes, pork, rice, and whole grain cereals, but dairy products, milled white flour, milled white rice, and most fruits contain little thiamine. Deficiency of thiamine can result in the clinical syndromes of beriberi or Wernicke encephalopathy. Beriberi is traditionally classified as 2 forms: dry beriberi, which is characterized by a symmetrical peripheral neuropathy, and wet beriberi, in which cardiac involvement predominates. Neuropathy in dry beriberi is progressive, with worsening weakness, muscle wasting, ambulation, ataxia, painful parasthesias, and loss of deep tendon reflexes. Edema is the hallmark symptom of wet beriberi, attributable to cardiomyopathy that progresses to congestive heart failure and death if untreated. Infantile beriberi generally occurs in breastfed children whose mothers have subclinical thiamine deficiency and is characterized by the sudden onset of shock in a 2- to 3-month-old previously well child. These symptoms may be preceded by a hoarse weak cry, poor feeding, and vomiting. Wernicke encephalopathy is characterized by the triad of ophthalmoplegia, nystagmus, and ataxia in addition to altered consciousness and has been reported with thiamine deficiency in infants and children, as well during a parenteral multivitamin preparation shortage.[21,22]

Thiamine deficiency may result from inadequate dietary intake, malabsorption, excessive loss, or defective transport of the vitamin. Mothers at risk for thiamine deficiency include those with a poor thiamine intake, alcohol abuse, gastrointestinal disease, hyperemesis gravidarum, and HIV/AIDS. Other populations at particularly high risk for the development of thiamine deficiency include children who follow fad diets, have anorexia nervosa, have undergone gastric bypass surgery, are undergoing chronic dialysis for kidney disease, are hospitalized in the pediatric intensive csre unit, with congenital heart disease, and potentially also receiving long-term parenteral nutrition.[21,23–26]

Several tests are used to detect thiamine deficiency. These include the thiamine-dependent enzyme, blood transketolase activation test at baseline and after added thiamine pyrophosphate (TPP)[27] or erythrocyte TPP concentration.[28] Infantile beriberi is treated with 50 to 100 mg of parenteral thiamine as a 1-time dose, withholding breastfeeding until maternal diet is supplemented with thiamine.[29] Beriberi in children is treated with 10 to 25 mg of parenteral thiamine once daily for 2 weeks followed by 5 to 10 mg orally daily for 1 month. When mild, beriberi can be treated with 10 mg of oral thiamine daily. Tolerable upper limits have not been established, but in high doses, interactions with chemotherapy agents or other high-dose vitamins have been reported.[4] Although rare, injections may cause hypersensitivity dermatitis, tenderness, tingling, pruritis, pain, weakness, sweating, nausea, gastrointestinal tract distress, restlessness, respiratory distress, pulmonary edema, vascular collapse, or even death.[4]

Riboflavin (Vitamin B$_2$)

Riboflavin is a precursor of the enzyme cofactors flavin mononucleotide (FMN) and flavin adenine dinucleotide (FAD), involved in in oxidation-reduction reactions integral to carbohydrate, protein, and fat metabolism. FAD is an essential component of the antioxidant enzymes glutathione reductase and xanthine oxidase. Riboflavin is found in abundance in animal protein (meat, dairy, and eggs) as well as green vegetables and fortified cereals. Riboflavin deficiency is generally accompanied by deficiencies of one or more other B complex vitamins, in part because of riboflavin's role in the metabolism of folate, pyridoxine, and niacin.[30,31] Signs and symptoms are nonspecific in the mildly deficient state but progress in severity to more characteristic symptoms, including pharyngitis, cheilosis, angular stomatitis, glossitis (magenta tongue), and seborrheic dermatitis with involvement of the nasolabilal folds, flexural area of extremities, and the genital area.

Children at risk for deficiency include the economically disadvantaged with limited dietary meat or dairy intake, but also include breastfed infants who have not yet weaned to cow milk. Ariboflavinosis has been described in protein-energy malnutrition states such as kwashiorkor and anorexia nervosa and prolonged malabsorptive disease such as celiac disease and short bowel syndrome. Riboflavin deficiency has been reported in patients with cystic fibrosis.[32] Additionally, children who have undergone bariatric surgery are at risk for thiamine deficiency.[33] Thyroid and adrenal insufficiency can impair the synthesis of riboflavin cofactors and may precipitate the deficiency state.

Deficiency can be directly assessed with a 24-hour urine collection for riboflavin or measurement of riboflavin in red blood cells (RBCs).[34,35] Deficiency can also be assessed indirectly by RBC glutathione reductase activity coefficient,[36,37] but the test is inaccurate in patients with glutathione reductase deficiency, gluclose-6-phosphate dehydrogenase (G6PD) deficiency, and β-thalassemia. Deficiency in children is treated with oral riboflavin, 1 mg, 3 times daily until signs of deficiency resolve. Infants may respond to 0.5 mg, twice weekly.

Although tolerable upper limits of dosing have not be established, doses greater than 400 mg daily may cause diarrhea, polyuria, and/or orange urine and exacerbate or precipitate acneiform eruptions.[38] High doses of riboflavin decrease the effectiveness of sulfonamide antibiotics.[4] Although more studies are necessary, riboflavin for migraine prophylaxis has been prescribed alone, 25 to 200 mg daily, or 400 mg daily with magnesium and the herb feverfew. The dosage of 25 mg alone has also been reported to acheive a 50% reduction in migraines in 44% of people studied.[39,40]

Niacin (Vitamin B₃)

Nicotinic acid and nicotinamide are the 2 vitamins commonly referred to as niacin. These 2 forms of niacin are chemically modified in the mitochondria to form the coenzymes NAD and NAD phosphate (NADP). Enzymes involved in oxidation-reduction reactions require the coenzymes NAD and NADP to accept or donate electrons. Unlike most WSVs, half of the body's niacin can be synthesized in the liver and kidney from tryptophan in a series of reactions dependent on riboflavin and pyridoxine. Animal protein (dairy, eggs, and meat), beans, and fortified cereals are excellent sources of niacin, and many of these are also good sources of tryptophan. However, sugars and high leucine content of some nonfortified grains may bind to niacin, reducing bioavailablity.[12]

Deficiency of niacin results in the clinical syndrome known as pellagra, or "rough skin" in Italian. Pellagra is characterized by the triad of diarrhea, dermatitis, and dementia, or in the case of advanced stages, it could extend to a tetrad that includes death. The gastrointestinal symptoms associated with niacin deficiency include glossitis, angular stomatitis, cheilitis, and diarrhea in up to one third to one half of patients.[41] The skin lesions in pellagra are quite characteristic, with painful erythema in areas of sun-exposed skin (dorsal surface of the hands, face, and neck), sparing the hair and nails, but that can progress to an exudatitve phase. Repeated sun exposure of the skin may result in vesicles coalescing into bullae, eventually becoming rough, hard, and scaly, giving pellagra its name.[42] This rash differs from the generalized dermatitis found in kwashiorkor that localizes to both sun-exposed and -unexposed skin. The early neuropsychiatric symptoms of

IV

pellagra may include insomnia, fatigue, nervousness, irritability, depression, mental dullness, apathy, and memory impairment. Untreated, these symptoms may progress to dementia and, ultimately, death.

With few exceptions, pellagra is a disease limited to malnourished children from developing countries. In the industrialized regions of the world, those at risk include homeless people, individuals with malabsorptive conditions such as Crohn disease, and people with nutritional self-deprivation states such as anorexia nervosa.[43,44] Pellagra has been reported in patients receiving long-term anticonvulsants and in Hartnup disease, a disorder of neutral amino acid transport resulting in tryptophan malabsorption. It has also been reported in the carcinoid syndrome from depleted tryptophan stores and in patients treated with isoniazid, 5-fluorouracil, or 6-mercaptopurine from inadequate conversion of tryptophan to niacin.[12,45,46]

Niacin status can be evaluated by 24-hour urinary excretion of niacin and its metabolite N_1-methylnicotinamide.[47] Red blood cell levels of NAD and NADP can be measured to determine whether the "niacin number" (NAD/NADP x 100) is deficient (ie, less than 130).[47–49] The treatment for pellagra in children is an oral dose of 50 to 100 mg nicotinamide, 3 times daily. Use of nicotinamide avoids the uncomfortable flushing associated with nicotinic acid therapy. Therapy should be continued until resolution of acute symptoms. High-dose niacin, as seen in energy drinks and energy shots, also causes a rush, with flushing.[10] Niacin is used to treat dyslipidemia in adults and children, with daily dosage of 20 to 40 mg/kg/day, up to 3 g. However, pharmacologic doses of niacin for treatment of dyslipidemia in children has been inadequately studied.[50] Adverse effects of pharmacologic doses of niacin include flushing, pruritis, nausea, vomiting, headache, vomiting, bloating, diarrhea, anorexia, peptic ulcer, and rarely, hepatotoxicity. Chronic administration can also impair glucose control and impair uric acid excretion.[4] Niacin can interfere with commonly administered drugs, such as insulin, oral diabetes drugs, nonsteroidal anti-inflammatory drugs, warfarin, and seizure medications by increasing either levels or risk for toxicity (see Table 21.2).

Pyridoxine (Vitamin B₆)

There are 3 naturally occurring forms of vitamin B_6: pyridoxine, pyridoxal, and pyridoxamine. These pyridines are activated to the coenzyme form by phosphorylation. Pyridoxal 5'-phosphate is the most ubiquitous form of the vitamin and is integral to a multitude of enzymes necessary for human amino acid and carbohydrate metabolism. It is required for the conversion of tryptophan to both niacin and serotonin. Similarly, vitamin B_6 is also required for the conversion of dopa to dopamine and as well the synthesis of the inhibitory neurotransmitter gamma-aminobutyric acid (GABA). Hematologically, pyridoxine is a necessary cofactor in the rate limiting step of heme biosynthesis. Foods rich in pyridoxine include bananas, fish, milk, yeast, eggs, and fortified cereals.

Isolated deficiency of pyridoxine is rare because of its interaction with other WSVs. Pyridoxine metabolism requires adequate levels of riboflavin, niacin, and zinc. Biosynthesis and metabolism of niacin and folate requires pyridoxine. As with other WSVs, children in resource-limited countries with marginal nutrition are at risk for deficiency.[51] In the 1950s, a manufacturing error in infant formula resulted in severe vitamin B_6 deficiency and seizures in a cohort of infants. Deficiency in childhood has been described in those with leukemia and chronic renal failure.[52,53] Mild deficiency of vitamin B_6 can result from the covalent binding of certain drugs (isoniazid, hydralazine, oral contraceptives, penicillamine, cycloserine, theophylline) to pyridoxal 5'-phosphate. The manifestations of pyridoxine deficiency are nonspecific and include seborrheic eruption on the face, scalp, neck, and shoulders; glossitis; angular stomatitis; cheilosis; irritability; depression; and confusion.

There are several rare vitamin B_6-dependency syndromes that include vitamin B_6-responsive anemia, xanthurenic aciduria, cystathionuria, and homocystinuria. Pyridoxine-dependent seizure disorder is a deficiency of alpha aminoadipic semialdolase dehyrodgenase (antiquitin) encoded by the gene ALDH7A1, an autosomal recessive disorder presenting with intractable seizures, because byproducts degrade pyridoxine, making it unavailable to function as a cofactor in the conversion of glutamic acid to the inhibitory neurotransmitter GABA.[54] Despite a normal serum vitamin B_6 level, the seizures in these infants respond to 10 to 500 mg of parenteral vitamin B_6. Oral folinic acid (3 to 5 mg/kg/day) can be added for pyridoxine-dependent seizures because of improved response in some patients. Maintenance pyridoxine therapy is required indefinitely, with doses as high as 15 to 18 mg/kg orally per day (maximum of 500 mg), well above the Recommended Dietary Allowance (RDA).[55] A pyridoxine-responsive seizure disorder has also been found to respond to pyridoxine, but discontinuation of the vitamin can occur later.[54] Additionally, a rare pyridoxal phosphate dependent seizure disorder caused by deficiency of pyridox(am)ine 5' phosphate oxidase

(PNPO), also presents with intractable seizures, hypoglycemia, and lactic acidosis. It is treated with 30 to 50 mg/kg/day of pyridoxal 5'-phosphate divided in 4 to 6 doses. A fourth seizure disorder, infantile spasms (West syndrome), can also be treated with pyridoxal 5'-phosphate and adreno-cortocotropic hormone. Because pyridoxal 5'-phosphate treats all these conditions, experts recommend that pyridoxine, pyridoxal 5'-phosphate and folate be given for retractable seizures in newborn infants, until biochemical and genetic testing allow final diagnosis and optimal treatment.[54]

Vitamin B_6 has been used at pharmacologic doses with little proof of efficacy to remedy the symptoms of carpal tunnel syndrome, depression, hyperoxaluria, and dysmenorrhea, among others.[56–61] High-dose vitamin B_6 has also been used to treat children with autism spectrum disorders, as plasma pyridoxine levels are high and pyridoxal 5'-phosphate concentrations are low in some of these children because of deficient activity of the enzyme, pyrodoxal kinase. A Cochrane review found data insufficient to recommend treatment of autism with vitamin B_6.[62] Despite the lack of evidence, vitamin B_6 continues to be used for many of the aforementioned conditions, including autism, and with a potential for toxicity when given in excess. When taken in excess on a chronic basis, vitamin B_6 can exacerbate or precipitate acneiform eruptions and cause a peripheral sensory neuropathy characterized by bilateral parasthesias, hyperaesthesia, limb pain, ataxia, somnulence, and poor coordination.[6] Nausea, vomiting, allergic reactions, breast soreness and enlargement, and increased risk of ulcerative colitis can be seen. The combination of high doses of both vitamin B_6 and vitamin B_{12} may result in a severe rosascea fulminans.[4]

Various methods have been used to assess vitamin B_6 status, including 24-hour urine assay for the pyridoxine metabolic product 4-pyridoxic acid or plasma pyridoxal 5'-phosphate, the predominant B_6 vitamer present in the plasma.[63] Children deficient in vitamin B_6 without neuritis should receive 5 to 25 mg/day of oral pyridoxine for 3 weeks followed by 1.5 to 2.5 mg/day orally in a multivitamin product. With peripheral neuropathy, the dosing is increased to 10 to 50 mg of oral pyridoxine for 3 weeks, then decreased to 1 to 2 mg/day. Vitamin B_6 therapy has been used to slow the development of nephropathy and vascular disease in adult diabetes, as higher plasma levels of vitamin B_6 protected against coronary artery disease in the Nurses Health Study and other studies.[64]

Folate

Folic acid carries hydroxymethyl and formyl groups necessary for the synthesis of purines and thymine which are required for DNA formation. The vitamin is necessary for RBC maturation and promotion of cellular growth in general. Total serum homocysteine is increased in the presence of folate deficiency in neonates.[65] Supplemental folate, taken alone or added to food, is better absorbed than folate normally within food, but many cereals, grains, and breads are now fortified with folate. Natural sources include fresh green vegetables, liver, yeast, and some fruits. Megaloblastic anemia is the primary sign of deficiency.

Low serum and RBC folic acid levels in women of childbearing potential increase the risk of fetal birth defects, particularly neural tube defects. Some evidence also supports maternal deficiency of either folic acid or vitamin B_{12} as independent risk factors for these defects.[66] Since identification of the first genetic risk factor for neural tube defects, a single nucleotide polymorphism (SNP) C677T of the 5,10–methylenetetrahydrofolate reductase,[67] work has proceeded to investigate the relationships between SNPs in folate metabolism pathways and occurrence of neural tube defects. C677T homozygosity in either mother or fetus increases fetal risk for neural tube defects. Many other SNPs in the folate pathway have been investigated and a small number have also been linked to neural tube defects.[68] Additionally, risk for stroke in children with the C677T allele may be double that of age-matched controls,[69] so studies to determine whether folate supplementation prevents recurrent stroke in this group are needed. Some additional data also support that lower periconceptual folate intake by pregnant women is associated with orofacial clefts and congenital heart disease in the fetus.[70,71] Recent studies found modest evidence for decrease in the prevalence of specific congenital heart defects, small-for-gestational-age infants, and preterm births after maternal ingestion of multivitamins with folate during pregnancy.[72,73] As far as adverse effects of folate, epidemiologic studies are coflicting as to whether higher-dose folate intakes during the second and third trimesters of pregnancy are linked to childhood atopy and asthma, but randomized trials are needed to address this concern.[74]

In contrast to the other WSVs, inadequate intake of folate in children and adolsecents is common. Greater fruit and vegetable consumption in adolescents can translate into higher plasma and RBC folate levels.[75] In one study of white preschool children of middle and upper socioeconomic status 2 to 5 years of age, the mean folate intake was consistently below recommended amounts.[76] Foods and beverages most commonly eaten were fruit drinks, carbonated drinks, 2% milk, and French fries, with folate intakes only 79% of recommended amounts.[77] The diets of US adolescents include greater consumption of soft drinks and noncitrus fruit juices and consumption of fruits and vegetables well below the recommended 7 to 9 servings per day, resulting in inadequate folate intake, especially in girls.[78] In a large European adolescent cohort, higher dietary intake of folate was beneficial. Biomarkers of folate and vitamin B_{12} were directly associated with serum polyunsaturated fatty acid levels and an overall better fasting lipid profile.[79]

Other patients at risk of folate deficiency are those with malabsorption syndromes, including Crohn disease, and patients with HIV infection.[80,81] Lower-than-recommended intake can be found in very low birth weight infants and is associated with poor weight and length gain.[82] In pediatric and adolescent patients on chronic dialysis, folate deficiency promotes erythropoietin resistance.[83] There are also inherited diseases of folate metabolism. Methylenetetrahydrofolate reductase deficiency was described in 4 siblings presenting with retarded psychomotor development, poor social contact, and seizures with low serum and RBC folate concentrations.[84] Cerebral folate deficiency is a disorder in which serum and RBC folate concentrations are normal, but folate transport from plasma to the central nervous system (CNS) is prevented by an inherited defect in CNS transporter or autoantibodies[85]; however, the disease is responsive to folinic acid treatment. In children with autism spectrum disorders, vitamin B_{12} and folinic acid have been studied as a treatment because of a previously identified dysfunctional folate-methionine metabolic pathway crucial for DNA synthesis, DNA methylation, and cellular redox balance. Although a subset of patients showed improvement in glutathione-mediated redox status,[6] a systematic reviews of the studies shows that they are underpowered and confounded with clinical heterogeneity that makes findings inconclusive.[86]

Adverse effects of folate deficieny include abdominal cramps, nausea, diarrhea, rash, altered sleep patterns, irritability, worsening of seizures, and worsening of B_{12} deficiency. Low serum folate indicates short-term deficiency, and low RBC folate indicates chronic folate deficiency. Measurement of 5-methyltetrahydrofolate, the principal circulating form of plasma folate, may be clinically useful,[85] as well as measurment of the serum concentration of homocysteine, which is elevated in folic acid deficiency. Folic acid deficiency is treated with daily administration of oral supplements of 0.1 mg in infants and 1.0 mg in children, followed by maintenance of 0.1 to 0.5 mg daily. Folic acid can also be given parenterally. Adverse interactions with other medications have been reported, including methotrexate, seizure medications, oral contraceptives, and trimethoprim.[4] Nonsteroidal anti-inflammatory drugs inhibit folate enzymes.

Cobalamin (Vitamin B$_{12}$)

Cobalamin functions as a coenzyme for a number of enzymes involved in RBC maturation and central nervous system development. Cobalamin and folate are necessary for the re-methylation of homocysteine to methionine by methionine synthase. Higher concentrations of cobalamin are found in colostrum compared with values in the third month of lactation. Levels of cobalamin and its binding protein in human milk are similar over the course of a day and in fore or hind milk.[87] Cobalamin is found in foods of animal origin only. Good sources of cobalamin are meat, fish, poultry, cheese, milk, eggs, and vitamin B$_{12}$-fortified soy milk. Signs and symptoms of deficiency include macrocytic megaloblastic anemia and neurologic problems (ataxia, muscle weakness, spasticity, incontinence, hypotension, vision problems, dementia, psychoses, and mood disturbances). Vitamin B$_{12}$ deficiency is accompanied by hyperhomocysteinemia, which is a reported risk factor for cardiovascular disease.[88] Higher biomarkers of folate and vitamin B$_{12}$ levels are associated with a better fasting lipid profile in adolescents[79] (see Folate). Vitamin B$_{12}$ and folate have been studied as a treatment for autism[86] (see Folate).

Breastfed infants of strict vegan mothers are at risk for vitamin B$_{12}$ deficiency. Maternal and newborn vitamin B$_{12}$ levels are highly correlated.[89] The prevalence of vitamin B$_{12}$ deficiency is as low as 6% in the United States but as high as 40% in Latin America, 50% in certain regions in India, and 70% of Sub-Saharan Africa or South Asia.[89] Maternal vitamin B$_{12}$ deficiency in pregnancy can result in a higher risk for gestational diabetes, pregnancy loss, fetal neural tube defects, fetal orofacial clefts, small-for-gestational-age, low birth weight, and/or intrauterine growth restriction.[89] Infant vitamin B$_{12}$ deficiency can present as impairments in growth, psychomotor function, and brain development and potentially also insulin resistance.[89] Vitamin B$_{12}$ combined with iron and folic acid supplementation during pregnancy increased maternal vitamin B$_{12}$ status, reduced the rate of fetal growth restriction, and increased infant vitamin B$_{12}$ levels.[89] In addition, it appears that maternal vitamin B_{12} supplementation improves infant temperament and intelligence and potentially decreases the risk for infant insulin resistance.[89]

Elevated plasma methylmalonic acid and total homocysteine are useful indicators of functional vitamin B_{12} deficiency in infants, and administration of either oral or intramuscular vitamin B_{12} can normalize urinary values of methylmalonic acid in vitamin B_{12}-deficient infants.[90] Megaloblastic anemia secondary to vitamin B_{12} deficiency in children consuming alternative diets has also been reported.[91] Other subjects at risk for B_{12} deficiency include those with surgical resections of the stomach and/or ileum attributable to gastric intrinsic factor deficiency. Patients with phenylketonuria on an unrestricted or relaxed diet are at risk for vitamin B_{12} deficiency.[92] Vitamin B_{12}-responsive inborn errors of metabolism exist, including transcobalamin II deficiency, homocysteinuria, and hereditary juvenile vitamin B_{12} deficiency caused by mutations in gastric intrinsic factor.[93,94] Imerslund-Grasbeck syndrome, a familial selective vitamin B_{12} malabsorption disorder, can be successfully treated by intramuscular administration of vitamin B_{12}. Maternal vitamin B_{12} deficiency has also been associated with neural tube defects in offspring.[95]

The diagnosis of cobalamin deficiency is made by determination of the serum cobalamin concentration. If serum concentration is borderline low, finding elevated plasma homocysteine and urinary methylmalonic acid would be confirmatory.[96,97] Treatment includes large doses of cobalamin given orally or, in the case of malabsorption syndromes, by periodic administration via the intramuscular or intranasal route. The dose for treatment of vitamin B_{12} deficiency in children is 30 to 50 µg intramuscularly, or alternatively, deep subcutaneously, daily for 2 weeks, followed by maintenance injection of 100 µg monthly. Energy drinks and "shots" contain vitamin B_{12} with variable amounts but can be greater than 8000% of the recommended daily value. Toxic reactions include urticaria, anaphylaxis, and exacerbation of acneiform eruptions. High-dose vitamin B_{12} in combination with pyridoxine may cause the severe skin lesion rosascea fulminans.[98] Drug interactions with corticosteroids and ibuprofen have been reported with vitamin B_{12}. Antiretroviral drugs may lower vitamin B_{12} levels.[4]

Vitamin C

Vitamin C is essential for many biological functions, including folate metabolism, collagen biosynthesis, bone formation, neurotransmitter synthesis, and iron absorption. Dietary sources include papaya, citrus fruits, tomatoes, cabbage, potatoes, cantaloupe, and strawberries. The RDA for vitamin C for adults was established on the basis of maintenance of near-maximal neutrophil concentration with minimal urinary excretion of ascorbate. Because similar data in infants were not available, the Adequate Intake (AI) for vitamin C in infants was based on mean vitamin C intake of breast-fed infants. RDAs for children and adolescents were estimated on the basis of relative body weight. Signs and symptoms of deficiency include fatigue, malaise, and lethargy, followed by abnormal hyperkeratiotic hair follicles and brittle, coiled hair. As the deficiency state progresses, peri-follicular hemorrhage, osmotic diarrhea, bleeding gums, ocular hemorrhages, and anemia occur, followed by the development of frank scurvy with painful bones, joint hemorrhage, and arthropathy.[12,99]

Intakes of vitamin C by school-aged children have been studied. After defining marginal vitamin C intake as less than 30 mg/day, 12% of boys and 13% of girls between 7 and 12 years of age as well as 14% of boys and 20% of girls between 14 and 18 years of age reported intakes of vitamin C as submarginal.[100] Children with low vitamin C intake tended to have greater energy-adjusted intakes of fat and saturated fat, and children with desirable vitamin C intakes consumed more high-vitamin C-containing fruit juice and whole milk, more high-vitamin C-containing containing vegetables, and more citrus fruits than children with low vitamin C intake.[100] In a group of children receiving long-term dialysis, dietary intake of vitamin C was less than 100% of RDA in most children not receiving supplementation.[101] Vitamin C is removed by dialysis, necessitating adequate intake in dialysis patients. Limited intake can result from unsupplemented parenteral nutrition, anorexia nervosa, ulcerative colitis, and Crohn disease. Although scurvy is rare in children, it is still reported particularly in children who ingest only well-cooked foods and few fruits or vegetables. Use of alcohol and tobacco can decrease vitamin C absorption and increase its metabolism. Low periconceptual intake of vitamins C and E has been associated with low birth weight.[102] Low levels of vitamin C during pregnancy in smokers or diabetics can increase pregnancy complications.[103,104] In newborn infants born to smokers in a randomized controlled trial of vitamin C during pregnancy, the infants exhibited better pulmonary function at birth and less wheezing through 1 year of age.[105] Vitamin C supplementation during pregnancy in women who smoked also prevented smoking-related methylation changes in placenta, cord blood, and newborn buccal samples.[106] Children with autism spectrum disorder who eat a restrictive diet can develop scurvy.[2,107] Vitamin C deficiency may play a role in oxidant stress in children

IV

with chronic renal disease, in children receiving hematopoietic stem cell transplants after chemotherapy, and in children with sickle cell anemia or thalassemia receiving multiple transfusions.[108,109] In addition to dietary deficiencies, a hereditary methemoglobinemia in infants that is responsive to vitamin C has been described. Vitamin C status is best assessed by measuring the concentration of ascorbate in blood leukocytes, considered a better measure of tissue reserves than plasma ascorbate.[110] In children, scurvy is treated with 100 mg of ascorbic acid administered 3 times daily for 1 week, then 100 mg daily for several weeks until tissue saturation is normal. The regimen may be administered intramuscularly, intravenously, or orally. High-dose vitamin C has been touted to prevent the common cold, but data are unsupportive unless a person is under extreme physcial stress. However, vitamin C may have a modest effect in reducing the duration, but not necessarily the severity, of the common cold in adults and children.[111] Excessive vitamin C may cause nausea, vomiting, esophagitis, abdominal cramps, constipation, headache, insomnia, and urinary stones. High doses of vitamin C can increase the blood levels of acetaminophen, aspirin, warfarin, and estrogens while decreasing levels of some antiviral medicines and decreasing enteral absorption of beta blockers.[4]

Other Water-Soluble Vitamins

Information on human needs for pantothenic acid is limited. Pantothenic acid is a component of CoA and is involved in many enzymatic reactions. Pantothenic acid is found in liver, yeast, egg yolks, fresh vegetables, whole grains, and legumes. Deficiency symptoms have not been characterized. In one survey, 49% of female adolescents and 25% of male adolescents consumed less than the recommended 4 mg/day.[112] However, average blood concentrations for both groups were in the normal range.

Biotin is the coenzyme for 5 mammalian carboxylases. Dietary sources include liver, egg yolks, soybeans, milk, and meat. Clinical biotin deficiency is characterized by hypotonia and severe exfoliative dermatitis. Biotin is now appreciated to play a role in epigenetics through gene repression complexes involved in DNA and histone methylation and in histone deacetylation.[20] Marginal biotin status has been documented during pregnancy, and research in animals suggests that this is potentially teratogenic and that biotin intakes during pregnancy may need to be at least 2 times the AI.[20] Symptomatic nutritional deficiency has been described in infants receiving total parenteral nutrition that was free of biotin and in children consuming undercooked eggs containing large amounts of avidin, a biotin-binding protein. However, children receiving long-term anticonvulsant therapy exhibit impaired biotin concentrations but not overt deficiency.[113] Inborn errors of metabolism that exhibit biotin dependency and various degrees of neurologic and dermatologic abnormalities include holocarboxylase synthetase deficiency, biotinidase deficiency, and a defect in biotin transport.[114] A biotin-thiamine–responsive basal ganglia disease has been described (see Thiamine).[19,20] Deficiency is diagnosed by measuring urinary biotin, urinary 3 hydroxyisovaleric acid, and lymphocyte proprionyl-CoA carboxylase. Expression of the potential biotin transporter SLC19A3 in leukocytes may prove to be a useful indicator of marginal biotin deficiency.[115] Biotin can also used as a clinical and research tool to determine RBC volume and survival.[116,117]

Conclusion

WSV deficiency states occur as a result of inadequate intake but can also be secondary to inborn errors of metabolism in which pharmacologic doses of WSVs may ameliorate signs of disease. The genetic basis for some diseases relating to WSVs have been delineated, and it is anticipated more genetic polymorphisms with disease potential will be identified in the future. Other research priorities include investigation of the global prevalence of WSV deficiencies, the role of WSVs in autism and cognitive development, the importance of nutrient-nutrient interactions, effects of excessive WSV ingestion, and the effects of age, gender, and genetics on WSV status in the pediatric age group.[118,119]

Summary Points:

- Supplemental WSVs are probably unnecessary for the healthy child older than 1 year who consumes a varied diet.

- Children at risk of WSV deficiencies may benefit from supplemental multivitamin preparations providing 50% to 100% of the RDA with minimal risks when given as recommended. At-risk children include those following a fad diet or a diet high in fat; those with anorexia, gastrointestinal tract malabsorptive diseases, chronic illess, history of bariatric surgery, HIV/AIDS, and obesity; and those receiving chemotherapeutic, antituberculosis, or anticonvulsant medications.

- Several gene polymorphisms and inherited metabolic defects can also least to deficiency states and have been described for thiamine, pyridoxine, folic acid, vitamin B_{12}, biotin, niacin, riboflavin, and vitamin C.

- Because of the interrelationships of WSV metabolic pathways, deficiencies of multiple WSVs can be seen simultaneously and must be considered.

- Symptoms of WSV deficiencies overlap and commonly include skin disorders, anemia, diarrhea, and imparied neurologic function.

References

1. Position of the American Dietetic Association and the Canadian Dietetic Association: nutrition for physical fitness and athletic performance for adults. *J Am Diet Assoc.* 1993;93(6):691–696

2. Malhi P, Venkatesh L, Bharti B, Singhi P. Feeding problems and nutrient intake in children with and without autism: a comparative study. *Indian J Pediatr.* 2017;84(4):283–288

3. Eisenberg DM, Davis RB, Ettner SL, et al. Trends in alternative medicine use in the United States, 1990–1997: results of a follow-up national survey. *JAMA.* 1998;280(18):1569–1575

4. Rogovik AL, Vohra S, Goldman RD. Safety considerations and potential interactions of vitamins: should vitamins be considered drugs? *Ann Pharmacother.* 2010;44(2):311–324

5. Lee AC, Kemper KJ. Homeopathy and naturopathy: practice characteristics and pediatric care. *Arch Pediatr Adolesc Med.* 2000;154(1):75–80

6. James SJ, Melnyk S, Fuchs G, et al. Efficacy of methylcobalamin and folinic acid treatment on glutathione redox status in children with autism. *Am J Clin Nutr.* 2009;89(1):425–430

7. Wilson K, Busse JW, Gilchrist A, Vohra S, Boon H, Mills E. Characteristics of pediatric and adolescent patients attending a naturopathic college clinic in Canada. *Pediatrics.* 2005;115(3):e338–e343

8. Boon HS, Cherkin DC, Erro J, et al. Practice patterns of naturopathic physicians: results from a random survey of licensed practitioners in two US States. *BMC Complement Altern Med.* 2004;4:14

9. 5-hour ENERGY. Available at: https://5hourenergy.com/facts/ingredients/. Accessed March 11, 2019

10. Dawodu A, Cleaver K. Behavioural correlates of energy drink consumption among adolescents: A review of the literature. *J Child Health Care.* 2017;21(4):446–462

11. Ogden CL, Flegal KM, Carroll MD, Johnson CL. Prevalence and trends in overweight among US children and adolescents, 1999–2000. *JAMA.* 2002;288(14):1728–1732

12. Jen M, Yan AC. Syndromes associated with nutritional deficiency and excess. *Clin Dermatol.* 2010;28(6):669–685

13. Kant AK. Reported consumption of low-nutrient-density foods by American children and adolescents: nutritional and health correlates, NHANES III, 1988 to 1994. *Arch Pediatr Adolesc Med.* 2003;157(8):789–796

14. Lee Y, Mitchell DC, Smiciklas-Wright H, Birch LL. Diet quality, nutrient intake, weight status, and feeding environments of girls meeting or exceeding recommendations for total dietary fat of the American Academy of Pediatrics. *Pediatrics.* 2001;107(6):E95

15. Tonstad S, Sivertsen M. Relation between dietary fat and energy and micronutrient intakes. *Arch Dis Child.* 1997;76(5):416–420

16. Nicklas TA, Myers L, O'Neil C, Gustafson N. Impact of dietary fat and fiber intake on nutrient intake of adolescents. *Pediatrics.* 2000;105(2):E21

17. Ishibashi S, Yokota T, Shiojiri T, et al. Reversible acute axonal polyneuropathy associated with Wernicke-Korsakoff syndrome: impaired physiological nerve conduction due to thiamine deficiency? *J Neurol Neurosurg Psychiatry.* 2003;74(5):674–676

18. Banka S, de Goede C, Yue WW, et al. Expanding the clinical and molecular spectrum of thiamine pyrophosphokinase deficiency: a treatable neurological disorder caused by TPK1 mutations. *Mol Genet Metab.* 2014;113(4):301–306

19. Brown G. Defects of thiamine transport and metabolism. *J Inherit Metab Dis.* 2014;37(4):577–585

20. Mock DM. Biotin: From Nutrition to Therapeutics. *J Nutr.* 2017;147(8):1487–1492

21. Hahn JS, Berquist W, Alcorn DM, Chamberlain L, Bass D. Wernicke encephalopathy and beriberi during total parenteral nutrition attributable to multivitamin infusion shortage. *Pediatrics.* Jan 1998;101(1):E10

22. Davis RA, Wolf A. Infantile beriberi associated with Wernicke's encephalopathy. *Pediatrics.* 1958;21(3):409–420

23. Towbin A, Inge TH, Garcia VF, et al. Beriberi after gastric bypass surgery in adolescence. *J Pediatr.* 2004;145(2):263–267

24. Hung SC, Hung SH, Tarng DC, Yang WC, Chen TW, Huang TP. Thiamine deficiency and unexplained encephalopathy in hemodialysis and peritoneal dialysis patients. *Am J Kidney Dis.* 2001;38(5):941–947

25. Shamir R, Dagan O, Abramovitch D, Abramovitch T, Vidne BA, Dinari G. Thiamine deficiency in children with congenital heart disease before and after corrective surgery. *JPEN J Parenter Enteral Nutr.* 2000;24(3):154–158

26. Winston AP, Jamieson CP, Madira W, Gatward NM, Palmer RL. Prevalence of thiamin deficiency in anorexia nervosa. *Int J Eat Disord.* 2000;28(4):451–454

27. Bayoumi RA, Rosalki SB. Evaluation of methods of coenzyme activation of erythrocyte enzymes for detection of deficiency of vitamins B1, B2, and B6. *Clin Chem.* 1976;22(3):327–335

IV

28. Talwar D, Davidson H, Cooney J, St JRD. Vitamin B(1) status assessed by direct measurement of thiamin pyrophosphate in erythrocytes or whole blood by HPLC: comparison with erythrocyte transketolase activation assay. *Clin Chem.* 2000;46(5):704–710

29. Reid DH. Acute infantile beriberi. *J Pediatr.* 1961;58:858–863

30. Powers HJ. Riboflavin (vitamin B-2) and health. *Am J Clin Nutr.* 2003;77(6): 1352–1360

31. McCormick DB. Two interconnected B vitamins: riboflavin and pyridoxine. *Physiol Rev.* 1989;69(4):1170–1198

32. McCabe H. Riboflavin deficiency in cystic fibrosis: three case reports. *J Hum Nutr Diet.* 2001;14(5):365–370

33. Pratt JS, Lenders CM, Dionne EA, et al. Best practice updates for pediatric/adolescent weight loss surgery. *Obesity (Silver Spring).* 2009;17(5):901–910

34. Floridi A, Palmerini CA, Fini C, Pupita M, Fidanza F. High performance liquid chromatographic analysis of flavin adenine dinucleotide in whole blood. *Int J Vitam Nutr Res.* 1985;55(2):187–191

35. Graham JM, Peerson JM, Haskell MJ, Shrestha RK, Brown KH, Allen LH. Erythrocyte riboflavin for the detection of riboflavin deficiency in pregnant Nepali women. *Clin Chem.* 2005;51(11):2162–2165

36. Tillotson JA, Baker EM. An enzymatic measurement of the riboflavin status in man. *Am J Clin Nutr.* 1972;25(4):425–431

37. Sauberlich HE, Judd JH Jr, Nichoalds GE, Broquist HP, Darby WJ. Application of the erythrocyte glutathione reductase assay in evaluating riboflavin nutritional status in a high school student population. *Am J Clin Nutr.* 1972;25(8):756–762

38. Schoenen J, Jacquy J, Lenaerts M. Effectiveness of high-dose riboflavin in migraine prophylaxis. A randomized controlled trial. *Neurology.* 1998;50(2): 466–470

39. Maizels M, Blumenfeld A, Burchette R. A combination of riboflavin, magnesium, and feverfew for migraine prophylaxis: a randomized trial. *Headache.* 2004;44(9):885–890

40. Schiapparelli P, Allais G, Castagnoli Gabellari I, Rolando S, Terzi MG, Benedetto C. Non-pharmacological approach to migraine prophylaxis: part II. *Neurol Sci.* 2010;31 Suppl 1:S137–139

41. Spivak JL, Jackson DL. Pellagra: an analysis of 18 patients and a review of the literature. *Johns Hopkins Med J.* 1977;140(6):295–309

42. Hegyi J, Schwartz RA, Hegyi V. Pellagra: dermatitis, dementia, and diarrhea. *Int J Dermatol.* 2004;43(1):1–5

43. Kertesz SG. Pellagra in 2 homeless men. *Mayo Clin Proc.* 2001;76(3):315–318

44. Pollack S, Enat R, Haim S, Zinder O, Barzilai D. Pellagra as the presenting manifestation of Crohn's disease. *Gastroenterology.* 1982;82(5 Pt 1):948–952

45. Darvay A, Basarab T, McGregor JM, Russell-Jones R. Isoniazid induced pellagra despite pyridoxine supplementation. *Clin Exp Dermatol.* 1999;24(3):167–169

46. Kaur S, Goraya JS, Thami GP, Kanwar AJ. Pellagrous dermatitis induced by phenytoin. *Pediatr Dermatol.* 2002;19(1):93

47. Jacobson EL, Jacobson MK. Tissue NAD as a biochemical measure of niacin status in humans. *Methods Enzymol.* 1997;280:221–230

48. Shah GM, Shah RG, Veillette H, Kirkland JB, Pasieka JL, Warner RR. Biochemical assessment of niacin deficiency among carcinoid cancer patients. *Am J Gastroenterol.* 2005;100(10):2307–2314

49. Fu CS, Swendseid ME, Jacob RA, McKee RW. Biochemical markers for assessment of niacin status in young men: levels of erythrocyte niacin coenzymes and plasma tryptophan. *J Nutr.* 1989;119(12):1949–1955

50. la Paz SM, Bermudez B, Naranjo MC, Lopez S, Abia R, Muriana FJ. Pharmacological effects of niacin on acute hyperlipemia. *Curr Med Chem.* 2016;23(25):2826–2835

51. Setiawan B, Giraud DW, Driskell JA. Vitamin B-6 inadequacy is prevalent in rural and urban Indonesian children. *J Nutr.* 2000;130(3):553–558

52. Pais RC, Vanous E, Hollins B, et al. Abnormal vitamin B6 status in childhood leukemia. *Cancer.* 1990;66(11):2421–2428

53. Mydlik M, Derzsiova K, Guman M, Hrehorovsky M. Vitamin B6 requirements in chronic renal failure. *Int Urol Nephrol.* 1992;24(4):453–457

54. Gospe SM, Jr. Neonatal vitamin-responsive epileptic encephalopathies. *Chang Gung Med J.* 2010;33(1):1–12

55. Baxter P. Pyridoxine-dependent seizures: a clinical and biochemical conundrum. *Biochim Biophys Acta.* 2003;1647(1-2):36–41

56. Findling RL, Maxwell K, Scotese-Wojtila L, Huang J, Yamashita T, Wiznitzer M. High-dose pyridoxine and magnesium administration in children with autistic disorder: an absence of salutary effects in a double-blind, placebo-controlled study. *J Autism Dev Disord.* 1997;27(4):467–478

57. Aufiero E, Stitik TP, Foye PM, Chen B. Pyridoxine hydrochloride treatment of carpal tunnel syndrome: a review. *Nutr Rev.* 2004;62(3):96–104

58. Williams AL, Cotter A, Sabina A, Girard C, Goodman J, Katz DL. The role for vitamin B-6 as treatment for depression: a systematic review. *Fam Pract.* 2005;22(5):532–537

59. Malouf R, Grimley Evans J. The effect of vitamin B6 on cognition. *Cochrane Database Syst Rev.* 2003(4):CD004393

60. Kaelin A, Casez JP, Jaeger P. Vitamin B6 metabolites in idiopathic calcium stone formers: no evidence for a link to hyperoxaluria. *Urol Res.* 2004;32(1):61–68

61. Proctor ML, Murphy PA. Herbal and dietary therapies for primary and secondary dysmenorrhoea. *Cochrane Database Syst Rev.* 2001(3):CD002124

62. Adams JB, George F, Audhya T. Abnormally high plasma levels of vitamin B6 in children with autism not taking supplements compared to controls not taking supplements. *J Altern Complement Med.* 2006;12(1):59–63

63. Bor MV, Refsum H, Bisp MR, et al. Plasma vitamin B6 vitamers before and after oral vitamin B6 treatment: a randomized placebo-controlled study. *Clin Chem.* 2003;49(1):155–161

64. Jain SK. Vitamin B6 (pyridoxamine) supplementation and complications of diabetes. *Metabolism.* 2007;56(2):168–171

65. Minet JC, Bisse E, Aebischer CP, Beil A, Wieland H, Lutschg J. Assessment of vitamin B-12, folate, and vitamin B-6 status and relation to sulfur amino acid metabolism in neonates. *Am J Clin Nutr.* 2000;72(3):751–757

66. Kirke PN, Molloy AM, Daly LE, Burke H, Weir DG, Scott JM. Maternal plasma folate and vitamin B12 are independent risk factors for neural tube defects. *Q J Med.* 1993;86(11):703–708

67. Botto LD, Yang Q. 5,10–Methylenetetrahydrofolate reductase gene variants and congenital anomalies: a HuGE review. *Am J Epidemiol.* 2000;151(9):862–877

68. van der Linden IJ, Afman LA, Heil SG, Blom HJ. Genetic variation in genes of folate metabolism and neural-tube defect risk. *Proc Nutr Soc.* 2006;65(2):204–215

69. Cardo E, Monros E, Colome C, et al. Children with stroke: polymorphism of the MTHFR gene, mild hyperhomocysteinemia, and vitamin status. *J Child Neurol.* 2000;15(5):295–298

70. Pei LJ, Zhu HP, Li ZW, et al. Interaction between maternal periconceptional supplementation of folic acid and reduced folate carrier gene polymorphism of neural tube defects. *Zhonghua Yi Xue Yi Chuan Xue Za Zhi.* 2005;22(3):284–287

71. Pei L, Zhu H, Zhu J, Ren A, Finnell RH, Li Z. Genetic variation of infant reduced folate carrier (A80G) and risk of orofacial defects and congenital heart defects in China. *Ann Epidemiol.* 2006;16(5):352–356

72. Liu S, Joseph KS, Luo W, et al. Effect of Folic Acid Food Fortification in Canada on Congenital Heart Disease Subtypes. *Circulation.* 2016;134(9):647–655

73. Zhang Q, Wang Y, Xin X, et al. Effect of folic acid supplementation on preterm delivery and small for gestational age births: a systematic review and meta-analysis. *Reprod Toxicol.* 2017;67:35–41

74. McStay CL, Prescott SL, Bower C, Palmer DJ. Maternal folic acid supplementation during pregnancy and childhood allergic disease outcomes: a question of timing? *Nutrients.* 2017;9(2):e123

75. Mielgo-Ayuso J, Valtuena J, Huybrechts I, et al. Fruit and vegetables consumption is associated with higher vitamin intake and blood vitamin status among European adolescents. *Eur J Clin Nutr.* 2017;71(4):458–467

76. Skinner JD, Carruth BR, Houck KS, et al. Longitudinal study of nutrient and food intakes of white preschool children aged 24 to 60 months. *J Am Diet Assoc.* 1999;99(12):1514–1521

77. Picciano MF, Smiciklas-Wright H, Birch LL, Mitchell DC, Murray-Kolb L, McConahy KL. Nutritional guidance is needed during dietary transition in early childhood. *Pediatrics.* 2000;106(1 Pt 1):109–114

78. Cavadini C, Siega-Riz AM, Popkin BM. US adolescent food intake trends from 1965 to 1996. *Arch Dis Child.* 2000;83(1):18–24

79. Iglesia I, Huybrechts I, Gonzalez-Gross M, et al. Folate and vitamin B12 concentrations are associated with plasma DHA and EPA fatty acids in European adolescents: the Healthy Lifestyle in Europe by Nutrition in Adolescence (HELENA) study. *Br J Nutr.* 2017;117(1):124–133

80. Jeejeebhoy KN. Clinical nutrition: 6. Management of nutritional problems of patients with Crohn's disease. *CMAJ.* 2002;166(7):913–918

81. Meira DG, Lorand-Metze I, Toro AD, Silva MT, Vilela MM. Bone marrow features in children with HIV infection and peripheral blood cytopenias. *J Trop Pediatr.* 2005;51(2):114–119

82. Sjostrom ES, Ohlund I, Ahlsson F, Domellof M. Intakes of Micronutrients are associated with early growth in extremely preterm infants. *J Pediatr Gastroenterol Nutr.* 2016;62(6):885–892

83. Bamgbola OF. Pattern of resistance to erythropoietin-stimulating agents in chronic kidney disease. *Kidney Int.* 2011;80(5):464–474

84. Tonetti C, Burtscher A, Bories D, Tulliez M, Zittoun J. Methylenetetrahydrofolate reductase deficiency in four siblings: a clinical, biochemical, and molecular study of the family. *Am J Med Genet.* 2000;91(5):363–367

85. Ramaekers VT, Rothenberg SP, Sequeira JM, et al. Autoantibodies to folate receptors in the cerebral folate deficiency syndrome. *N Engl J Med.* 2005;352(19): 1985–1991

86. Main PA, Angley MT, Thomas P, O'Doherty CE, Fenech M. Folate and methionine metabolism in autism: a systematic review. *Am J Clin Nutr.* 2010;91(6):1598–1620

87. Donangelo CM, Trugo NM, Koury JC, et al. Iron, zinc, folate and vitamin B_{12} nutritional status and milk composition of low-income Brazilian mothers. *Eur J Clin Nutr.* 1989;43(4):253–266

88. Chambers JC, Seddon MD, Shah S, Kooner JS. Homocysteine—a novel risk factor for vascular disease. *J R Soc Med.* 2001;94(1):10–13

89. Finkelstein JL, Layden AJ, Stover PJ. Vitamin B-12 and perinatal health. *Adv Nutr.* 2015;6(5):552–563

90. Specker BL, Miller D, Norman EJ, Greene H, Hayes KC. Increased urinary methylmalonic acid excretion in breast-fed infants of vegetarian mothers and identification of an acceptable dietary source of vitamin B-12. *Am J Clin Nutr.* 1988;47(1):89–92

91. Dagnelie PC, van Staveren WA, Hautvast JG. Stunting and nutrient deficiencies in children on alternative diets. *Acta Paediatr Scand Suppl.* 1991;374:111–118

92. Robinson M, White FJ, Cleary MA, Wraith E, Lam WK, Walter JH. Increased risk of vitamin B12 deficiency in patients with phenylketonuria on an unrestricted or relaxed diet. *J Pediatr.* 2000;136(4):545–547

93. Bibi H, Gelman-Kohan Z, Baumgartner ER, Rosenblatt DS. Transcobalamin II deficiency with methylmalonic aciduria in three sisters. *J Inherit Metab Dis.* 1999;22(7):765–772

94. Tanner SM, Li Z, Perko JD, et al. Hereditary juvenile cobalamin deficiency caused by mutations in the intrinsic factor gene. *Proc Natl Acad Sci U S A.* 2005;102(11):4130–4133

95. Steen MT, Boddie AM, Fisher AJ, et al. Neural-tube defects are associated with low concentrations of cobalamin (vitamin B12) in amniotic fluid. *Prenat Diagn.* 1998;18(6):545–555

96. Yetley EA, Coates PM, Johnson CL. Overview of a roundtable on NHANES monitoring of biomarkers of folate and vitamin B-12 status: measurement procedure issues. *Am J Clin Nutr.* 2011;94(1):297S–302S

97. Yetley EA, Pfeiffer CM, Phinney KW, et al. Biomarkers of vitamin B-12 status in NHANES: a roundtable summary. *Am J Clin Nutr.* 2011;94(1):313S–321S

98. Jansen T, Romiti R, Kreuter A, Altmeyer P. Rosacea fulminans triggered by high-dose vitamins B6 and B12. *J Eur Acad Dermatol Venereol.* 2001;15(5):484–485

99. Fain O. Musculoskeletal manifestations of scurvy. *Joint Bone Spine.* 2005;72(2): 124–128

100. Hampl JS, Taylor CA, Johnston CS. Intakes of vitamin C, vegetables and fruits: which schoolchildren are at risk? *J Am Coll Nutr.* 1999;18(6):582–590

101. Pereira AM, Hamani N, Nogueira PC, Carvalhaes JT. Oral vitamin intake in children receiving long-term dialysis. *J Ren Nutr.* 2000;10(1):24–29

102. Gadhok AK, Sharma TK, Sinha M, et al. Natural Antioxidant Vitamins Status in Pregnancies Complicated with Intrauterine Growth Restriction. *Clin Lab.* 2017;63(5):941–945

103. Juhl B, Lauszus FF, Lykkesfeldt J. Poor vitamin C status late in pregnancy is associated with increased risk of complications in type 1 diabetic women: a cross-sectional study. *Nutrients.* 2017;9(3):e186

104. McEvoy CT, Milner KF, Scherman AJ, et al. Vitamin C to Decrease the Effects of Smoking in Pregnancy on Infant Lung Function (VCSIP): Rationale, design, and methods of a randomized, controlled trial of vitamin C supplementation in pregnancy for the primary prevention of effects of in utero tobacco smoke exposure on infant lung function and respiratory health. *Contemp Clin Trials.* 2017;58:66–77

105. McEvoy CT, Schilling D, Clay N, et al. Vitamin C supplementation for pregnant smoking women and pulmonary function in their newborn infants: a randomized clinical trial. *JAMA.* 2014;311(20):2074–2082

106. Shorey-Kendrick LE, McEvoy CT, Ferguson B, et al. Vitamin C prevents offspring dna methylation changes associated with maternal smoking in pregnancy. *Am J Respir Crit Care Med.* 2017;196(6):745–755

107. Golriz F, Donnelly LF, Devaraj S, Krishnamurthy R. Modern American scurvy - experience with vitamin C deficiency at a large children's hospital. *Pediatr Radiol.* 2017;47(2):214–220

108. Amer J, Ghoti H, Rachmilewitz E, Koren A, Levin C, Fibach E. Red blood cells, platelets and polymorphonuclear neutrophils of patients with sickle cell disease exhibit oxidative stress that can be ameliorated by antioxidants. *Br J Haematol.* 2006;132(1):108–113

109. Zwolinska D, Grzeszczak W, Szczepanska M, Kilis-Pstrusinska K, Szprynger K. Vitamins A, E and C as non-enzymatic antioxidants and their relation to lipid peroxidation in children with chronic renal failure. *Nephron Clin Pract.* 2006;103(1):c12–c18

110. Thurnham DI. Micronutrients and immune function: some recent developments. *J Clin Pathol.* 1997;50(11):887–891

111. Douglas RM, Hemila H, Chalker E, Treacy B. Vitamin C for preventing and treating the common cold. *Cochrane Database Syst Rev.* 2007;(3):CD000980

112. Eissenstat BR, Wyse BW, Hansen RG. Pantothenic acid status of adolescents. *Am J Clin Nutr.* 1986;44(6):931–937

113. Krause KH, Bonjour JP, Berlit P, Kynast G, Schmidt-Gayk H, Schellenberg B. Effect of long-term treatment with antiepileptic drugs on the vitamin status. *Drug Nutr Interact.* 1988;5(4):317–343

114. Mardach R, Zempleni J, Wolf B, et al. Biotin dependency due to a defect in biotin transport. *J Clin Invest.* 2002;109(12):1617–1623

115. Vlasova TI, Stratton SL, Wells AM, Mock NI, Mock DM. Biotin deficiency reduces expression of SLC19A3, a potential biotin transporter, in leukocytes from human blood. *The Journal of nutrition.* 2005;135(1):42–47

116. Mock DM, Matthews NI, Zhu S, et al. Red blood cell (RBC) survival determined in humans using RBCs labeled at multiple biotin densities. *Transfusion.* 2011;51(5):1047–1057

117. Mock DM, Matthews NI, Zhu S, et al. Red blood cell (RBC) volume can be independently determined in vivo in humans using RBCs labeled at different densities of biotin. *Transfusion.* 2011;51(1):148–157

118. Bryan J, Osendarp S, Hughes D, Calvaresi E, Baghurst K, van Klinken JW. Nutrients for cognitive development in school-aged children. *Nutr Rev.* 2004;62(8):295–306

119. Viteri FE, Gonzalez H. Adverse outcomes of poor micronutrient status in childhood and adolescence. *Nutr Rev.* 2002;60(5 Pt 2):S77–S83

IV

Nutrient Delivery Systems

V

Chapter 22

Parenteral Nutrition

Introduction

Parenteral nutrition (PN) may be required as a supplement or as a complete substitute for enteral nutrition. This chapter reviews PN as a nutritional strategy to ensure appropriate growth and development for full term infants and children. For PN use in preterm infants, see Chapter 5: Nutritional Needs of the Preterm Infant.

Important Considerations Before Initiating Parenteral Nutrition

PN is a complex and expensive nutrition intervention. It is important to use PN only when enteral or oral routes are not feasible or are insufficient to meet nutrient needs. Whenever possible, enteral nutrition should be used and PN should be resorted to only when enteral feeding is not possible. Common indications for PN include prematurity, intestinal failure attributable to short bowel syndrome and other conditions, intractable diarrhea, intestinal dysmotility, surgical conditions precluding use of the gastrointestinal tract, oncologic conditions, and hematopoietic stem cell transplantation. When enteral nutrition is not feasible, PN should be started within 3 days of nil per os (NPO [nothing by mouth]) status for infants and within 5 days of NPO status for older children.[1] These guidelines may vary depending on the nutrition status and degree of gastrointestinal tract involvement with regard to ability to tolerate and absorb enteral feeds as well as the severity of the underlying disease. However, given the risks associated with PN, PN should not be initiated if the expected duration of nutrition support is less than 5 days. In pediatric patients, PN should not be initiated in the home setting; all pediatric patients should be admitted to the hospital for initiation and advancement of PN and should not be discharged on home PN until they are on a stable PN prescription.[1]

Contraindications

A functional gastrointestinal tract should be considered a contraindication to PN.

Prior to initiating PN, patients must be hemodynamically stable. If significant electrolyte or metabolic disturbances exist, they must be corrected with intravenous fluids or intravenous supplementation prior to initiation of PN. Food and medication allergies must be reviewed prior to initiating PN. Patients with allergies to egg, soybean, peanut, or fish may react to

PN components.[2] Rarely, allergies to PN components, such as amino acid solutions and multivitamin preparations, have been documented in patients without known food allergies.[2] Lack of appropriate venous access can be a rare contraindication. Depending on patient and family wishes, PN may be contraindicated in end-of-life care.

Access

PN can be administered through peripheral or central veins. Using standard intravenous catheters, only solutions with an osmolarity up to 900 mOsml/L can be safely infused into peripheral veins.[3,4] Hence, peripheral parenteral nutrition solutions are limited to a dextrose concentration of 10% to 12.5%, thus requiring a larger volume of fluid for adequate energy provision.[5] Peripheral veins can be used for short-term PN, which is usually associated with fewer complications. Central venous parenteral nutrition is usually reserved, by consensus, for patients who are or will be intolerant of enteral feedings for more than 2 weeks and for whom solutions with osmolarity >900 mOsm/L are necessary.[3] However, infants and young children may lack the peripheral venous access to enable peripheral PN to be used even for 2 weeks. Large central veins will tolerate solutions of higher osmolarity and glucose concentrations of up to 25% or higher. The tip of the central venous catheter is typically placed near the junction of the superior vena cava and the right atrium. Two techniques are commonly used for central venous catheter (CVC) placement: (1) a percutaneously inserted central catheter (PICC), positioned in an upper or lower extremity vein or external jugular vein, is advanced into the superior or inferior vena cava to lie at the junction of the right atrium and the large vein; or (2) a catheter is placed in a central location surgically via the jugular or subclavian veins. The second approach is largely used when a much longer duration of PN is required or percutaneous placement is not possible.

Writing the Parenteral Nutrition Prescription

Prior to initiating PN, consult a registered dietitian with expertise in PN support to help calculate macronutrient and micronutrient needs as well as a PN infusion pharmacist to ensure the safety and stability of the PN solution. Table 22.1[6,7,8] outlines the recommended doses of PN components for infants and children.

Table 22.1.

Components of Maintenance Parenteral Nutrition in Infants and Children

Base Components	Weight		
	<10 kg	*10–20 kg*	*>20 kg*
Fluid[6]	100–150 mL/kg	1000 mL + 50 mL/kg >10 kg	1500 mL + 20 mL/kg >20 kg
Calories	85%–90% of predicted from standard equation or patient history		
Dextrose GIR, mg/kg/minute (3.4 kcal/g)[7]	10–14	8–10	5–6
Protein, g/kg (4 kcal/g)[8]	2–3	1–2	0.8–1.5
Fat, g/kg (10 kcal/g)[a,8]	1–3	1–3	1–3
Electrolytes	**Infants and Toddlers**	**Children (<50 kg)**	**Adolescents (>50 kg)**
Sodium	2–5 mEq/kg		1–2 mEq/kg
Potassium	2–4 mEq/kg		1–2 mEq/kg
Chloride	As needed for acid-base balance		
Acetate	As needed for acid-based balance		
Minerals[8]	**Infants and Children (<50 kg)**		**Adolescents (>50 kg)**
Magnesium (125 mg/mEq)	0.3–0.5 mEq/kg		10–30 mEq/day
Calcium	0.5–4 mEq/kg		10–20 mEq/day
Phosphorus (31 mg/mmol)	0.5–2 mmol/kg		10-40 mmol/day

[a] Based on 20% lipid emulsion.

Continued

Table 22.1. *Continued*
Components of Maintenance Parenteral Nutrition in Infants and Children

Base Components	Weight		
	<10 kg	10–20 kg	>20 kg
Micronutrients[a,8]	Infants and Toddlers	Children (<40 kg)	Adolescents (>40 kg)
Multivitamin	Per manufacturer directions	Per manufacturer directions	Per manufacturer directions
Multitrace	Per manufacturer directions or dose individually	Per manufacturer directions or dose individually	Per manufacturer directions or dose individually
Zinc	50–250 mcg/kg/d	50–125 mcg/kg/d	2000–5000 mcg/day
Copper	20 mcg/kg/d	5–20 mcg/kg/d	200–500 mcg/day
Manganese	1 mcg/kg/d	1 mcg/kg/d	40–100 mcg/day
Chromium	0.2 mcg/kg/d	0.14–0.2 mcg/kg/d	5–15 mcg/day
Selenium	2 mcg/kg/d	1–2 mcg/kg/d	40–60 mcg/day
Heparin (optional)	0.5–1 U/mL	0.5–1 U/mL	0.5–1 U/mL

[a] Based on 20% lipid emulsion.

A dosing weight must be determined before writing the PN prescription. For patients with unreliable weight measurements and fluid shifts, a historical weight or usual body weight may be used as the dosing weight. As they gain weight, infants and young children may require frequent adjustments in dosing weight.

Energy, Protein, and Fluid Needs
Energy needs may be calculated using standard equations or based on that patient's previous enteral or oral nutrition intake. Critically ill children and

some hospitalized children may benefit from tailoring their PN prescription being tailored to reflect their measured resting energy expenditure (as measured by indirect calorimetry). Typically, patients on PN require 10% to 15% fewer calories than patients receiving enteral or oral feedings.

Protein needs vary by age and patient condition. Recommended Dietary Allowances can be used for establishing minimum protein needs. Higher protein needs may be indicated for critically ill patients and patients with specific medical conditions.

Fluid needs vary by patient condition. For patients without fluid restriction or diagnoses suggesting excessive fluid needs, the Holliday-Segar formula can be used to determine maintenance fluid needs.[6] Based on this formula, a child needs:

- 100 mL/kg for the first 10 kg of body weight
- 50 mL/kg for each kg of body weight between and 11 and 20 kg
- 20 mL/kg for each kg of additional body weight

If patients are tolerating enteral or oral feedings and require PN as partial nutrition support, begin by calculating their energy, protein, and fluid intake from enteral and oral feedings. Deduct this intake from PN energy and fluid goals prior to continuing with the PN prescription.

Macronutrients

PN is composed of 3 macronutrients: dextrose as a source of carbohydrates, an amino acid solution as a source of protein, and a lipid emulsion as a source of fat. The typical macronutrient distribution for infant and pediatric PN is 45% to 60% carbohydrate, 10% to 15% protein, and 25% to 40% fat.

Dextrose

Dextrose is the most common carbohydrate source used in PN solutions. Other carbohydrate sources have no advantage over dextrose and can produce serious complications in preterm infants. Consideration of the glucose infusion rate (GIR), calculated as mg of glucose provided per kg of body weight per minute, is important to prevent hyperglycemia and hypoglycemia. Goal GIR varies on the basis of age (Table 22.1). Excess glucose provision has been associated with intestinal failure associated liver disease (IFALD). In infants and in children prone to hypoglycemia, tapering PN for the last hour of infusion when infusions are not continuous but cycled may prevent hypoglycemia (see discussion of cycling below). Parenteral dextrose provides 3.4 kcal/g. Dextrose tolerance is usually monitored through urine or capillary blood glucose measurements.

Amino Acid Solution

Crystalline amino acids provide the nitrogen in PN solutions. The amino acid component of PN should be provided to support lean body mass and support the production of proteins that are essential for metabolism. Pediatric amino acid formulations are available to meet the needs of preterm infants, term infants, and children. Many brands are available and they vary not only in their amino acid profile but also in pH and potential for calcium-phosphate solubility in the PN solution (see Table 22.2). The available amino acid solutions are generally well tolerated. In addition, L-cysteine, which is conditionally essential in neonates, is added to the final mixture. Metabolic complications related to amino acids, such as azotemia

Table 22.2.
Parenteral Nutrition Solutions

Pediatric/Infant Parenteral Nutritional Solutions:

Aminosyn-PF: 10% (Hospira)
    https://www.rxlist.com/aminosyn-pf-10-drug.htm
Premasol: 6%,10% (Baxter)
    http://www.baxtermedicationdeliveryproducts.com/pdf/
PREMASOLPI6.14.pdf
Trophamine: 6%, 10% (BBraun)
    https://www.bbraunusa.com/en/products/b2/trophamine-
    glass500ml.html

Adult Parenteral Nutrition Solutions:

Aminosyn: 10% (Hospira)
    https://www.drugs.com/pro/aminosyn-10.html
Aminosyn II: 10%, 15% (Hospira)
    https://dailymed.nlm.nih.gov/dailymed/fda/fdaDrugXsl.
    cfm?setid=0936353b-88ab-4746-c881-cb0a4c7e6e2b&type=display
Clinisol 15% (Baxter)
    http://www.baxtermedicationdeliveryproducts.com/pdf/
CliniSol0719173182.pdf
FreAmine III: 10% (BBraun)
    https://medlibrary.org/lib/rx/meds/freamine-iii/
Plenamine 15% (BBraun)
    https://medlibrary.org/lib/rx/meds/plenamine-1/
Prosol 20% (Baxter)
    http://www.baxtermedicationdeliveryproducts.com/pdf/ProSolPI.pdf
Premasol, 6%, 10% (Baxter)
    http://www.baxtermedicationdeliveryproducts.com/pdf/
PREMASOLPI6.14.pdf
Travasol: 10% (500 mL, 1000 mL, 2000 mL) (Baxter)
    https://dailymed.nlm.nih.gov/dailymed/archives/fdaDrugInfo.
    cfm?archiveid=88932

and acidosis, have occurred when infants have received more than 4 g of protein equivalent per kg per day. For older, critically ill children, lack of adequate protein has been associated with respiratory failure, muscle weakness, and sepsis.[9] Protein requirements will vary with the age or weight of the patient, as depicted in Table 22.1. Parenteral amino acids provide 4 kcal/g.

Lipid Emulsion

Lipid is an essential component of PN as it is a concentrated source of energy and provides essential fatty acids. There are several types of lipid emulsions currently available. Intralipid is a soybean oil-based lipid emulsion. Long-term use has been strongly implicated in the development of IFALD.[10] If soybean oil-based lipid emulsion is used in the setting of intestinal failure or is expected to be used long-term, consider cycling PN and/ or reducing the lipid dose to 0.5 to 1 g·kg^{-1}·day^{-1} and monitoring for essential fatty acid deficiency. Smoflipid is a lipid emulsion containing soybean oil, medium-chain triglycerides, olive oil, and fish oil. Emerging data suggest that Smoflipid may be more hepatoprotective than standard soybean oil-based lipid emulsion.[11] Smoflipid is currently only approved by the US Food and Drug Administration (FDA) for use in children 16 years or older. A third type of lipid emulsion, Omegaven, is entirely fish oil-based and has been shown to potentially reverse some of the manifestations of IFALD.[12] However, Omegaven is not FDA approved and can only be obtained in the United States through a compassionate use protocol.

PN lipid emulsions may be mixed into the PN to make a 3-in-1 PN solution or may be infused separately while the dextrose and amino acids are compounded with the other ingredients to make a 2-in-1 PN solution. Such 3-in-1 solutions, also called total nutrient admixtures, may be preferred because of (1) simplified administration, which may prove to be cost effective; (2) less manipulation of the delivery system (reduced opportunity for contamination); and (3) lessened loss of vitamin A. One retrospective study of 3-in-1 solutions in infants younger than 1 year found them to be safe, efficacious, and cost-effective.[13] Although 3-in-1 solutions are widely and safely used in pediatrics, especially at home, iron is not compatible with 3-in-1 solutions, and patients who receive long-term 3-in-1 solutions will likely need iron supplementation.[14,15]

In pediatrics, 20% lipid emulsions are the most commonly used and provide 10 kcal/g of lipid, 2 kcal/mL of lipid emulsion, and 5 mL fluid/g of lipid. Twenty-percent intravenous fat has a lower phospholipid-to-triglyceride ratio than 10% intravenous emulsion. Because phospholipid is believed to inhibit lipoprotein lipase, the main enzyme for intravenous fat clearance, the 20% emulsion is cleared more efficiently and is preferable. In patients receiving 2-in-1 PN, the fluid volume provided by lipid should be taken into account and is especially important for patients with fluid restrictions. The typical dosing for PN lipid emulsions are 2 to 3 g·kg^{-1}·day^{-1} unless lipid minimization is indicated. Infusion rates of lipid emulsions should not exceed 0.15 g·kg^{-1}·hour^{-1}.[5] Tolerance of the lipid emulsion is monitored via serum triglycerides, which should ideally be maintained under 250 mg/dL.

Electrolytes, Micronutrients, and Additives

Electrolytes and Minerals
Electrolytes are an essential component of the PN prescription (see Table 22.1 for initial electrolyte dosing ranges). Close monitoring of serum electrolytes and adjusting the PN prescription accordingly is necessary to determine the appropriate electrolyte content of the nutrition prescription.

Micronutrients
Vitamins, minerals, and trace elements must be supplied in PN solutions unless patients are receiving adequate enteral feedings to meet their micronutrient needs. Metabolic complications have been described because of deficiencies and excesses of some of these micronutrients. Five trace elements are included in standard trace element preparations: zinc, copper, selenium, chromium, and manganese. Zinc deficiency is common in patients on PN without adequate supplementation.[16] The zinc dosage provided by trace element products may not meet the needs of patients with excess gastrointestinal losses; hence, additional zinc may need to be added to PN to prevent zinc deficiency.[16] Copper toxicity has been described in patients on PN with liver disease as hepatic excretion of copper may be impaired. Monitoring for toxicity is imperative for patients receiving long-term PN. However, the presence of liver disease does not automatically increase the risk of copper toxicity; low serum levels have been seen even in children with liver disease.[17] Hence, monitoring of serum levels is crucial. Serum selenium should be used to help guide selenium dosing. The symptoms of selenium deficiency occur only with extreme deficiency and symptoms of toxicity occur only when levels are 10-fold above normal.[18,19] Chromium and manganese are contaminants introduced during the production of PN and, thus, deficiency of these trace elements is uncommon. However, manganese toxicity has been reported.

Trace elements can be provided using trace element mixtures or by individually dosing trace elements. If using a trace element mixture, dose using the manufacturer's guidelines and monitor for micronutrient deficiencies and toxicities. Consider individually dosing trace elements if it will better meet the patient's trace element needs and prevent toxicity. Intravenous dose requirements for parenteral trace elements are not fully known. Guidelines from an expert panel for trace elements for parenteral use are shown in Table 22.1.

Pediatric intravenous multivitamin preparations are available and should be dosed according to the manufacturer's directions. After 11 years of age, consider using adult multivitamin products. Some adult products do not contain vitamin K. Consider adding vitamin K separately if using these products.

PN multivitamin/trace element products do not contain iron, and iron cannot be added to 3-in-1 PN solutions. When able, supplement iron via the enteral or oral route. If enteral or oral iron is not feasible or is not effective, consider IV iron infusions to be administered separately from PN.

In the United States, iodine is currently not supplied via PN trace element mixtures. Previously, iodine-containing disinfectants were used topically on patients receiving PN. However, these products are no longer standard of care.[20] Hence, monitoring of thyroid function in children receiving long-term PN is suggested to detect iodine deficiency.

Aluminum is an unfortunate contaminant of PN solutions. Preterm infants are most vulnerable to potential aluminum toxicity because of their immature renal function; this can lead to central nervous system toxicity or worsen metabolic bone disease.[8] The FDA mandated that 5 $mcg \cdot kg^{-1} \cdot day^{-1}$ should be the maximum amount tolerated and added that the aluminum content of PN should be stated on the label. Every effort should be made to minimize aluminum exposure in infants and children receiving PN.[8]

Other Additives

Carnitine

Carnitine is required for the optimal metabolism of fatty acids. Infants have a poorly developed capacity to synthesize and store carnitine. Some experts recommend carnitine supplementation (2.4–10 mg/kg/day in preterm and term infants), but the lack of carnitine in PN formulations has not been associated with any clinical deficiency syndrome, and the results of clinical studies of its addition to PN formulations have been contradictory.[21] Hence, carnitine may be added to the PN of children younger than 1 year.

HEPARIN

Heparin is sometimes added to PN at doses ranging from 0.5 to 1 units/mL of PN solution. Heparin is added with the dual intention of prolonging the life of the central venous catheter (by preventing occlusion/thrombosis) and improving tolerance of lipid emulsion, because heparin enhances lipoprotein lipase activity. There are also some data to suggest that the presence of heparin in PN solutions can be associated with fewer central line-associated bloodstream infections (CLABSIs). However, heparin causes bone loss by decreasing bone formation and also by increasing bone resorption.[22] There are also some data that suggest that the activity of heparin on lipid metabolism may not be truly beneficial.[23-25] Given these conflicting data, some authorities do not recommend the long-term use of heparin in PN.[3]

Other intravenous medications may be added to the PN solution. It is important to work closely with the PN infusion pharmacist to ensure the safety and stability of the PN prescription.

Implementing the PN Prescription

Once the goals for the PN prescription are decided, the initial PN prescription can be written. It is important to start PN with a lower macronutrient prescription and slowly increase over 3 to 7 days to the goal PN to prevent complications such as hyperglycemia and azotemia. The initial dextrose concentration of PN should be less than or equal to 10% dextrose. Increase by 2% to 5% dextrose daily to meet dextrose goal. Protein and lipid should be started at 1 to 2 g/kg and advanced as able to goal. Most institutions start with PN infusions over 24 hours and decrease the infusion time as able after the goal prescription is delivered.

Cycling PN to run for less than 24 hours per day has benefits for certain patients. Cycling helps promote patient independence by allowing freedom from PN for a few hours per day. Cycling is also hepatoprotective. When cycling the PN prescription, the prescriber must account for the increased GIR and ensure that it does not exceed the maximum recommended GIR for age and weight (Table 22.1). The lipid infusion rate should not exceed 0.15 g·kg^{-1}·hour^{-1}.[5] Infants and young children require a taper to prevent quick declines in serum glucose concentrations.

PN Order Forms

The American Society for Parenteral and Enteral Nutrition (ASPEN) recommends standardized order forms for PN orders so that prescribing errors are minimized. All PN components should be ordered in grams, milligrams, millimoles, or milliequivalents per kilogram or per day, not per liter. In addition to the PN components addressed previously and in Table 22.1, the PN order should also include: dosing weight, the location of the venous access device (central or peripheral), and parenteral nutrition indication.[8]

Monitoring

Clinical Status

All children who need to begin PN should be clinically assessed to ascertain nutritional status, including current nutritional intake and adequacy as well as fluid status. Accurate anthropometric measurements and calculation of appropriate z-scores are essential. Reliance on weight alone may be inaccurate in children requiring PN, including patients with fluid shifts and stool losses, edema, and organomegaly secondary to liver disease. Acute critical illness can also affect weight and fluid status. Hence, a complete nutrition assessment and continual monitoring of weight, mid-upper arm circumference, and triceps skinfold thickness and a nutrition-focused physical examination are important components of PN monitoring.

Laboratory Monitoring

During PN initiation and advancement to goal PN, monitoring of fluid and electrolyte status is crucial. This monitoring also continues to remain an integral part of the management of children receiving PN at home. Biochemical monitoring helps ensure tolerance to the various components of PN and also may protect against several complications. The initial monitoring of children on PN is outlined in Table 22.3.

Multiple micronutrient deficiencies have been described in children who are receiving home PN for intestinal failure. These deficiencies need to be identified and treated even if the child is growing well and exhibiting no symptoms of the deficiencies. Anemia, particularly iron-deficiency anemia, is almost universal. However, multiple vitamin and mineral deficiencies have been reported in the literature.[26,27] The ongoing monitoring of a child receiving PN at home is outlined in Figure 22.1.[28]

Complications (see Table 22.4)

Infectious Complications

CLABSIs can be life threatening and lead to significant morbidity and mortality. In the hospitalized patient, CVCs should be managed using a set of activities termed a "bundle" to prevent CLABSIs.[29] The elements of this

Table 22.3.

Suggested Laboratory Monitoring Schedule During Parenteral Nutrition in the Hospitalized Patient

Parameter	Prior to Initiation	Initial	Follow-up
CBC	Yes	Weekly	Weekly
CMP	Yes	Daily[a]	Weekly
Magnesium	Yes	Daily	Weekly
Phosphorus	Yes	Daily	Weekly
Triglycerides	Yes	Daily	Weekly
Direct bilirubin	As indicated[b]	As indicated[b]	As indicated[b]
Urinary glucose and ketones	As indicated[c]	As indicated[c]	As indicated[c]

CBC, complete blood cell count with auto differential count; CMP, comprehensive metabolic panel (sodium, potassium, carbon dioxide, chloride, blood urea nitrogen, creatinine, glucose, calcium, aspartate transaminase, alanine aminotransferase, albumin, alkaline phosphatase, total bilirubin).

[a] During the initial phase of ramping up of parenteral nutrition to goal parenteral nutrition and until both parenteral nutrition constituents and metabolic parameters are relatively stable.

[b] When there is a concern for cholestasis (ie) total bilirubin and/or alkaline phosphatase are elevated.

[c] When there is a concern for hyperglycemia (ie) in the initial phase of ramping up of dextrose concentrations in parenteral nutrition or when significant changes are made to the glucose infusion rate due to cycling or decreasing the number of hours that parenteral nutrition is being provided.

bundle include proper CVC insertion practices, rules on handling and maintenance of CVCs, and prompt removal of unnecessary CVCs.

In the patient receiving PN at home, a CLABSI can be caused either by improper catheter care and contamination or from bacterial translocation across the gut epithelium in children with short bowel syndrome or severe intestinal inflammation.[30] In patients with short bowel syndrome, in addition to immediate risks related to sepsis, CLABSIs are often associated with acute worsening of cholestasis and are an independent risk factor for IFALD.[31] Prompt evaluation and treatment of children with suspected CLABSI (ie, presence of fever in a child with a CVC) is vital to reduce morbidity and mortality. Children receiving PN at home with suspected CLABSI

Fig 22.1.

Suggested Laboratory Monitoring Schedule for Patient Receiving Parenteral Nutrition at Home (Adapted with permission from Smith et al[28])

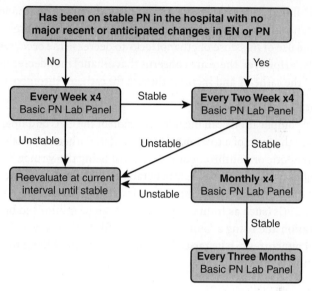

Basic PN Panel

Complete blood count with auto differential, Sodium, Potassium, CO_2, Chloride, Blood urea nitrogen, Creatinine, Glucose, Calcium, Magnesium, Phosphorus, ALT, Triglycerides, Albumin, Alkaline phosphatase, Direct bilirubin

PN Micronutrient Panel

Every 6 Months: Copper, Selenium, Zinc, Vitamins A, E, D, B12, Methylmalonic Acid,Homocysteine, Prothrombin time, Iron, Total Iron-Binding Capacity, RBC Folate; T4,TSH; Carnitine if < 1 year of age

Every 6 months: DEXA scan

ALT, alanine aminotransferase; DEXA, dual-energy x-ray absorptiometry; EN, enteral nutrition; PN, parenteral nutrition; RBC, red blood cell; T4, thyroxine; TSH, thyroid-stimulating hormone.

require hospital admission and monitoring; they should receive intravenous antibiotics while awaiting blood culture results.

Prevention of CLABSIs is a vital endeavor in children receiving PN at home. It is extremely important that CVCs at home are managed using another "bundle" to prevent CLABSIs. This bundle includes the use of sterile technique when the CVC is accessed; scrubbing the access points with appropriate products; and keeping the dressing dry, intact, and occlusive. All caregivers should be educated in all elements of CLABSI prevention.

The use of ethanol locks has gained significant traction in children receiving long-term PN delivered through a tunneled CVC. Typically, 70% ethanol is used to fill the CVC and retained for 4 to 6 hours (the time when the child is not receiving PN). At the end of the time, the ethanol is drawn out and discarded and the next bag of PN is started. The literature supports the use of this dose of ethanol locks to decrease the occurrence of CLABSIs.[32] However, there are concerns that ethanol may decrease the integrity of the catheter and increase the risk for catheter thrombosis.[33]

Mechanical Complications

Mechanical complications can include occlusion of the CVC or damage to the tubing in the form of a torn or broken catheter. Catheter occlusions can be thrombotic or nonthrombotic, with most being the former.[34,35] Nonthrombotic occlusions can be attributable to calcium precipitates. CVC occlusions can be treated using thrombolytic agents to restore patency. Damage to CVCs (such as from tears or breaks) can be minimized by caregiver education and using a "bundle" to care for the CVC. Many of these breaks and punctures can be repaired using repair kits and these may help preserve the CVC.

Metabolic Complications

A variety of metabolic complications are possible in children receiving PN. Some of these are directly related to a lack or excess of some component in PN. Others are related to the primary reason for the child receiving PN (such as dehydration). These complications are outlined in Table 22.4.

Refeeding syndrome can occur when PN is commenced. It is likely to occur in malnourished children who are started on PN that causes rapid or excessive infusion of dextrose. It can be prevented by understanding the likelihood of refeeding syndrome in malnourished patients and providing modest total overall energy when initiating PN and slowly increasing energy provision as tolerated to the goal PN prescription.

Liver Disease

IFALD is one of the most important contributors to the morbidity experienced by children with intestinal failure who receive long-term PN. The prevalence of IFALD is estimated to be up to 85% in neonates and 40% to 60% of infants who are receiving long-term PN for intestinal failure.[36] The cause of IFALD is multifactorial with key factors including prematurity and sepsis. Among the various components of PN, it is currently believed that the key role is played by soy-based intravenous lipid emulsions through excess phytosterols, predominance of proinflammatory omega-6 fatty

Table 22.4.
Complications of Parenteral Nutrition

Infectious
  Central line-associated bloodstream infections (sepsis)
    Bacterial, fungal

Mechanical
Complications following placement:
  Air embolism
  Pneumothorax, hemothorax, hydrothorax
  Perforation of an organ
  Pericardial effusion
Malposition:
  Arrhythmias, cardiac tamponade, Brachial plexus injury, diaphragmatic palsy
Thrombotic events and thrombophlebitis
Extravasation:
  Skin sloughing and subcutaneous injury
Mechanical catheter-related events:
  Crack or breakage of catheter; catheter occlusion

Metabolic
Acute metabolic
  Refeeding syndrome
  Dehydration/fluid overload
  Hyperglycemia/hypoglycemia
  Hypernatremia/hyponatremia
  Hyperkalemia/hypokalemia
  Hypermagnesemia/hypomagnesemia
  Hyperphosphatemia/hypophosphatemia
  Hypercalcemia/hypocalcemia
  Metabolic acidosis or alkalosis
  Azotemia
  Hyperlipidemia/essential fatty acid deficiency
  Deficiencies and toxicities of trace elements
Long-term metabolic
  Hepatobiliary dysfunction (cholestasis, steatosis, intestinal failure-associated liver disease)
  Metabolic bone disease (osteopenia to frank rickets or fractures)
  Renal disease (calculi, decrease in renal function)

acids, and antioxidant imbalance related to inadequate provision of alpha tocopherol.[37] Various strategies to prevent and treat IFALD include lipid minimization, cycling of PN, use of alternative lipids, prompt recognition and treatment of CLABSIs, prevention of CLABSIs (through meticulous CVC care and ethanol locks), and most importantly, aggressive optimization of enteral nutrition with concomitant decreases in the amount PN delivered to the patient.

Bone Disease

Metabolic bone disease is common in children receiving long-term PN. Approximately 40% of chronic PN patients have bone mineral density z-score <-2.[38,39] Significant predictors of lower bone mass include increasing age and lower height z-score.[38,39] Frequent monitoring of bone mineral density is recommended to prevent bone disease in patients receiving long-term PN.

Renal Disease

Renal calculi are common in patients with short bowel syndrome whether or not they are receiving PN.[40] Some groups have shown declines in renal function in children and adults receiving PN and suggest that this could be attributable to chronic dehydration in the majority of these patients.[40] Thus, frequent monitoring of laboratory tests and hydration status is an essential component of PN monitoring.

Long-Term Management

Home PN

Any child on stable PN in the hospital who is expected to continue on long-term PN should be considered for discharge. Children discharged home receiving PN should have a stable tunneled central venous line or PICC line. They should be on a stable PN prescription that should not require changes more often than weekly. The parents should undergo education about all aspects of the child's care and demonstrate competence before discharge. The discharging team should liaise with the home care agency and home PN pharmacy to ensure a seamless transition. Nurses should visit the home initially to ensure that parents are able to complete the PN cares safely, provide central line care, draw blood for PN laboratory tests, and to monitor the patient's weight. The frequency of nursing visits typically decreases over time as the patient becomes more stable and parents are more comfortable with cares.

In general, children receiving PN at home receive a 3-in-1 PN solution that is cycled to allow time off PN. While receiving PN at home, the child is monitored by the hospital PN team on a regular schedule, the frequency of which also decreases over time. Similarly, laboratory monitoring protocols should be in place to ensure that the child does not develop deficiencies or toxicities.

Cycling PN

Cyclic PN (or providing PN for only some part of the day with a rest period before starting PN again) is a strategy used for both in the prophylaxis and treatment of IFALD.[41] It also allows the child to be disconnected from the PN solution and tubing for a period of time each day. It is thought that the intermittent supply of nutrients (particularly glucose) allows more efficient substrate utilization with the rest period allowing metabolic unloading of the liver.[42] Cycling of PN is appropriate for children who will be on long-term PN (>1 month). The child must be able to tolerate shifts in glucose and fluid provision. In general, children need to be at least 2.5 kg in body weight and clinically stable and have stable endocrine, renal, hepatic, and cardiac function. Serum electrolytes and glucose should have been stable for 2 to 3 days before attempting cycling.[41] In general, continuous PN is gradually reduced in 2-hour increments. In infants, there may be a need to ramp up and ramp down PN during cycling (ie, provide PN at half the hourly rate for 30 minutes at the start and prior to the discontinuation of PN). Serum or urine glucose should be monitored during (to ensure that the child does not have hyperglycemia), and serum glucose should be monitored immediately after discontinuation of the infusion (to ensure that the child does not have hypoglycemia).

Enteral Feeding

Most children who are receiving PN at home can tolerate some enteral nutrition, and the majority of children with short bowel syndrome can expect to wean completely off PN. Every child who can tolerate enteral nutrition should be provided enteral nutrition to promote intestinal adaptation, minimize translocation of bacteria, and protect the liver.

Enteral nutrition is usually administered as a continuous infusion, gradually advancing the rate based on feeding tolerance, as evidenced by emesis and stool output. With increasing tolerance of enteral nutrition, PN can be weaned.

Other Considerations

The PN prescription is a complex one and, thus, is best managed by a nutrition support team. There is strong literature support for a multidisciplinary PN support team to aid in patient selection, assessment, and ongoing monitoring.[43] Interdisciplinary nutrition support teams consist of a physician, dietitian, pharmacist, and nurse.

Over the past several years, shortages of various components of the PN prescription have occurred. All PN products except dextrose and water have been in short supply at some point since 2010. Shortages further complicate the management of patients on PN, particularly long-term patients, with the youngest patients and patients who are fed solely parenterally being at the highest risk. PN shortages tend to be a dynamic issue with different components being short at various times. Shortages of PN components requires vigilance and a team approach to be able to meet the nutrient needs of patients requiring PN.

Approaches to interrupting PN therapy during drug administration differs from institution to institution and should be carefully discussed with pharmacy staff and the institution's parenteral nutrition committee. Acyclovir, amphotericin B, metronidazole, and trimethoprim-sulfamethoxazole are just a few of the drugs that are incompatible with PN solutions. Drugs may be given in the central catheter with 10% dextrose with the PN turned off. Bicarbonate also should not be given with the PN solution. Although ranitidine is compatible with PN solutions, no studies in infants and children have demonstrated that this is of any benefit. On the contrary, the association of the use of ranitidine and the increased risk of sepsis and necrotizing enterocolitis in neonates should be considered before any decision to use ranitidine is made.[44] Information about the compatibility of individual drugs with PN is available through the pharmacies of all major hospitals.

References

1. Worthington P, Balint J, Bechtold M, et al. When Is Parenteral Nutrition Appropriate? *JPEN J Parenter Enteral Nutr.* 2017;41(3):324–377

2. Hernandez CR, Ponce EC, Busquets FB, et al. Hypersensitivity reaction to components of parenteral nutrition in pediatrics. *Nutrition.* Nov-Dec 2016; 32(11–12):1303–1305

3. Boullata JI, Gilbert K, Sacks G, et al. A.S.P.E.N. clinical guidelines: parenteral nutrition ordering, order review, compounding, labeling, and dispensing. *JPEN J Parenter Enteral Nutr.* 2014;38(3):334–377

4. Dugan S, Le J, Jew RK. Maximum tolerated osmolarity for peripheral administration of parenteral nutrition in pediatric patients. *JPEN J Parenter Enteral Nutr.* 2014;38(7):847–851

5. Kaur S, Goraya JS, Thami GP, Kanwar AJ. Pellagrous dermatitis induced by phenytoin. *Pediatr Dermatol.* 2002;19(1):93

6. Holliday MA, Segar WE. The maintenance need for water in parenteral fluid therapy. *Pediatrics.* 1957;19(5):823–832

7. *How to Prescribe Parenteral Nutrition Therapy.* 2 ed. Silver Spring, MD: A.S.P.E.N.; 2014

8. Mirtallo J, Canada T, Johnson D, et al. Safe practices for parenteral nutrition. *JPEN J Parenter Enteral Nutr.* 2004;28(6):S39–70

9. Deitch EA, Ma WJ, Ma L, Berg RD, Specian RD. Protein malnutrition predisposes to inflammatory-induced gut-origin septic states. *Ann Surg.* 1990;211(5):560–567

10. Goulet OJ. Intestinal failure-associated liver disease and the use of fish oil-based lipid emulsions. *World Rev Nutr Diet.* 2015;112:90–114

11. Diamond IR, Grant RC, Pencharz PB, et al. Preventing the Progression of Intestinal Failure-Associated Liver Disease in Infants Using a Composite Lipid Emulsion. *JPEN J Parenter Enteral Nutr.* 2017;41(5):866–877

12. Venick RS, Calkins K. The impact of intravenous fish oil emulsions on pediatric intestinal failure-associated liver disease. *Curr Opin Organ Transplant.* 2011;16(3):306–311

13. Rollins CJ, Elsberry VA, Pollack KA, Pollack PF, Udall JN, Jr. Three-in-one parenteral nutrition: a safe and economical method of nutritional support for infants. *JPEN J Parenter Enteral Nutr.* 1990;14(3):290–294

14. Driscoll DF, Bhargava HN, Li L, Zaim RH, Babayan VK, Bistrian BR. Physicochemical stability of total nutrient admixtures. *Am J Health Syst Pharm.* 1995;52(6):623–634

15. Leung FY. Trace elements in parenteral micronutrition. *Clin Biochem.* 1995;28(6):561–566

16. Livingstone C. Zinc: physiology, deficiency, and parenteral nutrition. *Nutr Clin Pract.* Jun 2015;30(3):371–382

17. Corkins MR, Martin VA, Szeszycki EE. Copper levels in cholestatic infants on parenteral nutrition. *JPEN J Parenter Enteral Nutr.* 2013;37(1):92–96

18. Abdalian R, Fernandes G, Duerksen D, et al. Prescription of trace elements in adults on home parenteral nutrition: current practice based on the Canadian Home Parenteral Nutrition Registry. *JPEN J Parenter Enteral Nutr.* 2013;37(3): 410–415

19. Shenkin A. Selenium in intravenous nutrition. *Gastroenterology.* 2009;137 (5 Suppl):S61–69

20. Moukarzel AA, Buchman AL, Salas JS, et al. Iodine supplementation in children receiving long-term parenteral nutrition. *J Pediatr.* Aug 1992;121(2):252–254

21. Cairns PA, Stalker DJ. Carnitine supplementation of parenterally fed neonates. *Cochrane Database Syst Rev.* 2000(4):CD000950

22. Muir JM, Andrew M, Hirsh J, et al. Histomorphometric analysis of the effects of standard heparin on trabecular bone in vivo. *Blood.* 1996;88(4):1314–1320

V

23. Berkow SE, Spear ML, Stahl GE, et al. Total parenteral nutrition with intralipid in premature infants receiving TPN with heparin: effect on plasma lipolytic enzymes, lipids, and glucose. *J Pediatr Gastroenterol Nutr.* 1987;6(4):581–588

24. Peterson J, Bihain BE, Bengtsson-Olivecrona G, Deckelbaum RJ, Carpentier YA, Olivecrona T. Fatty acid control of lipoprotein lipase: a link between energy metabolism and lipid transport. *Proc Natl Acad Sci.* 1990;87(3):909–913

25. Spear ML, Stahl GE, Paul MH, Egler JM, Pereira GR, Polin RA. The effect of 15-hour fat infusions of varying dosage on bilirubin binding to albumin. *JPEN J Parenter Enteral Nutr.* 1985;9(2):144–147

26. Ubesie AC, Kocoshis SA, Mezoff AG, Henderson CJ, Helmrath MA, Cole CR. Multiple micronutrient deficiencies among patients with intestinal failure during and after transition to enteral nutrition. *J Pediatr.* 2013;163(6):1692–1696

27. Yang CF, Duro D, Zurakowski D, Lee M, Jaksic T, Duggan C. High prevalence of multiple micronutrient deficiencies in children with intestinal failure: a longitudinal study. *J Pediatr.* 2011;159(1):39–44 e31

28. Smith A, Feuling MB, Larson-Nath C, et al. Laboratory Monitoring of Children on Home Parenteral Nutrition. *JPEN J Parenter Enteral Nutr.* 2016: 0148607116673184

29. Centers for Disease Control and Prevention. Guidelines for the Prevention of Intravascular Catheter-Related Infections. 2011; https://www.cdc.gov/infectioncontrol/guidelines/bsi/index.html. Accessed July 17, 2017

30. Cole CR, Frem JC, Schmotzer B, et al. The rate of bloodstream infection is high in infants with short bowel syndrome: relationship with small bowel bacterial overgrowth, enteral feeding, and inflammatory and immune responses. *J Pediatr.* 2010;156(6):941–947, 947 e941

31. Ralls MW, Blackwood RA, Arnold MA, Partipilo ML, Dimond J, Teitelbaum DH. Drug shortage-associated increase in catheter-related blood stream infection in children. *Pediatrics.* Nov 2012;130(5):e1369–1373

32. Oliveira C, Nasr A, Brindle M, Wales PW. Ethanol locks to prevent catheter-related bloodstream infections in parenteral nutrition: a meta-analysis. *Pediatrics.* Feb 2012;129(2):318–329

33. Wales PW, Allen N, Worthington P, et al. A.S.P.E.N. clinical guidelines: support of pediatric patients with intestinal failure at risk of parenteral nutrition-associated liver disease. *JPEN J Parenter Enteral Nutr.* 2014;38(5):538–557

34. Fuhrman MP. Complication management in parenteral nutrition In: Matarese LE, Gottschlich MM, eds. *Contemporary Nutrition Support Practice.* St Louis, MO: WB Saunders; 2003:242–262

35. Haire WD, Herbst SL. Invited Review: Use of Alteplase (t-PA) for the Management of Thrombotic Catheter Dysfunction: Guidelines From a Consensus Conference of the National Association of Vascular Access Networks (NAVAN). *Nutr Clin Pract.* 2000;15(6):265–275

36. Lauriti G, Zani A, Aufieri R, et al. Incidence, prevention, and treatment of parenteral nutrition-associated cholestasis and intestinal failure-associated liver disease in infants and children: a systematic review. *JPEN J Parenter Enteral Nutr.* 2014;38(1):70–85

37. Diamond IR, Pencharz PB, Feldman BM, Ling SC, Moore AM, Wales PW. Novel lipid-based approaches to pediatric intestinal failure-associated liver disease. *Arch Pediatr Adolesc Med.* 2012;166(5):473–478

38. Diamanti A, Bizzarri C, Basso MS, et al. How does long-term parenteral nutrition impact the bone mineral status of children with intestinal failure? *J Bone Miner Metab.* 2010;28(3):351–358

39. Pichler J, Chomtho S, Fewtrell M, Macdonald S, Hill SM. Growth and bone health in pediatric intestinal failure patients receiving long-term parenteral nutrition. *Am J Clin Nutr.* 2013;97(6):1260–1269

40. Dudley J, Rogers R, Sealy L. Renal consequences of parenteral nutrition. *Pediatr Nephrol.* 2014;29(3):375–385

41. Nghiem-Rao TH, Cassidy LD, Polzin EM, Calkins CM, Arca MJ, Goday PS. Risks and benefits of prophylactic cyclic parenteral nutrition in surgical neonates. *Nutr Clin Pract.* 2013;28(6):745–752

42. Collier S, Crough J, Hendricks K, Caballero B. Use of cyclic parenteral nutrition in infants less than 6 months of age. *Nutr Clin Pract.* 1994;9(2):65–68

43. Force APMT, Delegge M, Wooley JA, et al. The state of nutrition support teams and update on current models for providing nutrition support therapy to patients. *Nutr Clin Pract.* 2010;25(1):76–84

44. Terrin G, Passariello A, De Curtis M, et al. Ranitidine is associated with infectious necrotizing enterocolitis, and fatal outcome in newborns. *Pediatrics.* 2012;129(1):e40–e50

V

Chapter 23

Enteral Feeding for Nutritional Support

Introduction

Pediatric patients who do not have adequate growth with oral intake may be supported by enteral nutrition for nutritional management depending on gastrointestinal digestive and absorptive capacity. Commonly used enteral tube feeding routes for nutritional support include nasogastric, gastrostomy, nasojejunal, gastrojejunal, and jejunostomy. Although both enteral and parenteral routes can be used to provide nutritional support to pediatric patients, enteral nutrition is preferred, because it is more "physiologic," less expensive, and easier to administer. Enteral nutrition produces fewer metabolic and infectious complications and better supports the integrity of the barrier function of the gastrointestinal tract. Enteral nutrition also allows for better physiologic control of electrolyte levels and serves as prophylaxis against stress-induced gastropathy and gastrointestinal (GI) tract hemorrhage. Enteral nutrition also can provide a more complete range of nutrients and other factors that potentially may be beneficial in certain clinical settings, including glutamine, long-chain polyunsaturated fatty acids, short-chain fatty acids, fiber, prebiotics, and probiotics. Finally, enteral nutrition provides a trophic effect on the gut by promoting pancreatic and biliary secretions as well as endocrine, paracrine, and neural factors that enhance the function and immunologic integrity of the intestine. Timely initiation of enteral nutrition also is important, with the greatest clinical benefits likely resulting from initiating early enteral nutrition within less than 72 hours of injury or admission. Within the setting of critical illness, however, enteral nutrition should not be initiated until the child achieves hemodynamic stability, thus minimizing the risk of bowel ischemia.[1]

Indications for Enteral Tube Feedings: Management of Nutrition-Related Disorders (Table 23.1)

Prematurity

A feeding method for preterm infants should be individualized on the basis of gestational age, birth weight, and medical status. Preterm infants present a unique nutritional challenge because of their GI tract immaturity, limited fluid tolerance, high nutrient requirements on a per-weight basis, immature renal function, and predisposition to specific metabolic and clinical complications, such as hyper- and hypoglycemia, bronchopulmonary dysplasia, necrotizing enterocolitis, and metabolic bone disease.

Table 23.1.
Conditions in Which Enteral Tube Feeding May Be Warranted[a]

Prematurity
Cardiorespiratory illness
Chronic lung disease
Cystic fibrosis
Congenital heart disease
Gastrointestinal tract disease and dysfunction
Inflammatory bowel disease
Short bowel syndrome
Biliary atresia
Gastroesophageal reflux disease
Protracted diarrhea of infancy
Chronic nonspecific diarrhea
Renal disease
Hypermetabolic states
Burn injury
Severe trauma or closed head injury
Cancer
Neurologic disease or cerebral palsy
Oral motor dysfunction
Inadequate spontaneous oral intake

[a] Modified from: Abad-Sinden, A, Sutphen J. Enteral nutrition. In: Walker WA, Goulet O, Kleinman RE, et al, eds. *Pediatric Gastrointestinal Disease: Pathophysiology, Diagnosis, Management.* 4th ed. Burlington, Ontario: BC Decker Inc; 2004:1981-1994

Because the coordination of sucking and swallowing appears at approximately 34 weeks of gestation, oro- or nasogastric feedings are routinely used before this time. These techniques may be useful beyond 34 weeks' gestation in selected infants who are unable to achieve and/or tolerate adequate oral feedings. Studies in preterm infants have suggested that minimal or trophic enteral feedings (2–8 mL/kg per day) administered soon after birth promote a gastrointestinal hormone response that mediates intestinal adaptation, promotes growth, and decreases hospital stay[2]; however, recent systematic reviews have concluded from the present evidence that early trophic feedings in preterm infants have little impact on feeding tolerance, growth, development, or length of hospital stay compared with enteral fasting during the first or second week of life.[3] Others have associated delayed onset and slower progression of enteral feedings with increased risk for necrotizing enterocolitis,[4] but this remains an area of controversy.[3] For further information, see Chapter 5: Nutritional Needs of the Preterm Infant.

Cardiorespiratory Illness

Infants with congenital heart disease (CHD) (see also Chapter 44: Cardiac Disease) are at significant nutritional risk. Growth failure resulting from inadequate intake and elevated energy expenditure may be caused by respiratory distress, increased metabolic needs, tissue hypoxia, impaired absorption, and protein-losing enteropathy. Because of their elevated nutritional needs and limited fluid tolerance, these infants often require high-energy–density formulas (Appendix C). Increased energy density formulas up to 30 kcal/oz have been used in these infants. Concentration of formula by increasing the formula-to-water ratio increases the renal solute load and may not allow enough free water for excretion of the renal solute load by immature kidneys. Additional energy may be provided through modular carbohydrate and/or fat supplementation. Consultation with a registered dietitian will guide customization of this recipe to safely meet an individual infant's needs. Infants with CHD often experience delayed gastric emptying, resulting in early satiety and/or gastroesophageal reflux disease (GERD).[5] Continuous nocturnal nasogastric feedings or 24-hour enteral feedings of infants, particularly those with acyanotic CHD, may result in significant catch-up growth.[6] Alternatively, providing intermittent oral feedings with nasogastric supplementation of the remainder of the required volume also may facilitate achievement of the nutritional goals.[7]

Infants and children with pulmonary disease often require enteral nutrition support during acute exacerbations of their primary lung disease as well as for nutritional rehabilitation of chronic secondary malnutrition. Growth failure in patients with neonatal chronic lung disease can be caused by hypoxia, hypercapnia, elevated metabolic rates, inefficient suck and swallow mechanisms, poor appetite, decreased intake, and recurrent emesis with decreased gastric motility. Children with cystic fibrosis (CF) (see also Chapter 46: Nutrition in Cystic Fibrosis) have increased energy needs and poor intake resulting from their lung disease, malabsorption, and chronic infection.[8] Nocturnal nasogastric feedings using elemental or polymeric nutrient formulas supplemented with pancreatic enzymes are used in children and adolescents with CF in whom conservative nutritional supplement measures have failed. Short-term nasogastric feedings have resulted in increased energy intake and significant weight gain for patients with CF, but long-term effectiveness may be limited by noncompliance. Gastrostomy feedings are more appropriate when long-term (beyond 3 months) infusions are required.[9]

Gastrointestinal Disease and Dysfunction

Pediatric patients with acute and chronic gastrointestinal tract disease and dysfunction often benefit from enteral feeding regimens (see Chapter 42: Nutritional Aspects of Chronic Autoimmune Inflammatory Bowel Diseases in Children). Growth failure in children with Crohn disease is causally related to inadequate nutrient intake, the increased energy requirements associated with chronic inflammation, and malabsorption. In addition to higher oral energy intake, the use of elemental and semi-elemental diets administered orally and/or nasogastrically may produce a significant improvement in nutritional status. Clinical remission of Crohn disease of the small bowel with the use of enteral nutrition has been reported and may be as effective as the use of corticosteroids, with the additional benefit of improved linear growth.[10]

The nutritional management of short bowel syndrome is particularly challenging and usually involves the artful implementation of both enteral and parenteral nutrition (see also Chapter 45: Nutrition in Children With Short Bowel Syndrome). Total parenteral nutrition often is used initially. As soon as possible after recovery from surgery, enteral feedings should begin at a slow, continuous rate and advanced as tolerated. The period of transition to complete enteral feedings may take weeks to years, depending on the length and function of the residual intestine. If the ileocecal valve is preserved, the outcome may be improved, but overall length and function of the remaining intestine are the most important determinants of intestinal adaptation. In the early stages of enteral nutrition support, and particularly in cases in which the formula is delivered directly into the small bowel distal to the ligament of Treitz, elemental or semi-elemental formulas are preferred to polymeric formulas.[11] Long-term parenteral nutrition for infants with short bowel syndrome can lead to parenteral nutrition-associated liver disease (PNALD), which is a significant cause of morbidity and mortality in infants and children with short bowel syndrome (see also Chapter 43: Liver Disease). Sepsis, small intestinal bacterial overgrowth, and absence of enteral intake are factors that increase the probability of PNALD. Enteral nutrition helps prevent and/or ameliorate hepatic disease in this situation. Cyclic (10 to 12 hours) customized parenteral nutrition with lipid minimization[12] plus continuous and/or intermittent enteral feedings and oral intake as tolerated, as well as the early identification and treatment of catheter-related infections, usually are the most successful strategies to avoid PNALD.[13] Eventual weaning of parenteral nutrition to full enteral nutrition is the major goal and often will allow for recovery of PNALD if the clinical course has not regressed to end-stage liver disease.[13]

When children with short bowel syndrome are fed enterally, they inevitably will have some degree of diarrhea. In general, diarrhea should be tolerated as long as there is adequate weight gain, appropriate electrolyte and fluid balance, and the absence of perineal complications from skin contact with fecal fluid.[14] Extra sodium should be provided if the serum sodium concentration is low. Measurement of urinary sodium excretion also may be useful in assessing body sodium status. Prevention and careful management of perineal skin breakdown and infection is important. In infants it is useful to monitor the number of diapers that have urine alone without fecal material as a measure of the adequacy of fluid balance. As the concentration or volume of formula is advanced, the maximum absorptive capability of the remaining intestine will be exceeded and typically an abrupt increase in stool output will occur, or the maximum rate of gastric emptying will be exceeded and emesis will occur. At this point, the feedings should be decreased and a variable amount of time should be allowed for the intestine to adapt to the increased intake. Judicious, often empirical, treatment of bacterial overgrowth with periodic antibiotics may facilitate the advancement of enteral feeding volumes.

Continuous feedings may provide the best nutrient absorption when the intestinal length is shortened, but it is important to allow a break of a few hours in both enteral and parenteral feedings each day. During this time, oral intake, especially in infants, should be encouraged to promote the development or maintenance of oral motor function (see Chapter 45: Nutrition in Children With Short Bowel Syndrome).

Several other illnesses affecting GI tract function and nutritional status usually can be managed successfully with enteral tube feedings. For selected infants and children who undergo surgery for whatever cause and who encounter difficulty feeding in the perioperative period, enteral nutrition can be a valuable adjunct to support nutritional needs and enhance recovery. Infants with biliary atresia frequently experience reduced intake associated with hepatic disease and infection. Nutritional support with nasogastric tube feedings using a semi-elemental or elemental formula rich in medium-chain triglycerides can promote energy and nitrogen balance in preparation for and after hepatic transplantation. Once the clinical condition of the infant or child is stable after transplantation, transition to a polymeric formula or an oral diet should be made. Infants with GERD and poor weight gain may benefit from continuous nasogastric tube feedings with improved weight gain, reduction or cessation of vomiting, and catch-up growth.[15] However, one should be cautious in attributing poor weight gain to GERD alone, and other underlying diseases, such as CF, should be ruled out with appropriate tests before embarking on aggressive enteral feeding regimens. Children with chronic nonspecific or protracted diarrhea and malnutrition also may benefit from continuous enteral tube feedings.

Renal Disease

Chronic renal failure in infants and children commonly results in growth failure and developmental delay, particularly in patients with congenital renal disease early in life.[16] The cause of growth failure is thought to be related to protein-energy malnutrition, renal osteodystrophy, chronic metabolic acidosis, and endocrine dysfunction. Despite aggressive medical management and specialized high–energy-density formulas, inadequate weight gain often persists. Early nutritional intervention can augment the effect of dialysis by improving anabolism and reducing nitrogen losses (see Chapter 40: Nutrition in Renal Disease).

Critical Illness and Hypermetabolic States

Patients with extensive trauma, head or spinal cord injury, burn injury, and hypermetabolic states, such as cancer, HIV infection, or sickle cell anemia (see Chapter 39: Nutrition for Children With Sickle Cell Disease and Thalassemia) often require specialized nutritional support. Children with advanced cancer (see Chapter 41: Nutritional Management of Children With Cancer) who are at high nutritional risk and who have minimal GI tract symptoms may be fed enterally via nocturnal or 24-hour nasogastric or gastrostomy tube feedings, depending on the extent of oral intake.[17] Enteral nutrition support is the preferred method for the nutritional support of children with uncomplicated trauma, such as severe head and spinal cord injuries, who have a significant elevation in their basal metabolic rates in the initial days following injury.[18] Enteral nutrition can be used to support infants and children with critical illness to meet their initial energy and protein needs. Careful consideration of nutrient needs in these patients will avoid the adverse consequences of overfeeding energy, including hyper-capnia, difficulty weaning from the ventilator, hepatotoxicity, hyperglyce-mia, and increased infection rates[18] (see Chapter 37: Nutrition of Children Who Are Critically Ill). Metabolic effects associated with burn wounds leading to malnutrition include an accelerated rate of energy expenditure, increased urine and wound nitrogen losses, and abnormal protein and glucose metabolism. Pediatric patients with burns greater than 20% total body surface area often are provided nutritional support using continuous enteral feedings.[19]

Neurologic Disease or Impairment

The specific nutritional requirements and feeding approach for neurologically impaired children are highly variable and depend on the degree of impairment, oral motor function, mobility, muscle control, and level of physical activity.[20] Children and infants with neurologic impairment, including Down syndrome, Prader-Willi syndrome, or myelomeningocele, may have decreased growth rates and motor activity compared with healthy children and, therefore, have lower energy needs.[21] Children with cerebral palsy generally are underweight for height and may have increased energy needs, particularly if they have spasticity, severe contractures, or choreoathetoid movements. Energy requirements of children with devastating neurologic disease may be less than those predicted based on standard methods of estimating energy requirements. Excessive energy intake may place the child at risk for aspiration. Obesity may compromise neuromuscular and respiratory function. The concerns of primary caregivers about lifting heavy children also must be considered. A children's multivitamin and mineral supplement, as well as additional protein, calcium, sodium, and iron supplements, may be needed for children with special needs with restricted volume intake to ensure that their protein, vitamin, and mineral requirements are being met.

Finally, one must remember to provide adequate water for children with neuromuscular disease. These children may not be able to communicate thirst to the caregiver. In an attempt to decrease the risk of aspiration or improve nutritional status, concentrated formulas often are used with a resultant decrease in water intake. Fluid balance is important in the pediatric patient who is fed by tube because several metabolic complications can be related to inadequate fluid intake. Fluid requirements can be estimated by calculating normal water requirements and adjusting for specific disease-related factors. Measurement of urine output, urine specific gravity and serum chemistries (electrolytes, BUN) may be useful to determine if fluid intake should be modified. Special consideration must be given to monitoring the fluid balance of children receiving high-energy, high-protein formulas and children with excess water loss resulting from emesis, diarrhea, fever, or polyuria[22] (see Chapter 36: Nutritional Support for Children With Developmental Disabilities).

V

Enteral Formula Selection for Children
1 to 13 Years of Age

When children are older, they often are more capable of expressing their own preferences for favorite foods. Few children will spontaneously decide that they prefer nutritional supplements to other favorite foods that they see other children eating and/or see advertised in the media. Before parents embark on a control struggle to force or tube feed a high-energy supplement to a thin child who does not want to eat, it is useful to first try commonly available high-energy foods that are appetizing. If these foods lead to adequate weight gain, they can be helpful. After the nutritional status improves, less energy-dense, "healthier" dietary options may be provided.

If it is not possible for a child to gain weight on his or her favorite energy-dense foods, enteral feedings should be started in a timely manner, optimally within the first 48 to 72 hours after injury or hospitalization, depending on the child's clinical status.[16] Foods should be offered first by mouth, preferably by a trusted caregiver. If the child refuses them, enteral tube feedings can be used. Formula selections for children younger than 1 year are discussed in Chapter 4: Formula Feeding of Term Infants. A variety of pediatric formulas are available. However, the composition of the formula may differ between retail and institution sources. Pediatric formulas can provide the recommended intakes of energy, protein, and micronutrients for most children 1 to 13 years of age (see Appendix M-1). Formulas with an energy density of approximately 1 kcal/mL are commonly used in children. Formulas with higher energy density (eg, 1.5 kcal/mL) are useful for children with increased metabolic needs or for those with fluid restrictions. Pediatric formulas with lower energy density (eg, 0.6–0.7 kcal/mL) are useful for children with reduced energy needs. The vitamin and mineral concentrations in 1000 to 1200 mL of most pediatric formulas meet or exceed 100% of the Recommended Dietary Allowances (RDAs) for children in this age range. "Predigested" or elemental formulas are only necessary when there is a cow milk or soy protein allergy or a deficiency in the digestive and/or absorptive process. Elemental formulas do not confer any advantage for the child with normal digestive function who does not have a milk or soy protein allergy. In the past, adult formulas were used for the nutritional support of children older than 1 year, because pediatric formulas were not available. The primary disadvantages of using adult formulas for young children are the elevated renal solute load and insufficient vitamin and mineral levels. In situations in which higher protein, mineral, or vitamin intakes are required, the addition of individual nutrient supplements may be warranted.

Enteral Formulas for Use in Children Older Than 13 Years: Standard Tube-Feeding Formulas

Standard adult tube-feeding formulas are available for children older than 13 years (Appendix M-1). These formulas, most of which are lactose free and low residue, vary in osmolality from 300 to 650 mOsm/kg and in energy density from 1.0 to 2.0 kcal/mL. Isotonic formulas that contain medium-chain triglyceride oil may be useful where there is a history of delayed gastric emptying, dumping syndrome, or osmotic diarrhea. Tube-feeding formulas with added fiber may be useful in the management of patients with chronic constipation and diarrhea. Although high-energy, high-nitrogen, hypertonic formulations are well tolerated by adults with elevated metabolic needs, they usually are not tolerated by children and may lead to diarrhea, emesis, abdominal distention, and delayed gastric empty-ing. Children and adolescents with markedly elevated energy and protein requirements attributable to severe malnutrition, trauma, or burn injury are best managed with high-energy density pediatric formulations (1.5 kcal/mL). Because of the elevated protein levels in these formulas, however, hydration status must be closely monitored. In this situation, fluid, protein, sodium, potassium, calcium, iron, and vitamin D needs should be estimated individually to meet nutrient needs. Judicious selection of laboratory tests can be used to monitor the adequacy of individual dietary nutrient intakes.

Peptide-Based and Elemental Formulas

Peptide-based (hydrolysate) and elemental formulas with predigested nutrients can be used for the nutritional support of pediatric patients with short bowel syndrome, inflammatory bowel disease, and/or food protein allergy/sensitivity (Appendix M). Peptide-based formulas may be used in the nutritional support of patients with cystic fibrosis, although the use of intact protein formulas with appropriate pancreatic enzyme administra-tion may be just as effective. Amino acid-based formulas may offer further protection from feeding intolerance over protein hydrolysate formulas in some children. However, there is a significant increase in cost to purchase amino acid-based formulas. Immunonutrition, the use of enteral formula supplemented with possible immune-modulating nutrients, such as glutamine, arginine, antioxidants, and omega-3 fatty acids, has been considered for use in critically ill pediatric patients. Data are limited on safety and efficacy, and there are no guidelines or standardized critical care formulas for pediatric patients[23,24] (see Chapter 37: Nutrition of Children Who Are Critically Ill).

Oral Supplements

Various flavored polymeric formulas may be used as oral supplements for pediatric patients. As noted previously, high-energy commercially available foods may be more palatable and affordable than specialized supplements for most children. The constant supervision required to enforce frequent intake of commercial supplements can be a source of considerable family conflict. Oral supplements mixed with milk, such as Carnation Breakfast Essentials (Nestlé Nutrition), may be better accepted by some children than are the lactose-free commercial supplements. Tips for increasing the nutrient and caloric density of foods are provided in Tables 23.2 and 23.3. Flavored polymeric formulas that contain intact proteins, long-chain fatty acids, and simple carbohydrates are usually marketed as oral supplements because of their palatability. These products, which have osmolalities ranging from 450 to 600 mOsm/kg, often are not sufficiently palatable for

Table 23.2.
Increasing the Nutrient Density of Foods

Use cream, whole milk, or evaporated whole milk instead of water for baking whenever possible.
Use liberal portions of butter, margarine, oil, and cheeses on vegetables, on breads, and in soups and hot cereals. Add sauces and gravies to foods.
Add sugar, jelly, or honey to toast and cereals. Use fruits canned in heavy syrup, or sweeten fresh fruits with added sugar.
Add skim milk powder or instant breakfast powder to regular whole milk for use as a beverage or for cooking. Add powdered milk to puddings, potatoes, soups, and cooked cereals.
Use thinly spread peanut butter or cheese on fruit or crackers. Make finger sandwiches with mayonnaise and avocado for meals or snacks.
Provide a variety of high-calorie salad dressings for addition to vegetables or other foods to increase caloric density.
Emphasize variety with all high-calorie foods to decrease flavor fatigue and increase exploratory behavior with foods.

Table 23.3.
Energy and Protein Content of Selected Energy-Dense Foods[a]

	Energy, kcal	Protein, g
Instant breakfast powder (1 packet)	130	5
Mixed with 1 cup whole milk	276	13
Powdered milk (1 tbsp)	25	3
Evaporated milk (1 tbsp)	20	1
Cheese (1 oz)	100	7
Peanut butter (1 tbsp)	95	4
Butter or margarine (1 tsp)	45	0[b]
Avocado (100 g)	160	2

[a] See also Appendix O.

[b] Not "spreads," which have a lot of air and water added and, therefore, are lower in kcal.

long-term voluntary supplementation for children. Examples of polymeric oral supplements are included in Appendix M-1. It is useful to remember that salt is an appetite stimulant and that the combination of salty foods with sugary fluids to slake the resultant thirst can stimulate oral intake and initiate insulin surges that may be useful to further increase appetite.

Blenderized Formulas

Commercially available "blenderized" formulas (such as Compleat Pediatric, Appendix M-1) may contain variable amounts of meats, fish, eggs, milk, cereal, fruits, vegetables, and vegetable oils, depending on the specific product. These formulas, which contain a moderate to high level of residue, have osmolalities usually ranging from 300 to 500 mOsm/kg. Blenderized feedings are beneficial for chronically ill patients who have normal digestive function and require long-term enteral nutrition; however, they may not be well tolerated by the malnourished pediatric patient with compromised gastrointestinal tract function. Newer, "more natural" food products may be deficient in one or more nutrients and should be administered with appropriate additional table foods and beverages to meet these micronutrient requirements.[25,26] Dietary nutrient intakes should be estimated individually to ensure the adequacy of dietary intake. Often, the "natural food" formulas are expensive, and their high viscosity may cause obstruction of pediatric enteral feeding tubes.

Blenderized feedings can be prepared at home from milk, juices, cereals, and baby food. Parents of neurologically impaired children who require long-term feeding through a gastrostomy tube are often interested in learning how to prepare blenderized feedings at home because of the economic and psychosocial advantages.[27,28] The help of a registered dietitian is important to ensure that adequate free water, macronutrient, and micronutrient concentrations are provided with these mixtures.

Formula Concentration and Supplementation With Use of Modular Components

Because of the unique and often elevated or reduced nutritional requirements of the enterally fed pediatric patient, modification of enteral formulas through either formula concentration, volume reduction, or supplementation with modular components is often necessary. The use of liquid formula concentrates or liquid modular products is usually the preferred modality for increasing formula concentration. Infant formula powder also may be used as a convenient and economical way to increase the caloric density of human milk and infant formulas. However, within the hospital setting, use of liquid formula concentrates and liquid modular components are preferred to minimize the risk of formula contamination (see Appendix M-2). It is important to remember that increasing formula concentration may lead to decreased oral food and beverage intake in patients who are voluntarily drinking the formula and may lead to vomiting if they prolong gastric emptying in patients who are being tube fed. Therefore, fluid and electrolyte balance must be monitored.

Tube Feeding

When the requirement for enteral nutrition support has been established, the optimal route for delivering nutrients must be determined.[29] Many practitioners recommend the placement of nasogastric or nasoduodenal feeding tubes when the estimated course of therapy will not exceed 3 months (a 6 French size tube is usually adequate). These tubes should be changed from one nostril to the other every 1 to 3 weeks to decrease associated sinus and ear disease. During upper respiratory tract infections, extra care should be taken to avoid airway compromise. Tube placement should be verified after episodes of emesis before restarting feedings.[30] If the risk of aspiration is low, gastric feedings are preferable, because they are more physiologic and easier to manage. Tubes made of polyurethane and silicone rubber are soft and pliable and may be left in place for longer time periods. Polyvinyl chloride tubes become stiff and nonpliable when left in place for more than a few days; however, they are useful for intestinal decompression or short-term feeding. They should be changed every 2 to 3 days to avoid skin necrosis or intestinal perforation.

Some feeding tubes made of polyurethane or silicone rubber have a tungsten or mercury weight at the tip that makes them useful for duodenal or jejunal feedings. Placement of transpyloric tubes can be greatly facilitated by the use of an intravenous prokinetic drug, such as metoclopramide. Children who require long-term tube feeding for longer than 3 months are potential candidates for placement of a gastrostomy tube. Despite the benefits and widespread use of gastrostomy tube feedings, some patients experience complications.[31,32] GERD, which may occur in neurologically disabled children or healthy infants after gastrostomy tube placement, may necessitate an operative antireflux procedure (eg, Nissen fundoplication).[33] Although the procedure is effective in reducing GERD, postoperative complications can be troublesome when high-volume, rapid-rate bolus feedings are provided too soon after surgery. Intractable retching episodes, dumping syndrome, continued problems with swallowing, impaired esophageal emptying, slow feeding, and gas bloating have all been reported with inappropriate feeding regimens. Controversy exists over the necessity of an antireflux procedure in neurologically impaired children who require a feeding gastrostomy tube.[34] A trial of nasogastric feedings to determine whether they are well tolerated without significant GERD before the placement of the gastrostomy tube can often help the clinician determine the need for a simultaneous fundoplication. During the trial of nasogastric feeding, documented pulmonary disease associated with GERD in the face of maximal medical therapy is an indication for a fundoplication when a subsequent gastrostomy tube placement is performed.

A common problem with gastrostomy tubes is inward migration of the standard gastrostomy tube through the ostomy site. The tip of the catheter may come in contact with the pylorus, where it can induce retching as it passes in and out of the gastric outlet. This problem can be minimized by firmly attaching the tube and placing a mark on the tube to detect inward migration. When a urinary catheter is used as a temporary gastrostomy tube, migration (caused by lack of an effective external bolster) remains a common problem. The low-profile gastrostomy button tube is a feeding device that can be used to form an effective 1-way valve at the gastrostomy site.[35] The button fits flush with the skin and attaches to commercial feeding tubes that lock onto the button in a variety of ways. Gastrostomy buttons generally do not migrate through the pylorus or cause retching and are less prone to accidental removal. Buttons may be placed in standard percutaneous gastrostomies after the site has matured. Newer devices that allow for percutaneous placement of a low-profile gastrostomy button at the time of the initial gastrostomy also are available.

To overcome problems related to gastric emptying and frequent GERD, transpyloric feedings offer potential benefit. Gastrojejunal feeding tubes can be placed through existing gastrostomies. If a modified (eg, urinary catheter) tube is used for gastrojejunal feedings, care must be exercised to be certain that retching or emesis has not moved the tip of the tube into the esophagus. Even commercial gastrojejunal feeding tubes can accidentally migrate retrograde into the esophagus when persistent emesis occurs. Retrograde continuous delivery of formula into the esophagus presents an extreme risk of aspiration. Nasal transpyloric tubes can be used but are relatively easily displaced and are uncomfortable as a long-term approach to enteral nutrition support. Operative direct feeding jejunostomies overcome these difficulties and may be indicated for selected patients. Patients with direct-feeding jejunostomies generally do not tolerate large bolus feedings over short intervals without experiencing dumping syndrome. Button adapters, by virtue of the large internal bolster, often are precluded for direct feeding jejunostomies.

The transition from enteral feeding to full oral feeding can be prolonged.[36] If infants and children are completely deprived of oral feeding during critical maturation phases, feeding refusal and oral aversion often occur when oral feedings are resumed.[37] Reinstituting oral feedings in children who have been fed exclusively by a gastrostomy tube for a long period of time can evoke a resistance response, such as gagging, choking, or vomiting. To preserve oral motor function during prolonged tube feedings, it is important to offer oral intake whenever possible. This approach may require interrupting the infusion to allow a sufficient amount of hunger to develop to facilitate oral intake. Generally, this method may require several hours. Experienced speech pathologists and occupational therapists can help provide oral motor stimulation exercises and feeding therapy for such children. Without frequent oral stimulation, infants can lose the suckle reflex within a few weeks, which severely limits their ability to control oral intake and may compromise language and oral motor development. They also may develop oral defensiveness as a result of prolonged absence of oral stimulation.

Continuous Versus Intermittent Enteral Feeding

Two methods are used for delivery of enteral feedings. Intermittent bolus feedings deliver the formula over a relatively short period of time similar to that for an oral feeding—10 to 20 minutes. This technique is simple, requires minimal supplies, and may facilitate the transition to home care. Generally, bolus feedings are used during the day and are not used at night because of the greater tendency for gastroesophageal reflux with the bolus feed. Gastric distension by bolus feeding can lead to a better gastrocolic reflex and aid the prevention of constipation, which is a frequent problem in tube-fed patients. When intermittent bolus feeding is not tolerated, a continuous infusion using an infusion pump may be effective. To improve patient mobility, a backpack pump may be of considerable benefit. Continuous feeding may be particularly beneficial when used for patients who have impaired absorption. In some situations, a combination of bolus feeding during the day and continuous feeding at night is beneficial.

Final Note of Caution

Specialized formulas are very expensive, and their cost can easily exceed the food budget of an entire family. Many patients have discovered that it is possible to buy large quantities of expensive elemental and other specialized formulas on the Internet from people who have "left-over" quantities that were prescribed for them. Although this can represent an enormous savings, it is important to remember that the bidder is depending on the integrity of the seller for Internet purchases from private individuals. Counterfeit nutritional products sold online pose the same problems that are encountered with counterfeit medications.

References

1. Canete A, Duggan C. Nutritional support of the pediatric intensive care unit patient. *Curr Opin Pediatr.* 1996;8(3):248–255

2. Meetze W, Valentine C, McGuigan JE, Conlon M, Sacks N, Neu J. Gastrointestinal priming prior to full enteral nutrition in very low birth weight infants. *J Pediatr Gastroenterol Nutr.* 1992;15(2):163–170

3. Morgan J, Bombel S, McGuire W. Early trophic feedings versus enteral fasting for very preterm or very low birth weight infants. *Cochrane Database Syst Rev.* 2013;(3):CD000504

4. Rozé JC, Ancel PY, Lepage P, et al. Nutrition EPIPAGE 2 study group and the EPIFLORE Study Group. Nutritional strategies and gut microbiota composition as risk factors for necrotizing enterocolitis in very-preterm infants. *Am J Clin Nutr.* 2017;106(3):821–830

5. Cavell B. Effect of feeding an infant formula with high energy density on gastric emptying in infants with congenital heart disease. *Acta Paediatr Scand.* 1981;70(4):513–516

6. Schwarz SM, Gewitz MH, See CC, et al. Enteral nutrition in infants with congenital heart disease and growth failure. *Pediatrics.* 1990;86(3):368–373

7. Abad-Sinden A, Sutphen A. Growth and nutrition. In: Emmanoullides GC, Riemenschneider TA, Allen HD, Gutgessel HP, eds. *Moss and Adams Heart Diseases in Infants, Children and Adolescents, Including the Fetus and Young Adult.* Philadelphia, PA: Williams & Wilkins; 2001:325–332

8. Schwarzenberg SJ, Hempstead SE, McDonald CM, et al. Enteral tube feeding for individuals with cystic fibrosis: Cystic Fibrosis Foundation evidence-informed guidelines. *J Cyst Fibros.* 2016;15(6):724–735

9. Corkins MR, Balint J, Bobo E, Plogsted S, Yaworski JA, eds. *The A.S.P.E.N. Pediatric Nutrition Support Core Curriculum.* 2nd ed. Gaithersburg, MD: ASPEN Publishers Inc; 2015

10. Critch J, Day A, Otley A, King-Moore C, Teitelbaum JE, H S. NASPGHAN IBD Committee. Use of enteral nutrition for the control of intestinal inflammation in pediatric Crohn disease. *J Pediatr Gastroenterol Nutr.* 2012;54(2):298–305

11. Olieman JF, Penning C, Ijsselstijn H, et al. Enteral nutrition in children with short-bowel syndrome: current evidence and recommendations for the clinician. *J Am Diet Assoc.* 2010;113(3):420–426

12. Cober MP, Teitelbaum DH. Prevention of parenteral nutrition-associated liver disease: lipid minimization. *Curr Opin Organ Transplant.* 2010;15(3):330–333

13. Javid PJ, Collier S, Richardson DeaJPS-. The role of enteral nutrition in the reversal of parenteral nutrition-associated liver dysfunction in infants. *J Pediatr Surg.* 2005;40(6):1015–1018

14. Samela K, Mokha J, Emerick K, Davidovics ZH. Transition to a tube feeding formula with real food ingredients in pediatric patients with intestinal failure. *Nutr Clin Pract.* 2017;32(2):277–281

15. Lightdale JR, Gremse DA, American Academy of Pediatrics, Section on Gastroenterology H, and Nutrition,. Gastroesophageal reflux: Management guidance for the pediatrician. *Pediatrics.* 2013;131(5):e1684–e1695

16. Spinozzi NS. Chronic renal disease. In: Queen Samour P, King Helm K, Lang CE, eds. *Handbook of Pediatric Nutrition.* Gaithersburg, MD: ASPEN Publishers Inc; 1999:385–394

17. Barale KV, Charuhas PM. Oncology and bone marrow transplant. In: Queen Samour P, King Helm K, Lang CE, eds. *Handbook of Pediatric Nutrition.* Gaithersburg, MD: ASPEN Publishers Inc; 1999:465–492

18. Chwals W. Overfeeding the critically ill child: fact or fantasy? *New Horizons.* 1994;2(2):147–155

19. Trocki O, Michelini JA, Robbins ST, Eichelberger MR. Evaluation of early enteral feeding in children less than 3 years old with smaller burns (8-25 percent TBSA). *Burns.* 1995;21(1):17–23

20. Romano C, van Wynckel M, Hulst J, et al. European Society for Paediatric Gastroenterology, Hepatology and Nutrition Guidelines for the evaluation and treatment of gastrointestinal and nutritional complications in children with neurological impairment. *J Pediatr Gastroenterol Nutr.* 2017;65(2):242–264

21. Cloud HH. Developmental disabilities. In: Queen Samour P, King Helm K, Lang CE, eds. *Handbook of Pediatric Nutrition.* Gaithersburg, MD: ASPEN Publishers Inc; 1999:293–314

22. Schwenk WF, Olson D. Pediatrics. In: Gottschlich MM, ed. *The Science and Practice of Nutrition Support: A Case-Based Core Curriculum.* Dubuque, IA: Kendall/Hunt Publishing Co; 2001:347–372

23. Heyland DK, Novak F, Drover JW, Jain M, Su X, Suchner U. Should immunonutrition become routine in critically ill patients? A systematic review of the evidence. *JAMA.* 2001;286(8):944–953

24. Briassoulis G, Filippou O, Hatzi E, Papassotiriou I, Hatzis T. Early enteral administration of immunonutrition in critically ill children: results of a blinded randomized controlled clinical trial. *Nutrition.* 2005;21(7-8):799–807

25. Vieira MM, Santos VF, Bottoni A, Morais TB. Nutritional and microbiological quality of commercial and homemade blenderized whole food enteral diets for home-based enteral nutritional therapy in adults. Published online December 1, 2016. *Clin Nutr.* 2018;37(1):177–181

26. Santos VF, Morais TB. Nutritional quality and osmolality of home-made enteral diets, and follow-up of growth of severely disabled children receiving home enteral nutrition therapy. *J Trop Pediatr.* 2010;56(2):127–128

27. Bobo E. Reemergence of blenderized tube feedings: exploring the evidence. *Nutr Clin Pract.* 2016;31(6):730–735

28. Epp L, Lammert L, Vallumsetla N, Hurt RT, Mundi MS. Use of blenderized tube feeding in adult and pediatric home enteral nutrition patients. *Nutr Clin Pract.* 2017;32(2):201–205

V

29. Singhal S, Baker SS, Bojczuk GA, Baker RD. Tube feeding in children. *Pediatr Rev.* 2017;38(1):23–34

30. Tsujimoto H, Tsujimoto Y, Nakata Y, Akazawa M, Kataoka Y. Ultrasonography for confirmation of gastric tube placement. *Cochrane Database Syst Rev.* 2017;(4):CD012083

31. Blumenstein I, Shastri YM, Stein J. Gastroenteric tube feeding: techniques, problems and solutions. *World J Gastroenterol.* 2014;20(26):8505–8524

32. Franken J, Mauritz FA, Stellato RK, Van der Zee DC, Van Herwaarden-Lindeboom MYA. The effect of gastrostomy placement on gastric function in children: a prospective cohort study. *J Gastrointest Surg.* 2017;21(7):1105–1111

33. Albanese CT, Towbin RB, Ulman I, Lewis J, Smith SD. Percutaneous gastrojejunostomy versus Nissen fundoplication for enteral feeding of the neurologically impaired child with gastroesophageal reflux. *J Pediatr.* 1993;123(3): 371–375

34. Stone B, Hester G, Jackson D, et al. Effectiveness of fundoplication or gastrojejunal feeding in children with neurologic impairment. *Hosp Pediatr.* 2017;7(3):140–148

35. Haijat T, Rahhal RM. Differences in durability, dislodgement, and other complications with use of low-profile nonballoon gastrostomy tubes in children. *Nutr Clin Pract.* 2017;32(2):219–224

36. Krom H, de Winter JP, Kindermann A. Development, prevention, and treatment of feeding tube dependency. *Eur J Pediatr.* 2017;176(6):683–688

37. Ramasamy M, Perman JA. Pediatric feeding disorders. *J Clin Gastroenterol.* 2000;30(1):34–46

Nutrition in Acute and Chronic Illness

Chapter 24

Assessment of Nutritional Status

Introduction

Assessment of nutritional status should be an integral part of the evaluation and management of all children with acute and chronic disease and is the primary step in the evaluation of all children whose growth differs from the norm.[1] A complete nutritional assessment includes the evaluation of dietary intake, physical examination, biochemical parameters, body size, and composition compared with age-appropriate norms, as available. During a prolonged hospital stay, nutritional disturbances can occur, particularly when oral intake is suspended or limited. This chapter discusses nutritional assessment methods and their practical application. For most patients, dietary history, physical examination, and longitudinal changes in height, weight, and relative weight, such as body mass index (BMI), are sufficient to assess nutritional status.

Assessment of Dietary Intake

Not all children eat normally, so a detailed diet history (including factors such as timing of meals, food choices, site [home or out of home], preparation, use of supplements) is important as an initial evaluation of intake. Children on a strict vegetarian diet may ingest inadequate amounts of protein, vitamin B_{12}, iron, or pyridoxine if meals are not properly planned (see also Chapter 11: Nutritional Aspects of Vegetarian Diets). Adolescents often skip meals, and athletic children may not consume adequate calories, or they may become involved in fad diets associated with some sports (see also Chapter 8: Adolescent Nutrition). Older children and adolescents may attempt weight loss by starvation, and anorexia nervosa or bulimia may develop (see also Chapter 38: Eating Disorders in Children and Adolescents). On the other hand, children may snack frequently throughout the day and consume large amounts of sugar-containing beverages and energy-dense snack foods; combined with sedentary behavior, this pattern may lead to obesity.

For a more quantitative evaluation of dietary intake, 3- to 5-day food records may be used. Tracking diet allows for an assessment of usual intake, which is important when trying to identify nutrient inadequacies and evaluate relationships between diet and biological parameters or chronic disease.[2] Ideally, the child and/or caregiver should be trained on how to estimate or measure food portions for the food records, and the dietary

VI

analysis is best performed by a registered dietitian. Some medications can cause nutritional disturbances (see Appendix G).

Clinical Assessment

Physical examination of the patient remains a valid method of nutritional assessment.[3] The current epidemic of childhood obesity has distorted perceptions of the normal appearance of children. Distinguishing wasting from stunting in the young child is also difficult. Obesity and wasting may not be obvious and must be confirmed using weight-for-length or BMI reference charts. Visual assessment is a useful screening test for gross changes in body composition by which edema, dehydration, excess or inadequate subcutaneous fat, and increase or decrease of the muscle mass can be detected. Some of the findings of vitamin and mineral deficiencies are listed in Tables 24.1 and 24.2. Deficiency of any trace substance can result in growth failure. The clinical signs and symptoms of specific vitamin or mineral deficiencies or toxic effects are usually not pathognomonic.

Growth Assessment

Anthropometric measurements are used to assess growth. If children are measured once, their "growth status" for age is assessed by comparing this measurement with the appropriate reference curve or table (Table 24.3; Appendix Q). If children are measured more than once, their growth status for age can be tracked over time. When sequential measurements are plotted on a growth chart, the growth trajectory or degree of "tracking" (ie, maintaining centile rank on the growth chart) can be evaluated. Growth velocity also can be assessed to determine whether their rate of growth is appropriate for age compared with growth velocity reference data (Table 24.3; Appendix Q). However, the intervals between measurements should be comparable to the intervals used to generate the reference data for valid comparisons. Growth assessment accuracy relies on good quality anthropometric measurements, so particular care should be taken to use the appropriate equipment and measurement techniques detailed later in this chapter (see Assessment Tools for Anthropometric Measurements by Age Group).

Table 24.1.

Signs and Symptoms of Vitamin Deficiency or Excess

Vitamin	Deficiency	Excess
A	Night blindness, xerophthalmia, keratomalacia, follicular hyperkeratosis	Scaly skin, bone pain, pseudotumor cerebri, hepatomegaly
C	Scurvy: capillary hemorrhage of gingiva, skin, bone, poor wound healing	"Rebound" deficiency after high intake
D	Rickets, osteomalacia	Constipation, renal stones, myositis ossificans, hypercalcemia
E	Hemolysis (in preterm infant), peripheral neuropathy	Suppresses hematologic response to iron in anemia
K	Bruising, bleeding	Jaundice
Thiamine	Beriberi: cardiomyopathy, peripheral neuropathy, and encephalopathy	None known
Riboflavin	Cheilosis, glossitis, angular stomatitis	None known
Niacin	Pellagra: dementia, diarrhea, and dermatitis	Flushing
Pyridoxine	Seizures, anemia, irritability	Neuropathy
Biotin	Dermatitis, alopecia, muscle pain	None known
Folate	Macrocytic anemia, stomatitis paresthesia, glossitis, neural tube defects of fetus	None known
B_{12}	Megaloblastic anemia, neuropathy, paresthesia, glossitis	None known

VI

Table 24.2.

Signs and Symptoms of Mineral Deficiency or Excess

Mineral	Deficiency	Excess
Aluminum	None known	Central nervous system disorder
Boron	Calcification abnormalities	None known
Calcium	Osteomalacia, tetany	Constipation, heart block, vomiting
Chloride	Alkalosis	Acidosis
Chromium	Diabetes (in animals)	None known
Cobalt	Vitamin B$_{12}$ deficiency	Cardiomyopathy
Copper	Anemia, neutropenia, osteoporosis, neuropathy, depigmentation of hair and skin	Cirrhosis, central nervous system effects, Fanconi nephropathy, corneal pigmentation
Fluoride	Dental caries	Fluorosis
Iodine	Goiter, cretinism	Goiter
Iron	Anemia, behavioral abnormalities	Hemosiderosis
Lead	None known	Encephalopathy, neuropathy, stippled red blood cells
Magnesium	Hypocalcemia, hypokalemia, tremor, weakness, arrhythmia	Weakness, sedation, hypotension, nausea, vomiting
Molybdenum	Growth retardation (in animals)	None known
Phosphorus	Rickets, neuropathy	Calcium deficiency
Potassium	Muscle weakness, cardiac abnormalities	Heart block
Selenium	Cardiomyopathy, anemia, myositis	Nail and hair changes, garlic odor
Sodium	Hypotension	Edema
Sulfur	Growth failure	None known
Zinc	Growth failure, dermatitis, hypogeusia, hypogonadism, alopecia, impaired wound healing	Gastroenteritis

Equally important is the use of appropriate reference growth curves and tables to interpret anthropometric measurements for growth status determination. Several considerations affect the appropriateness of reference data. First, it should be clear whether a growth curve or table is "descriptive," reference data that describe growth in a population of children, or "prescriptive," a growth standard that defines an optimal growth pattern.[4] For example, the reference values for children from birth to 2 years of age from the World Health Organization (WHO) Multicentre Growth Reference Study are based on a large, international sample of healthy, exclusively breastfed infants; therefore, the WHO growth charts are prescriptive. Differences between the WHO growth charts and other infant growth charts are attributable, in part, to the different patterns of growth associated with different feeding modes.[5] Other important features of a reference curve are (1) whether the sample is of sufficient size to capture the variability in the population at all ages; (2) whether appropriate statistical techniques were used to generate percentile distributions; (3) whether secular trends (eg, improvements in health care, obesity epidemic) may affect the applicability of older or current reference curves; and (4) the child's age and sex. Cutoffs for identifying high-risk small- and large-for-age infants and children will vary among growth curves for these reasons. See Table 24.3 for a summary of reference data.

Weight, length or stature, and head circumference (up to approximately 3 years of age) are the most common anthropometric measurements. Measures of relative weight, such as weight-for-length or BMI provide additional important information regarding growth and nutritional status. Other measures, such as mid-upper arm circumference and triceps skinfold thickness, also may be useful in the nutritional assessment of an infant or child.

Assessment Tools for Anthropometric Measurements by Age Group

Preterm Infants

Two types of growth curves used in the assessment of preterm infant growth are intrauterine curves and postnatal curves. Intrauterine growth curves[6-17] are generally accepted as the best available tool for growth assessment of preterm infants at birth and postnatally. These curves are created using cross-sectional birth data—that is, a different group of infants is

Table 24.3.

Resources for Growth and Nutrition Assessment by Age Group *(see also Appendix Q)*

Length/Stature, Weight, Head Circumference, and Relative Weight Growth Charts				
Age group	**Citation**	**Reference Measure**	**Age Range**	**Comments**
Preterm	**Citation:** Olsen et al 2010[16] Olsen et al 2015[30] **Web link:** https://www.aap.org/en-us/ Documents/GrowthCurves.pdf **Data source:** Preterm data: Large sample of US birth data (1998-2006), ethnically representative of US births, from Pediatrix Clinical Data Warehouse. Post-term data: WHO Child Growth Standards curves (Multicentre Growth Reference Study) (see below) **Web link:** For Olsen and WHO curves: http://www.pediatrix. com/workfiles/ NICUGrowthCurves7.30.pdf	Weight-for-age Length-for-age Head circumference-for-age BMI-for-age	23–41 wk gestational age (GA) 23–50 wk GA	• Only set of intrauterine growth curves with weight, length, head circumference and BMI-for-age created using the same data source for all curves • Sex-specific • 3rd to 97th percentiles • Reference (descriptive) data[a] Updated graphical version of Olsen and WHO weight, length, and head circumference growth curves: • Olsen curves from 23–38 wk GA • WHO curves from 39–50 wk GA

Citation: Fenton 2013[25] **Web link:** http://www.ucalgary.ca/fenton/2013chart **Data sources:** Preterm data for weight-for-age curves- based on pooled data from 6 countries (Germany, US, Canada, Australia, Scotland, Italy) Preterm data for length-for-age and head circumference-for-age curves- based on pooled data from 2 countries (US, Italy) Post-term data- WHO Child Growth Standards curves (Multicentre Growth Reference Study) (see below)	Weight-for-age Length-for-age Head circumference-for-age	22–50 wk GA	• Sex-specific • 3rd to 97th percentiles Preterm portion: • Intrauterine curves • Reference (descriptive) data[a] • Created from metanalysis Post-term portion: • Combination of cross-sectional national survey data and longitudinal data • Standard (prescriptive) data[b]

VI

Continued

Table 24.3. *Continued*

Resources for Growth and Nutrition Assessment by Age Group

Citation: Villar et al 2014[23] **Web link:** https://intergrowth21.tghn.org/newborn-size-birth/#ns1 **Data source:** INTERGROWTH-21st Project's Newborn Cross-Sectional Study newborns from 8 geographically defined urban populations worldwide with optimal growth conditions (2009–2014)	Weight-for-age Length-for-age Head circumference-for-age	33–43 wk GA	• Intrauterine growth • Sex-specific • 3rd to 97th percentiles • Standard (prescriptive) data[b] • Research quality measurements • Limited sample of preterm infants <36 wk GA given strict "healthy" inclusion criteria; not recommended for use in infants <36 wk GA • Provides gestation-specific estimate of size in newborns born at approximately 36–41 wk GA in NICU and newborn nursery (see text for discussion)

Citation / Data source	Measurements	GA	Notes
Citation: Villar et al 2015[35] **Web link:** https://intergrowth21.tghn.org/postnatal-growth-preterm-infants/#pg1 **Data source:** INTERGROWTH-21st Project's Preterm Postnatal Follow-up Study newborns from 8 geographically defined urban populations worldwide with optimal growth conditions (2009–2014)	Weight-for-age Length-for-age Head circumference-for-age	27-36 wk GA	• Postnatal growth • Sex-specific • 3rd to 97th percentiles • Standard (prescriptive) data[b] • Research quality measurements • Based on small dataset (n=201; by GA: 27-32 wk n=12; 33 wk n=16; 34-35 wk n=68; 36 wk n=105) • Given small numbers, these curves are not ready for use in the US at the present time
Citation: Williamson et al 2018[36] **Web link:** N/A **Data source:** Large sample of US birth and NICU data (2009-2013), sex and race breakdown representative of US NICUs, from Pediatrix Clinical Data Warehouse	BMI-for-age	24-36 wk GA at birth	Part of the "Olsen growth curves" set • Postnatal growth presented by Birth GA categories: 24-27 wk GA - 60 days of postnatal growth 28-31 wk GA - 45 days of postnatal growth 32-36 wk GA - 30 days of postnatal growth • Sex-specific • 3rd to 97th percentiles • Reference (descriptive) data[a]

VI

Continued

Table 24.3. *Continued*

Resources for Growth and Nutrition Assessment by Age Group

Age	Citation / Web link / Data source	Measurements	Recommendation	Notes
0 to 24 mo	**Citation:** WHO Multicentre Growth Reference Study 2006[26], and 2007[40] and de Onis et al 2006[5] **Web link:** https://www.cdc.gov/growthcharts/who_charts.htm#The%20WHO%20Growth%20Charts **Data source:** Cross-sectional and longitudinal data from the WHO Multicentre Growth Reference Study (MGRS), an international sample of healthy children with "optimal" conditions for growth (eg, breastfed)	Weight-for-age Length-for-age Head circumference-for-age Weight-for-length curves BMI-for-age	0 to 60 mo • Recommended by CDC for children <24 mo	• Full term infants (defined as 37–41 wk GA) and children • For newborns, do not provide gestation-specific assignment of size • Sex-specific • 2nd to 98th percentiles • Standard (prescriptive) data[b] • Research quality measurements
2 to 20 y	**Citation:** Kuczmarski et al 2000[38] (CDC 2000 growth charts) **Web link:** http://www.cdc.gov/growthcharts/clinical_charts.htm **Data source:** Strategic random sample of US children (1963–1994) based on multiple cross-sectional national survey data and longitudinal data from the Fels Research Institute	Stature-for-age curves Weight-for-age BMI-for-age Head circumference-for-age	0 to 20 y • Recommended by CDC for 2–20 y 0 to 36 mo • Used for 24–36 mo, as needed	• Sex specific • "Set 1": 5th to 95th percentiles • "Set 2": 3rd to 97th percentiles • Weight-for-age, BMI-for-age, and weight-for-length charts excluded data collected for children >6 y from 1988 to 1994 because of the increase in obesity prevalence

Incremental Growth Charts

Age group	Citation	Reference measure	Age range	Comments
0 to 24 mo	**Citation:** WHO Multicentre Growth Reference Study 2009[41] **Web link:** http://www.who.int/childgrowth/standards/en/ **Data source:** Longitudinal data from the WHO Multicentre Growth Reference Study (MGRS), an international sample of healthy children with "optimal" conditions for growth (eg, breastfed)	Weight increment and velocity Length increment and velocity Head increment and circumference velocity	0 to 24 mo	Sex-specific[b] • For ages 0–12 mo: increments of 1 mo for weight • For ages 0–24 mo: increments of 2 to 6 mo for weight and length • For ages 0–60 days: increments of 1 to 2 wk for weight • For ages 0 to 12 months: 2- and 3-month increments for head circumference • For ages 0 to 24 months: 4- and 6-month increments for head circumference • For ages 0–24 mo: 2 to 6 mo increments for length

VI

Continued

Table 24.3. *Continued*

Resources for Growth and Nutrition Assessment by Age Group

Age Group	Citation / Web link / Data source	Measurement	Age Range	Notes
2 to 18 years	**Citation:** Baumgartner et al 1986[43] **Web link:** http://www.ncbi.nlm.nih.gov/entrez/query.fcgi?cmd=Retrieve&db=PubMed&dopt=Citation&list_uids=3706184 **Data source:** Longitudinal US data from the Fels Longitudinal Study (1929–1978)	Weight velocity Length velocity Stature velocity	0 to 18 y 0 to 3 y 3 to 18 y	• Sex-specific • 3rd to 97th percentiles • For ages 0-12 mo: measurements at birth, 1, 3, 6, 9, 12 mo • For ages 1-18 y: increments of 6 mo
	Citation: Tanner and Davies 1985[45] **Web link:** http://www.ncbi.nlm.nih.gov/entrez/query.fcgi?cmd=Retrieve&db=PubMed&dopt=Citation&list_uids=3875704 **Data source:** 1977 National Center for Health Statistics growth charts data[50] were combined with data from other longitudinal studies	Height and height velocity	2 to ~14-19 y (depending on sex and stage of maturity)	• Sex-specific • 3rd to 97th percentiles • Curves for early, middle, and late maturers

	Height velocity	7 to 18 y	• Sex-specific • Ages 7 to 18 y • Race-specific • Curves for early, average and late maturing children • 3rd to 97th percentiles
Citation: Berkey 1993[44] **Web link:** http://www.ncbi.nlm.nih.gov/pubmed?term=Berkey%20Dockery%201993 **Data source:** Longitudinal data from a sample of US children participating in the Six Cities Study (1974–1989)			
	Annual height velocity	Females: 6 to 17 y Males: 6 to 19 y	• Sex specific • Curves for earlier, average and later maturing children • 3rd to 97th percentiles
Citation: Kelly et al. 2014[46] **Web link:** http://www.ncbi.nlm.nih.gov/pubmed/24601728 **Data Source:** Longitudinal data from a multi-ethnic sample of US children participating in the NICHD Bone Mineral Density in Childhood Study (2001 to 2010)			

Continued

VI

Table 24.3. *Continued*

Resources for Growth and Nutrition Assessment by Age Group

Other Anthropometric Measures		
Citation: WHO Multicentre Growth Reference Study 2007[40] **Web link:** http://www.who.int/childgrowth/standards/en/ **Data source:** Cross-sectional and longitudinal data from the WHO Multicentre Growth Reference Study, an international sample of healthy children with "optimal" conditions for growth (eg, breast-fed)	Arm circumference-for-age Triceps skinfold-for-age	3 mo to 5 y	• Sex-specific[b] • 3rd to 97th percentile
Citation: Addo and Himes 2010[47] **Web link:** http://www.ncbi.nlm.nih.gov/pubmed?term=Addo%20 Himes%202010 **Data source:** NHANES data same as that used for the CDC 2000 BMI-for-age curves[38]	Triceps and subscapular skinfold-for-age	1.5 to 20 y	• Sex-specific • Partly prescriptive because of exclusion of potentially obese children (same data set as CDC 2000 BMI curves) • 3rd to 97th percentiles

| **Citation:** Addo et al[48] **Web link:** http://www.ncbi.nlm.nih.gov/pubmed/27806975 **Data Source:** NHANES data same as that used for the CDC 2000 BMI-for-age curves[38] | Mid-upper arm circumference, upper arm fat area and upper arm muscle area for age | 1 to 20 y | • Sex-specific
• Partly prescriptive because of exclusion of potentially obese children (same data set as CDC 2000 BMI curves)
• 3rd to 97th percentiles |

[a] Most of the growth curves and tables included in this table are considered *reference* (or descriptive) data, because they describe growth of children who participated in a survey or convenience sample.

[b] The WHO child growth standards and the INTERGROWTH-21st Project curves are considered *standard* (or prescriptive) curves and tables, because they describe growth of a sample of children selected for optimal growth patterns (healthy, well-nourished, breastfed infants).

VI

measured *at birth* for each gestational age. Intrauterine growth curves represent intrauterine or fetal growth, which is considered the goal for preterm infant growth. Using birth data of preterm infants as an indicator of intrauterine growth is not perfect, because these infants are born smaller than if they had remained in utero,[13,18,19] but there is no method to *directly* measure fetal weight while still in utero. Thus, this method remains the best available option.[20–22]

There are many examples of intrauterine growth curves, but only some include weight, length, and head circumference.[8,10–12,14,16,23] For former preterm infants, growth measurements are plotted using corrected age, calculated by subtracting the number of weeks born before 40 weeks of gestation from the chronologic age for up to the first 3 years of life.[24]

There are 3 recent sets of intrauterine curves for weight, length, and head circumference-for-age from the INTERGROWTH-21st Project,[23] Fenton,[25] and Olsen et al[16] (Table 24.3). The INTERGROWTH-21st Project developed standard-type growth curves (from 33 to 43 wk GA at birth; the authors call these "International Newborn Size Standards") using carefully measured weights, lengths, and head circumferences, taken within 12 hours of birth, for more than 20 000 infants from 8 different countries living in optimal preterm conditions (detailed elsewhere).[23] These curves are intended to complement the WHO growth curves[26] and used similar methods. Their sampling strategy targeting healthy, low-risk infants resulted in a limited number of preterm infants born between 33 and 36 weeks' gestational age (n=210 for weight), and thus, the INTERGROWTH-21st intrauterine curves are not recommended for use in infants <36 weeks' gestational age. Intrauterine curves based on very preterm infants (born <33 weeks gestational age; n=112) were published in a correspondence by the INTERGROWTH-21st Project authors[27] but provide an even less robust standard because of the very small sample size and are also not recommended for use.

The 2013 Fenton curves[25] (Table 24.3; Appendix Q-2.1, Q-2.2) are sex-specific and combine intrauterine and postnatal curves ranging from 22 to 50 weeks. Like the 2003 version,[10] the 2013 Fenton curves[25] were created from a metanalysis of published growth data. For the preterm portion of the curves, data from 6 studies representing 6 countries (Canada, Germany, Australia, Scotland, Italy, United States) were used depending on the growth measure: the weight-for-age curves used data from all 6 studies; the length-for-age and head circumference-for-age curves used data from 2 studies (Italian and US data). The WHO growth curves were used for older infants.[26] The preterm (metanalysis) and term/post-term (WHO) curves were connected and manually smoothed to remove the disjunction between the 2 curves, as a means of following preterm infants to older ages.[25,28]

The 2010 intrauterine growth curves from Olsen et al[16] (Table 24.3; Appendix Q-3.1, Q-3.2, Q-3.4, Q-3.5) were created and validated using a large sample of US infants born at 23 to 41 weeks' gestational age between 1998 and 2006 that represents the racial distribution of US births. An updated graphical version of the 2010 Olsen curves (Table 24.3; Appendix Q-4.1, Q-4.2) consolidated weight, length, and head circumference onto the same graph (ranging from 24–38 wk). The WHO growth curves[26] (from 39–50 wk) are included on these same graphs as a means of following preterm infants to older ages, without any manual smoothing of the curves.[29] The Olsen and Fenton curves are similar between approximately 23 and 36 weeks (Olsen data included in Fenton dataset).[25]

The Olsen curves also include BMI-for-age[30] (Table 24.3; Appendix Q-3.3, Q-3.6) in addition to weight, length, and head circumference-for-age curves, and all curves were created and validated from the same reference dataset. These BMI-for-age curves are intended for use in conjuction with weight, length, and head circumference-for-age curves to identify and quantify disproportionate growth in weight and length in preterm infants (see BMI for details).

Postntatal growth curves[31–33] are also used to assess preterm infant growth. These curves are created using longitudinal data, in which one group of infants is measured at birth and repeated measurements are obtained over time. As a result, postnatal curves illustrate *actual* growth (ie, descriptive curves), not *ideal* growth (prescriptive curves). Patterns of growth in preterm infants differ from full-term infants.[34] Two well-known examples of preterm postnatal curves include the curves from Ehrenkranz et al based on data from 1994–1995[31] and the Infant Health and Development Program (IHDP) curves for low birth weight and extremely low birth weight infants based on data from 1984–1985.[32,33] Postnatal curves are used to compare the growth of a preterm infant to that of other preterm infants and, therefore, may serve as useful adjunct assessment tools to intrauterine growth curves.

In 2015, the INTERGROWTH-21st Project published standard (ie, "prescriptive") postnatal growth curves for preterm infants[35] (Table 24.3), based on preterm infants from 8 countries growing in optimal pre- and post-term conditions (eg, good maternal health and nutrition conditions; gestational age confirmed by ultrasonography; breastfed; without congenital malformations, fetal growth restriction, or severe postnatal illness). These curves are intended to complement the WHO growth curves and used similar

VI

methods. The strengths of the INTERGROWTH 21st postnatal curves are that they are based on research-quality (versus clinical) growth measurements, carefully defined statistical methods, and a geographically and ethnically diverse sample. Currently, there are no comparable postnatal curves for the growth assessment of preterm infants. As noted previously, a major limitation of the INTERGROWTH-21st postnatal growth curves is the small sample of infants on which they are based (1446 observations from 201 individuals [girls and boys combined]; by GA: 33 wk, n=16 infants; 34–35 wk, n=68 infants; 36 wk, n=105 infants) and the dearth of extremely preterm infants in this sample (27–32 wk, n=12 infants; <27 wk, n=0 infants).[35] Given the small sample size and pooled international sample used, research is needed to evaluate the use of these curves, in particular in the United States. These curves are not included in Appendix Q.

In 2018, Williamson et al published a set of postnatal BMI-for-age growth curves[36] (Table 24.3; selected Figure and Tables in Appendix Q-5.1–Q-5.3) as an adjunct to the Olsen weight, length, head circumference and BMI-for-age intrauterine (cross-sectional) growth curves.[16,30] These BMI longitudinal curves provide clinicians data on how preterm infants' body proportionality (weight relative to length) changes over time in the NICU. As expected postnadir, these curves (representing actual growth) remained consistently below the intrauterine curves (representing optimal growth) and varied by gestational age and sex (Appendix Q-5.1). Further, the most preterm infants (24–27 weeks' gestational age at birth) showed the most rapid increase in BMI back toward birth percentiles compared with the more mature preterm infants.[36] These postnatal BMI longitudinal curves provide an adjunct tool to the intrauterine curves for a more comprehensive assessment of growth in preterm infants.

Currently, there are no widely used reference data for growth velocity, circumferences, or skinfold measurements for preterm infants at birth or postnatally, although clinical research studies are starting to emerge.[37,38] See Table 24.3 for a summary of reference data.

Infants and Toddlers (Full-Term to <24 mo)

The CDC recommends the use of the WHO Multicentre Growth Reference Study growth curves[28] (Table 24.3; Appendix Q-1.1–Q-1.6) for children younger than 24 months (regardless of diet) in place of the currently used CDC 2000 growth curves.[39,40] These charts are available online (Table 24.3) and include weight-for-age, length-for-age, head circumference-for-age; weight-for-length (recommended for children ages 0-24 months), and

BMI-for-age curves. The WHO growth curves are based on an international sample of healthy children (singleton and full-term at birth) living in "optimal" conditions to support growth (eg, breastfed, nonsmoking environment).[26,40] Thus, the WHO curves are growth *standard* curves (or prescriptive) versus the growth *reference* (or descriptive) CDC 2000 curves, which describe the size and growth of US children between 1963 and 1994 on the basis of a combination of cross-sectional national survey data and longitudinal data from the Fels Research Institute.[4,22,39,40] Unlike the sample in the WHO Multicentre Growth Reference Study, the infants used to create the CDC 2000 growth curves were predominantly fed cow milk-based formula.

The WHO growth curves for children younger than 24 months were developed using a combination of longitudinal (birth to 23 months) and cross-sectional data (birth data for infants who did not meet the feeding and maternal nonsmoking criteria and additional cross-sectional data for 18 to 24 months) collected between 1997 and 2003.[41] The CDC and the American Academy of Pediatrics (AAP) recommend using the 2.3rd and 97.7th percentiles of the WHO growth curves (labeled as 2nd and 98th on the curves, or 2 standard deviations above and below the median) to identify children with potentially suboptimal growth in the first 24 months after birth.[40] The INTERGROWTH-21st newborn curves[23] (see Preterm Infants section for details; Table 24.3; Appendix Q-6.1–Q-6.6) provide another *standard*-type growth curves option for older newborn infants. In particular, these curves offer a gestation-specific assignment of size at birth for full-term and near full-term infants (approximately 36 or more weeks' gestational age), whereas the WHO curves at birth are not gestation-specific because of the wide range of gestational ages included in their definition of "full term" (37–41 weeks). Therefore, the INTERGROWTH-21st newborn curves allow for a gestational age-specific assignment of small and large for gestational age in newborn infants with gestational age of approximately 36 to 41 weeks.

The WHO Multicentre Growth Reference Study also provided norms for growth velocity (for weight, length, and head circumference; see Growth Velocity) in table format (selected tables in Appendix Q-7.1–Q-7.14) and arm circumference-for-age and triceps skinfold-for-age (3 to 24 months) in both curve and table formats (selected curves in Appendix Q-8.1, Q-8.2, Q-9.1, Q-9.2).[41,42] See the sections on anthropometric measurement and clinical body composition for details on arm circumference and triceps skinfold, respectively. See Table 24.3 for a summary of reference anthropometric data.

Children (>24 months)

The CDC and the AAP recommend the use of the CDC 2000 growth charts (Table 24.3; Appendix Q-1.7–Q-1.10) for children 2 to 20 years of age.[39,40] These are available online (Table 24.3) and include growth curves for weight-for-age, length/stature-for-age, BMI-for-age, weight-for-length, and head circumference-for-age (for use from 24 to 36 months of age, as needed). The CDC charts, published in 2000, are based on a series of large cross-sectional surveys conducted from 1963 to 1994. As a result, the CDC growth curves are reference growth curves and *describe* the growth in strategically sampled US children over this time period.[39] The weight-for-age, weight-for-length, and BMI-for-age curves excluded the data for children older than 6 years collected from 1988 to 1994 because of the increase in obesity prevalence during this time frame. Consequently, these 3 curves are partly prescriptive. Generally, the CDC 2000 curves allow for the comparison of one child's growth to that of a large reference population of other children.

Two sets of CDC 2000 growth charts are available for use (Table 24.3). Set 1 provides curves that span from the 5th to the 95th percentiles and are most commonly used in the clinical setting to classify and monitor over time the growth of children; set 2 provides curves that span from the 3rd and 97th percentiles and are helpful in the growth assessment of children whose growth falls at the extremes.[43]

Growth velocity reference data based on US children are available for children >24 months of age[44–47] (see Growth Velocity). Other sources of reference data for nutritional assessment include the WHO Multicentre Growth Reference Study for arm circumference-for-age and triceps skinfold-for-age for children up to 5 years of age.[41] Norms for triceps skinfold-for-age, mid-upper arm circumference-for-age, upper arm fat area-for-age, and upper arm muscle area-for-age for children 1 to 20 years of age[48,49] are available using the same subset of US survey data from which the CDC 2000 BMI charts were constructed. See the sections on anthropometric measurements and clinical body composition for details on arm circumference and triceps skinfold, respectively. See Table 24.3 for a summary of reference data.

Growth Velocity

Growth increments can be sensitive indicators of nutritional status, because they reflect the recent state of the infant. Growth increments are determined as the change in weight (or length/height or head circumference) divided by the time interval. Growth increments are sensitive to the time interval between measurements because growth occurs as a series of intermittent small or large spurts,[50] which vary in magnitude according to age, sex, maturational status, and season. Comparison of a growth increment based on a longer or shorter interval than that used in the reference curve may overestimate or underestimate incremental growth status. In addition, the accuracy of growth increments is dependent on the accuracy and precision of the 2 measurements on which it is calculated, each with its own measurement error. Therefore, growth increments should be based on accurate growth measurements, carefully calculated, and compared with reference values based on similar time intervals.

Growth velocity standards for young children are available from the WHO Multicentre Growth Study (Table 24.3). These standards are presented in table format for children 0 to 24 months of age (see Appendix Q-7.1–Q-7.14 for selected tables). Weight growth velocity reference data are available in 1-mo increments (birth to 12 months of age), in 2- to 6-month increments (birth to 24 months of age), and in 1- and 2-week increments (birth to 60 days of age). Length velocity values are available in 2- to 6-month increments (birth to 24 months of age). Head circumference velocity values are available in 2- to 3-month increments (birth to 12 months of age) and in 4- to 6-month increments (birth to 24 months of age). Clinicians are encouraged to use the interval that most closely approximates the time elapsed between the child's measurements. Because of the variability in growth velocity over time as discussed previously, a growth assessment should always consider achieved growth (ie, size-for-age, as discussed earlier in this chapter) when interpreting growth velocity values.[42]

Growth velocity reference data based on US children are also available for older age groups (Table 24.3). Baumgartner et al[44] published sex-specific weight and length/height velocity tables for children 0 to 18 years of age based on longitudinal measurements obtained in the Fels Longitudinal Study. Tanner and Davies[46] created height velocity curves and tables that are specific to sex and stage of maturity. They combined data from the US 1977 growth charts[51] with longitudinal data from other studies. Sex- and race-specific height velocity centiles are available from Berkey et al[45] for children 7 to 18 years of age based on data collected in a large US multicenter study conducted between 1974 and 1989 and more recently from Kelly et al for children 5 to 18 years of age collected between 2001 and 2009.[47]

VI

Anthropometric Measurements

Length or Stature

Length or stature is the most useful indicator of linear growth status. Recumbent length is measured in infants and children younger than 2 years and in children 2 to 3 years of age who are unable to stand unsupported. Devices for measuring length and stature should be appropriately calibrated and accurate to 0.1 cm. Two people are required to accomplish this measurement. The measuring table or board should consist of a fixed headboard, a movable footboard, and a rule attached at one side. The infant should be positioned with the body flat and the midline centered on the board. Interfering hair adornments should be removed. One measurer should hold the crown of the infant's head firmly against the headboard with the external auditory meatus and the lower margin of the eye orbit aligned perpendicular to the table. When measuring a preterm infant, it is often necessary to gently untuck its chin (from the chest) to position the head properly. The second measurer gently flattens the infant's knees to fully extend the legs and grips both ankles of the infant with one hand. The footboard is then guided gently to the feet such that the feet are pointing upward and positioned flat on the footboard in order to obtain the measurement. The recumbent length should be recorded to the nearest 0.1 cm.

Stature, or standing height, is measured in children older than 2 years. A wall-mounted device should be used with a headboard that glides at a 90° angle to the wall. The use of measuring devices attached to beam balance scales is discouraged, because accurate measurement cannot be achieved. Measurements are made with the child's feet bare and interfering hair adornments removed. The child should stand erect, and if possible, with the heels, buttocks, shoulders, and head touching the measuring device, and the arms down and relaxed at his or her side. The heels should be as close together as possible with the feet at a 60-degree angle. The head should be positioned with the child looking ahead and the external auditory meatus and lower margin of the orbit aligned horizontally. Children should be told to make themselves "as tall as possible with their heels on the ground." Asking them to take a deep breath often helps to improve posture and stand as tall as possible. The headboard is then gently glided to the top of the crown and stature is recorded to the nearest 0.1 cm.

For both length and stature, measurements are best obtained when the child is relaxed and cooperative. Accurate measurement is particularly important for calculating growth velocity. Reference values for length, stature, and growth velocity are shown in Appendix Q. Reference values for length and stature are also available for preterm infants (Appendix Q). See Table 24.3 for a summary of reference growth data.

When possible, the parents' stature should be obtained to determine the influence of genetics on growth. If only one parent is available, the maternal stature is more valuable for comparison. There are 2 approaches to estimating the influence of heredity on stature. The parent-specific adjustment for evaluation of recumbent length and stature of children[52] uses a table of values, whereby an adjustment value at each age is given for mid-parental height. The adjustment value is added to the measured height or length, and this value is plotted on the growth chart to obtain the parent-specific percentile. For example, because children of tall parents are generally tall for their age, a short child with tall parents would have a negative adjustment value and his or her "adjusted height" would be less than his or her measured height. A tall child with tall parents would have no adjustment to his or her actual height. The "adjusted height" can be plotted on a growth chart to separate the estimated genetic contribution from other factors, such as malnutrition or disease, which may affect height. In children with cystic fibrosis, parent-adjusted heights are more strongly associated with the child's lung function than unadjusted heights.[53] The alternative approach for children 2 to 9 years of age is to estimate the child's adult height on the basis of the following formula[54]:

For boys: $$\frac{[\text{father's height} + (\text{mother's height} + 5 \text{ inches or } 13 \text{ centimeters})]}{2}$$

For girls: $$\frac{[\text{mother's height} + (\text{father's height} - 5 \text{ inches or } 13 \text{ centimeters})]}{2}$$

The estimated adult height is plotted on the growth chart to determine a target percentile. The child's current height percentile is compared with his or her target percentile as an estimate of genetic versus other factors influencing the child's growth status. Both the mid-parental height adjustment and the adult height prediction methods are based on studies of people of European origin, and it is unknown whether further adjustment is needed for other population ancestry groups. The mid-parental height adjustment is more difficult to use, because it requires the use of published tables that are age, sex, and height specific. However, this method accounts for the fact that the association between child's height and mid-parental height varies with age.

Estimating Length/Stature From Knee Height

For children who are unable to stand unsupported, such as those with severe cerebral palsy, spina bifida, and other conditions with which they are wheelchair bound or bedridden, stature can be estimated by the use of prediction equations based on lower leg length measurements.[55] Lower leg length is measured from the heel to the superior surface of the knee. Prediction equations for stature are given in Table 24.4. Two caveats of this approach are (1) there are differences in limb length relative to stature that cluster within population ancestry groups (people of Asian ancestry have shorter lower legs and people of African ancestry have longer legs relative to stature than those of European ancestry); and (2) nonambulatory children can have stunted growth of lower limbs. Prediction equations for height have also been developed using ulna length, measured from the tip of the elbow to the ulnar styloid.[56]

Weight

Various types of scales (infant scales, beam-balance scales, and digital scales) are available to measure body weight. Scales need to be regularly calibrated to maintain accuracy. Scales should be zeroed before a measurement is obtained. Infants should be weighed with clothing and diaper removed; if this is not possible, the infant may be weighed in a clean diaper after the scale is zeroed with a clean diaper on it. Children should be weighed in light clothing or examination gowns with shoes removed. Reference data for body weight are included in Appendix Q. Reference values for infant weight gain are now available (Appendix Q), but attention should be given to the time interval between measurements when using these reference charts (see Growth Velocity for details). See Table 24.3 for a summary of reference data.

Measures of Relative Weight

Weight relative to length/stature provides a more complete picture of nutritional status than weight or length alone. It is useful for identifying children whose weight is appropriate for their age, yet their weight may be low or high relative to their length/stature. Likewise, for very short or tall children, relative weight is a good indicator of whether body weight is appropriate for size. The relationship between weight and length/stature changes as a function of age and sexual maturation. Weight-for-length measurement is recommended for full-term infants through 2 years of age, although BMI may be a better indicator of excess relative weight in infants younger than 6 months.[57] BMI is recommended for children 2 years and older. The ideal relative weight measure for preterm infants continues to be investigated[58–61]; use of BMI curves has been proposed in these infants.[30]

Table 24.4.

Prediction of Stature (cm) From Knee Height

Without Cerebral Palsy[54]

Males	6–18 y	White	[Knee Height (cm) x 2.22] + 40.54
		African American	[Knee Height (cm) x 2.18] + 39.60
	19–60 y	White	[Knee Height (cm) x 1.88] + 71.85
		African American	[Knee Height (cm) x 1.79] + 73.42
Females	6–18 y	White	[Knee Height (cm) x 2.15] + 43.21
		African American	[Knee Height (cm) x 2.02] + 46.59
	19–60 y	White	[Knee Height (cm) x 1.87] – [Age (years) x 0.06] + 70.25
		African American	[Knee Height (cm) x 1.86] – [Age (years) x 0.06] + 68.10

With Cerebral Palsy[119]

| All | 0–12 y | All | [Knee Height (cm) x 2.69] + 24.2 |

Weight for Length

For infants, the relationship of weight to length can be used to differentiate stunted growth from wasting and is independent of age. Stunting frequently is constitutional but can also be caused by malnutrition, chronic illness, and genetic or endocrine abnormalities. Stunting typically results in a child who is small for age but has a body weight proportional to length. Wasting results from acute or subacute nutritional deprivation and can be caused by medical conditions, such as diarrhea or malabsorption, in which body weight is depleted out of proportion to length, resulting in a low weight-for-length/height. The currently accepted index is the weight-for-length percentile or z-score based on the WHO growth charts (0 to 2 years of age). Reference values for weight in relation to length are shown in Appendix Q-1.2, Q-1.5. See Table 24.3 for a summary of reference data. The WHO BMI charts also are used to screen for overnutrition and undernutrition. A comparative study of nearly 74 000 full-term infants found consistent agreement between BMI and weight-for-length from 6 months of age onward. However, at 2 months of age, BMI was a better predictor of subsequent obesity at 2 years than was weight-for-length.[57]

BMI

BMI is the most widely used screening measure of adiposity. BMI is calculated as weight in kg divided by the square of height in meters (kg/m^2). It can also be calculated by dividing the weight in lb by the square of height in inches, multiplied by 703 ($lb/in^2 \times 703$). The calculated BMI is then plotted on the WHO BMI curve for children <2 years of age (Appendix Q-1.3, Q-1.6) and on the CDC 2000 BMI-for-age growth curve for children >2 years of age (Table 24.3; Appendix Q-1.8, Q-1.10). There is no accepted definition of underweight, overweight, or obesity for children <2 years of age. For children >2 years of age, a BMI-for-age less than the 5th percentile is considered "underweight," the 5th to less than the 85th percentile is considered "healthy weight," the 85th to less than the 95th percentile is considered "overweight," and ≥95th percentile is considered "obese."[62] All children followed by a physician should have their BMI calculated and plotted periodically. If the child begins to cross percentile lines (upward) on the BMI-for-age chart, the family can be counseled early about prevention of obesity.[63]

For children with BMI levels that exceed the 97th percentile, it is difficult to describe the degree of obesity and to monitor trends in treatment. To address this problem, charts are available that use "percentage" of the 95th percentile for age and sex from the CDC 2000 charts to characterize the degree of obesity.[64,65] This method is a good indicator of the degree of excess adiposity assessed by dual energy x-ray absorptiometry.[66]

For preterm infants, BMI-for-age (Table 24.3; Appendix Q-3.3, Q-3.6) has been proposed as the best overall measure to capture relative weight across gestational ages and in both sexes.[30,67,68] Gender-specific BMI-for-age intrauterine growth curves are available based on the data from US infants used to create and validate the 2010 Olsen curves.[16,30] These BMI-for-age curves are intended for use in conjuction with weight, length, and head circumference-for-age curves to identify and quantify disproportionate growth in weight and length in preterm infants. Two recent studies tested BMI measured *at or near birth* as a proxy of body fat in preterm infants and found that it is not a good proxy at this early timepoint.[60,61] However, most preterm infants have little body fat and are not disproportionate in size at birth. Further evaluation of BMI-for-age in preterm infants as a measure of disproportionality and/or proxy for body fat postnatally is needed.

Head Circumference

Head circumference is a proxy measure for brain growth and a useful screening tool for identification of hydrocephalus until approximately 3 years of age, when head growth slows. Head circumference is measured with a narrow and nonstretchable measuring tape with interfering hair adornments removed. The tape is positioned on the forehead just above the supraorbital ridges, and wrapped around the occiput so that the maximum circumference is obtained, keeping the tape level on both sides; it is a good practice to move the tape slightly up and down to ensure maximum circumference. The tape should have sufficient tension to press the hair against the skull, and head circumference is recorded to the nearest 0.1 cm. Reference values from birth to 2 years of age are shown in Appendix Q-1.2, Q-1.5. Reference values for preterm infants are shown in Appendix Q-2.1, Q-2.2, Q-3.2, Q-3.5, Q-4.1, Q-4.2. See Table 24.3 for a summary of reference data.

Mid-arm Circumference

Mid-upper–arm circumference is an indicator of soft tissue growth in all ages. The right arm is measured at its mid-point using a flexible, nonstretchable tape measure. The upper arm midpoint is marked midway between the acromion (shoulder) and the olecranon (elbow) on the vertical axis of the upper arm between the lateral and medial surface of the arm with the arm bent at a right angle. For the actual circumference measurement, the arm should hang loosely at the side with the tape passed around the arm at the level marked and perpendicular to the long axis of the arm.

The tape is positioned so that it touches but does not compress the skin or alter the contour of the arm. Reference values from the WHO Multicentre Growth Reference Study for children 3 months to 5 years of age are presented as curves in Appendix Q-8.1, Q-8.2, Q-9.1, Q-9.2. See Table 24.3 for a summary of reference data. Arm circumference values for US children, ages 2 to 20 years, are also presented in Appendix Q-8.3.[49] These reference ranges are based on the same group of children used to create the CDC 2000 BMI charts. They are particularly useful in situations when it is not possible to obtain a BMI measurement for nutritional assessment, as in the case of the critically ill child.[69]

Nutritional Assessment Through the Measurement of Body Composition

Body composition assessment, depending on the method used, can provide information about the fat, lean, and bone tissue compartments. Fat is an indicator of energy stores and varies with overnutrition and undernutrition. Lean mass is composed of organs (not including bone) and skeletal muscle and is representative of protein stores in the body. Like fat, protein can be used for energy, but all protein in the body is present as functional tissue, so its utilization potentially results in a decrease in the functional body mass. Bone is the primary reservoir for calcium, and adequate bone accretion during childhood is important for lifelong skeletal health. Many methods of measuring body composition exist; however, few are used clinically and some are not practical in infants and/or children because of safety, feasibility, and availability. Some methods offer easy measurement of fat and fat-free mass accompanied by reference data so they can enhance the surveillance of the nutritional status of children. However, body composition methods vary in underlying assumptions and are not standardized, so methods need to be selected with care, and results from different methods are not interchangeable. Most body composition methods are research tools; understanding them is important for interpreting the pediatric nutrition literature, so they are summarized below. A few body composition assessment methods are now more widely available for clinical application. These will be reviewed separately.

Research Body Composition Assessment Techniques

Hydrodensitometry

The oldest method of estimating the fat and fat-free mass compartments in the human body is hydrodensitometry, introduced in 1942 by Albert Behnke.[70] Hydrodensitometry, or underwater weighing, is based on Archimedes' principle, which observes that the weight of an object completely immersed in water, relative to its weight in air, is proportional to the weight of the volume of water displaced. Because 1 mL of water has a mass of 1 g, the difference between the mass in air and the mass under water (in g) is equivalent to the volume (in mL) of the object. Body density is then calculated as mass divided by volume. Corrections are needed for the volume of air in the lungs and intestines and for the density of air and water. With the assumption that the density of fat and the lean tissue are essentially constant, calculation of the proportion of each is possible when the density of the whole body is known. The Siri formula[71] is most widely used for estimating the proportion of fat in the body as follows:

$$\text{Siri}^{70} \quad \% \text{ body fat} = (4.95/\text{Body Density} - 4.50) \times 100$$

Hydrodensitometry requires that the individual is capable of being completely submerged in water long enough to take the measurements. This is not feasible for younger children, infants, hospitalized patients, or individuals with cognitive or physical disabilities. Also, the method assumes a constant density of fat-free mass; however, the hydration of fat-free mass decreases and bone density increases through the course of childhood. This results in small errors in the estimation of fat-free mass and fat mass during childhood.[72] Newer methods using this principle with air rather than water displacement have been developed (see Air-Displacement Plethysmography).

Total Body Potassium

The body cell mass represents the fat-free intracellular space of the body. This is the most metabolically active cellular compartment of the body, because it includes organs and muscles.[73] Because potassium is located in the intracellular fluids, body cell mass can be estimated by measuring total body potassium in a specially designed scintillation chamber or whole-body potassium counter.[74,75] Potassium (^{40}K), a naturally occurring stable isotope in human tissue, occurs as a very small percentage (0.0118%) of the nonradioactive ^{39}K also present in the body. The whole-body potassium counter measures the gamma rays emitted by ^{40}K to determine whole-body content of ^{40}K. The method assumes a constant ratio of intracellular fluid to body cell mass, so body cell mass is estimated as: total body K (mmol) x 0.0083. This technique is noninvasive but not practical because (1) it is not widely available and requires an entirely lead-shielded room; (2) it requires isolation in a special chamber for 30 to 60 minutes; and (3) it is not sufficiently sensitive to measure infants or small children who have little lean body mass and relatively fewer radioactive disintegrations per unit of time than do adults.

Total Body Water
The nonfat compartment of the body is largely composed of water, so determination of the body's water content can easily be used to estimate total body fat and fat-free mass.[76] Stable isotopes of water, deuterium (^2H), or oxygen 18 (O^{18}) are naturally occurring and can be consumed orally in small concentrations to determine the total body water space. Following collection of a baseline biological specimen, administration of a small oral dose of ^2H or O^{18}, an equilibration period of a few hours, and a subsequent specimen collection, total body water can be estimated based on the change in concentration of the isotope within a body fluid, such as serum, urine, or saliva. The method is safe and noninvasive and involves minimal participant burden and can be used in a variety of natural settings as well as hospitalized infants and children. However, analysis of specimens to determine isotopic concentration is primarily performed in research laboratories, so it is of little usefulness clinically. In adults, the water content of lean body mass is relatively constant (72.3%), but in infants and children, the hydration of lean tissues changes with age.[77,78] Lean tissue hydration also increases with obesity.[79] These factors influence the accuracy of total body water and body composition estimates in infants and children using this technique.

Neutron Activation
In vivo neutron activation analysis is the technique used to measure the elemental composition of the body.[80] The human body comprises more than 60 elements. Just 4 elements constitute 95% of the body's composition: oxygen (65%), carbon (18%), hydrogen (10%), and nitrogen (3%). Other elements that contribute to the composition of the total body in proportions greater than 0.05% are: sodium, potassium, phosphorus, chlorine, calcium, magnesium, and sulfur. The neutron activation method involves a whole-body chamber within which the subject receives a low dose of neutron irradiation. The neutrons interact with body tissues to excite the targeted

element, creating unstable isotopes that emit gamma radiation. A whole-body gamma radiation counter measures the energy emitted and the decay rate to determine the total quantity of the element in the body. The resulting information is used to understand the elemental composition of the body and can also be used to estimate other body compartments based on the known contribution of elements to target tissues. For example, total body nitrogen can be used to estimate lean body mass, and total calcium content can be used to estimate bone mass. This method is completely impractical for use in infants and children because of the risks involved and the very small number of neutron activation chambers available worldwide.

Imaging Technologies

Imaging methods, such as quantitative computed tomography (QCT) and magnetic resonance imaging (MRI), have created new opportunities for understanding the growth and development of body compartments. QCT is an x-ray based technique that relies on the attenuation characteristics of a tissue, determined by the tissue density and chemical composition, to determine the size and density of an organ or tissue compartment.[81] For example, QCT images of the mid-section can be used to determine verte-bral trabecular density[82] or the cross-sectional area of subcutaneous and intra-abdominal fat.[83] MRI uses a powerful magnetic field combine with radio frequency pulses specific to hydrogen to generate signals that can be converted to detailed images of organs and tissues. MRI is safer to use than QCT, because it does not involve radiation exposure. It has been used to estimate the volume of intra-abdominal adipose tissue, as well as intermus-cular adipose tissue, the size of skeletal muscles, and volume of internal organs.[84] Magnetic resonance spectroscopy is a further technological development that has led to breakthroughs in such areas as measurement of intramyocellular and intrahepatic lipid fractions.[85] Of note, both MRI and QCT are costly techniques that require cooperation. Sedation may be required for infants and children to complete these tests, making it undesir-able for many research applications.

Clinical Assessment Tools for Body Composition Assessment

Skinfold Thickness Measurements

Total or regional body fat can be estimated using skinfold thickness, a tech-nique that can be easily performed in the clinical setting or at the bedside. With proper training, this technique is safe, reasonably accurate, rapid, and inexpensive. Skinfold thickness is determined using spring-loaded calipers at standardized measurement sites. The use of Holtain (Holtain, LTD, Cyrmych, UK) or Lange (Cambridge Instruments, Silver Spring, MD) calipers is recommended. Measurements are obtained on the right side, if possible. The triceps skinfold thickness is often measured, because it is an easily accessible site and is generally representative of energy status. When combined with an arm circumference measurement, mid-upper arm fat area and muscle area can be estimated.

To measure triceps skinfold thickness, the child should be upright with his or her right arm hanging down in a relaxed position. The fold of fat and skin is lifted away from the underlying triceps muscle at the same level of the mid-upper arm, where the arm circumference is measured (midway between the acromion and the olecranon with the arm bent at a right angle). While holding the tissue in place, the calipers are placed over the skinfold and released so that they exert a constant pressure on the subcutaneous fat fold. The reading should be taken 3 seconds after releasing the caliper's handles. The subscapular skinfold thickness is a measure of fat stores on the trunk of the body. It is obtained by lifting a skinfold on an inferior lateral diagonal below the inferior angle of the scapula. A strong advantage of these skinfold thickness measures is the availability of excellent pediatric reference data[41,48] (see Table 24.3; Appendix Q-9.1, Q-9.2). In addition, prediction equations to estimate total body fat using triceps and subscapular skinfold thickness can be used.[86,87] Additional equations have been published using 4 skinfold thickness measures—the triceps, biceps, subscapular, and suprailiac skinfolds.[86,88,89] The primary disadvantages of measuring skinfold thickness is the inability to get accurate measurements in obese individuals and the training required to get reproducible measurements.

Air-Displacement Plethysmography

The newest, rapid, noninvasive method for measuring fat and fat-free mass of the total body in infants and children is air-displacement plethysmography.[90–92] The method measures the volume of air displaced by the body. The air displacement plethysmograph contains 2 chambers of known volume; 1 for the patient and the other for measuring changes in pressure as the diaphragm connecting the 2 chambers oscillates. These pressure changes are accurately measured, and displaced volume is determined by invoking Boyle's law, which states that volume and pressure are inversely related. Corrections are made for lung volume and for noncompressible regions around the body, such as hair, and microconvection of air at the skin surface. Because the individual's weight is known and volume is measured, density can be calculated. Body density is then used to estimate the fat and fat-free mass compartments (as in hydrodensitometry). Two versions of this instrument exist at the present time; the Bod Pod (Life Measurement Inc, Concord, CA) is used to measure children and adults, and the Pea Pod is designed for infants weighing up to 8 kg. These instruments are more user-friendly than underwater weighing and can be more easily used in obese individuals than some other clinically available body composition methods. The primary limitations are: (1) it requires the individual to be sealed into a chamber, limiting its use in patients requiring electronic monitoring or continuous infusions; and (2) it involves assumptions about the hydration and mineral composition of fat-free mass. For infants, it is a preferred method because it is safe, rapid, and valid, does not require sedation, and tolerates movement.[93,94]

Dual-Energy X-ray Absorptiometry

Dual-energy x-ray absorptiometry (DXA) is rapidly becoming the preferred method for body composition determination and can be used in infants, children, and adults. The technique uses very low-energy x-rays and measures the attenuation of the x-rays as they pass through tissues of different density.[95] For a given x-ray energy level, tissues such as fat, muscle, and bone have unique attenuation properties. The attenuation is a function of a constant specific to that tissue and the tissue mass. The use of 2 energy beams of different intensity allows for determination of 2 tissue compartments. As the x-ray beam passes over soft tissue regions, the respective masses of lean and fat tissues are determined. As the beam passes over regions that also include bone, the algorithm solves for bone versus soft tissue, assuming that the composition of soft tissue surrounding the bone is similar to the adjacent soft tissue of muscle and fat. In this manner, DXA is able to estimate the mass of lean, fat, and bone mineral from a whole-body DXA scan.[76,96]

Although DXA is widely used as a body composition assessment tool in children, it is not a well-validated technique. Differences between DXA manufacturers and changes in software specifications can have a significant impact on body fat measurements.[97,98] Comparisons of fat estimates by DXA to measurements of a 4-compartment model, an approach that combines total body water, bone mass, and body density measurements, show a systematic bias in pediatric samples such that fatness is overestimated in obese children.[99,100] The increased hydration and lower density of lean mass in obesity may account for this pattern. Because DXA model type and software specifications affect body composition results in children, DXA body composition should not be considered a "gold standard." Despite these limitations, the recent publication of reference values for percent body fat, lean body mass, fat mass index (fat mass (kg) divided by height (m²)) and lean body mass index (lean body mass (kg) divided by height (m²)) from the National Health and Nutrition Examination Survey[101–103] for children 8 years and older has the potential to increase the clinical utility of DXA body composition assessment. DXA can also be used to estimate visceral adipose tissue from whole body scans. This method has been validated in children and adults.[104,105]

DXA is more widely used for the assessment of bone mass and density. Total body and regional DXA scans of the lumbar spine, proximal femur, and forearm are commonly used to determine bone mineral density (BMD) in adults; total body less head and lumbar spine DXA scans are the preferred scan sites for children, although the lateral distal femur scan is an optimal site for children with contractures or metal implants that preclude other scan sites.[106] The spine provides an index of the density of trabecular bone, and the total body scan is largely cortical bone. In addition, total body scans can generate an estimate of total body calcium. Of note, BMD by DXA is not an authentic volumetric density measure, because DXA is a 2-dimensional imaging technique that is not capable of determining the thickness of bone. BMD by DXA is often referred to as areal BMD, because it is based on bone mineral content (BMC) divided by bone area from the 2-dimensional projection. As children grow, BMC increases and bone size increases in 3 dimensions. As a consequence, age-related changes in areal-BMD are largely growth dependent and only partly reflect volumetric BMD changes.[107]

Abnormalities in bone mineral accretion can be attributable to a primary disorder, such as osteogenesis imperfecta, or to secondary disorders, such as preterm birth or diseases associated with inflammation, malabsorption, altered dietary intake, reduced physical activity, or use of medications affecting bone mineral metabolism, such as glucocorticoids.[108] In addition to calcium and vitamin D, other nutrients that may be associated with bone density include vitamin K, phosphorus, zinc, magnesium, and protein intake.[109,110] DXA has several advantages: it is safe (radiation exposure equivalent to background radiation), accurate, reproducible, rapid, and widely available. For children and adolescents, excellent reference data are now available for BMC, BMD,[111] and body composition.[101–103] Limitations of DXA are: (1) it cannot be performed in pregnant females or individuals with indwelling hardware within scan regions; (2) most DXA devices have an upper weight limit, so total body and spine scans cannot be acquired in very obese individuals; (3) it requires cooperation without movement for short time periods (depending on the scan); and (4) it assumes a constant tissue composition of fat, lean, and bone.

Bioelectrical Impedance Analysis

Bioelectrical impedance analysis (BIA) is a portable, inexpensive method of body composition that is often used in survey type research studies and is becoming somewhat popular in settings such as exercise programs. The method is based on the principle that electrical currents are conducted through the water and electrolytes in the body. The impedance to electrical flow is directly proportional to the amount of lean tissue present; prediction equations translate the measured resistance to estimates of fat and fat free mass. The prediction equations were developed by validation studies that compared BIA to measures of body composition derived from other techniques, such as hydrodensitometry and/or total body water measurement by isotope dilution in adults. The validity of the prediction equations is not always well established and may vary as a function of ethnicity[112] obesity status,[113] age,[114] or health condition.[115] BIA does not measure bone mass.

BIAs come in several forms. The original devices used 4 electrodes, 2 placed on the hand and 2 placed on the foot. Devices with 8 electrodes have also been used. Because these designs allow flexibility in the placement location of the electrodes, they can be used to assess total and appendicular body composition.[116] There are now foot-to-foot analyzers, hand-to-hand analyzers,[117] and a model that combines both.[112]

Small changes in body water, such as normal diurnal variation, appear to make significant differences in the estimate of lean body mass. For models using electrodes, proper placement of the source and detectors electrodes is critical and can be problematic in very small children. The changing water content and distribution of the lean body mass of growing children should cause the impedance to change progressively with age, making this method extremely difficult to calibrate for children.[78] Various modifications are being made to these instruments in an attempt to enhance their precision.

Multifrequency BIA and bioelectrical impedance spectroscopy operate on principles similar to single-frequency BIA. The difference resides in the frequencies. At low frequency (<5 kHz), the impedance to current flow is an index of extracellular water, because this frequency does not penetrate the cell membrane. At higher frequencies, the cell membrane no longer acts as a

VI

capacitor, and the intracellular water also conducts current, thereby reducing impedance at higher frequencies. Thus, total body water and extracellular water are estimated by impedance, and intracellular water is derived from these 2 measures. As with single-frequency BIA devices, prediction equations are needed to convert the measured impedance to body water and body composition estimates. Typically, these prediction equations are based on healthy individuals with normal nutritional status and may not be applicable to patients outside the age range, those with health conditions that affect fluid balance, or those at the extremes of nutritional status. They also fail to account for variability in the contribution of bone mass to fat-free mass. Thus, although promising, these methods are not yet sufficiently accurate for use in monitoring individual clinical patients but may be useful for studying group characteristics.[118]

Laboratory Assessment

The initial laboratory assessment of nutritional status includes the measurement of hematologic status and protein nutrition. The absence of anemia may not exclude nutritional deficiencies, such as iron, folate, and vitamin B_{12} deficiencies. Red blood cell size is valuable in the differential diagnosis of anemias. Albumin concentration is a better measure of protein nutrition than is serum globulin concentration, because its biologic half-life is shorter (approximately 20 days). A low albumin concentration occurs with malnutrition, in liver disease, or when albumin is lost from the body in large amounts, as in nephrosis, protein-losing enteropathy, burns, or surgical drains. The so-called visceral proteins synthesized by the liver (such as retinol-binding protein with a half-life of 12 hours, transthyretin [prealbumin] with a half-life of 1.9 days, and transferrin with a half-life of 8 days) have shorter half-lives than does albumin, and their concentrations are better indicators of shorter-term protein status (ie, anabolism or catabolism) than is the serum albumin concentration. Serum concentrations of essential amino acids may be lower than those of nonessential amino acids, and 3-methyl histidine excretion is increased during states of protein insufficiency. Other abnormalities of protein depletion include a decreased creatinine concentration and decreased hydroxyproline excretion. Values for protein status may or may not reflect the degree of nutritional deficiency. In simple starvation (marasmus), a tendency to maintain the circulatory pool of visceral proteins at the expense of somatic protein is evident. The blood urea nitrogen concentration tends to decrease during starvation; however, in patients in whom water intake is restricted, such as those with anorexia nervosa, the serum concentration may be elevated.

Serum sodium concentration is frequently decreased in malnutrition as the result of dilution, because total body water is physiologically increased during starvation. This value is seldom lower than 133 mEq/L, however. The dilution effect can also be seen with hematologic parameters, such as hematocrit and hemoglobin concentrations. Immunologic abnormalities, such as loss of delayed hypersensitivity, fewer T-lymphocytes, and changes in lymphocyte response to in vitro stimulation by phytohemagglutinin, are sometimes helpful clinical measurements of nutritional status.

Assays of specific nutrients can be helpful in the assessment of the nutritional status of an individual, but their usefulness is limited by their wide variation within normal groups and the lack of easy availability of many of the vitamin assays. Normal values for some of these biochemical measurements are shown in Table 24.5. Other vitamins, such as biotin and niacin, as well as essential fatty acids, can be measured, but these measurements are seldom clinically indicated. Assessment of the concentrations of minerals, such as calcium, magnesium, phosphorus, iodine, copper, and selenium, is readily available in most laboratories and sometimes is important to measure as part of the nutritional assessment.

VI

Table 24.5.

Normal Values: Biochemical Measurement of Specific Nutritional Parameters

Test	Age	Normal Range Male	Normal Range Female
Protein, blood			
Serum albumin, g/dL[a]	Day 0–5	2.6–3.6	2.6–3.6
	Day 6–30	2.8–4.0	2.8–4.0
	1–6 mo	3.1–4.2	3.1–4.2
	7–11 mo	3.3–4.3	3.3–4.3
	1–3 y	3.5–4.6	3.5–4.6
	4–6 y	3.5–5.2	3.5–5.2
	7–19 y	3.7–5.6	3.7–5.6
	20+ y	3.5–5.0	3.5–5.0
Retinol binding protein, mg/dL[b]		3.0–6.0	3.0–6.0
Blood urea nitrogen, mg/dL[a]	0–2 y	2.0–19.0	2.0–19.0
	3–12 y	5.0–17.0	5.0–17.0
	13–18 y	7.0–18.0	7.0–18.0
	19–20 y	8.0–21.0	8.0–21.0
	21+ y	9.0–20.0	7.0–17.0
Transferrin, mg/dL[a]		180–370	180–370
Prealbumin, mg/dL[a]	0–11 mo	6.0–21.0	6.0–21.0
	1–5 y	14.0–30.0	14.0–30.0
	6–9 y	15.0–33.0	15.0–33.0
	10–13 y	20.0–36.0	20.0–36.0
	14+ y	22.0–45.0	22.0–45.0
Protein, urine			
Creatinine/height index		>0.9	>0.9

Table 24.5. *Continued*

Normal Values: Biochemical Measurement of Specific Nutritional Parameters

Test	Age	Normal Range	
		Male	**Female**
3-methyl histidine, nmol/mg creatinine[a]	Day 1–6	81–384	81–384
	Day 7–8 wk	75–430	75–430
	9 wk–12 mo	142–377	142–377
	13 mo–3 y	134–647	134–647
	4+ y	93–323	93–323
Creatinine (24-h), mg/d[b]	0–2 y	NA	NA
	3–8 y	140–700	140–700
	9–12 y	300–1300	300–1300
	13–17 y	500–2300	400–1600
	18–50 y	1000–2500	700–1600
Hydroxyproline index		>2	>2
Vitamin A			
Serum or plasma retinol, μg/dL[b]	0–1 mo	18–50	18–50
	2 mo–12 y	20–50	20–50
	13 y–17 y	26–70	26–70
	18+ y	30–120	30–120
Vitamin D			
25-OH-D$_3$, ng/mL[a]		>20	>20
1-25-OH-D$_3$, pg/mL[b]		15–75	15–75
Folic acid			

Continued

VI

Table 24.5. *Continued*

Normal Values: Biochemical Measurement of Specific Nutritional Parameters

		Normal Range	
Test	**Age**	**Male**	**Female**
Serum folate, ng/mL[a]	0–1 y	7.2–22.4	6.3–22.7
	2–3 y	2.5–15.0	1.7–15.7
	4–6 y	0.5–13.0	2.7–14.1
	7–9 y	2.3–11.9	2.4–13.4
	10–12 y	1.5–10.8	1.0–10.2
	13–17 y	1.2–8.8	1.2–7.2
	18+ y	2.8–13.5	2.8–13.0
Red blood cell folate, ng/mL[b]		280–903	280–903
Vitamin K			
Prothrombin time, sec[a]	0–5 mo	NA	NA
	6+ mo	11.7–13.2	11.7–13.2
Vitamin E			
Serum or plasma α-tocopherol, mg/L[a]	0–1 mo	1.0–3.5	1.0–3.5
	2–5 mo	2.0–6.0	2.0–6.0
	6–12 mo	3.5–8.0	3.5–8.0
	2–12 y	5.5–9.0	5.5–9.0
	13+ y	5.5–18.0	5.5–18.0
Vitamin C			
Plasma vitamin C, mg/dL[b]		0.4–2.0	0.4–2.0
Vitamin B_{12}			
Serum vitamin B_{12}, pg/mL[a]	0–1 y	293–1208	228–1514
	2–3 y	264–1216	416–1209
	4–6 y	245–1078	313–1407
	7–9 y	271–1170	247–1174
	10–12 y	183–1088	197–1019
	13–17 y	214–865	182–820
	18+ y	199–732	199–732

Table 24.5. *Continued*

Normal Values: Biochemical Measurement of Specific Nutritional Parameters

Test	Age	Normal Range Male	Normal Range Female
Iron			
Hematocrit, %[a]	Day 0	42.0–60.0	42.0–60.0
	Day 1–29	45.0–65.0	45.0–65.0
	1–2 mo	31.0–55.0	31.0–55.0
	3–5 mo	29.0–41.0	29.0–41.0
	6–12 mo	33.0–39.0	33.0–39.0
	2–5 y	34.0–40.0	34.0–40.0
	6–11 y	35.0–45.0	35.0–45.0
	12–17 y	37.0–49.0	36.0–46.0
	18+ y	41.0–52.0	36.0–46.0
Hemoglobin, g/dL[a]	Day 0	13.5–19.5	13.5–19.5
	Day 1–29	14.5–22.0	14.5–22.0
	1–2 mo	10.0–18.0	10.0–18.0
	3–5 mo	9.5–13.5	9.5–13.5
	6–12 mo	10.5–13.5	10.5–13.5
	2–5 y	11.5–13.5	11.5–13.5
	6–11 y	11.5–15.5	11.5–15.5
	12–17 y	13.0–16.0	12.0–16.0
	18+ y	13.5–17.0	12.0–16.0
Serum ferritin, ng/mL[b]	0–6 mo	6–400	6–430
	7–35 mo	12–57	12–60
	3–14 y	14–80	12–73
	15–19 y	20–155	12–90
	20–29 y	38–270	12–114

Continued

VI

Table 24.5. *Continued*

Normal Values: Biochemical Measurement of Specific Nutritional Parameters

		Normal Range	
Test	Age	Male	Female
Serum iron, μg/dL[b]	0–6 wk	100–250	100–250
	7 wk–11 mo	40–100	40–100
	1 yr–10 y	50–120	50–120
	11+ y	50–170	30–160
Serum total iron binding capacity, μg/dL[b]	0–2 mo	59–175	59–175
	3 mo–17 y	250–400	250–400
	18+ y	240–450	240–450
Serum transferrin saturation, %[b]		20–50	20–50
Serum transferrin, mg/dL[a]		180–370	180–370
Erythrocyte porphyrin (whole blood), μg/dL[b]		0–35	0–35
Zinc			
Serum zinc, μg/dL[a]	0–16 y	66–144	66–144
	17+ y	75–291	65–256
Phosphorus			
Serum phosphate, mg/dL[a]	Day 0–11 mo	4.8–8.2	4.8–8.2
	1–3 y	3.8–6.5	3.8–6.5
	4–6 y	4.1–5.4	4.1–5.4
	7–11 y	3.7–5.6	3.7–5.6
	12–13 y	3.3–5.4	3.3–5.4
	14–15 y	2.9–5.4	2.9–5.4
	16–20 y	2.7–4.7	2.7–4.7
	21+ y	2.5–4.5	2.5–4.5

Table 24.5. *Continued*

Normal Values: Biochemical Measurement of Specific Nutritional Parameters

Test	Age	Normal Range Male	Normal Range Female
Calcium			
Serum total calcium, mg/dL[a]	Day 0	6.9–9.4	6.9–9.4
	Day 1–6	8.0–11.4	8.0–11.4
	Day 7–13	8.0–11.2	8.0–11.2
	Day 14–29	9.3–10.9	9.3–10.9
	1 mo	9.3–10.7	9.3–10.7
	2 mo	9.3–10.6	9.3–10.6
	3–4 mo	9.2–10.5	9.2–10.5
	5–11 mo	9.2–10.4	9.2–10.4
	1–3 y	8.7–9.8	8.7–9.8
	4–20 y	8.8–10.1	8.8–10.1
	21+ y	8.4–10.2	8.4–10.2
Serum ionized calcium, mmol/L[a]	Day 0	1.07–1.27	1.07–1.27
	Day 1–1 y	1.00–1.17	1.00–1.17
	2–4 y	1.21–1.37	1.21–1.37
	5–17 y	1.15–1.34	1.15–1.34
	18+ y	1.12–1.3	1.12–1.3
Magnesium			
Serum magnesium, mg/dL[a]	0–20 y	1.5–2.5	1.5–2.5
	21+ y	1.6–2.3	1.6–2.3

Continued

VI

Table 24.5. *Continued*

Normal Values: Biochemical Measurement of Specific Nutritional Parameters

Test	Age	Normal Range Male	Female
Copper			
Serum copper, μg/dL[b]	0–6 mo	20–70	20–70
	7 mo–18 y	90–190	90–190
	19+ y	70–140	80–155
Selenium			
Serum selenium, μg/L[b]		23–190	23–190

NA indicates not available.

[a] Laboratory values from the clinical laboratories at Children's Hospital of Philadelphia (2011).

[b] Laboratory values retrieved from ARUP laboratories at http://www.aruplab.com/ (June 27, 2011).

References

1. Fomon SM. *Nutritional Disorders of Children: Prevention, Screening, and Followup.* Bethesda: Department of Health and Human Services; 1977. DHEW Publication No. HSA 77–5104

2. Gibson RS. Measuring food consumption of individuals. In: *Principles of Nutritional Assessment.* 2nd ed. Oxford, England: University Press; 2005:41–64

3. Baker JP, Detsky AS, Wesson DE, et al. Nutritional assessment: a comparison of clinical judgement and objective measurements. *N Engl J Med.* 1982;306(16): 969–972

4. Cameron N. The use and abuse of growth charts. In: Johnston F, Zemel B, Eveleth P, eds. *Human Growth in Context.* London, England: Smith Gordon and Company, Limited; 1999:65–74

5. de Onis M, Onyango AW, Borghi E, Garza C, Yang H, S WMGR. Comparison of the World Health Organization (WHO) Child Growth Standards and the National Center for Health Statistics/WHO international growth reference: implications for child health programmes. *Public Health Nutr.* Oct 2006;9(7): 942–947

6. Alexander GR, Himes JH, Kaufman RB, Mor J, Kogan M. A United States national reference for fetal growth. *Obstet Gynecol.* 1996;87(2):163–168

7. Arbuckle TE, Wilkins R, Sherman GJ. Birth weight percentiles by gestational age in Canada. *Obstet Gynecol.* 1993;81(1):39–48

8. Babson SG, Benda GI. Growth graphs for the clinical assessment of infants of varying gestational age. *J Pediatr.* 1976;89(5):814–820

9. Bonellie S, Chalmers J, Gray R, Greer I, Jarvis S, Williams C. Centile charts for birthweight for gestational age for Scottish singleton births. *BMC Pregnancy Childbirth.* 2008;8:5

10. Fenton TR. A new growth chart for preterm babies: Babson and Benda's chart updated with recent data and a new format. *BMC Pediatr.* 2003;3(1):13

11. Kramer MS, Platt RW, Wen SW, et al. A new and improved population-based Canadian reference for birth weight for gestational age. *Pediatrics.* 2001;108(2):E35

12. Lubchenco LO, Hansman C, Boyd E. Intrauterine growth in length and head circumference as estimated from live births at gestational ages from 26 to 42 weeks. *Pediatrics.* 1966;37(3):403–408

13. Lubchenco LO, Hansman C, Dressler M, Boyd E. Intrauterine growth as estimated from liveborn birth-weight data at 24 to 42 weeks of gestation. *Pediatrics.* 1963;32:793–800

14. Niklasson A, Albertsson-Wikland K. Continuous growth reference from 24th week of gestation to 24 months by gender. *BMC Pediatr.* 2008;8:8

15. Oken E, Kleinman KP, Rich-Edwards J, Gillman MW. A nearly continuous measure of birth weight for gestational age using a United States national reference. *BMC Pediatr.* Jul 8 2003;3:6

16. Olsen IE, Groveman SA, Lawson ML, Clark RH, Zemel BS. New intrauterine growth curves based on United States data. *Pediatrics.* 2010;125(2):e214–e224

17. Riddle WR, DonLevy SC, Qi XF, Giuse DA, Rosenbloom ST. Equations to support predictive automated postnatal growth curves for premature infants. *J Perinatol.* 2006;26(6):354–358

18. Bukowski R, Gahn D, Denning J, Saade G. Impairment of growth in fetuses destined to deliver preterm. *Am J Obstet Gynecol.* 2001;185(2):463–467

19. Doubilet PM, Benson CB, Wilkins-Haug L, Ringer S. Fetuses subsequently born premature are smaller than gestational age-matched fetuses not born premature. *J Ultrasound Med.* 2003;22(4):359–363

20. Ehrenkranz RA. Estimated fetal weights versus birth weights: should the reference intrauterine growth curves based on birth weights be retired? *Arch Dis Child Fetal Neonatal Ed.* 2007;92(3):F161–F162

21. Moyer-Mileur LJ. Anthropometric and laboratory assessment of very low birth weight infants: the most helpful measurements and why. *Semin Perinatol.* 2007;31(2):96–103

22. Rao SC, Tompkins J. Growth curves for preterm infants. *Early Hum Dev.* 2007;83(10):643–651

23. Villar J, Cheikh Ismail L, Victora CG, et al. International standards for newborn weight, length, and head circumference by gestational age and sex: the Newborn Cross-Sectional Study of the INTERGROWTH-21st Project. *Lancet.* 2014;384(9946):857–868.

VI

24. Engle WA, American Academy of Pediatrics Committee on F, Newborn. Age terminology during the perinatal period. *Pediatrics*. 2004;114(5):1362–1364

25. Fenton TR, Kim JH. A systematic review and meta-analysis to revise the Fenton growth chart for preterm infants. *BMC Pediatr*. 2013;13:59

26. WHO Child Growth Standards based on length/height, weight and age. *Acta Paediatr Suppl*. 2006;450:76–85

27. Villar J, Giuliani F, Fenton TR, et al. INTERGROWTH-21st very preterm size at birth reference charts (Correspondence). *Lancet*. 2016;387(10021):844–845

28. Fenton TR, Nasser R, Eliasziw M, Kim JH, Bilan D, Sauve R. Validating the weight gain of preterm infants between the reference growth curve of the fetus and the term infant. *BMC Pediatr*. 2013;13:92

29. Olsen IE, Lawson ML, Clark RH, Spitzer AR. An alternate perspective on creating NICU growth charts (comment). *BMC Pediatr*. 2013;13:59

30. Olsen IE, Lawson ML, Ferguson AN, et al. BMI curves for preterm infants. *Pediatrics*. 2015;135(3):e572–e581

31. Ehrenkranz RA, Younes N, Lemons JA, et al. Longitudinal growth of hospitalized very low birth weight infants. *Pediatrics*. 1999;104(2 Pt 1):280–289

32. Guo SS, Roche AF, Chumlea WC, Casey PH, Moore WM. Growth in weight, recumbent length, and head circumference for preterm low-birthweight infants during the first three years of life using gestation-adjusted ages. *Early Hum Dev*. 1997;47(3):305–325

33. Guo SS, Wholihan K, Roche AF, Chumlea WC, Casey PH. Weight-for-length reference data for preterm, low-birth-weight infants. *Arch Pediatr Adolesc Med*. 1996;150(9):964–970

34. Casey PH, Kraemer HC, Bernbaum J, Yogman MW, Sells JC. Growth status and growth rates of a varied sample of low birth weight, preterm infants: a longitudinal cohort from birth to three years of age. *J Pediatr*. 1991;119(4):599–605

35. Villar J, Giuliani F, Bhutta ZA, et al. Postnatal growth standards for preterm infants: the Preterm Postnatal Follow-up Study of the INTERGROWTH-21(st) Project. *Lancet Glob Health*. 2015;3(11):e681–691

36. Williamson AL, Derado J, Barney B, et al. Longitudinal BMI growth curves for surviving preterm NICU infants based on a large US sample. *Pediatrics*. 2018;142(3):e20174169

37. Daly-Wolfe KM, Jordan KC, Slater H, Beachy JC, Moyer-Mileur LJ. Mid-arm circumference is a reliable method to estimate adiposity in preterm and term infants. *Pediatr Res*. 2015;78(3):336–341

38. Ashton JJ, Johnson MJ, Pond J, et al. Assessing the growth of preterm infants using detailed anthropometry. *Acta Paediatr*. 2017;106(6):889–896

39. Kuczmarski RJ, Ogden CL, Grummer-Strawn LM, et al. CDC growth charts: United States. *Adv Data*. 2000(314):1-27

40. Grummer-Strawn LM, Reinold C, Krebs NF. Use of World Health Organization and CDC growth charts for children aged 0–59 months in the United States. *MMWR Recomm Rep*. 2010;59(RR-9):1–15

41. WHO Multicentre Growth Reference Study Group. WHO Child Growth Standards: Head circumference-for-age, arm circumference-for-age, triceps skinfold-for-age and subscapular skinfold-for-age: Methods and development. 2007. Accessed June 9, 2011

42. WHO Multicentre Growth Reference Study Group. WHO Child Growth Standards: Growth velocity based on weight, length and head circumference: Methods and development. 2009. Accessed June 9, 2011

43. Centers for Disease Control and Prevention. Clinical Growth Charts. Available at: http://www.cdc.gov/growthcharts/clinical_charts.htm#Summary. Accessed June 9, 2011

44. Baumgartner RN, Roche AF, Himes JH. Incremental growth tables: supplementary to previously published charts. *Am J Clin Nutr*. 1986;43(5):711–722

45. Berkey CS, Dockery DW, Wang X, Wypij D, Ferris B, Jr. Longitudinal height velocity standards for U.S. adolescents. *Stat Med*. 1993;12(3-4):403–414

46. Tanner JM, Davies PS. Clinical longitudinal standards for height and height velocity for North American children. *J Pediatr*. 1985;107(3):317–329

47. Kelly A, Winer KK, Kalkwarf H, et al. Age-based reference ranges for annual height velocity in US children. *J Clin Endocrinol Metab*. 2014;99(6):2104–2112

48. Addo OY, Himes JH. Reference curves for triceps and subscapular skinfold thicknesses in US children and adolescents. *Am J Clin Nutr*. 2010;91(3):635–642

49. Addo OY, Himes JH, Zemel BS. Reference ranges for midupper arm circumference, upper arm muscle area, and upper arm fat area in US children and adolescents aged 1-20 y. *Am J Clin Nutr*. Jan 2017;105(1):111–120.

50. Lampl M, Thompson AL, Frongillo EA. Sex differences in the relationships among weight gain, subcutaneous skinfold tissue and saltatory length growth spurts in infancy. *Pediatr Res*. 2005;58(6):1238–1242

51. Hamill PV, Drizd TA, Johnson CL, Reed RB, Roche AF. NCHS growth curves for children birth-18 years. United States. *Vital Health Stat 11*. 1977(165):i–iv, 1–74

52. Himes JH, Roche AF, Thissen D, Moore WM. Parent-specific adjustments for evaluation of recumbent length and stature of children. *Pediatrics*. 1985;75(2): 304–313

53. Zhang Z, Shoff SM, Lai HJ. Incorporating genetic potential when evaluating stature in children with cystic fibrosis. *J Cyst Fibros*. 2010;9(2):135–142

54. Tanner JM, Goldstein H, Whitehouse RH. Standards for Children's Height at Age 2 to 9 years allowing for height of Parents. *Arch Dis Child*. 1970;45(244):819

55. Chumlea WC, Guo SS, Steinbaugh ML. Prediction of stature from knee height for black and white adults and children with application to mobility-impaired or handicapped persons. *J Am Diet Assoc*. 1994;94(12):1385–1388, 1391; quiz 1389–1390

56. Gauld LM, Kappers J, Carlin JB, Robertson CF. Height prediction from ulna length. *Dev Med Child Neurol*. 2004;46(7):475–480

57. Roy SM, Spivack JG, Faith MS, et al. Infant BMI or weight-for-length and obesity risk in early childhood. *Pediatrics*. 2016;137(5):e20153492

VI

58. Cole TJ, Henson GL, Tremble JM, Colley NV. Birthweight for length: ponderal index, body mass index or Benn index? *Ann Hum Biol.* 1997;24(4):289–298

59. Olsen IE, Lawson ML, Meinzen-Derr J, et al. Use of a body proportionality index for growth assessment of preterm infants. *J Pediatr.* 2009;154(4):486–491

60. Ramel SE, Zhang L, Misra S, Anderson CG, Demerath EW. Do anthropometric measures accurately reflect body composition in preterm infants? *Pediatr Obes.* 2017;12(Suppl 1):72–77

61. Villar J, Puglia FA, Fenton TR, et al. Body composition at birth and its relationship with neonatal anthropometric ratios: the newborn body composition study of the INTERGROWTH-21st project. *Pediatr Res.* 2017;82(2): 305–316

62. Centers for Disease Control and Prevention. About BMI for Children and Teens. Available at: http://www.cdc.gov/healthyweight/assessing/bmi/childrens_bmi/about_childrens_bmi.html#How%20is%20BMI%20calculated>. Accessed June 15, 2011

63. Krebs NF, Jacobson MS. Prevention of pediatric overweight and obesity. *Pediatrics.* 2003;112(2):424–430

64. Flegal KM, Wei R, Ogden CL, Freedman DS, Johnson CL, Curtin LR. Characterizing extreme values of body mass index-for-age by using the 2000 Centers for Disease Control and Prevention growth charts. *Am J Clin Nutr.* 2009;90(5):1314–1320

65. Gulati AK, Kaplan DW, Daniels SR. Clinical tracking of severely obese children: a new growth chart. *Pediatrics.* 2012;130(6):1136–1140

66. Freedman DS, Butte NF, Taveras EM, et al. BMI z-Scores are a poor indicator of adiposity among 2- to 19-year-olds with very high BMIs, NHANES 1999–2000 to 2013–2014. *Obesity (Silver Spring).* 2017;25(4):739–746

67. Benn RT. Some mathematical properties of weight-for-height indices used as measures of adiposity. *Br J Prev Soc Med.* 1971;25(1):42–50

68. Cole TJ, Green PJ. Smoothing reference centile curves: the LMS method and penalized likelihood. *Stat Med.* 1992;11(10):1305–1319

69. Mehta NM, Compher C, Directors ASPENBo. A.S.P.E.N. Clinical Guidelines: nutrition support of the critically ill child. *JPEN J Parenter Enteral Nutr.* 2009;33(3): 260–276

70. Lohman TG. Skinfolds and body density and their relation to body fatness: a review. *Hum Biol.* 1981;53(2):181–225

71. Siri W. The gross composition of the body. In: Tobias C, Lawrence JH, ed. *Advances in Biological and Medical Physics.* Vol 4. New York: Academic Press; 1956: 239–280

72. Wells JC, Williams JE, Chomtho S, et al. Pediatric reference data for lean tissue properties: density and hydration from age 5 to 20 y. *Am J Clin Nutr.* 2010;91(3): 610–618

73. Heymsfield SB, Wang Z, Baumgartner RN, Ross R. Human body composition: advances in models and methods. *Annu Rev Nutr.* 1997;17:527–558

74. Forbes GB, Schultz F, Cafarelli C, Amirhakimi GH. Effects of body size on potassium-40 measurement in the whole body counter (tilt-chair technique). *Health Phys.* 1968;15(5):435–442

75. Remenchik AP, Miller CE, Kessler WV. Body composition estimates derived from potassium measurements. ANL-7461. *ANL Rep.* 1968:73–90

76. Ellis KJ. Human body composition: in vivo methods. *Physiol Rev.* 2000;80(2):649–680

77. Schoeller D. Hydrometry. In: Roche A, Heymsfield SB, Lohman TG, ed. *Human Body Composition*. Champaign, IL: Human Kinetics; 1996:25–43

78. Wells JC, Fuller NJ, Dewit O, Fewtrell MS, Elia M, Cole TJ. Four-component model of body composition in children: density and hydration of fat-free mass and comparison with simpler models. *Am J Clin Nutr.* 1999;69(5):904–912

79. Haroun D, Wells JC, Williams JE, Fuller NJ, Fewtrell MS, Lawson MS. Composition of the fat-free mass in obese and nonobese children: matched case-control analyses. *Int J Obes (Lond).* 2005;29(1):29–36

80. Ellis L. Whole-body counting and neutron activation analysis. In: Roche AF, Lohman TG, eds. *Human Body Composition*. Champaign, IL: Human Kinetics; 1996:45–61

81. Heymsfield SB, Fulenwider T, Nordlinger B, Barlow R, Sones P, Kutner M. Accurate measurement of liver, kidney, and spleen volume and mass by computerized axial tomography. *Ann Intern Med.* 1979;90(2):185–187

82. Gilsanz V. Bone density in children: a review of the available techniques and indications. *Eur J Radiol.* 1998;26(2):177–182

83. Goran MI, Bergman RN, Gower BA. Influence of total vs. visceral fat on insulin action and secretion in African American and white children. *Obes Res.* 2001;9(8):423–431

84. Lee SY, Gallagher D. Assessment methods in human body composition. *Curr Opin Clin Nutr Metab Care.* 2008;11(5):566–572

85. Shen W, Liu H, Punyanitya M, Chen J, Heymsfield SB. Pediatric obesity phenotyping by magnetic resonance methods. *Curr Opin Clin Nutr Metab Care.* 2005;8(6):595–601

86. Wendel D, Weber D, Leonard MB, et al. Body composition estimation using skinfolds in children with and without health conditions affecting growth and body composition. *Ann Hum Biol.* 2017;44(2):108–120

87. Slaughter MH, Lohman TG, Boileau RA, et al. Skinfold equations for estimation of body fatness in children and youth. *Hum Biol.* 1988;60(5):709–723

88. Brook CG. Determination of body composition of children from skinfold measurements. *Arch Dis Child.* 1971;46(246):182–184

89. Durnin J, Rahaman M. The assessment of the amount of fat in the human body from measurements of skinfold thickness. *Br J Nutr.* 1967;21:681–689

90. Dempster P, Aitkens S. A new air displacement method for the determination of human body composition. *Med Sci Sports Exerc.* 1995;27(12):1692–1697

VI

91. Dewit O, Fuller NJ, Fewtrell MS, Elia M, Wells JC. Whole body air displacement plethysmography compared with hydrodensitometry for body composition analysis. *Arch Dis Child.* 2000;82(2):159–164

92. Fields DA, Gilchrist JM, Catalano PM, Gianni ML, Roggero PM, Mosca F. Longitudinal body composition data in exclusively breast-fed infants: a multicenter study. *Obesity (Silver Spring).* 2011;19(9):1887–1891

93. Ellis KJ, Yao M, Shypailo RJ, Urlando A, Wong WW, Heird WC. Body-composition assessment in infancy: air-displacement plethysmography compared with a reference 4-compartment model. *Am J Clin Nutr.* 2007;85(1): 90–95

94. Hawkes CP, Zemel BS, Kiely M, et al. Body Composition within the First 3 Months: Optimized Correction for Length and Correlation with BMI at 2 Years. *Horm Res Paediatr.* 2016;86(3):178–187

95. Laskey MA. Dual-energy X-ray absorptiometry and body composition. *Nutrition.* 1996;12(1):45–51

96. Prentice A. Application of dual energy x-ray absorptiometry and related techniques to the assessment of bone and body composition. In: Davies PaCT, ed. *Body Composition Techniques in Health and Disease. Society for the Study of Human Biology Symposium 36.* Cambridge: Cambridge University Press; 1995:1–13

97. Pearson D, Horton B, Green DJ. Cross calibration of Hologic QDR2000 and GE Lunar Prodigy for whole body bone mineral density and body composition measurements. *J Clin Densitom.* 2011;14(3):294–301

98. Shypailo RJ, Butte NF, Ellis KJ. DXA: can it be used as a criterion reference for body fat measurements in children? *Obesity (Silver Spring).* 2008;16(2):457–462

99. Sopher AB, Thornton JC, Wang J, Pierson RN, Jr., Heymsfield SB, Horlick M. Measurement of percentage of body fat in 411 children and adolescents: a comparison of dual-energy X-ray absorptiometry with a four-compartment model. *Pediatrics.* 2004;113(5):1285–1290

100. Wells JC, Haroun D, Williams JE, et al. Evaluation of DXA against the four-component model of body composition in obese children and adolescents aged 5-21 years. *Int J Obes (Lond).* 2010;34(4):649–655

101. Ogden CL, Li Y, Freedman DS, Borrud LG, Flegal KM. Smoothed percentage body fat percentiles for U.S. children and adolescents, 1999–2004. *Natl Health Stat Report.* 2011(43):1–7

102. Weber DR, Moore RH, Leonard MB, Zemel BS. Fat and lean BMI reference curves in children and adolescents and their utility in identifying excess adiposity compared with BMI and percentage body fat. *Am J Clin Nutr.* 2013;98(1): 49–56

103. Kelly TL, Wilson KE, Heymsfield SB. Dual energy X-Ray absorptiometry body composition reference values from NHANES. *PLoS One.* 2009;4(9):e7038

104. Bosch TA, Dengel DR, Kelly AS, Sinaiko AR, Moran A, Steinberger J. Visceral adipose tissue measured by DXA correlates with measurement by CT and is associated with cardiometabolic risk factors in children. *Pediatr Obes.* 2015;10(3): 172–179

105. Micklesfield LK, Goedecke JH, Punyanitya M, Wilson KE, Kelly TL. Dual-energy X-ray performs as well as clinical computed tomography for the measurement of visceral fat. *Obesity (Silver Spring).* 2012;20(5):1109–1114

106. Crabtree NJ, Arabi A, Bachrach LK, et al. Dual-energy X-ray absorptiometry interpretation and reporting in children and adolescents: the revised 2013 ISCD Pediatric Official Positions. *J Clin Densitom.* 2014;17(2):225–242

107. Wren TA, Liu X, Pitukcheewanont P, Gilsanz V. Bone acquisition in healthy children and adolescents: comparisons of dual-energy x-ray absorptiometry and computed tomography measures. *J Clin Endocrinol Metab.* 2005;90(4):1925–1928

108. Leonard MB, Zemel BS. Current concepts in pediatric bone disease. *Pediatr Clin North Am.* 2002;49(1):143–173

109. Bounds W, Skinner J, Carruth BR, Ziegler P. The relationship of dietary and lifestyle factors to bone mineral indexes in children. *J Am Diet Assoc.* 2005;105(5): 735–741

110. Jesudason D, Clifton P. The interaction between dietary protein and bone health. *J Bone Miner Metab.* 2011;29(1):1–14

111. Zemel BS, Kalkwarf HJ, Gilsanz V, et al. Revised reference curves for bone mineral content and areal bone mineral density according to age and sex for black and non-black children: results of the bone mineral density in childhood study. *J Clin Endocrinol Metab.* 2011;96(10):3160–3169

112. Haroun D, Croker H, Viner RM, et al. Validation of BIA in obese children and adolescents and re-evaluation in a longitudinal study. *Obesity (Silver Spring).* 2009;17(12):2245–2250

113. Sluyter JD, Schaaf D, Scragg RK, Plank LD. Prediction of fatness by standing 8-electrode bioimpedance: a multiethnic adolescent population. *Obesity (Silver Spring).* 2010;18(1):183–189

114. Clasey JL, Bradley KD, Bradley JW, Long DE, Griffith JR. A new BIA equation estimating the body composition of young children. *Obesity (Silver Spring).* 16 2011

115. Puiman PJ, Francis P, Buntain H, Wainwright C, Masters B, Davies PS. Total body water in children with cystic fibrosis using bioelectrical impedance. *J Cyst Fibros.* 2004;3(4):243–247

116. Kriemler S, Puder J, Zahner L, Roth R, Braun-Fahrlander C, Bedogni G. Cross-validation of bioelectrical impedance analysis for the assessment of body composition in a representative sample of 6- to 13-year-old children. *Eur J Clin Nutr.* 2009;63(5):619–626

117. Erceg DN, Dieli-Conwright CM, Rossuello AE, Jensky NE, Sun S, Schroeder ET. The Stayhealthy bioelectrical impedance analyzer predicts body fat in children and adults. *Nutr Res.* 2010;30(5):297–304

118. Buchholz AC, Bartok C, Schoeller DA. The validity of bioelectrical impedance models in clinical populations. *Nutr Clin Pract.* 2004;19(5):433–446

119. Stevenson RD. Use of segmental measures to estimate stature in children with cerebral palsy. *Arch Pediatr Adolesc Med.* 1995;149(6):658–662

VI

Chapter 25

Pediatric Feeding and Swallowing Disorders

Introduction

Feeding is an extremely complex activity that involves a variety of unique inputs and requires some very precise skills. A commonly overlooked aspect of feeding is the cultural background. These are the particular tastes and activities associated with meals that are unique to a family unit and are dependent on the family's history and experiences.[1] Then there are the children themselves, who have a unique personality with taste and texture preferences that often change as the child matures.[2] These factors are layered with the biology and physiology involved in feeding and then swallowing. There are a variety of precisely timed steps involved in feeding and swallowing and therefore, many potential opportunities for subtle dysfunction. Feeding problems are never as simple as just biology/anatomy or solely behavioral but instead have multiple components involved.[3]

A variety of disciplines are involved in assessing and treating children with feeding disorders.[4] Because the different specialties all have a different focus, they have viewed these disorders differently. When the literature is reviewed, the nomenclature and approaches vary greatly by the specific discipline that authored it. To bring clarity to this issue, a multidisciplinary task force has published a consensus definition and conceptual framework for pediatric feedings disorders.[5]

Pediatric Feeding Disorder

The consensus definition of a pediatric feeding disorder (PFD) is "impaired oral intake that is not age-appropriate and is associated with medical, nutritional, feeding skill, and/or psychosocial dysfunction."[5] Note the importance of age and the developmental feedings skills in this definition, which also include the importance of meeting nutritional needs via oral intake. The method by which a child is fed, as well the particular content of the feedings, vary greatly over time. Symptoms of a PFD must be present for at least 2 weeks; symptoms present for less than 3 months are considered an acute PFD, and those that persist for longer than 3 months are considered a chronic PFD.

From the definition, there are 4 domains of a PFD: medical, nutritional, feeding skills, and psychosocial. The medical domain includes anatomic, neurologic, and developmental issues that may lead to inflammation in the areas involved in feeding. The nutritional domain of PFD includes altered intake that affects nutritional status. The domain of feeding skills refers to the lack the development of normal feeding skills that may be attributable to a medical issue or just an adverse or delayed feeding exposure. Once the appropriate developmental window is missed, then it is very difficult to establish a normal pattern of feeding. The psychosocial domain includes the complex interactions between the child and his or her caregivers and the overall social situation.

Sensory Intake Issues That May or May Not Be Associated With PFD

There are some children in whom a PFD is attributable to a sensory issue. They limit their intake based on appearance, smell, texture, taste, or temperature of the offered food.[3] This can range from the "picky eating," which does not qualify as a feeding disorder, to malnutrition resulting from the extremely limited intake. Many children are "neophobes" who have a reluctance to try something new, which, again, may not be a feeding disorder. Selective eating behavior is correlated with sensory sensitivity and also a component of anxiety.[6] Thus, children with these issues are a blend of medical and psychosocial domains. The specifics of the sensory issue can manifest as texture aversion in children who lacked exposure during the appropriate developmental window. These issues are also commonly observed in children with autism spectrum disorder who may have very limited diets because of narrow acceptable sensory choices. The approach to these issues is normally multidisciplinary with behavioral and/or nutritional interventions.

Oral Motor Difficulties and PFD

Another group of children with PFD is characterized by oral motor difficulties. These children are often assessed and treated by speech and language pathologists who can intervene with therapies to improve strength and coordination of the oral motor skills.[4]

Summary of PFD

Even when the initial intake issue has resolved, the learned behaviors associated with that issue often persist. These feeding difficulties require a behavioral treatment approach.[4] There are outpatient multidisciplinary teams for feeding problems at many major medical centers. There are also a handful of intensive inpatient feeding disorder programs available, but these tend to be expensive and far from home for many families with these issues.

Swallowing Disorders

Swallowing is primarily an involuntary response. Difficulty swallowing leads to a feeding problem resulting from avoidance of intake. Significant inflammation of the esophagus leads to odynophagia, which can also result in reduced intake. Esophageal inflammation may result from significant gastroesophageal reflux, eosinophilic esophagitis (allergic etiology), or a variety of other etiologies. Some children have had a traumatic swallowing event that may result in an ongoing fear of swallowing (globus hystericus).[3]

The evaluation for swallowing issues varies depending on the age and history of the patient. Therefore, the crucial initial step is obtaining a thorough history. Often, the next step is an upper gastrointestinal tract contrast study to delineate the anatomy and grossly assess the motility of the upper gastrointestinal tract. Many children with these issues are seen in consultation with a pediatric gastroenterologist. There may be a need for an esophagogastroduodenoscopy for examination and biopsy of the enteric mucosa. A pH probe to quantify reflux may be recommended. Some patients may need an esophageal motility study to evaluate for dysmotility of the upper gastrointestinal tract.

Dysphagia

The primary mode of nutrition intake is by mouth for most children. However, safely swallowing food is a very complex task that requires highly complex neuromuscular coordination. The oropharynx is the common entry point for both nutrition and breathing. If one of the many complex steps involved in safe swallowing is dysfunctional, there is a risk of aspiration. During early embryologic development, the tubular structures that develop into the intestinal and respiratory tracts are among the first to be formed. A bud off of the foregut at 3.5 to 4 weeks' gestation becomes the trachea.[7] A variety of developmental errors can occur during this process and lead to less-than-complete separation of the intestinal and respiratory tracts, with a resulting laryngeal cleft, tracheoesophageal fistula, and other congenital anomalies that predispose to aspiration.

Even in the absence of congenital anomalies of the upper gastrointestinal and/or respiratory tracts, swallowing disorders can occur. The coordination between breathing and swallowing is very complex and involves of number of distinct motor activities that can be adversely affected by a variety of structural or neuromuscular disorders. Swallowing has 3 distinct phases.[8] The voluntary oral phase includes chewing the food and moving it to the back of the mouth. The subsequent pharyngeal phase is involuntary and

VI

requires several timed steps. The soft palate and uvula lift to protect the nasal passages. The muscles around the larynx contract, and the epiglottis folds over to protect the airway. Breathing stops for a moment, and the food or fluid moves toward the esophagus. The third phase, the esophageal phase, is also involuntary. The upper esophageal sphincter opens, and once the food enters the esophagus, it is propelled by organized peristalsis toward the stomach.

Dysphagia is a general term for any difficulty transitioning food/liquids from the mouth to the esophagus. Dysphagia can result in a variety of medical issues including the potential for aspiration.[9] Other children may present with recurrent pneumonias attributable to dysphagia.[10] Dysphagia is observed at high frequency in children with neurologic issues, such as cerebral palsy or neuromuscular diseases.[11] Children with these orders need a comprehensive evaluation because of their high risk of dysphagia. Dysphagia is commonly assessed by speech-language pathologists, often in conjunction with radiologists or another specialist. The most commonly utilized studies to assess feeding and swallowing are the videofluoroscopic swallow study or the fiberoptic endoscopic evaluation of swallowing.[12] There are various levels of dysphagia, from complete dysphagia of all food textures to dysphagia only with thin liquids.

Dysphagia Therapy

The appropriate intervention depends on the cause and degree of dysphagia. Some children require gastrostomy feedings and avoidance of oral intake, and others benefit from therapy to improve their feedings skills. There is very little experimental evidence to guide the therapies for dysphagia. A Cochrane review of children with neurologic diagnoses and dysphagia did not find enough high-level evidence to support the effectiveness of oral sensorimotor or lip strengthening interventions.[13] The prognosis depends on the etiology of the dysphagia and potential for developmental progress.

One of the primary interventions used to treat dysphagia has been to thicken feedings. Although this technique is widely used, there are surprisingly few studies documenting effectiveness of thickening feedings. One study in infants from 2 weeks to 14 months of age with documented dysphagia found that thickened feedings resulted in fewer respiratory symptoms and that the infants had increased oral intake.[14] A systemic review found 6 studies that supported the use of thickened feedings for children with dysphagia.[15] The same review found 16 studies that did not document any significant adverse effects. However, adverse events have been reported with the use of thickened feeding in preterm and newborn infants.[16] In May 2011, the US Food and Drug Administration issued a report of 15 preterm infants who developed necrotizing enterocolitis (NEC) after using a thickening agent.[17] The gastrointestinal tract in preterm infants may not have a fully developed mucosal barrier. There is no clear etiology by which the thickeners lead to NEC at this time.

All of the thickening agents commercially available now have labels warning against use in early infancy. The general recommendation is that thickeners should not be used until the risk of NEC is minimal at 44 weeks' postmenstrual age.[17]

Apart from nasogastric feeding that bypasses the oral cavity and esophagus, there are few alternatives to thickening formula that allow continued oral feedings. One potential method to deal with dysphagia would be the use of slow-flow nipples to slow the bottle feedings to a point at which feedings would be safe. When nipple flow rates have been studied, the measured flow rates are extremely variable and are not consistent from nipple to nipple within the same type.[18,19] Another approach has been a side-lying position for feedings rather than the normal "cradle" position. There are only a few small studies with mixed results on this approach.[20-23]

Summary

Appropriate evaluation and therapy for pediatric swallowing disorders require input from multiple disciplines. The evaluation begins with a complete history that then informs the subsequent more invasive evaluation. Thickeners for dysphagia are currently not recommended for preterm and newborn infants.

References

1. Harris G. Development of taste and food preferences in children. *Curr Opin Clin Nutr Metab Care.* 2008;11(3):315–319

2. Lupton D. *Food, the Body and the Self.* Thousand Oaks, CA: Sage Publications; 1996

3. Bryant-Waugh R, Markham L, Kreipe RE, Walsh BT. Feeding and eating disorders in childhood. *Int J Eat Disord.* 2010;43(2):98–111

4. Silverman AH. Interdisciplinary care for feeding problems in children. *Nutr Clin Pract.* 2010;25(2):160–165

5. Goday PS, Huh SY, Silverman A, et al. Pediatric feeding disorder: consensus definition and conceptual framework. *J Pediatr Gastroenterol Nutr.* 2019;68(1): 124–129

6. Farrow CV, Coulthard H. Relationships between sensory sensitivity, anxiety and selective eating in children. *Appetite.* 2012;58(3):842–846

7.   Sadler TW. *Langman's Medical Embryology.* Philadelphia, PA: Williams & Wilkins; 2011

8.   Corkins MR, McKown CG, Gosa MM. Mechanics of nutrient intake. In: Corkins MR, ed. *The A.S.P.E.N. Pediatric Nutrition Support Core Curriculum.* 2nd ed. Silver Spring, MD: American Society for Parenteral and Enteral Nutrition; 2015

9.   Mercado-Deane MG, Burton EM, Harlow SA, et al. Swallowing dysfunction in infants less than 1 year of age. *31.* 2001(423–428)

10. Serel Arslan S, Demir N, Karaduman AA. Both pharyngeal and esophageal phases of swallowing are associated with recurrent pneumonia in pediatric patients. Epub December 15, 2016. *Clin Respir J.* 2018;12(2):767–771

11. van den Engel-Hoek L, de Groot IJ, de Swart BJ, Erasmus CE. Feeding and swallowing disorders in pediatric neuromuscular diseases: an overview. *J Neuromuscul Dis.* 2015;2(4):357–369

12. Arvedson JC, Lefton-Greif MA. Instrumental assessment of pediatric dysphagia. *Semin Speech Lung.* 2017;38(2):135–146

13. Morgan AT, Dodrill P, Ward EC. Interventions for oropharyngeal dysphagia in children with neurological impairment. *Cochrane Database Syst Rev.* 2012;(10):CD009456

14. Krummrich P, Kline B, Krival K, Rubin M. Parent perception of the impact of using thickened fluids in children with dysphagia. *Pediatr Pulmonol.* 2017;52(11): 1486–1494

15. Gosa MM, Schooling T, Coleman J. Thickened liquids as a treatment for children with dysphagia and associated adverse effects. *Infant Child Adolesc Nutr.* 2011;3(6):344–350

16. Clarke P, Robinson MJ. Thickening milk feedings may cause necrotising enterocolitis. *Arch Dis Child Fetal Neonatal Ed.* 2004;89(3):F280

17. Abrams SA. Be cautious in using thickening agents for preemies. *AAP News.* 2011;32(7):23

18. Pados BF, Park J, Thoyre SM, Estrem H, Nix WB. Milk flow rates from bottle nipples used after hospital discharge. *MCN Am J Matern Child Nurs.* 2016;41(4): 237–243

19. Jackman KT. Go with the flow: choosing a feeding system for infants in the neonatal intensive care unit and beyond based on flow performance. *Newborn Infant Nurs Rev.* 2013;13(1):31–34

20. Clark L, Kennedy G, Pring T, Hird MI-. Improving bottle feeding in preterm infants: investigating the elevated side-lying position. *Infant.* 2007;3(4):354–358

21. Thoyre SM, Holditch-Davis D, Schwartz TA, Melendez Roman CR, Nix WB. Coregulated approach to feeding preterm infants with lung disease. *Nurs Res.* 2012;61(4):242–251

22. Park J, Thoyre SM, Knafl GJ, Hodges EA, Nix WB. Efficacy of semielevated side-lying positioning during bottle-feeding of very preterm infants. *J Perinat Neonat Nurs.* 2014;28(1):69–79

23. Dawson JA, Myers LR, Moorhead A, et al. A randomised trial of two techniques for bottle feeding preterm infants. *J Paediatr Child Health.* 2013;49(6):462–466

Chapter 26

Malnutrition/Undernutrition/Failure to Thrive

Introduction

Past editions of *Pediatric Nutrition* have included a chapter titled "Failure to Thrive." Yet, failure to thrive as a diagnostic "label" has been viewed as inappropriate for some time. Parents do not appreciate the term "failure," and health care professionals know that this is a vague descriptive term that provides no distinct diagnostic direction. In support of this position is this statement from the 7th edition of the handbook: "Failure to thrive (FTT) is an imprecise, archaic term that refers to children whose growth is significantly lower than the norms for their age and gender," and the editors go on to assert that the underlying cause of "failure to thrive" is malnutrition.[1]

Definition and Epidemiology

This chapter focuses on malnutrition and, specifically, undernutrition in upper/middle- and high-income (UMHI) countries. For a description of this topic in low- and middle-income countries, see Chapter 10: Pediatric Global Nutrition.

It is now well recognized that in UMHI countries, there is a significant prevalence of undernutrition among children of all ages associated with underlying disease (such as inflammatory processes[2]) and in those hospitalized for subacute and chronic illnesses. A 2008 review of malnutrition in hospitalized pediatric patients from UMHI countries between 1990 and 2008 found that the prevalence ranged from 6.1% to 32%.[3] However, the diagnosis/definition of malnutrition varied greatly from study to study in the review. Among the 6 countries where rates were reported, 5 different definitions of malnutrition were used. A single children's hospital in the United States reported 35% of its patients were acutely malnourished in 1976, and the same hospital in 1992 reported that 24.5% of its patients were acutely malnourished and 27.3% were chronically malnourished.[4,5] These prevalence rates were based on measurements obtained on a single day. Other studies have published rates up to 51%.[6,7] These prevalence rates are based on children examined for concomitant malnutrition. In contrast, the US 2010 Healthcare Cost and Utilization Project (HCUP) claims for pediatric malnutrition found that discharge codes for malnutrition were filed for 2.8% of children younger than 1 year and 1.5% of children from 1 to 17 years of age.[8] These data would indicate a significant rate of underdiagnosis of undernutrition in hospitalized children. Another estimate of the potential magnitude of malnutrition among children in the United States comes from data identifying children as having a "special health care need" from the US Department of Health and Human Services.[9] These children are defined as "those who have or are at increased risk for a chronic physical, developmental, behavioral, or emotional condition and who also require heath and health-related services of a type or amount beyond that of children generally." Fourteen percent of children in the United States currently fulfill this definition.[9]

A definition of malnutrition/undernutrition incorporating the concept of a contributing disease process, along with non-illness–related malnutrition/undernutrition, was developed and subsequently endorsed by the American Academy of Pediatrics. The formal definition of pediatric malnutrition/undernutrition is an imbalance between nutrient requirements and intake. This results in cumulative deficits of energy, protein, or micronutrients that negatively affect growth, development, and other relevant outcomes.[10] The practical results of the nutrient intake imbalance and nutrient deficit is characterized by the underlying history and measurable physical parameters. These were organized into separate documented domains by the new definition. The definition includes the domains of anthropometric parameters, etiology and chronicity of malnutrition, mechanisms of pathogenesis, and developmental/functional outcomes. Figure 26.1 provides a framework for understanding the relationships between the various factors to be considered.

Using this framework, the parameters that most reliably predict malnutrition were the anthropometric measurements of weight, height/length, body mass index (BMI), and mid-upper arm circumference (MUAC).[10] The MUAC was a parameter that has not been measured routinely in many pediatric facilities. However, the literature indicates it is a good proxy for weight and avoids inaccurate determinations of nutritional status in patients with fluid shifts and edema. Significant edema that effects reproducibility and the absence of reference standards for infants from birth to 6 months are limitations.[11–14] These studies also documented that MUAC is a good predictor of malnutrition related mortality. The anthropometric parameters need to be obtained with careful attention to the appropriate techniques.

The use of z-scores, or the standard deviations from the median value of each anthropometric parameter at each age, is now routinely recommended for evaluating the anthropometric measurements of examined patients. The use of z-scores has been recommended by the World Health Organization

Figure 26.1.
Key domains for defining pediatric malnutrition

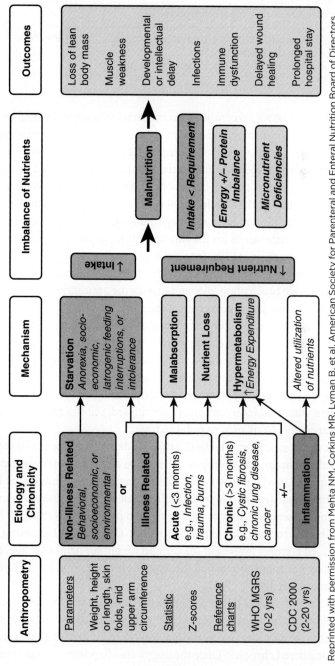

Reprinted with permission from Mehta NM, Corkins MR, Lyman B, et al. American Society for Parenteral and Enteral Nutrition Board of Directors. Defining pediatric malnutrition: a paradigm shift toward etiology-related definitions. *JPEN J Parenter Enteral Nutr.* 2013;37(4):460–481.[10]

Table 26.1.
Electronic Resources for Anthropometrics

http://www.cdc.gov/growthcharts/computer_programs.htm http://www.peditools.org http://www.who.int/childgrowth/software/en/

(WHO) since 1977.[15] Percentile reference standards are less useful in defining the state of malnutrition in pediatric patients. Less than the third percentile could be barely or far below the percentile. The z-scores are mathematically continuous and therefore quantitative. The definition is based on anthropometrics using the growth curves of the WHO for children younger than 2 years (supine length) and the Centers for Disease Control and Prevention (CDC) for children 2 to 20 years of age (standing height).[10] In the past, obtaining z-score values for the various anthropometrics was extremely difficult, but electronic applications are now available that can quickly derive the appropriate z-score (Table 26.1). Ideally, electronic medical records should be able to calculate, plot and display the appropriate z-scores for all of the measured anthropometrics (Tables 26.2 and 26.3).

A multisociety task force has created a document of malnutrition indicators on the basis of an extensive literature review that are in accord with those used in low- and middle-income countries (see Chapter 10: Pediatric Global Nutrition).[16] A more accurate diagnosis of malnutrition/undernutrition is made on 2 data points separated over time; however, to ensure that children who need intervention are not missed, criteria can be based on measurements from a single point in time.

For children with special health care needs, some of the parameters are difficult to obtain, and therefore, alternative anthropometric determinations may be used (ie, crown-rump length, arm span), although the lack of reference standards and reproducibility limit their usefulness. An important consequence of chronic undernutrition in children is stunting (see also Chapter 10: Pediatric Global Nutrition). Children with stunting have decreased z-scores for height for age and weight for height for age, but their BMI may not appear abnormal, because the malnutrition has affected both height and weight.

On the basis of US National Center for Health Statistics standard guidelines, if the disease process or state of undernutrition is less than 3 months in duration, it is considered acute, and if greater than 3 months, it is considered chronic.[17] Once the diagnosis of undernutrition is made, it

Table 26.2.
Diagnostic Z-scores, Single Encounter

	Mild Malnutrition	Moderate Malnutrition	Severe Malnutrition
Weight for height z-score	−1 to −1.9 z-score	−2 to −2.9 z-score	−3 or greater z-score
BMI for age z-score	−1 to −1.9 z-score	−2 to −2.9 z-score	−3 or greater z-score
Length/height z-score	No data	No data	−3 z-score
Mid-upper arm circumference	Greater than or equal to −1 to −1.9 z-score	Greater than or equal to −2 to −2.9 z-score	Greater than or equal to −3 z-score

Reprinted with permission from Becker P, Nieman Carney L, Corkins MR, et al. Consensus statement of the academy of nutrition and dietetics/american society for parenteral and enteral nutrition: indicators recommended for the identification and documentation of pediatric malnutrition (undernutrition). *Nutr Clin Pract.* 2015;30(1):147-161.[16]

Table 26.3.
Diagnostic Z-scores, Multiple Encounters

	Mild Malnutrition	Moderate Malnutrition	Severe Malnutrition
Weight gain velocity (<2 years of age)	Less than 75% of the norm for expected weight gain	Less than 50% of the norm for expected weight gain	Less than 25% of the norm for expected weight gain
Weight loss (2–20 years of age)	5% usual body weight	7.5% usual body weight	10% usual body weight
Deceleration in weight for length/height z-score	Decline of 1 z-score	Decline of 2 z-score	Decline of 3 z-score
Inadequate nutrient intake	51%–75% estimated energy/protein need	26%–50% estimated energy/protein need	≤25% estimated energy/protein need

Reprinted with permission from Becker P, Nieman Carney L, Corkins MR, et al. Consensus statement of the Academy of Nutrition and Dietetics/American Society for Parenteral and Enteral Nutrition: Indicators recommended for the identification and documentation of pediatric malnutrition (undernutrition). *Nutr Clin Pract.* 2015;30(1):147–161.[16]

should be formally stated in the medical record and include the degree of malnutrition, followed by the related disease that led to the malnutrition, and then the supporting evidence. For instance: moderate malnutrition related to congenital heart disease as evidenced by a BMI z-score of −2.5.

Prevalence

The new definition of malnutrition was published in 2013 and is just now working its way into the pediatric literature. Therefore, there are variety of studies that use their own definition of malnutrition in the literature. The majority of the published studies have looked at the rate of malnutrition among hospitalized children. As cited earlier, a review published in 2008 found a range from 6.1% to 32%.[3] The studies were from 6 different countries and used 5 different definitions. Investigators from Boston Children's Hospital have published 2 "snapshot" studies in which they evaluated the rate of malnutrition on a single specified day in its facility.[4,5] In 1976, these investigators found that 35% were acutely malnourished and 47% chronically malnourished. When they looked again in 1992, they found 24.5% were acutely malnourished and 27.3% chronically malnourished. Other studies have published rates up to 51%.[6,7]

These prevalence numbers are all from studies evaluating for malnutrition. They must be contrasted with the numbers from actual claims data. The 2010 HCUP claims for pediatric malnutrition found that discharge codes for malnutrition were filed for 2.8% of children younger than 1 year of age and 1.5% of children from 1 to 17 years of age.[8] These data would indicate a significant rate of underdiagnosis in hospitalized children, because when carefully evaluated, the published rates are at least double the amounts coded for.

Etiology

The historical approach to determining the cause of underweight or malnourishment in children was to divide causes into "organic" and "nonorganic." However, social, behavioral, and environmental causes are often present in children with underlying illness, so that approach is now considered obsolete. In a recent study, the majority of patients admitted to the hospital with a primary diagnosis of poor weight gain improved with behavioral interventions and were not found to have concomitant underlying chronic illness.[18] However, in this same study, children with concomitant medical/surgical disorders were hospitalized longer and gained weight

Table 26.4.

Prevalence of Malnutrition Based on Underlying Disease Type

Disease	Prevalence
CNS disease	40%
Infectious disease	34.5%
Cystic fibrosis	33.3%
CVS disease	28.6%
Oncology	27.3%
GI disease	23.6%
Multiple diagnoses	43.8%

CNS, central nervous system; CVS, cyclical vomiting syndrome; GI, gastrointestinal.

Reprinted with permission from: Pawellek I, Dokoupil K, Koletzko B. Prevalence of malnutrition in paediatric hospital patients. *Clin Nutr.* 2008;27(1):72–76.[6]

more slowly. On the other hand, it is also important to recognize the high prevalence of malnutrition in children who have an underlying chronic medical condition. Pawellek et al published their respective rates of malnutrition based on the underlying disease category (Table 26.4).[6]

Another study that evaluated children hospitalized more than once with "failure to thrive" and risk factors for readmission found that among those readmitted for failure to thrive, 40.8% of them had at least 1 complex chronic condition and 16.4% had 2 or more.[19] An underlying disease not only predisposes a child to malnutrition but also makes it harder to treat.

As the framework presented in Figure 26.1 suggests, non-illness–related undernutrition has the potential to affect the growth and development of children. Parental social, emotional, and behavioral risks leading to malnutrition in the infant and child include[20]:

- Parental depression, stress, marital strife, divorce
- Parental history of abuse as a child
- Developmental delay and psychological problems in the parent(s)
- Young and single mothers without social supports
- Domestic violence
- Alcohol or other substance abuse
- Previous child abuse in the family

- Social isolation and/or poverty
- Parents with inadequate adaptive and social skills
- Parents who are overly focused on career and/or activities away from home
- Failure to adhere to medical regimens
- Lack of knowledge of normal growth and development

Long-Term Outcomes

Pooled data from multiple international studies found that children with mild to moderate malnutrition had a 2.2 times greater chance of mortality.[21] Beyond the mortality concerns are the long-term consequences on the patient's health and development. Evidence suggests that metabolic programming occurring during the first 1000 days of life affects health later in life during adulthood.[22] Brain development also is occurring at a rapid rate during this early period and can be significantly affected by maternal health and postnatal infant/child nutritional status, with potential long-term consequences on cognition.[23-25]

Few prospective longitudinal cohort-controlled studies are available to examine the long- term effects of undernutrition on behavioral, emotional, cognitive, and long-term health outcomes. One prospective cohort study on the island of Mauritius followed 1559 children from 3 to 11 years of age.[26] Physical findings of malnutrition or anemia were assessed at 3 years of age. The children were then followed for 8 years with outcomes adjusted for psychosocial confounders. Children with 3 indicators of malnourishment at age 3 years had a 15.3-point decrease in IQ at 11 years of age. It is acknowledged, however, that these children largely remained in the same social/ecological and family environment throughout their childhoods and that it is impossible to control for all the effects of these social/ecological factors on cognitive development and IQ. Evidence of the value of early nutritional intervention in malnourished infants and children also comes from the Carolina Abecedarian Project,[27] in which 122 children from a region with a high prevalence of poverty Appalachia were randomly assigned to 2 groups from 1972 to 1977. Sixty-five children received an educational intervention that included 2 meals and a snack, and the other 57 received free formula for 15 months plus standard public education and school lunch. Males in the intervention group had a lower BMI during childhood that persisted into adulthood. The same males had a lower prevalence of risk factors for cardiovascular disease and metabolic syndrome when they were in their mid-30s. These outcomes were not observed in the female subjects in the intervention group.

Short-Term Outcomes

A variety of studies show detrimental short-term health-related outcomes in children with malnutrition. What is generally lacking are studies that demonstrate the value of intervention. However, these would clearly be difficult studies to design from an ethical standpoint. One study found that, of children presenting to a single children's hospital emergency department, 24.5% of malnourished children required admission, compared with 16.6% of adequately nourished children.[28] The malnourished children had an increased prevalence of respiratory infections and fractures. A prospective, multicenter study from European pediatric hospitals also found children who were moderately to severely malnourished had a significantly longer length of stay (1.6 versus 1.3 days).[29] Another study documented that pediatric patients who were malnourished prior to surgery had double the number of postoperative days that they remained hospitalized and a significantly higher rate of infectious complications.[7] Children with congenital heart disease and malnutrition that underwent surgery had an intensive care stay 1.4 days longer and were on mechanical ventilation 17 hours longer.[30]

The 2010 HCUP data, which probably underestimate malnourished children, found that children for whom malnutrition was coded had a significantly longer length of stay: 9.7 versus 3.8 days.[8] A key outcome from these data is that the mean hospital costs were also significantly different: $55 255 for malnourished patients versus $17 309 for those with good nutritional status.

Evaluation

The causes of malnutrition/undernutrition fall into 1 of 3 broad categories: inadequate intake, excessive losses, or increased metabolism. The evaluation of a child with malnutrition begins with a complete social and medical history of both child and parents. This will indicate whether there is an underlying disease process that could be reasonably expected to be the cause of malnutrition. The history can also indicate whether the reported nutrient intake even reaches the level needed to support the child's well-being or whether there are symptoms that indicate a potential source of nutrient loss.

Next is a thorough physical examination, which would include the anthropometrics that are used to determine whether malnutrition/undernutrition is present. The examiner should look for any characteristics of a disease process that could lead to malnutrition as well as any findings consistent with malnutrition (anthropometric and others). Some of the more common findings of malnutrition include temporal wasting, loss of subcutaneous fat pads, and changes in the skin, hair, and nails.[31] An additional component of the examination is to observe a feeding. This can identify whether the child has a behavioral issue with eating and allow observation of the parent-child interaction.[20]

Further evaluation then must be guided by the findings from the history and physical examination. The report by Larson-Nath et al on children admitted to the hospital with poor weight gain found that testing tended to be negative, and they recommended a trial of "feeding and following for weight gain" as the first step.[18] A working group that examined definitions of malnutrition in pediatrics found no evidence to support any laboratory test being diagnostic for malnutrition and found that the only evidence-informed way to evaluate nutritional status is to regularly and accurately measure the child's anthropometrics.[10] Thus, the first priority for children with no historical or physical indicators is a period of close observation, with frequent assessments.[20] This observation can be performed on an outpatient basis if there is the capacity to closely and frequently follow the infant or child over time, but it may require hospitalization for more challenging cases.

Treatment

The first intervention is nutrition repletion. However, repletion must be provided with caution in children with moderate to severe malnutrition, because there is a risk of the patient developing refeeding syndrome. Refeeding syndrome is the shift in phosphate, potassium, and magnesium that accompanies the metabolic shift to a fed state.[32] Refeeding syndrome can have serious and life-threatening results. The safest approach is to monitor electrolytes, including phosphorus, potassium, and magnesium, frequently and provide supplemental phosphorus and potassium, along with appropriate vitamins.

If the gastrointestinal tract is functional (motility, absorption, and digestion are intact), oral or enteral feeding is the preferred route for nutritional rehabilitation. If significant gastrointestinal tract compromise is present because of an underlying medical or surgical condition, it may be necessary on rare occasions to use parenteral nutrition. There is wide variation in the possible approaches to feeding the patient. The ideal would be to start by providing the patient a standard diet with documentation of the intake and monitoring for weight gain.[33] If there is known underlying disease that could affect intake by altering taste, appetite, or gastrointestinal motility, then nasogastric feedings may be the first intervention. Nasogastric feedings may also be indicated in known disorders with increased metabolic needs. This approach allows for documentation of weight gain with better caloric intake.

Malnutrition is associated with immune dysfunction (see also Chapter 35: Nutrition and Immunity). In patients with severe acute malnutrition, Trehan et al demonstrated decreased mortality and improved weight gain compared with controls when the children were started on prophylactic antibiotics at diagnosis.[34] The use of prophylactic antibiotics in milder acute or chronic forms of malnutrition has not been studied and is not recommended.

If malnutrition is attributable to parental or caregiver neglect, then reporting to the local child protective services agency is required.[20] Such a report can result in providing the family the resources and interventions that will be in the child's best interests.

Summary

Malnutrition is common among infants and children with concomitant medical or surgical disorders. Psychosocial factors are present in the majority of patients who present with a diagnosis of undernutrition. A diagnosis of undernutrition/malnutrition is based primarily on patient anthropometrics and an evaluation that includes a complete family and patient history and physical examination of the infant or child. Malnutrition has both short- and long-term consequences for the child. Poverty remains the most significant social risk factor for developing malnutrition in infancy and childhood. For children with malnutrition not related to underlying illness, addressing environmental and familial psychosocial factors and a trial of observed feeding of an appropriate diet for age remain the optimal approach.

References

1. American Academy of Pediatrics, Committee on Nutrition. Failure to thrive. In: Kleinman RE, Greer FR, eds. *Pediatric Nutrition*. 7th ed. Elk Grove Village, IL: American Academy of Pediatrics; 2013:663–700

2. Jensen GL. Inflammation as the key interface of the medical and nutrition universes: a provocative examination of the future of clinical nutrition and medicine. *JPEN J Parenter Enteral Nutr*. 2006;30(5):453–463

3. Joosten KFM, Hulst JM. Prevalence of malnutrition in pediatric hospital patients. *Curr Opin Pediatr*. 2008;20(5):590–596

4. Merritt RJ, Suskind RM. Nutritional survey of hospitalized pediatric patients. *Am J Clin Nutr*. 1979;32(6):1320–1325

5. Hendricks KM, Duggan C, Gallagher L, et al. Malnutrition in hospitalized pediatric patients. *Arch Pediatr Adolesc Med*. 1995;149(10):1118–1122

6. Pawellek I, Dokoupil K, Koletzko B. Prevalence of malnutrition in paediatric hospital patients. *Clin Nutr*. 2008;27(1):72–76

7. Secker DJ, Jeejeebhoy KN. Subjective global nutritional assessment for children. *Am J Clin Nutr*. 2007;85(4):1083–1089

8. Abdelhadi RA, Bouma S, Bairdain S, et al. Characteristics of hospitalized children with a diagnosis of malnutrition: United States, 2010. *J Parent Enteral Nutr*. 2016;40(5):623–635

9. US Deparment of Health and Human Services, Health Resources and Services Administration, Maternal and Child Health Bureau. *The National Survey of Children with Special Health Care Needs Chartbook 2005-2006*. Rockville, MD: US Department of Health and Human Services; 2007

10. Mehta NM, Corkins MR, Lyman B, et al. American Society for Parenteral and Enteral Nutrition Board of Directors. Defining pediatric malnutrition: a paradigm shift toward etiology-related definitions. *JPEN J Parenter Enteral Nutr*. 2013;37(4):460–481

11. Myatt M, Khara T, Collins S. A review of methods to detect cases of severely malnourished children in the community for their admission into community-based therapeutic care programs. *Food Nutr Bull*. 2006;27(3 Suppl):S7–S23

12. Alam N, Wojtyniak B, Rahaman MM. Anthropometric indicators and risk of death. *Am J Clin Nutr*. 1989;49(5):884–888

13. Briend A, Maire B, Fontaine O, Garenne N. Mid-upper arm circumference and weight-for-height to identify high-risk malnourished under-five children. *Matern Child Nutr*. 2012;8(1):130–133

14. Chen LC, Chowdhury A, Huffman SL. Anthropometric assessment of energy-protein malnutrition and subsequent risk of mortality among preschool aged. *Am J Clin Nutr*. 1980;33(8):1836–1845

VI

15. Waterlow JC, Buzina R, Keller W, Lane JM, Nichaman MZ, Tanner JM. The presentation and use of height and weight data for comparing the nutritional status of groups of children under the age of 10 years. *Bull World Health Organ.* 1977;55(4):489–498

16. Becker P, Nieman Carney L, Corkins MR, et al. Consensus statement of the academy of nutrition and dietetics/american society for parenteral and enteral nutrition: indicators recommended for the identification and documentation of pediatric malnutrition (undernutrition). *Nutr Clin Pract.* 2015;30(1):147–161

17. National Center for Health Statistics. Health, United States, 2017: With Special Feature on Mortality. Hyattsville, MD: National Center for Health Statistics; 2018.

18. Larson-Nath C, St Clair N, Goday PS. Hospitalization for failure to thrive. *Clin Pediatr (Phila).* 2017;57(2):212–219

19. Puls HT, Hall M, Bettenhausen J, et al. Failure to thrive hospitalizations and risk factors for readmission to children's hospitals. *Hosp Pediatr.* 2016;6(8):468–475

20. Block RW, Krebs NF, American Academy of Pediatrics, Committee on Child Abuse and Neglect, Committee on Nutrition. Failure to thrive as manifestation of child neglect. *Pediatrics.* 2005;116(5):1234–1237

21. Schroeder DG, Brown KH. Nutritional status as a predictor of child survival: summarizing the association and quantifying its global impact. *Bull World Health Organ.* 1994;72(4):569–579

22. Adair LS, Fall CHD, Osmond C, et al. COHORTS Group. Associations of linear growth and relative weight gain during early life with adult health and human capital in countries of low and middle income: findings from five birth cohort studies. *Lancet.* 2013;382(9891):525–534

23. Wachs TD, Georgieff MK, Cusick S, McEwen BS. Issues in the timing of integrated early interventions: contributions from nutrition, neuroscience, and psychological research. *Ann N Y Acad Sci.* 2014;1308:89–106

24. Prado EL, Dewey KG. Nutrition and brain development in early life. *Nutr Rev.* 2014;72(4):267–284

25. Monk C, Georgieff MK, Osterholm EA. Research review: maternal prenatal distress and poor nutrition-mutually influencing risk factors affecting infant neurocognitive development. *J Child Psychol Psychiatry.* 2013;54(2):115–130

26. Liu J, Raine A, Venables PH, Dalais C, Mednick SA. Malnutrition at age 3 years and lower cognitive ability at age 11 years. *Arch Pediatr Adolesc Med.* 2003;157(6):593–600

27. Campbell F, Conti G, Heckman JJ, et al. Early childhood investments substantially boost adult health. *Science.* 2014;343(6178):1478–1485

28. Wyrick S, Hester C, Sparkman A, et al. What role does body mass index play in hospital admission rates from the pediatric emergency department? *Pediatr Emerg Care.* 2013;29(9):974–978

29. Hecht C, Weber M, Grote V, et al. Disease associated malnutrition correlates with length of hospital stay in children. *Clin Nutr.* 2015;34(1):53–59

30. Courtney-Martin G, Kosar C, Campbell A, et al. Plasma aluminum concentrations in pediatric patients receiving long-term parenteral nutrition. *JPEN J Parenter Enteral Nutr.* 2015;39(5):578–585

31. Green Corkins K. Nutrition-focused physical examination in pediatric patients. *Nutr Clin Pract.* 2015;30(2):203–209

32. Pulcini CD, Zettle S, Srinath A. Refeeding syndrome. *Pediatr Rev.* 2016;37(12): 516–523

33. Derumeaux-Burel H MM, Morin L, Boirie Y. Prediction of resting energy expenditure in a large population of obese children. *Am J Clin Nutr.* 2004;80(6): 1544–1550

34. Trehan I, Goldbach HS, LaGrone LN, et al. Antibiotics as part of the management of severe acute malnutrition. *N Engl J Med.* 2013;368(5):425–435

VI

Chapter 27

Chronic Diarrheal Disease

Introduction

Infants and children with chronic or persistent diarrhea continue to pose a significant medical challenge. Aggressive oral rehydration programs have significantly decreased diarrheal morbidity and mortality in developing countries. Oral rehydration solutions developed in the 1960s revolutionized the care of adults and children with severe acute diarrhea. Nevertheless, the World Health Organization (WHO) notes that diarrheal diseases are the second leading cause of childhood mortality, globally accounting for about 500 000 deaths/year. Diarrhea (ie, repeated episodes) is still a leading cause of malnutrition in children younger than 5 years.[1]

This chapter focuses on chronic diarrheal states in resource-rich countries. For chronic diarrhea in children from resource-limited countries, many excellent resources exist.[2,3] The following discussion first describes the pathophysiological basis for diarrhea, outlines an approach to clinical and laboratory evaluation, highlights disorders of particular relevance in pediatrics, and provides general guidance with respect to treatment and prevention.

Definitions and Pathophysiology

Patients or their parents often report the presence of diarrhea when stools are looser than expected or are frankly watery. A widely accepted definition of diarrhea is a stool weight greater than 10 g/kg/day in infants and toddlers[4] and greater than 200 g/day in older children.[5] Typically, this will translate into loose or watery stools occurring >3 times per day.[5] Cross-sectional studies of healthy young children 1 to 4 years of age in high-income[6] and low-income[7] countries found an average stool weight of 5 and 15 g/kg/day, respectively. Normal stool volume thresholds should, therefore, be used to raise concern but not define a pathologic condition.

The World Health Organization (WHO) defines persistent diarrhea as a diarrheal episode lasting >14 days.[1] Chronic diarrhea has generally been defined as lasting >4 weeks.[5,8] For clinical purposes, there is little utility in categorizing diarrheas as persistent versus chronic. Diarrheal episodes lasting greater than 2 to 4 weeks are commonly referred to as chronic and should prompt an evaluation.

The etiologies of chronic diarrhea can be divided by pathophysiology into 5 distinct but often overlapping mechanisms. The first is osmotic diarrhea, or more accurately, substrate-induced diarrhea, secondary to the failure to absorb a luminal solute and thereby resulting in luminal retention or secretion of water. Osmotic diarrhea can result from either congenital or acquired conditions and most often occurs from the failure to absorb a dietary carbohydrate, such as lactose. Carbohydrates may be malabsorbed either because of absolute disaccharidase deficiency or relative disaccharidase deficiency from decreased surface area related to surgical resection or villus injury. Carbohydrate malabsorption may also occur because of an complete inability to transport selected carbohydrates (as in glucose-galactose malabsorption) or a relative transport deficiency because the absorptive capacity of the intestine for that sugar may be overwhelmed by excessive dietary intake (eg, fructose and sorbitol) or because of decreased surface area. Osmotic diarrhea typically ceases with elimination of the offending solute from the diet.

The second form, secretory diarrhea, which more accurately may be referred to as abnormal electrolyte transport-related diarrhea, occurs when there is excessive electrolyte secretion into the intestinal lumen and/or inadequate electrolyte absorption from the intestinal lumen into the body. The net result of excessive electrolytes in the lumen is the osmotic retention or secretion of water into the lumen. A variety of both endogenous and exogenous substances, often called "secretagogues," can stimulate fluid and electrolyte secretion or inhibit sodium absorption across the intestinal epithelium. Typically, secretagogues affect ion transport in the large and small bowel both by inhibiting sodium and chloride absorption and by stimulating chloride secretion. A classical pathological secretagogue, cholera toxin, induces the massive water and solute losses that occur following infection with the pathogen *Vibrio cholerae*. Other examples include congenital disorders with identified genetic mutations that affect gut epithelial ion transport.[9] This form of diarrhea typically persists even with cessation of oral intake.

The third form of chronic diarrhea results from rapid transit of the luminal contents of the intestine. This results in decreased total resident time of the luminal contents, reducing the necessary time for fluid absorption required to produce solid fecal matter and subsequently resulting in passage of a liquid stool. The most common example of this form of diarrhea presents in the first few years of life as "toddler's diarrhea" or functional diarrhea (see below). In patients with this type of diarrhea, rapid transit may ensue because of an ineffective switch in motility from a fasting to a fed response to food.[10]

Excess fat in the stool may also result in diarrhea, because fat maldigestion may produce excess stool weight, but typically will not cause hypovolemia. These stools are typically greasy or oily but may also be loose or watery because of bacterial metabolism of triglycerides, producing free fatty acids that may induce secretion in the colon.[11] Pancreatic insufficiency is the most common cause of fat maldigestion.

Inflammation is the fifth pathophysiologic mechanism. This often encompasses components of the prior mechanisms because of the influence of inflammation on villus function and gut motility. The etiologies range from acute viral enteritis to chronic small and large bowel inflammation seen in chronic inflammatory bowel disease (IBD), Crohn disease, and ulcerative colitis. Increased serum proteins, mucus, and blood may also be found in the stool.

Evaluation of the Infant and Child With Persistent Diarrhea

History and Physical Examination

It is important initially to define the character of the diarrhea using criteria such as age of onset, frequency, volume, duration, characteristics of the stool, and relationship to feeding or dietary intake. A prospective 3- to 5-day history of dietary intake, stool pattern, and associated symptoms is helpful. Also important is the presence or absence of persistent fever, abdominal pain, weight loss, rash, fatigue, vomiting, joint pain, or oral ulcers among other extraintestinal symptoms. Important historical features include family history, cultural influences on feeding, travel, and preschool/school exposures.

The physical examination begins with the documentation of weight, height, and head circumference, plotted on a standardized reference growth chart. The examination should focus on evidence of chronic disease and nutrient deficiency, such as rickets in vitamin D deficiency, abdominal distension with loss of subcutaneous tissue in cases of severe malabsorption in celiac disease, or perianal dermatitis in zinc deficiency. The physical examination should include a perianal examination.

Examination of Stool Sample

Confirmation of the cause of chronic diarrhea requires evaluation of a fresh stool sample, ideally one that has been collected in a way that separates urine from stool, and for infants in diapers, using a method to prevent the stool water from soaking into the diaper. Macroscopic inspection of the

VI

stool gives information on consistency and color. The stool can also be tested for the presence of occult blood and lactoferrin or calprotectin (enzymes released from neutrophils).[12] The presence of neutrophil-derived enzymes are expected with significant mucosal inflammation seen in invasive bacterial disease and chronic ulcerative colitis and argues against viral or malabsorptive diarrheas. Techniques for analysis of the stool sample for malabsorbed fat using Sudan/Oil Red O stains are available in clinical laboratories. When pancreatic insufficiency is suspected, a spot stool sample can be sent for elastase activity, which correlates well with exocrine pancreatic function.[13] When quantitative assessment of fat malabsorption is desired (when spot testing is equivocal and identifying steatorrhea is important), 3-day quantitative collections can be performed,[13] and this is coupled with a 4-day history of dietary fat intake. A coefficient of fat malabsorption more than 5% (of ingested dietary fat) is generally abnormal after 3 years of age (up to 20% fat malabsorption may be normal in early infancy, and up to 10% from 10 months to 3 years of age). Unabsorbed carbohydrates in the stool can be detected by reagent tablets for reducing sugars. Note that sucrose is not a reducing sugar. A stool pH <5.5 suggests fermentation of carbohydrates. Breastfed healthy infants will often have traces of reducing sugar and fat in the stool.

Analysis of the stool for electrolyte content and osmolarity may be helpful in distinguishing osmotic from a secretory diarrhea. Osmotic diarrhea is usually present if the osmolar gap (serum osmolarity − 2 [stool sodium + stool potassium]) is >100, and secretory diarrhea needs to be strongly considered if the gap is <50,[14] although very high purging volumes may make these cut points less relevant. Direct measurement of stool osmolality of a fresh specimen can confirm if purposeful dilution or urine contamination is suspected (the stool osmolality will be significantly less than 290 mOsm/kg). Loss of serum protein from the mucosal surface can be confirmed by determining the fecal content of alpha-1-antitrypsin, a large-molecular weight serum protein that is resistant to proteolytic degradation in the gastrointestinal tract.

To exclude ongoing infection as a contributing factor to chronic diarrhea, it is appropriate to culture the stool for enteric pathogens. Bacterial infections from organisms such as *Yersinia*, *Shigella*, and *Salmonella* species may develop into chronic illness and can be evaluated for by routine stool culture. Additionally, some stool cultures may include testing for diarrhea-causing

Aeromonas and *Plesiomonas* species.[15] *Clostridium difficile* toxin/polymerase chain reaction (PCR) assay should be performed in patients >1 year of age, because this infection is being increasingly recognized in the community.[16] Antigen detection for *Giardia* and *Cryptosporidium* species is more sensitive and specific than routine microscopy-based "ova and parasite" examinations and, therefore, may be helpful if these infections are suspected.[17] Viral gastroenteritis does not usually cause diarrhea for more than 14 days. However, notable exceptions are in infants, and severe cases should be broadly evaluated for infectious agents, including cytomegalovirus (CMV),[18] which is treatable.

Screening Laboratory Blood Studies

An analysis of blood or serum constituents is individualized according to the clinical situation and degree of concern for malabsorption, malnutrition, and inflammatory disease. A routine complete blood cell count with indices addresses issues of anemia as well as iron, vitamin B_{12}, and folate sufficiency. An elevated platelet count may indicate iron or vitamin E deficiency and, more commonly, intestinal inflammation, because platelets are acute phase reactants. Characteristic alterations of red cell morphology are seen in abetalipoproteinemia. Erythrocyte sedimentation rate and C-reactive protein support the possibility of intestinal inflammation but are nonspecific.

Serum immunoglobulins are measured specifically, with special emphasis on immunoglobulin A (IgA). To screen for celiac disease, the specific IgA anti-tissue transglutaminase antibody has replaced the role of less specific anti-gliadin antibodies. Elevated tissue transglutaminase IgA antibody (TTG) has a high specificity for celiac disease of greater than 95% and a sensitivity of up to 96%, but a low total serum IgA level may result in a false-negative test result. IgA anti-endomysial antibody performs similarly to TTG but is more expensive.[19] Low serum albumin and prealbumin concentrations reflect low dietary protein intake and/or protein loss.

Serum calcium, phosphorus, and alkaline phosphatase concentrations should be determined, along with concentrations of one or more of the fat-soluble vitamins—A, D, E, and K—if fat malabsorption or deficiency is suspected. Serum vasoactive intestinal peptide (VIP) and/or urinary concentrations of the catecholamines homovanilmandelic and vanilmandelic acids should be obtained when chronic diarrhea appears to be secretory and particularly if serum potassium and bicarbonate are abnormal.

Sweat Test
The analysis of sweat sodium and/or chloride by iontophoresis should be performed in all infants and toddlers with growth failure and diarrhea as well as any child with suspected or documented steatorrhea to exclude cystic fibrosis. A genotypic analysis for the known mutations in cystic fibrosis can also be performed on a sample of blood (and in most states is part of the newborn screening process). The nutritional support of children with cystic fibrosis is discussed in detail in Chapter 46: Nutrition in Cystic Fibrosis.

The Fasting Trial
A fasting trial can be informative for a diagnosis in chronic diarrheal disorders. To undertake a formal fasting trial, oral or enteral intake is interrupted for 24 to 48 hours, including all noncritical oral or enteral medications. A fasting trial can be quite burdensome to patients and families, so clinicians should end the trial as soon as critical information is collected. Fasting periods are also an appropriate management strategy when stool output is massive, so that fluid losses may be mitigated during aggressive fluid resuscitation. Diagnostically, it is useful to confirm the presence of a secretory diarrheal state. Liquid stools will continue during a fast in most secretory diarrheal states, and stool electrolyte analysis during this phase of assessment can point toward particular conditions (eg, elevated stool chloride in congenital chloride diarrhea).[20]

Breath Hydrogen Analysis
The hydrogen breath test is a noninvasive test that can be used to examine for carbohydrate malabsorption. The test requires commensal hydrogen-producing enteric bacterial flora and generally is not valid after recent antibiotic use. When an oral carbohydrate is given, it is either digested and absorbed normally or it reaches the bacterial flora of the cecum and colon intact and is fermented to produce hydrogen gas that is absorbed and excreted in the breath. Analysis of breath hydrogen concentrations that reveals an increase of >20 ppm from the fasting baseline suggests carbohydrate malabsorption or bacterial overgrowth. The test is performed with oral lactose (for suspected lactase deficiency) or sucrose (for suspected sucrase-isomaltase deficiency).

Imaging
The value of radiologic studies for the evaluation of chronic diarrhea is generally limited. A plain radiograph of the abdomen may reveal constipation, dilated blind loops of bowel, or calcifications of the biliary or pancreatic

system. Abdominal ultrasonography may also be used to assess for pancreatic echogenicity, indicative of fatty replacement sometimes seen in cystic fibrosis or Shwachman-Diamond syndrome. Oral contrast studies and computed tomography scans with contrast are routine for the evaluation of inflammatory bowel disease, identifying, in particular, areas of small bowel disease not viewable by endoscopy. Magnetic resonance enterography has been recognized also as an important imaging modality in IBD, because it may demonstrate intestinal inflammation without exposure to radiation.

Endoscopic Procedures
When chronic diarrhea cannot be explained by an infectious disease or a specific dietary source, endoscopic assessment with mucosal biopsies is appropriate. Endoscopy may reveal duodenal villous blunting and intraepithelial lymphocytes in celiac disease or evidence of ileal or colonic inflammation in infectious colitis or IBD. Small bowel biopsy during endoscopy also may show evidence of duodenitis in parasitic infections. Routine staining of tissue samples may be supplemented by electron microscopy, to examine for congenital enteropathies such as microvillus inclusion disease, or biochemical analysis of the biopsy sample, which might reveal the lack of a disaccharidase activity. Normal histology in the face of clinically significant watery diarrhea that does not resolve with a fasting trial suggests a defect in ion transport or endogenous production of secretory hormone. When a congenital enteropathy is suspected, special stains such as MOC31 (EPCAM) for tufting enteropathy, CD10 or villin for microvillus inclusion disease, and chromogranin (enteroendocrine aplasia) are useful additions to standard hematoxylin and eosin staining of intestinal tissue biopsies.

Genetic Testing
Several monogenic disorders result in significant and potentially life-threatening chronic diarrhea. These conditions almost always (although not exclusively) manifest in the first 3 months of life. In these cases, parallel genetic testing in addition to dietary manipulations, stool and serum testing, and endoscopy is helpful to identify a specific genetic cause. In some patients, initial clinical evaluations or a family history of an identified monogenic condition may point to increased suspicion of a known enteropathy. Examples include the very high stool chloride seen in SLC26A3 mutations (congenital chloride diarrhea) or the characteristic epithelial tufts seen on biopsy in EPCAM mutations (tufting enteropathy). In these cases, targeted genetic sequencing (Sanger sequencing) for suspected genes or specific genetic panels (eg, congenital diarrhea gene panel), which test

for known and relatively more common monogenic conditions, are a useful initial step. However, over the past few years the advent of next-generation sequencing technologies has meant that the cost and speed of whole exome or whole genome sequencing has revolutionized the diagnosis of suspected Mendelian genetic conditions. Therefore, in cases of suspected congenital enteropathy where the diagnosis based on clinical evaluation is unclear, it is now appropriate and helpful to have whole-exome sequencing (WES) performed, if available, to identify a possible causative genetic mutation. If WES analysis reveals a previously unreported gene variant, functional testing in a specialized center is required to confirm that it is a causative mutation for the enteropathy.

Differential Diagnosis of Chronic Diarrhea

A comprehensive review of the many disorders that cause chronic diarrhea is beyond the scope of this chapter. In Table 27.1, the major conditions are listed as either commonly associated with normal growth or those expected to be complicated by growth failure or failure to thrive. Inappropriate nutritional management of any of these disorders, however, can lead to weight loss and growth failure. Highlights for common and/or important conditions are provided here.

Diarrhea Without Malnutrition or Hypovolemia

Functional (Toddler's) Diarrhea

Functional diarrhea is the most common form of diarrhea in the first 3 years of life.[21] The Rome IV Committee defined functional diarrhea as present when all of the following criteria are met: daily painless, recurrent passage of 4 or more large, unformed stools; symptoms lasting more than 4 weeks; onset between 6 and 60 months of age; and no growth failure/malnutrition if caloric intake is adequate. Symptoms typically resolve by the time affected children are school age.[8] Transit time of enteral contents may be especially short, and parents frequently describe undigested food remnants in the stool. Excessive sorbitol-containing fruit juice consumption (eg, prune, pear, or apple) has been reported in children with functional diarrhea.[22] The American Academy of Pediatrics (AAP) policy statement on fruit juice in pediatrics discourages any fruit juice consumption in infants younger than 12 months, very limited consumption in toddlers, and recommends against the use of fruit juice in the treatment of dehydration or the management of diarrhea.[23]

Table 27.1.

Chronic Diarrhea in Childhood

Diarrhea Without Failure to Thrive
Functional diarrhea
Irritable bowel syndrome—diarrhea predominant
Substrate-induced diarrhea
- Excessive juice
- Disaccharide intolerance: lactose, sucrose
- Laxative use
- Caregiver-induced (Munchausen by proxy)

Infectious enteritis[a]
- Parasitic: *Giardia, Strongyloides, Cryptosporidium, Cyclospora* species
- Bacteria: *Salmonella, Yersinia, Aeromonas, Plesiomonas* species
- Small-bowel bacterial overgrowth

Overflow diarrhea from constipation

Diarrhea With Growth Failure/Malnutrition
Pancreatic insufficiency-steatorrhea
- Cystic fibrosis
- Shwachman-Diamond syndrome

Disorders of lipid digestion, absorption, or transport
- Abetalipoproteinemia
- Chylomicron retention disease
- DGAT1 deficiency
- Intestinal lymphangiectasia

Enterocyte structural disorders
- Microvillus inclusion disease
- Tufting disease

Reduced small intestinal surface area
- Short-bowel syndrome
- Malnutrition

Disorders of ion transporter
- Congenital chloride diarrhea
- Congenital sodium diarrhea

Substrate-induced
- Glucose-galactose malabsorption
- Congenital lactase deficiency
- Sucrase-isomaltase deficiency
- Enteric anendocrinosis

Inflammatory villus injury
- Post-gastroenteritis diarrhea with malabsorption
- Celiac disease[b]
- Dietary protein induced enteropathy: milk, soy, egg, fish[b]
- Allergic eosinophilic gastroenteropathy[b]
- Autoimmune enteritis
- Crohn disease
- Blind loop/pseudo-obstruction
- Whipple enteropathy
- Ischemic, radiation enteropathy
- Graft-versus-host disease

Endogenous secretogogue
- Hormonal diarrhea
- Bile acid malabsorption

[a] Chronic infection may also present with weight loss, depending on the severity and length of the infection.

[b] Milder forms of these conditions may not be associated with malnutrition.

Toddlers will do best eating a balanced diet with fruit juice limited to less than 4 ounces per day. Diarrhea often resolves with the acquisition of successful bowel toilet training, which allows greater duration of rectal retention.

Lactose Malabsorption

Lactose is a major dietary constituent for most children, because it is the primary carbohydrate of all mammalian milks other than the sea lion.[24] Lactose is a major source of energy and facilitates intestinal absorption of calcium and magnesium.[25] It is hydrolyzed by the mucosal brush-border disaccharidase lactase to glucose and galactose. Lactase activity decreases, in many species, under genetic control after weaning. Approximately 70% of the world's adult population has lactase nonpersistence. Age of onset varies among populations, with one fifth of Hispanic, Asian, and black children developing lactose malabsorption before 5 years of age. White children typically do not lose lactase function until after 5 years of age and often much later, during later teen years or beyond. Molecular studies have elucidated differences in messenger RNA expression among races that might explain population-based variations in lactase activity. Congenital lactase deficiency is exceedingly rare.[26]

As lactase activity decreases, dietary lactose is incompletely digested and induces an osmotic secretion of electrolytes and fluid in the distal small bowel. As the lactose reaches the bacterial flora of the distal bowel, it is fermented to hydrogen, methane, and carbon dioxide. This allows the diagnosis by breath hydrogen and methane analysis and also contributes to the child's sense of discomfort from gas and increased flatus. The fermentation of lactose also produces volatile fatty acids that are absorbed across the colonic epithelium as an energy source. It is important to distinguish between lactose malabsorption, a laboratory finding, and lactose intolerance, a set of symptoms accompanying the malabsorption of lactose. Symptoms and laboratory evidence of malabsorption may be poorly correlated.[27]

The first step in the treatment of lactose malabsorption involves eliminating lactose from the diet to determine whether symptoms resolve. A gradual reintroduction of lactose-containing foods can help determine the threshold for tolerance of lactose in the diet. Lactose-reduced milks are commonly available, as are lactase tablets, which are taken before ingesting lactose-containing foods. A number of probiotics to enhance lactose tolerance are under investigation, but none have demonstrated reproducible

What the AAP Says About Lactose[28]

1. Lactose intolerance is a common cause of abdominal pain in older children and teenagers.
2. Lactose intolerance attributable to primary lactase deficiency is uncommon before 2 to 3 years of age in all populations; when lactose malabsorption becomes apparent before 2 to 3 years of age, other etiologies must be sought.
3. Evaluation for lactose intolerance can be achieved relatively easily by dietary elimination and challenge. More formal testing is usually noninvasive, typically with fecal pH in the presence of watery diarrhea and hydrogen breath testing.
4. If lactose-free diets are used for treatment of lactose intolerance, the diets should include a good source of calcium and/or calcium supplementation to meet daily recommended intakes.
5. Treatment of lactose intolerance by elimination of milk and other dairy products is not usually necessary given newer approaches to lactose intolerance, including use of partially digested products (such as yogurts, cheeses, products containing *Lactobacillus acidophilus*, and pretreated milks). Evidence that avoidance of dairy products may lead to inadequate calcium intake and consequent suboptimal bone mineralization makes these important as alternatives to milk. Dairy products remain principle sources of protein and other nutrients that are essential for growth in children.

Pediatrics. 2006;118(3):1279–1286

beneficial effects on symptoms. The heating and fermentation of many cheeses reduce lactose content, and yogurt is also lower in lactose than fluid milk. It is important to make sure that lactose limited diets have adequate calcium from either lactose limited cow milk and cow milk products or calcium-fortified alternative milks.

Infectious Colitis and Enteritis

A variety of bacterial and parasitic pathogens may cause chronic diarrhea. *Salmonella* species may cause chronic diarrhea.[29] *Salmonella* infections are a common cause of foodborne intestinal disease reported to the Centers for Disease Control and Prevention each year[30] (see also Chapter 51: Food Safety: Infectious Disease). The infection is usually contracted from exposure to food of animal origin related to poultry, eggs, beef, and dairy products. Nontyphoidal *Salmonella* organisms typically cause gastroenteritis with diarrhea, abdominal cramping, and fever. *Salmonella* organisms are generally detected in routine stool culture for up to 5 weeks but may be excreted in stool for >1 year in 5% of patients.[29] Antibiotic therapy for uncomplicated nontyphoidal *Salmonella* serotypes is not indicated, because it does not shorten the disease duration and may prolong the duration of excretion of bacteria in the stool. Antibiotics are appropriate, however, in infants younger than 3 months or with immunosuppressive diseases, given the increased risk for invasive disease (bacteremia, osteomyelitis, abscess, meningitis) in these populations.[30]

Yersinia enterocolitica may cause chronic diarrhea but less commonly than *Salmonella* organisms in US children. Infection typically occurs via exposure to food products, specifically pork (major *Yersinia* reservoir) and dairy products. Diarrheal stool may contain blood, mucus, and leukocytes, and symptoms may mirror appendicitis or ileal Crohn disease because of inflammation of the terminal ileum. Antibiotics should be used for patients with severe symptoms.[31]

Other causes of bacterial chronic diarrhea include *Aeromonas* and *Plesiomonas* species. *Aeromonas*, long considered a normal commensal organism, may in fact be an uncommon cause of chronic diarrhea. Symptoms are persistent in approximately one third of patients. Antibiotics are recommended in complicated *Aeromonas* infections.[32] *Pleisomonas* species can be found in fish, shellfish, cats, and dogs. It can uncommonly cause chronic secretory diarrhea. Again, antibiotic treatment is reserved for severe infection.[33]

The protozoa *Giardia intestinalis* and *Cryptosporidium* species may affect immunocompetent as well as immunodeficient children and adolescents. Both infections may affect the duodenum and upper small bowel, leading to mild villous blunting, disaccharidase deficiency, and resultant osmotic-type and/or secretory diarrhea. Malabsorption of fat, protein, and carbohydrates may occur. Both infections are linked to contaminated water and may be associated with child care centers, exposure to wild animals, or recent travel to developing countries. Symptomatic giardiasis should be treated even in immunocompetent children.[34] *Cryptosporidium* infection is generally self-resolving in immunocompetent hosts. Immunocompromised children found to be infected should be treated.[35] Nutritional support is particularly important during such cases of enteritis.

Irritable Bowel Syndrome
Irritable bowel syndrome (IBS) may affect up to 3% of school-aged children,[36] and about one third of this group may have the diarrhea-predominant form (IBS-D).[37] The Rome IV Committee defines IBS-D as

a change of stool consistency along with abdominal pain for least 4 days/month for 2 months.[36] These patients do not have rectal bleeding, anemia, weight loss, or fever. Celiac disease should be ruled out. Treatment is often challenging; there is some limited evidence to support the use of probiotics, peppermint oil, elimination diets, and behavioral treatments.[36]

Diarrhea With Growth Failure/Malnutrition

Postgastroenteritis Diarrhea With Malabsorption

Uncommonly, after a severe episode of infectious gastroenteritis, children in resource-rich countries can go on to have a clinical syndrome similar to environmental enteric dysfunction (EED) endemic in resource-limited locations. The mechanisms that give rise to this syndrome are not well understood. Allergic sensitization is unlikely to play a role,[38] and lactase deficiency seems uncommon.[39] Pathologically, one may see patchy villus blunting and a nonspecific inflammatory infiltrate in the lamina propria.[40] To prevent malnutrition, special diets (eg, low fat, diluted formula) should be avoided, and elemental nutrition should not be needed. Probiotics may play a role in the management of the postgastroenteritis syndrome.[41]

Celiac Disease (Gluten-Sensitive Enteropathy)

Celiac disease is an immune-mediated enteropathy that occurs with gluten ingestion in a genetically susceptible individual. With its prevalence in adults and children approaching 1% worldwide, celiac disease has become a more commonly diagnosed disorder.[19] The gluten-induced injury causes varying changes in the small intestinal mucosa, from increased intra-epithelial lymphocytes to complete villus atrophy. The IgA antibody to tissue transglutaminase is detected in serum of affected children and serves as a highly specific screening test.[19] The diagnosis is confirmed by small-bowel biopsy, obtained by esophagogastroduodenoscopy. Treatment is by complete elimination of gluten-containing foods—wheat, barley, and rye. Gluten-free foods are now readily marketed, and parents of children with celiac disease are instructed to read the labels of processed foods carefully. Anti-tissue transglutaminase antibody testing is repeated 6 to 8 months after the start of the gluten-free diet, and a decrease in serum concentrations is usually seen if the patient is adhering to the diet. Relative to the general population, the risk of developing celiac disease is higher in children with type 1 diabetes mellitus, Williams syndrome, trisomy 21, and autoimmune disorders of the thyroid gland.[42]

Short-Bowel Syndrome (see also Chapter 45: Short Bowel Syndrome)

Short-bowel syndrome (SBS) is the consequence of small bowel resection and the resulting severe nutrient malabsorption that occurs with loss of mucosal surface area. It is seen after surgical intervention for long-segment necrotizing enterocolitis, midgut volvulus, acute ischemic injury, small-bowel aganglionosis, gastroschisis, and diffuse Crohn disease of the small bowel. The best prognosis is for children in whom the ileum and ileocecal valve can be preserved.[43]

In the initial postoperative period following loss of a significant length of small bowel, total parenteral nutrition is used. The early initiation of enteral feedings maximizes enteric hormonal stimulation and adaptation of the residual bowel by elongation, hypertrophy, and reduction in peristaltic rate.

The greatest potential for recovery is when SBS is acquired in infancy, because postnatal intestinal growth is greatest in infancy and toddlerhood. The normal absorptive surface area at birth is approximately 950 cm^2, increasing to 7500 cm^2 in the adult. As noted, enteral feedings are begun as soon as possible to minimize the mucosal atrophy that can occur with long fasting periods. Initial feedings usually contain a protein hydrolysate or amino acids, lipid as a combination of medium-chain and long-chain triglycerides, and carbohydrate as glucose polymers; constituents that are most efficiently digested and absorbed when surface area is limited.[43]

Inflammatory Bowel Disease

The nutritional consequences of diffuse small bowel IBS (Crohn disease) can be devastating. Affected children generally present with abdominal pain, diarrhea, and anorexia. Combined with increased enteric loss of protein, zinc, and blood across the inflamed or ulcerated mucosa, the result is weight loss, reduced growth rate, delayed puberty, and anemia unresponsive to dietary iron. These effects are further complicated when active disease occurs during puberty, when nutritional needs for growth are increased, and by the use of anti-inflammatory and growth-inhibiting corticosteroid therapy. For further discussion of nutritional support in patients with IBS, see Chapter 42: Nutrition in the Management of Chronic Autoimmune Inflammatory Bowel Diseases.

Allergic Enteropathy

Allergic enteropathy, or eosinophilic enteropathy, associated with growth failure/malnutrition, vomiting, and diarrhea, should be distinguished from allergic colitis occurring in otherwise healthy and thriving infants. As in allergic colitis, allergic enteropathy is induced by food proteins, with the most common being cow milk protein. In allergic enteropathy, however, there is small-intestinal mucosal damage resulting in malabsorption of protein, carbohydrate, and fat.[44] The enteropathy resolves with elimination of the responsible protein. Protein hydrolysate and sometimes amino acid-based formulas are used as nutritional sources for these children. Food protein-induced enterocolitis syndrome (FPIES) is related but distinct, because exposure to antigen causes an acute clinical syndrome of vomiting, diarrhea, and sometimes severe hypovolemia and shock. The offending antigens are most often milk and soy proteins. However, cereal proteins may also be triggers, promoting recent consensus guidelines that recommend first foods in infants with FPIES should be fruits or vegetables and not rice, oats, or other cereals.[45]

Congenital Enteropathies

Congenital diarrheas and enteropathies are rare, monogenic disorders that present early in life <6 months of age) and mostly result from defects in intestinal epithelial cell function. Congenital enteropathies are typically associated with life-threatening dehydrating diarrhea, feeding intolerance, and malabsorption and require significant dietary and therapeutic interventions including specialized formulas or parenteral nutrition to sustain appropriate growth and electrolyte and nutrient balance. These disorders can be broadly classified into 5 major categories reflective of a common pathophysiology, although there remains overlap between a number of these categories. These disorders include: (1) disorders of epithelial nutrient or electrolyte transport such as glucose-galactose malabsorption (*SLC5A1*); (2) disorders of epithelial enzymes and metabolism such as sucrase-isomaltase deficiency (SI); (3) disorders of epithelial structure and trafficking such as microvillus inclusion disease (MYO5B); (4) disorders of enteroendocrine dysfunction such as enteroendocrine dysplasia (NEUROG3); and (5) autoimmune enteropathies such as immunodysregulation polyendocrinopathy enteropathy X-linked syndrome (IPEX, FOXP3).

Summary

Chronic diarrhea in childhood can result from many different causes that often must be defined before definitive treatment can be initiated. Particular attention should be paid to growth measurements to distinguish between chronic diarrhea with or without associated growth failure/malnutrition. Understanding the basic pathophysiologic mechanisms of diarrhea—osmotic, secretory, intestinal dysmotility, fatty, and inflammatory—may also aid in making a diagnosis. Nutrition support is the mainstay of treatment in children with an undefined cause of chronic diarrhea. Throughout the evaluation process, appropriate nutrition must be provided to meet the child's needs, enterally or parentally if necessary, to facilitate healing and good health.

References

1. World Health Organization. Diarrhoeal disease. Available at: http://www.who.int/mediacentre/factsheets/fs330/en/. Accessed December 14, 2017

2. Moore SR. Update on prolonged and persistent diarrhea in children. *Curr Opin Gastroenterol.* 2011;27(1):19–23

3. Fagundes-Neto U. Persistent diarrhea: still a serious public health problem in developing countries. *Gastroenterol Rep.* 2013;15(9):345

4. Vanderhoof JA. Chronic diarrhea. *Pediatr Rev.* 1998;19(12):418–422

5. Fine KD, Schiller LR. AGA technical review on the evaluation and management of chronic diarrhea. *Gastroenterology.* 1999;116(6):1464–1486

6. Weaver LT, Steiner H. The bowel habit of young children. *Arch Dis Child.* 1984;59(7):649–652

7. Myo-Khin, Thein-Win-Nyunt, Kyaw-Hla S, Thein-Thein-Myint, Bolin TD. A prospective study on defecation frequency, stool weight, and consistency. *Arch Dis Child.* 1994;71(4):311–313

8. Benninga MA, Faure C, Hyman PE, St James Roberts I, Schechter NL, Nurko S. Childhood functional gastrointestinal disorders: neonate/toddler. *Gastroenterology.* February 15, 2016: doi: 10.1053/j.gastro.2016.1002.1016

9. Canani RB, Castaldo G, Bacchetta R, Martín MG, Goulet O. Congenital diarrhoeal disorders: advances in this evolving web of inherited enteropathies. *Nat Rev Gastroenterol Hepatol.* 2015;12(5):293–302

10. Fenton TR, Harries JT, Milla PJ. Disordered small intestinal motility: a rational basis for toddlers' diarrhoea. *Gut.* 1983;24(10):897–903

11. Tiruppathi C, Balasubramanian KA, Hill PG, Mathan VI. Faecal free fatty acids in tropical sprue and their possible role in the production of diarrhoea by inhibition of ATPases. *Gut.* 1983;24(4):300–305

12. Sherwood RA. Faecal markers of gastrointestinal inflammation. *J Clin Pathol.* 2012;65(11):981–985

13. Beharry S, Ellis L, Corey M, Marcon M, Durie P. How useful is fecal pancreatic elastase 1 as a marker of exocrine pancreatic disease? *J Pediatr.* 2002;141(1):84–90

14. Thomas PD, Forbes A, Green J, et al. Guidelines for the investigation of chronic diarrhoea. 2nd ed. *Gut.* 2003;52(Suppl 5):v1–v15

15. Kaiser L, Surawicz CM. Infectious causes of chronic diarrhoea. *Best Pract Res Clin Gastroenterol.* 2012;26(5):563–571

16. Adams DJ, Eberly MD, Rajnik M, Nylund CM. Risk factors for community-associated *Clostridium difficile* infection in children. *J Pediatr.* 2017;186:105–109

17. Bruijnesteijn van Coppenraet LES, Wallinga JA, Ruijs GJHM, Bruins MJ, Verweij JJ. Parasitological diagnosis combining an internally controlled real-time PCR assay for the detection of four protozoa in stool samples with a testing algorithm for microscopy. *Clin Microbiol Infect.* 2009;15(9):869–874

18. Sue PK, Salazar-Austin NM, McDonald OG, Rishi A, Cornish TC, Arav-Boger R. Cytomegalovirus enterocolitis in immunocompetent young children: a report of two cases and review of the literature. *Pediatr Infect Dis J.* 2016;35(5):573–576

19. Fasano A, Catassi C. Clinical practice. Celiac disease. *N Engl J Med.* 2012;367(25): 2419–2426

20. Wedenoja S, Höglund P, Holmberg C. Review article: the clinical management of congenital chloride diarrhoea. *Aliment Pharmacol Ther.* 2010;31(4):477–485

21. van Tilburg MAL, Hyman PE, Walker L, et al. Prevalence of functional gastrointestinal disorders in infants and toddlers. *J Pediatr.* 2015;166(3):684–689

22. Lifshitz F, Ament ME, Kleinman RE, et al. Role of juice carbohydrate malabsorption in chronic nonspecific diarrhea in children. *J Pediatr.* 1992;120(5): 825–829

23. Heyman MB, Abrams SA, American Academy of Pediatrics, Section on Gastroenterology H, and Nutrition,, Committee on Nutrition. Fruit juice in infants, children, and adolescents: current recommendations. *Pediatrics.* 2017;139(6):e20170967

24. Pilson ME, Kelly AL. Composition of the milk from *Zalophus californianus*, the California Sea Lion. *Science.* 1962;135(3498):104–105

25. Schuette SA, Knowles JB, Ford HE. Effect of lactose or its component sugars on jejunal calcium absorption in adult man. *Am J Clin Nutr.* 1989;50(5):1084–1087

26. Bayless TM, Brown E, Paige DM. Lactase non-persistence and lactose intolerance. *Curr Gastroenterol Rep.* 2017;19(5):23

27. Hammer HF, Petritsch W, Pristautz H, Krejs GJ. Evaluation of the pathogenesis of flatulence and abdominal cramps in patients with lactose malabsorption. *Wien Klin Wochenschr.* 1996;108(6):175–179

28. Heyman MB, American Academy of Pediatrics, Committee on Nutrition. Lactose intolerance in infants, children, and adolescents. *Pediatrics.* 2006;118(3):1279–1286

29. Marzel A, Desai PT, Goren A, et al. Persistent infections by nontyphoidal *Salmonella* in humans: epidemiology and genetics. *Clin Infect Dis.* 2016;62(7): 879–886

30. Centers for Disease Control and Prevention. Information for Healthcare Professionals: Salmonella. Available at: https://www.cdc.gov/salmonella/general/technical.html. Accessed December 19, 2017

31. Centers for Disease Control and Prevention. Information for Health and Laboratory Professionals: Yersinia. Available at: https://www.cdc.gov/yersinia/healthcare.html. Accessed December 19, 2017

VI

32. Parker JL, Shaw JG. Aeromonas spp clinical microbiology and disease. *J Infect.* 2011;62(2):109–118

33. Khan AM, Faruque AS, Hossain MS, Sattar S, Fuchs GJ, Salam MA. Plesiomonas shigelloides-associated diarrhoea in Bangladeshi children: a hospital-based surveillance study. *J Trop Pediatr.* 2004;50(6):354–356

34. American Academy of Pediatrics. *Giardia intestinalis* (formerly *Giardia lamblia* and *Giardia duodenalis*) Infections. In: Kimberlin DK, Brady MT, Jackson MA, Long SS, eds. *Red Book: 2018 Report of the Committee on Infectious Diseases.* 31st ed. Itasca, IL: American Academy of Pediatrics; 2018:352–355

35. American Academy of Pediatrics. Cryptosporidiosis. In: Kimberlin DK BM, Jackson MA, Long SS, ed. *Red Book: 2018 Report of the Committee on Infectious Diseases.* 31st ed. Itasca, IL: American Academy of Pediatrics; 2018:304–307

36. Hyams JS, Di Lorenzo C2 SM, Shulman RJ4, Staiano A5, van Tilburg M6. Functional isorders: children and adolescents. *Gastroenterology.* Epub February 15, 2016. doi: 2010.1053/j.gastro.2016.2002.2015

37. Rajindrajith S, Devanarayana NM. Subtypes and Symptomatology of Irritable Bowel Syndrome in Children and Adolescents: A School-based Survey Using Rome III Criteria. *J Neurogastroenterol Motil.* 2012;18(3):298–304

38. Gibbons T, Fuchs GJ. Chronic enteropathy: clinical aspects. *Nestle Nutr Workshop Ser Pediatr Program.* 2007;59:89–101

39. Boudraa G, Benbouabdellah M, Hachelaf W, Boisset M, Desjeux JF, Touhami M. Effect of feeding yogurt versus milk in children with acute diarrhea and carbohydrate malabsorption. *J Pediatr Gastroenterol Nutr.* 2001;33(3):307–313

40. Thomas AG, Phillips AD, Walker-Smith JA. The value of proximal small intestinal biopsy in the differential diagnosis of chronic diarrhoea. *Arch Dis Child.* 1992;67(6):741–743

41. Gaón D, García H, Winter L, et al. Effect of *Lactobacillus* strains and *Saccharomyces boulardii* on persistent diarrhea in children. *Medicina (Mex).* 2003;63(4):293–298

42. Hill ID, et al. J. Pediatr. Gastroenterol. Nutr. 40. Guideline for the diagnosis and treatment of celiac disease in children: recommendations of the North American Society for Pediatric Gastroenterology, Hepatology and Nutrition. *J Pediatr Gastroenterol Nutr.* 2005;40(1):1–19

43. Duggan CP, Jaksic T. Pediatric intestinal failure. *N Engl J Med.* 2017;377(7):666–675

44. Iyngkaran N, Yadav M, Boey CG, Lam KL. Severity and extent of upper small bowel mucosal damage in cow's milk protein-sensitive enteropathy. *J Pediatr Gastroenterol Nutr.* 1988;7(5):667–674

45. Nowak-Węgrzyn A, Chehade M, Groetch ME, et al. International consensus guidelines for the diagnosis and management of food protein-induced enterocolitis syndrome: Executive summary-Workgroup Report of the Adverse Reactions to Foods Committee, American Academy of Allergy, Asthma & Immunology. *J Allergy Clin Immunol.* 2017;4(139):1111–1126.e1114

Chapter 28

Oral Therapy for Acute Diarrhea

Introduction

Although significant global efforts in diarrhea treatment and prevention have reduced annual deaths from 4.6 million in the 1970s to roughly half a million currently,[1] diarrheal illness and accompanying dehydration remain major causes of preventable childhood deaths in the world. The cholera epidemic in Yemen in 2017 and the childhood mortality that occurred as a result speak to the severe consequences of untreated cholera even in the 21st century. Reduction of the morbidity and mortality from diarrhea through the use of oral rehydration solutions (ORSs) continues to be a major goal of the United Nations Children's Fund (UNICEF) and the World Health Organization (WHO) as one of the critical strategies for saving children's lives. Because of its simplicity, great effectiveness, and low cost, ORSs are an ideal treatment for use in both resource-limited and resource-rich nations. In resource-limited countries, ORSs have played a major role in reducing the estimated number of deaths from diarrhea in children younger than 5 years by more than half. Although the death rate from diarrheal illness in resource-rich countries like the United States is low, diarrheal illness still accounts for a substantial proportion of preventable childhood deaths and a large proportion of the morbidity and the expense associated with pediatric care. Although the advent of effective vaccines against rotavirus has greatly reduced the burden of that etiology of childhood diarrhea,[2] oral therapy for acute diarrhea remains a cornerstone of therapy.[3-5] Indeed, several trials have confirmed that even in industrialized countries in appropriately identified subjects, ORS is at least as effective, if not more so, than intravenous rehydration.[6,7]

Physiologic Principles

The physiologic basis of ORS is simple and extraordinarily elegant. A combination of sodium with simple organic molecules, such as glucose, in the lumen of the small intestine can promote the absorption of water.[8] In concert with the transport of a glucose molecule, a sodium molecule is also brought from the luminal side of the membrane to the interior of the cell via SGLT-1. This sodium ion is subsequently transferred out of the enterocyte by the action of Na-K ATPase into the adjacent capillaries and, thus, into the circulation. Water follows the movement of sodium along a concentration gradient, with the net result being absorption of sodium and water.

VI

Fig 28.1.
Solute-coupled sodium absorption

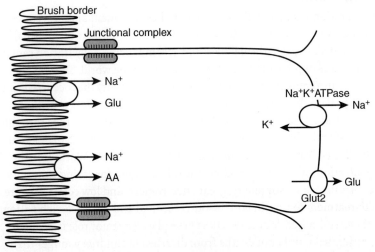

Reprinted from: Lo Vecchio A, Vandenplas Y, Benninga M, et al. An international consensus report on a new algorithm for the management of infant diarrhoea. *Acta Paediatr.* 2016;105(8):e384-e389

Alternative carrier solutes (eg, amino acids) also work as glucose cotransporters (Figure 28.1).

The earliest clinical studies of solutions that take advantage of the cotransport system were performed in patients with cholera.[9] Glucose-sodium cotransport system remains intact in all types of infectious diarrhea. This fact makes oral therapy appropriate for use in any kind of enteric infection in which dehydration is an end result. The other components of ORSs include potassium and chloride to replace stool losses and base, usually in the form of citrate, to replace stool losses, combat acidosis, and act as an additional cotransport molecule.

Many fluids that have traditionally been recommended for the treatment of diarrhea and dehydration are inappropriate, are nonphysiologic, and may actually worsen the condition. For example, juices such as apple or white grape juice have a high osmolality related to their high sugar content and contain virtually no sodium and very little potassium, thus increasing the risk of hyponatremia. Table 28.1 lists the composition of some currently available ORSs. Some of the frequently used inappropriate fluids are listed for comparison. Particular attention should be paid to the osmolality of the fluids. In general, solutions with osmolality lower than serum

Table 28.1.

Composition of Fluids Frequently Used in Oral Rehydration Compared With Fluids Not Recommended for Oral Rehydration

Solution	Glucose/ CHO, g/L	Sodium, mEq/L	HCO_3^-, MEq/L	Potassium, mEq/L	Osmolality, mmol/L	CHO/ Sodium
Pedialyte[a] (Abbott Laboratories)	25	45	30	20	250	3.1
Enfalyte (Mead Johnson)	30	50	34	25	200	
Pediatric Electrolyte[b] (Nutramax)	25	45	20	30	250	3.1
WHO ORS, 2002[c] (reduced osmolarity)	13.5	75	10	20	245	1.0
WHO ORS, 1975, (original formulation)	20	90	10	20	311	1.2
Cola[d]	126	2	13	0.1	750	1944
Apple juice[d]	125	3	0	32	730	1278
Gatorade[d]	45	20	3	3	330	62.5

CHO indicates carbohydrate; HCO_3^-, bicarbonate; WHO, World Health Organization.

[a] Mainly for maintenance therapy; may be used for rehydration therapy in mildly dehydrated patients.

[b] This formulation is supplied to many retail establishments to which they apply their company name.

[c] Best for rehydration therapy; may be used during the maintenance phase with adequate access to free water in the form of human milk, infant formula, or diluted juices.

[d] Cola, juice, and Gatorade are shown for comparison only; they are not recommended for use (as is the case for energy drinks, vitamin waters, gelatin desserts, and other fluids that do not contain glucose and sodium in appropriate concentrations).

VI

(approximately 285–290 mOsm/L) make the most effective ORSs if the ratio of glucose to sodium is maintained near one.

A large randomized trial among well-nourished children with minimal or no dehydration attributable to mild gastroenteritis showed that the provision of dilute apple juice as maintenance fluid was associated with fewer treatment failures, including a lower need for subsequent intravenous fluids, compared with a commercially available ORS.[10] Of note, only 42% of the subjects had a history of diarrhea (whereas 94% had vomiting) and 68% had no evidence of dehydration. The results confirm that children without dehydration can be treated with an increase in the intake of their usual fluids and that some children dislike the taste of ORS. Because juice intake has been associated with chronic diarrhea and encouraging juice is contrary to the usual advice about feeding during acute diarrhea (see below), routine treatment of gastroenteritis with juice is not recommended.

The Search for a More Effective ORS

Although ORSs have an impressive record of success, they remain under-utilized in the United States.[11] One hypothesized reason for underuse of ORSs has been their lack of antidiarrheal properties. Initial efforts to create ORSs that would decrease stool volume and output focused on the addition of other sodium cotransport molecules, such as the amino acids glycine, alanine, and glutamine. However, these solutions proved to be no more effective than ORSs[12] and had some potentially dangerous adverse effects, perhaps related to their higher osmolarity.[13] Similarly, studies of complex carbohydrates (starches) from cereals were undertaken. Starches do not contribute significantly to the osmotic content of the solution and yield individual glucose molecules at the brush border of the small intestine. Several studies demonstrated that cereal-based ORSs reduce the volume of stools and the duration of diarrheal illness in cholera infections, although not necessarily in the case of noncholera diarrhea.[14,15] When cereal-based solutions were compared with the combination of glucose-based solutions and the early reinstitution of feeding, the differences between the 2 approaches disappeared,[16] so cereal-based ORSs have not replaced the easier-to-prepare glucose ORSs.

In 2002, WHO and UNICEF formally endorsed the global use of an ORS of reduced osmolarity (245 mmol/L vs the original WHO ORS of 311 mmol/L). This newer ORS contains 75 mEq/L of sodium and 75 mmol/L of glucose to maintain a 1:1 molar ratio for effective rehydration.[17,18]

Reduced-osmolarity ORSs are more effective in replacing fluid and electrolyte losses compared with the standard WHO ORS.[14,15] A meta-analysis of
clinical trials in children in resource-limited countries showed that these
solutions resulted in less need for supplemental intravenous fluids, less
vomiting, and a slight reduction in stool output compared with the standard WHO ORS.[19]

Zinc Supplementation

Zinc supplementation during acute and chronic diarrhea has been shown
to reduce diarrhea duration and stool frequency and decrease the chances
of persistent diarrhea, especially in children with malnutrition.[20] The WHO
recommends zinc supplementation (20 mg/day for 10–14 days for children
6 months and older, and 10 mg/day for children younger than 6 months)
in combination with ORS for children with acute diarrhea. The precise
dose of supplemental zinc that is most effective is unclear and currently
under study. Trials of zinc supplementation in resource-rich countries,
where dietary intake and bioavailability of zinc is presumably higher than
in resource-limited countries, have failed to show an advantage of zinc
supplementation.[20,21]

Probiotics

Probiotics are defined as "live microorganisms that, when administered in
adequate amounts, confer a health benefit on the host."[22] Numerous studies
have suggested that probiotics may have a positive effect on enterocyte and
mucosal immune system health as well as modulation of the microbiota,
although these studies have been marked by several different intestinal
models and myriad different probiotic species. Clinical data supporting the
use of probiotics have also been plagued by different interventions and study
designs. A 2010 Cochrane review found that probiotic supplementation
was associated with a mean reduction of diarrhea duration of 24.76 hours
(95% confidence interval [CI], 15.9–33.6 hours; n=4555; trials=35) and a
59% reduction in the risk of diarrhea lasting ≥4 days (relative risk, 0.41;
95% CI, 0.32–0.53; n=2853; trials=29).[23] *Saccharomyces boulardii* as a treatment for acute childhood diarrhea was evaluated in a meta-analysis and was
also found to be effective in reducing the duration of diarrhea and odds of
diarrhea on days 3 and 4 of illness.[24] Evidence also suggests that probiotics,
specifically *Lactobacillus rhamnosus* or *Saccharomyces boulardii*, may help reduce
the incidence of antibiotic-associated diarrhea in children.[25]

In general, although many trials have been performed with a variety
of probiotic species, the American Academy of Pediatrics and other

VI

policy-making groups have not generally endorsed their routine use in children with diarrhea because of concerns with study designs, methodologic quality of some trials, uncertainty about dosage and effective species, and limited cost-effectiveness data. Although probiotics tend to be safe interventions, they should be used with caution in children with altered immunity, increased intestinal permeability, or indwelling central venous catheters.[26]

Early, Appropriate Feeding

For many years, clinicians have recognized that a return to an age-appropriate and healthy diet early in the course of diarrheal illness is superior to the outdated practice of "resting the gut" by providing only clear liquids or dilute milks.[27] Appropriate feeding is the component of oral therapy that has the potential for the greatest effect on stool volume and duration. In addition, the appetite of the infant and child is generally better maintained, and intestinal repair can occur.

Successful feeding trials have been conducted using human milk, dilute or full-strength animal milk or animal milk formulas, dilute and full-strength lactose-free formulas, and mixed diets of staple foods with milk. Data from multiple studies support the use of lactose-containing milks during diarrhea, especially if given with complex carbohydrates.[31] In general, the change to a lactose-free formula should be made only if the stool output increases on a milk-based diet or if the child has persistent diarrhea.[3] Semisolid and solid foods that have proven to be effective in controlled trials include rice, wheat, peas, potatoes, chicken, and eggs.

Oral Therapy for Diarrhea

In addition to the use of a physiologically sound ORS and early, appropriate feeding, effective oral therapy requires a thoughtful parental education component. When possible, explaining to the parent that the child's diarrhea is likely to continue, regardless of therapy, for 3 to 7 days can be extremely helpful. Parents who understand that hydration is the primary concern, not the duration of the diarrheal stool, will generally be more comfortable managing the child's illness at home. Emphasizing that ORS replaces fluid and electrolyte losses but does not stop diarrhea may result in less disappointment and discouragement for the parents. A positive approach to teaching parents includes pointing out the degree of control that parents retain when the child receives ORS compared with the loss of that control that results when intravenous solutions are used. In addition, parents are often reassured to know that ORSs are less painful, have fewer complications, and are just as effective as intravenous therapy. Finally, most parents greatly desire to feed their child, particularly when the child appears to be hungry and thirsty, and this should be encouraged. The following management guidelines are based on the severity of the child's condition.

Children With Diarrhea and No Dehydration

If no dehydration develops, which is the case in the great majority of diarrhea cases in the United States, continued age-appropriate feeding is the only therapy required. Nonweaned infants should receive human milk or continue use of regular, nondiluted formula. Weaned infants and children should have their regular nutritionally balanced diet continued, emphasizing complex carbohydrates (such as rice, wheat, and potatoes), meats (especially chicken), and the child's regular milk or formula. Diets high in simple sugars and fats should be avoided. The "BRAT" diet (bananas, rice, applesauce, tea, and toast) should be avoided, because it is not a balanced diet and is low in energy and critical micronutrients.[28]

Children With Mild or Moderate Dehydration

After dehydration is corrected (Table 28.2), appropriate feeding should begin, using the guidelines in the previous paragraph. The most convenient method for carrying out rehydration is to divide the total volume deficit by 4 and aim to deliver this volume of fluid during each of the 4 hours of the rehydration phase. A teaspoon or 5-mL syringe can be used for the initial administration of fluid, especially if the child is vomiting. The parent is instructed to administer at least 1 teaspoon (5 mL) of solution each minute. Having a clock with a sweep second hand available is useful. Although this rate of fluid delivery may appear slow, 5 mL per minute results in an hourly intake of 300 mL. In a 10-kg infant, this is equivalent to 30 mL/kg. Children larger than 15 to 20 kg can receive 2 teaspoons, or 10 mL, per minute and achieve a similar volume of fluid intake. In general, this rate of fluid administration is more than adequate to replace the entire calculated volume deficit within a 4-hour period.

During rehydration, in the clinical setting, the volume of stool and emesis should be carefully recorded and added to the hourly quantity of fluid to be administered. After 1 or 2 hours of successful rehydration using a syringe or teaspoon, most infants and children will be able to take the fluid ad libitum. On rare occasions, a child will not cooperate in taking the

Table 28.2.
Fluid Therapy Chart

Degree of Dehydration	Signs	Fluids	Feeding
Mild[a]	Slightly dry mucous membranes, increased thirst	ORS, 50–60 mL/kg[b]	Breastfeeding, undiluted lactose-free formula, full-strength cow milk, or lactose-containing formula
Moderate	Sunken eyes, sunken fontanelle, loss of skin turgor, dry mucous membranes	ORS, 80–100 mL/kg[b]	Same as above
Severe	Signs of moderate dehydration plus 1 or more of the following: rapid thready pulse, cyanosis, rapid breathing, delayed capillary refill time, lethargy, coma	Intravenous or intraosseous isotonic fluids (0.9% saline solution or lactated Ringer solution), 40 mL/kg per hour until pulse and state of consciousness return to normal, then 50–100 mL/kg of ORS based on remaining degree of dehydration.[c]	Begin after clinically improved and ORS has started

[a] If no signs of dehydration are present, rehydration phase may be omitted. Proceed with maintenance therapy and replacement of ongoing losses.

[b] First 4 hours, repeat until no signs of dehydration remain. Replace ongoing stool losses and vomitus with oral rehydration solution (ORS), 10 mL/kg for each diarrheal stool and 5 mL/kg for each episode of vomiting.

[c] While parenteral access is being sought, nasogastric infusion of ORS may be begun at 30 mL/kg per hour, provided airway protective reflexes remain intact.

solution from a syringe (this is most often the case with toddlers) or may be too exhausted to remain awake during the administration of fluid. In these cases and after carefully establishing that airway protective reflexes are intact, a soft 5F polymeric silicone nasogastric tube may be placed by the health care provider into the lumen of the stomach. The ORS may then be administered via the nasogastric tube at approximately 5 to 10 mL/kg per minute. This method has been widely used in resource-limited countries, has proved quite successful in resource-rich countries[29] and can be encouraged with appropriate education of caregivers.[30]

Children With Severe Dehydration

Children with severe dehydration, which is a shock or near shock-like condition, should be treated as a true medical emergency. A large-bore catheter should be used for the infusion of lactated Ringer solution, normal saline solution, or similar solution, and boluses of 20 to 40 mL/kg should be administered until signs of shock resolve. Fluid and electrolyte resuscitation may require more than 1 intravenous site, and the use of alternate access sites, including venous cutdown, femoral vein, or intraosseous locations, may be needed. As the level of consciousness improves, oral rehydration therapy can be instituted. Hydration status must be frequently reassessed to monitor the effectiveness of the therapy. When rehydration is complete, feeding is continued as described for children without dehydration.

Common Concerns About Oral Rehydration Solutions in the United States

Refusal to Take ORS

One of the most common complaints about ORSs from children and their parents in the United States is the salty taste. However, children who are truly dehydrated rarely refuse an ORS, because they usually crave salt and water. By recognizing that ORS may not be required in children with mild diarrhea and no dehydration, the problem of refusal could be greatly reduced.[10] Methods to try to increase ORS intake have included the use of flavoring in ORSs, which does not alter the composition of fluid and electrolytes but improves taste. Flavored ORSs are now the most popular forms of ORSs sold in North America. Another effective technique to increase intake is to freeze the ORS in an ice-pop form, but the volume of ORSs included in these commercial preparations are minimal (2–3 ounces). Newly available ORSs (flavored with nonsugar sweeteners such as sucralose) have

VI

not, in limited studies, shown appreciable improvements compared with standard ORSs.[31]

Vomiting

Vomiting, which is commonly associated with acute diarrhea, can make oral rehydration therapy more challenging, but almost all children with vomiting can be treated successfully with an ORS. Correction of fluid and electrolyte deficits with a balanced electrolyte ORS can help speed recovery from vomiting. As vomiting decreases, the ORS can be administered in larger volumes. Supplemental medical therapy for emesis with ondansetron or other antiemetics seems to make oral rehydration more successful, with lower rates of hospitalization and need for intravenous rehydration.[32]

(A precautionary note must be made about vomiting, which can be evidence of bowel obstruction. For this reason, efforts should be made to eliminate the possible diagnosis of bowel obstruction on a clinical basis before proceeding with an ORS. In a patient who may have an obstructive or other acute process, immediate vascular access must be gained, a surgical consultation must be obtained, and the child should be kept without oral fluids or food.)

Hypernatremia

ORSs were originally developed to treat dehydration resulting from cholera, in which stool losses of sodium are substantial. In resource-rich countries like the United States, concerns have been expressed about the risk of hypernatremia with the use of solutions containing 90 mEq/L of sodium in infants and children whose diarrhea results from noncholera organisms. In the presence of mature, functioning kidneys, the earlier 90-mEq sodium solution and newer 75-mEq sodium solution are both safe and extremely effective in children with a wide range of initial serum sodium concentrations and are effective treatments for hypernatremia.[4] In contrast, when liquids with little sodium such as juices, sodas, or water (Table 28.1) are used, the risk of hyponatremia is very real. Of greater importance than the sodium concentration is the ratio of sodium to glucose (or other cotransport molecule), which should be close to 1.

Failure of Therapy

Failure of ORS occurs when the net output over a 4- to 8-hour period exceeds net intake or when clinical indicators of dehydration are worsening rather than improving. Before determining that ORS has failed in a child, a review of the treatment guidelines should be made with the parents or other

caregiver. Often, treatment failures and unnecessary intravenous line placement can result from lack of understanding or failure to encourage staff or
parents to continue to administer adequate volumes of ORS.

References

1. Liu L, Oza S, Hogan D, et al. Global, regional, and national causes of under-5
   mortality in 2000–15: an updated systematic analysis with implications for the
   Sustainable Development Goals. *Lancet.* 2016;388(10063):3027–3035

2. Desai R, Curns AT, Steiner CA, Tate JE, Patel MM, Parashar UD. All-cause
   gastroenteritis and rotavirus-coded hospitalizations among US children,
   2000–2009. *Clin Infect Dis.* Aug 2012;55(4):e28–34

3. Lo Vecchio A, Vandenplas Y, Benninga M, et al. An international consensus
   report on a new algorithm for the management of infant diarrhoea. *Acta
   Paediatr.* 2016;105(8):e384–389

4. King CK, Glass R, Bresee JS, Duggan C, Centers for Disease C, Prevention.
   Managing acute gastroenteritis among children: oral rehydration, maintenance,
   and nutritional therapy. *MMWR Recomm Rep.* 2003;52(RR-16):1–16

5. American Academy of Pediatrics Provisional Committee on Quality
   Improvement Subcommittee on Acute Gastroenteritis. Practice parameter: the
   management of acute gastroenteritis in young children. *Pediatrics.* 1996;97:
   424–436

6. Spandorfer PR, Alessandrini EA, Joffe MD, Localio R, Shaw KN. Oral versus
   intravenous rehydration of moderately dehydrated children: a randomized,
   controlled trial. *Pediatrics.* 2005;115(2):295–301

7. Atherly-John YC, Cunningham SJ, Crain EF. A randomized trial of oral vs
   intravenous rehydration in a pediatric emergency department. *Arch Pediatr
   Adolesc Med.* 2002;156(12):1240–1243

8. Field M. Intestinal ion transport and the pathophysiology of diarrhea. *J Clin
   Invest.* 2003;111(7):931–943

9. Greenough WB, III. The human, societal, and scientific legacy of cholera. *J Clin
   Invest.* 2004;113(3):334–339

10. Freedman SB, Willan AR, Boutis K, Schuh S. Effect of Dilute Apple Juice and
    Preferred Fluids vs Electrolyte Maintenance Solution on Treatment Failure
    Among Children With Mild Gastroenteritis: A Randomized Clinical Trial. *JAMA.*
    2016;315(18):1966–1974. doi: 1910.1001/jama.2016.5352

11. Reis EC, Goepp JG, Katz S, Santosham M. Barriers to use of oral rehydration
    therapy. *Pediatrics.* 1994;93(5):708–711

12. Bhan MK, Mahalanabis D, Fontaine O, Pierce NF. Clinical trials of improved oral
    rehydration salt formulations: a review. *Bull World Health Organ.* 1994;72(6):
    945–955

13. Santosham M, Burns BA, Reid R, et al. Glycine-based oral rehydration solution:
    reassessment of safety and efficacy. *J Pediatr.* 1986;109(5):795–801

14. CHOICE Study Group. Multicenter, randomized, double-blind clinical trial to evaluate the efficacy and safety of a reduced osmolarity oral rehydration salts solution in children with acute watery diarrhea. *Pediatrics*. 2001;107(4):613–618

15. Alam NH, Majumder RN, Fuchs GJ, CHOICE Study group. Efficacy and safety of oral rehydration solution with reduced osmolarity in adults with cholera: a randomised double-blind clinical trial. *Lancet*. 1999;354(9175):296–299

16. Fayad IM, Hashem M, Duggan C, et al. Comparative efficacy of rice-based and glucose-based oral rehydration salts plus early reintroduction of food. *Lancet*. 1993;342(8874):772–775

17. Duggan C, Fontaine O, Pierce NF, et al. Scientific rationale for a change in the composition of oral rehydration solution. *JAMA*. 2004;291(21):2628–2631

18. World Health Organization. *Oral rehydration salts (ORS): A new reduced osmolarity formulation*. Geneva: WHO; 2002

19. Kim Y, Hahn S, Garner P. Low osmolarity oral rehydration solution for treating diarrhoea-associated dehydration in children [Cochrane Review]. 2001; Issue 2

20. Lazzerini M, Wanzira H. Oral zinc for treating diarrhoea in children. *Cochrane Database Syst Rev*. 2016(12) CD005436

21. Patro B, Szymanski H, Szajewska H. Oral zinc for the treatment of acute gastroenteritis in Polish children: a randomized, double-blind, placebo-controlled trial. *J Pediatr*. 2010;157(6):984–988 e981

22. Sanders ME. Probiotics: definition, sources, selection, and uses. *Clin Infect Dis*. 2008;46 Suppl 2:S58–61; discussion S144–151

23. Allen SJ, Martinez EG, Gregorio GV, Dans LF. Probiotics for treating acute infectious diarrhoea. *Cochrane Database Syst Rev*. 2010(11):CD003048

24. Feizizadeh S, Salehi-Abargouei A, Akbari V. Efficacy and safety of Saccharomyces boulardii for acute diarrhea. *Pediatrics*. 2014;134(1):e176–191

25. Goldenberg JZ, Lytvyn L, Steurich J, Parkin P, Mahant S, Johnston BC. Probiotics for the prevention of pediatric antibiotic-associated diarrhea. *Cochrane Database Syst Rev*. 2015(12):CD004827

26. Kunz AN, Noel JM, Fairchok MP. Two cases of Lactobacillus bacteremia during probiotic treatment of short gut syndrome. *J Pediatr Gastroenterol Nutr*. 2004;38(4):457–458

27. Duggan C, Nurko S. "Feeding the gut": the scientific basis for continued enteral nutrition during acute diarrhea. *J Pediatr*. 1997;131(6):801–808

28. Duro D, Duggan C. The BRAT for acute diarrhea in children: Should it be used? *Pract Gastroenterol*. 2007;6:60–88

29. Gremse D. Effectiveness of nasogastric rehydration in hospitalized children with diarrhea. *J Pediatr Gastroenterol Nutr*. 1995;21:145–148

30. Freedman SB, Keating LE, Rumatir M, Schuh S. Health care provider and caregiver preferences regarding nasogastric and intravenous rehydration. *Pediatrics*. 2012;130(6):e1504–1511

31. Hurt RT, Vallumsetla N, Edakkanambeth Varayil J, et al. A pilot study comparing 2 oral rehydration solutions in patients with short bowel syndrome receiving home parenteral nutrition: a prospective double-blind randomized controlled trial. *Nutr Clin Pract.* 2017;32(6):814-819

32. Fedorowicz Z, Jagannath VA, Carter B. Antiemetics for reducing vomiting related to acute gastroenteritis in children and adolescents. *Cochrane Database Syst Rev.* 2011(9):CD005506

VI

Chapter 29

Inborn Errors of Metabolism

Introduction

Metabolism may be defined as the sum of chemical processes through which food is converted into other molecules and energy. Although there are some variations in metabolism that are benign, an inborn error of metabolism (IEM) is defined as an inherited defect in the structure or function of a key protein in a metabolic pathway that is clinically significant, causing human disease.[1] These diseases involve processes of energy production; the anabolism and catabolism of fats, carbohydrates, or amino acids; the synthesis and degradation of complex macromolecules; synthesis of enzyme cofactors; the transport of substances across cell membranes; and the detoxification of cellular wastes. The spectrum of cardinal features, age of clinically apparent symptoms, morbidity, mortality, and types of currently used therapies vary widely across this diverse group of disorders.

Inheritance

Each individual IEM occurs rarely, with population incidences ranging from 1:2500 births for hemochromatosis to only a few single case reports of other disorders. Collectively, the total incidence of IEM in the population is approximately 1:1000 births. Most IEMs are autosomal-recessive diseases attributable to single-gene defects encoded by nuclear DNA. A few IEMs are inherited in an autosomal-dominant pattern, and a small fraction are X-linked disorders, exhibiting a more severe phenotype in hemizygous males than in heterozygous females. Still other IEMs are attributable to alterations in the mitochondrial DNA and are inherited through maternal lineage.

Newborn Screening for IEMs

For many IEMs, although signs and symptoms may not be present in the immediate neonatal period, damage nonetheless occurs, either as a result of a critical shortage of enzyme product or accumulation of deleterious compounds in the brain or other organs and in body fluids. In some cases, recognition of the disease and early institution of therapy can significantly alter the morbidity and mortality of these initially occult disorders. As a result, newborn screening tests have been developed. Each state has a newborn screening system to identify at-risk children and coordinated follow-up to confirm the diagnosis. This screening consists of both bedside testing (ie, critical congenital heart disorders and hearing loss) and blood testing. All states perform blood spot testing shortly after birth. The blood spots are used to screen for many disorders, including aminoacidopathies such as phenylketonuria, several disorders of fatty acid oxidation and organic acid metabolism, galactosemia, biotinidase deficiency, hypothyroidism, congenital adrenal hyperplasia, hemoglobinopathies, cystic fibrosis, and some other types of IEMs. Currently in the United States, the Advisory Committee on Heritable Disorders in Newborns and Children, a federal advisory committee, makes recommendations to the Secretary of Health and Human Services with respect to a recommended uniform screening panel (RUSP).[2] As of February 2017, the RUSP consisted of 34 disorders. States use the RUSP and their own state laws, mandates, and public health resources to develop their screening programs. More information about newborn screening is available from the American Academy of Pediatrics publication, *Medical Genetics in Pediatric Practice*,[1] and a searchable database with state-specific information can be found at http://www.babysfirsttest.org. Newborn screening has been awarded a place in the "top ten" public health successes by the Centers for Disease Control and Prevention. Across the United States, newborn screening programs screen more than 95% of babies each year in an effort to provide each baby in every state the chance to have a healthy start, regardless of gender, birth location, ethnicity, or socioeconomic status. The American College of Medical Genetics and Genomics has developed a series of ACT sheets to aid primary care providers in the newborn screening process and to help direct care for children with an abnormal screen.[3] Newsteps, a web-based resource of the Association of Public Health Laboratories, maintains an up-to-date list of state screening programs and resources for newborn screening (https://newsteps.org).

Key elements to a successful screening program are rapid transit of specimens to the newborn screening laboratory, timely specimen testing and identification of abnormal results, notification of health care providers, follow-up with a definitive confirmatory assay, and the initiation of effective treatment to be conducted in consultation with a multidisciplinary center specializing in IEM therapy. Patients with abnormal results, especially when the disease in question may have acute manifestations, should be referred promptly to a metabolic disease center that can further evaluate the potential disorder. If the patient is at risk of acute or severe illness, immediate consultation with a physician specializing in metabolic disorders either in person or by telephone for diagnosis and treatment options should be undertaken. Each state has a plan in place for patient referral for abnormal newborn screens. If a primary care provider is unsure of how to arrange for tertiary care support, the state follow-up group can provide this information. Precise and early diagnosis is essential so that effective therapies can be instituted safely and the family receives proper counseling and education. Recommendations for dealing with newborn screening results in the primary care setting have been published by the American Academy of Pediatrics in a clinical report.[4]

Evaluation for IEM

For IEMs for which there is newborn screening, the first "sign" of the IEM could be a positive newborn screen. However, newborn screening is a screening process, not diagnostic testing, and for some IEMs, there is no newborn screening test available. Therefore, whether or not a newborn infant's screen is positive, an IEM should be suspected whenever an infant has persistent vomiting or decreased feeding, altered mental status, or an acute catastrophic illness following a period of normal behavior and feeding. An IEM should also be considered when an infant or child of any age has lethargy or coma, recurrent seizures, jaundice, growth failure, unusual body odor, developmental delay, hyperammonemia, hypoglycemia, metabolic acidosis, or a family history of recurrent illness or unexplained deaths in siblings. Because there is an important physiologic relationship between some IEMs and nutrition, symptoms of certain IEMs may present following important developmental steps in nutrition, including first exposure to catabolism (either in the neonatal period or later with longer periods of sleep or acute intercurrent childhood illness), increased protein intake (eg, when changing from human milk to formula or solid foods), or exposure to carbohydrate (eg, exposure to galactose in milk or fructose from fruit).

The steps and timing of the evaluation are tempered, in part, by the acuity of the problem and by the presentation. Algorithms for evaluation of patients with these signs and symptoms have been published.[5,6] If an IEM is suspected, early consultation with a metabolic specialist for advice regarding the appropriate diagnostic evaluation is strongly advised.

Emergency Therapy for a Suspected or Known IEM

Therapy should be initiated as soon as an IEM is diagnosed, or in the case of an infant in an acutely decompensated state, instituted as soon as such a disorder is suspected. After appropriate blood, urine, and cerebrospinal fluid samples have been obtained for diagnostic evaluation, but prior to a definitive diagnosis being made, immediate nonspecific therapy should include restriction of dietary protein and fat intake with aggressive administration of intravenous dextrose to prevent or reduce catabolism. Although this initial approach is not ideal for every known IEM, it is appropriate for the most common IEMs that may be life threatening, including urea cycle defects, amino acid disorders, organic acid disorders, or fatty acid disorders.

The key to acute nonspecific therapy is the reversal of catabolism and the promotion of anabolism. In some cases, care can provided locally, and for the most critically ill or those for whom rare medications are needed, treatment will require care at a tertiary care center by a metabolic multidisciplinary team with access to orphan drugs. Intravenous fluids should contain at least 10% dextrose and be administered at double the usual maintenance rate to provide energy and to promote urinary excretion of toxic metabolites. Severe acidosis (pH <7.1) should be treated with sodium bicarbonate infusion. Hyperammonemia, if not immediately responsive to intravenous fluid therapy and ammonia scavenger medications (eg, benzoate and phenylacetate), should be treated by hemodialysis. Not all hospitals are able to administer ammonia scavengers; thus, an elevated ammonia level should initiate transport of the patient to a facility with this medication option. Insulin infusions have been used to prevent hyperglycemia and promote anabolism when giving large amounts of glucose for metabolic decompensation in such disorders as maple syrup urine disease, disorders of fatty acid oxidation, and organic acidemias.[7]

Enteral feedings will also promote anabolism and may be safely given if the protein content is restricted and as appropriate for the specific condition suspected and the fat content is managed as appropriate (ie, avoiding lipids completely when certain conditions are suspected and giving increased medium-chain triglycerides for other conditions). Multivitamins should also be provided in this situation. Prolonged or overrestriction of protein and/or fat can lead to severe iatrogenic complications. Collaboration with a specialized multidisciplinary team is important, even before a definitive diagnosis is made.

Once the diagnosis of a specific IEM has been made, therapy should be tailored to the specific disorder. Therapy for IEMs is rapidly evolving, and specialists in metabolic disease and contemporary medical literature should be consulted for new advances. Therapy for any inherited metabolic disease is based on the pathophysiologic effects of the disease. For many IEMs attributable to a single-enzyme defect, disease-associated pathology is caused by accumulation of an immediate or remote precursor of the impaired reaction. The accumulated substrate may have direct toxic effects or may secondarily impair other critical biochemical reactions. For instance, elevation of phenylalanine in phenylalanine hydroxylase deficiency correlates with the pathology associated with untreated phenylketonuria (PKU). For other disorders, symptoms may be caused by a deficiency of a critical reaction product. Finally, the substrate of the deficient reaction may be converted to an alternative product via little-used pathways. These secondary metabolites may, in themselves, be toxic. For example, succinylacetone, a product of alternative metabolism of fumarylacetoacetic acid, accumulates in the disease tyrosinemia type 1, inhibits certain steps in heme synthesis, and causes symptoms mimicking porphyria. Disease-specific therapy may, therefore, include attempts to limit the accumulation of substrate, enhance the excretion of toxic substrate or secondary metabolites, restore the supply of an essential product, or inhibit alternative metabolism of the substrate. Other therapeutic approaches may include stabilization of the impaired enzyme to improve residual activity, replacement of deficient enzymatic cofactors, induction of enzyme production, enzyme replacement, or even correcting the defect at the level of the abnormal gene (gene therapy).

Nutritional Therapy Using Medical Foods

Manipulation of precursors and limitation of substrates that lead to toxic metabolites form a major portion of the available therapies for many IEMs. Disorders that involve the intermediary metabolism of protein, carbohydrate, or lipids are most responsive to treatment with medical nutritional therapy. In the specialized diets designed for IEM, the intake of precursor nutrients is severely limited, balancing the normal requirements for these nutrients against their potential toxicities. The necessary restriction of usually consumed foods is associated with significant risk for nutritional deficiency. For example, the elimination of dairy products, as is necessary in the treatment of galactosemia and for many disorders of amino acid and organic acid metabolism, is associated with risk of calcium deficiency and consequent osteoporosis. Overrestriction of even a single essential (or conditionally essential) amino acid can cause growth restriction and other complications. Furthermore, dietary protein or fat restriction is associated with risks of iron-deficiency anemia, vitamin B_{12} deficiency, and deficiency of essential polyunsaturated fatty acids. Commercially available medical foods for the treatment of IEMs support normal growth and development by supplying a complete complement of dietary macro- and micronutrients required in the context of restricted intake of normal foods. For IEMs requiring dietary protein restriction, a variety of low-protein food products (pastas, breads, baking mixes, etc) that mimic normal foodstuffs are available to provide needed energy and improve the palatability and appeal of the restricted diet. However, all medical foods are, by design, nutritionally incomplete and, therefore, are not to be used without the guidance of trained specialists. Purchase of these products from their manufacturers typically requires physician authorization.

Medical foods are therapeutic agents specifically designed for the treatment of IEMs, not unlike prescription pharmaceuticals. These medical foods are quite expensive, with the wholesale cost of disease-specific infant medical food formulas up to 2.5 times the retail cost of standard infant formula and the cost of foods modified to be low in protein 2 to 8 times the retail price of typical foodstuffs. Medical foods are regulated under food statutes, not as prescription drugs. Consequently, insurance reimbursement for medical foods in the United States is inconsistent, creating significant financial hardship for those who do not benefit from coverage stipulated by state legislative mandate or support through Medicaid. All 50 states practice newborn screening for as many as 40 different disorders, yet as of 2016, only 35 states have mandated insurance coverage for medical foods in the treatment of these disorders.[8] Additionally, these mandates vary in their scope with differences in the specific disorders covered, the types of food included in the coverage, copay and deductible requirements, and age restrictions. Several medical professional organizations, including the American Academy of Pediatrics, have endorsed reimbursement for medical foods and low-protein products, yet barriers to treatment coverage remain.[9] Federal legislation that would require uniform national insurance coverage for the treatment of screenable disorders has been proposed.

Education of the family and patient regarding the pathophysiology of the disorder and the rationale for dietary therapy is essential. Families must be taught to prepare medical formulas and implement a feeding schedule, design daily menus, and track the intake of protein, fat, or carbohydrate, depending on the specific disorder. Family support and ongoing clinical supervision of therapy adherence are critical components of effective implementation of these complex regimens. There is little room for spontaneity with this type of therapeutic food lifestyle. Restaurants are generally not an option as a source of a complete meal. The constant need to count dietary macronutrient content and the lack of any preprepared quick meal options are challenging to any family's commitment to dietary treatment.

For some IEMs, families must also be taught to recognize the signs and symptoms of impending metabolic decompensation and to institute emergency procedures, including the administration of a generally more restrictive "sick" diet. The successful implementation of a satisfactory diet during a period of relative health does not ensure that the diet is appropriate during periods of metabolic decompensation. The increased metabolic stress of even minor illness associated with increased energy requirements and increased catabolism of endogenous energy sources frequently necessitate further restriction or even elimination of dietary protein intake in individuals with aminoacidopathies or organic acidemias. Families must be encouraged to contact health care providers during these minor illnesses. The additionally restricted diet may not be adequate to prevent further metabolic derangement, and its use requires supervision; because it is nutritionally incomplete, it may contribute to malnutrition if used for more than a couple of days. Illnesses that would normally be manageable at home in typical children may trigger the need for hospitalization in patients with an IEM. Intravenous hydration, nutrition, and in some IEMs, administration of special medications play major roles in correcting the acutely decompensated state.

Other Nutritional Therapies

Some IEMs are or may be vitamin or cofactor responsive. Cofactor supplementation may be an adjunct to therapy with medical foods for some of the IEMs listed in Table 29.1. For other IEMs, cofactor administration may be the mainstay of treatment. Cofactor dependency can be determined empirically through controlled trials of vitamin supplementation with monitoring of laboratory studies and clinical response. For instance, a subset of individuals with PKU (20%–40% of patients, depending on the specific population) respond to treatment with sapropterin dihydrochloride, a synthetic version of tetrahydrobiopterin cofactor.[10] Oral sapropterin is administered daily over 4 to 6 weeks while dietary phenylalanine intake is kept relatively constant; a substantial and sustained decrease in blood phenylalanine concentration measured weekly indicates sapropterin responsiveness. For some IEMs, such as maple syrup urine disease, cofactor dependency may be assessed through in vitro assays of enzyme function in the presence and absence of cofactor. The goal of cofactor therapy may be to stabilize a poorly functional enzyme, to overcome a block in cofactor binding, or to correct a block in cofactor metabolism that results in secondary metabolic derangement.

Therapy for other select IEMs is presented in Table 29.2. The treatment of several of these IEMs is based on dietary avoidance of substrate, but

VI

Table 29.1.

Select Inborn Errors of Metabolism Treated With Commercially Available Medical Foods

IEM	Modify or Restrict	Vitamin or Cofactor Responsive	Other Therapies
Phenylketonuria	Phenylalanine	<1% of cases are attributable to biopterin synthetic defect and require biopterin supplementation. Sapropterin dihydrochloride treatment lowers blood phenylalanine in an additional 20% to 40% of PKU patients.	Supplemental tyrosine or other large neutral amino acids
Tyrosinemia type I	Phenylalanine, tyrosine, methionine	No	Nitisinone
Tyrosinemia type II	Phenylalanine, tyrosine	No	
Maple syrup urine disease	Leucine, valine, isoleucine	Some cases are thiamine responsive	Optimize valine and isoleucine levels to ensure the leucine level remains in the normal range
Isovaleric acidemia	Leucine	No	Supplemental carnitine and glycine
Methylmalonic acidemia	Isoleucine, valine, methionine, threonine	Some cases are attributable to defect in cobalamin metabolism	Supplemental carnitine

Propionic acidemia	Isoleucine, valine, threonine		Supplemental carnitine
Homocystinuria	Methionine	Some cases are pyridoxine responsive	Supplemental folate, betaine (converts homocysteine to methionine)
Ornithine transcarbamylase deficiency	Protein	No	Supplemental citrulline, benzoate, phenylacetate, phenylbutyrate
Citrullinemia	Protein	No	Supplemental arginine, benzoate, phenylacetate, phenylbutyrate
Glutaric aciduria type I	Lysine, tryptophan	Possible role for riboflavin	Supplemental carnitine
Long-chain fatty acid oxidation disorders	Dietary long-chain fatty acids		Avoid fasting, supplement with medium-chain triglyceride oil

VI

Table 29.2.
Therapy of Other Select IEM

IEM	Modify or Restrict	Vitamin or Cofactor Responsive	Other Therapies
Biotinidase deficiency	None	Biotin	
Familial hypophosphatemic rickets	None	1,25-dihydroxy-vitamin D	Phosphorus
Acrodermatitis enteropathica	None	Zinc	
Pyruvate dehydrogenase deficiency	Low-carbohydrate, high-fat diet	Possibly thiamine responsive	Alkali therapy
Galactosemia (transferase deficiency)	Galactose, lactose		Lactose-free infant formula
Glycogen storage diseases	Lactose, fructose, sucrose		Frequent feedings, complex starches, high-protein diet
Fructosemia (fructose-1,6-bisphosphatase or aldolase deficiency)	Fructose		Frequent glucose feedings in bisphosphatase deficiency
Medium-chain acyl-CoA dehydrogenase deficiency			Avoid fasting, possible supplemental carnitine

Barth syndrome (X-linked 3-methyl-glutaconic aciduria)	None	Pantothenic acid	
Cystinosis	None	None	Cysteamine, phosphate, potassium, vitamin D, alkali
Alpha-aminoadipic semialdehyde dehydrogenase deficiency (pyridoxine responsive epilepsy)		Pyridoxine	
Cerebral folate deficiency	None	Folinic acid	
Creatine synthesis disorders	None	Creatine	
Thiamine-responsive megaloblastic anemia syndrome	None	Thiamine	

VI

for these disorders, supplementation with medical foods is not required. For instance, the treatment of galactosemia includes avoidance of dietary galactose, which is primarily found in the disaccharide, lactose (milk sugar) in dairy products. In infancy, this dietary restriction is easy to accomplish, because the affected infant may be fed lactose-free soy-based formula. As the child ages, however, avoidance of dairy products, especially in baked goods and processed foods, is more difficult. Families must be taught to read food labels and to contact manufacturers of prepared foods to determine whether foodstuffs contain galactose. Families should assume that all new foods contain galactose until proven otherwise and should be encouraged to seek other hidden sources of galactose in over-the-counter and prescription medications.

Fructose ingestion must be strictly avoided by individuals with either hereditary fructose intolerance or fructose 1,6-bisphosphatase deficiency. Ingestion of fruits, fruit juices, or any food product sweetened with fructose-containing sweetener (eg, high-fructose corn syrup in baked goods and soda) can trigger potentially life-threatening episodes of abdominal pain, vomiting, metabolic acidosis, and electrolyte disturbance. Individuals with fructose 1,6-bisphosphatase deficiency are also intolerant of fasting, because this enzyme participates in gluconeogenesis. In mannose phosphate isomerase deficiency (congenital disorder of glycosylation type 1b), a rare disease that impairs glycosylation of cellular proteins and lipids, some aspects of the disorder, including protein-losing enteropathy and other gastrointestinal symptoms improve with addition of mannose to the diet.[11]

In type 1 glycogen storage disease, glycogenolysis during fasting is impaired because glucose-6-phosphate cannot be converted to glucose. Consumption of nonglucose carbohydrates (fructose, galactose) leads to excessive glycogen storage or shunting through alternative pathways to form lactate, uric acid, or triglycerides. Frequent feedings during infancy, overnight enteral tube feedings, and after 1 year of age, the administration of uncooked cornstarch as a slowly released source of glucose are key to the prevention of hypoglycemia and preservation of liver function. In other forms of glycogen storage disease involving the liver, gluconeogenesis is intact. Amino acids can serve as precursors for endogenous glucose production, and a high-protein diet (3 g/kg per day) is recommended.

Fatty acid oxidation disorders are caused by deficiencies in multiple genes involved in the metabolism of fats to energy. In medium-chain acyl-coenzyme A dehydrogenase deficiency, the most common disorder of fatty acid oxidation identified via newborn screening, prevention of fasting eliminates the body's need to metabolize stored body fat for energy, reduces the accumulation of toxic partially oxidized fatty acids, and reduces the risk of secondary findings that can include hyperammonemia and hypoglycemia. Infants with disorders of long-chain fatty acid oxidation, such as very long-chain acyl-coenzyme A dehydrogenase deficiency or trifunctional protein deficiency, are more sensitive to fasting, which can result in hypoglycemia, metabolic acidosis, liver dysfunction, or cardiomyopathy. Dietary long-chain fatty acid intake must be restricted; provision of medium-chain triglycerides provides a fuel source that bypasses the block in fatty acid oxidation.[12]

Prevention of micronutrient deficiencies is another important aspect of nutritional therapy for IEMs. These deficiencies may be direct effects of certain IEMs or may be a consequence of dietary restrictions. As previously mentioned, intakes of calcium (as in galactosemia), iron, and vitamin B_{12} (as in disorders requiring low protein diets) can be inadequate when necessary restrictions are implemented. Zinc and selenium deficiencies are also potential problems in organic acidemias and other disorders that require protein-restricted diets. Severe dietary fat restriction for disorders of fatty acid metabolism or the administration of nutritionally incomplete synthetic medical foods may lead to deficiencies of essential polyunsaturated fatty acids. Multivitamin preparations with minerals should be prescribed to all patients on altered diets who are not receiving most of their nutrition from micronutrient-fortified medical foods. All patients receiving nutritional therapy must be periodically assessed for nutrient deficiencies.

Other Therapeutic Modalities

Nutritional therapy, although important, is only one modality used for many of the disorders of intermediary metabolism. Other, nonnutritional therapies include pharmacologic agents such as alkali to reduce metabolic acidosis, benzoate and phenylacetate to provide "metabolic sinks" (ie, alternative pathways for metabolite excretion) for ammonia in urea cycle disorders, vitamin D and phosphorus supplementation in hypophosphatemic rickets, and cysteamine to enhance cellular cystine release in the lysosomal storage disease cystinosis. A rare form of congenital megaloblastic anemia is completely corrected with thiamine supplementation. Treatment with pyridoxine or folinic acid (a non-methylated form of folic acid) is critical to the prevention of convulsions in alpha-aminoadipic semialdehyde dehydrogenase deficiency (formerly known as pyridoxine responsive epilepsy) or cerebral folate deficiency, respectively. Rare disorders of creatine synthesis present with seizures, abnormal involuntary movements, and expressive speech delay; creatine supplementation may improve symptoms dramatically.

For a few disorders, enzyme replacement therapies are available. In Gaucher disease, a lysosomal storage disease, repetitive intravenous infusions of purified enzyme is used to gradually reduce the amount of stored glucocerebroside, reversing some of the pathophysiologic changes and improving the quality of life. Similar enzyme replacement strategies are now clinically available for a variety of lysosomal storage diseases including Pompe disease, Fabry disease, and several mucopolysaccharidoses. For other disorders, use of enzyme replacement therapies are being explored in clinical trials, including a pegylated recombinant phenylalanine ammonia-lyase for PKU treatment.

Organ transplantation has been performed in several IEMs. The most common transplanted organs are bone marrow and liver. Bone marrow or stem cell transplantation has been used in many lysosomal storage disorders, such as the mucopolysaccharidoses, in attempts to provide a tissue that is capable of metabolizing the stored material. Liver transplantation has been performed in tyrosinemia type 1 to prevent hepatocellular carcinoma, a known complication of the disease, and to correct the primary defect. With the use of nitisinone, liver transplantation is now required only for a minority of patients with tyrosinemia, although lifelong monitoring for hepatocellular carcinoma is recommended. Fewer than 5% of children placed on nitisinone before 2 years of age developed hepatocellular carcinoma.[13] Liver transplantation has also been used successfully for urea cycle disorders, maple syrup urine disease, and some organic acidemias.[14] A successful graft may have a profound effect on the health of an individual with an IEM. However, liver transplantation does not reverse previous neurologic or organ damage or biochemical alterations not directly resolved by provision of normal liver biochemistry, which may remain significant. For example, complications from metabolic stroke affecting basal ganglia of individuals with methylmalonic acidemia remain significant, even after liver transplant. The infusion of hepatocytes into the portal vein for engraftment into liver may also hold promise as a treatment for many liver enzyme deficiencies, such as urea cycle disorders.[15]

Permanent replacement of the mutant gene with the correct DNA sequence in the somatic cells of an individual with an IEM is a very attractive potential future treatment modality. Research centers around the world are actively investigating gene therapy as a treatment for a wide variety of

IEMs. Using contemporary DNA transfer methods, achieving stable, physiologically significant gene expression still continues to be the major limiting factor in clinical gene therapy trials. Issues of treatment toxicity using certain gene transfer technologies have also slowed the progress of moving gene therapy from the laboratory to the clinical bedside. However, success using gene therapy to treat hemophilia,[16] inherited immunodeficiencies,[17] congenital retinopathies,[18] and X-linked adrenoleukodystrophy[19] in humans has provided renewed promise that gene therapy may be a viable treatment option for treatment of IEM in the future.

Conclusion

Regardless of the specific therapy plan, successful treatment of IEMs requires a multidisciplinary approach to include the expertise of the metabolic physician, metabolic dietitian, clinical nurse, genetic counselor, and social worker backed up by a full complement of medical specialists and

---

AAP

AAP Recommendations on Reimbursement for Foods for Special Dietary Use[9]

1. All foods for special dietary use with accepted benefit for treatment of a medical condition should be reimbursed as a medical expense, provided the costs are over and above usual foods. Individual and family financial barriers to obtaining these foods should be removed.

2. All states should enact legislation that would require health insurance policy providers to reimburse all foods for special dietary use with accepted medical benefit recommended by a physician to prevent death and serious disability or to foster normal growth and development.

3. All expenses for medical equipment and medical supplies necessary for the delivery of foods for special dietary use should be reimbursed.

4. Reimbursement for foods for special dietary use should be mandatory for the following:

   a. Any medical condition for which specific dietary components or the restriction of specific dietary components is necessary to treat a physical, physiologic, or pathologic condition resulting in inadequate nutrition.

   b. An inherited metabolic disorder, including but not limited to disorders of carbohydrate metabolism, lipid metabolism, vitamin metabolism, mineral metabolism, or amino acid and nitrogen metabolism.

   c. A condition resulting in impairment of oral intake that affects normal development and growth.

   Pediatrics. 2003;111(5):1117-1119

VI

---

ancillary services. Education of the family, genetic counseling, and family support are all essential components. Genetic counseling teaches the family about the risks associated with future pregnancies and demystifies the concepts of dysfunctional genes being passed from asymptomatic carrier to affected child. The availability and implications of prenatal diagnosis for IEMs are also explained. Heterozygote detection and the ethical issues of sharing that information within a family or with future mates are other issues that may be addressed by counseling. Support for the family needs to ensure availability of coping mechanisms for dealing with a member who may have significant restrictions in developmental capacity or who has extraordinary needs for care. Educational goals include the successful implementation of the diet and the need for immediate intervention during metabolic crises. Additional online educational resources for patients and families are listed in Table 29.3.

Nutritional therapies will continue to be the cornerstone of treatment for most IEM in the foreseeable future. The lessons learned with several IEMs, especially PKU, emphasize the need for lifelong therapy in all these disorders. The necessity of "diet for life" has been affirmed by multiple groups.[20-22] This necessity, therefore, requires a long-term commitment from parents, patient, and health care providers to implement and maintain the appropriate dietary therapy. The needs of an individual for energy, protein, and cofactors change with age and body mass. Therapeutic diets must be established and reevaluated at regular intervals to allow for the most normal growth and development possible. The adequacy of nutritional therapy must be assessed periodically through combinations of diet record review, anthropometric assessment, and laboratory testing. Cooperation of the patient, family, and the metabolic clinic as a dedicated team throughout the life of the patient is essential for successful treatment of an IEM.

Table 29.3.

Selected Resources Related to Newborn Screening and Inborn Errors of Metabolism

NEWBORN SCREENING	
Baby's First Test http://www.babysfirsttest.org	A clearinghouse that provides current educational and family support and services information, materials, and resources about newborn screening at local, state, and national levels. Resources for health professionals include links to the ACMG ACT Sheets and Algorithms, a database with state-specific information (screening and treatment resources), and a checklist for communicating with families about out-of-range newborn screening results.
Recommended Uniform Screening Panel (RUSP) https://www.hrsa.gov/advisorycommittees/mchbadvisory/heritabledisorders/recommendedpanel	The RUSP is a list of disorders that are screened at birth and recommender by the Secretary of the Department of Health and Human Services (HHS) for state to screen as part of their state universal screening program. This HHS website includes the RUSP, as well as supporting documentation and communication from the Advisory Committee on Heritable Disorders in Children.
Newsteps https://newsteps.org	This web-based resource of the Association of Public Health Laboratories (APHL) maintains an up-to-date list of state screening programs and resources for newborn screening.
INBORN ERRORS OF METABOLISM AND GENETICS	
GeneReviews https://www.ncbi.nlm.nih.gov/books/NBK1116/	GeneReviews provides clinically relevant information about inherited conditions, including inborn errors of metabolism. Each condition-specific chapter reviews diagnosis, management, and genetic counseling.
Genetics Home Reference https://ghr.nlm.nih.gov/	This website provides consumer-friendly information about the effects of genetic variation on human health, including IEM.

Continued

VI

Table 29.3. *Continued*

Selected Resources Related to Newborn Screening and Inborn Errors of Metabolism

INBORN ERRORS OF METABOLISM AND GENETICS *Continued*	
Medical Genetics in Pediatric Practice. Saul RA, ed. American Academy of Pediatrics; 2013 http://ebooks.aappublications.org/content/medical-genetics-in-pediatric-practice	This resource includes practice-focused information, including genetics and testing basics, indications for genetic testing and/or consultation, and case-based examples.
Inborn Metabolic Diseases – Diagnosis and Treatment, 6th edition. Saudubray JM, et al, eds. Springer; 2012. E-book for purchase: http://www.springer.com/us/book/9783642157202	This textbook includes information about diagnosis and management of inborn errors of metabolism, as well as metabolic pathways and pathophysiology involved in inborn errors of metabolism.
Management Guidelines • https://www.nature.com/gim/journal/v16/n2/full/gim2013157a.html • https://www.guidelines.gov/summaries/summary/50488/updated-webbased-nutrition-management-guideline-for-pku-an-evidence-and-consensus-based-approach?q=pku • https://www.guidelines.gov/summaries/summary/48859/nutrition-management-guideline-for-maple-syrup-urine-disease-an-evidence-and-consensusbased-approach?q=msud	A number of evidence-based management guidelines have been published, including guidelines for diagnosis and management of PKU, nutritional management of PKU, and nutritional management of maple syrup urine disease (MSUD): • Phenylalanine hydroxylase deficiency: diagnosis and management guideline (https://www.nature.com/gim/journal/v16/n2/full/gim2013157a.html) • Updated, web-based nutrition management guideline for PKU: an evidence and consensus based approach (https://www.guidelines.gov/summaries/summary/50488/updated-webbased-nutrition-management-guideline-for-pku-an-evidence-and-consensus-based-approach?q=pku) • Nutrition management guideline for maple syrup urine disease: an evidence- and consensus-based approach (https://www.guidelines.gov/summaries/summary/48859/nutrition-management-guideline-for-maple-syrup-urine-disease-an-evidence-and-consensusbased-approach?q=msud)
Orphanet http://www.orpha.net	Orphanet is a resource with information about rare diseases, including IEMs. It includes information in various languages.

ADVOCACY AND FAMILY SUPPORT ORGANIZATIONS	
NORD – National Organization for Rare Disorders https://rarediseases.org/	NORD is a patient advocacy organization for individuals with rare diseases and the organizations that serve them. Activities include patient advocacy, patient and professional education, patient assistance program, research support, international partnerships, and mentorship for patient organizations.
Global Genes https://globalgenes.org/	Global Genes is a rare disease patient advocacy organization. Resources include advocacy, research, and tools for individuals and organizations.
National PKU Alliance (NPKUA) https://www.npkua.org	The NPKUA works to improve the lives of families and individuals associated with phenylketonuria (PKU) through research, support, education, and advocacy, while ultimately seeking a cure. Resources include patient education materials, research grants, and information about US clinics.
Genetic Alliance http://www.geneticalliance.org/	The mission of Genetic Alliance is to engage individuals, families, and communities to transform health.
PROFESSIONAL ORGANIZATIONS	
American College of Medical Genetics and Genomics (ACMG) https://www.acmg.net/	The mission of ACMG is to develop and sustain genetic and genomic initiatives in clinical and laboratory practices, education, and advocacy.
American Academy of Pediatrics (AAP) https://www.aap.org	The AAP is an organization of pediatricians committed to the optimal physical, mental, and social health and well-being for all infants, children, adolescents, and young adults.
Genetic Metabolic Dietitians International (GMDI) http://gmdi.org/	The mission of GMDI is to provide standards of excellence and leadership in nutrition therapy for genetic metabolic disorders through clinical practice, education, advocacy, and research.
Society for Inherited Metabolic Disorders (SIMD) http://www.simd.org/	SIMD aims to increase knowledge of and promote research in inborn errors of metabolism in humans and to stimulate interactions between clinicians and investigators in inborn errors of metabolism.

References

1. American Academy of Pediatrics, Committee on Genetics. *Medical Genetics in Pediatric Practice*. Saul RA, ed. Elk Grove Village, IL: American Academy of Pediatrics; 2013

2. US Department of Health and Human Services, Health Resource Services Admnistration. Advisory Committee on Heritable Disorders in Newborns and Children. Available at: https://www.hrsa.gov/advisorycommittees/mchbadvisory/heritabledisorders/index.html. Accessed May 31, 2017

3. American College of Medical Genetics. Newborn screening ACT sheets and confirmatory algoritims. Available at: http://www.ncbi.nlm.nih.gov/books/NBK55827. Accessed August 13, 2013

4. American Academy of Pediatrics, Newborn Screening Authoring Committee. Newborn screening expands: recommendations for pediatricians and medical homes—implications for the system. *Pediatrics*. 2008;121(1):192–217

5. Saudubray JM, Baumgartner MR, Walter J. *Inborn Metabolic Diseases: Diagnosis and Treatment*. 6th ed. Berlin, Germany: Springer; 2016

6. Gallagher RC, Greene CL. Inborn errors of metabolism in the neonate. In: Bajaj L, Berman S, eds. *Berman's Pediatric Decision Making*. 5th ed. Philadelphia, PA: Elsevier/Mosby; 2011:684–686

7. Prietsch V, Lindner M, Zschocke J, Nyhan WL, Hoffmann GF. Emergency management of inherited metabolic diseases. *J Inherit Metab Dis*. 2002;25(7): 531–543

8. Wilson K, Charmchi P, Dworetzky B. *State Statutes and Regulations on Dietary Treatment of Disorders Identified through Newborn Screening*. Boston, MA: Center for Advancing Health Policy and Practice, Boston University School of Public Health; 2016

9. Greer FR, American Academy of Pediatrics, Committee on Nutrition. Reimbursement for foods for special dietary use. *Pediatrics*. 2003;111(5 Pt 1): 1117–1119

10. Levy H, Burton B, Cederbaum S, Scriver C. Recommendations for evaluation of responsiveness to tetrahydrobiopterin (BH(4)) in phenylketonuria and its use in treatment. *Mol Genet Metab*. 2007;92(4):287–291

11. Sparks S, Krasnewich D. Congenital disorders of n-linked glycosylation and multiple pathway overview. *GeneReviews*. 2005 (updated January 2017); Available at: https://www.ncbi.nlm.nih.gov/books/NBK1332. Accessed February 9, 2019

12. Gillingham MB, Scott B, Elliott D, Harding CO. Metabolic control during exercise with and without medium-chain triglycerides (MCT) in children with long-chain 3-hydroxy acyl-CoA dehydrogenase (LCHAD) or trifunctional protein (TFP) deficiency. *Mol Genet Metab*. 2006;89(1-2):58–63

13. Holme E, Lindstedt S. Nontransplant treatment of tyrosinemia. *Clin Liver Dis*. 2000;4(4):805–814

14. Oishi K, Arnon R, Wasserstein MP, Diaz GA. Liver transplantation for pediatric inherited metabolic disorders: considerations for indications, complications, and perioperative management. *Pediatr Transplant.* 2016;20(6):756–769

15. Meyburg J, Das AM, Hoerster F, et al. One liver for four children: first clinical series of liver cell transplantation for severe neonatal urea cycle defects. *Transplantation.* 2009;87(5):636–641

16. Baruteau J, Waddington SN, Alexander IE, Gissen P. Gene therapy for monogenic liver diseases: clinical successes, current challenges and future prospects. *J Inherit Metab Dis.* 2017;40(4):497–517

17. Kuo CY, Kohn DB. Gene therapy for the treatment of primary immune deficiencies. *Curr Allergy Asthma Rep.* 2016;16(5):39

18. Jacobson SG, Cideciyan AV, Ratnakaram R, et al. Gene therapy for leber congenital amaurosis caused by RPE65 mutations: safety and efficacy in 15 children and adults followed up to 3 years. *Arch Ophthalmol.* 2012;130(1):9–24

19. Cartier N, Hacein-Bey-Abina S, Bartholomae CC, et al. Hematopoietic stem cell gene therapy with a lentiviral vector in X-linked adrenoleukodystrophy. *Science.* 2009;326(5954):818–823

20. Camp KM, Parisi MA, Acosta PB, et al. Phenylketonuria Scientific Review Conference: state of the science and future research needs. *Mol Genet Metab.* 2014;112(2):87–122

21. Vockley J, Andersson HC, Antshel KM. Phenylalanine hydroxylase deficiency: diagnosis and management guideline. *Genet Med.* 2014;16(2):188–200

22. Singh RH, Rohr F, Frazier D, et al. Recommendations for the nutrition management of phenylalanine hydroxylase deficiency. *Genet Med.* 2014;16(2): 121–131

VI

Chapter 30

Nutrition Therapy for Children and Adolescents With Type 1 and Type 2 Diabetes Mellitus

Introduction

Since the discovery of insulin in 1921, tremendous progress has been made in understanding the pathophysiology of diabetes mellitus, comorbidities observed, and management paradigms. Improvements in insulin types, insulin delivery systems and glucose monitoring devices have not only advanced the care of patients with diabetes but also highlighted the importance of nutritional management, which remains a cornerstone of treatment. Providing guidance on appropriate dietary intake for children with type 1 or type 2 diabetes mellitus is an essential component to any successful diabetes program. This chapter reviews the most accepted and evidenced-based practices for nutritional management of diabetes mellitus in children.

Background: Diabetes Mellitus in Children

Type 1 Diabetes Mellitus

Type 1 diabetes mellitus (T1D) is an autoimmune disorder that results in the destruction of pancreatic beta cells and eventual insulin deficiency. T1D affects approximately 0.3% of all individuals in the United States, although the incidence of the disease is slowly increasing both in the United States[1] and worldwide.[2] Individuals with T1D are dependent on insulin to avoid acute and chronic complications of the disease.

Prior to the discovery and pharmacologic application of insulin therapy, management of diabetes mellitus primarily consisted of restricting intake of carbohydrate in the diet, but the disease was most often fatal in early life. Once techniques to isolate and purify insulin derived from animals (mainly pigs and cows) were developed, insulin therapy became the mainstay of treatment. Still, availability and allergic responses limited treatment. The emergence of recombinant DNA technology provided a plentiful supply of a bioequivalent form of human insulin that essentially eliminated the risks of allergic reactions. Analogues of insulin that varied in their onset and duration of action were designed by substituting amino acids within the insulin peptide that effectively changed the bioavailability of the insulin protein once delivered into the subcutaneous tissue. As newer insulins arrived, nutritional therapies and meal plans were designed around their use to better accommodate the lifestyle of the individual patient. Insulin pump therapy further revolutionized insulin delivery and provided greater flexibility in meal planning.

Current nutritional management for patients with T1D is centered on an understanding of the nutritional composition of foods, particularly carbohydrates, in order to use present-day insulins effectively. The general goal is for these patients is to consume well-balanced diets that promote a healthy weight, provide essential vitamins and minerals, and reduce risks of future cardiovascular disease.

Type 2 Diabetes Mellitus

The incidence of type 2 diabetes mellitus (T2D) in children has become more frequent over the past 2 decades, mirroring the increase in pediatric obesity observed globally. T2D accounts for the majority of new cases of diabetes among American Indian/Alaska Native, African American, and Hispanic adolescents in the United States.[3] The overall prevalence of T2D in US adolescents increased approximately 30% from 2001 to 2009 and remains highest in adolescents from these ethnic backgrounds (prevalence of 1 in 1000).[1] Pediatric T2D, similar to adult T2D, encompasses a spectrum of disease continuum that is rooted in insulin resistance. Insulin resistance is driven by the cascade of metabolic derangements stemming from increased visceral adiposity in a genetically at-risk population. As insulin resistance increases, progressive stress on beta cells to maintain euglycemia occurs. Disordered glucose metabolism eventually occurs in individuals who experience some degree of beta cell failure or loss.

Similar to children with T1D, an understanding of nutrition is a critical component of disease management in pediatric patients with T2D. Strategies that promote a healthy weight by improving diet quality, reducing unnecessary and unhealthy carbohydrates, and enhancing insulin sensitivity through physical activity are cornerstones of nutritional therapy. A number of pharmaceutical agents that improve glycemic control through a variety of mechanisms are approved for use in adults. Only metformin, a biguanide that enhances insulin sensitivity, is approved for use in children. Insulin therapy is also frequently required in children (and adults). Thus, the use of insulin in this population of children also requires a working knowledge of carbohydrate content of foods if meal coverage is being provided.

Reducing Risks of Microvascular and Macrovascular Complications

Present-day glycemic targets and glycosylated hemoglobin (HbA1c) goals for children and adults emerged primarily from the Diabetes Care and Complications Trial (DCCT) and its follow-up study, the Epidemiology of Diabetes Intervention and Complications (EDIC) trial. These studies demonstrated that intensive insulin administration to maintain euglycemia rather than the prior standard of care (2 injections per day) was superior with respect to improving glycemic control, lowering HbA1c concentrations, and decreasing risks of both micro- and macrovascular complications.[4,5] Achieving tighter glycemic goals must be balanced with avoidance of hypoglycemic events.

General and Disease-Specific Principles for Nutritional Management of Children With Diabetes Mellitus

The primary goals of treatment for all forms of pediatric diabetes mellitus remain: (1) maintaining glucose concentrations in a physiologically normal range; (2) minimizing episodes of hypoglycemia and; (3) allowing for normal growth and development, both physical and emotional. To achieve these goals, current nutrition recommendations for children and adolescents with diabetes mellitus are rooted in the same principles as those established for all healthy children and adolescents without diabetes. There is no evidence to recommend an ideal percentage of calories from carbohydrate, protein, and fat for people with diabetes. Individualized meal plans should emphasize a wide variety of healthy food choices to meet the recommended nutrient intakes for essential vitamins and minerals, energy, and fiber and to provide for normal growth and development.[6-8]

Strategies for nutrition therapy may be based on individual, cultural, and family needs. Examples of such interventions include reducing energy and fat intake, carbohydrate counting, simplified meal plans, healthy food choices, individualized meal planning strategies, exchange lists, insulin-to-carbohydrate ratios, physical activity, and behavioral strategies. Nutrition recommendations should be practical and comprehensible to families and patients, and the relationship between food and blood glucose should be emphasized. Routine monitoring of diet and utilization of food records are important interventions to assist with improving diet quality and detecting nutrient deficiencies. Cultural and traditional food practices, food

VI

Table 30.1.
General Nutrition Recommendations for Children With Diabetes Mellitus

- Consultation with a dietitian to develop/discuss the medical nutrition plan is encouraged, as part of initial team education and on referral, as needed; generally requires a series of sessions over the initial 3 months after diagnosis, then at least annually, with young children requiring more frequent reevaluations.
- Evaluate height, weight, BMI, and nutrition plan annually.
- Energy intake should be adequate for growth and restricted if a child becomes overweight.

preferences, family eating schedules, economic considerations, school and child care menus, willingness to change, and physical activity patterns should be taken into consideration when working with patients and families. Guidelines for managing specific cultural foods and practices are being increasingly described and used in different communities.[9,10] A summary of general guidelines is provided in Table 30.1.

Beyond the standard nutrition guidelines for healthy children, evidence-based nutrition therapy has emerged as a critical component in the management of diabetes in children, adolescents, and young adults.[11,12] Nutrition therapy should balance blood glucose goals with avoiding hypoglycemia and should promote a healthy lipid profile and blood pressure.[13,14] Achieving adequate control of blood glucose is likewise essential for normal growth and development.[14] In addition to normal linear growth, healthy weight gain should be part of routine follow-up. Strategies to reduce calories should be implemented if the child becomes overweight or is overweight or obese at time of diagnosis.[15,16] Energy needs can be evaluated by tracking weight gain, body mass index (BMI), and growth patterns on pediatric growth charts from the Centers for Disease Control and Prevention (CDC).[17]

Nutritional Deficits Among Children With Diabetes Mellitus

Despite current guidelines and food availability, children with diabetes mellitus in the United States have significant deficits in several aspects of their dietary intake. The intake of saturated and total fat is higher and fiber intake is lower among children with T1D compared with healthy controls.[18,19] Vitamin D deficiency (25 hydroxy-vitamin D < 50 nmol/L) is associated with children with T1D[20,21] and in obese children with insulin resistance.[22] The prevalence of overweight among children with T1D appears to be increasing, as 22.6% of children with T1D were categorized as overweight (ie, BMI at 85th–95th percentile) compared with only 16.1% of a matched control population.[23] Among 5529 adolescents with T1D registered in the Type 1 Diabetes Exchange, 22.9% were categorized as being overweight, and an additional 13.1% were obese.[24] Overweight among this population of patients with diabetes mellitus may suggest disordered eating,[25,26] which can further affect glycemic control. These data highlight the importance of emphasizing a global, healthy approach to nutrition, focusing on the quality of food, not just the quantity.

Guidelines for Medical Nutritional Management of T1D and T2D

Evidence-Based Nutrition Principles and Recommendations for T1D and T2D

Nutrition therapy for T1D and T2D should be based on available evidence and current standards of medical care. The American Diabetes Association (ADA) publishes clinical practice recommendations annually that include nutrition therapy in addition to position statements.[13,14,27] The Academy of Nutrition and Dietetics has compiled a vast evidence analysis library for medical nutrition therapy for T1D and T2D (www.andeal.org). Recommendations for macro- and micronutrients and other pertinent nutrition therapy for children with T1D and T2D are summarized in Table 30.2.

Individual Nutrient Considerations

Carbohydrate

Among patients with diabetes, the primary determinants of postprandial glucose concentrations are total carbohydrate intake, type of carbohydrate, and the dose and timing of insulin administration (in patients on insulin). Therefore, providing education that allows for proper matching of insulin to carbohydrate intake to obtain target postprandial blood glucose control is recommended.[28] In addition, the amount of fat and protein in a meal can affect glycemic response and should be factored in when determining the bolus insulin dose and delivery, which will be discussed later in this chapter.

Given the flexibility in current management strategies (ie, basal-bolus insulin therapy), it is also important to monitor carbohydrate quality to avoid excess energy intake from "empty" calorie carbohydrates (eg,

Table 30.2.

Specific Recommendations for Nutrition Management of T1D in Children[6,14,27]

- The mix of dietary carbohydrate, protein, and fat may be adjusted to meet the metabolic goals and individual preferences of the person with T1D. There is no ideal percentage of calories from carbohydrate, protein, and fat for people with diabetes.
- Monitoring carbohydrate, whether by carbohydrate counting, choices, or experience-based estimation, remains a key strategy in achieving glycemic control. High-protein and high-fat foods may require additional insulin and dosing strategies.
- For individuals with T1D, the use of the glycemic index and glycemic load may provide a modest additional benefit for glycemic control over that observed when total carbohydrate is considered alone.
- Saturated fat intake should be <7% of total calories.
- Reducing intake of trans fatty acids lowers low-density lipoprotein and increases high-density lipoprotein concentrations; therefore, intake of trans fatty acids should be minimized.
- Routine supplementation with antioxidants, such as vitamins E and C and beta-carotene, is not advised because of lack of evidence of efficacy and concerns related to long-term safety.
- Individualized meal planning should include optimization of food choices to meet RDA/DRI for all micronutrients.

nondiet soda, juice, sweets, snacks). The Recommended Dietary Allowance (RDA)/Dietary Reference Intake (DRI) of carbohydrate for children and adolescents ≥1 year of age is 45% to 65% of total energy requirements. Diets that contain less than 130 g of carbohydrate for children older than 1 year may not provide adequate glucose as fuel for the central nervous system without relying on gluconeogenesis from ingested protein and fat. Low-carbohydrate diets can restrict intake of essential nutrients, energy, and fiber found in whole grains, fruits, vegetables, dried peas and beans, legumes, nuts and seeds, and low-fat milk and yogurt.[6,8,11,13,27,29] Adoption of these strategies provides for normal growth, development, and weight gain in this population.

Sucrose

Intake of up to 35% of total calories from sucrose (glucose + fructose), or table sugar, has not been shown to have a negative effect on glycemic response or HbA1c outcomes in children and adolescents when compared with isocaloric, lower-sucrose diets.[30-32] Foods containing sucrose may be substituted for other carbohydrates in the meal plan or, if consumed in addition to the meal plan, should be covered with insulin. However, sucrose-containing foods typically provide additional calories from fats and are frequently devoid of essential nutrients. Sucrose and fructose in the form of high-fructose corn syrup found in sugar-sweetened beverages should be avoided because of the potential for excessive energy intake and worsening of cardiometabolic risk profile. Nutrition therapy strategies should focus on consuming these foods in moderation in the context of a healthy, well-balanced diet.

Protein

In individuals with T1D and T2D, protein intake is based on the RDA for all children and adolescents. Nutrition therapy should emphasize lean protein sources that are low in saturated fat, such as fish, poultry, lean cuts of meat, low-fat dairy products, dried peas, beans, and legumes.[33] Typical protein intakes in children in the United States have minimal effects on blood glucose. However, ingestion of a high-protein meal in patients with T1D may cause greater glycemic excursions than would be expected.[34] In people with T2D, ingested protein can increase endogenous insulin response while not increasing blood glucose and, therefore, should not solely be used to treat hypoglycemia or prevent hypoglycemia overnight.[35] In adults with micro or macroalbuminuria, a reduction of protein below the usual intake has not been shown to alter the rate of glomerular filtration rate decline, cardiovascular risk factors, or glycemic measures.[27]

Fat

The increased risk of cardiovascular disease in people with T1D and T2D warrants an emphasis on a diet low in saturated fat as part of nutritional therapy, as outlined by the National Cholesterol Education Program and the American Heart Association, for all children and adolescents. These guidelines include reductions in trans-fatty acids, saturated fats, and total dietary cholesterol along with interventions to reduce blood pressure (ie, low-sodium diets). The American Heart Association Step 2 diet is indicated as initial therapy for elevated lipids in addition to optimizing glucose control.[14,36]

Less than 7% of daily caloric intake should come from saturated fat, dietary cholesterol should amount to <200 mg/day, and intake of trans-fatty acids should be minimized. Saturated fatty acids are found in fatty and processed meats, butter, lard, shortening, hydrogenated fats, coconut, palm and palm kernel oils, cocoa butter, and high-fat dairy products. Added trans-fatty acids are primarily found in stick margarine and processed and commercially prepared foods. Dietary cholesterol is only found in foods of animal origin.

Healthier fats, including monounsaturated and polyunsaturated fats, are the favored sources of dietary fats in patients with diabetes because of their relative cardioprotective profile compared with saturated fats and trans-fatty acids,[37] Sources of mono- and polyunsaturated fats include olive, canola, peanut, corn, safflower, sunflower, and soy oils; olives; nuts and nut butters; seeds; avocados; and soft-tub or spray margarines.

Diets high in omega-3 fatty acids (fish and seafood) compared with omega-6 fatty acids had no detrimental effects on blood glucose, and both diets improved lipoprotein profiles and improved insulin sensitivity in adults with T2D.[38] As recommended for the general public, eating 2 or more servings of fish per week (with the exception of commercially fried fish filets) is recommended to provide an excellent source of omega-3 polyunsaturated fatty acids (eicosapentaenoic acid [EPA] and docosahexaenoic acid [DHA]) and omega-3 alpha-linolenic acid (ALA). Evidence does not support using omega-3 supplements for people with diabetes for prevention or treatment of cardiovascular events.[14] Marine sources of omega-3 polyunsaturated fatty acids are salmon, albacore tuna, herring, sardines, mackerel, trout, and anchovies. Omega-3 polyunsaturated fatty acids can also be found in flax seeds and oil, chia seeds, various nuts, and canola and soybean oil, although larger amounts of these plant-derived sources are needed to achieve the same lipid-lowering effect as marine-derived sources.[39,40]

Micronutrients

Several individual micronutrients have previously been proposed as potential adjunctive therapies in patients with diabetes mellitus. Chromium supplementation in adults with diabetes mellitus has not consistently demonstrated a glycemic benefit, but studies have been limited by small study size and other study design issues.[41,42] Additional concerns regarding potential toxicity associated with chromium supplementation should preclude its routine use, especially in the pediatric population. Routine supplementation of antioxidants, vitamins E and C, and beta-carotene cannot be recommended because of a lack of evidence for benefit and concerns regarding long-term safety.[27,33] Although low serum 25-hydroxyvitamin D concentrations are globally associated with children and adolescents with T1D,[21,43,44] no cause-and-effect relationship has been established. Moreover, the vitamin D status of children with T1D and T2D appears to be no different from that of children without diabetes.[45] Vitamin D supplementation can, therefore, be considered in children and adolescents with T1D, particularly if they are not meeting the RDA of 600 IU vitamin D per day. In summary, there is no clear evidence of benefit from vitamin or mineral supplementation in people with diabetes mellitus (compared with the general population) who do not have underlying deficiencies.[27] Supplementation with micronutrients is not necessary if a well-balanced, healthy diet is consumed.

Sodium

Current sodium intake guidelines for healthy children and adolescents are the same as for the general, nonhypertensive population (less than 2300 mg/day). For individuals with hypertension, a reduction to 1500 mg/day of sodium is recommended. The majority of the sodium in the American diet today comes from processed and convenience foods, restaurant meals, and fast foods. Using fresh or frozen ingredients or low- or no-sodium packaged foods in preparing meals is a way to decrease sodium in the diet.[6,13,14,27]

Nutritive and Nonnutritive Sweeteners

Nutritive and nonnutritive sweeteners are considered safe for use by children with diabetes mellitus when consumed within the daily intake levels established by the Food and Drug Administration (FDA). Nutritive sweeteners approved by the FDA include sugar alcohols (polyols), erythritol, isomaltose, lactitol, maltitol, mannitol, sorbitol, xylitol, tagatose, and hydrogenated starch hydrolysates. These sweeteners contain approximately 2 kcal/g, which is half the calories of nutritive sweeteners, such as sucrose. Subtraction of half the sugar alcohol grams from the total carbohydrate in grams is advised when reading food labels and calculating the total carbohydrate from the Nutrition Facts Panel (see Fig 30.1). Sugar alcohols may cause diarrhea, especially in children.

Seven nonnutritive sweeteners have been approved by the FDA for use in the United States: acesulfame potassium, aspartame, neotame, saccharin, sucralose, luo han guo fruit extract (monk fruit), and stevia.[46] The safety of all of these sweeteners has been rigorously evaluated and confirmed, and they may be consumed by children and adolescents with diabetes mellitus and women during pregnancy.[27,47] An ADI (Acceptable Daily Intake) has been approved for all nonnutritive sweeteners by the FDA. Consumption of nonnutritive sweeteners does not increase blood glucose concentration or affect insulin response in adults, although no similar data are available

Fig. 30.1.
Reading a Food Label for Carbohydrates

Nutrition Facts

Serving Size ½ cup (114g)
Servings Per Container 4

Amount Per Serving

Calories 90	Calories from Fat 30

	% Daily Value*
Total Fat 3g	**5%**
Saturated Fat 0g	**0%**
Cholesterol 0mg	**0%**
Sodium 300mg	**13%**
Total Carbohydrate 13g	**4%**
Dietary Fiber 3g	**12%**
Sugars 3g	
Protein 3g	

Vitamin A 80%	•	Vitamin C 60%
Calcium 4%	•	Iron 4%

*Percent Daily Values are based on a 2,000 calorie diet.
Your daily values may be higher or lower depending on
your caloric needs:

	Calories:	2,000	2,500
Total Fat	Less than	65g	80g
Sat Fat	Less than	20g	25g
Cholesterol	Less than	300mg	300mg
Sodiuum	Less than	2,400mg	2,400mg
Total Carbohydrate		300g	375g
Dietary Fiber		25g	30g

Calories per gram:
Fat 9 • Carbohydrate 4 • Protein 4

in children. Because foods containing nonnutritive sweeteners may still contain carbohydrates (and calories), careful reading of food labels is always recommended.

Fiber

The recommended fiber intake for children with diabetes is based on the DRI for all children and adolescents: 14 g/1000 kcal, or approximately 19 to 38 g of fiber/day. In children with T1D, a higher fat and lower fiber intake in all youth using insulin pumps were associated with an A1c level of ≥8.5%.[48] However, the effect of fiber supplementation on glycemic control remains unclear. In a small study of children with T1D, the addition of a 20-g fiber supplement (wheat dextrin) resulted in no differences in postprandial mean blood glucose excursions or in rates of hypoglycemia.[49] In the Treatment Options for Type 2 Diabetes in Adolescents and Youth (TODAY) trial, females who decreased their saturated fat intake and/or increased their fiber intake had lower HbA1c at month 24 of the study.[50] Whether the dose or type of fiber has more of an effect and the relative effect of decreasing fat in the diet remain to be determined in future studies.

Fiber from whole foods also appears to have a beneficial effect on serum cholesterol and other cardiovascular disease risk factors in adults. Dietary fiber is found in whole grains, fruits, vegetables, dried peas, beans, legumes, nuts, and seeds. Soluble fiber sources should be emphasized, because studies in people without diabetes show that diets high in total and soluble fiber (7–13 g) can reduce total cholesterol concentration by 2% to 3% and low-density lipoprotein cholesterol concentration by up to 7%.[13,27,51,52] Potent sources of soluble fiber include oatmeal, oat cereal, lentils, apples, oranges, pears, oat bran, strawberries, nuts, flaxseeds, beans, dried peas, blueberries, psyllium, cucumbers, celery, and carrots.

Carbohydrate Counting Basics, Reading Food Labels

Carbohydrates are primarily classified as "sugars" (previously referred to as simple sugars) and "starches" (previously referred to as complex carbohydrates). Most foods contain carbohydrates. Those most commonly considered foods to have significant amounts of carbohydrates include grains (bread, rice, pasta, and cereal); fruits (fresh, canned, and dried fruit and fruit juice); starchy vegetables (potatoes, corn, peas, and winter squash); milk and yogurt; dried peas, beans, and legumes; desserts; sweetened drinks; and snack foods.

Carbohydrate counting has become increasingly common as insulin regimens have become more flexible, allowing patients to base their rapid-acting insulin dose on the amount of carbohydrates consumed. Counting carbohydrates gives children and adolescents flexibility in food choices as well as freedom to adjust their eating schedule according to individual circumstances and preferences. Accuracy in the ability to effectively count carbohydrates improves glycemic outcomes.[53] Therefore, family members and other care providers should be acquainted with this approach to maintain euglycemia. As children grow older and become more independent, it should not be assumed that they are able to count carbohydrates accurately. Care providers should continue to partner with adolescents on carbohydrate choices and counting during this time. Frequent visits with a registered dietitian can help reinforce carbohydrate counting strategies on their own as well as basic nutrition principles. It is also imperative that healthy diets are maintained and assessed periodically, as focusing exclusively on carbohydrates can lead to diets that are high in fat and deficient in many nutrients.

There are 2 methods to count carbohydrates: counting *grams* of carbohydrate, as listed on food labels, or a simplified method commonly referred to as carbohydrate *choices, units,* or *exchanges*. One carbohydrate choice/unit/exchange equals 12 to 15 g of total carbohydrates. To calculate carbohydrate choices/units/exchanges, divide the grams of total carbohydrates by 15 to determine how many carbohydrate units are in the food. There are many education materials with food lists showing either method that patients can use when counting carbohydrates. Counting in carbohydrate grams is advantageous when utilizing intensive insulin regimens with multiple daily injections or an insulin pump as it allows for better precision with the insulin dose. Other methods of meal planning, specifically the "exchange food lists," also incorporate carbohydrate counting. Each of these methods can be successfully used to manage the carbohydrate load in diabetes mellitus.[54]

When reading a food label for carbohydrates, it is important to emphasize 2 points: the *serving size* in household measures and the *total carbohydrate* in grams. The grams of sugar in food are included in the total carbohydrate and need not be counted separately. In Fig 30.1, the serving size is ½ cup and the total carbohydrate is 13 g. If a patient needed 1 unit of rapid-acting insulin per 15 g of carbohydrate, he or she would use this information to help determine the insulin dose, which would be approximately 1 unit of rapid-acting insulin for 1 serving (½ cup) of this food item. The serving size is also commonly underestimated, overlooked, or ignored, because many children or teenagers may not pay attention to the amount of food they are eating and, therefore, will underdose insulin. Frequent follow-up visits and reinforcement of these issues are helpful. Additionally, assisting caregivers as well as patients to learn how to interpret the other information on the food label can help them to make healthier food selections. A list of common food items and their associated carbohydrate content are outlined in Table 30.3.

Glycemic Index and Glycemic Load

Although the primary determinants of postprandial glucose response are the total amount of carbohydrates consumed and available insulin, a number of other factors may influence the glycemic response to food. These factors include the type of sugar (glucose, fructose, sucrose, lactose), type of starch (amylase, amylopectin, resistant starch), cooking and food processing (degree of starch gelatinization, particle size, cellular form), food form, and other food components such as fat and natural substances (lectins, phytates, tannins, and starch-protein and starch-lipid combinations) that can slow digestion.

The glycemic index (GI) is one tool to account for the relative differences in effect of carbohydrate on postprandial plasma glucose concentrations. The GI for a particular carbohydrate is calculated by comparing the relative area under the 2-hour postprandial glucose curve of 50 g of the proposed digestible carbohydrate to 50 g of a reference food, either glucose or white bread. Pure glucose is the standard comparative carbohydrate, with a GI of 100. The GI, therefore, ranks carbohydrates on a scale from 0 to 100 according to the extent to which they increase blood glucose concentrations after eating. It is important to note that the GI does not measure how *rapidly* blood glucose increases. Low-GI foods are defined as less than 55, moderate-GI foods are 55 to 70, and high-GI foods are greater than 70. Foods containing little or no carbohydrate (such as meat, poultry, fish, eggs, cheese, fats and oils, wine, beer, spirits, and most nonstarchy vegetables) do not have a GI. The glycemic load (GL) takes into consideration the amount of carbohydrate in the portion actually consumed.

The use of the GI as a means of controlling postprandial blood glucose or weight remains controversial as foods are rarely consumed alone. In addition, selecting foods according to their GI is not necessarily an indicator of healthy food choices. Addition of fat or protein with carbohydrate may further reduce the postprandial glycemic increase because of delayed gastric emptying.

Table 30.3.

Amount of Carbohydrates in Typical Food Groups/Items[98]

One carbohydrate unit or choice or exchange = 15 g of total carbohydrate

Starches: 15 g carbohydrate equals:

- One slice bread or dinner roll (whole wheat, rye, white, or pumpernickel)
- One 6-inch tortilla, chapati, roti, or injera bread
- One waffle or pancake (the size of a slice of bread)
- ¼ large bagel
- ½ English muffin, pita, hot dog bun, hamburger bun, or naan bread
- ½ cup cooked cereal or ¾ cup most dry cereals
- One small egg roll or spring roll, one medium meat samosa, or ½ vegetable samosa
- One 4-inch rice or corn patty (baked)
- ⅓ cup cooked rice or pasta (wheat, egg, or rice noodles)
- ½ cup cooked mung bean or chow Mein noodles
- ½ cup cooked peas, corn, sweet potato, white potato, taro, plantains, or legumes (dried beans, peas, or lentils, including dal or chole)
- 1 cup winter squash
- 31 (¾ oz) pretzel sticks
- 18 (1 oz) potato chips or tortilla chips
- 3 cups popped popcorn
- 4 to 6 crackers

Fruit: 15 g carbohydrate equals:

- One small fresh fruit (the size of a tennis ball)
- ½ cup mango, 1 cup papaya, or ½ grapefruit
- ½ cup canned fruit (packed in its own juice)
- ½ cup orange juice or apple juice
- ⅓ cup grape, cranberry, or prune juice
- 1 cup melon or berries
- 17 small grapes

- ¼ cup dried fruit
- 2 tablespoons raisins or craisins
- 3 dried figs

Milk: 12–15 g carbohydrate equals:
- 1 cup (8 oz) fat-free or low-fat milk or buttermilk
- 1 cup fat-free yogurt (plain)
- 6–8 oz light yogurt
- 1 cup (8 oz) soy milk

Nonstarchy vegetables: 15 g carbohydrate equals:
- 1½ cups most vegetables (except potato, peas, corn, squash) such as:
  o Green beans
  o Broccoli
  o Carrots
  o Cauliflower
  o Tomatoes
  o Cucumber
  o Celery
  o Asparagus
  o Cabbage and green leafy vegetables
  o Zucchini

Note: 1 cup lettuce or raw spinach equals 1 g of carbohydrate

Other: 15 g carbohydrate equals:
- 2-inch square of cake or brownie
- 2 small cookies
- 2 fortune cookies
- ½ cup ice cream or frozen yogurt
- ½ cup sherbet or sorbet
- ¼ cup rice pudding or kheer
- 1 tablespoon syrup, molasses, jam, jelly, sugar, or honey
- 1 tablespoon sweet-and-sour sauce

VI

Several studies have evaluated the use of a GI-specific diet and its effect on glycemic outcomes and diet composition. Children with T1D who consume a low-GI meal plan do not appear to have more limited food choices or a worse macronutrient diet composition compared with children who follow a traditional carbohydrate exchange diet.[55,56] Several studies have demonstrated modest benefits with respect to HbA1c,[55] mean blood glucose levels as assessed by continuous glucose monitoring,[57] mean capillary glucose measurements,[58] and postprandial capillary glucose measurements[59] in children with T1D consuming low- or moderate-GI diets.

Each of these studies evaluating the effect of low-GI diets in children and adolescents with T1D has been difficult to interpret, given the inter- and intravariability among individuals and study groups, along with inconsistent definitions of GI used.[60,61] A meta-analysis from 2003 concluded that use of a low-GI diet results in a modest but significant reduction in medium-term glycemic control.[62] Conversely, GI was found to be an unreliable guide for the effect of food on blood sugar levels in healthy adults and was influenced by individual differences in baseline measures of HbA1c, markers of insulin resistance, and insulin secretory capacity.[63] The American Diabetes Association 2017 *Standards of Medical Care* neither endorses nor dissuades the use of GI and GL in adults with diabetes.[13]

Low-Carbohydrate Diets in Patients With T1D and T2D

Low-%–40% energy from carbohydrate) and very low-carbohydrate diets (21–70 g/day) for the treatment of T1D and T2D have become increasingly visible on various media outlets. Although there is some evidence that low-carbohydrate diets can promote weight loss in adults with obesity and improve glycemic control in adults with T2D, there is insufficient evidence to support the use of these diets in children with T1D. The adoption of such diets may lead to poor energy levels, psychological comorbidities, and potentially contribute to the development of eating disorders.[64] Intake of healthy carbohydrates while restricting unnecessary empty calorie carbohydrates remains an important dietary principle in children with T1D. In obese adolescents, there may be an advantage to a very low-carbohydrate diet as compared with a low-fat diet in reducing risk for development of T2D.[65]

Hypoglycemia

Hypoglycemia in children with diabetes mellitus, defined as a blood glucose concentration less than 70 mg/dL, may result from a combination of excess insulin administration, decreased food intake, or increased physical activity. Hypoglycemia should always be treated immediately, and patients and family members need to be educated on signs and symptoms of low blood glucose concentration as well as appropriate treatment. Patients with diabetes mellitus should always carry a source of carbohydrate with them when away from home to treat hypoglycemia in addition to their blood glucose meter. The goal of treatment is to achieve rapid normalization of blood glucose without consuming excess carbohydrate and resultant rebound hyperglycemia.

Hypoglycemia should be treated with an appropriate amount of carbohydrate to increase blood glucose concentrations to a safe range in approximately 10 to 15 minutes. Glucose or sucrose is the preferred treatment while fructose is less desirable.[66] As a rule of thumb, 15 g of carbohydrate will increase the blood glucose approximately 30 to 50 mg/dL, but individual differences can occur. Blood glucose measurement should be repeated 15 minutes after treatment, and more carbohydrate should be consumed if it remains low. Once blood glucose concentration returns to normal, a meal or snack may be consumed to prevent recurrence of hypoglycemia, especially if continued physical activity is expected. A proposed treatment algorithm for hypoglycemia is listed in Table 30.4.

Table 30.4.

Treatment of Hypoglycemia[13]

1. Test blood glucose
2. If blood glucose is 51 mg/dL to 70 mg/dL, eat or drink 15–20 g of carbohydrate. If blood glucose is less than 50 mg/dL, eat or drink 30 g of carbohydrate. Each of the following equals 15 g of carbohydrate:
   - 3 to 4 glucose tablets
   - 1/2 cup (4 oz) regular soft drink (soft drink with sugar) or fruit juice
   - 1 small box of raisins
   - 1 cup (8 oz) skim milk
   - 1 tablespoon of honey or sugar
   - 1 small tube (15 g) of glucose gel
3. Wait 15 minutes before eating anything else. Then, retest blood glucose.
4. Repeat these steps until blood glucose is between 70 mg/dL and 100 mg/dL. It should be at least 100 mg/dL if:
   • the individual is going to drive.
   • the individual is going to exercise—this includes housework, yard work, running, jumping, or other physical activity.
   • the next meal is more than an hour away.

VI

Carbohydrate Adjustments for Exercise and/or Increased Physical Activity in Patients With T1D

Exercise remains an important component to overall treatment plans in all children with diabetes mellitus. However, precautionary measures to avoid either hyperglycemia or hypoglycemia during or after exercise need to be made. For most children, a decrease in insulin administration or the consumption of extra carbohydrate may be necessary to avoid hypoglycemia during or after exercise. The use of insulin pump therapy and "peakless" insulins has improved convenience in reducing insulin administration.

For managing exercise strictly with dietary changes, the type, duration, and intensity of exercise as well as the initial blood glucose concentration dictate the amount of carbohydrate required. Patients should be instructed to monitor their blood glucose before, during, and after exercise to establish patterns. New sports or activities frequently may result in different blood glucose patterns, and therefore, more frequent monitoring is recommended once again until patterns are established. A general starting guideline is to consume 15 g of carbohydrate for every 30 to 60 minutes of physical activity (Table 30.5).

Meal Planning Strategies Using Intensive Insulin Therapy Versus Fixed Insulin Doses in T1D

Intensive insulin therapy is defined as multiple daily injections or continuous subcutaneous insulin infusion (insulin pump therapy). The basal-bolus approach consists of a once- or twice-daily long-acting insulin given as background or basal insulin, while frequent doses of rapid-acting insulin are given throughout the day to correct hyperglycemia and to "cover" dietary carbohydrate. Basal-bolus plans allow people with diabetes mellitus the freedom to eat normally and not according to their insulin action time as was previously necessary with older insulin types. In children and adolescents, this method provides them with a more normal approach to eating and can help improve quality of life.[28] Meal and snack insulin doses should be adjusted to match carbohydrate intake.

The overall quality of the child's diet as well as protein and fat content must not be overlooked when using this approach, because excess energy intake will lead to weight gain. Several recent studies have shown that fat and protein also effect postprandial glucose, particularly when consumed in large amounts.[34,67-74] Large amounts of protein (≥75 g consumed alone)

Table 30.5.

Guidelines for Carbohydrate Intake When Exercising to Prevent Low Blood Glucose

Duration of Exercise	Exercise Intensity	Grams of Carbohydrate Needed Prior to Exercise		
		Blood Glucose <90 mg/dL	Blood Glucose 90–150 mg/dL	Blood Glucose 150–250 mg/dL
15–30 min	Mild Moderate Hard	15 15 15	0–15 15 15	0 0–15 0–15
30–60 min	Mild Moderate Hard	15–30 15–45 30–45	15–30 15–30 15–30	0–15 15 15–30
60–90 min	Mild Moderate Hard	15–45 30–45 30–60	15–45 30–45 30–45	15–30 30–45 30–45
>90 min	Mild, moderate, or hard	Follow guidelines for 60–90 min of activity. Check blood glucose and consume 15 g of carbohydrate for every 30 min of exercise.		

Adapted from Franz/American Diabetes Association.[99]

VI

significantly increases postprandial blood glucose levels 3 to 5 hours after consumption in people with T1D using intensive insulin therapy. High-fat meals can cause delayed gastric emptying, resulting in lower blood glucose 1 to 2 hours after eating and hyperglycemia thereafter. High-fat/high-protein meals may require more insulin than low-fat/low-protein meals with identical carbohydrate content. The use of continuous glucose monitors allow patients to identify such patterns in their blood glucose responses to specific foods so that they can adjust insulin doses accordingly. The use of dual-wave bolus (the amount of insulin delivered via an insulin pump is split over time, according to the macronutrient mix of the meal) and square-wave bolus (amount of insulin delivered evenly over a specified time period, used with gastroparesis or with extended periods of eating such as buffets) via insulin pumps is another effective tool to manage blood glucose levels when eating high-fat/high-protein foods.

Comprehensive nutrition education and counseling by the health care team on the relationship between food and blood glucose concentration, interpretation of blood glucose patterns, and nutrition-related insulin adjustment is important for optimal care. Registered dietitians should follow up with parents and patients at least annually for reinforcement of basic carbohydrate counting, especially if they experience deterioration in glycemic control, as well as healthy eating review. Accuracy in the ability to count carbohydrates among parents of children with T1D is associated with lower HbA1c values.[53] The use of meal-specific carbohydrate ratios was one of several factors associated with improved control among children with T1D from the Type 1 Diabetes Exchange.[75] Moreover, dietary quality correlates with knowledge of carbohydrates in adolescents with T1D,[76] suggesting that greater knowledge of foods containing carbohydrates results in a better overall diet.

Fixed Insulin Doses

Fixed insulin doses may also be used in intensive diabetes management, but carbohydrate, fat, and protein amounts must also be fixed and distributed throughout the day to optimize glycemic control and avoid hypoglycemia. Similar to basal bolus therapy, this strategy also relies on matching carbohydrate intake to insulin administration to effectively maintain glucose concentrations in a normal range while avoiding hypoglycemia.

Therapy for T2D and Prediabetes

Therapeutic data from children with T2D, compared with those from children with T1D, are far more limited, but the same principles (lifestyle modification in conjunction with pharmacologic intervention) have been adopted.[77,78] Recommendations from the AAP clinical practice guideline for management of T2D are shown in the text box. Reducing risk for development of T2D in children with prediabetes is based on the same principles of weight reduction and improving insulin sensitivity in treatment of T2D. Dietary modification, as part of a lifestyle modification program, has been shown to be an effective means of decreasing BMI, markers of insulin resistance, and other metabolic abnormalities (dyslipidemia, hypertension) commonly observed in obese children without T2D. Children meeting diagnostic criteria for T2D should be treated with metformin as a first-line pharmacologic agent (with or without insulin) along with adopting lifestyle modifications, including dietary changes and increased physical activity. Although lifestyle modification is still considered a critical component of treatment in pediatric T2D, in a multicenter trial of treatment options for T2D in adolescents, the combined intervention of metformin with an intensive lifestyle intervention program was not superior to metformin alone with respect to the rate of progression to glycemic failure (HbA1c >8% or inability to wean from insulin).[79] Additional trials investigating other classes of pharmaceutical agents are underway, but none are currently approved for use in children.[80] At this time, it is still accepted that attention to lifestyle modification, including dietary changes, should remain an important, adjunctive component of therapy for T2D.

Given the strong association of obesity and insulin resistance as inherent risk factors for pediatric T2D, recommendations are aimed at weight loss and increased physical activity to improve insulin sensitivity. The goals of management are to (1) achieve euglycemia and HbA1c targets; (2) achieve appropriate weight and normal linear growth; and (3) reduce comorbidities (dyslipidemia, hypertension) that are frequently present. Dietary modifications in all forms of pediatric diabetes, but particularly prediabetes and T2D, should be a family-based effort.[82] Scheduled meal times with the entire family are integral to establishing healthy eating behaviors. Parents should serve as models for healthy eating behavior and oversee portion sizes for their children in conjunction with guidance from a dietitian. Efforts should focus on reductions in total and saturated fat intake, increasing

AAP Recommendations for Treatment of Type 2 Diabetes Mellitus[81]

1. Clinicians must ensure that insulin therapy is initiated for children and adolescents with TD2DM who are ketotic or in diabetic ketoacidosis and in whom the distinction between T1DM and T2DM is unclear; and, in usual cases should initiate insulin therapy for patients:
   a. who have random venous or plasma blood glucose concentrations ≥250 mg/dL; or
   b. whose HbA1c is >9%
2. In all instances, clinicians should initiate a lifestyle modification program, including nutrition and physical activity, and start metformin as first-line therapy for children and adolescents at the time of diagnosis of TD2DM.
3. The committee suggests that clinicians monitor HBA1c concentrations every 3 months and intensify treatment if treatment goals for blood glucose and HbA1c concentrations are not being met.
4. The committee suggests that clinicians advise patients to monitor finger-stick blood glucose concentrations in those who:
   a. are taking inulin or other medications with a risk of hypoglycemia; or
   b. are initiating or changing their diabetes treatment goals; or
   c. have not met treatment goals; or
   d. have intercurrent illness
5. The committee suggests that clinicians incorporate the Academy of Nutrition and Dietetics Pediatric Weight Management Evidence Based Nutrition Practice Guidelines in the nutrition counseling of patients with T2DM both at the time of diagnosis and as part of ongoing management.
6. The committee suggests that clinicians encourage children and adolescents with T2DM to engage in moderate-to-vigorous exercise for at least 60 minutes daily and to limit nonacademic screen time to less than 2 hours per day.

Pediatrics. 2013;131(2):364–382

fiber intake, and targeting calorie intake goals that result in a healthy BMI. Similar to recommendations for children with exogenous obesity, juices and other sugar-based soft drinks should be eliminated and replaced with lower-energy beverages.[83,84] Increased energy expenditure through physical activities that are enjoyable for the child promotes improved insulin sensitivity and is needed, in combination with dietary changes, to achieve weight loss. Specific recommendations from an expert committee on therapy in pediatric obesity can also be applied to the pediatric T2D or prediabetes population (Table 30.6).

Table 30.6.
Evidence-Based Initial Lifestyle Interventions to Treat Pediatric Obesity[15]

- Eliminate sugar-sweetened beverages of all kinds, including fruit juices
- Increase intake of water or skim milk
- Eat a healthy breakfast daily
- Strive for 5 total fruits and vegetables daily at a minimum
- Set short-term attainable goals for incremental changes
- Eat family meals together as much as possible
- Limit eating out at restaurants, particularly fast food
- Limit portion size
- Limit intake of saturated and trans fats
- Encourage consumption of skim and low-fat milk in place of whole milk and increase consumption of calcium
- Encourage physical activity for at least 1 hour each day
- Limit computer/tablet/television screen time to no more than 2 hours per day

Special Situations and Chronic Diseases Associated With Diabetes Mellitus in Children

Nutrition Management in the School and Child Care Setting for Children Requiring Insulin

Children and adolescents with diabetes mellitus need assistance with managing their blood glucose concentrations at school and in child care.[85] School nurses play a critical role, along with other school personnel, in assisting and supervising blood glucose monitoring, insulin administration, treatment of hypoglycemia, and meal plans.

Federal laws that protect children with diabetes mellitus include Section 504 of the Rehabilitation Act of 1973 (Pub L No. 93-112) and the Individuals with Disabilities Education Act (Pub L No. 108-446 [originally the Education for All Handicapped Children Act of 1975, Pub L No. 94-142]) and the Americans with Disabilities Act (Pub L No. 101-336). Diabetes mellitus is considered to be a disability under these laws; therefore, it is illegal for schools and/or child care centers to discriminate against children with diabetes mellitus. Any school that receives federal funding or any facility considered open to the public must reasonably accommodate the special needs of children with diabetes mellitus. Federal law requires an individualized assessment for any child with diabetes mellitus. The required accommodations should be documented in a written plan developed under the applicable federal law, such as a Section 504 Plan or individualized

VI

education program (IEP). An individualized diabetes medical management plan (DMMP) should be developed by the student's diabetes health care team with input from the parent or guardian. The DMMP should address the information about the student's meal/snack schedule. For young children, instructions should be given for when food is provided during school parties and other activities.

Celiac Disease

Celiac disease is an autoimmune disorder that occurs more frequently in individuals with preexisting T1D. Large-scale registries from the United States, Germany, Austria, the United Kingdom, and Australia found prevalence rates of celiac disease of 1.9% to 7.7% in children with T1D.[86] Reduction in growth rates and weight gain often accompany children with both T1D and celiac disease. In addition, individuals with T1D and celiac disease are at a higher risk for poor bone mineral density, which can lead to fractures and hypoglycemia as adults.[87]

Care providers must be well versed on the intricacies of the gluten-free diet and celiac disease in relation to its influence on nutritional status and metabolic control in children and adolescents with diabetes mellitus. Frequent visits with patients and families as well as other caregivers are necessary to ensure comprehension because of the complexity of the gluten-free diet. Children with celiac disease who carefully follow a well-balanced, healthy gluten-free diet have the same nutrition requirements as other children once the intestinal mucosa is healed. Consultation with a registered dietitian experienced in managing both diabetes and celiac disease is strongly recommended.[13] A detailed discussion of celiac disease is found in Chapter 27: Chronic Diarrheal Disease, but principles of screening and treatment are outlined in Table 30.7.

Nutrition Recommendations for Cystic Fibrosis-Related Diabetes Mellitus in Children and Adolescents (see also Chapter 46: Nutrition in Cystic Fibrosis)

Cystic fibrosis-related diabetes (CFRD) has become the most common comorbidity in people with cystic fibrosis as the population ages. CFRD occurs in approximately 20% of adolescents with cystic fibrosis, with an incidence of approximately 3% per year beginning in the teenage years but has been observed at all ages, including infants.[88] The etiology of diabetes in cystic fibrosis is not related to either T1D or T2D; however, there are some shared similarities. It is primarily caused by insulin insufficiency resulting from scarring and fibrosis of beta cells, although fluctuating levels of insulin

Table 30.7.

Recommendations for Screening and Treatment of Celiac Disease in Children With T1D[14,100]

- Children with T1D should be screened for celiac disease by measuring serum concentrations of immunoglobulin (Ig) A and anti-tissue transglutaminase antibodies, or, with IgA deficiency, screening can include measuring IgG tissue transglutaminase antibodies or IgG deamidated gliadin peptide antibodies. These should be obtained soon after the diagnosis of T1D has been made and repeated at 2 and 5 years thereafter.
- Testing should be repeated in children with growth failure, failure to gain weight, weight loss, diarrhea, flatulence, abdominal pain, or signs of malabsorption or in children with frequent unexplained hypoglycemia or deterioration in glycemic control.
- Children with positive antibodies should be referred to a gastroenterologist for evaluation with endoscopy and biopsy.
- Children with biopsy-confirmed celiac disease should be placed on a gluten-free diet and have consultation with a dietitian experienced in managing both diabetes and celiac disease.

resistance related to acute and chronic illness also contribute to glycemic state.[89]

Nutrition therapy for CFRD differs significantly from that for T1D and T2D,[90] specifically with regard to requirements for energy, fat, protein, sodium, and supplemental vitamins and minerals. Adequate energy intake to maintain the recommended BMI for children and adolescents is critical for health and survival.[91] Normalization of blood glucose concentration is essential to optimize nutrient metabolism and to improve BMI and lean body mass.[92]

The diagnosis of CFRD does not change the standard cystic fibrosis nutrition recommendations. Energy intake should almost never be restricted. The high-energy eating pattern does not replace the need for healthy, nutrient-dense food intake, and most people with cystic fibrosis will need routine vitamin and mineral supplementation because of malabsorption. Appetite can be highly variable from day to day in people with cystic fibrosis, necessitating the use of oral high-energy supplements and/or enteral tube feedings to meet energy requirements in some patients.[93] For these reasons, meal plans are not practical. The use of carbohydrate counting and insulin-to-carbohydrate ratios in conjunction with the cystic fibrosis eating pattern to guide insulin therapy are essential to optimize blood glucose control.[90] Insulin regimens can be individualized to allow for adequate glycemic control for frequent meals or enteral feedings overnight.

The risk of hypoglycemia in CFRD is no different from insulin-treated patients with T1D or T2D. Absorption of fat-free carbohydrates is not compromised in patients with cystic fibrosis. Therefore, low blood glucose concentrations should be treated with fat-free carbohydrate sources that do not require pancreatic enzyme replacement.

Eating Disorders in Children and Adolescents With Diabetes *(see also Chapter 38: Eating Disorders in Children and Adolescents)*
Eating disorders are common among adolescents with T1D and negatively affect glycemic control.[94] Historically, 10% of females with T1D meet *Diagnostic and Statistical Manual of Mental Disorders* criteria for an underlying eating disorder while an additional 14% had symptoms but did not reach diagnostic threshold.[95] This may be an underestimate, however, as more recent data revealed that 38% of female and 16% of male adolescents with T1D exhibit symptoms of disordered eating.[96] Bulimia is the most common eating disorder in females with T1D, with insulin omission (diabulimia) used as an additional method to lose weight.

Diabetes and eating disorders both involve attention to food and weight, and therefore, it is not uncommon for patients to use their diabetes to conceal their eating disorder. Foods being labeled as "good" or "bad" can lead to guilt or anxiety surrounding eating, which can result in behaviors of disordered eating.[96] Concurrent depression and/or emotional dysregulation are additional risk factors for bulimia in this population.[97] Technological advances in diabetes such as insulin pumps and continuous glucose monitoring, although helpful in managing diabetes, may also allow for misuse in those with body dissatisfaction.

The combination of diabetes mellitus and an eating disorder can lead to serious or even fatal consequences (diabetic ketoacidosis, electrolyte disturbances, cardiac conduction abnormalities, edema); therefore, timely identification and appropriate treatment is imperative. Ideally, patients diagnosed with both diabetes mellitus and an eating disorder will be referred to a team of providers who are comfortable treating both diseases and are knowledgeable regarding diabetes management, given the differences that may exist between the treatment approaches.

The American Diabetes Association recommends screening for disordered eating behaviors when patients reach early adolescence.[14] Several tools for use in the adolescent T1D population have been developed and validated, such as the Diabetes Eating Problem Survey[25] and Screen for Early Eating Disorder Signs.[26] Nonspecific signs such as unintentional weight gain or loss or a sudden worsening of HbA_{1c} may also be indicators of a concomitant eating disorder and should be factored into individual patient screening.

Summary/Conclusion

Treatment of diabetes mellitus in children is a complex task, but ultimately is centered on the approach to nutrition, insulin when indicated, and a healthy lifestyle. Although a focus on careful carbohydrate counting is integral to insulin delivery and glycemic control for patients with T1D, many of the other fundamental principles of healthy nutrition apply to children with T1D or T2D. A team approach, capitalizing on the expertise of pediatric dietitians, psychologists, nurses, and physicians can best assist children and their families overcome challenges in their care and reach their therapeutic goals. Table 30.8 provides additional educational resources for care providers, patients, and families.

Table 30.8.
Resources for Nutrition Education

Academy of Nutrition and Dietetics	http://www.eatrightstore.org *Choose Your Foods: Food Lists for Diabetes* (English and Spanish versions) *Eating Healthy with Diabetes: Easy Reading Guide* *Match Your Insulin to Your Carbs*
American Academy of Pediatrics	https://www.healthychildren.org/english/healthy-living/nutrition/pages/default.aspx
American Diabetes Association	http://www.shopdiabetes.org/Categories/8-Diabetes-Books.aspx *The Complete Guide to Carbohydrate Counting*, 3rd ed *Diabetes Carbohydrate and Fat Gram Guide*, 4th ed *Diabetic Carb-Smart Essentials* *Eat Out, Eat Well* *Diabetic Meal Planning Essentials* http://www.shopdiabetes.org/Categories/48-Carb-Counting.aspx

Continued

Table 30.8. *Continued*
Resources for Nutrition Education

Diabetes and Celiac Disease	Diabetes and Celiac Disease: *Academy of Nutrition and Dietetics Pocket Guide to Gluten-Free Strategies for Clients with Multiple Diet Restrictions, 2nd Ed.* http://www.eatrightstore.org/product/F7393595-5A17-4C63-9469-270E6F9E3B1A *Counting Gluten Free Carbohydrates* www.nbdiabetes.org/sites/default/files/documents/Carb_Counting_GF_a.doc Gluten Free Recipes For People with Diabetes *https://nationalceliac.org/gluten-free-recipes-old/ Gluten Free Recipes for People with Diabetes:*
Cystic Fibrosis Related Diabetes	*Managing Cystic Fibrosis-Related Diabetes (CFRD): An Instruction Guide for Patients and Families.* 6th ed: https://www.cff.org/Life-With-CF/Daily-Life/Cystic-Fibrosis-related-Diabetes/Managing-CFRD.pdf
US Department of Agriculture National Nutrient Database for Standard Reference	http://www.nal.usda.gov/fnic/foodcomp/search/
National Institute of Diabetes and Digestive and Kidney Diseases (NIDDK)	http://diabetes.niddk.nih.gov/dm/pubs/eating_ez/index.aspx

References

1. Dabelea D, Mayer-Davis EJ, Saydah S, et al. Prevalence of type 1 and type 2 diabetes among children and adolescents from 2001 to 2009. *JAMA.* 2014;311(17):1778–1786

2. Patterson C, Guariguata L, Dahlquist G, Soltesz G, Ogle G, Silink M. Diabetes in the young - a global view and worldwide estimates of numbers of children with type 1 diabetes. *Diabetes Res Clin Pract.* 2014;103(2):161–175

3. Writing Group for the SfDiYSG, Dabelea D, Bell RA, et al. Incidence of diabetes in youth in the United States. *JAMA.* 27 2007;297(24):2716–2724

4. Diabetes C, Complications Trial Research G, Nathan DM, et al. The effect of intensive treatment of diabetes on the development and progression of long-term complications in insulin-dependent diabetes mellitus. *N Engl J Med.* 1993;329(14):977–986

5. Nathan DM, Cleary PA, Backlund JY, et al. Intensive diabetes treatment and cardiovascular disease in patients with type 1 diabetes. *N Engl J Med.* 2005;353(25):2643–2653

6. US Department of Health and Human Services, Office of Disease Prevention and Health Promotion. Dietary Guidelines for Americans. 2015; 8th:http://health.gov/dietaryguidelines/2015/guidelines/

7. Chiang JL, Kirkman MS, Laffel LM, Peters AL, Type 1 Diabetes Sourcebook A. Type 1 diabetes through the life span: a position statement of the American Diabetes Association. *Diabetes Care.* 2014;37(7):2034–2054

8. National Institute of Health, Office of Dietary Supplements. Dietary Reference Intakes (DRI). Available at: https://ods.od.nih.gov/Health_Information/Dietary_Reference_Intakes.aspx. Accessed June 30, 2019

9. Sunni M, Brunzell C, Kyllo J, Purcell L, Plager P, Moran A. A picture-based carbohydrate-counting resource for Somalis. *J Int Med Res.* 2017;46(1):219-224

10. Sunni M, Brunzell C, Nathan B, Moran A. Management of diabetes during Ramadan: practical guidelines. *Minnesota Med.* 2014;97(6):36–38

11. Smart CE, Annan F, Bruno LP, et al. ISPAD Clinical Practice Consensus Guidelines 2014. Nutritional management in children and adolescents with diabetes. *Pediatr Diabetes.* 2014;15 Suppl 20:135–153

12. Evert AB, Boucher JL, Cypress M, et al. Nutrition therapy recommendations for the management of adults with diabetes. *Diabetes Care.* 2013;36(11):3821–3842

13. American Diabetes A. 4. Lifestyle Management. *Diabetes Care.* 2017;40(Suppl 1): S33–S43

14. Siscovick DS, Barringer TA, Fretts AM, et al. Omega-3 polyunsaturated fatty acid (fish oil) supplementation and the prevention of clinical cardiovascular disease: a science advisory from the American Heart Association. *Circulation.* 2017;135(15):e867–e884

15. Styne DM, Arslanian SA, Connor EL, et al. Pediatric obesity-assessment, treatment, and prevention: an Endocrine Society Clinical Practice Guideline. *J Clin Endocrinol Metab.* 2017;102(3):709–757

16. Hoelscher DM, Kirk S, Ritchie L, Cunningham-Sabo L. Position of the Academy of Nutrition and Dietetics: interventions for the prevention and treatment of pediatric overweight and obesity. *J Acad Nutr Diet.* 2013;113(10):1375–1394

17. Centers for Disease Control and Prevention. Clinical Growth Charts. Available at: http://www.cdc.gov/growthcharts/clinical_charts.htm. Accessed June 30, 2019

18. Mehta SN, Volkening LK, Quinn N, Laffel LM. Intensively managed young children with type 1 diabetes consume high-fat, low-fiber diets similar to age-matched controls. *Nutr Res.* 2014;34(5):428–435

VI

19. Overby NC, Flaaten V, Veierod MB, et al. Children and adolescents with type 1 diabetes eat a more atherosclerosis-prone diet than healthy control subjects. *Diabetologia*. 2007;50(2):307–316

20. The NS, Crandell JL, Lawrence JM, et al. Vitamin D in youth with Type 1 diabetes: prevalence of insufficiency and association with insulin resistance in the SEARCH Nutrition Ancillary Study. *Diabet Med*. 2013;30(11):1324–1332

21. Svoren BM, Volkening LK, Wood JR, Laffel LM. Significant vitamin D deficiency in youth with type 1 diabetes mellitus. *J Pediatr*. 2009;154(1):132–134

22. Kelly A, Brooks LJ, Dougherty S, Carlow DC, Zemel BS. A cross-sectional study of vitamin D and insulin resistance in children. *Arch Dis Child*. 2011;96(5):447–452

23. Liu LL, Lawrence JM, Davis C, et al. Prevalence of overweight and obesity in youth with diabetes in USA: the SEARCH for Diabetes in Youth study. *Pediatr Diabetes*. 2010;11(1):4–11

24. Minges KE, Whittemore R, Weinzimer SA, Irwin ML, Redeker NS, Grey M. Correlates of overweight and obesity in 5529 adolescents with type 1 diabetes: The T1D Exchange Clinic Registry. *Diabetes Res Clin Pract*. 2017;126:68–78

25. Markowitz JT, Butler DA, Volkening LK, Antisdel JE, Anderson BJ, Laffel LM. Brief screening tool for disordered eating in diabetes: internal consistency and external validity in a contemporary sample of pediatric patients with type 1 diabetes. *Diabetes Care*. 2010;33(3):495–500

26. Powers MA, Richter S, Ackard D, Craft C. Development and validation of the Screen for Early Eating Disorder Signs (SEEDS) in persons with type 1 diabetes. *Eating Disord*. 2016;24(3):271–288

27. Evert AB, Boucher JL, Cypress M, et al. Nutrition therapy recommendations for the management of adults with diabetes. *Diabetes Care*. 2014;37 Suppl 1:S120–143

28. Group DS. Training in flexible, intensive insulin management to enable dietary freedom in people with type 1 diabetes: dose adjustment for normal eating (DAFNE) randomised controlled trial. *BMJ*. 2002;325(7367):746

29. Academy of Nutrition and Dietetics Evidence Analysis Library. Available at: https://www.andeal.org. Accessed March 11, 2019

30. Loghmani E, Rickard K, Washburne L, Vandagriff J, Fineberg N, Golden M. Glycemic response to sucrose-containing mixed meals in diets of children of with insulin-dependent diabetes mellitus. *J Pediatr*. 1991;119(4):531–537

31. Schwingshandl J, Rippel S, Unterluggauer M, Borkenstein M. Effect of the introduction of dietary sucrose on metabolic control in children and adolescents with type I diabetes. *Acta Diabetol*. 1994;31(4):205–209

32. Rickard KA, Cleveland JL, Loghmani ES, Fineberg NS, Freidenberg GR. Similar glycemic responses to high versus moderate sucrose-containing foods in test meals for adolescents with type 1 diabetes and fasting euglycemia. *J Am Diet Assoc*. 2001;101(10):1202–1205

33. Smart C, Aslander-van Vliet E, Waldron S. Nutritional management in children and adolescents with diabetes. *Pediatr Diabetes*. 2009;10 Suppl 12:100–117

34. Smart CE, Evans M, O'Connell SM, et al. Both dietary protein and fat increase postprandial glucose excursions in children with type 1 diabetes, and the effect is additive. *Diabetes Care.* 2013;36(12):3897–3902

35. Gannon MC, Nuttall JA, Damberg G, Gupta V, Nuttall FQ. Effect of protein ingestion on the glucose appearance rate in people with type 2 diabetes. *J Clin Endocrinol Metab.* 2001;86(3):1040–1047

36. Maahs DM, Dabelea D, D'Agostino RB, Jr., et al. Glucose control predicts 2-year change in lipid profile in youth with type 1 diabetes. *J Pediatr.* 2013;162(1): 101–107 e101

37. Franz MJ, Powers MA, Leontos C, et al. The evidence for medical nutrition therapy for type 1 and type 2 diabetes in adults. *J Am Diet Assoc.* 2010;110(12): 1852–1889

38. Karlstrom BE, Jarvi AE, Byberg L, Berglund LG, Vessby BO. Fatty fish in the diet of patients with type 2 diabetes: comparison of the metabolic effects of foods rich in n-3 and n-6 fatty acids. *Am J Clin Nutr.* 2011;94(1):26–33

39. Prasad K. Flaxseed and cardiovascular health. *J Cardiovasc Pharmacol.* 2009;54(5): 369–377

40. Saremi A, Arora R. The utility of omega-3 fatty acids in cardiovascular disease. *Am J Ther.* 2009;16(5):421–436

41. Althuis MD, Jordan NE, Ludington EA, Wittes JT. Glucose and insulin responses to dietary chromium supplements: a meta-analysis. *Am J Clin Nutr.* 2002;76(1): 148–155

42. Balk EM, Tatsioni A, Lichtenstein AH, Lau J, Pittas AG. Effect of chromium supplementation on glucose metabolism and lipids: a systematic review of randomized controlled trials. *Diabetes Care.* 2007;30(8):2154–2163

43. Borkar VV, Devidayal, Verma S, Bhalla AK. Low levels of vitamin D in North Indian children with newly diagnosed type 1 diabetes. *Pediatr Diabetes.* 2010;11(5):345–350

44. Janner M, Ballinari P, Mullis PE, Fluck CE. High prevalence of vitamin D deficiency in children and adolescents with type 1 diabetes. *Swiss Med Wkly.* 2010;140:w13091

45. Wood JR, Connor CG, Cheng P, et al. Vitamin D status in youth with type 1 and type 2 diabetes enrolled in the Pediatric Diabetes Consortium (PDC) is not worse than in youth without diabetes. *Pediatr Diabetes.* 2016;17(8):584–591

46. Baker-Smith CM, de Ferranti SD, Cochran WJ, Bhatia JJS. American Academy of Pediatrics, Committee on Nutrition, Section on Gastroenterology, Hepatology, and Nutrition. Policy statement: The use of nonnutritive sweeteners in children. *Pediatrics.* 2019:in press

47. Fitch C, Keim KS, Academy of Nutrition and Dietetics. Position of the Academy of Nutrition and Dietetics: use of nutritive and nonnutritive sweeteners. *J Acad Nutr Diet.* 2012;112(5):739–758

VI

48. Katz ML, Mehta S, Nansel T, Quinn H, Lipsky LM, Laffel LM. Associations of nutrient intake with glycemic control in youth with type 1 diabetes: differences by insulin regimen. *Diab Technol Ther.* 2014;16(8):512–518

49. Nader N, Weaver A, Eckert S, Lteif A. Effects of fiber supplementation on glycemic excursions and incidence of hypoglycemia in children with type 1 diabetes. *Int J Pediatr Endocrinol.* 2014;2014(1):13

50. Kriska A, El Ghormli L, Copeland KC, et al. Impact of lifestyle behavior change on glycemic control in youth with type 2 diabetes. *Pediatr Diabetes.* 2018;19(1): 36–44

51. Wheeler ML, Dunbar SA, Jaacks LM, et al. Macronutrients, food groups, and eating patterns in the management of diabetes: a systematic review of the literature, 2010. *Diabetes Care.* 2012;35(2):434–445

52. Dahl WJ, Stewart ML. Position of the Academy of Nutrition and Dietetics: Health Implications of Dietary Fiber. *J Acad Nutr Diet.* 2015;115(11):1861–1870

53. Mehta SN, Quinn N, Volkening LK, Laffel LM. Impact of carbohydrate counting on glycemic control in children with type 1 diabetes. *Diabetes Care.* 2009;32(6):1014–1016

54. Smart CE, Ross K, Edge JA, King BR, McElduff P, Collins CE. Can children with Type 1 diabetes and their caregivers estimate the carbohydrate content of meals and snacks? *Diab Med.* 2010;27(3):348–353

55. Gilbertson HR, Brand-Miller JC, Thorburn AW, Evans S, Chondros P, Werther GA. The effect of flexible low glycemic index dietary advice versus measured carbohydrate exchange diets on glycemic control in children with type 1 diabetes. *Diabetes Care.* 2001;24(7):1137–1143

56. Gilbertson HR, Thorburn AW, Brand-Miller JC, Chondros P, Werther GA. Effect of low-glycemic-index dietary advice on dietary quality and food choice in children with type 1 diabetes. *Am J Clin Nutr.* 2003;77(1):83–90

57. Rovner AJ, Nansel TR, Gellar L. The effect of a low-glycemic diet vs a standard diet on blood glucose levels and macronutrient intake in children with type 1 diabetes. *J Am Diet Assoc.* 2009;109(2):303–307

58. Nansel TR, Gellar L, McGill A. Effect of varying glycemic index meals on blood glucose control assessed with continuous glucose monitoring in youth with type 1 diabetes on basal-bolus insulin regimens. *Diabetes Care.* 2008;31(4):695–697

59. Ryan RL, King BR, Anderson DG, Attia JR, Collins CE, Smart CE. Influence of and optimal insulin therapy for a low-glycemic index meal in children with type 1 diabetes receiving intensive insulin therapy. *Diabetes Care.* 2008;31(8):1485–1490

60. Vega-Lopez S, Ausman LM, Griffith JL, Lichtenstein AH. Interindividual variability and intra-individual reproducibility of glycemic index values for commercial white bread. *Diabetes Care.* 2007;30(6):1412–1417

61. Pi-Sunyer FX. Glycemic index and disease. *Am J Clin Nutr.* 2002;76(1):290S–298S

62. Brand-Miller J, Hayne S, Petocz P, Colagiuri S. Low-glycemic index diets in the management of diabetes: a meta-analysis of randomized controlled trials. *Diabetes Care.* 2003;26(8):2261–2267

63. Matthan NR, Ausman LM, Meng H, Tighiouart H, Lichtenstein AH. Estimating the reliability of glycemic index values and potential sources of methodological and biological variability. *Am J Clin Nutr.* 2016;104(4):1004–1013

64. de Bock M, Lobley K, Anderson D, et al. Endocrine and metabolic consequences due to restrictive carbohydrate diets in children with type 1 diabetes: An illustrative case series. *Pediatr Diabetes.* 2018;19(1):129–137

65. Gow ML, Garnett SP, Baur LA, Lister NB. The effectiveness of different diet strategies to reduce type 2 diabetes risk in youth. *Nutrients.* 2016;8(8):e486

66. Husband AC, Crawford S, McCoy LA, Pacaud D. The effectiveness of glucose, sucrose, and fructose in treating hypoglycemia in children with type 1 diabetes. *Pediatr Diabetes.* 2010;11(3):154–158

67. Bell KJ, Toschi E, Steil GM, Wolpert HA. Optimized mealtime insulin dosing for fat and protein in type 1 diabetes: application of a model-based approach to derive insulin doses for open-loop diabetes management. *Diabetes Care.* 2016;39(9):1631–1634

68. Bell KJ, Smart CE, Steil GM, Brand-Miller JC, King B, Wolpert HA. Impact of fat, protein, and glycemic index on postprandial glucose control in type 1 diabetes: implications for intensive diabetes management in the continuous glucose monitoring era. *Diabetes Care.* 2015;38(6):1008–1015

69. Campbell MD, Walker M, King D, et al. Carbohydrate Counting at Meal Time Followed by a Small Secondary Postprandial Bolus Injection at 3 Hours Prevents Late Hyperglycemia, Without Hypoglycemia, After a High-Carbohydrate, High-Fat Meal in Type 1 Diabetes. *Diabetes Care.* 2016;39(9):e141–e142

70. Paterson MA, Smart CE, Lopez PE, et al. Influence of dietary protein on postprandial blood glucose levels in individuals with Type 1 diabetes mellitus using intensive insulin therapy. *Diabet Med.* 2016;33(5):592–598

71. Neu A, Behret F, Braun R, et al. Higher glucose concentrations following protein- and fat-rich meals - the Tuebingen Grill Study: a pilot study in adolescents with type 1 diabetes. *Pediatr Diabetes.* 2015;16(8):587–591

72. Garcia-Lopez JM, Gonzalez-Rodriguez M, Pazos-Couselo M, Gude F, Prieto-Tenreiro A, Casanueva F. Should the amounts of fat and protein be taken into consideration to calculate the lunch prandial insulin bolus? Results from a randomized crossover trial. *Diabetes Technol Ther.* 2013;15(2):166–171

73. Lodefalk M, Aman J, Bang P. Effects of fat supplementation on glycaemic response and gastric emptying in adolescents with Type 1 diabetes. *Diabet Med.* 2008;25(9):1030–1035

74. Wolpert HA, Atakov-Castillo A, Smith SA, Steil GM. Dietary fat acutely increases glucose concentrations and insulin requirements in patients with type 1 diabetes: implications for carbohydrate-based bolus dose calculation and intensive diabetes management. *Diabetes Care.* 2013;36(4):810–816

75. Campbell MS, Schatz DA, Chen V, et al. A contrast between children and adolescents with excellent and poor control: the T1D Exchange clinic registry experience. *Pediatr Diabetes.* 2014;15(2):110–117

VI

76. Bansal N, Cuttler L, O'Riordan MA, Koontz MB. Dietary quality in adolescents with type 1 diabetes. *Diabetes Care.* 2013;36(8):e113

77. ISPAD Clinical Practice Consensus Guidelines 2014 Compendium: Type 2 diabetes in the child and adolescent. *Pediatr Diabetes.* 2015;16(5):392

78. Nadeau KJ, Anderson BJ, Berg EG, et al. Youth-Onset Type 2 Diabetes Consensus Report: Current Status, Challenges, and Priorities. *Diabetes Care.* 2016;39(9):1635–1642

79. Group TS, Zeitler P, Hirst K, et al. A clinical trial to maintain glycemic control in youth with type 2 diabetes. *N Engl J Med.* 2012;366(24):2247–2256

80. Nambam B, Silverstein J, Cheng P, et al. A cross-sectional view of the current state of treatment of youth with type 2 diabetes in the USA: enrollment data from the Pediatric Diabetes Consortium Type 2 Diabetes Registry. *Pediatr Diabetes.* 2017;18(3):222–229

81. Copeland KC, Silverstein J, Moore KR, et al. Clinical practice guideline: Management of newly diagnosed type 2 Diabetes Mellitus (T2DM) in children and adolescents. *Pediatrics.* 2013;131(2):364–382

82. Wrotniak BH, Epstein LH, Paluch RA, Roemmich JN. Parent weight change as a predictor of child weight change in family-based behavioral obesity treatment. *Arch Pediatr Adolesc Med.* 2004;158(4):342–347

83. American Academy of Pediatrics, Committee on Nutrition, Council on Sports Medicine and Fitness. Sports drinks and energy drinks for children and adolescents: are they appropriate? *Pediatrics.* 2011;127(6):1182–1189

84. Heyman MB, Abrams SA, Section On Gastroenterology H, Nutrition, Committee On N. Fruit Juice in Infants, Children, and Adolescents: Current Recommendations. *Pediatrics.* 2017;139(6)

85. Jackson CC, Albanese-O'Neill A, Butler KL, et al. Diabetes care in the school setting: a position statement of the American Diabetes Association. *Diabetes Care.* 2015;38(10):1958–1963

86. Craig ME, Prinz N, Boyle CT, et al. Prevalence of celiac disease in 52,721 youth with type 1 diabetes: international comparison across three continents. *Diabetes Care.* 2017;40(8):1034–1040

87. Thong EP, Wong P, Dev A, Ebeling PR, Teede HJ, Milat F. Increased prevalence of fracture and hypoglycaemia in young adults with concomitant type 1 diabetes mellitus and coeliac disease. *Clin Endocrinol.* 2018;88(1):37–43

88. Moran A, Dunitz J, Nathan B, Saeed A, Holme B, Thomas W. Cystic fibrosis-related diabetes: current trends in prevalence, incidence, and mortality. *Diabetes Care.* 2009;32(9):1626–1631

89. Moran A, Doherty L, Wang X, Thomas W. Abnormal glucose metabolism in cystic fibrosis. *J Pediatr.* 1998;133(1):10–17

90. Moran A, Brunzell C, Cohen RC, et al. Clinical care guidelines for cystic fibrosis-related diabetes: a position statement of the American Diabetes Association and a clinical practice guideline of the Cystic Fibrosis Foundation, endorsed by the Pediatric Endocrine Society. *Diabetes Care.* 2010;33(12):2697–2708

91. Stallings VA, Stark LJ, Robinson KA, et al. Evidence-based practice recommendations for nutrition-related management of children and adults with cystic fibrosis and pancreatic insufficiency: results of a systematic review. *J Am Diet Assoc.* 2008;108(5):832–839

92. Moran A, Pekow P, Grover P, et al. Insulin therapy to improve BMI in cystic fibrosis-related diabetes without fasting hyperglycemia: results of the cystic fibrosis related diabetes therapy trial. *Diabetes Care.* 2009;32(10):1783–1788

93. Borowitz D, Baker RD, Stallings V. Consensus report on nutrition for pediatric patients with cystic fibrosis. *J Pediatr Gastroenterol Nutr.* 2002;35(3):246–259

94. Neumark-Sztainer D, Patterson J, Mellin A, et al. Weight control practices and disordered eating behaviors among adolescent females and males with type 1 diabetes: associations with sociodemographics, weight concerns, familial factors, and metabolic outcomes. *Diabetes Care.* 2002;25(8):1289–1296

95. Jones JM, Lawson ML, Daneman D, Olmsted MP, Rodin G. Eating disorders in adolescent females with and without type 1 diabetes: cross sectional study. *BMJ.* 2000;320(7249):1563–1566

96. Hanlan ME, Griffith J, Patel N, Jaser SS. Eating disorders and disordered eating in type 1 diabetes: prevalence, screening, and treatment options. *Curr Diabetes Rep.* 12 2013

97. Young-Hyman DL, Peterson CM, Fischer S, Markowitz JT, Muir AB, Laffel LM. Depressive symptoms, emotion dysregulation, and bulimic symptoms in youth with type 1 diabetes: varying interactions at diagnosis and during transition to insulin pump therapy. *J Diabetes Sci Technol.* 2016;10(4):845–851

98. American Diabetes Association, Academy of Nutrition and Dietetics. Choose Your Foods: Food Lists for Diabetes. Chicago, IL: Academy of Nutrition and Dietetics; 2014:64

99. Franz M. *Nutrition, physical activity, and diabetes.* In: Devlin JT, Schneider SH, Kriska A, eds. *Handbook of Exercise in Diabetes.* Alexandria, VA: American Diabetes Association; 2002:321-327

100. North American Society for Pediatric Gastroenterology, Hepatology and Nutrition. NASPGAN Clinical Guide for Pediatric Celiac Disease. Available at: https://clinical.celiac.org/. Accessed March 27, 2019

VI

Chapter 31

Hypoglycemia in Infants and Children

Introduction and Definition of Hypoglycemia

Hypoglycemia is a surrogate marker for harmfully low levels of energy in the central nervous system (CNS). However, the degree and duration of low plasma glucose that can cause CNS damage in infants and children are uncertain. Important determinants of CNS energy sufficiency include the efficiency of the transport of glucose into the brain, the need of brain cells for energy, and the availability of alternative energy sources. Serum glucose concentrations do not accurately measure any of these processes.[1,2] This is particularly important in hyperinsulinism, because there is diminished availability of alternative substrates for the brain. Glucose is transported from the circulation across the blood-brain barrier, and such transport may vary depending on the availability and efficiency of specific glucose transporters. GLUT-1 is the major transporter of glucose across the blood-brain barrier, but other transporters are important for the entry of glucose into neurons and glial cells.[3] A rare genetic exemplar is that children with a defective copy of one GLUT-1 gene may have severe symptomatic CNS glucose deficiency with normal circulating serum glucose concentrations.[4] Energy utilization in the CNS varies depending on the activation state of neural tissues. Seizure activity, for instance, rapidly depletes neurons of energy even when peripheral plasma glucose concentration is normal.[5] Alternative substrates, such as ketones, lactate, and perhaps, free fatty acids and amino acids, also support the energy needs of the brain.[1,6,7] These substrates circulate in the plasma in concentrations that are dependent on the metabolic state of the child and, in general, cross the blood-brain barrier assisted by specific transporters.[8] Because of the potential differences in glucose transport to the brain, the utilization rate by neural tissues, and the availability of alternative energy substrates, plasma glucose concentration is not a precise measure of CNS cellular energy supply.

Variation in measurement of circulating glucose can further confound this problem. Early studies used whole blood glucose measures. Human red blood cell concentrations of glucose are about half those of plasma. Therefore, measures of whole blood glucose are 10% to 15% lower than the plasma or serum glucose measurement commonly obtained in automated analyzers. If the hematocrit concentration is higher than adult norms, as occurs in ill neonates, whole blood glucose measures may be even lower. In addition, blood samples obtained for the assay of glucose must be maintained on ice, analyzed rapidly, and/or protected from glycolysis by the addition of fluoride. Glycolytic degradation of glucose is more rapid in the neonate than in adult blood and can markedly decrease measured blood glucose in unprotected samples stored at room temperature.[9]

Acceptable plasma glucose concentrations in the newborn infant remains an ongoing area of discussion, particularly in the first 48 hours of life.[10] The main concern remains identifying the concentration of peripheral glucose in the neonate that is associated with a poor developmental outcome.[11] However, there is a reasonable correlation among these statistical, epidemiologic, and acute experimental approaches to this problem, which gives some assurance that for most infants, plasma glucose concentrations commonly accepted as normal are clinically sound. Although the patterns of cerebral injury and neurodevelopmental outcomes are well described,[12] it is likely for the newborn infant that neuroglycopenia cannot be defined by a single numerical value, as the interactions among glycemic exposure, alternative cerebral fuels, other perinatal stressors, and neuronal function are complex and infant specific.[2] In a study of 404 infants at 2 years of age, it was found that hypoglycemia (defined as plasma glucose <47 mg/dL) was common (53% of infants), but not associated with neurosensory impairment (relative risk [RR], 0.95; 95% confidence interval [CI], 0.75–1.20; $P = .07$) or processing difficulty (defined by an executive function score) (RR, 0.92; 95% CI, 0.56–1.51; $P = .74$).[2] Follow-up of these same infants at 4.5 years of age found that hypoglycemia was still not associated with neurosensory impairment but was now associated with increased risk of low executive function (RR, 2.32; 95% CI, 1.17–4.69) and poor visual motor function (RR, 3.67; 95% CI, 1.15–11.69).[13] Infants at the highest risk as children were exposed to severe, recurrent, or clinically undetected (diagnosed by continuous interstitial glucose monitoring) hypoglycemia. This study has been corroborated by a recent report of schooling difficulties in 4th graders with neonatal hypoglycemia.[14]

Operational thresholds for neonates (plasma glucose concentrations at which clinical interventions should be considered) based on available data have been determined by a number of consensus statements and reviews, including those of the American Academy of Pediatrics (AAP) and the Pediatric Endocrine Society.[1,10,11,15–17] These are summarized in Table 31.1. The AAP has concluded that routine monitoring of plasma glucose concentration is not necessary in a term infant with a normal pregnancy and delivery.[10] The ranges of glucose concentrations in Table 31.1 are based on the age of the infant and provide a margin of safety that takes into consideration infants who are at risk for hypoglycemia or have hypoglycemia with or

Table 31.1.

Operational Thresholds for Hypoglycemia in Newborn Infants at Various Times After Birth, Including Preterm Infants[a,b]

- <4 hours, plasma glucose 25–50 mg/dL (1.4–2.2 mmol/L)
- 4–24 hours, plasma glucose 35–45 mg/dL (1.9–2.5 mmol/L)
- 24–48 hours, plasma glucose 45–50 mg/dL (2.5–2.8 mmol/L)
- >48 hours, plasma glucose 6070 mg/dL (3.3–3.9 mmol/L

Adapted from data in Thornton,[1] Adamkin,[10] Boluyt,[11] Stanley et al,[15] Adamkin and Polin,[16] and Rozance.[17]

[a] Risk factors include: those associated with maternal metabolism (intrapartum administration of glucose, terbutaline, ritodrine, propanolol, oral hypoglycemic agents, infant of a diabetic mother); those associated with neonatal problems (perinatal hypoxia-ischemia, infection, hypothermia, hyperviscosity, erythroblastosis fetalis, congenital cardiac disease, prematurity); intrauterine growth restriction; hyperinsulinism; endocrine disorders; and inborn errors of metabolism.

[b] Ranges reflect lower values for normal term infants, and a higher values for symptomatic infants, or asymptomatic infants at risk for hypoglycemia.

without symptoms. It is also consistent with the idea that neuroglycopenia cannot be defined by a single numerical value, as discussed previously.[2] The same operational thresholds have been suggested for term and preterm neonates.[10] The Pediatric Endocrine Society has suggested that guidelines for the first 48 hours of life should not be extended further into the neonatal period, because there is a physiologic shift after the 48-hour phase of newborn "transitional hypoglycemia," and that higher blood glucoses should be maintained thereafter (above 70 mg/dL in those at risk for hyperinsulinism or fatty acid oxidation disorders and >60 mg/dL in those at less risk).[1] Infants with hyperinsulinism or fatty acid oxidation disorders should be maintained at blood glucose concentrations of 70 mg/dL or greater, because they are almost entirely dependent on CNS glucose transport for brain energy. Identifying these infants is immensely important, because they are at risk of CNS damage at levels of blood glucose considered "normal" in newborn infants in the first 24 to 48 hours of life.

Clinical Manifestations of Hypoglycemia

Signs and symptoms of hypoglycemia can be broadly divided into those resulting from neuroglycopenia and those from adrenergic responses to hypoglycemia. The early signs of hypoglycemia are usually adrenergic and include sweating, weakness, tachycardia, tremor, hunger, paresthesias, pallor, anxiety or nervousness, nausea, and palpitations. Prolonged

VI

hypoglycemia may lead to more symptoms of neuroglycopenia, including lethargy, dizziness, irritability, mental confusion, behavior that is out of character, blurred vision, difficulty speaking, loss of coordination, and in its extreme, seizures, coma, and death. These signs and symptoms are less obvious or absent in infants and young children. The nonspecific signs of hypoglycemia in newborn and young infants may be manifested by irritability, jitteriness, feeding difficulties, lethargy, apnea, cyanosis, bradycardia, tachypnea, abnormal cry, hypothermia, hypotonia, apathy, and seizures. These signs are not specific for hypoglycemia and are also the early manifestations of other severe newborn disorders (sepsis, congenital heart disease, ventricular hemorrhage, respiratory distress syndrome, and aspiration). With repeated or prolonged episodes of hypoglycemia, the threshold for autonomic symptoms decreases compared with the neuroglycopenic symptoms. As a result, the infant develops severe hypoglycemia with little or no warning, a condition called hypoglycemia unawareness, or hypoglycemia-associated autonomic failure (HAAF).[1,18]

Etiology of Hypoglycemia

Neonates
In newborn infants, the differential diagnosis of hypoglycemia initially can be guided but not limited by birth weight (Table 31.2). If the newborn infant remains hypoglycemic after the first 48 hours of life, then causes of prolonged neonatal hypoglycemia, such as perinatal stress-induced hyperinsulinism or hypopituitarism, and causes of permanent neonatal hypoglycemia, such as congenital hyperinsulinism or inborn errors of metabolism, should be considered.[19,20]

Children
The most common type of hypoglycemia in children is insulin-induced hypoglycemia in individuals with type 1 diabetes mellitus. In other children, hypoglycemia can be categorized as ketotic fasting hypoglycemia, hypoketotic fasting hypoglycemia, or reactive or postprandial hypoglycemia. Postprandial hypoglycemia in young children is often associated with metabolic dumping syndrome (as occurs after fundal plication procedures), but in adolescents, it may be associated with obesity and high-carbohydrate eating habits (Table 31.3). This categorization generally aids in diagnosis but should not limit clinical judgment. Mild reactive hypoglycemia is common in the otherwise healthy adolescent population and is not considered a disease.

Table 31.2.
Causes of Hypoglycemia in Newborn Infants

Perinatal Stress (low glucose stores and/or increased glucose utilization as a result of stress-induced hyperinsulinism)
  Prematurity
  Birth asphyxia/ischemia; C-section delivery for fetal distress
  Maternal preeclampsia or hypertension
  Hypothermia
  Meconium aspiration syndrome
  Infection

Small for gestational age (SGA)
  Primary failure to produce and store glycogen

Appropriate for gestational age (AGA)
  Endocrine deficiency:
  • Hypopituitarism/growth hormone deficiency
  • Cortisol/ACTH deficiency
  • ACTH unresponsiveness
  Depletion of glycogen stores in congenital heart failure/congenital heart disease
  Inborn errors of carbohydrate, protein, and lipid metabolism
  Hyperinsulinism attributable to:
  • Alloimmune hemolytic disease of the newborn after exchange transfusion
  • Perinatal asphyxia
  • Maternal intrapartum treatment with glucose or with antihyperglycemia agents, such as sulfonylureas
  • Malposition of an umbilical catheter

Large for gestational age (LGA): hyperinsulinism
  Infant of a diabetic mother
  Beckwith-Wiedemann syndrome
  Gene mutations causing congenital hyperinsulinism (persistent hyperinsulinemic hypoglycemia of infancy [PHHI])[a] including:
  • SUR1 (sulphonylurea receptor type 1) inactivating gene mutation
  • KIR 6.2 (inward-rectifying potassium channel) inactivating gene mutation
  • SCHAD (short-chain L-3-hydroxyacyl-CoA dehydrogenase enzyme) inactivating gene mutation
  • GK (glucokinase) activating gene mutation
  • GDH (glutamate dehydrogenase) activating gene mutation
  • HNF4A (hepatocyte nuclear factor 4 alpha gene) inactivating gene mutation
  • HNF1A (hepatocyte nuclear factor 1 alpha gene) inactivating gene mutation
  • MCT1 (monocarboxylate transporter 1) activating gene mutation
  • SLC16A1 gene (solute carrier family 16, member 1)
  • UCP2 gene (uncoupling protein 2

[a] Because these disorders can be of variable severity and may not always present at birth, they are not invariably associated with fetal overgrowth.

VI

Table 31.3.
Causes of Hypoglycemia in Children

Ketotic Fasting Hypoglycemia
  Accelerated starvation ("ketotic hypoglycemia")
  Endocrine deficiencies: growth hormone (GH), ACTH/cortisol, hypopituitarism (ACTH/cortisol and GH)
  Metabolic defects:
    Disorders of carbohydrate metabolism:
    Glycogen synthase deficiency
    Type III glycogen storage disease (amylo-1,6-glucosidase deficiency)
    Type VI glycogen storage disease (phosphorylase deficiency)
    Type IX glycogen storage disease (phosphorylase kinase deficiency)
    Defects in gluconeogenesis: pyruvate carboxylase deficiency, PEPCK deficiency, fructose 1-6-biphosphatase deficiency
  Disorders of protein metabolism (organic acidemias) examples:
    Maple syrup urine disease (branched-chain ketoacid decarboxylase deficiency)
    Methylmalonic acidemia
  Miscellaneous:
    Salicylate intoxication
    Reye syndrome
    Ethanol intoxication
    Malaria
    Diarrhea
    Malnutrition
    Jamaican vomiting sickness (ingestion of unripe ackee fruit)

Hypoketotic Fasting Hypoglycemia
  Glycogen storage disease type 1 (glucose-6-phosphatase deficiency)
  Tyrosinemia
  Disorders of fatty oxidation and ketone synthesis:
    Carnitine transport and metabolism
    Beta-oxidation cycle
    Electron transfer
    HMG-CoA synthase or lyase deficiency
  IGF-1, IGF-2 excess
  Insulinoma
  Sulfonylurea or other insulin secretagogue ingestion
  Exogenous insulin administration
  Congenital hyperinsulinism (See Table 31.2)

Reactive or Postprandial Hypoglycemia:
  "Metabolic dumping syndrome" (ie, post fundoplication procedures)
  Galactosemia
  Fructose intolerance (fructose-1-phosphate aldolase deficiency)

PEPCK indicates phosphoenolpyruvate carboxykinase; HMG, 3-hydroxy-3-methylglutaryl IGF, insulin-like growth factor.

Evaluation of Hypoglycemia

Neonates

The history and physical examination are often revealing. Gestational age and birth weight; maternal health, including history of diabetes or glucose intolerance; and medications may guide diagnosis, prognosis, and therapy. Most hypoglycemic infants who are large for gestational age are hyperinsulinemic, although rare disorders of macrosomia and overgrowth with severe hypoglycemia and low insulin levels have been traced to activating mutations in the molecular pathway that controls insulin effects.[20,21] Most hyperinsulinemic infants are born to women with diabetes, and the hypoglycemia and hyperinsulinemia are of relatively short duration (24 hours to a few days).[22] Other rare transient causes of hyperinsulinism include Beckwith-Wiedemann syndrome, characterized by macrosomia, large tongue, omphalocele/umbilical hernia, visceromegaly, and horizontal grooves on ear lobes.[23] Persistent hyperinsulinism and hypoglycemia require careful genetic and physiologic evaluation and management planning. Genetic hyperinsulinism because of mutations in genes controlling insulin release, including beta-cell potassium channels, glucokinase, and glutamate dehydrogenase genes, must always be considered, although it is rare (1:50 000 children, except in inbred populations). These disorders require immediate intervention and continued and definitive therapy. Many infants born preterm or small for gestational age are unable to produce enough glucose through glycogenolysis and gluconeogenesis to meet the needs of their relatively large brains. These infants may respond with increased glucose when sufficient fat is included in their diet to alter the hepatocellular ratio of nicotinamide adenine dinucleotide (NAD) to reduced nicotinamide adenine dinucleotide (NADH) in favor of gluconeogenesis.[24] Recently, it has been postulated that infants with transitional hypoglycemia may have a lower glucose threshold set point for insulin release as is likely during fetal life.[15] Some of these infants may also have prolonged hyperinsulinism, and the etiology may be a prolonged reset of this physiologic hyperinsulinism.[25] Normal-weight infants are most likely to have an endocrine deficiency disorder or an inborn error of carbohydrate or fatty acid metabolism. Prolonged neonatal jaundice, microphallus in a boy, or facial midline anomalies might suggest hypopituitarism. However, a mutation in the transcription factor FOXA2 has been reported in an infant with both hypopituitarism, craniofacial abnormalities, and hyperinsulinism, so evaluation of all of these infants requires sophisticated endocrine and genetic consultation.[26] Hepatomegaly might suggest a genetic disorder of glycogen synthesis or release. Metabolic disorders may present in the immediate neonatal period or somewhat later. Metabolic disorders that cause acidosis may manifest as hyperventilation that is misdiagnosed as pneumonia or reactive airway disease or may be misdiagnosed as overwhelming sepsis in the first months of life. A history of unusual odors may be a clue in maple syrup urine disease, isovaleric acidemia, 3-methylcrotonyl coenzyme A carboxylase deficiency, and glutaric acidemia type II. Many states now perform neonatal screening for these disorders so that diagnosis is made early, often before the infants are symptomatic (see also Chapter 29: Inborn Errors of Metabolism).

Children

Birth weight, history of neonatal complications, age of onset, and frequency of symptoms can aid in diagnosis. Symptoms of hypoglycemia at birth or during the neonatal period might point to hypopituitarism or hyperinsulinism; prolonged neonatal jaundice might suggest cortisol and/or thyroid deficiency. The temporal relationship of symptoms to food intake may aid in diagnosis. Hypoglycemia that occurs within about 2 hours of eating is considered reactive. It may be observed in dumping syndrome, which is more common after a fundoplication, in obese individuals with overactive insulin response to carbohydrate, and very rarely in individuals with galactosemia or hereditary fructose intolerance. The specific content of feedings and relationship to onset of symptoms as well as food intolerance or aversion may guide the diagnosis, as may the usual laboratory evaluation. Early dumping syndrome, which occurs within 60 minutes of feeding, is characterized by postprandial irritability, diaphoresis, abdominal pain, and diarrhea. Late dumping syndrome presents with hypoglycemia 1 to 4 hours after the feeding and may present without other systemic symptoms.[27]

Symptomatic hypoglycemia that appears approximately 4 hours after eating more commonly occurs in defects of glycogenolysis or in hyperinsulinism. Hypoglycemia that occurs 10 to 12 hours after feedings suggests a defect of gluconeogenesis or fatty acid oxidation but may also represent hyperinsulinism.

A potential drug exposure should be sought in all children with hypoglycemia. Insulin, hypoglycemic agents, and alcohol are often implicated. Erratic episodes of hypoglycemia may be a warning of fabricated or induced illness by caregivers (formerly known as Munchausen syndrome by proxy).[28]

Findings from the physical examination suggestive of growth hormone deficiency or hypopituitarism are short stature or growth failure, microphallus, midline defects (cleft lip and palate, single central incisor), and optic nerve hypoplasia (in septo-optic dysplasia). Hepatomegaly is usually present in glycogen storage diseases, disorders of gluconeogenesis, galactosemia, hereditary fructose intolerance, disorders of fatty acid oxidation and carnitine metabolism, and tyrosinemia type 1. Increased pigmentation may be present in Addison disease. Disorders of fatty acid oxidation may cause cardiomyopathy.

Laboratory Investigation of Unexplained Hypoglycemia

Glucose meters for self-monitoring of plasma glucose concentration are calibrated to normal blood or plasma glucose ranges and adult ranges for hypoglycemia (50 mg/dL or less plasma glucose). Readings may be influenced by hematocrit, because meters are calibrated to read plasma glucose within an adult range of hematocrit, and plasma glucose concentration is higher than whole blood glucose concentration.

Even the most accurate meters are not consistently reliable at low blood glucose concentrations. Hence, a glucose meter value below 45 mg/dL should be confirmed by a laboratory glucose value. If appropriate additional laboratory studies are obtained at the same time, this laboratory plasma glucose value may serve as a "critical" or diagnostic sample. It may be necessary to perform a monitored fast of 8 to 24 hours, depending on the age of the child. Fasting may induce cerebral edema in a child with a fatty acid oxidation defect. This should be ruled out before performing the fast by determination of nonfasting plasma acylcarnitines and urinary acylglycines.[29] Table 31.4 outlines the protocol that can be used for the monitored diagnostic fasting evaluation and lists potential laboratory tests to send with the "critical blood sample."

In addition, it is important to remember that a "safety fast" to determine whether treatment is effective or whether an infant or child can go for some hours between feeding and can be discharged from hospital is quite different from a diagnostic fast and does not require the full blood sample evaluation described in this table. A stable normal blood glucose after an appropriate fast of 6 hours in a neonate or longer in an older child, depending on age, indicates that treatment is effective and the child should be "safe" on discharge. Although still in the research phase, continuous interstitial glucose monitoring may at some point be used to detect and treat episodes of asymptomatic hypoglycemia.[30,31]

Table 31.4.
Monitored Fasting for Diagnostic Evaluation of Hypoglycemia

If blood glucose reaches 45 mg/dL or less, select the following
studies based on clinical judgment in the appropriate tube for your
laboratory:
Glucose
Insulin
C-peptide
Beta-hydroxybutyrate
Free fatty acids
Cortisol
Growth hormone
Lactate: free-flowing blood
Pyruvate: free-flowing blood
NH3: free-flowing blood[a]
Carnitine and acylcarnitine panel[a]
Free T4 and TSH[a]
Urine sample for organic acids and amino acids[a]
IGF-1[a]
IGF-2[a]

Before starting the monitored fast, confirm that appropriate blood tubes are ready and
labeled for these tests; some must be obtained on ice and in special tubes. After sending
the blood sample, administer 30 µg/kg of glucagon intravenously or subcutaneously, and
obtain blood for glucose concentration at 10, 15, 20, and 30 minutes. If the blood glucose
has not increased with glucagon, administer 2 mL/kg of 25% glucose intravenously and
feed or treat with a continuous glucose infusion as possible.

T4 indicates thyroxine; TSH, thyroid-stimulating factor.

[a] These tests do not need to be drawn during the hypoglycemic event.

Differential Diagnosis of Hypoglycemia

Neonates

Hyperinsulinism
In the neonate, the diagnostic challenge is to ensure that the child does not
have persistent hyperinsulinism. This disorder carries a worse prognosis
than other causes of hypoglycemia for several reasons. First, high insulin
concentrations will make alternative brain fuels like ketones, lactate, and
free fatty acids unavailable so that the need of the CNS for glucose will be
greater than in other types of hypoglycemia.[32,33] Second, at least one of the
disorders associated with hyperinsulinism (glutamate dehydrogenase-
activating mutations leading to hyperinsulinemia and hyperammonemia)
involves metabolic pathways common to the brain so that the underlying

disorder may separately interfere with neuronal function and development.[34] Last, hypoglycemia from hyperinsulinism is often quite difficult to control, requiring large quantities of glucose (>10–12 mg/kg/minute, intravenously) and additional therapeutic agents, such as diazoxide, octreotide, and sirolimus, which have their own toxicities.[33,35–37] In many children, either partial or total pancreatectomy is necessary for control of blood glucose concentration. The decision about surgery and the type of surgery requires sophisticated techniques to assess the etiology of the hyperinsulinism and the nature of the pancreatic involvement. Once congenital hyperinsulinism is confirmed or suspected, transfer to a specialist is prudent. Diagnosis should be suspected if the need for glucose is greater than 10 to 12 mg/kg per minute and the child's hypoglycemia is not relieved by physiologic cortisol supplementation. Plasma insulin concentration must be determined at the same time as the glucose concentration. Insulin concentrations obtained at the time of hypoglycemia are generally higher than anticipated for hypoglycemia (>2 µU/mL), but many assays designed to measure adult insulin concentrations will not be able to detect concentrations this low and will report no measurable insulin in plasma, even in infants suffering from hyperinsulinism.

Other Etiologies of Hypoglycemia

Cortisol deficiency can be difficult to diagnose in neonates who often do not respond to hypoglycemia with elevations in cortisol but can respond to adrenocorticotropic hormone (ACTH) testing. However, treatment with cortisol should rapidly ameliorate the hypoglycemia. The underlying etiology is usually panhypopituitarism. Absence of ketonemia is indicative of hyperinsulinism, except in rare disorders of ketogenesis, activating mutations along the insulin action pathway, or in congenital hypopituitarism in many cases. Neonates have a high renal threshold for ketones and may have normal ketogenesis with hypoglycemia without measurable ketonuria.[38] Ketonuria in a newborn infant with hypoglycemia suggests either glycogen storage disease type III or rare genetic organic acidemias. Urinary organic acid determination is critical to determine the presence of abnormal ketoacids. If available, the rapid bedside meter and strip method for checking serum levels of beta-hydroxybutyrate can be diagnostically useful.

Children

The laboratory differential diagnosis can be initially guided by the presence or absence of ketonuria or ketonemia.

VI

Ketotic Hypoglycemia

Ketoacids in normal fasting individuals include beta-hydroxybutyrate, measured in plasma with specific reagent strips and a meter or (preferred) by a reference laboratory, and acetoacetate, measured in urine as "ketones" on a test strip. Acetoacetate is quite labile and will not persist in a stored plasma sample unless handled very carefully, but beta-hydroxybutyrate is more stable. In the presence of adequate ketosis, if the urine organic acids do not show an abnormal diagnostic pattern and there is no hepatomegaly, the following diagnoses should be considered: accelerated starvation, growth hormone or cortisol deficiency, and glycogen synthase deficiency. "Accelerated starvation" (previously termed ketotic hypoglycemia) is a diagnosis of exclusion and should be made when the other causes of ketotic hypoglycemia have been ruled out. Children with this disorder are typically underweight for height. Hypoglycemia usually occurs after 12 to 24 hours of fasting and is associated with a normal metabolic response to hypoglycemia with ketonuria, low plasma alanine concentration, normal lactate and pyruvate concentrations, suppressed insulin, and elevated growth hormone and cortisol concentrations. The response to glucagon administration is blunted at the time of hypoglycemia, because hepatic and other glycogen stores have been used for energy.[39]

The presence of a large liver should point to the diagnosis of glycogen storage disease and disorders of gluconeogenesis. The diagnosis of glycogen synthase deficiency should be confirmed at the molecular level after an oral glucose tolerance test demonstrates initial hyperglycemia, followed by hypoglycemia at 3 to 4 hours.[40] The urine organic or amino acid pattern should give the diagnosis in the case of disorders of organic acid or amino acid metabolism and these diagnoses should also be confirmed at the molecular level. A plasma cortisol concentration less than 10 µg/dL during hypoglycemia suggests cortisol/ACTH deficiency. A low plasma growth hormone concentration should raise suspicion of growth hormone deficiency/hypopituitarism, but low growth hormone and cortisol levels are sometimes found in normal individuals following persistent or frequent hypoglycemia (HAAF).

Hypoketotic Hypoglycemia

Insulin should be undetectable during hypoglycemia. In hyperinsulinism, insulin inhibits ketone production and lipolysis, and ketone and free fatty acid concentrations are inappropriately low during hypoglycemia. The plasma insulin concentration will be inappropriately high during hypoglycemia (>2 μU/mL). A positive response to glucagon (30 μg/kg, subcutaneously or intravenously) with an increment in plasma glucose of at least 30 mg/dL (1.7 mmol/L), despite severe hypoglycemia, is also diagnostic of hyperinsulinism.[41] However, some children with hyperinsulinism have required a larger dose of glucagon (up to 1 mg) to elicit significant glycogenolysis. Typically, the intravenous glucose rate required to maintain normoglycemia is 2 to 4 times greater than the glucose production rate (6–8 mg/kg/minute in a newborn infant, 4–6 mg/kg/minute in a slightly older child, and 1–2 mg/kg/minute in an adult). The reason for the differences in glucose production rate is evident in Fig 31.1, which demonstrates that to maintain euglycemia, glucose production rate must equal glucose utilization rate. As the relative brain size compared with body weight decreases with age, the relative glucose utilization rate per kg of body weight also decreases.[42]

In hyperinsulinism, plasma cortisol and growth hormone concentrations may be normal or inappropriately low if the hypoglycemia occurs gradually or is recurrent (blunted counter-regulatory response). A low C-peptide concentration associated with elevated insulin concentrations suggests exogenous insulin administration.

Imaging of the pancreas with computerized axial tomography or ultrasonography is very rarely sensitive enough to identify an insulinoma and cannot visualize focal adenomatous hyperplasia or diffuse beta-cell hyperplasia. Positron emission tomography (PET) using ^{18}F dihydroxyphenylalanine (DOPA) as a marker has proved very useful in localization and in making this diagnostic distinction but is presently available at only a few specialized centers.[33,43]

Preoperative pancreatic catheterization is no longer a first-line diagnostic tool, but intraoperative histopathologic studies can be helpful to confirm localization of focal lesions. Mutational analysis can be helpful in the diagnosis of focal hyperinsulinism and in defining a genetic etiology.

If the plasma insulin concentration is adequately suppressed with hypoketotic hypoglycemia, a fatty acid oxidation defect or a stimulatory mutation in the insulin transduction pathway should be suspected. A diagnostic pattern is often seen in the concentrations of urine organic acids and acylglycine and plasma acylcarnitine in fatty acid oxidation disorders.[29]

VI

Fig 31.1.

Total glucose rate of disappearance (Rd) (mmol/min) as a function of body weight from infancy to adulthood (n = 141; body weights range from 0.6 to 94 kg). The data points represent mean values for subjects with brain sizes in kg of 0.14 (0.070–0.20); 0.37 (0.22–0.40); 0.44 (0.40–0.57); 0.0, 1.2, 1.3, and 1.4, respectively.

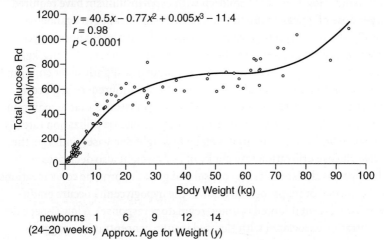

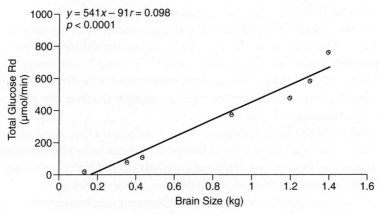

Reprinted with permission from Haymond MW, Sunehag A. Controlling the sugar bowl. Regulation of glucose homeostasis in children. *Endocrinol Metab Clin North Am.* 1999;28(4):663-694.

Treatment of Hypoglycemia

Infants and Young Children

A pragmatic management plan is not based on outcome measures but depends on the clinical picture, including laboratory-determined plasma glucose concentration and signs and symptoms.[1]

If the plasma glucose concentration is between 35 and 45 mg/dL (1.9-2.5 mmol/L) and the neonate is able to feed, then breastfeeding or formula feeding or 5% dextrose administration by nipple is appropriate. Use of oral dextrose gel is supported by prospective studies.[44,45] If the neonate is very symptomatic and unable to feed, intravenous glucose with 5% to 12.5% dextrose at a rate of 4 to 6 mg/kg/minute[-1] should be initiated. If the plasma glucose concentration is between 25 and 34 mg/dL (1.4-1.9 mmol/L), intravenous glucose with 5% to 12.5% dextrose at a rate of 6 to 8 mg/kg/minute[-1] should be started regardless of symptoms, and oral feedings should be allowed as tolerated.[46]

If the plasma glucose concentration is less than 25 mg/dL (1.4 mmol/L), it is appropriate to administer a minibolus of 2 mL/kg of 10% dextrose (200 mg/kg) over 5 to 10 minutes, followed by an infusion rate of 6 to 8 mg/kg/minute[-1]. It has been argued that a minibolus given over 1 minute could cause hyperosmolar cerebral edema, because it exceeds glucose uptake capacity and might, if the dose is large enough, induce excessive insulin secretion, worsening the hypoglycemia.[47–49] The glucose infusion rate can be calculated with the following formula:

$$\text{glucose (mg/kg/min}^{-1}) = (\%\text{glucose in solution} \times 10) \times (\text{rate of infusion per hour}) / (60 \times \text{weight [kg]})$$

The glucose concentration should be monitored every 30 minutes. Therapy should be intensified if hypoglycemia is not corrected by the initial measures. Maintenance of blood glucose at greater than 60 to 70 mg/dL is reasonable for neuroprotection, although no outcome data support this consensus approach.[1] The glucose infusion rate should be increased to achieve euglycemia with the minimal concentration of glucose required. Infusions at rates greater than 15 mg/kg/minute[-1] should be administered by a central venous catheter, except in emergency situations. The glucose infusion rate should be gradually reduced rather than abruptly terminated to avoid reactive hypoglycemia.

VI

If euglycemia is not maintained with a dextrose infusion rate above 15 mg/kg/minute^{-1}, the use of corticosteroids should be considered. Although it will not be effective in hyperinsulinism, hydrocortisone administered at a dose of 5 mg/kg/day, intravenously or orally, divided every 12 hours, or prednisone administered at a dose of 1 to 2 mg/kg/day, orally, as a temporizing measure can be useful. Gradual decrease should be attempted once euglycemia is achieved. Glucagon may be given in a dose of 30 μg/kg at the time of hypoglycemia to assess glycogenolysis. A response of more than 30 mg/dL at 30 minutes is confirmatory of hyperinsulinism.[41]

The consensus aim for neuroprotection, although there are no supportive outcome data, should be to maintain plasma glucose concentrations above 70 mg/dL (3.9 mmol/L) in infants and young children with persistent hyperinsulinism or other disorders in which alternative brain energy substrates are not available. This may require glucose infusion rates of higher than 20 mg/kg/minute^{-1}, in addition to frequent enteral feedings. A central venous catheter and a nasogastric tube or a gastrostomy tube may be necessary. Pharmacologic agents should be added to normalize the carbohydrate intake and decrease insulin secretion.[33,35,36] Diazoxide (10–20 mg/kg per day in 2–3 divided oral doses) with added chlorothiazide or furosemide if the patient is edematous (7–10 mg/kg per day in 2 divided oral doses) is recommended for the initial treatment. The response is variable depending on the underlying etiology of the hyperinsulinism. If the response is suboptimal or the adverse effects of fluid retention and cardiac failure from diazoxide are significant, nifedipine could be the next choice in management, at a dose of 0.25 to 2.5 mg/kg/day, orally, divided every 8 hours. A very limited number of hyperinsulinemic young children have responded to nifedipine, but this drug is not often effective. Monitoring of blood pressure is mandatory. More effective agents given by infusion or injection include octreotide, which is a somatostatin analogue, and glucagon. Both can cause tachyphylaxis at high doses. They should be used when the orally administered drugs have not been effective and if the infant or young child remains glucose-infusion dependent. Some argue to use both concurrently, because glucagon may stimulate insulin secretion. Glucagon has specific benefit in neonates who are hyperinsulinemic and may be infused at a rate of approximately 5 to 10 μg/kg/hour. Glucagon may be a useful adjunct as a child is being prepared for management in an experienced referral center. Prolonged glucagon usage in this manner could be associated with proteolysis and skin rashes as seen in the glucagonoma syndrome. Octreotide can be given at a rate of 5 to 20 µg/kg/day in an intravenous or subcutaneous infusion. If octreotide is effective as an infusion, it can be converted to a chronic parenteral therapy, administered by subcutaneous injection 3 times a day. Tachyphylaxis often occurs, preventing it from being used chronically. In addition, it has been associated with necrotizing enterocolitis.

Although experience with sirolimus has been somewhat more limited, it has been very effective in some children who have not been candidates for surgery and have not responded well to diazoxide or octreotide.[36,37]

The criteria for successful medical management of hyperinsulinism are a feeding regimen acceptable to the family with normal plasma glucose concentrations after reasonable periods of fasting (at least 6 hours in newborn infants, 8 hours for slightly older infants). Failure of pharmacologic therapy in a period of a few days to weeks should lead to surgical treatment with either a localized or a near-total (95%–99%) pancreatectomy.[32,33] Recurrent hypoglycemia is to be avoided as much as possible because of its long-term deleterious effects on neurologic functioning.

Older Children

Acute hypoglycemia associated with a mismatch between insulin administration and insulin need in children with diabetes mellitus should be treated on the basis of the severity of hypoglycemia. If the child is alert and able to drink or eat safely, treatment with 10 to 20 g of rapidly available carbohydrate in the form of fruit juice, sweetened drink, candy, or specially prepared glucose tablets is adequate for initial therapy. The response usually lasts less than 2 hours, so it should be followed by a mixed snack containing carbohydrate, fat, and protein or a scheduled meal. In children who require the assistance of another person to treat hypoglycemia, gel preparations of carbohydrate are available that can be administered orally and are effective as long as swallowing is preserved. Buccal absorption of carbohydrate is minimal. Children who are unable to eat or drink by mouth or are comatose or seizing should immediately receive a subcutaneous or intramuscular injection of glucagon of 0.02 to 0.03 mg/kg to a maximum of 1 mg. Families should be taught how much glucagon to prepare and administer for such emergencies, and the dosage should be changed as the child gains weight. Children respond within 15 minutes and then should be encouraged to eat, because the effect of the glucagon is relatively short lived, and nausea and vomiting are common adverse effects of both hypoglycemia and glucagon administration.

VI

In the emergency department or hospital, regardless of the cause of hypoglycemia, if the child is unable to drink or eat after critical blood samples are obtained, 25% dextrose (2–3 mL/kg) should be administered intravenously. The infusion of 25% dextrose should be followed by a continued infusion of 10% dextrose initially, at a rate of 6 to 8 mg/kg/minute⁻¹, to avoid rebound hypoglycemia and maintain normoglycemia. The plasma glucose concentration should be monitored, and the infusion rate should be adjusted to maintain a concentration >80 mg/dL (4.5 mmol/L). Children with hyperinsulinism will require higher rates of infusion. Long-term treatment is similar to that in the neonate (see previous section).

In disorders of fatty acid oxidation, a glucose infusion rate of 10 mg/kg/minute⁻¹, by stimulating insulin release and inhibiting lipolysis, reverses the acute metabolic disorder.[31] Long-term treatment of endocrine deficiency disorders and genetic metabolic disorders should be specific for the disorder.

Treatment and prevention of ketotic hypoglycemia, or "accelerated starvation," consists of educating parents to avoid prolonged periods of fasting and offer a bedtime snack consisting of both carbohydrate and protein. During an intercurrent illness, carbohydrate-rich drinks should be given at frequent intervals. Parents are instructed to test urine or blood for ketones. Ketonuria and ketonemia precede hypoglycemia by several hours.

Frequent feedings with glucose protect children with types 1 and 3 glycogen storage diseases from hypoglycemia and reduces hepatomegaly. Intermittent or continuous glucose can be provided during the day, and continuous glucose can be provided during the night by a nasogastric or gastrostomy tube. After 6 to 8 months of age, the infantile gut has matured to the point that it can digest uncooked cornstarch. Feedings of uncooked starch (1.75–2.5 g) can be given intermittently, because it is slowly absorbed into the circulation, acting like a continuous source of glucose. It is given in water or artificially flavored drinks. Carbohydrate sources should only be glucose or glucose polymers. Blood glucose monitoring allows the creation of a successful feeding regimen.[50] A new longer-acting preparation of waxy maize cornstarch, available commercially, has been shown to have a more prolonged effect in these children and may be the agent of choice.[51] Uncooked cornstarch at bedtime may help to prevent hypoglycemia in other groups of children, including children receiving insulin for diabetes.[52]

Children with metabolic dumping syndrome causing reactive hypoglycemia can be treated with an alpha-glucosidase inhibitor like acarbose (12.5–50 mg) before each feeding to slow carbohydrate absorption.[27]

Hereditary fructose intolerance is treated with elimination of fructose and sucrose. Fructose 1,6-diphosphatase deficiency is treated by elimination of fructose and sucrose and avoidance of prolonged fasting. During intercurrent illness, intravenous glucose may be necessary to arrest catabolism. Galactosemia is treated by elimination of galactose from the diet.

Summary

Hypoglycemia is the result of an alteration in the metabolic and hormonal interrelationships that balance glucose absorption, release, and production with glucose utilization. Symptomatic hypoglycemia is caused by decreased CNS energy levels (neuroglycopenia) and is reflected somewhat imperfectly in measures of blood sugar. It is the health care professional's task to recognize the signs and symptoms of hypoglycemia, document hypoglycemia using laboratory tests, and obtain appropriate studies to identify the etiology. Initial symptomatic treatment of hypoglycemia will preserve brain function, but long-term management depends on identification of the cause of the energy imbalance.

References

1. Thornton P, Stanley CA, DeLeon DD, et al. Recommendations from the Pediatric Endocrine Society for evaluaton of persistent hypoglycemia in neonates, infants, and children. *J Pediatr.* 2015;167(2):238–245

2. McKinlay CJD, Alsweiler JM, Ansell JM, et al. Neonatal glycemia and neurodevelopmental outcomes at 2 years. *N Engl J Med.* 2015;373(16):1507–1518

3. McEwen B, Reagan L. Glucose transporter expression in the central nervous system: relationship to synaptic function. *Eur J Pharmacol.* 2004;490(1-3):13–24

4. Wang D, Pascual JM, Yang H, et al. Glut-1 deficiency syndrome:clinical and therapeutic aspects. *Ann Neurol.* 2005;57(1):111–118

5. Fujikawa D, Vannucci RC, Dwyer BE, Wasterlain CG. Generalized seizures deplete brain energy reserves in normoxemic newborn monkeys. *Brain Res.* 1988;454(1-2):51–59

6. Settergren G, Lindblad BS, Persson B. Cerebral blood flow and exchange of oxygen, glucose, ketone bodies, lactate, pyruvate and amino acids in infants. *Acta Paediatr Scand.* 1976;65(3):343–353

7. Vannucci R, Vannucci S. Hypoglycemic brain injury. *Semin Neonatol.* 2001;6(2):147–155

8. Mason G, Petersen KF, Lebon V, Rothman DL, Shulman GI. Increased brain monocarboxylic acid transport and utilization in type 1 diabetes. *Diabetes.* 2005;55(4):929–934

VI

9. Ramachandran TS. Disorders of carbohydrate metabolism. *Emedicine. Medscape. com.* December 11, 2017. Available at: https://emedicine.medscape.com/article/1183033-overview. Accessed February 9, 2019

10. Adamkin DH, American Academy of Pediatrics, Committee on Fetus and Newborn. Clinical report: postnatal glucose homeostasis in late-preterm and term infants. *Pediatrics.* 2011;127(3):575–578

11. Boluyt N, van Kempen A, Offringa M. Neurodevelopment after neonatal hypoglycemia: a systematic review and design of an optimal future study. *Pediatrics.* 2006;117(6):2231–2243

12. Burns CM, Rutherford MA, Boardman JP, Cowan FM. Patterns of cerebral injury and neurodevelopmental outcomes after symptomatic neonatal hypoglycemia. *Pediatrics.* 2008;122(1):65–74

13. McKinlay CJD, Alsweiler JM, Anstice NS, et al. Association of neonatal glycemia with neurodevelopmental outcomes at 4.5 years. *JAMA Pediatr.* 2017;171(10): 972–983

14. Kaiser JR, Bai S, Gibson N, et al. Association between transient newborn hypocglycemia and fourth-grade achievement test proficiency: a population-based study. *JAMA Pediatr.* 2015;169:913–921

15. Stanley CA, Rozance PJ, Thornton PS, et al. Revaluating "transitional neonatal hypoglycemia": Mechanism and implications for management. *J Pediatr.* 2015;166(6):e1520–e1525

16. Adamkin DH, Polin RA. Imperfect advice: neonatal hypoglycemia. *J Pediatr.* 2016;176:195–196

17. Rozance PJ. Management and outcome of neonatal hypoglycemia. *UptoDate.com.* Available at: https://www.uptodate.com/contents/management-and-outcome-of-neonatal-hypoglycemia. Accessed February 9, 2019

18. Cryer P. Mechanisms of hypoglycemia-associated autonomic failure and its component syndromes in diabetes. *Diabetes.* 2005;54(12):3592–3601

19. De Leon DD, Stanley CA. Mechanisms of disease: advances in diagnosis and treatment of hyperinsulinism in neonates. *Nat Clin Pract Endocrinol Metab.* 2007;3(1):57–68

20. Hussain K, Challis B, Rocha N, et al. An activating mutation of AKT2 and human hypoglycemia. *Science.* 2011;334(6055):474

21. Leiter SM, Parker VER, Welters A, et al. Hypoinsulinaemic hypoketotic hypoglycaemia due to mosaic genetic activation of PI3-kinase. *Eur J Endocrinol.* 2017;177(2):175–186

22. Nold J, Georgieff M. Infants of diabetic mothers. *Pediatr Clin North Am.* 2004;51(3):619–637

23. Shuman C, Beckwith JB, Weksberg R. Beckwith-Wiedemann syndrome. In: Pagon RA, Bird TD, Dolan CR, Stephens K, eds. *GeneReviews.* Seattle, WA; 2000. Updated 2010

24. Sabel K, Olegård R, Mellander M, Hildingsson K. Interrelation between fatty acid oxidation and control of gluconeogenic substrates in small-for-gestational-age (SGA) infants with hypoglycemia and normoglycemia. *Acta Paediatr Scand.* 1982;71(1):53–61

25. Hoe F, Thornton PS, Wanner LA, Steinkrauss L, Simmons RA, Stanley CA. Clinical features and insulin regulation in infants with a syndrome of prolonged neonatal hyperinsulinism. *J Pediatr.* 2006;148(2):207–212

26. Giri D, Vignola ML, Gualtieri A, et al. Novel FOXA2 mutation causes hyperinsulinism, hypopituitarism with craniofacial and endoderm-derived organ abnormalities. *Hum Mol Genet.* 2017;26(22):4315–4326

27. Ng DD, Ferry R.J. Jr, Kelly A, Weinzimer SA, Stanley CA, Katz LE. Acarbose treatment of postprandial hypoglycemia in children after Nissen fundoplication. *J Pediatr.* 2001;139(6):877–879

28. Giurgea I, Ulinski T, Touati G. Factitious hyperinsulinism leading to pancreatectomy: severe forms of Munchausen syndrome by proxy. *Pediatrics.* 2005;116(1):e145–e148

29. Vianey-Liaud C, Divry P, Gregersen N, Mathieu M. The inborn errors of mitochondrial fatty acid oxidation. *J Inherit Metab Dis.* 1987;10(Suppl 1):159–200

30. McKinlay CJD, Chase JG, Dicson J, Harris DL, Alsweiler JM, Harding JE. Continuous glucose monitoring in neonates: a review. *Matern Health Neonatol Perinatol.* 2017;3:18

31. Galderisi A, Facchinetti A, Steil GM, et al. Continuous glucose monitoring in preterm infants: A randomized controlled trial. *Pediatrics.* 2017;140(4):e20171162

32. Arnoux J-B, Verkarre V, Saint-Martin C. Congenital hyperinsulinism: current trends in diagnosis and therapy. *Orphanet J Rare Dis.* 2011;6:63

33. Aynsley-Green A, Hussain K, Hall J, et al. Practical management of hyperinsulinism in infancy. *Arch Dis Child Fetal Neonatal Ed.* 2000;82(2):F98–F107

34. Raisen D, Brooks-Kayal A, Steinkrauss L, Tennekoon GI, Stanley CA, Kelly A. Central nervous system hyperexcitability associated with glutamate dehydrogenase gain of function mutations. *J Pediatr.* 2005;146(3):388–394

35. Hussain K, Aynsley-Green A, Stanley CA. Medications used in the treatment of hypoglycemia due to congenital hyperinsulinism of infancy (HI). *Pediatr Endocrinol Rev.* 2004;2(Suppl 1):163–167

36. Senniappan S, Alexandrescu S, Tatevian N, et al NEJM-. Sirolimus therapy in infants with severe hyperinsulinemic hypoglycemia. *N Engl J Med.* 2014;370(12):1131–1137

37. Banerjee I, De Leon D, Dunne MJ. Extreme caution on the use of sirolimus for the congenital hyperinsulinism in infancy patient. *Orphanet J Rare Dis.* 2017;12(1):70

38. Warshaw J, Curry E. Comparison of serum carnitine and ketone body concentrations in breast- and formula-fed newborn infants. *J Pediatr.* 1980;97(1):122–125

VI

39. Bodamer OA, Hussein K, Morris AA, et al. Glucose and leucine kinetics in idiopathic ketotic hypoglycemia. *Arch Dis Child.* 2006;91(6):483–486

40. Bachrach B, Weinstein DA, Orho-Melander M, Burgess A, Wolfsdorf JI. Glycogen synthase deficiency (glycogen storage disease type 0) presenting with hyperglycemia and glycosuria: report of three new mutations. *J Pediatr.* 2002;140(6):781–783

41. Finegold D, Stanley C, Baker L. Glycemic response to glucagon during fasting hypoglycemia: an aid in the diagnosis of hyperinsulinism. *J Pediatr.* 1980;96(2):257–259

42. Haymond MW, Sunehag AL. Controlling the sugar bowl. Regulation of glucose homeostasis in children. *Endocrinol Metab Clin North Am.* 1999;28(4):663–694

43. Hussain K, Seppänen M, Näntö-Salonen K, et al. The diagnosis of ectopic focal hyperinsulinism of infancy with (18F)-dopa positron emission tomography. *J Clin Endocrinol Metab.* 2006;91(8):2839–2842

44. Weston PJ, Harris DL, Battin M, Brown J, Hegarty JE, Harding JE. Oral dextrose for the treatment of hypoglycaemia in newborn infants (review). *Cochrane Database Syst Rev.* 2016;(5):011027

45. Harris DL, Gamble GD, Weston PJ, Harding JE. What happens to blood glucose concentrations after oral treatment of neonatal hypoglycemia? *J Pediatr.* 2017;190:136–141

46. Cornblath M. Neonatal hypoglycemia. In: Donn SM, Fisher CW, eds. *Risk Management Techniques in Perinatal and Neonatal Practice.* Armonk, NY: Futura; 1996

47. Cowett R, Farrag H. Neonatal glucose metabolism. In: Cowett R, ed. *Principles of Perinatal-Neonatal Metabolism.* New York, NY: Springer-Verlag; 1998:683–722

48. Farrag RM. Hypoglycemia in the newborn, including infant of a diabetic mother. In: Lifshitz F, ed. *Pediatric Endocrinology.* New York, NY: Marcel Dekker; 2003:541–574.

49. Mehta A. Prevention and management of neonatal hypoglycaemia. *Arch Dis Child Fetal Neonatal Ed.* 1994;70(1):F54–F59

50. Wolfsdorf JI, Crigler JFJ. Cornstarch regimens for nocturnal treatment of young adults with type 1 glycogen storage disease. *Am J Clin Nutr.* 1997;65(5):1507–1511

51. Ross KM, Brown LM, Corrado MM, et al. Safety and efficacy of chronic extended release cornstarch therapy for glycogen storage disease type I. *JIMD Rep.* 2016;26:85–90

52. Kaufman FR, Devgan S. Use of uncooked cornstarch to avert nocturnal hypoglycemia in children and adolescents with type 1 diabetes. *J Diabetes Complications.* 1996;10(2):84–87

Chapter 32

Dyslipidemia

Introduction

Coronary artery disease and blood cholesterol levels are associated. Although the incidence of coronary artery disease has been declining in the United States, it remains the leading cause of death in adults in the United States and most industrialized countries. The familial occurrence of coronary heart disease has been known since the 19th century; however, the risk factors have been better delineated over the past 4 decades. The Framingham study[1] and subsequent studies have identified the following risk factors for coronary heart disease:

1. Family history
2. Male sex
3. Elevated serum total cholesterol level
4. Reduced level of high-density lipoprotein cholesterol (HDL-C)
5. Elevated level of low-density lipoprotein cholesterol (LDL-C)
6. Elevated level of triglycerides
7. Hypertension
8. Cigarette smoking
9. Diabetes mellitus
10. Lack of physical activity

Not all investigators agree that an elevated level of plasma triglycerides is an independent risk factor for coronary heart disease. Although a direct correlation is evident in univariate analysis, this effect is diminished when the influences of obesity, diabetes mellitus, total cholesterol, and HDL-C are removed,[1] suggesting hypertriglyceridemia may be a marker for the insulin resistance observed in obesity.

The American Academy of Pediatrics (AAP) endorses the findings and recommendations of the National Heart Lung and Blood Institute (NHLBI) Expert Panel on Integrated Guidelines for Cardiovascular Health and Risk Reduction in Children and Adolescents.[2] The Expert Panel included guidance on all pediatric risk factors for future cardiovascular disease, including dyslipidemia. With respect to the evidence relating dyslipidemia and cardiovascular disease, the Expert Panel reported that:

1. Certain inborn or acquired diseases accompanied by hypercholesterolemia are associated with premature atherosclerosis.
2. Serum cholesterol levels are higher, on average, in people with coronary heart disease.

3. People with high serum cholesterol levels develop coronary heart disease more often and at a younger age than those with normal levels.

4. The mortality rate from coronary heart disease in different countries varies in relation to the average blood cholesterol values (and with dietary fat and animal protein intake).

5. Experimentally induced hypercholesterolemia in animals is associated with atherosclerotic deposits.

6. Atherosclerotic plaques contain lipids similar in composition to that in the blood.

Evidence that atherosclerosis begins in childhood includes the following:

1. In autopsies of black and white males and females between 15 and 19 years of age, the coronary arteries showed fatty streaks in 71% to 83% and raised atherosclerotic lesions in 7% to 22%.[3]

2. When bodies of US soldiers who died at a mean age of 22 years were examined, 77% of those from the Korean Conflict[4] and 45% of those from the Vietnam War[5] had evidence of coronary vessel atherosclerosis.

3. US adolescents who died of nonatherosclerotic causes show atherosclerotic changes of a magnitude directly related to postmortem LDL-C plus very low-density lipoprotein cholesterol (VLDL-C) levels and inversely related to HDL-C levels.[6]

4. Clustering of risk factors results in increased atherosclerotic burden in adolescents and young adults.[7]

These findings underpin the clinical guidelines for screening for and treatment of dyslipidemia in children and adolescents who are at subsequent increased risk of cardiovascular disease.

Lipoproteins

Lipoproteins are necessary to make fats soluble so they can be transported in the plasma. All lipoproteins contain an outer polar layer of phospholipid, unesterified cholesterol, and protein (called apoprotein). The inner, nonpolar core contains cholesterol ester and triglyceride in varying proportions. The types of lipoproteins are:

1. Chylomicrons, which are formed from dietary fat and enter the plasma via the thoracic duct. Chylomicrons are removed from the blood by the activity of lipoprotein lipase (LPL) with the fatty acids, stored in adipose tissue as triglyceride, or catabolized by the liver. They do not form other lipoproteins.

2. VLDLs (also called prelipoproteins), which are formed from dietary glucose and nonesterified fatty acids in the liver and are then secreted into the plasma. The outer surface of VLDLs contains apoproteins B-100 and E. The LPL on capillary endothelium of adipose tissue and cardiac and skeletal muscle partially metabolizes the VLDLs to nonesterified fatty acids for storage or for energy, leaving a remnant. The apoprotein E allows the remnant to be taken up by the liver. Several types of hyper-lipoproteinemia have been identified.[8,9]

3. LDL-C, which is formed in the liver from VLDL remnants containing apoprotein B-100. LDL-C is an important source of cholesterol for peripheral tissues. An important step in the regulation of cholesterol metabolism is the attachment of LDL-C to receptor sites on cell surfaces (LDLR).[10]

4. HDL-C, which is secreted by the liver and small intestine and is important in helping to remove cholesterol from cells (high levels are protective, up to a point; low levels are a strong risk factor for coronary heart disease).

Hyperlipidemia

Historically, there have been numerous approaches to the classification of lipid disorders. For practical clinical purposes, it is most useful to classify dyslipidemia in 2 major categories: genetic and lifestyle-related dyslipidemias. This dichotomy is not perfect, because every dyslipidemia tends to have both a genetic and a lifestyle (diet and physical activity) component. However, this classification approach identifies the major component and distinguishes genetic dyslipidemias from secondary dyslipidemias, such as those related to lifestyle factors or other disease processes.

Genetic Dyslipidemias

The most important genetic dyslipidemia is familial hypercholesterolemia (FH). This is a dominant genetic disorder. In homozygous FH, the LDL-C is very high (>500 mg/dL) and is associated with substantial elevation of risk for atherosclerotic cardiovascular disease, which can occur in the first decade of life. The prevalence of homozygous FH is 1:300 000 to 1 million individuals.[11,12] Children with homozygous FH most often present with xanthomas appearing as early as 6 months of age and are often identified by dermatologists after referral for this skin condition.

The heterozygous form of FH has a prevalence of 1:250 individuals. In the pediatric age range, there are usually no outward manifestations as the xanthomas tend to occur in adulthood. In heterozygous FH, the LDL-C is usually >190 mg/dL but <500 mg/dL; in childhood, an LDL-C of 160 mg/dL or greater may also be suggestive of heterozygous FH, particularly in the setting of a family history of significantly elevated cholesterol or premature coronary artery disease. Individuals with heterozygous familial hypercholesterolemia are at increased lifetime risk of atherosclerotic cardiovascular disease, which can occur as early as the twenties but is more common in the age range from 30 to 60 years.[13]

The underlying genetic defect in familial hypercholesterolemia is one of a family of genes related to the LDL receptor structure, function, or metabolism.[10] When LDL-C cannot attach to the LDL receptor on the cell membrane, then cholesterol is not internalized in the cell and cholesterol synthesis is not suppressed by the normal feedback mechanism. The most recent set of genetic abnormalities discovered are related to the PCSK9 gene. This represents the system that is involved in the metabolism of the LDL receptor.[14] When there is a loss of function mutation, metabolism of the LDL receptor is slowed, leading to an increased number of functional receptors. These individuals have lower circulating LDL-C. In Mendelian randomization analysis, those with loss-of-function mutations have greatly reduced lifetime risk of atherosclerotic cardiovascular disease.[15] Individuals with PCSK9 gain of function abnormalities have more rapid metabolism of the LDL receptor, higher circulatory LDL-C, and increased lifetime risk of cardiovascular disease.

There are other genetic disorders of cholesterol that are much less common. These disorders include genetic defects that result in very elevated serum levels of triglycerides, including type 1 hyperlipoproteinemia.[16] In this disorder, the triglycerides are primarily chylomicron-rich triglycerides because of the loss of activity of LPL. This enzyme is responsible for hydrolysis and removal of chylomicrons from the blood. Patients with this type of dyslipidemia may present with pancreatitis and abdominal pain; cardiovascular disease is not a typical feature.

Lifestyle-Related Dyslipidemia

These secondary forms of dyslipidemia are related to lifestyle factors or other disease processes, including obesity, diabetes, chronic renal disease, liver disease, and endocrine disorders, such as hypothyroidism. These

Table 32.1.
Causes of Secondary Hypercholesterolemia

Exogenous	Storage Diseases
Drugs: Oral contraceptives, corticosteroids, isotretinoin (Accutane), thiazides, anticonvulsants, beta-blockers, anabolic steroids Alcohol Obesity	Glycogen storage diseases Sphingolipidoses **Obstructive Liver Diseases** Biliary atresia Biliary cirrhosis
Endocrine and Metabolic Hypothyroidism Diabetes mellitus Lipodystrophy Pregnancy Idiopathic hypercalcemia	**Chronic Renal Diseases** Nephrotic syndrome **Others** Anorexia nervosa Progeria Collagen vascular disease Klinefelter syndrome

secondary forms of dyslipidemia should be considered in children and adolescents presenting with lipid abnormalities and are outlined in Table 32.1.

The most prevalent form of this dyslipidemia is a result of obesity and is often referred to as atherogenic dyslipidemia. Patients with atherogenic dyslipidemia have elevated serum triglycerides and low HDL-C.[16] Adults with atherogenic dyslipidemia are at increased risk of coronary heart disease, but the role of this constellation of lipid abnormalities in early atherosclerosis in children is less clear.[17] The most effective treatment for this lipid disorder is change in diet and physical activity, resulting in improvement in the BMI percentile.

Prevention of Atherosclerosis and Prudent Lifestyle and Diet
The AAP has endorsed NHLBI recommendations about the risks of atherosclerosis and the avoidance of known cardiovascular risk factors during childhood and adolescence, including cigarette smoking and secondary smoke exposure, inadequate physical activity, and suboptimal diet.[2] Dietary approaches to prevent hypertension, abnormal lipid levels, and diabetes mellitus are emphasized. Dietary advice should be tailored to the age of the child both in approach and in daily caloric consumption.

Breastfeeding is emphasized in infancy. After 1 year of age, a varied diet is advised to best ensure nutritional adequacy. Decreased consumption of saturated fats, cholesterol, and sodium and increased intake of mono-unsaturated and polyunsaturated fats are also recommended (Table 32.2). When there is a concern about obesity or a family history of cardiovascular disease, reduced-fat milk can be considered starting at 12 months of age. It has been shown that decreasing fat intakes in infants' diets can be done safely.[18] Approximately 50% of the calories in the diet of the exclusively breastfed infant comes from the fat content of the milk. As solids are introduced during the first and second years of life, the percentage of calories in the diet contributed by fat should decrease.

At age 2 to 3 years, if only 30% of total calories are derived from fat, for some infants, the protein content would have to provide 15% or more of calories for the diet to meet the recommended dietary allowances for minerals.

Table 32.2.
Serving Sizes in Food Groups

Bread, Cereal, Rice, and Pasta Group (Grains Group)—Whole Grain and Refined 1 slice bread About 1 cup of ready-to-eat cereal 1 cup of cooked cereal, rice, or pasta
Vegetable Group 1 cup raw, leafy vegetables 1/2 cup of other vegetables—cooked or raw 1 cup vegetable juice
Fruit Group 1 medium apple, banana, orange, pear 1 cup chopped, cooked, or canned fruit 1 cup fruit juice
Milk, Yogurt, and Cheese Group (Milk Group) 2 cups fat free milk or yogurt 1 oz of natural cheese (such as cheddar) 2 oz of processed cheese (such as American)
Meat, Poultry, Fish, Dry Beans, Eggs, and Nuts Group (Meat and Beans Group) 2–3 oz of cooked lean meat, poultry, or fish 1/2 cup of cooked dry beans or 1/2 cup of tofu counts as 1 oz of lean meat 2 oz of soy burger or 1 egg counts as 1 oz of lean meat 2 tbsp of peanut butter or 1/3 cup of nuts counts as 1 oz of meat

Early childhood, therefore, should be considered a transition period during which the fat and cholesterol content of the diet should gradually decrease to the recommended amounts. Particular care should be taken to avoid excessive intake of total calories, which may lead to obesity. Early recognition and treatment of obesity and hypertension, a regular exercise program, and counseling about the dangers of smoking are recommended for all children older than 2 years. The suggested optimal total fat intake is approximately 30% of calories for children older than 2 years, with less than 10% of calories in the diet coming from saturated fat.[19] Care should also be taken to avoid excessive restriction of calories and fat in the diet, which can result in malnutrition and growth failure. The consumption of lower-fat dairy products and lean meats; critical sources of protein, iron, and calcium; and grains, cereals, fruits, and vegetables should be encouraged in this transition period, starting at 1 year of age and throughout childhood and adolescence (see also Appendix P: Saturated and Polyunsaturated Fat and Cholesterol Content of Common Foods).

For children 2 years and older, the NHLBI Expert Panel on Integrated Guidelines for Cardiovascular Health and Risk Reduction in Children and Adolescents and the AAP offer the following specific recommendations[2] (Tables 32.2, 32.3, and 32.4):

1. Nutritional adequacy should be achieved by eating a variety of foods.
2. Energy (calories) should be adequate to support growth and to reach or maintain desirable body weight and avoid obesity development.
3. The following intake pattern is recommended: saturated fatty acids, less than 10% of total energy intake (serum cholesterol appears most responsive to dietary saturated fatty acids); total fat, averaged over several days, no less than 25% of total calories and no more than 30% of calories; and dietary cholesterol, less than 300 mg/day.
4. Carbohydrate content of the diet should be 55% to 60% of the calories, of which the majority should be complex carbohydrates. Fiber is an important dietary constituent that can improve blood cholesterol levels. Protein should provide 10% to 15% of dietary calories.

This diet is similar to the diet recommended by the American Heart Association for moderate reduction of serum cholesterol levels. Similarly composed diets may also be useful in controlling obesity.

VI

Table 32.3.
Diets for Control of Cholesterol[a]

Nutrient	Recommended Intake		
	Population Diet	More Restrictive Diet Focus on lowering LDL-C	Focus on Lowering Triglycerides
Total fat	Average of no more than 30% of total calories and no less than 25%	Same as Population Diet	Same as Population Diet
Saturated fatty acids	Less than 10% of total calories	Less than 7% of total calories	Less than 7% of total calories
Polyunsaturated fatty acids	Up to 10% of total calories	Same as Population Diet	Same as Population Diet
Monounsaturated fatty acids	Remaining dietary fat calories	Same as Population Diet	Same as Population Diet
Cholesterol	Less than 300 mg/day	Less than 200 mg/day	Less than 200 mg/day
Carbohydrates	About 55% of total calories	Same as Population Diet	Decrease sugar intake
Protein	About 15% of total calories	Same as Population Diet	Same as Population Diet
Calories	To promote growth and development	Same as Population Diet	Same as Population Diet

[a] Adapted from NHLBI Integrated Guidelines.[2]

Table 32.4.

Number of Servings from Each of the Food Groups That Should Be Taken for the Population Diet[a]

FOOD GROUPS	Children 2 to 6 y, Women, Some Older Adults (About 1600 kcal)	Older Children, Teen Girls, Active Women, Most Men, Active Men (About 2200 kcal)	Teen Boys, Active Men (About 2800 kcal)
Bread, cereal, rice, and pasta group (grains group)—especially whole grain	6	9	11
Vegetable group	3	4	5
Fruit group	2 or 3	2 or 3	2 or 3
Meat, poultry, fish, dry beans, eggs, and nut groups, (meat and beans group—preferably lean or low fat)	2, for a total of 5 oz	2, for a total of 6 oz	3, for a total of 7 oz

[a] Based on Dietary Guidelines for Americans 2015. US Department of Agriculture, US Department of Health and Human Services. Available at: http://health.gov/dietaryguidelines/

Screening for Hyperlipidemia

The AAP has endorsed individualized and universal approaches to screening and treating children (older than 2 years) and adolescents for dyslipidemia, depending on the age of the child. It should be noted that screening on the basis of family history (individualized approach) has been shown to miss many children with elevated total and LDL-C levels.[20] Although many children with the most elevated LDL-C and the highest risk of early cardiovascular disease have a genetic dyslipidemia, the family history is often unobtainable, incomplete, or modified by statin therapy. This has led to the recommendation for universal screening for children 9 to 11 years of age (before the transient pubertal changes in lipids and lipoproteins) by the NHLBI, the National Lipid Association, and the AAP as incorporated into *Bright Futures: Guidelines for Health Supervision of Infants, Children, and Adolescents*, in addition to the previously advised selective screening approach based on personal and family history.[2,21,22] This strategy is directed at the identification of children with heterozygous familial hypercholesterolemia.

A nonfasting, non-HDL-C level can be used to evaluate a child's lipid status by 9 to 11 years of age and before the onset of puberty. This is determined by subtracting the HDL-C from the total cholesterol and has been found to be a useful risk indicator in adults and children, whether or not they are in a fasting state. If the non-HDL-C is ≥145 mg/dL, then a fasting lipid panel should be obtained. Fig 32.1 presents an algorithm for screening and initiating therapy.

In a fasting lipid profile, levels of total cholesterol, HDL-C, and triglycerides are determined; the LDL-C level is calculated from these values. In some laboratories, LDL-C can be measured directly, regardless of fasting state. Interpretations of cholesterol levels are provided in Table 32.5 for children and adolescents. Appropriate examinations or tests for secondary causes of hypercholesterolemia should be performed before considering treatment (Table 32.1).

Treatment

Therapy should be initiated after the diagnosis of hyperlipidemia is confirmed by 2 separate serum lipid profiles performed at least 2 weeks apart. Dietary therapy is the first mode of treatment in almost all instances, whether or not elevations are attributable to a genetic cause; exceptions include extremely elevated LDL or triglyceride levels suggestive of a

Fig 32.1.

Classification, education, and follow-up based on LDL-cholesterol (LDL-C) from National Cholesterol Education Program [NCEP][4]). To convert mg/dL to mmol/L, multiply by 0.02586.

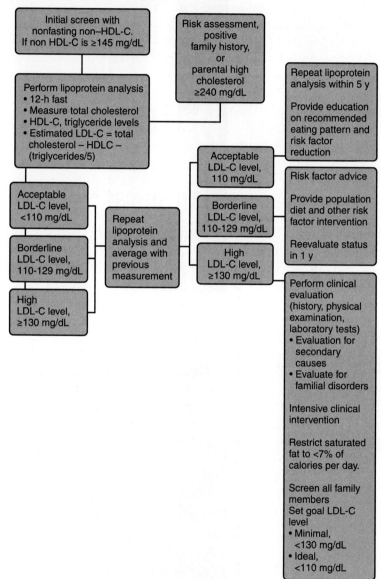

Table 32.5.
Interpretation of Cholesterol Levels for Children and Adolescents[a]

Term	Total Cholesterol, mg/dL	LDL Cholesterol, mg/dL	HDL Cholesterol, mg/dL	Non-HDL Cholesterol, mg/dL	Triglycerides, mg/dL
Acceptable	<170	<110	>45	<120	<90
Borderline	170–199	110–129	40–44	120–144	90–129
High	>200	>130	(Low) <40	≥145	≥130

[a] From National Cholesterol Education Program (NCEP).[2] To convert g/dL to mmol/L, multiply by 0.02586.

homozygous genetic lipid condition. A 3-day dietary record is helpful for suggesting changes; this record should be representative of the child's usual intake, including both weekdays and weekend days. Consultation with a registered dietitian is very helpful.

The population diet (Table 32.2) suggests an average intake of saturated fatty acids less than 10% of total calories, total fat 25% to 30% of calories, and cholesterol less than 300 mg/day. The polyunsaturated fatty acids constitute up to 10% and the monounsaturated fatty acids 10% to 15% of the total calories. The 2015 Dietary Guidelines for Americans can be a useful guide to a healthful diet for children older than 2 years and adolescents.[19]

Avoidance of smoking, the value of exercise, attaining weight appropriate for age and height, and correction of or treatments for other risk factors are also emphasized. If, after 3 months of diet intervention, desired lipid levels are not achieved, a more restrictive diet is initiated. Intake of saturated fatty acids is reduced to approximately 7% of the caloric intake and intake of cholesterol is reduced to less than 200 mg/day. For most children and adolescents with hypertriglyceridemia, a diet lower in carbohydrates, particularly refined carbohydrates low in fiber, high in glycemic index, with restricted saturated fat, is effective (Table 32.3). In contrast, for the rare patient with type 1 hyperlipoproteinemia, characterized by severely elevated triglycerides (>1000 mg/dL), dietary fat must be severely restricted to achieve lower plasma triglyceride concentrations.

The NHLBI Expert Panel on Integrated Guidelines for Cardiovascular Health and Risk Reduction for Children and Adolescents,[2] which has been endorsed by the AAP, recommend that after an adequate trial of diet therapy has been completed (6 months to 1 year), drug therapy should be considered in children 10 years or older (except in extreme circumstances, see below) under the following conditions:

1. If LDL-C remains greater than 4.9 mmol/L (190 mg/dL); or
2. If LDL-C remains greater than 4.1 mmol/L (160 mg/dL) **and** there is a positive family history of cardiovascular disease before age 55 years; **or** 2 or more other risk factors for cardiovascular disease are present.
3. Statin therapy can be considered at younger ages (~8 years) in the setting of particularly concerning family history or severely elevated LDL-C levels.

The optimal goal of drug therapy is to achieve an LDL-C level to approach 2.85 mmol/L (110 mg/dL). In some circumstances, however, a target of 130 mg/dL for LDL-C may be appropriate. Hydroxymethylglutaryl-CoA reductase inhibitors (statins) are now first-line therapy in children and adolescents with elevated LDL-C, on the basis of randomized clinical trial data in children with familial hypercholesterolemia.[21,23] Multiple short-term studies of the use of hydroxymethylglutaryl-CoA reductase inhibitors in adolescents have shown their efficacy, acceptability, and safety.[24-27] Because the long-term effects of these drugs are reported only in 1 small follow-up study, monitoring of baseline liver function and creatine kinase and the assessment for clinical signs of myositis should be performed throughout childhood and adolescence. Statins have been shown to result in a higher incidence of type 2 diabetes mellitus in randomized clinical trials in adult populations; little is known about this risk in the pediatric population, but some type of surveillance may be reasonable. Bile acid sequestrants have been shown to be safe and effective, lowering LDL- cholesterol levels by as much as 18%, but are often difficult to take because they come in a powder or large pills, and adverse effects include constipation and bloating, result-ing in low adherence.[28] Ezetimibe, which blocks cholesterol absorption in the gastrointestinal tract, can also be used in children and adolescents.[21] However, ezetimibe has not been extensively studied in pediatric patients. Niacin is not generally recommended for use in children because of adverse effects, including flushing and headaches, and lack of efficacy for preven-tion of cardiovascular disease in adults.

Summary

Elevated levels of LDL-C are an important risk factor for development of atherosclerotic cardiovascular disease. Both genetic and lifestyle factors can contribute to elevated LDL-C. Screening should primarily focus on identify-ing children with genetic dyslipidemias, particularly heterozygous familial hypercholesterolemia, which occurs in approximately 1:250 individuals. All children should have their lipids tested with either a nonfasting non-HDL-C or a fasting lipid profile once between the ages of 9 and 11 years. Children with heterozygous familial hypercholesterolemia often have an LDL-C >190 mg/dL. Screening will also identify individuals with hyperlipidemia attributable to lifestyle factors (usually high triglycerides and low HDL-C). These dyslipidemias are often seen in children and adolescents with excess weight who will benefit from improved lifestyle.

Treatment of dyslipidemia should usually start with changes in diet to reduce intake of saturated fat, simple sugars, and cholesterol. If, after a trial of dietary therapy, the LDL-C remains elevated, then treatment with a medication should be considered in children age 10 years and older, and rarely at younger ages in extreme cases. If medications are used, dietary therapy should be continued, because it may allow use of a lower dose of medication. Children and adolescents on drug therapy for elevated LDL-C should be monitored for both safety and efficacy. When treatment with medication is not successful, then referral to a lipid specialist should be considered.

References

1. Kannel WB, Castelli WP, Gordon T. Cholesterol in the prediction of atherosclerotic disease. New perspectives based on the Framingham study. *Ann Intern Med.* 1979;90(1):85–91

2. National Heart, Lung, and Blood Institute Expert Panel. Integrated guidelines for cardiovascular health and risk reduction in children and adolescents. *Pediatrics.* 2011;128(Suppl 5):S213–S256

3. Strong JP, McGill HC, Jr. The pediatric aspects of atherosclerosis. *J Atherosclerosis Res.* 1969;9(3):251–265

4. Enos WF, Jr., Beyer JC, Holmes RH. Pathogenesis of coronary disease in American soldiers killed in Korea. *JAMA.* 1955;158(11):912–914

5. McNamara JJ, Molot MA, Stremple JF, Cutting RT. Coronary artery disease in combat casualties in Vietnam. *JAMA.* 1971;216(7):1185–1187

6. Strong JP, Malcom GT, McMahan CA, et al. Prevalence and extent of atherosclerosis in adolescents and young adults: implications for prevention from the Pathobiological Determinants of Atherosclerosis in Youth Study. *JAMA.* 1999;281(8):727–735

7. Berenson GS, Srinivasan SR, Bao W, Newman WP, III, Tracy RE, Wattigney WA. Association between multiple cardiovascular risk factors and atherosclerosis in children and young adults. The Bogalusa Heart Study. *N Engl J Med.* 1998;338(23):1650–1656

8. Fredrickson DS, Goldstein JL, Brown MS. The familial hyperlipoproteinemias. In: Stanbury JB, Wyngaarden JB, Fredrickson DS, eds. *The Metabolic Basis of Inherited Disease.* 4th ed. New York, NY: McGraw-Hill Book Co; 1978:604–655

9. Havel RJ, Kane JP. Introduction: structure and metabolism of plasma lipoproteins. In: Scriver CR, Beaudet AL, Sly WS, Valle D, eds. *The Metabolic Basis of Inherited Disease.* 6th ed. New York, NY: McGraw-Hill Book Co; 1989:1129–1138

10. Goldstein JL, Brown MS. The LDL receptor defect in familial hypercholesterolemia. Implications for pathogenesis and therapy. *Med Clin North Am.* 1982;66(2):335–362

11. Sjouke B, Kusters DM, Kindt I, et al. Homozygous autosomal dominant hypercholesterolaemia in the Netherlands: prevalence, genotype-phenotype relationship, and clinical outcome. *Eur Heart J.* 2015;36(9):560–565

VI

12. Sánchez-Hernández RM, Civeira F, Stef M, et al. Homozygous familial hypercholesterolemia in Spain: prevalence and phenotype-genotype relationship. *Circ Cardiovasc Genet.* 2016;9(6):504–510

13. Gidding SS, Champagne MA, de Ferranti SD, et al. American Heart Association Atherosclerosis, Hypertension, and Obesity in Young Committee of Council on Cardiovascular Disease in Young, Council on Cardiovascular and Stroke Nursing, Council on Functional Genomics and Translational Biology, and Council on Lifestyle and Cardiometabolic Health. The agenda for familial hypercholesterolemia: a scientific statement from the American Heart Association. *Circulation.* 2015;132(22):2167–2192

14. Benjannet S, Rhainds D, Essalmani R, et al. NARC-1/PCSK9 and its natural mutants: zymogen cleavage and effects on the low-density lipoprotein (LDL) receptor and LDL cholesterol. *J Biol Chem.* 2004;279(47):48865–48875

15. Cohen JC, Boerwinkle E, Mosley TH, Jr,, Hobbs HH. Sequence variations in PCSK9, low LDL, and protection against coronary heart disease. *N Engl J Med.* 2006;354:1264–1272

16. Kwiterovitch PO, Jr. Recognition and management of dyslipidemia in children and adolescents. *J Clin Endocrinol Metab.* 2008;93:4200–4209

17. Morrison JA, Glueck CJ, Wang P. Childhood risk factors predict cardiovascular disease, impaired fasting glucose plus type 2 diabetes mellitus, and high blood pressure 26 years later at a mean age of 38 years: the Princeton-lipid research clinics follow-up study. *Metabolism.* 2012;61(4):531–540

18. Simell O, Niinikoski H, Viikari J, Rask-Nissila L, Tammi A, Ronnemaa T. Cardiovascular disease risk factors in young children in the STRIP baby project. *Ann Med.* 1999;31(Suppl 1):55–61

19. US Department of Health and Human Services, US Department of Agriculture. Dietary Guidelines for Americans, 2015–2020. 2015; Available at: http://health.gov/dietaryguidelines/2015/guidelines/. Accessed February 11, 2019

20. Ritchie SK, Murphy ECS, Ice C, et al. Universal versus targeted blood cholesterol screening among youth: the CARDIAC Project. *Pediatrics.* 2010;126(2):260–265

21. Daniels SR, Gidding SS, de Ferranti SD. Pediatric aspects of familial hypercholesterolemias: recommendations from the National Lipid Association Expert Panel on Familial Hypercholesterolemia. *J Clin Lipidol.* 2011;5(3 Suppl):S30–S37

22. American Academy of Pediatrics. Bright Futures: Prevention and health promotion for infants, children, adolescents, and their families. Available at: https://brightfutures.aap.org/Pages/default.aspx. Accessed February 9, 2018

23. McCrindle BW, Urbina EM, Dennison BA, et al. Drug therapy of high-risk lipid abnormalities in children and adolescents: a scientific statement from the American Heart Association Atherosclerosis, Hypertension, and Obesity in Youth Committee, Council of Cardiovascular Disease in the Young, with the Council on Cardiovascular Nursing. *Circulation.* 2007;115(14):1948–1967

24. Stein EA, Illingworth DR, Kwiterovich PO, Jr, et al. Efficacy and safety of lovastatin in adolescent males with heterozygous familial hypercholesterolemia: a randomized controlled trial. *JAMA*. 1999;281(2):137–144

25. McCrindle BW, Ose L, Marais AD. Efficacy and safety of atorvastatin in children and adolescents with familial hypercholesterolemia or severe hyperlipidemia: a multicenter, randomized, placebo-controlled trial. *J Pediatr*. 2003;143(1):74–80

26. deJongh S, Ose L, Szamosi T, et al. Simvastatin in Children Study Group. Efficacy and safety of statin therapy in children with familial hypercholesterolemia: a randomized, double-blind, placebo-controlled trial with simvastatin. *Circulation*. 2002;106(17):2231–2237

27. Wiegman A, Hutten BA, de Groot E, et al. Efficacy and safety of statin therapy in children with familial hypercholesterolemia: a randomized controlled trial. *JAMA*. 2004;292(3):331–337

28. Stein EA, Marais AD, Szamosi T, et al. Colesevelam hydrochloride: efficacy and safety in pediatric subjects with heterozygous familial hypercholesterolemia. *J Pediatr*. 2010;156(2):231–236.e231–e233

VI

Chapter 33

Pediatric Obesity

Introduction

Pediatric obesity has increased significantly over the last 4 decades and is a prevalent problem among youth today. Obesity prevalence among 2- to 19-year-old US children continues to increase across most age groups, with the overall rates of obesity increasing from 17.3% in 2013–2014 to 18.5% in 2015–2016,[1,2] with increasing risks of comorbidities such as dyslipidemia and hypertension associated with excess adiposity. The increase in pediatric obesity is occurring worldwide.[3] Given the burden of pediatric obesity on child health as well as associated health care costs, it has been recognized as an urgent public health priority.[4,5] Unfortunately, the public health approach to the epidemic has been largely unsuccessful to date. Understanding the pathophysiology of obesity involves an appreciation of the complexity of the regulation of energy balance, the mechanisms driving hunger and satiety, and the gene-environment interaction (epigenetics) potentially driving the epidemic. It is also important to understand the role of excess adiposity, ectopic fat, and adipocyte dysfunction in the development of obesity-related comorbidities. Obesity prevention is aimed at optimizing energy balance to support healthy growth and development without accumulation of excess adipose tissue. Once energy balance is altered toward fat accumulation, treatment is directed at identifying and reversing factors that contribute to energy excess and optimizing factors that contribute to energy expenditure. An awareness of the complexity of the dysregulation of energy balance is crucial to devising prevention and treatment strategies. As effective obesity treatment through lifestyle interventions has proven more and more challenging, the emphasis of many pediatricians and policy makers has shifted toward obesity prevention.[6]

Adipose Tissue: An Organ

Obesity may be defined functionally as a maladaptive increase in adipose tissue. Adipose tissue is the major organ system involved in energy regulation and accounts for up to 25% of body weight in a person of normal weight.[7] White adipose tissue is also an important secretory organ that has roles in immune response, blood pressure control, hemostasis, bone mass, and thyroid and reproductive functions, through the synthesis and secretion of hormones called adipokines.[8] It also functions as an insulating and structural element in the body. Excess accumulation of white adipose

VI

tissue results in obesity, and products of the increased visceral storage depot drain directly into the portal system, exacerbating obesity-related metabolic comorbidities. In addition to increased adiposity, when children become obese, ectopic fat deposition occurs, with accumulation of triglycerides within nonadipose tissue, such as the liver, muscles, pancreas, and heart, compromising organ structure and function.[9] Both brown and white adipocytes are derived from fibroblasts. Brown adipose tissue is found only in mammals, and its primary function is to produce heat by nonshivering thermogenesis.[10] White adipose tissue is made up of both adipocytes (25%–60%) and nonadipocytes, including fibroblastic preadipocytes, endothelial cells, mast cells, and macrophages.[11] Adipocytes are key regulators of energy balance. Other factors important for energy balance are genetics, physical activity, nutrition, and environmental and behavior influences. Environmental and behavior influences include the state of overall health, medication use, composition of intestinal microflora,[12] and psychological/emotional factors that influence food intake and energy expenditure. All of these factors are operative in the overall energy balance equation.[7]

Pathophysiology

Energy Balance

The accumulation of stored energy as adipose tissue is caused by intake in excess of energy expenditure. A small excess of energy intake relative to expenditure will, over time, lead to a gradual but substantial increase in body weight. For example, an individual increasing daily energy intake by 150 kcal above daily energy expenditure would consume an excess of 55 000 kcal per year and could gain approximately 15 pounds per year. Despite the potentially large effects of small imbalances in energy intake versus expenditure, complex integrated control mechanisms ensure that adults maintain a relatively constant body weight, and most children tend to grow steadily along individualized weight percentiles for age, with little conscious effort to regulate energy intake or expenditure.[13,14] In addition, the high rate of recidivism to previous levels of adiposity after a period of weight loss in obese children and adults, and the tendency for individuals to maintain a relatively stable body weight over long periods of time despite wide variations in caloric intake, provide empiric evidence that body weight is regulated and that energy intake and expenditure are not independent processes but are regulated by complex interlocking control mechanisms.[13,15]

However, data generated from studies of energy homeostasis in adults must be applied cautiously to children. Unlike adults, children accrue both fat mass and fat-free mass as they grow, and the magnitude and composition of this weight gain is more age and gender dependent. A simplified overview of this complex system controlling energy balance is shown in Fig 33.1, illustrating the interaction of the hypothalamus, brainstem, gut hormones, and adipose tissue that regulate body weight and energy intake and expenditure. Input to the hypothalamus from energy stores and hunger signals are integrated with efferent output regarding feeding behavior, satiety, insulin secretion, and autonomic regulation of adipocytokines, including leptin secreted by adipose tissue. These molecules directly or indirectly affect the hypothalamus, from which outflow tracts affect energy expenditure.

Hypothalamus and Energy Homeostasis

Within the hypothalamus, the arcuate nucleus (ARC) responds to signals regarding energy stores from the gut, adipose tissue, pancreas, and other parts of nervous system by increasing or decreasing the expression of the potent orexigens and anorexigens[16] (Fig 33.1). Orexigenic peptides that increase food intake and decrease energy expenditure include neuropeptide Y (NPY) and agouti-related peptide (AgRP). Anorexigenic peptides that decrease food intake and reduce body weight include pro-opiomelanocortin (POMC) and cocaine- and amphetamine-related transcript (CART).[17,18] Gut hormones, such as cholecystokinin (CCK), ghrelin, and peptide YY (PYY), and vagal nerve signals also input information at the hypothalamic level to regulate hunger and satiety.[18] The ARC interacts with the brainstem via the dorsal vagus complex that includes the dorsal vagal motor nucleus (receives signals from visceral organs via the vasovagal reflex), the nucleus tractus solitarius (taste, afferent signals from visceral organs), and the area postrema, which is outside the blood-brain barrier and receives physiologic signals from molecules/hormones in the blood (controls nausea and vomiting).

In addition, central alpha-adrenergic stimulation results in increased food intake and decreased energy expenditure (orexiant effect), whereas beta-adrenergic and dopaminergic stimulation have anorexiant effects and increase energy expenditure. Peripheral alpha-adrenergic stimulation inhibits lipolysis, whereas peripheral beta-adrenergic stimulation is lipolytic.[19,20]

Fig 33.1.

The brain integrates long-term energy balance through integration of peripheral signals[a]

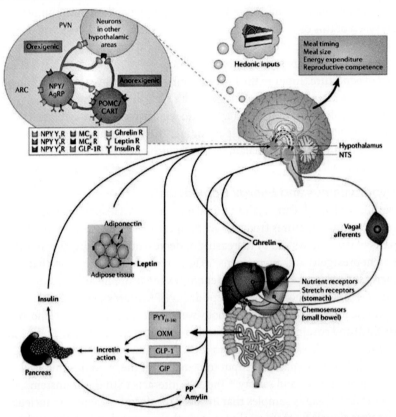

[a] Peripheral signals relating to long-term energy stores are produced by adipose tissue (leptin) and the pancreas (insulin). Feedback relating to recent nutritional state takes the form of absorbed nutrients, neuronal signals (PVN), and gut peptides. Neuronal pathways, primarily by way of the vagus afferent nerve, relate information about the stomach distention and chemical and hormonal milieu in the upper small bowel to the NTS within the dorsal vagal complex. Hormones released by the gut have incretin-, hunger-, and satiety-stimulating actions. The incretin horones GLP-1, GIP, and potentially OXM improve the response of the endocrine pancrease to absorbed nutrients. GLP-1 and potentially OXM also reduce food intake. Ghrelin is released by th stomach and stimulates appetite. Gut hormones stimulating satiety include CCK released from the gut to feedback by way of the vagus nerve. OXM and PYY are released from the lower gastrointestinal tract and PP is released from the islets of Langerhans.

PVN indicates vagus nerve and other neuronal pathways; NTS, nucleus of the tractus solitarius; GLP-1, glucagon-like peptide 1; GIP, gastric inhibitory polypeptide; OXM, oxyntomodulin; CCK, cholecystokinin; PYY, peptide YY; PP, pancreatic polypeptide.

Reprinted with permission from Badman MK, Flier JS. The gut and energy balance: visceral allies in the obesity wars. *Science.* 2005;307(5717):1909–1914

Leptin is secreted from adipose tissue and provides a signal linking fat mass to food intake and energy expenditure (Fig 33.1 and Fig 33.2). Leptin binds to cells in the ARC of the hypothalamus to affect the expression of

Fig 33.2.

The effects of leptin in states of energy excess and energy deficiency[a]

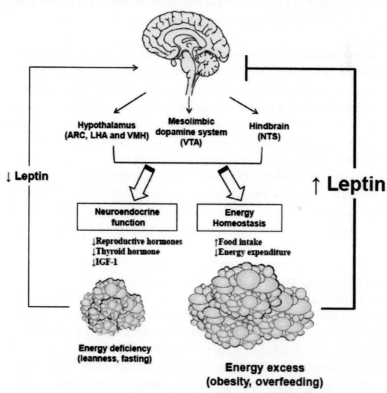

[a] In states of energy deficiency such as fasting, circulating leptin levels decrease. As a result, food intakes increase due to increased expression of orexigenic neuropeptides and decreased expression of anorexigenic neuropeptides. In addition, the decline of leptin modulates mesolimibic dopamine system and hindbrain circuits to increase food intake, and also has effects on neuroendocrine function and sympathetic nervous system to decrease energy expenditure. In states of energy exess such as obesity and overfeeding, leptin levels increase; however, leptin effects in the CNS are somewhat blunted due to leptin resistance. Leptin enhances weight loss maintenance in obesity by suppressing food intake and increasing energy expenditure.

ARC indicates arcuate nucleus; CNS, central nervous system; IGF, insulin-like growth factors; LHA, lateral hypothalamic area; NTS, nucleus solitary tract; VMH, ventromedial hypothalamus; VTA, ventral tegmental area.

Reprinted with permission from Park HK, Ahima RS. Physiology of leptin: energy homeostasis, neuroendocrine function and metabolism. *Metabolism*. 2015;64(1):24–34.

POMC,[21] producing alpha-, beta-, and gamma-melanocyte–stimulating hormones. These peptides signal target neurons in the lateral hypothalamus that express the melanocortin receptors MC3R and MC4R, which results in a decrease in food intake and increase in energy expenditure.[22] Leptin is increased in the fasting state and elevated in typical exogenous obesity, which is associated with a state of leptin resistance.[23] Leptin also exerts a permissive effect on puberty and has effects on the thyroid hormone axis as well. In rare genetic states of leptin deficiency, leptin can be used as therapy.[23]

Insulin inhibits release of free fatty acids from adipocytes. In obesity, adipose tissue becomes resistant to insulin, and release of free fatty acids (FFAs) increases. This increase in FFAs is associated with the development of insulin resistance in peripheral muscle and liver.[24] Studies have also indicated a central role for insulin action.[16] Rodent data show that insulin binds to insulin receptors in the brain to suppress hepatic glucose production.[25]

Gut peptides (Fig 33.1) play an important role in both long- and short-term energy regulation.[26,27] PYY is produced in the distal gut and increases for several hours after a meal to reduce appetite.[28] Pancreatic polypeptide (PP) is increased after a meal secondary to vagal stimulation and release of CCK and reduces food intake.[29] Glucagon-like peptide 1 (GLP-1) is produced in the ileum in response to ingested carbohydrates and fat; it stimulates the islet cells in the pancreas to secrete insulin and has been shown to reduce appetite and body weight.[30] Oxyntomodulin (OXM) has been shown to reduce food intake and body weight[31] and to improve glucose homeostasis. OXM increases after gastric bypass surgery.[32] OXM is secreted postprandially by the gut endocrine cells (L-cells) in the small intestine together with GLP-1 and PYY. Ghrelin is a peptide produced by the gastric mucosal X/A-like cells of the gastric fundus.[33] Ghrelin stimulates NPY and AGRP in the ARC, causing increased food intake and reduced energy expenditure, and is suppressed by eating.[34,35] There is some evidence that anticipating a meal can enhance ghrelin suppression after a meal, indicating a possible cognitive link in peptide secretion.[36] CCK is released in the blood as a result of the presence of fat or protein in the duodenum and suppresses appetite by delaying gastric emptying.[37]

The Microbiome
The microbiome has also been implicated in the etiology of obesity. Proposed mechanisms include increased energy production from dietary

constituents, modification in gut PYY and glucagon-like peptide secretion, and alteration of intestinal barrier permeability.[38] The human gut is colonized by trillions of bacteria, 90% of which are in the phyla *Bacteroidetes* and *Firmicutes*. These bacteria affect which nutrients are absorbed in the gut, contributing to weight gain. *Firmicutes* create more energy from dietary constituents than *Bacteroidetes*. Both obese humans and mice fed a high-fat diet have been found to have relatively more *Firmicutes* than *Bacteroidetes*; furthermore, this characteristic can be transferred from one mouse to another by transplanting the microbiota.[39,40] In addition, gut bacteria break down carbohydrates to produce short chain fatty acids, which can stimulate enteric hormones such as GLP-1.[41] Future research will further elucidate the impact of the microbiota on energy balance.

Role of Adipokines and Inflammation

Adipocytes produce inflammatory cytokines and acute-phase proteins, and obesity can be considered a low-grade inflammatory state.[42] Macrophages migrate into adipose tissue, and tumor necrosis factor-alpha (TNF-alpha) secreted by adipocytes stimulates the production of monocyte chemoattractant protein 1 (MCP-1).[43] Adipose tissue is an important endocrine organ, secreting adipokines such as adiponectin and leptin.[44] As stated earlier, leptin is typically increased in exogenous obesity, a state of leptin resistance. Increased leptin contributes to the low grade inflammatory state, by stimulating interleukin-6 and TNF-alpha proinflammatory cytokines.[44,45] Inflammatory factors have been found in children with obesity as young as 3 years old.[46] Adiponectin, however, is decreased in exogenous obesity, and is anti-inflammatory, insulin-sensitizing, anti-atherogenic, and anti-diabetic in its effects.[47] Obesity is also associated with systemic inflammation, with elevations of C-reactive protein (CRP) as well.

VI

Lifestyle intervention has shown reductions in low-grade inflammation and macrophage infiltration in adipose tissue, and in reduction of inflammatory cytokines.[48,49] In obesity, increased inflammatory cytokine production and inflammation occur in nonalcoholic fatty liver disease and nonalcoholic steatohepatitis,[50] and in skeletal muscle.[51] Proinflammatory cytokines are produced in the hypothalamus in animals fed diets high in calories and dietary fat, causing resistance to both insulin and leptin.[52] In addition, adipokines produced by the adipocytes play a role in regulation of blood pressure, lipid metabolism, hemostasis, appetite and energy balance, immunity, insulin sensitivity, and angiogenesis.[53]

Genetics

Genetic differences in predisposition to obesity or excess fat storage clearly exist. Twin studies of pairs raised together versus apart have shown that genetic components of obesity to account for 30% to 70% of body mass index (BMI) variation between individuals. Moreover, monozygotic twins have a fat mass concordance rate of 80%, compared with 40% in dizygotic twins.[54,55]

Body weight is a polygenic trait and is highly heritable, with estimates of genetic contribution to BMI ranging from 64% to 84%, and contribution to body fatness and fat distribution ranging from 30% to 70%.[56] However, lifestyle factors, such as diet, physical activity, stress, and sleep cycles may modify DNA expression through DNA methylation and histone acetylation (epigenetic changes). These changes, once made, are lifelong and heritable, and thus have important implications for prevention of obesity through early intervention.[57]

Familial and animal studies were used to identify genes associated with childhood obesity, before the onset of genome-wide association studies. Several rare familial syndromes of childhood obesity (eg, Prader Willi, Bardet Biedl, Alstrom), as well as monogenic mutations causing childhood-onset obesity, were identified.[54] One of these monogenic forms of childhood obesity is caused by mutations of the *MC4R* gene and is associated with increased hunger, decreased satiety, and increased total body fat. Unlike most other forms of monogenic obesity, individuals with *MC4R* mutations do not have an intellectual disability. Affected children tend to be tall, and mutations can show both dominant and recessive inheritance. *MC4R* mutations are the most common monogenic cause of obesity in childhood, although they are still rare.[58]

The advent of genome-wide association studies performed in large groups of individuals has allowed for the identification of genetic variants involved in the more common forms of obesity. One of the earliest obesity loci identified, *FTO* (fat mass- and obesity-associated gene), located on chromosome 16, has been identified in adults and children.[59] Studies have identified significant genetic influences on resting metabolic rate, feeding behavior, food preferences, and changes in energy expenditure that occur in response to overfeeding.[60] The *FTO* gene mutations are associated with increased total and fat dietary intake[61,62] as well as with diminished satiety and/or increased feeling of hunger in children.[63] Almost 100 BMI loci have been identified by genome-wide association studies.[54]

The monogenic and syndromic forms of obesity illustrate the pivotal role of genetics in the control of body weight.[58,64,65] These syndromes with obesity must be differentiated from the more common polygenic form of obesity and should be considered in the differential diagnosis of obesity in children 5 years and younger.[66]

Assessment

Although direct assessment of adiposity can be accomplished using hydrodensitometry (underwater weighing), air displacement plethysmography, or dual-energy x-ray absorptiometry, these are primarily research tools. In clinical practice, BMI (weight [kg]/height^2 [m^2]) is used as a surrogate measure of adiposity that correlates well with direct measures of body fatness within a population.[67,68] The US Preventive Services Task Force (USPSTF) recently recommended screening children $\geq$6 years for obesity,[69] a recommendation endorsed by the AAP. However, the recent joint statement of the Endocrine Society, Pediatric Endocrine Society, and European Society of Endocrinology recommended that BMI obesity screening begin at 2 years of age.[70] Current definitions of overweight and obesity are based on population norms from the National Health and Nutrition Examination Survey I (NHANES I), which were determined before the current obesity epidemic began. Children between 2 and 18 years of age with a BMI between the 85th and 95th percentile for age and gender based on NHANES I (1971–1974) data are categorized as "overweight." Children 2 to 18 years of age with a BMI greater than the 95th percentile or BMI >30 kg/m^2 (whichever is smaller) are categorized as "obese."[71] For children from birth to 2 years of age, the weight-for-recumbent length percentiles should be used for evaluating weight relative to linear growth.[71] Weight-for-length greater than the 97.7th percentile is considered the equivalent of obesity (+2 SD) in this age group.[71] In the United States, the CDC and AAP recommend that providers use the World Health Organization (WHO) growth charts for children younger than 2 years and the Centers for Disease Control and Prevention (CDC) growth charts for children 2 to 18 years of age.[72–74] The WHO growth charts for 0 to 2 years of age also include BMI charts (see Chapter 24: Nutritional Assessment, and Appendix Q). Because of the increased prevalence of severe obesity in the pediatric age range, additional subcategories have been developed to classify the top extremes of obesity: class I is BMI 95% to 120% of the 95th percentile, class II is BMI 120% to 140% of the 95th percentile, and class III is BMI above 140% of the 95th percentile.[75] These

VI

new categories have been incorporated into growth charts for severely obese children as well.[76]

Although the use of WHO or CDC growth charts are recommended for all children, there is some evidence to suggest that differences in body composition by race and ethnicity exist. Adipose tissue has its own growth curve, and calculations based on skinfold measurements illustrate the gender dimorphism in adiposity. Boys and girls have similar growth patterns until 9 years of age, with percentage of body fat peaking for boys at 11 years of age but continuing to increase for girls throughout adolescence. Median percentage of body fat at 18 years of age for boys is 17.0% and for girls is 27.8%.[77]

African American children have somewhat less fat, and Hispanic and Southeast Asian children have a higher percentage of body fat than do white children at the same BMI.[78–83] It should also be noted that body fat distribution at any given level of body adiposity may constitute an independent risk factor for adiposity-related morbidity.[84,85]

Measurement of skinfold thickness has been a standard method of nutritional assessment. Skinfold measurements correlate with total body fat lipid levels, blood pressure, plasma glucose, and insulin levels as well as insulin resistance and indicators of inflammation.[86–89] However, because it is difficult to produce reliable and reproducible measurements and there are no reference standards or criteria for treatment, the AAP does not recommend measurement of skinfold thicknesses for routine clinical use[71] (see Chapter 24: Nutritional Assessment). Measuring waist circumference provides a better estimate of visceral adiposity in children than does BMI.[71] Waist circumference can also predict insulin resistance, blood pressure, and lipid levels[90–93] but may be no better than BMI measurements for this purpose.[94] The AAP currently does not recommend routine use of waist circumference in the office setting until more clinical experience with its use is available.[71]

Epidemiology of Pediatric Obesity

Using the data from the National Health and Nutrition Examination Surveys (NHANES) from 1963 through 2014, the National Center for Health Statistics describes trends in pediatric obesity in the United States among 2- to 19-year-olds (Fig 33.3). In 2011–2014, 17% of children 2 to 19 years of age had BMI ≥95th percentile (classified as obese), and the prevalence of extreme obesity (≥120% of the sex-specific 95th percentile) was 5.8%.[1] The obesity prevalence increased during the 25-year period among 12- to

Fig 33.3.

Prevalence of obesity in US children and adolescents aged 2 to 19 years from 1963 through 2014

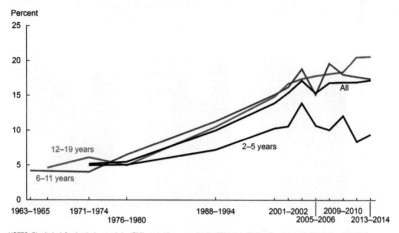

Figure. Trends in obesity among children and adolescents aged 2–19 years, by age: United States, 1963–1965 through 2013–2014

NOTES: Obesity is defined as body mass index (BMI) greater than or equal to the 95th percentile from the sex-specific BMI-for-age 2000 CDC Growth Charts.
SOURCES: NCHS, National Health Examination Surveys II (ages 6–11) and III (ages 12–17); and National Health and Nutrition Examination Surveys (NHANES) I–III, and NHANES 1999–2000, 2001–2002, 2003–2004, 2005–2006, 2007–2008, 2009–2010, 2011–2012, and 2013–2014.

From: https://www.cdc.gov/nchs/data/hestat/obesity_child_13_14/obesity_child_13_14.pdf

VI

19-year-olds. CDC data show the obesity rates by sex (Fig 33.4), as well as by race (Fig 33.5), the latter of which demonstrates the increased prevalence of obesity in minority populations. The geographic distribution of obesity shows an increased prevalence in the southeast United States (https://www.stateofobesity.org/children1017/). Using the most recent 2016 data of the NHANES, Skinner et al have shown the prevalence of pediatric obesity among 2- to 19-year-olds has further increased to 18.5% with an overweight prevalence of 35%.[2]

Influence of the Life Cycle on Pediatric Obesity

The Barker Hypothesis, originating in publications during the 1980s and 1990s and summarized by Barker himself,[95] led to what is now called the Developmental Origins of Health and Disease (DOHAD). This approach,

Fig 33.4.

Prevalence of obesity among youth aged 2 to 19 years, by sex and age, United States, 2015–2016

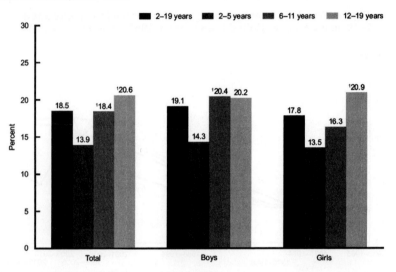

[1] Significantly different from those aged 2–5 years.

Note: Access data table for figure at: https://www.cdc.gov/nchs/data/databriefs

Source: NCHS, National Health and Nutrition Examination Survey, 2015–2016.

Reprinted from Hales CM, Carroll MD, Fryar CD, Ogden CL. Prevalence of obesity among adults and youth: United States, 2015–2016. *NCHS Data Brief.* 2017 Oct;(288):1-8

which originally emerged from early epidemiologic studies of birth and death records, focuses on the significance of events early in human development, which affect later health and disease as well as adult morbidity and mortality. The concept of the childhood onset of adult disease points to the importance of disease prevention from the preconceptual period throughout pregnancy and early infancy and into childhood. Thus, the fetal period and the first 2 years of life may be critical periods for the programming of obesity and related behaviors. The long-term impacts of both under- and overnutrition in the prenatal period on pediatric obesity have been well described.

Prenatal Undernutrition

In addition to Barker's work, Ravelli et al also examined adults conceived during the Dutch "Winter Hunger," of 1944-1945 and compared their long-term health to those conceived before or after the famine.[96,97] They

Fig 33.5.

Prevalence of obesity among youth aged 2 to 19 years, by sex and race and Hispanic origin: United States 2015–2016

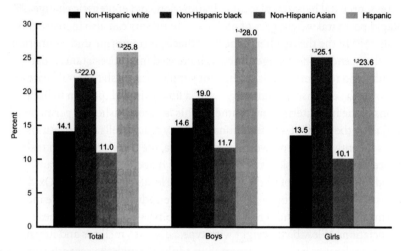

¹ Significantly different from non-Hispanic Asian persons.
² Significantly different from non-Hispanic white persons.
³ Significantly different from non-Hispanic black persons.
Note: Access data table for figure at: https://www.cdc.gov/nchs/data/databriefs/db288_table.pdf#4.
Source: NCHS, National Health and Nutrition Examination Survey, 2015–2016.
Reprinted from Hales CM, Carroll MD, Fryar CD, Ogden CL. Prevalence of obesity among adults and youth: United States, 2015–2016. *NCHS Data Brief.* 2017 Oct;(288):1–8

VI

determined that the prevalence of impaired glucose tolerance was highest in infants with low birth weights who were in utero while mothers were exposed to the famine during the last 2 trimesters of pregnancy. These studies suggested that there is environmental programming in the prenatal period for disease risk in humans.

Maternal risk factors during pregnancy are particularly highlighted as precursors of later disease. Maternal obesity is one of the strongest and best predictors of childhood obesity.[98] Diabetes in pregnancy results in increased risk of childhood obesity and diabetes,[99] as does maternal smoking.[100] Low birth weight (small for gestational age or preterm birth) can also be a marker of increased risk of later obesity, insulin resistance, type 2 diabetes mellitus, hypertension, and cardiovascular disease.[101,102]

Hypothesized mechanisms for the association of low birth weight and increased metabolic and cardiovascular disease risk have included the "thrifty phenotype," postnatal accelerated or catch-up growth, oxidative stress, prenatal hypoxia, placental dysfunction, and epigenetic changes.[103] Rapid postnatal weight gain of underweight infants can also increase this risk.[104,105] In the thrifty phenotype hypothesis, intrauterine undernutrition results in endocrine changes, such as increased insulin resistance, that would tend to divert a limited nutrient supply to nourish the fetal heart and brain at the expense of somatic growth, a life-saving adaptation to limitations of the intrauterine environment. This is accomplished by permanently reducing the number and functional capacity of islet cells. If the fetus is subsequently born into a world of abundance, the increased insulin resistance increases the risk of obesity and type 2 diabetes mellitus, because the child is unable to adapt to the higher glucose levels[105-107] (Fig 33.6). Oxidative stress[108] and prenatal hypoxia[109] have also been advanced as possible mechanisms for creating insulin resistance in low birth weight infants. These associations of low birth weight with type 2 diabetes mellitus and impaired glucose tolerance have been reported in adults through the seventh and eighth decades of life.[110-112]

Prenatal Overnutrition
Macrosomia at birth, indicative of fetal overnutrition, is associated with increased deposition of body fat in childhood and increased risk of obesity[113-115] and the metabolic syndrome.[116] The infant of a mother with diabetes is a model for the influences of fetal overnutrition on postnatal adiposity. Exposure of the fetus to high ambient glucose concentrations stimulates fetal hyperinsulinism, increases fat deposition, and results in macrosomia. This alters the developing neuroendocrine system in a manner that favors deposition of stored calories as fat as well as insulin resistance.[117] In studies controlled for the effects of maternal adiposity, being an infant of a mother with diabetes is still associated with an increased risk of obesity, independent of maternal adiposity before or during pregnancy.[118-120]

Epigenetic mechanisms may be responsible for the ability of the intrauterine environment to affect chronic disease states, such as obesity.[121] Gene-environment interactions result in methylation changes and post-translational histone modifications, which can cause alterations in gene transcription. These changes are heritable, thus programming later disease.[122,123] For example, animal studies have demonstrated transmission to the next generation of programmed phenotypes of diabetes based on maternal gestational diabetes.[124]

Fig 33.6.

The original diagrammatic representation of the thrifty phenotype hypothesis

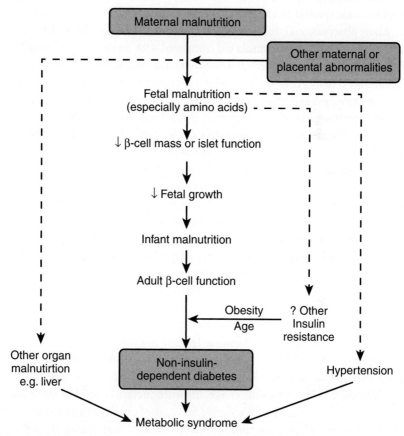

Reprinted with permission from Hales CN, Barker DJ. The thrifty phenotype hypothesis. *Br Med Bull.* 2001;60:5–20

Newborn/Infancy

Infant weight gain has shown a positive association with subsequent obesity.[125–127] Upward crossing of 2 weight-for-length percentiles on the CDC 2000 growth curves in the first 6 months of life is associated with the highest prevalence of obesity 5 and 10 years later.[125] There have also been reports that formulas with higher protein levels are associated with increased infant weight gain. In one study, feeding infants formula containing a lower amount of protein resulted in slower weight gain and lower weight status at 24 months of age.[128] However, in a recent systematic review of this literature, some studies showed decreased weight in low-protein formula fed infants at 6 to 12 months of age, but only 1 of 12 randomized control trials showed an effect on BMI by 6 years of age.[129]

Many observational studies suggest an increased risk of obesity in children who have been formula fed compared with those who have been breastfed.[130] Exclusively breastfed children have been found to have lower mean BMI z-scores than children who were never breastfed, and this may be explained in part by weight gain in infancy.[131] However, any casual association based on these observational studies is unclear. At least 3 studies of siblings who were discordant for breastfeeding status have been performed.[132–134] Two concluded that formula feeding increased the risk of obesity, and the third did not find any association. Another study found that breastfeeding was associated with reduced obesity at 3 years of age compared with formula feeding (7% vs 13%, respectively) and that the sum of triceps and subscapular skinfolds was increased for formula-fed infants.[135] Using pooled data from 4 contemporary cohort studies, a recent publication found that full breastfeeding for <3 months versus ≥3 months increased the odds for being in a rapid growth pattern group in the first 6 years of life, which may persist into adulthood.[136] Again, causative data are lacking. Breastfeeding has also been associated with delayed introduction of solid foods; 8% of breastfeeding mothers introduced solid foods before 4 months of age, compared with 33% of formula-feeding mothers. In addition, the timing of the introduction of solids to infants is also thought to influence their obesity risk. Among formula-fed infants and those who stopped breastfeeding before 4 months of age, the introduction of solid foods before 4 months was associated with a sixfold increase of obesity at 3 years of age.[135] However, a European clinical trial did not find that timing of solid food introduction predicted anthropometric measurements at 24 months of age.[137] A recent systematic review has also concluded that there is limited evidence that introducing complementary food and beverages before 4 months of age is associated with higher odds of overweight/obesity.[138]

Toddler/Preschool Years

Obesity in the young child is associated with significant risk of adult obesity. In one study, more than 50% of obese 3- to 6-year-olds became obese adults.[139] Accelerated weight gain in preschool children has been associated with higher baseline fat intakes and inappropriately large portion sizes.[140] For children 2 to 3 years of age with BMI between the 85th and 95th percentiles, as little as 1 extra sweetened drink a day (eg, juice, soda, fruit drink) doubled their risk of having a BMI greater than the 95th percentile in the following year.[141] At 5 to 6 years of age, body fat normally declines to a minimum, referred to as the point of adiposity rebound, before increasing again until the onset of adolescence. Adiposity rebound before 5 years of age is associated with an increased risk of adult obesity.[142]

In a study of TV time, children as young as 3 years watched an average of 1.7 hours/day. For each 1-hour increase in viewing, they had increased intake of sugar-sweetened beverages, fast food, red and processed meat, total energy intake, and percentage of energy from trans fatty acids. Increased TV time was also associated with lower fruit and vegetable, calcium, and fiber intakes.[143]

Parental obesity is the major predictor of overweight and obesity in this age group. In addition to the strong genetic influence, poor lifestyle choices by parents have a negative influence on the nutrition and activity level of the child. In a large nationally representative sample of 4-year-olds, obesity prevalence was reduced from 24.5% to 14.3% in households in which the following routines were maintained: (1) eating the evening meal (dinner) as a family 6 to 7 times/week; (2) obtaining >10.5 hours of night-time sleep/day; and (3) limiting screen/viewing time (television/video/DVD) to 2 hours or less/day.[144] Preschool children with active parents are more likely to be active than those with sedentary parents, and a low level of physical activity in this age group has been associated with increased subcutaneous fat by first grade.[145] The type of child care can also influence BMI. A toddler cared for in someone else's home is more likely to have a higher BMI than a child cared for in a center or in their own home by someone other than their parent.[146] A recent review of the literature found evidence for a relationship between child care and pediatric obesity, with the most "risky" environment being informal care by a relative or nonrelative. However, the relationships are multifaceted, with many covariates.[147]

School Age

School age is also a period when many eating, physical activity, and sedentary habits are established or reinforced (see Chapter 9: School Nutrition). The effect of parental and family behavior on child behavior remains significant. However, entering school can result in increased exposure to additional obesity risk factors. Exposure to foods competing with school lunches begins in elementary school and escalates through high school.[148] In a study of Florida public middle schools, 99% of participants reported having a snack vending machine in school, 89% a beverage vending machine, and 88% reported having both.[149] Sugar-sweetened beverages can add to total energy consumption and enhance weight gain,[150] and juice consumption of more than 12 oz/day has also been linked to overweight.[151] The AAP recommends that children 7 to 18 years of age should limit their juice consumption to 8 to 12 oz/day, and children 6 years and younger should limit juice to 4 to 6 oz/day.[152]

Many children eat both breakfast and lunch at school. School breakfast and lunch choices may be limited in elementary school. In its 2010 report *School Meals: Building Blocks for Healthy Children*, the Institute of Medicine (now National Academy of Medicine) recommended that the US Department of Agriculture (USDA) adopt standards for menu planning, including increasing the amount and variety of fruits, vegetables, and whole grains; setting a minimum and maximum level of calories; and focusing more on reducing saturated fat and sodium.[153] Mid-morning snacks are often encouraged, and after-school programs usually provide a snack. This means that the majority of a school-aged child's calorie intake may occur outside the home, and parents may be unaware of the quality or quantity of the food consumed. In a study of 8- to 10-year-old African American girls, greater low-fat food preparation at home was related to lower consumption of total fat.[154] Access to screen time is an issue, and snacking increases with hours of television watched, and this effect is magnified in families with one or both parents who are overweight.[155]

Adolescence
During adolescence, parents continue to be responsible to supply a healthy food environment, but adolescents make their own specific choices of food. Increased weight during adolescence not only increases the risk of diabetes during adolescence but also affects risk for adult obesity as well as adult complications. There is a normal increase in insulin resistance at the onset of puberty, peaking at mid–puberty, coinciding with peak height velocity and decreasing to almost prepubertal levels by the completion of puberty. Insulin resistance and BMI are strongly correlated throughout puberty.[88] Obesity increases the risk of insulin resistance and impaired glucose tolerance, a precursor of type 2 diabetes mellitus.[156] In one study, up to 21% of obese adolescents had impaired glucose tolerance,[157] and in another, impaired glucose tolerance was identified in 35% of adolescents with both obesity and a positive family history of type 2 diabetes mellitus.[158] Data from the US National Longitudinal Study of Adolescent Health showed that adolescents with obesity were significantly more likely to have incident severe obesity as an adult, compared with adolescents with normal weight

or overweight (hazard ratio of 16).[159] Elevated BMI in adolescence, even with normalization of weight as an adult, has an independent association with the onset of coronary artery disease in young adulthood (30 years of age).[160]

Children and adolescents 6 to 17 years of age are recommended to get at least 60 minutes of physical activity daily, most of which should be moderate to vigorous aerobic exercise.[161,162] Only 35.8% of high school students met a threshold of 60 minutes of exercise on 5 days/week in 2005. Girls, older adolescents, minority adolescents, and disadvantaged teenagers are less likely to meet this baseline requirement.[161] The most recent obesity clinical practice guidelines published by the Endocrine Society in 2017 recommended that physicians support decreasing inactivity time, with a minimum of 20 minutes of moderate to vigorous physical activity daily, with a goal of 60 minutes.[70] Adolescents with obesity have been found to have limited exercise tolerance because of the greater oxygen demand of their excess body mass. Exercise recommendations for these adolescents should be tailored to allow for activities that can be sustained without fatigue caused by lactate accumulation.[163]

Obesity prevention does not contribute to eating disorders in adolescents. However, some adolescents may misinterpret the need for healthy eating and engage in unhealthy eating patterns such as fad diets and skipping meals, which can lead to eating disorders.[164] The AAP clinical report on eating disorders provides guidance to pediatricians and identifies certain behaviors associated with obesity and eating disorders in teenagers, such as dieting, weight talk, and weight teasing. The clinical report encourages the use of motivational interviewing to bring about behavioral change and encourages family meals and the importance of a healthy body image[164] (see Chapter 38: Eating Disorders in Children and Adolescents).

Comorbidities of Obesity

Obesity adversely affects every organ system. Obesity in childhood constitutes a risk factor for adiposity-related adult morbidity and mortality, even if childhood obesity does not persist. In 40- to 50-year follow-up studies of obese and lean adolescents, adolescent obesity was a powerful predictor of mortality, cardiovascular disease, colorectal cancer, gout, and arthritis, irrespective of body fatness at the time that the morbidity was diagnosed.[165] In a 2016 follow-up study of up to 44 years in 2.3 million adolescents (16–19 years of age), Twig et al showed that adult rates of death from cardiovascular causes were related to adolescent BMI percentile.[166] Not only did they find significantly increased adult cardiovascular mortality in overweight and obese adolescents, but they also found increased adult mortality in the adolescents with BMI in the 50th to 75th percentile, which is considered within the normal BMI range.

Obesity is associated with increased risk for cardiovascular disease risk. Obesity and insulin resistance are associated with metabolic dyslipidemia, a pattern of increased triglycerides, lower high-density lipoprotein cholesterol (HDL-C), and increased concentration of small, dense low-density lipoprotein cholesterol (LDL-C) particles, known to be atherogenic.[167] In a systematic review and meta-analysis of the literature including 63 studies, Friedemann et al concluded that there was increased cardiovascular disease risk factors even in school-aged children with overweight and obesity. Elevated BMI was associated with elevated blood pressure, abnormal lipids, and increased left ventricular mass.[168] Data from the Bogalusa Heart Study showed the tracking of childhood dyslipidemia to adulthood and the association of this dyslipidemia with surrogate markers of atherosclerosis.[169,170] The NHLBI Expert Panel guidelines recommend screening blood pressure by auscultation annually and checking nonfasting non-HDL-cholesterol or fasting lipid screening for all children 9 to 11 years of age (to identify children with genetic dyslipidemias) and for all children with BMI ≥85th percentile for age and sex who are ≥2 years of age.[171] Congestive heart failure resulting from obesity has occurred in morbidly obese adolescents and is thought to result from high metabolic activity of excessive fat, which increases total blood volume and cardiac output and leads to left ventricular dysfunction. Pulmonary hypertension caused by upper airway obstruction can also can lead to signs and symptoms of cardiac failure.[172,173] Other comorbidities that require attention and action include pseudotumor cerebri, slipped capital femoral epiphysis (SCFE), Blount disease, obstructive sleep apnea, nonalcoholic steatohepatitis (NASH), cholelithiasis, polycystic ovarian syndrome (PCOS), and type 2 diabetes mellitus. These comorbidities give urgency to the need to institute prevention and early intervention as well as diagnosis and treatment of pediatric obesity.[174]

Pseudotumor cerebri is defined as increased intracranial pressure with papilledema and normal cerebrospinal fluid in the absence of ventricular enlargement. Pseudotumor has been associated with obesity but may also occur in children with normal weight.[175] The presentation may range from an incidental finding of papilledema on funduscopic examination to headaches, vomiting, blurred vision, or diplopia. Loss of peripheral visual fields and reduction in visual acuity may be present at diagnosis.[176] Neck, shoulder, and back pain have also been reported.[176] Treatment of pseudotumor cerebri includes acetazolamide, ventriculoperitoneal shunt in severe cases, and weight loss.[175,177] Pseudotumor is a diagnosis of exclusion after other causes of increased intracranial pressure are eliminated.[172] Matthews et al recently published the largest study to date of pseudotumor cerebri during childhood.[178] This prospective study found that most cases occurred in children older than 7 years, and in this group, pseudotumor was more common in girls and with increased age and overweight. They found that more than 80% of 12- to 15-year-old cases could be attributed to obesity.[178]

SCFE is a slipping of the femoral epiphysis through the zone of hypertrophic cartilage cells, which are under the influence of gonadal hormones and growth hormone.[179] Fifty to 70% of patients with SCFE are obese.[180] Patients can present with a limp or complaints of groin, thigh, or knee pain. Hips should be examined, and radiographs of both hips should be obtained, because bilateral slips can occur. Medial and posterior displacement of the femoral epiphysis is seen through the growth plate relative to the femoral neck.[181] Treatment requires surgical pinning of the hip.[172] In a recent retrospective study, investigators studied all children presenting to their institution between 1998 and 2005, measured their BMI percentile, and followed them until closure of the bilateral proximal femoral physes.[182] Patients with a BMI ≥95th percentile were significantly more likely to present with bilateral disease, with the prevalence of bilateral SCFE in this study 40%.

The diagnosis of Blount disease involves the identification of bowing of the tibia and femur, affecting 1 or both knees. This condition results from the overgrowth of the medial aspect of the proximal tibial metaphysis. Obesity has been reported in two thirds of patients with Blount disease,[183] and the risk of Blount disease is increased by vitamin D deficiency.[184] Treatment requires surgical correction and weight loss.

Obstructive sleep apnea (OSA) is commonly associated with obesity. This condition is defined as a disorder of breathing during sleep characterized by prolonged partial upper airway obstruction or intermittent complete obstruction that disrupts normal ventilation during sleep and normal sleep patterns.[185] Symptoms can include night-time awakening, restless sleep, difficulty awakening in the morning, daytime sleepiness, napping, enuresis, decreased concentration and memory, and poor school performance.[186] Night-time polysomnography is the diagnostic procedure of choice to make this diagnosis. If left untreated, children can have pulmonary hypertension, systemic hypertension, and right-sided heart failure.[185] Weight gain, hypertrophy of the tonsils and adenoids, and intercurrent upper respiratory infections can provoke symptoms. Studies in children have shown

VI

a significant association between the presence of mild to moderate OSA and increased insulin resistance and cardiometabolic risk.[187] Results from the Bogalusa Heart Study suggest that pediatric obesity is associated with increased OSA risk as an adult.[188]

NASH is suspected when elevated liver enzymes are found in the context of fatty liver identified by ultrasonography or other imaging techniques in the absence of other causes of liver disease. It is a progressive form of nonalcoholic fatty liver disease (NAFLD). NAFLD is defined by having liver fat >5% of liver weight (not caused by consumption of alcohol) and is associated with insulin resistance.[189] NAFLD has been found to be more prevalent in Hispanic children.[190] Twenty to 25% of obese children have been found to have evidence of steatohepatitis.[191] The definitive diagnosis is by liver biopsy in which evidence of inflammatory infiltrates and fibrosis can be seen; however, biopsy is not often not considered clinically indicated because it does not change treatment. NASH can progress to cirrhosis and end-stage liver disease.[192] Weight loss reduces fatty infiltration and may decrease fibrosis. Current AAP recommendations are to screen children with BMI ≥85th percentile for age and sex for NAFLD biannually with aspartate aminotransferase ad alanine aminotransferase measurements[193] (see Chapter 43: Liver Disease).

Risk of cholelithiasis is higher for people of Hispanic ethnicity and increases with BMI.[194] Cholelithiasis symptoms in children include abdominal pain and tenderness, with diagnosis made by ultrasonography and appropriate laboratory studies.

PCOS is a condition characterized by hyperandrogenism, menstrual irregularities/ovulatory dysfunction, and polycystic ovaries.[195] Pediatric obesity and overweight are associated with increased odds of PCOS in adolescents.[196] Clinical signs and symptoms include oligomenorrhea or amenorrhea, hirsutism, acne, polycystic ovaries, and obesity. There is some evidence that girls with premature adrenarche are at risk of PCOS.[197] A recent study comparing obese adolescent girls with PCOS versus obese adolescent girls without PCOS found that girls with PCOS had increased insulin resistance by hyperinsulinemic euglycemic clamp, greater carotid intima-media thickness, stiffer arteries, a more atherogenic lipoprotein cholesterol distribution, and increased free fatty acids, which are markers of cardiovascular disease risk.[198]

Increased obesity among children has led to a significant increase in the prevalence type 2 diabetes mellitus (T2D) during childhood. Obesity leads to insulin resistance and a compensatory increase in insulin secretion.

However, a loss of first-phase insulin secretion and relative insulin deficiency lead to hyperglycemia. Diabetes mellitus can be diagnosed by HbA1c, oral glucose tolerance test, fasting glucose, and/or random glucose in criteria established by the American Diabetes Association (ADA). T2D disproportionately affects minority and socially stressed youth and has a strong genetic component. The ADA recommends screening asymptomatic children with BMI ≥85th percentile and with 1 or more additional risk factors for elevated glucose levels. Risk factors include maternal history of diabetes mellitus or gestational diabetes, first- or second-degree relative with T2D, high-risk race/ethnicity, and signs of or conditions associated with insulin resistance (acanthosis nigricans, hypertension, dyslipidemia, PCOS, or small for gestational age or low birth weight).[199] Symptoms include polyuria, polydipsia, and nocturia, and unlike adults, youth with T2D present not infrequently with diabetic ketoacidosis. The TODAY study was the first multicenter, randomized clinical trial of T2D in youth.[200] This landmark 5-year study demonstrated higher rates of failure of metformin therapy and a more rapid decline in beta cell function in youth[200] with T2D than has been observed in adults.[201,202] In addition, significant numbers of youth with T2D had diabetes complications already present at baseline and even more had such complications at follow-up. First-line treatment for T2D is lifestyle modification through diet and exercise. Currently, the only medications approved by the US Food and Drug Administration (FDA) for T2D in youth are insulin and metformin.

Obesity and T2D have been associated with mental health disorders, such as depression and anxiety.[193,203,204] Obesity is associated with stigma and shame, and children are often bullied by peers. Stigma and shame can lead to isolation and depression as well.[205] The AAP recommends screening children with obesity for mental health disorders.[193]

Metabolic syndrome is a cluster of component cardiometabolic risk factors known to convey increased risk for cardiovascular disease and T2D in adults. The component risk factors include central obesity, elevated blood pressure, elevated triglyceride levels, decreased HCL-C, increased LDL-C, and hyperglycemia.[172] The pathophysiologic origins of this condition lie in insulin resistance and related adipose tissue dysfunction. There has been much controversy as to how and even whether to define the metabolic syndrome in children. However, in a recent clinical report, the AAP recommended that pediatricians not focus on a particular definition or specific cut-points of cardiometabolic risk factors, because most of these risks lie on a continuum.[206] The focus for intervention should be on screening youth

VI

and identifying those with clustering of risk factors. Comorbid conditions, such as NAFLD, OSA, mental health disorders, and PCOS, should also be screened for and treated.

Prevention of Childhood Obesity

Although community, family, and individual change is crucial in obesity prevention and treatment, the interaction of the complex array of factors that result in either healthy or unhealthy weight can be illustrated by the ecologic model of predictors of childhood overweight in Fig 33.7. This model can serve as a tool for identifying partners and highlighting opportunities for change and can be used in a 360-degree assessment for an individual child/family or community. In addition, a recent AAP policy statement stressed the importance of screening children for food insecurity, as 21% of children live in households without consistent access to adequate food.[207] Recommendations for obesity prevention and treatment can be found in the 2015 AAP clinical report "The Role of the Pediatrician in Primary Prevention of Obesity."[72]

Fig 33.7.
Ecological model of predictors of childhood overweight

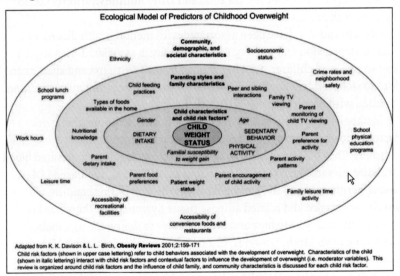

Reprinted with permission from Davison KK, Birch LL. Childhood overweight: a contextual model and recommendations for future research. *Obes Rev.* 2001;2(3):159–171.

The 2012 Institute of Medicine report "Accelerating Progress in Obesity Prevention: Solving the Weight of the Nation" established 5 goals for obesity prevention for the United States and emphasized the importance of obesity prevention in the pediatric population.[208] Goal 1 is to make physical activity an integral and routine part of daily life and includes a recommendation to adopt physical activity requirements for licensed child care providers. Goal 2 is to create food and beverage environments that ensure that healthy food and beverage options are the routine and easy choice and includes a recommendation to increase the availability of lower-calorie and healthier food and beverage options for children in restaurants. Goal 3 is to transform messages about physical activity and nutrition that surround Americans in their environment and specifically recommends implementation of common standards for marketing foods and beverages to children and adolescents. Goal 4 is to expand the role of health care providers, insurers, and employers and recommends that standards or practice include routine screening of BMI, counseling, and behavioral interventions for children and adolescents. Goal 5 is to make schools a national focal point for obesity prevention. Schools should be required to provide quality physical education and opportunities for physical activity. There should be strong nutritional standards for all foods and beverages sold or provided in schools. Thus, prevention of childhood obesity remains a public health priority, because obesity is the most prevalent chronic health condition in the pediatric population. Although, as noted in the report, many constituents of the society need to be mobilized to address this problem, pediatric primary care practice has a unique role to play and is an integral part of the solution.

Health-promotion efforts should aim at removing sugar-sweetened beverages from children's diets. There is significant evidence of a strong association between dietary sugars, particularly those in sugar-sweetened beverages (SSBs) and an increase in pediatric adiposity.[209,210] The ideal beverage for children at all meals and during the day is water, whereas low-fat or fat-free, preferably unflavored, milk also has an important place in the diet of children beginning at 12 months of age. Fruit juice (100% juice only) should not be consumed before 1 year of age and should limited after that. Eating fruit should be encouraged over consumption of fruit juice. Recently, multiple health organizations have issued statements focused on the dangers of added sugars in the diet, which are estimated to constitute 16% of calories consumed by American children.[211] Added sugars (sugars that are ingredients in produced or processed foods or those eaten separately or added at the table) are associated with increased hypertension,[212,213]

VI

dyslipidemia,[214,215] and in those who are overweight, insulin resistance.[216,217] The 2015 Dietary Guidelines for Americans recommended that added sugars constitute less than 10% of calories consumed.[162] Similarly, the World Health Organization recommended limiting sugar intake to less than 10% of total calories, with increased benefits of decreasing to less than 5%. In its recent scientific statement, the American Heart Association recommended that children 2 years and older eat ≤25 g (6 teaspoons) of added sugars per day. Children younger than 2 years should avoid added sugars completely.[211]

One of the places where children can be exposed to energy-dense and nutrient poor drinks is at school. The 2012 Institute of Medicine Report stated that children consume 35% to 40% of their daily energy in school.[208] As outlined in the AAP policy statement "Snacks, Sweetened Beverages, Added Sugars, and Schools,"[148] food is available at school in 3 different venues: federally funded school meal programs, competitive items sold outside of school meals (vending machines, school meals, etc), and foods available in informal settings, such as bake sales, fundraisers, and school parties. The statement advocates for pediatricians to become more involved in local schools and use their roles to promote foods with increased nutritional value, variety, appropriate portion sizes, and high quality.[148]

To address obesity prevention effectively in clinical practice, pediatricians should become familiar with the complex and interconnected factors that lead to excessive weight gain.[218] They should understand how these factors converge in a developmental fashion and how they create important periods for preventive intervention. This intervention includes screening for food insecurity among children and families, as mentioned earlier.[207] By better understanding the environmental determinants of obesity, including those that they cannot control, pediatric practitioners can improve their ability to provide recommendations that are relevant to their patients and their families.

Most prevention strategies that can be used in pediatric practice have not been rigorously tested through scientific research. However, preliminary evidence, indirect evidence, and inferences from other settings provide clues to recommend evidence-informed approaches, especially those with low risk for a negative health effect or those with known health benefits. Although the prevention messages are similar for all, counseling should be tailored to the child's developmental stage as well as the socioeconomic, cultural, and psychological characteristics of the family.

Pediatric practice is critical in identifying children who are early on the path to become obese by calculating BMI and plotting it on percentile charts at every health care visit. Although the USPSTF recommends screening for obesity starting at 6 years of age,[219] the Endocrine Society and the AAP recommend BMI screening for overweight/obesity starting at 2 years of age.[70,193] Children at risk can also be identified through the nutrition, sedentary, and physical activities questions that are part of the *Bright Futures: Guidelines for Health Supervision of Infants, Children, and Adolescents* templates as well as through family history.

Education and advice alone are likely to be ineffective in most cases for obesity prevention. Pediatricians should, therefore, become familiar with other forms of interventions that they can apply to obesity prevention, such as behavior modification techniques, environment control approaches, or the promotion of improved parenting skills. They should also become familiar with the resources available in the area they are serving so that they are better suited to help each individual family.

Nutrition is a key aspect of obesity prevention. Promotion of a diet rich in foods with low caloric density (vegetables, fruits, whole grain, low-fat dairy products, lean meats, lean fish, legumes) and poor in foods with high caloric density (fat-rich meats, fried foods, baked goods, sweets, cheeses, oil-based sauces) is likely to contribute to the prevention of obesity (see Appendix P).

Recent AAP statements also address limiting pediatric screen use, which includes television, video games, texting, computer use not related to school, and other forms of electronic entertainment or communications. These guidelines discourage screen use other than video chatting for children before 18 to 24 months.[220,221] Promotion of active play, lifestyle, family-based, or sport-based moderate to vigorous physical activity for a total of 60 minute per day on most days is likely to contribute to the prevention of obesity.

Prevention of childhood obesity should start by promoting healthy maternal weight beginning in the prenatal period, smoking cessation before pregnancy, appropriate gestational weight gain and diet, breastfeeding, and appropriate weight gain in infancy. The next steps are the transition to healthier foods with weaning, elimination of sedentary entertainment, active play for physical activity, and parental role modeling of healthy dietary and physical activity behaviors. The AAP has recommended a staged approach to prevention and treatment of pediatric obesity including the following elements: prevention at the office level, prevention at the community level, structured weight management, comprehensive weight management, and tertiary care/hospital management of obesity and comorbidities[193] (Fig 33.8).

Fig 33.8—Part 1.

Assessment and management of pediatric obesity

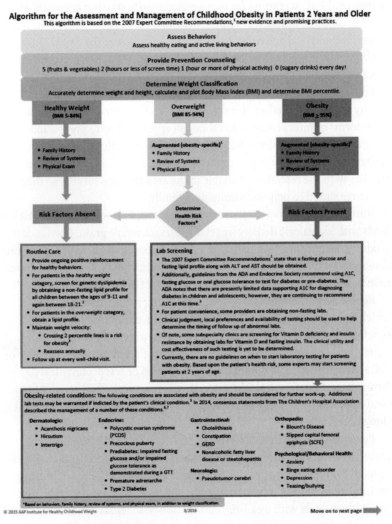

Algorithm for the Assessment and Management of Childhood Obesity in Patients 2 Years and Older
This algorithm is based on the 2007 Expert Committee Recommendations,[1] new evidence and promising practices.

Assess Behaviors
Assess healthy eating and active living behaviors

Provide Prevention Counseling
5 (fruits & vegetables) 2 (hours or less of screen time) 1 (hour or more of physical activity) 0 (sugary drinks) every day!

Determine Weight Classification
Accurately determine weight and height, calculate and plot Body Mass Index (BMI) and determine BMI percentile.

Healthy Weight (BMI 5-84%)	Overweight (BMI 85-94%)	Obesity (BMI ≥ 95%)
• Family History • Review of Systems • Physical Exam	Augmented (obesity-specific)[1] • Family History • Review of Systems • Physical Exam	Augmented (obesity-specific)[1] • Family History • Review of Systems • Physical Exam

Risk Factors Absent ← **Determine Health Risk Factors[a]** → **Risk Factors Present**

Routine Care
• Provide ongoing positive reinforcement for healthy behaviors.
• For patients in the *healthy weight* category, screen for genetic dyslipidemia by obtaining a non-fasting lipid profile for all children between the ages of 9-11 and again between 18-21.[2]
• For patients in the *overweight* category, obtain a lipid profile.
• Maintain weight velocity:
  • Crossing 2 percentile lines is a risk for obesity[4]
  • Reassess annually
• Follow up at every well-child visit.

Lab Screening
• The 2007 Expert Committee Recommendations[1] state that a fasting glucose and fasting lipid profile along with ALT and AST should be obtained.
• Additionally, guidelines from the ADA and Endocrine Society recommend using A1C, fasting glucose or oral glucose tolerance to test for diabetes or pre-diabetes. The ADA notes that there are presently limited data supporting A1C for diagnosing diabetes in children and adolescents; however, they are continuing to recommend A1C at this time.[3]
• For patient convenience, some providers are obtaining non-fasting labs.
• Clinical judgment, local preferences and availability of testing should be used to help determine the timing of follow up of abnormal labs.
• Of note, some subspecialty clinics are screening for Vitamin D deficiency and insulin resistance by obtaining labs for Vitamin D and fasting insulin. The clinical utility and cost effectiveness of such testing is yet to be determined.
• Currently, there are no guidelines on when to start laboratory testing for patients with obesity. Based upon the patient's health risk, some experts may start screening patients at 2 years of age.

Obesity-related conditions: The following conditions are associated with obesity and should be considered for further work-up. Additional lab tests may be warranted if indicted by the patient's clinical condition.[5] In 2014, consensus statements from The Children's Hospital Association described the management of a number of these conditions.[6,7]

Dermatologic:
• Acanthosis nigricans
• Hirsutism
• Intertrigo

Endocrine:
• Polycystic ovarian syndrome (PCOS)
• Precocious puberty
• Prediabetes: Impaired fasting glucose and/or impaired glucose tolerance as demonstrated during a GTT
• Premature adrenarche
• Type 2 Diabetes

Gastrointestinal:
• Cholelithiasis
• Constipation
• GERD
• Nonalcoholic fatty liver disease or steatohepatitis

Neurologic:
• Pseudotumor cerebri

Orthopedic:
• Blount's Disease
• Slipped capital femoral epiphysis (SCFE)

Psychological/Behavioral Health:
• Anxiety
• Binge eating disorder
• Depression
• Teasing/bullying

[a] Based on behaviors, family history, review of systems, and physical exam, in addition to weight classification.

© 2015 AAP Institute for Healthy Childhood Weight   8/2016   **Move on to next page** ▶

From AAP Institute for Healthy Childhood Weight, 2016. Available at: https://ihcw.aap.org/Documents/Assessment%20%20and%20Management%20of%20Childhood%20Obesity%20Algorithm_FINAL.pdf

Fig 33.8—Part 2.

Assessment and management of pediatric obesity

Management and Treatment Stages for Patients with Overweight or Obesity

- Patients should start at the least intensive stage and advance through the stages based upon the response to treatment, age, BMI, health risks and motivation.
- An empathetic and empowering counseling style, such as motivational interviewing, should be employed to support patient and family behavior change.[8,9]
- Children age 2 – 5 who have obesity should not lose more than 1 pound/month; older children and adolescents with obesity should not lose more than an average of 2 pounds/week.

Stage 1 Prevention Plus

Where/By Whom: Primary Care Office/Primary Care Provider
What: Planned follow-up themed visits (15-20 min) focusing on behaviors that resonate with the patient, family and provider. Consider partnering with dietician, social worker, athletic trainer or physical therapist for added support and counseling.
Goals: Positive behavior change regardless of change in BMI. Weight maintenance or a decrease in BMI velocity.[4]
Follow-up: Tailor to the patient and family motivation. Many experts recommend at least monthly follow-up visits. After 3 – 6 months, if the BMI/weight status has not improved consider advancing to Stage 2.

Stage 2 Structured Weight Management

Where/By Whom: Primary Care Office/Primary Care Provider with appropriate training
What: Same intervention as Stage 1 while including more intense support and structure to achieve healthy behavior change.
Goals: Positive behavior change. Weight maintenance or a decrease in BMI velocity.
Follow-up: Every 2 - 4 weeks as determined by the patient, family and physician. After 3 – 6 months, if the BMI/weight status has not improved consider advancing to Stage 3.

Stage 3 Comprehensive Multi-disciplinary Intervention

Where/By Whom: Pediatric Weight Management Clinic/Multi-disciplinary Team
What: Increased intensity of behavior changes, frequency of visits, and specialists involved. Structured behavioral modification program, including food and activity monitoring, and development of short-term diet and physical activity goals.
Goals: Positive behavior change. Weight maintenance or a decrease in BMI velocity.
Follow-up: Weekly or at least every 2 – 4 weeks as determined by the patient, family, and physician. After 3 – 6 months, if the BMI/weight status has not improved consider advancing to Stage 4.

Stage 4 Tertiary Care Intervention

Where/By Whom: Pediatric Weight Management Center/Providers with expertise in treating childhood obesity
What: Recommended for children with BMI ≥ 95% and significant comorbidities if unsuccessful with Stages 1 - 3. Also recommended for children > 99% who have shown no improvement under Stage 3. Intensive diet and activity counseling with consideration of the use of medications and surgery.
Goals: Positive behavior change. Decrease in BMI.
Follow-up: Determine based upon patient's motivation and medical status.

References
1. Barlow S, Expert Committee. Expert committee recommendations regarding prevention, assessment, and treatment of child and adolescent overweight and obesity: Summary report. *Pediatrics.* 2007;120(4):S164-S192.
2. US Department of Health and Human Services. Expert panel on integrated guidelines for cardiovascular health and risk reduction in children and adolescents: Full report. 2012.
3. American Diabetes Association. Classification and diagnosis of diabetes. Sec 2. In Standards of Medical Care in Diabetes – 2015. *Diabetes Care* 2015;38(Suppl 1):S8-S16.
4. Taveras EM, Rifas-Shiman SL, Sherry B, et al. Crossing growth percentiles in infancy and risk of obesity in childhood. *Arch Pediatr Adolesc Med.* 2011;165(11):993-998.
5. Copeland K, Silverstein J, Moore K, et al. Management of newly diagnosed type 2 Diabetes Mellitus (T2DM) in children and adolescents. *Pediatrics.* 2013;131(2):364-382.
6. Estrada E, Eneli I, Hampl S, et al. Children's Hospital Association consensus statements for comorbidities of childhood obesity. *Child Obes.* 2014;10(4):304-317.
7. Haemer MA, Grow HM, Fernandez C, et al. Addressing prediabetes in childhood obesity treatment programs: Support from research and current practice. *Child Obes.* 2014;10(4):292-303.
8. Preventing weight bias: Helping without harming in clinical practice. Rudd Center for Food Policy and Obesity website. http://biastoolkit.uconnruddcenter.org/
9. Resnicow K, McMaster F, Bocian A, et al. Motivational interviewing and dietary counseling for obesity in primary care: An RCT. *Pediatrics.* 2015;134(4): 649-657.

This algorithm was developed by the American Academy of Pediatrics Institute for Healthy Childhood Weight (Institute). The Institute serves as a translational engine, moving policy and research from theory into practice in healthcare, communities, and homes. The Institute gratefully acknowledges the shared commitment and support of its Founding Sponsor, Nestlé.

From AAP Institute for Healthy Childhood Weight, 2016. Available at: https://ihcw.aap.org/Documents/Assessment%20%20and%20Management%20of%20Childhood%20Obesity%20Algorithm_FINAL.pdf

Prevention—Primary Care Provider

Universal attention to age-appropriate healthy nutrition and activity should be part of every child's primary care. The AAP Clinical Decision Support 10 chart[193] recommends using the following mnemonic:

5 **Eat at least 5 servings of fruits and vegetables each day**

2 **Limit screen time unrelated to school to 2 hours or less each day**

1 **Hour or more of moderate to vigorous physical activity every day and 20 minutes of vigorous activity at least 2 times/week**

0 **Sweetened beverages; use water and low-fat milk instead of sugar sweetened drinks**

Additional preventive measures should be taken with children with a BMI between the 85th and 94th percentiles. In addition to the prevention message earlier, families should be encouraged to (1) eat a daily breakfast; (2) limit meals outside the home; (3) have family meals 5 to 6 times/week; and (4) allow the child to self-regulate at meals without overly restrictive behavior.

The goal should be weight maintenance with subsequent growth resulting in a decreased BMI. Follow-up visits should occur monthly. After 3 to 6 months, if there is no improvement in BMI/weight, move to the next stage.

Prevention: Community

Community factors that can be improved to decrease the prevalence of obesity through various measures to improve the environment include: (1) improving access to healthy foods by increasing availability of and safe access to supermarkets; (2) encouraging farmers markets to accept SNAP (Supplemental Nutrition Assistance Program, formerly known as Food Stamps) benefits and food coupons from the Special Supplemental Nutrition Program for Women, Infants, and Children (WIC) (see Chapter 49: Preventing Food Insecurity); (3) creating incentives for corner markets and vendors to carry healthier foods; and (4) increasing availability of healthier foods at public venues. Strategies to limit unhealthy foods in communities by limiting fast food outlets and restricting availability of unhealthy foods at public venues should be implemented. Communities can influence point-of-purchase decision making by incentivizing restaurants to provide healthier food options; requiring menu labeling (nutrition information including calories), smaller portion sizes, lower fat and salt content of foods; increasing access to safe drinking water to replace sugar-sweetened beverages; and encouraging family-friendly and healthy vending machine policies. Communities can also promote healthier eating using media campaigns and considering tax strategies that discourage consumption of energy-dense but nutrient-poor foods.

Physical activity in the community can be promoted by building and maintaining infrastructure for safe indoor and outdoor activity, improving access to safe recreational facilities, creating and promoting youth athletic leagues, encouraging walking and biking, and reducing transit fares.

Schools are important locations where improvements in healthy eating and activity can occur by implementing the recently issued USDA rules for healthier school meals that follow the 2015 Dietary Guidelines for Americans, which include reducing the availability of competitive energy-dense, nutrient-poor foods sold in schools (including fundraisers) and providing healthier vending machine food and drink choices.[148] This is also reviewed in the AAP policy statement, "Snacks, Sweetened Beverages, Added Sugars, and Schools."[148] Physical education opportunities should be increased, and active recess should be promoted. Physical activity should be incorporated into the school day and in after-school programs.

Pediatricians are in a unique position to influence healthy behaviors of families and patients in the community. Physicians' offices can support healthy eating among the office staff and provide guides to sources of healthy foods in the community including nutrition services provided through federal, state, and local health and nutrition agencies (see Chapter 49: Preventing Food Insecurity). Vending in hospitals and clinic sites can include healthier snacks and menu labeling. Healthy eating and physical activity can be promoted in the office with posters, brochures, and health-related magazines. TV and video can be limited in waiting rooms, and families can be provided with resources for after-school/family activities to try at home. Physicians can institute employee wellness programs in their practices; encourage physical activity for employees, patients, and families through events; and provide lists of community activities for family participation. More in-depth strategies and examples for community intervention can be found on the AAP obesity website under the heading Policy Tool at: https://ihcw.aap.org/Pages/popot.aspx.

VI

Treatment of Pediatric Obesity

Structured Weight Management (Primary Care Provider With Appropriate Training)

Structured weight management is for children for whom prevention was not successful, for children with a BMI from the 85th through 94th percentile, and for children with BMI greater than the 95th percentile. Counseling should build on all previous messages and include (1) a plan for utilization of a balanced macronutrient diet emphasizing a low amount of energy-dense foods; (2) increased structured daily meals and snacks; (3) supervised active play of at least 60 minutes/day; (4) screen time limited to 1 hour or less/day; and (5) increased monitoring (screen time, physical activity, dietary intake, restaurant logs) by provider, patients, and family.

For young children, the goal is weight maintenance, resulting in a decreasing BMI as age increases and the child grows in height. In children 2 to 11 years of age, weight loss should not exceed 1 lb (0.5 kg) per month or an average of 2 pounds (1.0 kg) per week in older overweight/obese children and adolescents. Follow-up visits should occur monthly, and if no improvement in BMI is observed after 3 to 6 months, the patient should be advanced to a more comprehensive, multidisciplinary intervention.

In 2017, the USPSTF published its findings that among 42 pediatric obesity lifestyle-based intervention trials to lose weight, those with approximately 26 hours or more of contact were successful in losing excess weight compared with usual care after 6 to 12 months. Interventions with ≥52 hours of contact showed increased improvements in blood pressure compared with controls.[222]

Comprehensive Multidisciplinary Intervention—Weight Management Clinic With Multidisciplinary Team (Expert Committee)[193]

Intervention is built on previous stages and includes (1) structured behavioral modification program, including food and activity monitoring and development of short-term diet and physical activity goals; and (2) involvement of primary caregivers/families for behavioral modification in children younger than 12 years and training of primary caregivers/families for all children. Goals are weight maintenance or gradual weight loss until BMI reaches less than the 85th percentile, not to exceed 1 lb (0.5 kg) per month in children 2 to 5 years of age or 2 pounds (1.0 kg) per week in older obese children and adolescents, as mentioned previously. Evidence suggests that younger obese children respond better to lifestyle modification than older adolescents,[223] so intervention should occur early. Further, the child does not have to achieve a normal BMI to obtain benefit. Weight loss and BMI reduction of 5% to 10% can result in metabolic improvements.[224] A multidisciplinary team, including a mental health professional, nutritionist, exercise specialist, and medical provider, should be included in the treatment.[193] Frequent office visits with weekly visits for at least 8 to 12 weeks have been shown to be most efficacious,[193] although not always feasible.

Tertiary Care Interventions—Hospital Based With Expertise in Childhood Obesity for Selected Patients

This intervention is recommended for children with BMI greater than the 95th percentile with significant comorbidities unsuccessful with previous stages and children with BMI greater than the 99th percentile who have shown no improvement under comprehensive multidisciplinary intervention. It is especially relevant to children demonstrating 1 or more comorbidities associated with obesity. This intervention involves a multidisciplinary team with expertise in childhood obesity, operating under a designated protocol, and may involve continued diet and activity counseling, consideration of possible additions such as meal replacements, very low-calorie diet, medication, and surgery.

The expert committee also recommended techniques such as motivational interviewing and/or brief focused negotiation to help families and patients increase motivation and confidence that they can accomplish lifestyle change.[193] Cognitive behavioral therapy has also been used in treatment of childhood obesity with promising results.[225]

For every child, a detailed history and physical examination should be performed to assess each child for current obesity-related morbidities and for birth history or family history that suggests risk of such morbidities. Anthropometric data should be plotted on height and weight velocity charts as well as standard BMI curves. For those with severe obesity (BMI ≥99th percentile for age and sex), new growth charts showing a child's BMI as a percentage of the 95th percentile allows for better tracking of progress.[76]

Treatment Strategies

The time required to significantly reduce adiposity can be estimated to be 1 year during normally rapid weight gain periods, such as adolescence, and 2 years during periods of slower weight gain. One to 2 years of weight maintenance will reduce excess weight-for-height by approximately 20% in a growing child.

VI

If gradual growth in stature in accordance with the child's weight is not possible because the child is already obese by adult standards (ie, body mass is so great that BMI will still be greater than the 85th percentile, even if weight remains stable until adult stature is achieved), then a weight-loss regimen, as outlined later, should be considered.

Therapeutic weight reduction is usually indicated for the child with evidence of current adiposity-related morbidity. Any therapeutic regimen should involve the entire family as well as the child's school. Frequent physical examination of the child and monitoring of school performance should be included.

Dietary Intervention
Recommendations for changes in diet should never be presented in a negative manner. The emphasis should be on healthy eating and the value of good nutrition, and, if at all possible, the child and the entire family should follow the same nutritional plan. This allows the parents to provide a healthy nutritional environment for the whole family, reduce food triggers, and allow for positive role modeling. If appropriate, the significance of any evident reduction in morbidity (eg, lowering of blood pressure or cholesterol) can be reinforced. Reasonable goals in the form of behavioral change that are achievable by the next visit should be set jointly with provider, family, and child. The composition of the diet should contain the recommended amounts of protein, essential fatty acids, vitamins, and minerals and should be low in saturated fats.[226] Fiber intake should be encouraged, and simple sugars should be reduced. The USDA website (www. Choosemyplate.gov) can provide families with food group information, tips, and recipes to use at home. Parents and adult caregivers should understand the important role they play in the development of proper eating habits in children. Parents' food preferences, the quantities and variety of foods in the home, and the parents' eating behavior and physical activity patterns all determine how supportive the home environment is to the child.

Weight reduction will occur only if energy expenditure exceeds energy intake in a consistent manner. A 300- to 400-kcal/day energy deficit should result in weight loss of approximately 1 lb (0.5 kg) per week. This can be determined by assessing dietary history or as calculated on the basis of a formula relating anthropometry to energy expenditure (eg, the Harris-Benedict equation).[227] A reduction in soft drinks/soda, sports drinks, or juice could accomplish this goal, as could reduction in eating fast food. Weight reduction, per se, causes decreased energy expenditure. This phenomenon, plus the ongoing loss of metabolic mass, necessitates periodic downward adjustments of energy intake to sustain ongoing weight loss unless there is ongoing increase in aerobic activity and increase in lean body mass.

Activity/Exercise

Exercise will promote increased muscle mass, thereby raising total metabolic rate, and reduce visceral adipose tissue mass, which may independently lower the risk of hyperlipidemia and diabetes mellitus. *However, the energy cost of even vigorous exercise is low when compared with the calorie content of many foods and snacks.* For example, walking at 3 miles/hour for 1 hour consumes approximately 200 kcal, approximately the same amount contained in a 1¾-oz bag of potato chips. Food should not be used as an incentive to exercise. Clinicians should encourage children to participate in organized or individual sports (stressing participation, not watching from the bench) and advocate for better community- and school-based activity programs.

Television, Screen Time

Food constitutes the most heavily advertised product on children's TV in the United States. Adiposity was significantly correlated with time spent watching TV but not with time spent watching videos,[228] suggesting that the bulk of the positive association of TV watching and adiposity is attributable to the fact that approximately 60% of advertising that is devoted to food.[229]

Pharmacotherapy

For adolescents with severe obesity in whom behavioral intervention is not successful, weight loss medications can be used. The Agency for Healthcare Research and Quality performed a systematic evidence review for the USPSTF.[222] Orlistat (Xenical [Roche Pharmaceuticals, Nutley, NJ]) is the only drug approved by the FDA for weight loss for the pediatric age group, specifically in children older than 12 years. The mechanism of action is by decreasing intestinal lipase activity, which results in decreased hydrolysis of dietary fat and, thus, allows approximately 30% of the fat ingested to pass through the gut undigested.[230] The most common adverse effects are gastrointestinal,[222] with loose stools, flatulence, and oily discharge. These effects make orlistat less appealing as a therapeutic option. Inhibition of pancreatic lipase also causes loss of fat-soluble vitamins (A, D, E, and K) in the stool, and vitamin supplementation is recommended.[231,232] Studies have shown small weight loss effects (BMI reduction <1 (~5–7 lb),[222] and its use needs to be combined with a structured weight-management program.[233] The use of lipase inhibitors has not been well studied in adolescents. Initial studies of lipase inhibitors as part of weight-reduction therapy in obese adolescents

VI

have reported that all patients experienced some gastrointestinal adverse effects and that 1 in 3 found them intolerable.[234] Lipase-inhibitor therapy in adolescents provoked significant reductions in circulating concentrations of vitamin D, even when they were provided with vitamin supplements.[235] Because of the possible effects of impaired vitamin D absorption on the extensive bone mineralization that occurs in adolescence, the use of any therapy that inhibits such absorption should be thoroughly investigated before it is prescribed for teenagers.

Metformin has been used off label for weight loss, and like orlistat, has been associated with small decreases in excess weight, on the magnitude of −0.86 kg/m².[222] Most studies have been of limited duration and did not show significant improvement of serum glucose, lipids, or blood pressure.[222] However, metformin is only approved by the FDA for treatment of T2D and not for weight loss during childhood. Metformin is also associated with gastrointestinal adverse effects, such as abdominal pain and bloating, which can decrease compliance.

Bariatric Surgery

Bariatric surgery has been increasing in adolescents in the last several years as the only method that has proven effective to date to treat subjects with a BMI greater than 50 kg/m². The most common laparoscopic bariatric procedures are Roux-en-Y gastric bypass surgery, laparoscopic adjustable gastric banding, and sleeve gastrectomy. There is extensive experience with adult gastric bypass surgery. Briefly, a 15- to 30-mL gastric pouch is created surgically, just below the gastroesophageal junction, and is then anastomosed to the jejunum. The least invasive and most reversible procedure is an adjustable gastric banding, in which a prosthetic band with an adjustable inner diameter is placed around the proximal stomach, restricting food entry to the volume of a small proximal gastric pouch. The band is connected to a subcutaneous port into which saline can be injected to alter the inner diameter of the band, thus requiring close follow-up with a physician and perhaps resulting in earlier detection of any complications. Sleeve gastrectomy is the newest bariatric procedure in which the goal is to reduce the stomach to about 25% of its original size by surgical removal of a large portion of the stomach following the major curve. The open edges are then attached together to form a sleeve or tube with a banana shape.

Current expert opinion recommendations for guidelines and criteria needed to deliver safe and effective bariatric surgical specialty care to adolescents have been published.[236,237] It is appropriate to consider bariatric surgery in some extremely obese adolescents, particularly those with obesity-related comorbidities, with the caveat that long-term follow-up and monitoring is needed. Agreed on criteria for pediatric bariatric surgery include the following[238-240]:

1. The adolescent has attained at least 95% of adult height.
2. The adolescent has a BMI ≥35 with major obesity-related comorbidities (T2D, moderate to severe obstructive sleep apnea, pseudotumor cerebri) or a BMI of ≥40 with mild comorbidities.
3. Severe obesity and comorbidities persist despite a formal program of lifestyle modification and weight management.
4. The adolescent demonstrates commitment to comprehensive medical and psychological evaluation before and after surgery.
5. The adolescent demonstrates the ability to adhere to postoperative nutrition guidelines.
6. Psychological evaluation confirms the decisional capacity of the adolescent to provide informed consent and the adolescent is willing to do so.
7. The female adolescent agrees to avoid pregnancy for at least 1 year.

The Teen-LABS study[240] was a significant multicenter national study of 242 adolescents undergoing bariatric surgery (n=161 Roux-en-Y gastric bypass, and n=67 sleeve gastrectomy). Participants' mean age was 17 years, with a mean BMI of 53 kg/m². Seventy-five percent of participants were female and 72% were white. Three-year postoperative data were published by Inge et al in 2016, showing that participants' mean weight decreased by 27% to 28% in those who underwent gastric bypass and 26% in those who underwent gastric sleeve. Importantly, 95% of adolescents with T2D, 74% of those with elevated blood pressure, and 66% of those with dyslipidemia at baseline achieved remission by 3 years after surgery. Nutritional deficiencies are a known complication of bariatric surgery. In Teen-LABS, nutritional deficiencies were more common in those who underwent bypass surgery but still needed to be monitored in all surgery recipients. At 3 years, 57% had low ferritin levels. Other deficiencies included vitamin B_{12} and vitamin A. In addition, as a result of the surgery, 13% required 1 additional intra-abdominal procedure or more. Surgical complications are an additional risk. Thus, adolescents undergoing surgery must be monitored carefully with ongoing follow-up after surgery with their bariatric program.

The long-term effects of bariatric surgery in adolescent populations have not been well characterized. Further studies are also needed to evaluate the long-term data regarding long-term weight loss, late complications, and mortality. The Teen-LABS cohort will likely continue to be followed over time and provide valuable outcome data. Five-year postoperative data were published in 2019 showing ongoing benefit of bariatric surgery to this adolescent cohort.[241]

Overview of Therapeutic Options

Long-term studies of weight-reduced children and adults have shown that 80% to 90% return to their previous weight percentiles. Weight loss maintenance is difficult for reasons noted in the pathophysiology section of this chapter. Obese children and their families must recognize that maintenance of a reduced degree of body fatness requires change that will need to become incorporated into the child's and family's life. Diets extremely low in calorie content or with unusual distributions of calories as fat, protein, and carbohydrate may precipitate cardiac arrhythmias, severe electrolyte disturbances, or other morbidities. As many as 80% of children using unsupervised diets obtained from popular magazines have been found to suffer from weakness, headaches, fatigue, nausea, constipation, nervousness, dizziness, poor concentration, dysmenorrhea, and/or fainting. Children on a supervised diet must also be closely monitored for treatment-associated psychological morbidities. Bariatric surgery is a viable option for some obese adolescents, particularly those with serious morbidity.

Therapeutic intervention should emphasize the need for participation of the entire family and lifelong attention to, and benefits of, a healthy lifestyle as well as ongoing positive reinforcement and family and community support.

Resources

o   We Can! (contains dietary recommendations, physical activity recommendations, monitoring tools)
    http://wecan.nhlbi.nih.gov/

o   Dietary Guidelines for Americans (provides dietary recommendations for children older than 2 years and adults)
    http://www.cnpp.usda.gov/dietaryguidelines.htm

o   Choose My Plate (contains dietary recommendations to the public based on Dietary Guidelines for Americans)
    http://www.choosemyplate.gov/

o   MyPlate, MyWins campaign (helps families find healthy eating solutions for everyday life)
    https://www.choosemyplate.gov/myplate-mywins

o   AAP Institute for Health Childhood Weight
    https://ihcw.aap.org

o   BAM! (contains dietary recommendations, physical activity recom-
     mendations, monitoring tools)
     Document3https://www.cdc.gov/bam/index.html
o   Exercise is Medicine (contains recommendations for physicians to
     include physical activity prescription as part of their practice)
     https://www.exerciseismedicine.org/support_page.php/
     health-care-providers/
o   Healthychildren.org (contains dietary recommendations, physi-
     cal activity recommendations, tips to change home environment,
     parenting skills advices)
     http://www.healthychildren.org/
o   WebMD (contains interactive content for children, teens, and
     parents)
     www.fit.webmd.com
o   "Change Talk: Childhood Obesity" (AAP Web and mobile app to
     train practitioners in motivational interviewing for behavior
     change)
     http://ihcw.aap.org/resources
o   Mindless eating (contains tips to change home environment)
     http://www.mindlesseating.org/
o   Calorie King (online and book to calculate calorie-content of foods)
     http://www.calorieking.com/

References

1.   Ogden CL, Carroll MD, Lawman HG, et al. Trends in obesity prevalence among
     children and adolescents in the United States, 1988–1994 through 2013–2014.
     JAMA. 2016;315(21):2292–2299

2.   Skinner AC, Ravanbakht SN, Skelton JA, Perrin EM, Armstrong SC.
     Prevalence of obesity and severe obesity in US children, 1999–2016. *Pediatrics.*
     2018;141:e20173459

3.   Lobstein T, Jackson-Leach R, Moodie ML, et al. Child and adolescent obesity:
     part of a bigger picture. *Lancet.* 2015;385(9986):2510–2520

4.   Institute of Medicine, Food and Nutrition Board. *Preventing Obesity: Health in the
     Balance.* Washington, DC: National Academies Press; 2005

5.   Kumanyika SK, Obarzanek E, Stettler N, et al. Population-based prevention
     of obesity; the needs for comprehensive promotion of healthful eating,
     physical activity, and energy balance: a scientific statement from American
     Heart Association Council on Epidemiology and Prevention, Interdisciplinary
     Committee for Prevention. *Circulation.* 2008;118(4):428–464

VI

6. Institute of Medicine, Committee on Obesity Prevention Policies for Young Children. *Early Childhood Obesity Prevention Policies.* Washington, DC: National Academies Press; 2011

7. Rosen ED, Spiegelman BM. Adipocytes as regulators of energy balance and glucose homeostatsis. *Nature.* 2006;444(7121):847–853

8. Trayhurn P. Endocrine and signaling role of adipose tissue: new perspectives on fat. *Acta Physiol Scand.* 2005;184(4):285–293

9. Lettner A, Roden M. Ectopic fat and insulin resistance. *Curr Diab Rep.* 2008;8(3): 185–191

10. Cannon B, Nedergarard J. Brown adipose tissue; function and physiological significance. *Physiol Rev.* 2004;84(1):277–359

11. Divoux A, Tordjman J, Lacasa D, et al. Fibrosis in human adipose tissue: composition, distribution, and link with lipid metabolism and fat mass loss. *Diabetes Care.* 2010;59(11):2817–2825

12. Vael C, Verhulst SL, Nelen V, Goossens H, Desager KN. Intestinal microflora and body mass index during the first three years of life: an observational study. *Gut Pathog.* 2011;3(1):8

13. Muller MJ, Bosy-Westphal A, Heymsfield SB. Is there evidence for a set point that regulates human body weight? *F1000 Med Rep.* 2010;2:59

14. American Academy of Pediatrics, Committee on Nutrition. Pediatric obesity. In: Kleinman RE, Greer FR, eds. *Pediatric Nutrition Handbook.* Elk Grove Village, IL: American Academy of Pediatrics; 2009:733–782

15. Spiegelman BM, Flier JS. Obesity and the regulation of energy balance. *Cell.* 2001;104(4):531–543

16. Roh E, Song DK, Kim MS. Emerging role of the brain in the homeostatic regulation of energy and glucose metabolism. *Exp Mol Med.* 2016;48:e216

17. Andino LM, Ryder DJ, Shapiro A, et al. POMC overexpression in the ventral tegmental area ameliorates dietary obesity. *J Endocrinol.* 2011;210(2):199–207

18. Korner J, Leibel RL. To eat or not to eat how the gut talks to the brain. *N Engl J Med.* 2003;349(10):926–927

19. Wellman P. Modulation of eating by central catecholamine systems. *Curr Drug Targets.* 2005;6(2):191–199

20. Saper C, Chou T, Elmquist J. The need to feed: homeostatic and hedonic control of eating. *Neuron.* 2002;36(2):199–211

21. Baker M, Gaukrodger N, Mayosi BM, et al. Association between common polymorphisms of the proopiomelanocortin gene and body fat distribution; a family study. *Diabetes.* 2005;54(8):2492–2449

22. Yeo GS, Farooqi IS, Challis BG, Jackson RS, O'Rahilly S. The role of melanocortin signaling in the control of body weight: evidence from human and murine genetic models. *QJM.* 2000;93(1):7–14

23. Park HK, Ahima RS. Physiology of leptin: energy homeostasis, neuroendocrine function and metabolism. *Metabolism.* 2015;64(1):24–34

24. Kovacs P, Stumvoll M. Fatty acids and insulin resistance in muscle and liver. *Best Pract Res Clin Endocrinol Metab.* 2005;19(4):625–635

25. Obici S, Feng Z, Karkanias G, Baskin DG, Rossetti L. Decreasing hypothalamic insulin receptors causes hyperphagia and insulin resistance in rats. *Nat Neurosci.* 2002;5(6):566–572

26. Small CJ, Bloom SR. Gut hormones and the control of appetite. *Trends Endocrinol Metab.* 2004;15(6):259–263

27. Strader AD, Woods SC. Gastrointestinal hormones and food intake. *Gastroenterology.* 2005;128(1):175–191

28. Batterham RL, Cowley MA, Small CJ, et al. Gut hormone PYY3-36 physiologically inhibits food intake. *418.* 2002;6898(650–654)

29. Howarth FC, Al Kitbi MK, Hameed RS, Adeghate E. Pancreatic peptides in young and elderly Zucker type 2 diabetic fatty rats. *JOP.* 2011;12(6):567–573

30. Zander M, Madsbad S, Madsen JL, Holst JJ. Effect of 6 week course of glucagon like peptide 1 on glycemic control, insulin sensitivity, and beta cell function in type 2 diabetes a parallel group study. *Lancet.* 2002;359(9309):824–830

31. Wynne K, Park AJ, Small CJ, et al. Subcutaneous oxyntomodulin reduces body weight in overweight and obese subjects: a double-blind, randomized, controlled trial. *Diabetes.* 2005;54(8):2390–2395

32. Laferrère B, Swerdlow N, Bawa B, et al. Rise of oxyntomodulin in response to oral glucose after gastric bypass surgery in patients with type 2 diabetes. *J Clin Endocrinol Metab.* 2010;95(8):4071–4076

33. Ariyasu H, Takaya K, Tagami T, et al. Stomach is a major source of circulating ghrelin, and feeding state determines plasma ghrelin-like immunoreactivity levels in humans. *The Journal of clinical endocrinology and metabolism.* 2001;86(10): 4753–4758

34. Schwarz NA, Rigby BR, La Bounty P, Shelmadine B, Bowden RG. A review of weight control strategies and their effects on the regulation of hormonal balance. *J Nutr Metab.* 2011;2011:237932

35. Koliaki C, Kokkinos A, Tentolouris N, Katsilambros N. The effect of ingested macronutrients on postprandial ghrelin response: a critical review of existing literature data. *Int J Pept.* 2010;2010:710852

36. Ott V, Friedrich M, Zemlin J, et al. Meal anticipation potentiates postprandial ghrelin suppression in humans. *Psychoneuroendocrinology.* 2012;37(7):1096–1100

37. Kisseleff HR, Carretta JC, Geleibter A, Pi-Sunyer FX. Cholecystekinin and stomach distension combine to reduce food intake in humans. *Am J Physiol Regul Integr Comp Physiol.* 2003;285(5):R992–R998

38. Musso G, Gambino R, Cassader M. Obesity, diabetes, and gut microbiota: the hygiene hypothesis expanded? *Diabetes Care.* 2010;33(10):2277–2284

39. Komaroff AL. The microbiome and risk for obesity and diabetes. *JAMA.* 2017;317(4):355–356

40. Turnbaugh PJ, Ley RE, Mahowald MA, Magrini V, Mardis ER, Gordon JI. An obesity-associated gut microbiome with increased capacity for energy harvest. *Nature.* 2006;444(7122):1027–1031

VI

41. Tolhurst G, Heffron H, Lam YS, et al. Short-chain fatty acids stimulate glucagon-like peptide-1 secretion via the G-protein-coupled receptor FFAR2. *Diabetes.* 2012;61(2):364–371

42. Lumeng CN, Saltiel AR. Inflammatory links between obesity and metabolic disease. *J Clin Invest.* 2011;121(6):2111–2117

43. Wellen KE, Hotamisligil GS. Obesity-induced inflammatory changes in adipose tissue. *J Clin Invest.* 2003;112(12):1785–1788

44. Poretsky L, ed. *Pediatric Obesity - Etiology, Pathogenesis, and Treatment.* 2nd ed. Cham, Switzerland: Humana Press, Springer International Publishing; 2018

45. Margetic S, Gazzola C, Pegg GG, Hill RA. Leptin: a review of its peripheral actions and interactions. *Int J Obes Relat Metab Disord.* 2002;26(11):1407–1433

46. Skinner AC, Steiner MJ, Henderson FW, Perrin EM. Multiple markers of inflammation and weight status: cross-sectional analyses throughout childhood. *Pediatrics.* 2010;125(4):e801–e809

47. Shehzad A, Iqbal W, Shehzad O, Lee YS. Adiponectin: regulation of its production and its role in human diseases. *Hormones (Athens).* 2012;11(1):8–20

48. Bruun JM, Helge JW, Richelsen B, Stallknecht B. Diet and exercise reduce low grade inflammation and macrophage infiltration in adipose tissue but not in skeletal muscle in severely obese subjects. *Am J Physiol Endocrinol Metab.* 2006;290(5):e961–e967

49. Balagopal P, George D, Patton N, et al. Lifestyle-only intervention attenuates the inflammatory state associated with obesity: a randomized controlled study in adolescents. *J Pediatr.* 2005;146(3):342–348

50. Fabbrini E, Magkos F, Mohammed BS, et al. Intrahepatic fat, not visceral fat, is linked with metabolic complications of obesity. *Proc Natl Acad Sci U S A.* 2009;106(36):15430–15435

51. Saghizadeh M, Ong JM, Garvey WT, Henry RR, Kern PA. The expression of TNF alpha by human muscle. Relationship to insulin resistance. *J Clin Invest.* 1996;97(4):1111–1116

52. Thaler JP, Schwartz MW. Minireview: inflammation and obesity pathogenesis: the hypothalamus heats up. *Endocrinology.* 2010;151(9):4109–4115

53. Trayhurn P, Wood IS. Adipokines; inflammation and the pleiotrophic role of white adipose tissue. *Br J Nutr.* 2004;92(3):347–355

54. Chesi A, Grant SF. The genetics of pediatric obesity. *Trends Endocrinol Metab.* 2015;26(12):711–721

55. Min J, Chiu DT, Wang Y. Variation in the heritability of body mass index based on diverse twin studies: a systematic review. *Obes Rev.* 2013;14(11):871–882

56. Alegría-Torres JA, Baccarelli A, Bollati V. Epigenetics and lifestyle. *Epigenomics.* 2011;3(3):267–277

57. Choquet H, Meyre D. Genetics of obesity: what have we learned? *Curr Genomics.* 2011;12(3):169–179

58. Farooqi IS, Yeo GS, Keogh JM, et al. Dominant and recessive inheritance of morbid obesity associated with melanocortin 4 receptor deficiency. *J Clin Invest.* 2000;106(2):271–279

59. Frayling TM, Timpson NJ, Weedon MN, et al. A common variant in the FTO gene is associated with body mass index and predisposes to childhood and adult obesity. *Science*. 2007;316(5826):889–894

60. Cecil JE, Tavendale R, Watt P, Hetherington MM, Palmer CN. An obesity-associated FTO gene variant and increased energy intake in children. *N Engl J Med*. 2008;359(24):2558–2566

61. Timpson NJ, Emmett PM, Frayling TM, et al. The fat mass- and obesity-associated locus and dietary intake in children. *Am J Clin Nutr*. 2008;88(4):971–978

62. Wardle J, Carnell S, Haworth CM, Farooqi IS, O'Rahilly S, Plomin R. Obesity associated genetic variation in FTO is associated with diminished satiety. *J Clin Endocrinol Metab*. 2008;93(9):3640–3643

63. Stutzmann F, Cauchi S, Durand E, et al. Common genetic variation near MC4R is associated with eating behaviour patterns in European populations. *Int J Obes (Lond)*. 2009;33(3):373–378

64. Huvenne H, Dubern B, Clement K, Poitou C. Rare genetic forms of obesity: clinical approach and current treatments in 2016. *Obes Facts*. 2016;9(3):158–173

65. Perrone L, Marzuillo P, Grandone A, del Giudice EM. Chromosome 16p11.2 deletions: another piece in the genetic puzzle of childhood obesity. *Ital J Pediatr*. 2010;36:43

66. Chung WK, Leibel RL. Molecular physiology of syndromic obesities in humans. *Trends Endocrinol Metab*. 2005;16(6):267–272

67. Pietrobelli A, Faith MS, Allison DB, Gallagher D, Chiumello G, Heymsfield SB. Body mass index as a measure of adiposity among children and adolescents: a validation study. *J Pediatr*. 1998;132(2):204–210

68. Reilly JJ, Dorosty AR, Emmett PM. Identification of the obese child: adequacy of the body mass index for clinical practice and epidemiology. Avon Longitudinal Study of Pregnancy and Childhood Study Team. *Int J Obes Relat Metab Disord*. 2000;24(12):1623–1627

69. Grossman DC, Bibbins-Domingo K, Curry SJ, Barry MJ, Davidson KW, Doubeni CA. Screening for obesity in children and adolescents: US Preventive Services Task Force recommendation statement. *JAMA*. 2017;317(23):2417–2426

70. Styne DM, Arslanian SA, Connor EL, et al. Pediatric obesity—assessment, treatment, and prevention: an Endocrine Society Clinical Practice Guideline. *J Clin Endocrinol Metab*. 2017;102(3):709–757

71. Krebs N, Himes J, Jacobson D, Nicklas TA, Guilday P, Styne DM. Assessment of child and adolescent overweight and obesity. *Pediatrics*. 2007;120(Suppl 4):S193–S228

72. Daniels SR, Hassink SG, American Academy of Pediatrics, Committee on Nutrition. The role of the pediatrician in primary prevention of obesity. *Pediatrics*. 2015;136(1):e275–e292

73. World Health Organization. WHO Child Growth Standards Based on Length/Height, Weight and Age. *Acta Paediatr Suppl*. 2006;450:76–85

VI

74. Centers for Disease Control and Prevention. Use of World Health Organization and CDC growth charts for children aged 0–59 months in the United States. *MMWR Recomm Rep.* 2010;59(RR-09):1–15

75. Flegal KM, Shepherd JA, Looker AC, et al. Comparisons of percentage body fat, body mass index, waist circumference, and waist-stature ratio in adults. *Am J Clin Nutr.* 2009;89(2):500–508

76. Gulati AK, Kaplan DW, Daniels SR. Clinical tracking of severely obese children: a new growth chart. *Pediatrics.* 2012;130(6):1136–1140

77. Laurson KR, Eisenmann JC, Welk GJ. Body fat percentile curves for U.S. children and adolescents. *Am J Prev Med.* 2011;41(4 Suppl 2):S87–S92

78. Ellis KJ, Abrams SA, Wong WW. Monitoring childhood obesity: assessment of the weight/height index. *Am J Epidemiol.* 1999;150(9):939–946

79. Ehtisham S, Crabtree N, Clark P, Shaw N, Barrett T. Ethnic differences in insulin resistance and body composition in United Kingdom adolescents. *J Clin Endocrinol Metab.* 2005;90(7):3963–3969

80. Wang J, Thornton JC, Burastero S, et al. Comparisons for body mass index and body fat percent among Puerto Ricans, blacks, whites and Asians living in the New York City area. *Obes Res.* 1996;4(4):377–384

81. Sisson SB, Katzmarzyk PT, Srinivasan SR, et al. Ethnic differences in subcutaneous adiposity and waist girth in children and adolescents. *Obesity (Silver Spring).* 2009;17(11):2075–2081

82. Liu A, Byrne NM, Kagawa M, et al. Ethnic difference in the relationship between body mass index and percentage body fat among Asian children from different backgrounds. *Br J Nutr.* 2011;106(9):1390–1397

83. Borrud LG, Flegal KM, Looker AC, Everhart JE, Harris TB, Shepherd JA. Body composition data for individuals 8 years of age and older: U.S. population, 1999–2004. *Vital Health Stat 11.* 2010;(250):1–87

84. Bjorntorp P. Classification of obese patients and complications related to the distribution of surplus fat. *The American journal of clinical nutrition.* 1987;45 (5 Suppl):1120–1125.

85. Bjorntorp P. Possible mechanisms relating fat distribution and metabolism. In: Bouchard C, Johnston FE, eds. *Fat Distribution During Growth and Later Health Outcomes.* New York, NY: Alan R. Liss Inc; 1988:175–191

86. Chu NF, Rimm EB, Wang DJ, Liou HS, Shieh SM. Relationship between anthropometric variables and lipid levels among school children: the Taipei Children Heart Study. *Int J Obes Relat Metab Disord.* 1998;22(1):66–72

87. Hansen SE, Hasselstrøm H, Grønfeldt V, Froberg K, Andersen LB. Cardiovascular disease risk factors in 6–7-year-old Danish children: the Copenhagen School Child Intervention Study. *Prev Med.* 2005;40(6):740–746

88. Moran A, Jacobs DR, Jr., Steinberger J, et al. Insulin resistance during puberty: results from clamp studies in 357 children. *Diabetes.* 1999;48(10):2039–2044

89. Sikram NK, Misra A, Pandey RM, Dwivedi M, Luthra K. Adiponectin, insulin resistance, and C-reactive protein in postpubertal Asian Indian adolescents. *Metabolism.* 2004;53(10):1336–1341

90. Brambilla P, Bedogni G, Moreno LA, et al. Crossvalidation of anthropometry against magnetic resonance imaging for the assessment of visceral and subcutaneous adipose tissue in children. *Int J Obes (Lond)*. 2006;30(1):23–30

91. Lee S, Bacha F, Gungor N, Arslanian SA. Waist circumference is an independent predictor of insulin resistance in black and white youths. *J Pediatr*. 2006;148(2):188–194

92. Maffeis C, Pietrobelli A, Grezzani A, Provera S, Tatò L. Waist circumference and cardiovascular risk factors in prepuberal children. *Obes Res*. 2001;9(3):179–187

93. Savva SC, Tornaritis M, Savva ME, et al. Waist circumference and waist to height ratio are better predictors of cardiovascular disease risk factors in children than body mass index. *Int J Obes Relat Metab Disord*. 2000;24(11): 1453–1458

94. Kotlyarevska K, Wolfgram P, Lee JM. Is waist circumference a better predictor of insulin resistance than body mass index in U.S. adolescents? *J Adolesc Health*. 2011;49(3):330–333

95. Barker DJ. Obesity and early life. *Obes Rev*. 2007;8(Suppl 1):45–49

96. Ravelli AC, van der Meulen JH, Michels RP, et al. Glucose tolerance in adults after prenatal exposure to famine. *Lancet*. 1998;351(9097):173–177

97. Ravelli AC, van der Meullen JH, Osmond C, Barker DJ, Bleker OP. Infant feeding and adult glucose tolerance, lipid profile, blood pressure, and obesity. *Arch Dis Child*. 2000;82(3):248–252

98. Parsons TJ, Power C, Logan S, Summerbell CD. Childhood predictors of adult obesity: a systematic review. *Int J Obes Relat Metab Disord*. 1999;23(Suppl 8): S1–S107

99. Crume TL, Ogden L, Daniels S, Hamman RF, Norris JM, Dabelea D. The impact of in utero exposure to diabetes on childhood body mass index growth trajectories: the EPOCH study. *J Pediatr*. 2011;158(6):941–946

100. Pryor LE, Tremblay RE, Boivin M, et al. Developmental trajectories of body mass index in early childhood and their risk factors: an 8-year longitudinal study. *Arch Pediatr Adolesc Med*. 2011;165(10):906–912

101. Barker D, Eriksson J, Forsen T, Osmond C. Fetal origins of adult disease: strength of effects and biological basis. *Int J Epidemiol*. 2002;31(6):1235–1239

102. Barker D, Osmond C, Forsen T, Kajantie E, Eriksson JG. Trajectories of growth among children who have coronary events as adults. *N Engl J Med*. 2005;353(17): 1802–1809

103. Luo Z, Xiao L, Nuyt A. Mechanisms of developmental programming of the metabolic syndrome and related disorders. *World J Diabetes*. 2010;1(3):89–98

104. Bhargava S, Sachdev H, Fall C, et al. Relation of serial changes in childhood body mass index to impaired glucose tolerance in young adulthood. *N Engl J Med*. 2004;350(9):865–875

105. Cianfarani S, Germani D, Branca F. Low birthweight and adult insulin resistance: the "catch-up growth" hypothesis. *Arch Dis Child Fetal Neonatal Ed*. 1991;81(1):F71–F73

VI

106. Hales CN, Barker DJ. Type 2 (non-insulin-dependent) diabetes mellitus: the thrifty phenotype hypothesis. *Diabetologia*. 1992;35(7):595–601

107. Lucas A. Programming by early nutrition: an experimental approach. *J Nutr*. 1998;128((2 Suppl)):401S–406S

108. Luo ZC, Fraser WD, Julien P, et al. Tracing the origins of "fetal origins" of adult diseases: programming by oxidative stress? . *Med Hypotheses*. 2006;66(1):38–44

109. Zhang L. Prenatal hypoxia and cardiac programming. *J Soc Gynecol Investig*. 2005;12(1):2–13

110. Rich-Edwards JW, Colditz GA, Stampfer MJ, Willett WC, Gillman MW, Hennekens CH. Birthweight and the risk for type II diabetes mellitus in adult women. *Ann Intern Med*. 1999;130(4 Pt 1):278–284

111. Phillips DI, Barker DJ, Hales CN, Hirst S, Osmond C. Thinness at birth and insulin resistance in adult life. *Diabetologia*. 1994;37(2):150–154

112. Hales C, Barker D, Clark PM, et al. Fetal and infant growth and impaired glucose tolerance at age 64. *BMJ*. 1991;303(6809):1019–1022

113. Schaefer-Graf UM, Pawliczak J, Passow D, et al. Birth weight and parental BMI predict overweight in children from mothers with gestational diabetes. *Diabetes Care*. 2005;28(7):1734–1740

114. Vohr BR, McGarvey ST. Growth patterns of large-for-gestational-age and appropriate-for-gestational-age infants of gestational diabetic mothers and control mothers at age 1 year. *Diabetes Care*. 1997;20(7):1066–1072

115. Gillman MW, Rifas-Shiman R, Berkey CS, Field AE, Colditz GA. Maternal gestational diabetes, birth weight, and adolescent obesity. *Pediatrics*. 2003;111(3): e221–e226

116. Boney CM, Verma A, Tucker R, Vohr BR. Metabolic syndrome in childhood: association with birth weight, maternal obesity, and gestational diabetes mellitus. *Pediatrics*. 2005;115(3):e290–e296

117. Pettitt DJ, Baird HR, Aleck KA, Bennett PH, Knowler WC. Excessive obesity in offspring of Pima Indian women with diabetes during pregnancy. *N Engl J Med*. 1983;308(5):242–245

118. Plagemann A. Perinatal programming and functional teratogenesis: impact on body weight regulation and obesity. *Physiol Behav*. 2005;86(5):661–668

119. Pettitt DJ, Knowler WC, Bennett PH, Aleck KA, Baird HR. Obesity in offspring of diabetic Pima Indian women despite normal birth weight. *Diabetes Care*. 1987;10(1):76–80

120. Pettitt DJ, Aleck KA, Baird HR, Carraher MJ, Bennett PH, Knowler WC. Congenital susceptibility to NIDDM. Role of intrauterine environment. *Diabetes*. 1988;37(5):622–628

121. Godfrey KM, Sheppard A, Gluckman PD, et al. Epigenetic gene promoter methylation at birth is associated with child's later adiposity. *Diabetes*. 2011;60(5): 1528–1534

122. Calkins K, Devaskar SU. Fetal origins of adult disease. *Curr Probl Pediatr Adolesc Health Care*. 2011;41(6):158–176

123. Devaskar SU, Thamotharan M. Metabolic programming in the pathogenesis of insulin resistance. *Rev Endocr Metab Disord.* 2007;8(2):105–113

124. Pinney SE, Simmons RA. Metabolic programming, epigenetics, and gestational diabetes mellitus. *Curr Diab Rep.* 2012;12(1):67–74

125. Taveras EM, Rifas-Shiman SL, Sherry B, et al. Crossing growth percentiles in infancy and risk of obesity in childhood. *Arch Pediatr Adolesc Med.* 2011;165(11): 993–998

126. Ong KK, Loos RJ. Rapid infancy weight gain and subsequent obesity: systemic reviews and hopeful suggestions. *Acta Paediatr.* 2006;95(8):904–908

127. Druet C, Stettler N, Sharp S, et al. Prediction of childhood obesity by infancy weight gain: an individual-level meta-analysis. *Paediatr Perinat Epidemiol.* 2012;26(1):19–26

128. Koletzko B, von Kries R, Closa R, et al. Lower protein in infant formula is associated with lower weight gain up to age 2 y: a randomized clinical trial. *Am J Clin Nutr.* 2009;89(6):1836–1845

129. Patro-Golab B, Zalewski BM, Kouwenhoven SM, et al. Protein concentration in milk formula, growth, and later risk of obesity: a systematic review. *J Nutr.* 2016;146(3):551–564

130. Owen CG, Martin RM, Whincup PH, Smith GD, Cook DG. Effect of infant feeding on the risk of obesity across the life course: a quantitative review of published evidence. *Pediatrics.* 2005;115(5):1367–1377

131. Van Rossem L, Taveras E, Gillman M, et al. Is the association of breastfeeding with child obesity explained by infant weight change? *Int J Pediatr Obes.* 2011;6 (2-2):e415–e422

132. Nelson MC, Gordon-Larsen P, Adair LS. Are adolescents who were breast-fed less likely to be overweight? Analyses of sibling pairs to reduce confounding. *Epidemiology.* 2005;16(2):247–253

133. Metzger MW, McDade TW. Breastfeeding as obesity prevention in the United States: a sibling difference model. *Am J Hum Biol.* 2010;22(3):291–196

134. Gillman MW, Rifas-Shiman SL, Berkey CS, et al. Breast-feeding and overweight in adolescence: within-family analysis [corrected]. *Epidemiology.* 2006;17(1): 112–114

135. Huh SY, Rifas-Shiman SL, Taveras EM, Oken E, Gillman MW. Timing of solid food introduction and risk of obesity in preschool-aged children. *Pediatrics.* 2011;127(3):e544–e551

136. Rzehak P, Oddy WH, Mearin ML, et al. WP10 Working Group of the Early Nutrition Project. Infant feeding and growth trajectory patterns in childhood and body composition in young adulthood. *Am J Clin Nutr.* 2017;106(2):568–580

137. Grote V, Schiess SA, Closa-Monasterolo R, et al. European Childhood Obesity Trial Study, Group. The introduction of solid food and growth in the first 2 y of life in formula-fed children: analysis of data from a European cohort study. *Am J Clin Nutr.* 2011;94(6 Suppl):1785S–1793S

VI

138. English LK, Obbagy JE, Wong YP. Timing of introduction of complementary foods and beverages and growth, size, and body composition: a systematic review. *Am J Clin Nutr.* 2019;109(Suppl):935S–955S

139. Whitaker RC, Wright JA, Pepe MS, Seidel KD, Dietz WH. Predicting obesity in young adulthood from childhood and parental obesity. *N Engl J Med.* 1997;337(13):869–873

140. Orlet Fisher J, Rolls BJ, Birch LL. Children's bite size and intake of an entrée are greater with large portions than with age-appropriate or self-selected portions. *Am J Clin Nutr.* 2003;77(5):1164–1170

141. Welsh JA, Cogswell ME, Rogers S, Rockett H, Mei Z, Grummer-Strawn LM. Overweight among low-income preschool children associated with the consumption of sweet drinks: Missouri, 1999–2002. *Pediatrics.* 2005;115(2): e223–e229

142. Whitaker RC, Pepe MS, Wright JA, Seidel KD, Dietz WH. Early adiposity rebound and the risk of adult obesity. *Pediatrics.* 1998;101(3):e5–e8

143. Miller SA, Taveras EM, Rifas-Shiman SL, Gillman MW. Association between television viewing and poor diet quality in young children. *Int J Pediatr Obes.* 2008;3(3):168–176

144. Anderson SE, Whitaker RC. Household routines and obesity in US preschool-aged children. *Pediatrics.* 2010;125(3):420–428

145. Moore LL, Lombardi DA, White MJ, Campbell JL, Oliveria SA, Ellison RC. Influence of parents' physical activity levels on activity levels of young children. *J Pediatr.* 1991;118(2):215–219

146. Benjamin S, Rifas-Shiman S, Taveras E, et al. Early child care and adiposity at ages 1 and 3 years. *Pediatrics.* 2009;124(2):555–562

147. Alberdi G, McNamara AE, Lindsay KL, et al. The association between childcare and risk of childhood overweight and obesity in children aged 5 years and under: a systematic review. *Eur J Pediatr.* Oct 2016;175(10):1277–1294

148. American Academy of Pediatrics, Council on School Health, Committee on Nutrition. Snacks, sweetened beverages, added sugars, and schools. *Pediatrics.* 2015;135(3):575–583

149. Park S, Sappenfield WM, Huang Y, Sherry B, Bensyl DM. The impact of the availability of school vending machines on eating behavior during lunch: the Youth Physical Activity and Nutrition Survey. *J Am Diet Assoc.* 2010;110(10): 1532–1536

150. Berkey CS, Rockett HR, Field AE, Gillman MW, Colditz GA. Sugar-added beverages and adolescent weight change. *Obes Res.* 2004;12(5):778–788

151. Dennison BA, Rockwell HL, Baker SL. Excess fruit juice consumption by preschool-aged children is associated with short stature and obesity. *Pediatrics.* 1997;99(1):15–22

152. Heyman MB, Abrams SA, Section on Gastroenterology, Hepatology, and Nutrition, Committee on Nutrition. Fruit juice in infants, children, and adolescents: current recommendations. *Pediatrics.* 2017;139(6):e20170967

153. Institute of Medicine, Food and Nutrition Board. *Building Blocks for Healthy Children*. Washington, DC: National Academies Press; 2010

154. Cullen KW, Baranowski T, Klesges LM, et al. Anthropometric, parental, and psychosocial correlates of dietary intake of African-American girls. *Obes Res.* 2004;12(Suppl):20S–31S

155. Francis LA, Lee Y, Birsch LL. Parental weight status and girls' television viewing, snacking, and body mass indexes. *Obes Res.* 2003;11(1):143–151

156. Li C, Ford ES, Zhao G, Mokdad AH. Prevalence of pre-diabetes and its association with clustering of cardiometabolic risk factors and hyperinsulinemia among US adolescents: NHANES 2005–2006. *Diabetes Care.* 2009;32(2):342–347

157. Sinha R, Fisch G, Teague B, et al. Prevalence of impaired glucose tolerance among children and adolescents with marked obesity. *N Engl J Med.* 2002;346(11): 802–810

158. Wiegand S, Maikowski U, Blankenstein O, Biebermann H, Tarnow P, Grüters A. Type 2 diabetes and impaired glucose tolerance in European children and adolescents with obesity—a problem that is no longer restricted to minority groups. *Eur J Endocrinol.* 2004;151(2):199–206

159. The NS, Suchindran C, North KE, Popkin BM, Gordon-Larsen P. Association of adolescent obesity with risk of severe obesity in adulthood. *JAMA.* 2010;304(18): 2042–2047

160. Tirosh A, Shai I, Afek A, et al. Adolescent BMI trajectory and risk of diabetes versus coronary disease. *N Engl J Med.* 2011;364(14):1315–1325

161. US Department of Health and Human Services. *2008 Physical Activity Guidelines for Americans*. ODPHP Publication No. U0036. Washington, DC: US Department of Health and Human Services; 2008

162. US Department of Health and Human Services, US Department of Agriculture. *2015–2020 Dietary Guidelines for Americans*. Washington, DC: US Department of Health and Human Services; 2015

163. Norman AC, Drinkard B, McDuffie JR, Ghorbani S, Yanoff LB, Yanovski JA. Influence of excess adiposity on exercise fitness and performance in overweight children and adolescents. *Pediatrics.* 2005;115(6):e690–e696

164. Golden NH, Schneider M, Wood C. Preventing obesity and eating disorders in adolescents. *Pediatrics.* 2016;138(3):e20161649

165. Must A, Jacques PF, Dallal GE, Bajema CJ, Dietz WH. Long-term morbidity and mortality of overweight adolescents. A follow-up of the Harvard Growth Study of 1922 to 1935. *N Engl J Med.* 1992;327(19):1350–1355

166. Twig G, Yaniv G, Levine H, et al. Body-Mass Index in 2.3 Million Adolescents and Cardiovascular Death in Adulthood. *N Engl J Med.* 2016;374(25):2430–2440

167. Ginsberg HN, Zhang YL, Hernandez-Ono A. Regulation of plasma triglycerides in insulin resistance and diabetes. *Arch Med Res.* 2005;36(3):232–240

168. Friedemann C, Heneghan C, Mahtani K, Thompson M, Perera R, Ward AM. Cardiovascular disease risk in healthy children and its association with body mass index: systematic review and meta-analysis. *BMJ.* 2012;345:e4759

VI

169. Li S, Chen W, Srinivasan SR, et al. Childhood cardiovascular risk factors and carotid vascular changes in adulthood: the Bogalusa Heart Study. *JAMA.* 2003;290(17):2271–2276

170. Magnussen CG, Venn A, Thomson R, et al. The association of pediatric low- and high-density lipoprotein cholesterol dyslipidemia classifications and change in dyslipidemia status with carotid intima-media thickness in adulthood evidence from the cardiovascular risk in Young Finns study, the Bogalusa Heart study, and the CDAH (Childhood Determinants of Adult Health) study. *J Am Coll Cardiol.* 2009;53(10):860–869

171. Expert Panel on Integrated Guidelines for Cardiovascular Health and Risk Reduction in Children and Adolescents, National Heart, Lung and Blood Institute. Expert panel on integrated guidelines for cardiovascular health and risk reduction in children and adolescents: summary report. *Pediatrics.* 2011;128(Suppl 5):S213–S256

172. Hassink S. *Pediatric Obesity: Prevention, Intervention, and Treatment Strategies for Primary Care.* Elk Grove Village, IL: American Academy of Pediatrics; 2006

173. Alpert MA. Obesity cardiomyopathy: pathophysiology and evolution of the clinical syndrome. *Am J Med Sci.* 2001;321(4):225–236

174. Field AE, Cook NR, Gillman MW. Weight status in childhood as a predictor of becoming overweight or hypertensive in early adulthood. *Obes Res.* 2005;13(1): 163–169

175. Faz G, Butler IJ, Koenig MK. Incidence of papilledema and obesity in children diagnosed with idiopathic "benign" intracranial hypertension: case series and review. *J Child Neurol.* 2010;25(11):1389–1392

176. Lessell S. Pediatric pseudotumor cerebri (idiopathic intracranial hypertension). *Surv Ophthalmol.* 1992;37(3):155–166

177. Distelmaier F, Sengler U, Messing-Juenger M, Assmann B, Mayatepek E, Rosenbaum T. Pseudotumor cerebri as an important differential diagnosis of papilledema in children. *Brain Dev.* 2006;28(3):190–195

178. Matthews YY, Dean F, Lim MJ, et al. Pseudotumor cerebri syndrome in childhood: incidence, clinical profile and risk factors in a national prospective population-based cohort study. *Arch Dis Child.* 2017;102(8):715–721

179. Kempers MJ, Noordam C, Rouwe CW, Otten BJ. Can GnRH-agonist treatment cause slipped capital femoral epiphysis? *J Pediatr Endocrinol Metab.* 2001;14(6):729–734

180. Wilcox PG, Weiner DS, Leighley B. Maturation factors in slipped capital femoral epiphysis. *J Pediatr Orthop.* 1988;8(2):196–200

181. Busch MT, Morrissy RT. Slipped capital femoral epiphysis. *Orthop Clin North Am.* 1987;18(4):637–647

182. Aversano MW, Moazzaz P, Scaduto AA, Otsuka NY. Association between body mass index-for-age and slipped capital femoral epiphysis: the long-term risk for subsequent slip in patients followed until physeal closure. *J Child Orthop.* 2016;10(3):209–213

183. Dietz WH, Gross WL, Kirkpatrick JA. Blount disease (tibia vara): another skeletal disorder associated with childhood obesity. *J Pediatr.* 1982;101(5):735–737

184. Montgomery CO, Young KL, Austen M, Jo CH, Blasier RD, Ilyas M. Increased risk of Blount disease in obese children and adolescents with vitamin D deficiency. *J Pediatr Orthop.* 2010;30(8):879–882

185. Marcus CL, Brooks LJ, Ward SD, et al. American Academy of Pediatrics, Subcommittee on Obstructive Sleep Apnea Syndrome. Technical report: diagnosis and management of childhood obstructive sleep apnea syndrome. *Pediatrics.* 2012;130(3):e714–e755

186. Gozal D. Sleep-disordered breathing and school performance in children. *Pediatrics.* 1998;102(3 Pt 1):616–620

187. Watson SE, Li Z, Tu W, et al. Obstructive sleep apnoea in obese adolescents and cardiometabolic risk markers. *Pediatr Obes.* 2014;9(6):471–477

188. Bazzano LA, Hu T, Bertisch SM, et al. Childhood obesity patterns and relation to middle-age sleep apnoea risk: the Bogalusa Heart Study. *Pediatr Obes.* 2016;11(6): 535–542

189. Ahmed MH, Barakat S, Almobarak AO. Nonalcoholic fatty liver disease and cardiovascular disease: has the time come for cardiologists to be hepatologists? *J Obes.* 2012;2012:483135

190. Schwimmer JB, Deutsch R, Kahen T, Lavine JE, Stanley C, Behling C. Prevalence of fatty liver in children and adolescents. *Pediatrics.* 2006;118(4):1388–1393

191. Tazawa Y, Noguchi H, Nishinomiya F, Takada G. Serum alanine aminotransferases activity in obese children. *Acta Paediatr.* 1997;86(3):238–241

192. Harrison SA, Diehl AM. Fat and the liver—a molecular overview. *Semin Gastrointest Dis.* 2002;13(1):3–6

193. Barlow SE, Expert Committee. Expert committee recommendations regarding the prevention, assessment, and treatment of child and adolescent overweight and obesity: summary report. *Pediatrics.* 2007;120(Suppl 4):S164–S192

194. Mehta S, Lopez ME, Chumpitazi BP, Mazziotti MV, Brandt ML, Fishman DS. Clinical characteristics and risk factors for symptomatic pediatric gallbladder disease. *Pediatrics.* 2012;129(1):e82–e88

195. Anderson AD, Solorzano CM, McCartney CR. Childhood obesity and its impact on the development of adolescent PCOS. *Semin Reprod Med.* 2014;32(3):202–213

196. Christensen SB, Black MH, Smith N, et al. Prevalence of polycystic ovary syndrome in adolescents. *Fertil Steril.* 2013;100(2):470–477

197. Ibanez L, Dimartino-Nardi J, Potau N, Saenger P. Premature adrenarche— normal variant or forerunner of adult disease? *Endocrin Rev.* 2000;21(6):671–696

198. Patel SS, Truong U, King M, et al. Obese adolescents with polycystic ovarian syndrome have elevated cardiovascular disease risk markers. *Vasc Med.* 2017;22(2):85–95

199. American Diabetes Association. 2. Classification and diagnosis of diabetes: standards of medical care in diabetes—2018. *Diabetes Care.* 2018;41(Suppl 1): S13–S27

VI

200. Zeitler P, Hirst K, Pyle L, et al. A clinical trial to maintain glycemic control in youth with type 2 diabetes. *N Engl J Med*. 2012;366(24):2247–2256

201. TODAY Study Group. Effects of metformin, metformin plus rosiglitazone, and metformin plus lifestyle on insulin sensitivity and beta-cell function in TODAY. *Diabetes Care*. 2013;36(6):1749–1757

202. Matthews DR, Cull CA, Stratton IM, Holman RR, Turner RC. UKPDS 26: Sulphonylurea failure in non-insulin-dependent diabetic patients over six years. UK Prospective Diabetes Study (UKPDS) Group. *Diab Med*. 1998;15(4):297–303

203. Nemiary D, Shim R, Mattox G, Holden K. The relationship between obesity and depression among adolescents. *Psychiatr Ann*. 2012;42(8):305–308

204. Silverstein J, Cheng P, Ruedy KJ, et al. Depressive symptoms in youth with type 1 or type 2 diabetes: results of the Pediatric Diabetes Consortium Screening Assessment of Depression in Diabetes Study. *Diabetes Care*. Dec 2015;38(12): 2341–2343

205. Pont SJ, Puhl R, Cook SR, Slusser W, American Academy of Pediatrics Section on Obesity, Obesity Society. Stigma experienced by children and adolescents with obesity. *Pediatrics*. 2017;140(6):e20173034

206. Magge SN, Goodman E, Armstrong SC, Committee on Nutrition, Section on Endocrinology, Section on Obesity. The metabolic syndrome in children and adolescents: shifting the focus to cardiometabolic risk factor clustering. *Pediatrics*. 2017;140(2):e20171603

207. American Academy of Pediatrics, Council on Community Pediatrics, Committee on Nutrition. Promoting food security for all children. *Pediatrics*. 2015;136(5): e1431–e1438

208. Institute of Medicine, Food and Nutrition Board, Committee on Accelerating Progress in Obesity Prevention. *Accelerating Progress in Obesity Prevention: Solving the Weight of the Nation*. Washington, DC: National Academies Press; 2012

209. de Ruyter JC, Olthof MR, Seidell JC, Katan MB. A trial of sugar-free or sugar-sweetened beverages and body weight in children. *N Engl J Med*. 2012;367(15): 1397–1406

210. Ebbeling CB, Feldman HA, Chomitz VR, et al. A randomized trial of sugar-sweetened beverages and adolescent body weight. *N Engl J Med*. 2012;367(15): 1407–1416

211. Vos MB, Kaar JL, Welsh JA, et al. Added sugars and cardiovascular disease risk in children: a scientific statement from the American Heart Association. *Circulation*. 2017;135(19):e1017–e1034

212. Chen L, Caballero B, Mitchell DC, et al. Reducing consumption of sugar-sweetened beverages is associated with reduced blood pressure: a prospective study among United States adults. *Circulation*. 2010;121(22):2398–2406

213. Perez-Pozo SE, Schold J, Nakagawa T, Sanchez-Lozada LG, Johnson RJ, Lillo JL. Excessive fructose intake induces the features of metabolic syndrome in healthy adult men: role of uric acid in the hypertensive response. *Int J Obes (Lond)*. 2010;34(3):454–461

214. Lee AK, Binongo JN, Chowdhury R, et al. Consumption of less than 10% of total energy from added sugars is associated with increasing HDL in females during adolescence: a longitudinal analysis. *Journal of the American Heart Association*. 2014;3(1):e000615

215. Lustig RH, Mulligan K, Noworolski SM, et al. Isocaloric fructose restriction and metabolic improvement in children with obesity and metabolic syndrome. *Obesity (Silver Spring)*. 2016;24(2):453–460

216. Wang JW, Mark S, Henderson M, et al. Adiposity and glucose intolerance exacerbate components of metabolic syndrome in children consuming sugar-sweetened beverages: QUALITY cohort study. *Pediatr Obes*. 2013;8(4):284–293

217. Welsh JA, Sharma A, Cunningham SA, Vos MB. Consumption of added sugars and indicators of cardiovascular disease risk among US adolescents. *Circulation*. 2011;123(3):249–257

218. Ogden CL, Carroll MD, Kit BK, Flegal KM. Prevalence of childhood and adult obesity in the United States, 2011–2012. *JAMA*. 2014;311(8):806–814

219. US Preventive Services Task Force. Screening for Obesity in Children and Adolescents: US Preventive Services Task Force Recommendation Statement. *JAMA*. 2017;317(23):2417–2426

220. American Academy of Pediatrics, Council on Communications and Media. Media and young minds. *Pediatrics*. 2016;138(5):e20162591

221. American Academy of Pediatrics, Media CoCa. Media use in school-aged children and adolescents. *Pediatrics*. 2016;138(5):e20162592

222. O'Connor EA, Evans CV, Burda BU, Walsh ES, Eder M, Lozano P. Screening for obesity and interventions for weight management in children and adolescents: a systematic evidence review for the U.S. Preventive Services Task Force. *JAMA*. 2017;317(23):2427–2444

223. Danielsson P, Kowalski J, Ekblom O, Marcus C. Response of severely obese children and adolescents to behavioral treatment. *Arch Pediatr Adolesc Med*. 2012;166(12):1103–1108

224. Knowler WC, Barrett-Connor E, Fowler SE, et al. Reduction in the incidence of type 2 diabetes with lifestyle intervention or metformin. *N Engl J Med*. 2002;346(6):393–403

225. Moens E, Braet C, Van Winckel M. An 8-year follow-up of treated obese children: children's, process and parental predictors of successful outcome. *Behav Res Ther*. 2010;48(7):626–633

226. American Heart Association, Nutrition Committee. Diet and lifestyle recommendations revision 2006: a scientific statement from the American Heart Association Nutrition Committee. *Circulation*. 2006;114(1):82–96

227. Roza AM, Shizgal HM. The Harris Benedict equation reevaluated: resting energy requirements and the body cell mass. *Am J Clin Nutr*. 1984;40(1):168–182

228. Hernandez B, Gortmaker SL, Colditz GA, Peterson KE, Laird NM, Parra-Cabrera S. Association of obesity with physical activity, television programs and other forms of video viewing among children in Mexico city. *Int J Obes Relat Metab Disord*. 1999;23(8):845–854

VI

229. Borzekowski DL, Robinson TN. The 30-second effect: an experiment revealing the impact of television commercials on food preferences of preschoolers. *J Am Diet Assoc.* 2001;101(1):42–46

230. Sjöström L, Rissanen A, Andersen T, et al. Randomised placebo-controlled trial of orlistat for weight loss and prevention of weight regain in obese patients. *Lancet.* 1998;352(9123):167–172

231. Finer N, James WP, Kopelman PG, Lean ME, Williams G. One-year treatment of obesity: a randomized, double-blind, placebo-controlled, multicentre study of orlistat, a gastrointestinal lipase inhibitor. *Int J Obes Relat Metab Disord.* 2000;24(3):306–313

232. Hill JO, Hauptman J, Anderson JW, et al. Orlistat, a lipase inhibitor, for weight maintenance after conventional dieting: a 1-y study. *Am J Clin Nutr.* 1999;69(6): 1108–1116

233. Butryn ML, Wadden TA, Rukstalis MR, et al. Maintenance of weight loss in adolescents: current status and future directions. *J Obes.* 2010;2010:789280

234. Ozkan B, Bereket A, Turan S, Keskin S. Addition of orlistat to conventional treatment in adolescents with severe obesity. *Eur J Pediatr.* 2004;163(12):738–741

235. McDuffie JR, Calis KA, Booth SL, Uwaifo GI, Yanovski JA. Effects of orlistat on fat-soluble vitamins in obese adolescents. *Pharmacotherapy.* 2002;22(7):814–822

236. Michalsky M, Kramer RE, Fullmer MA, et al. Developing criteria for pediatric/adolescent bariatric surgery programs. *Pediatrics.* 2011;128(Suppl 2):S65–S70

237. Hsia DS, Fallon SC, Brandt ML. Adolescent bariatric surgery. *Arch Pediatr Adolesc Med.* 2012;166(8):757–766

238. August GP, Caprio S, Fennoy I, et al, Endocrine Society. Prevention and treatment of pediatric obesity; an Endocrine Society clinical practice guideline based on expert opinion. *J Clin Endocrinol Metab.* 2008;93(12):4576–4599

239. Inge TH, Krebs NF, Garcia VF, et al. Bariatric surgery for severely overweight adolescents: concerns and recommendations. *Pediatrics.* 2004;114(217–223)

240. Inge TH, Courcoulas AP, Jenkins TM, et al. Teen Labs Consortium. Weight loss and health status 3 years after bariatric surgery in adolescents. *N Engl J Med.* 2016;374(2):113–123

241. Inge TH, Courcoulas AP, Jenkins TM, et al. Five-year outcomes of gastric bypass in adolescents as compared with adults. *N Engl J Med.* 2019;380(22):2136–2145

Chapter 34

Food Allergy

Introduction

Adverse reactions to foods may result from immunologic (*food allergy*) and nonimmunologic responses.[1,2] Food allergy is defined as an "adverse health effect arising from a specific immune response that occurs reproducibly on exposure to a given food."[1] Food allergy affects 4% to 8% of children in the United States, although rates of parent-perceived allergies are significantly higher.[3-5] It is not clear whether the discordance of self-perceived allergy compared with true allergy is the result of lay perceptions regarding any adverse response to a food being an "allergy," or simply incorrect self-diagnosis, but the discordance indicates the need for a physician diagnosis to avoid unnecessary dietary avoidance. Food allergies can be severe and potentially fatal,[6] also indicating the need for careful diagnostic assessments and appropriate education regarding allergen avoidance and treatment of reactions.

There are a number of adverse reactions to foods that are not allergies. Toxins or pharmacologically active components of the diet account for a number of nonimmune adverse reactions, such as food poisoning. Food intolerance is another adverse reaction not involving the immune system. A common example is lactose intolerance caused by lactase insufficiency. Symptoms include abdominal discomfort, bloating, and loose stools from a reduced ability to digest lactose. Examples of adverse reactions to foods are shown in Table 34.1. This chapter focuses on food allergies. Although celiac

Table 34.1.
Examples of Adverse Reactions to Foods[66]

Intolerance
Lactose intolerance (from lactase deficiency)
Caffeine (jitteriness)
Tyramine in aged cheeses (migraine)
Toxins
Bacterial food poisoning (*Staphylococcus aureus, Salmonella* species, *Clostridium botulinum*, etc)
Scombroid (from spoilage of dark-meat fish, may mimic allergy)
Food allergy (immune responses)
IgE-mediated
Non–IgE-associated
Mixed IgE/non-IgE (eosinophilic gastrointestinal disease, atopic dermatitis)
Neurologic and psychological/psychiatric
Auriculotemporal syndrome (facial flush with salivation)
Gustatory rhinitis (rhinorrhea from spicy foods)
Anorexia nervosa and food aversions

VI

disease involves an immune response to gluten, it is not generally considered among food allergies and is not discussed in this chapter (see Chapter 27: Chronic Diarrhea).

Pathophysiology

Immune responses to foods are a normal phenomenon resulting in oral tolerance.[7] Normal responses include the production of immunoglobulin (Ig) G antibodies directed at food proteins. In contrast, aberrant immune responses to food proteins can result in food allergies. It is conceptually and diagnostically helpful to consider food-allergic disorders by immunopathology as to whether they are or are not associated with detectable food-specific IgE antibodies. Disorders with an acute onset of symptoms following ingestion are typically mediated by IgE antibodies. Food-specific IgE antibodies bind to high-affinity IgE receptors on tissue mast cells and blood basophils, a state termed *sensitization*. Reexposure to the food proteins results in binding and cross-linking of allergen-specific IgE antibodies, initiating signal transduction pathways that result in the release of mediators, such as histamine. The release of mediators then results in symptoms that may affect the skin, gastrointestinal tract, respiratory tract, and cardiovascular system. Another group of food-allergic disorders affecting primarily the gastrointestinal tract, such as food protein-induced enteropathy and food protein-induced enterocolitis, are subacute or chronic and are mediated primarily by T lymphocytes and not IgE antibodies. Atopic dermatitis and eosinophilic gastrointestinal disorders are a third group of chronic disorders that may be associated with food allergies and are variably associated with detectable IgE antibody (IgE associated/cell-mediated disorders).

Food Allergens

Most relevant food allergens are water-soluble glycoproteins that are 10 to 70 kD in size and relatively stable to heat, acid, and proteases. The foods accounting for most significant allergic reactions are cow milk, egg, peanut, tree nuts (ie, cashew, walnut, hazel, Brazil, etc), fish, Crustacean shellfish, wheat, and soy. However, more than 170 foods are described to have caused allergic reactions in some individuals, and seeds, such as sesame seeds, appear to represent emerging potent allergens. Certain fruits and vegetables typically cause mild reactions, such as oral pruritus, presumably because the causal proteins are labile and do not enter the bloodstream intact after digestion. Sensitivity to these proteins is most often the result of initial reactivity to homologous proteins in pollens (pollen-food related syndrome). For example, a protein in Birch pollen is homologous with a protein in raw apple. Heating the apple denatures this protein, so affected children can tolerate apple juice or sauce without symptoms.

Although many botanically related proteins share regions of homology and may show cross-reactivity on allergy testing, clinical evidence of cross-reactivity is not as common.[8] For example, peanut is a legume, and most people with peanut allergy have IgE antibodies that recognize proteins in other legumes, such as peas and string beans. This phenomenon leads to positive allergy test results for these other legumes. However, 95% of children with peanut allergy tolerate most other beans. The rate of clinically relevant cross-reactivity varies by food. There are high rates of allergy among fish and among shellfish (>50%) but no significant cross-reactivity between finned fish and shellfish. There are low rates of cross-reactivity among grains (<20%). Although many children with peanut or tree nut allergy may be allergic to multiple related foods, this is not a consistent finding. A child may be allergic, for example, to cashew and pistachio but not to other tree nuts. Some physicians suggest avoidance of food "families" to avoid misidentification or cross-contact of allergens that could result in reactions; for example, some may suggest avoiding all tree nuts if there is an allergy to any. Some tree nuts have homologous proteins, such as walnut with pecan, cashew with pistachio, and hazel with almond.

Allergic reactions to food additives, such as colors or preservatives, are uncommon. Food additives derived from natural sources contain proteins that may trigger allergic reactions.[2] These include colors derived from paprika, seeds (annatto, a red food coloring), and insects (carmine from cochineal). Chemical additives are not likely to cause IgE-associated allergic reactions, but some may cause adverse reactions, including symptoms that are allergy-like, or may invoke immune responses. Tartrazine (yellow #5) is a synthetic color that has been extensively investigated because of concerns that it may trigger hives, allergic reactions, and asthma. However, well-conducted studies have generally not validated these concerns. Like tartrazine, many other synthetic colors have not been proven to cause allergic reactions; however, some of these chemicals have rarely been associated with rashes. Sulfites can, in sensitive people, induce asthma and very rarely cause more significant allergic-like responses.

VI

Prevalence

There are no comprehensive studies to confirm the rate of food allergy.[5] The rates appear to vary geographically, likely as a result of genetics and environment/diet. An Australian study that focused solely on egg, peanut, and sesame allergies estimated a rate higher than 10% among 1-year-olds.[9] Food allergy is estimated to affect 4% to 8% of children in the United States and appears to be increasing in prevalence.[3] A study from the Centers for Disease Control and Prevention (CDC) reporting the results of the National Health Interview Survey suggested an 18% increase in prevalence of food allergy from 1997–2007.[10] Studies of peanut allergy in children suggest almost a tripling in prevalence in just over a decade,[11] with multiple studies worldwide indicating that more than 1% and possibly over 2% of school-aged children are affected.[9,11–13] The reasons for the apparent increase remain unclear, but theories include changes in food processing, timing of introduction of foods (either too early or too late in infancy and childhood), alterations in other components of the diet, such as fats or vitamins, and the "hygiene hypothesis" that lack of farm living and control of infection has resulted in immune dysregulation.[14,15] Genetic risk factors for food allergy include a family or personal history of atopic disorders (asthma, atopic dermatitis, allergic rhinitis, food allergy).

Clinical Disorders

The clinical manifestations of food allergy are diverse and result from underlying immune mechanisms and their effects on particular target organs. Food allergy may present as an acute reaction with a sudden onset of stereotypical symptoms, such as hives or respiratory compromise; as an increase in chronic symptoms, such as exacerbation of atopic dermatitis; or as a chronic disease in which recognition of symptom patterns suggests a food allergy. Specific disorders are summarized by pathophysiology in Table 34.2.

IgE-Mediated Food Allergies

IgE-mediated food-allergic reactions typically occur within minutes and rarely beyond an hour following ingestion of a triggering food. The organ system/systems affected and the specific symptoms additionally define these reactions. *Urticaria* and/or *angioedema*, pruritus, and flushing are common skin manifestation of food allergy, either alone or in combination with other symptoms. *Contact urticaria* describes lesions that occur at

Table 34.2.

Clinical Disorders Associated With Food Allergy According to Pathophysiology[66]

IMMUNOPATHOLOGY/DISORDER
IgE antibody-associated Urticaria/angioedema Oral allergy syndrome (pollen-related) Anaphylaxis Food-associated, exercise-induced anaphylaxis Onset of isolated symptoms (wheeze, abdominal pain, vomiting, etc)
IgE antibody-associated/cell-mediated, chronic Atopic dermatitis Eosinophilic gastroenteropathies
Non–IgE-associated Dietary protein enterocolitis Dietary protein proctitis Dietary protein enteropathy Contact dermatitis Pulmonary hemosiderosis

the site of direct contact with the food that may not induce a reaction when ingested.

Pollen-food allergy syndrome (oral allergy syndrome) is a form of allergy confined primarily to direct contact with raw fruits and vegetables in the oropharynx.[2] Initial sensitization to pollen proteins may result in symptoms when homologous proteins, in particular fruits/vegetables, are ingested, as described previously. This type of allergy is probably the most common of all food allergies and requires exposure to pollen seasons to develop. Symptoms are usually limited to the oropharynx with pruritus and mild angioedema, but progression to a systemic reaction may occur. Causal proteins are presumably heat-labile, because cooking the food typically abolishes reactions.

Although chronic asthma and allergic rhinitis are not typically solely attributable to food allergy, the same symptoms may accompany systemic food-allergic reactions.[1] Inhalation of airborne allergenic food proteins may also induce respiratory reactions when stable proteins become aerosolized during cooking or processing, such as boiling milk.[16]

Food-induced anaphylaxis is a serious systemic allergic reaction that is rapid in onset and may cause death.[17] Symptoms vary and may affect any combination of organ systems among the skin, respiratory tract, gastrointestinal tract, and cardiovascular system. Symptoms may include an aura of "impending doom." Life-threatening symptoms include laryngeal edema, severe asthma, and cardiovascular compromise. Serum tryptase elevation associated with mast cell activation is often not detected during food-associated anaphylaxis. Reactions may follow a biphasic course, with initial symptoms waning and recurrence of severe symptoms 1 to 2 hours later or longer. Fatal reactions appear to be more common in teenagers and young adults, possibly because of risk-taking behaviors. Victims typically have a diagnosed food allergy and asthma and delay treatment with epinephrine despite significant symptoms during a reaction. *Food-associated, exercise-induced anaphylaxis* is a syndrome in which anaphylaxis only occurs if exercise follows ingestion of a causal food that is otherwise tolerated.

Mixed IgE-/non-IgE–Associated Food Allergies (Atopic Dermatitis/Eosinophilic Gastrointestinal Disease)

Studies using double-blind, placebo-controlled oral food challenges show that approximately 1 in 3 young children with moderate to severe *atopic dermatitis* has a food allergy.[18] There is controversy about the role of foods in chronic rash.[1] There is agreement that children with moderate to severe atopic dermatitis are at increased risk of having immediate-type food-allergic reactions. When there is food-responsive dermatitis, food-specific IgE antibody is usually detectable to the trigger foods. However, food-responsive disease has also been documented in children without IgE detectable to the causal food; therefore, cell-mediated mechanisms are likely involved. Because of the chronic nature of the disorder and its waxing and waning course, it is difficult to associate symptoms with particular foods by history. Studies in children identify that more than 90% of reactions, whether acute anaphylaxis or flares of eczema, are attributed to "major" allergens, including peanut, milk, egg, tree nuts, wheat, soy, fish, and shellfish.[19] Removal of food allergen from the diet to treat atopic dermatitis should be undertaken with caution, because doing so carries potential nutritional and immunologic risks, including development of anaphylaxis upon reexposure to the food (noted to occur in 19% in 1 study[20]).

Allergic eosinophilic esophagitis/gastroenteritis is a group of disorders characterized by eosinophilic inflammation in the gastrointestinal tract. Symptoms overlap those of other gastrointestinal disorders and may include dysphagia, vomiting, diarrhea, and malabsorption. Almost all children are food responsive, although it may be difficult to identify the offending food, and implicated foods may or may not be associated with evidence of IgE antibody.[21]

Non-IgE–Mediated Disorders

These disorders may also affect various target organs.[1,2] In regard to skin manifestations, contact dermatitis, a type IV hypersensitivity response, may occur from contact with foods. A rare pulmonary disorder affecting infants, Heiner syndrome or milk-induced pulmonary hemosiderosis, is associated with precipitating (IgG) antibodies to cow milk. Symptoms include anemia, pulmonary infiltrates, recurrent pneumonia, and growth failure, which resolve with milk elimination.

Several non-IgE mediated disorders of the gastrointestinal tract affect primarily infants.[1,2] *Food protein-induced proctocolitis* is characterized by mucous and blood in stools. Patients are usually breastfed infants, and the bleeding usually resolves with maternal exclusion of cow milk. The infant is otherwise well. Foods other than milk are sometimes implicated. Empiric dietary exclusion is commonly instituted. If rectal biopsy is performed, eosinophilic inflammation is observed. The disorder is not associated with detectable IgE antibody to milk and typically resolves by 1 year of age.[22] Infants with *food protein-induced enteropathy* experience diarrhea, poor growth, and edema attributable to hypoproteinemia caused by malabsorption when ingesting the causal food. A dramatic form of non-IgE mediated gastrointestinal food allergy is *food protein-induced enterocolitis syndrome*, mediated by T lymphocytes.[22] Onset is usually in infancy and is characterized by a symptom complex of profuse vomiting and heme-positive diarrhea, failure to thrive, and potentially dehydration and shock during chronic ingestion of the causal protein. These infants also may develop acidemia and methemoglobinemia and present with symptoms mimicking sepsis, including an elevated peripheral polymorphonuclear leukocyte count. Cow milk and soy are most often responsible, but grains, such as rice and oat, and poultry are common solid food triggers. Among those with reactions to cow milk, there is an increased risk of reactions to soy. Ingestion of the causal protein after resolution of symptoms may lead to a delayed (about 2 hours) recurrence of symptoms that may be severe and include shock. Resolution of the allergy usually occurs in 2 to 3 years, but readministration of the causal protein can trigger severe reactions and is typically undertaken under controlled settings with an intravenous line in place to administer hydration, steroids, and ondansetron.

VI

Diagnosis

The clinical evaluation of an adverse reaction to food requires a careful history and physical examination to determine the type of adverse response, whether potentially IgE or non-IgE associated.[2] Important factors to consider include the types of symptoms, the chronicity and reproducibility of the symptoms, and alternative explanations for symptoms. If symptoms indicate a nonimmune etiology, additional evaluation can be directed to the specific suspicion. For example, lactose intolerance may be confirmed by dietary elimination and challenge. For chronic disorders, such as atopic dermatitis and eosinophilic gastroenteritis, the identification of suspect foods is difficult, because food is ingested throughout the day and symptoms are often chronic with a waxing and waning course. Symptom diaries are helpful but rarely diagnostic. In addition, individuals with these disorders are often sensitized to multiple foods, many of which may not be causing illness. Care in selecting and interpreting the tests is paramount, and consideration of the previously reviewed epidemiology and pathophysiology of food allergies is helpful for test selection and interpretation.

After a history is obtained, tests for food-specific IgE antibodies may be performed. The test modalities include skin prick tests, performed using a probe to introduce food protein to the superficial skin layer, or serum tests. The tests have similar performance characteristics. They are generally very sensitive (~75%–95%) and modestly specific (~30%–60%).[1,2,23] Skin prick tests are used on rash-free skin while the patient is avoiding antihistamines; intradermal skin tests should not be used. Although commercial extracts are available for performing skin prick tests for many foods, fresh extracts, particularly when testing fruits and vegetables for which proteins are prone to degradation, may be more sensitive. If IgE antibody specific for the food protein is present, a wheal and flare will occur that is compared with positive (histamine) and negative (saline) controls. The skin prick test is available to allergists and has advantages of immediate results and low cost.

A more widely available test is a serum test for food-specific IgE antibodies. There are 3 commercial manufacturers of the test[24]; results between them vary, probably because the reagents have slight differences in the proteins displayed. Previous generation tests used radioactivity (radioallergosorbent test [RAST]), but these assays are no longer used. Like skin prick tests, the serum IgE tests are generally comprised of proteins extracted from the food being tested, representing numerous proteins. However, immune responses against digestion-stable proteins are more likely to represent true allergies than ones against heat- and digestion-labile food proteins. Tests have emerged to measure specific IgE against various component proteins in food. The best studied test is for peanut protein. IgE binding to the peanut protein Ara h 2, a stable protein, is associated with clinical allergy, and IgE binding to Ara h 8, a labile pollen-related protein, is not generally associated with reactions.[25,26] Component testing is commercially available for a limited number of foods.

A positive skin prick test or serum IgE test result merely indicates that food-specific IgE is present, a state termed *sensitization*. Sensitization is not equivalent to a diagnosis of clinical allergy.[1,2,23] Increasingly larger wheal diameters or increasing concentrations of IgE antibodies are associated with increasingly higher probability that the test reflects clinical allergy. In a limited number of studies of a few foods in infants and/or children, diagnostic values associated with very high ($\geq$95%) predictive values for reactions have been determined, although not universally confirmed.[26]

Food-specific IgE may be detected despite tolerance of a food or may remain detectable but typically declines as a food allergy resolves. Obtaining "panels" of food allergy tests without consideration of history is not a good practice, because numerous irrelevant positive results may result, creating confusion and anxiety.[1,2,23] History is key for test selection and interpretation. Food-specific IgE test results are expected to be negative when the pathophysiology of the response is consistent with non-IgE–mediated reactions. However, acute anaphylactic reactions may also occasionally occur despite a negative test result, so caution is needed when evaluating a patient with a convincing history but a negative test result. Neither the size of the skin prick test reaction nor concentration of IgE in serum usefully predicts the type or severity of reaction.

The atopy patch test, which is performed by placing the food allergen on the skin under occlusion for 48 hours and assessing for a delayed rash at 24 to 72 hours, has been tested for diagnosing non–IgE-mediated disorders, but studies have so far shown no predictive value for identifying foods triggering food protein-induced enterocolitis and very limited value in identifying causal foods in eosinophilic esophagitis.[1,2,23] Other tests have been touted for the diagnosis of food allergy but have never been found useful in blinded studies. These tests, which are not recommended, include measurement of IgG$_4$ antibody, provocation-neutralization (diluted liquid extracts of foods placed under the tongue or injected to diagnose and treat various symptoms), and applied kinesiology (muscle strength testing).[23] A

VI

AAP

AAP Summary of IgE Test Characteristics and Limitations[23]

- Treatment decisions for infants and children with allergy should be made on the basis of the appropriate diagnosis and identification of causative allergens, which may be identified through directed specific IgE testing.
- Allergy tests for specific IgE must be selected and interpreted in the context of a clinical presentation; test relevance may vary according to the patient's age, allergen exposure, and performance characteristics of the test.
- Positive specific IgE test results indicate sensitization, which is not equivalent to clinical allergy. Large panels of indiscriminately performed screening tests may, therefore, provide misleading information.
- Tests for specific IgE may be influenced by cross-reactive proteins that may or may not have clinical relevance to disease.
- Increasingly higher levels of specific IgE (higher concentrations on serum tests or skin prick test wheal size) generally correlate with an increased risk of clinical allergy.
- Specific IgE test results typically do not reflect severity of allergies.
- Tests for allergen-specific IgG antibodies are not helpful for diagnosing allergies.
- Consultation with a board-certified allergist-immunologist should be considered, because test limitations often warrant additional evaluation to confirm the role of specific allergens.

Pediatrics. 2012;129(1):193–197

---

clinical report from the American Academy of Pediatrics (AAP) on the topic of allergy testing emphasized the benefits and limitations of the tests and provides additional recommendations as summarized in the text box.[23]

For evaluation of chronic diseases such as atopic dermatitis and eosinophilic esophagitis, improvement of symptoms during dietary elimination of suspected foods provides presumptive evidence of causality. Elimination diets can be undertaken by removing foods suspected to be causing symptoms, removing all but a selected group of foods that are rarely allergenic (oligoantigenic diet), or giving an elemental diet consisting only of a hypoallergenic extensively hydrolyzed formula or a nonallergenic amino acid-based formula. The elemental diet provides the most definitive trial but is difficult for children and teenagers to follow. The type of elimination diet selected will depend on *a priori* reasoning concerning offending foods on the basis of history and epidemiology, and, when appropriate, the results of tests for IgE antibody. The length of trial depends on the type of symptoms, but 1 to 6 weeks is usually the range required. Consultation with a dietitian may be needed to ensure nutritional sufficiency of trial diets. For breastfed infants, maternal dietary elimination is required. When a food to which IgE has been demonstrated is removed from the diet during a chronic disorder, it is possible for reintroduction to induce severe reactions[20]; therefore, guidance from an allergist is prudent.

When history and IgE testing have not confirmed an allergy, or when the development of tolerance is suspected, an oral food challenge may be required to confirm clinical allergy.[1,2,23] An oral food challenge is performed by feeding gradually increasing amounts of the suspected food under medical observation.[27] Oral food challenges are performed either openly, in which the patient and physician know the food being tested is being ingested, or blinded, by camouflaging the food in a carrier food. The double-blind placebo-controlled food challenge is least prone to bias and is considered the "gold standard." Briefly, this format of oral food challenge has a third party develop 2 feedings that are identical in taste/texture but only 1 contains the test allergen. The oral food challenge is randomized such that true or placebo doses are given, for example, on separate days, and the patient and observer are not aware of the content. The oral food challenge can be used to evaluate any type of adverse response. For non–IgE-mediated reactions, the oral food challenge is usually the only means of diagnosis. Feeding tests, particularly in IgE-mediated reactions and enterocolitis syndrome, can induce severe reactions. The supervising clinician, usually an allergist, must have medications and supplies for resuscitation immediately available to manage reactions. Negative challenges should always be followed by a supervised open feeding of a relevant portion of the tested food in its commonly prepared state.

Treatment

Dietary Avoidance

The mainstay of treatment is avoidance of the food and preparation for treatment in the event of an accidental ingestion leading to an allergic reaction. Most formula-fed infants who are allergic to standard cow milk formulas will tolerate a formula labeled "hypoallergenic" for infants with milk allergy (eg, an extensively hydrolyzed, casein-based formula).[28] If the infant is reactive to these cow milk-derived formulas, an amino acid-based formula should be tolerated. Alternatively, a soy-based formula may be selected, because it is usually tolerated among infants with IgE-mediated cow milk allergy, although soy may present a higher risk for infants with enterocolitis syndrome.[29] Foods in the maternal diet may trigger reactions in a highly sensitive breastfed infant who is allergic to the particular food allergen, in which case maternal avoidance of the allergen may be required.

For children on limited diets, nutritional counseling and growth monitoring is recommended.[1,30] In the United States, labeling laws require plain English disclosure of the "major" food allergens—milk, egg, wheat, soy, peanut, tree nuts, fish, and shellfish (see Chapter 50.II: Federal Regulation of Food Labeling). The specific type of food is required to be named for categorical types (eg, cod, shrimp, walnut). Currently, additional potent allergens, such as sesame, are not included in the laws. Advisory labels (ie, "may contain peanut") are not regulated, are increasingly common, and reflect variable risks.[31] Strict avoidance, therefore, requires avoidance of products with advisory labeling. Cross-contamination and errors in restaurants are an additional obstacle, so it is imperative that individuals notify and discuss their allergy with restaurant personnel, who may need some coaching about situations in which foods may become contaminated with allergens, such as in fryers, in shared bowls, on cutting boards, etc.[32,33] For children, dietary management in schools can be difficult, because food sharing, school projects using foods, parties, lack of on-site medical personnel, and other issues arise.[34] Ingestion, rather than skin or air exposure, is the primary concern for avoidance,[35] although attention should be paid to avoid fumes of allergens (eg, boiling milk, steaming shellfish) and, for adolescents, passionate kissing when a partner recently consumed the allergen.[36]

Although strict avoidance is generally advised, there is a growing body of literature indicating that, in some cases, this may not be necessary. Approximately 70% of children with allergic reactions to milk products or egg can tolerate these foods when they are heated extensively—for example, baked into muffins or breads.[37] It is presumed that heating these particular foods results in conformational changes in the proteins, allowing ingestion for people with a milder form of the allergy, probably a phenotype that is also more likely to resolve the allergy. Adding such foods to the diet can improve quality of life and nutrition, but the effect on the natural course of allergy is not well studied. However, evidence suggests that immune responses to the addition of these foods are similar to those seen during successful active immunotherapy—for example, an increase in food-specific IgG antibodies is noted, and some suppression of IgE responses is also

> ### Candidates for Prescription of
> ### Self-Injectable Epinephrine and Dosing[1,17]
>
> Self-injectable epinephrine should be prescribed for children with:
> - Prior systemic allergic reactions
> - Food allergy and asthma
> - Food allergy to peanut, tree nut, fish, or shellfish
>   (and considered for any IgE-mediated food allergy)

observed, and there is some indication of accelerated tolerance. However, caution is advised with this approach, because some children experience anaphylaxis to the heated products.

Medical Management

In the event of an allergic reaction, antihistamines may be required to reduce itching and rash. However, for children experiencing more severe symptoms of anaphylaxis with respiratory and/or cardiovascular symptoms, additional therapies are required.[17] Self-injectable epinephrine should be prescribed for those at risk of anaphylaxis, as described in national guidelines and an AAP clinical report, as summarized in the text box.[1,17] Epinephrine dosing for first aid management of anaphylaxis is ideally 0.01 mg per kg (injected intramuscularly using the 1:1000 concentration). Fixed-dose epinephrine autoinjectors are available in 0.1-, 0.15-, and 0.3-mg doses in the United States (and 0.5-mg doses outside the United States). Dosing can be individualized to avoid underdosing as children grow, for example, by prescribing the 0.3-mg dose for those weighing more than 25 kg.[17] It is essential to periodically review the indications and technique of administration of self-injectable epinephrine. Patients must be instructed to seek prompt transportation (ie, ambulance, calling 911) to an emergency facility for treatment of anaphylaxis and remain under observation (>4 hours), because recurrence of severe symptoms is possible. Individuals with potential shock should remain prone; rising upright without proper treatment has rarely been reported to result in death as a result of the "empty ventricle syndrome." Patients should obtain medical jewelry identifying their allergy and be reminded to update expired epinephrine injectors. An important component of the school or camp management of food allergy is to have a clear written emergency plan in place,[38] medications readily available, and

VI

school personnel trained in recognizing and treating reactions.[34] Teenagers are at special risk of fatal reactions, probably because of risk-taking behaviors. It is, therefore, important to encourage education of the affected teenager, school staff, and his or her friends about the allergy and when to treat with epinephrine.[39]

The emotional toll of living with food allergy should not be neglected. Various studies have identified a serious effect on quality of life as well as increased anxiety.[40-42] Children with food allergies may be subjected to bullying as well.[43,44] Therefore, discussion of the psychosocial factors involved with management, ensuring that families are coping appropriately and not overly isolating themselves, and considering mental health referral are important components of management.

Natural History

Most children (approximately 85%) lose their sensitivity to most allergenic foods (egg, milk, wheat, soy) within the first 3 to 10 years of life.[45] In contrast, allergy to peanut, tree nuts, and seafood is rarely lost. Approximately 20% of peanut-allergic children younger than 2 years and 5% to 10% of those with tree nut allergy may achieve tolerance by school age.[45] Tolerance is typically determined by repeated testing, with reduced food-specific IgE antibodies possibly indicating resolution and with physician-supervised oral food challenges.

Prevention

Early approaches for prevention of food allergy, espoused by the AAP in 1998, focused on having infants avoid allergenic foods.[46,47] These approaches included recommendations to delay the introduction of cow's milk until 1 year, eggs until 2 years, and peanuts, nuts, and fish until 3 years of age. It also recommended using hypoallergenic formula until 6 months of age if human milk was not available. This approach was based partly on studies demonstrating that infants ingesting hypoallergenic forms of cow milk formula and delaying introduction of allergens had less atopic dermatitis than those following unrestricted diets.[46] However, epidemiologic and observational studies published after 2000 suggested that delayed ingestion was not protective and may allow more time for sensitization by routes such as skin or respiratory exposure, while mechanisms of oral tolerance are circumvented by a lack of ingestion.[48-50] In 2008, an AAP clinical report rescinded earlier advice about delaying introduction of allergenic foods and summarized data on atopy prevention through diet.[51]

Subsequent to the 2008 report, specifically regarding the timing of introduction of allergenic foods, the Learning Early About Peanut (LEAP) study directly addressed the possibility that early peanut ingestion might reduce the risk of developing peanut allergy.[52] LEAP randomly assigned 640 infants between 4 and 11 months of age with severe eczema and/or egg allergy to consume or avoid peanut-containing foods until 60 months of age. Mean age of randomization was 7.8 ± 1.7 months, but only 18% (116 infants) of the total cohort were younger than 6 months at the time of the first peanut introduction. At the time of the random assignment, 90% of infants had received formula. The study excluded infants with large (>4 mm) positive skin prick test results to peanut, assuming many were already allergic, and stratified the enrolled infants as having a peanut skin test wheal of 0 mm (not sensitized) or having one that was 1 to 4 mm in diameter. In the intention-to-treat (ITT) population with negative skin prick test results (n=530), the prevalence of peanut allergy at 60 months of age was 13.7% in the avoidance group versus 1.9% in the early consumption group ($P < .001$; relative risk reduction, 86.1%), and among those in the skin prick test positive result group (n=98), the prevalence of peanut allergy was 35.3% in the avoidance group and 10.6% in the consumption group ($P = .004$; relative risk reduction, 70%). Follow-up studies indicated that the approach was long lasting and did not adversely affect breastfeeding or nutrition.[53,54] On the basis of these results, an expert panel advised peanut introduction as early as 4 to 6 months of age in infants at high risk (with severe eczema and/or egg allergy, similar to the study).[55] Given that the pathophysiology of protection is likely to be similar for lower-risk infants and on the basis of additional studies in an unselected population,[56] the guidelines extrapolated earliest times of peanut introduction based on the degree of risk (Table 34.3). The preventive effect of early introduction is not lost if the infant is introduced to peanut later than the "earliest" ages described, but the opportunity to add peanut to the diet before sensitization/allergy occurs could decrease as the infant ages without ingesting it. The guidelines describe using infant-safe forms of peanut, providing prescribed amounts to the group at highest risk, and offering allergy evaluations, including serum peanut-specific IgE tests, skin tests, and or oral food challenges, depending on test results and risk assessments.

VI

Table 34.3.
Guidelines for Early Introduction of Peanut[55]

Infant Clinical Criteria	Recommendations	Earliest Age of Peanut Introduction
Guideline #1: Severe eczema, egg allergy, or both	Strongly consider evaluation by serum IgE or skin prick testing, and if necessary, an oral food challenge. On the basis of test results, introduce infant safe peanut-containing foods.	4–6 mo
Guideline #2: Mild to moderate eczema	Introduce infant-safe peanut-foods.	Around 6 mo
Guideline #3: No eczema or any food allergy	Introduce infant-safe peanut-containing foods.	Age appropriate and in accordance with family preferences and cultural practices

See Togias et al[55] for full discussion of criteria, screening tests, and modality of introduction of peanut.

AAP Recommendations for
Food Allergy Prevention Through Diet[64]

- There is lack of evidence that maternal dietary allergen restrictions during pregnancy or lactation play a significant role in the prevention of food allergy.
- There is no evidence that any duration of breastfeeding prevents or delays food allergy in infants and children.
- There is very limited evidence that partially or extensively hydrolyzed formula prevents food allergy including cow milk allergy in infants and children, even in those at high risk for allergic disease.
- There is no evidence that delaying the introduction of allergenic foods beyond 4 to 6 months prevents food allergy, including peanut, eggs, and fish.
- There is evidence that the early introduction of infant-safe forms of peanut reduces the risk for peanut allergies (see Table 34.3). Data are less clear for the timing of introduction of egg.

Pediatrics. 2019;143(4):e20190281

As a result of the publication of the LEAP trial[52,54] and other additional reports,[55,57-63] the AAP revised its clinical report in 2019 with new recommendations for dietary interventions for the prevention of food allergy.[64]

Summary

Food allergy is common and appears to be increasing. An accurate diagnosis of food allergy requires rational use of the available diagnostic tests, relying heavily on clinical history for test selection and interpretation and recognizing that a physician-supervised oral food challenge is often required. Current management requires avoidance and reactionary treatment in the event of symptoms. An opportunity to prevent peanut allergy by early introduction has been recommended. In addition, studies are underway for improved therapies using strategies such as oral, sublingual, or epicutaneous immunotherapy, anti-IgE antibodies, and others that may provide more definitive therapy in the future.[65,66]

VI

References

1. Boyce JA, Assa'ad A, Burks AW, et al. Guidelines for the diagnosis and management of food allergy in the United States: Summary of the NIAID-Sponsored Expert Panel Report. *J Allergy Clin Immun.* 2010;126(6):1105–1118

2. Sampson HA, Aceves S, Bock SA, et al. Food allergy: a practice parameter update-2014. *J Allergy Clin Immun.* 2014;134(5):1016–1025.e1043

3. Gupta RS, Springston EE, Warrier MR, et al. The prevalence, severity, and distribution of childhood food allergy in the United States. *Pediatrics.* 2011;128(1): e9–e17

4. Sicherer SH. Epidemiology of food allergy. *J Allergy Clin Immun.* 2011;127(3): 594–602

5. Sicherer SH, Allen K, Lack G, Taylor SL, Donovan SM, Oria M. Critical issues in food allergy: a National Academies Consensus Report. *Pediatrics.* 2017;140(2): e20170194

6. Umasunthar T, Leonardi-Bee J, Hodes M, et al. Incidence of fatal food anaphylaxis in people with food allergy: a systematic review and meta-analysis. *Clin Exp Allergy.* 2013;43(12):1333–1341

7. Berin MC, Shreffler WG. Mechanisms underlying induction of tolerance to foods. *Immunol Allergy Clin North Am.* 2016;36(1):87–102

8. Sicherer SH. Clinical implications of cross-reactive food allergens. *J Allergy Clin Immunol.* 2001;108(6):881–890

9. Osborne NJ, Koplin JJ, Martin PE, et al. Prevalence of challenge-proven IgE-mediated food allergy using population-based sampling and predetermined challenge criteria in infants. *J Allergy Clin Immunol.* 2011;127(3):668–676

10. Branum AM, Lukacs SL. Food allergy among children in the United States. *Pediatrics.* 2009;124(6):1549–1555

11. Sicherer SH, Munoz-Furlong A, Godbold JH, Sampson HA. US prevalence of self-reported peanut, tree nut, and sesame allergy: 11-year follow-up. *J Allergy Clin Immun.* 2010;125(6):1322–1326

12. Bunyavanich S, Rifas-Shiman SL, Platts-Mills TA, et al. Peanut allergy prevalence among school-age children in a US cohort not selected for any disease. *J Allergy Clin Immunol.* 2014;134(3):753–755

13. Nwaru BI, Hickstein L, Panesar SS, et al. Prevalence of common food allergies in Europe: a systematic review and meta-analysis. *Allergy.* 2014;69(8):992–1007

14. du Toit G, Tsakok T, Lack S, Lack G. Prevention of food allergy. *J Allergy Clin Immun.* 2016;137(4):998–1010

15. Allen KJ, Koplin JJ. Prospects for Prevention of food allergy. *J Allergy Clin Immunol Pract.* 2016;4(2):215–220

16. Roberts G, Lack G. Relevance of inhalational exposure to food allergens. *Curr Opin Allergy Clin Immunol.* 2003;3(3):211–215

17. Sicherer SH, Simons FE, Section On A, Immunology. Epinephrine for First-aid Management of Anaphylaxis. *Pediatrics.* 2017;139(3)

18. Sicherer SH, Sampson HA. Food hypersensitivity and atopic dermatitis: pathophysiology, epidemiology, diagnosis, and management. *J Allergy Clin Immunol.* 1999;104(3 Pt 2):S114–S122

19. Ellman LK, Chatchatee P, Sicherer SH, Sampson HA. Food hypersensitivity in two groups of children and young adults with atopic dermatitis evaluated a decade apart. *Pediatr Allergy Immunol.* 2002;13(4):295–298

20. Chang A, Robison R, Cai M, Singh AM. Natural history of food-triggered atopic dermatitis and development of immediate reactions in children. *J Allergy Clin Immunol Pract.* 2016;4(2):229–236 e221

21. Liacouras CA, Furuta GT, Hirano I, et al. Eosinophilic esophagitis: updated consensus recommendations for children and adults. *J Allergy Clin Immun.* 2011;128(1):3-20 e26

22. Ravelli A, Villanacci V, Chiappa S, Bolognini S, Manenti S, Fuoti M. Dietary protein-induced proctocolitis in childhood. *Am. J Gastroenterol.* 2008;103(10): 2605–2612

23. Sicherer SH, Wood RA, Immunology SA. Allergy testing in childhood: using allergen-specific IgE tests. *Pediatrics.* 2012;129(1):193–197

24. Hamilton RG, Williams PB. Human IgE antibody serology: a primer for the practicing North American allergist/immunologist. *J Allergy Clin Immunol.* 2010;126(1):33–38

25. Sicherer SH, Wood RA. Advances in diagnosing peanut allergy. *J Allergy Clin Immunol Pract.* 2013;1(1):1–13

26. Chokshi NY, Sicherer SH. Interpreting IgE sensitization tests in food allergy. *Expert Rev Clin Immunol.* 2016;12(4):389–403

27. Nowak-Wegrzyn A, Assa'ad AH, Bahna SL, Bock SA, Sicherer SH, Teuber SS. Work Group report: oral food challenge testing. *J Allergy Clin Immun.* 2009;123 (6 Suppl):S365–S383

28. Fiocchi A, Schunemann HJ, Brozek J, et al. Diagnosis and Rationale for Action Against Cow's Milk Allergy (DRACMA): a summary report. *J Allergy Clin Immunol.* 2010;126(6):1119–1128

29. Nowak-Wegrzyn A, Chehade M, Groetch ME, et al. International consensus guidelines for the diagnosis and management of food protein-induced enterocolitis syndrome: Executive summary-Workgroup Report of the Adverse Reactions to Foods Committee, American Academy of Allergy, Asthma & Immunology. *J Allergy Clin Immunol.* 2017;139(4):1111–1126 e1114

30. Nowak-Wegrzyn A, Groetch M. Nutritional aspects and diets in food allergy. *Chem Immunol Allergy.* 2015;101:209–220

31. Marchisotto MJ, Harada L, Kamdar O, et al. Food Allergen Labeling and Purchasing Habits in the United States and Canada. *J Allergy Clin Immunol Pract.* 2017;5(2):345–351 e342

32. Ahuja R, Sicherer SH. Food-allergy management from the perspective of restaurant and food establishment personnel. *Ann Allergy Asthma Immunol.* 2007;98(4):344–348

VI

33. Bailey S, Albardiaz R, Frew AJ, Smith H. Restaurant staff's knowledge of anaphylaxis and dietary care of people with allergies. *Clin Exp Allergy*. 2011;41(5): 713–717

34. Sicherer SH, Mahr T, American Academy of Pediatrics Section on A, Immunology. Management of food allergy in the school setting. *Pediatrics*. 2010;126(6):1232–1239

35. Fleischer DM, Perry TT, Atkins D, et al. Allergic reactions to foods in preschool-aged children in a prospective observational food allergy study. *Pediatrics*. 2012;130(1):e25–32

36. Simonte SJ, Ma S, Mofidi S, Sicherer SH. Relevance of casual contact with peanut butter in children with peanut allergy. *J Allergy Clin Immunol*. 2003;112(1):180–182

37. Leonard SA, Caubet JC, Kim JS, Groetch M, Nowak-Wegrzyn A. Baked milk- and egg-containing diet in the management of milk and egg allergy. *J Allergy Clin Immunol Pract*. 2015;3(1):13–23

38. Wang J, Sicherer SH, Section Allergy and Immunology. Guidance on completing a written allergy and anaphylaxis emergency plan. *Pediatrics*. 2017;139(3) e20164005

39. Marrs T, Lack G. Why do few food-allergic adolescents treat anaphylaxis with adrenaline?—Reviewing a pressing issue. *Pediatr Allergy Immunol*. 2013;24(3):222–229

40. Ravid NL, Annunziato RA, Ambrose MA, et al. Mental health and quality-of-life concerns related to the burden of food allergy. *Psychiatr Clin North Am*. 2015;38(1):77–89

41. Herbert L, Shemesh E, Bender B. Clinical Management of Psychosocial Concerns Related to Food Allergy. *J Allergy Clin Immunol Pract*. 2016;4(2):205–213

42. Shemesh E, D'Urso C, Knight C, et al. Food-allergic adolescents at risk for anaphylaxis: a randomized controlled study of supervised injection to improve comfort with epinephrine self-injection. *J Allergy Clin Immunol Pract*. 2017;5(2):391–397 e394

43. Shemesh E, Annunziato RA, Ambrose MA, et al. Child and parental reports of bullying in a consecutive sample of children with food allergy. *Pediatrics*. 2013;131(1):e10–e17

44. Annunziato RA, Rubes M, Ambrose MA, Mullarkey C, Shemesh E, Sicherer SH. Longitudinal evaluation of food allergy-related bullying. *J Allergy Clin Immunol Pract*. 2014;2(5):639–641

45. Savage J, Sicherer S, Wood R. The Natural History of Food Allergy. *J Allergy Clin Immunol Pract*. 2016;4(2):196–203

46. Zeiger RS, Heller S, Mellon MH, Forsythe AB, O'Connor RD, Hamburger RN. Effect of combined maternal and infant food-allergen avoidance on development of atopy in early infancy: a randomized study. *J Allergy Clin Immunol*. 1989;84(1):72–89

47. American Academy of Pediatrics, Committee on Nutrition. Hypersensitivity to food. In: Kleinman RE, Greer FR, eds. *Pediatric Nutrition Handbook*. 4th ed. Elk Grove Village, IL: American Academy of Pediatrics; 1998:257–266

48. Du Toit G, Katz Y, Sasieni P, et al. Early consumption of peanuts in infancy is associated with a low prevalence of peanut allergy. *J Allergy Clin Immunol*. 2008;122(5):984–991

49. Nwaru BI, Erkkola M, Ahonen S, et al. Age at the introduction of solid foods during the first year and allergic sensitization at age 5 years. *Pediatrics*. 2010;125(1):50–59

50. Zutavern A, Brockow I, Schaaf B, et al. Timing of solid food introduction in relation to eczema, asthma, allergic rhinitis, and food and inhalant sensitization at the age of 6 years: results from the prospective birth cohort study LISA. *Pediatrics*. 2008;121(1):e44–e52

51. Greer FR, Sicherer SH, Burks AW, American Academy of Pediatrics Committee on N, American Academy of Pediatrics Section on A, Immunology. Effects of early nutritional interventions on the development of atopic disease in infants and children: the role of maternal dietary restriction, breastfeeding, timing of introduction of complementary foods, and hydrolyzed formulas. *Pediatrics*. 2008;121(1):183–191

52. Du Toit G, Roberts G, Sayre PH, et al. Randomized trial of peanut consumption in infants at risk for peanut allergy. *N Engl J Med*. 2015;372(9):803–813

53. Feeney M, Du Toit G, Roberts G, et al. Impact of peanut consumption in the LEAP Study: Feasibility, growth, and nutrition. *J Allergy Clin Immun*. 2016;138(4):1108–1118

54. Du Toit G, Sayre PH, Roberts G, et al. Effect of avoidance on peanut allergy after early peanut consumption. *N Engl J Med*. 2016;374(15):1435–1443

55. Togias A, Cooper SF, Acebal ML, et al. Addendum guidelines for the prevention of peanut allergy in the United States: Report of the National Institute of Allergy and Infectious Diseases-sponsored expert panel. *J Allergy Clin Immun*. 2017;139(1):29–44

56. Perkin MR, Logan K, Tseng A, et al. Randomized trial of introduction of allergenic foods in breast-fed infants. *N Engl J Med*. 2016;374(18):1733–1743

57. Lodge CJ, Tan DJ, Lau MX, et al. Breastfeeding and asthma and allergies: a systematic review and meta-analysis. *Acta Paediatr*. 2015;104(467):38–53

58. Kramer MS, Kakuma R. Maternal dietary antigen avoidance during pregnancy or lactation, or both, for preventing or treating atopic disease in the child. *Evid Based Child Health*. 2014;9(2):447–483

59. Fiocchi A, Pawankar R, Cuello-Garcia C, et al. World Allergy Organization-McMaster University Guidelines for Allergic Disease Prevention (GLAD-P): Probiotics. *World Allergy Organ J*. 2015;8(1):4

60. Cuello-Garcia CA, Fiocchi A, Pawankar R, et al. World Allergy Organization-McMaster University Guidelines for Allergic Disease Prevention (GLAD-P): Prebiotics. *World Allergy Organ J*. 2016;9:10

VI

61. Boyle RJ, Ierodiakonou D, Khan T, et al. Hydrolysed formula and risk of allergic or autoimmune disease: systematic review and meta-analysis. *BMJ.* 2016;352:i974

62. Osborn DA, Sinn JK, Jones LJ. Infant formulas containing hydrolysed protein for prevention of allergic disease and food allergy. *Cochrane Database Syst Rev.* 2017;(3):CD003664

63. Kramer MS, Kakuma R. Optimal duration of exclusive breastfeeding. *Cochrane Database Syst Rev.* 2012;(8):CD003517

64. Greer FR, Sicherer SH, Burks AW, American Academy of Pediatrics, Committee on Nutrition, Section on Allergy and Immunology. The effects of early nutritional interventions on the development of atopic disease in infants and children: the role of maternal dietary restriction, breastfeeding, hydrolyzed formulas, and timing of introduction of allergenic complementary foods. *Pediatrics.* 2019;143(4):e20190281

65. Wood RA. Food allergen immunotherapy: current status and prospects for the future. *J Allergy Clin Immunol.* 2016;137(4):973–982

66. Sicherer SH, Sampson HA. Food allergy: A review and update on epidemiology, pathogenesis, diagnosis, prevention, and management. *J Allergy Clin Immunol.* 2018;141(1):41–58

Chapter 35

Nutrition and Immunity

Introduction

Nutrition plays an integral role in the development and function of the immune system. Malnutrition resulting from energy or specific nutrient deficiencies impairs the immune system and leads to functional abnormalities in cell mediated immunity, the complement system, phagocyte function, cytokine production, mucosal secretory antibody responses, and antibody affinity.

Nutrient-immune interactions are of special concern in infants because of an increased vulnerability of the developing immune system. Early in life, systemic humoral immunity is strongly dependent on transplacental acquisition of maternal immunoglobulin G (IgG), and specific mucosal immune responses rely heavily on secretory immunoglobulin A (sIgA) supplied via human milk. This reliance on maternal factors is attributable to the paucity of production of those immunoglobulin isotypes during early infancy, the decreased repertoire of antibody-binding specificities during that period, and the slow development of antibody responses to polysaccharide antigens during the first 2 to 3 years of life.

Nutritional status influences the immune system at different levels. Subclinical or marked micronutrient deficiencies may reduce the circulating levels and functional capacity of key immune cells and proteins. Specific micronutrient deficiencies, such as essential fatty acids, folate, zinc, and vitamin A, cause mucosal lesions or reduce mucosal integrity, thus increasing susceptibility to infections. As nutritional health influences immune status, immunodeficiencies may, in turn, compromise nutritional health. This chapter discusses nutrient-immune interactions, including a discussion of human milk and immunity, the microbiome, and developmental and acquired immunodeficiency in 3 related but separate sections.

Nutrition And Immunity: Immune System Interactions

Micronutrients

Micronutrients work in synergy to support different components of the immune system, including physical barriers, cellular responses, and antibody production (Table 35.1).[1] Even in mild cases of nutrient deficiency, the immunologic effects of a deficiency may precede the onset of clinical symptoms of the nutrient deficiency.[2] Unfortunately, much of the evidence on the effects of nutritional deficiency on immune competence is based largely

Table 35.1.
Summary of Action of Micronutrients on Immune Function

Epithelial Barriers	Cellular Immunity	Antibody Production
Vitamin A	Vitamin A	Vitamin A
Vitamin C	Vitamin B_6	Vitamin B_6
Vitamin E	Vitamin B_{12}	Vitamin B_{12}
Zinc	Vitamin C	Vitamin D
	Vitamin D	Vitamin E
	Vitamin E	Folic acid
	Folic acid	Zinc
	Iron	Copper
	Zinc	Selenium
	Copper	Nucleotides
	Selenium	LCPUFAs
	Nucleotides	
	LCPUFAs	

LCPUFA indicates long-chain polyunsaturated fatty acid.
Modified from Maggini, 2007.[1]

on data from severely malnourished individuals, cell culture experiments, animal models, and clinical trials with adult or elderly subjects.

A number of vitamins, minerals, and other dietary ingredients are marketed and sold in the United States for their putative immune system-enhancing properties. Given the high rates of common infectious diseases (eg, common cold, influenza) among young children, parents may choose to use such supplements. General pediatricians need to be familiar with the scientific evidence regarding individual nutrients and dietary supplement ingredients. The following described micronutrients have demonstrated direct modulation of immune function and continue to be studied widely.

Fat-Soluble Vitamins *(see also Chapter 21.I: Fat-Soluble Vitamins)*

Vitamin A
In developing countries, vitamin A supplementation of deficient children reduces overall mortality and morbidity.[3,4] Vitamin A deficiency leads to decreased phagocytic and oxidative burst activity, reduced natural killer cell activity, and altered production of interferon. In addition, there is altered integrity of the mucosal epithelium in the eye and the respiratory and gastrointestinal tracts.[1,5] However, there is no direct evidence that vitamin A supplementation benefits immune function of vitamin A-replete children.

Vitamin D

Vitamin D$_3$ has significant effects on both innate and acquired immunity.[6] Most cells of the immune system, except B lymphocytes, express vitamin D receptors.[1] Under physiological conditions, vitamin D$_3$ plays an active role in immune responses and may also contribute to reducing the risk of autoimmune responses. Vitamin D$_3$ enhances monocyte differentiation into macrophages but suppresses monocyte differentiation into dendritic cells while enhancing a tolerogenic phenotype and function of dendritic cells. Vitamin D$_3$ down-regulates the expression of toll-like receptors and induces production of antimicrobial peptides in vitro by monocytes and dendritic cells, thus, enhancing microbial killing.[7] Vitamin D$_3$ also influences acquired immunity by increasing regulatory T cell differentiation, decreasing T helper cell differentiation, and affecting specific cytokines leading to decreased homing to lymph nodes, plasma cell development, antibody secretion, and memory B cell differentiation.[6] Again, there is little evidence to support vitamin D supplementation of vitamin D-replete children to support immune function.

Vitamin E

Vitamin E, as a strong lipid-soluble antioxidant and among other functions, protects membrane lipids against the effects of free radicals and lipid peroxidation. Animal studies have demonstrated that vitamin E deficiency decreases lymphocyte proliferation, natural killer (NK) cell activity, specific antibody production, and phagocytosis by neutrophils.[8] Although high-dose vitamin E supplements can improve immune function in healthy elderly subjects,[1] it is unclear whether they are effective in children. Vitamin E supplements did not affect tetanus antibody titers in 2-month-old infants or neutrophil function in preterm infants.[9]

Water-Soluble Vitamins (see also Chapter 21.II: Water-Soluble Vitamins)

Vitamin C

Neutrophils maintain high concentrations of vitamin C in vivo,[10] and vitamin C may chemically inactivate histamine.[11] Vitamin C also stimulates interferon production in vitro when incubated with cultured mouse cells and in vivo when administered to mice. A recent review discussed the complementarity between zinc-related immune functions and vitamin C, in both innate and adaptive immunity.[12] Despite these documented biological effects, a comprehensive meta-analysis indicates that high-dose vitamin

C (1 g or more daily) does not reduce the incidence of the common cold, although it may slightly reduce the duration of the infection.[13] Five of the 11 studies evaluated in this meta-analysis were conducted in children, and the results in this subset were consistent with the overall finding. There is no evidence that high-dose vitamin C supplements have any general immunologic benefit for pediatric populations.

B Vitamins

Moderate to severe deficiencies of vitamin B_6, vitamin B_{12}, or folate suppress immune responses in adult humans and animal models.[3] Vitamin B_{12} deficiency may occur in breastfed infants of vegan mothers who consume no animal products[14] or in vegan children without a supplemental source of vitamin B_{12}. A human study of vitamin B_{12}-deficient patients showed a decreased number of lymphocytes with a high CD4+/CD8+ ratio and suppressed NK cell activity, with reversal of these effects after supplementation.[1] Vitamin B_6 supplementation improves some immune functions in vitamin B_6-deficient humans and experimental animals. A possible mechanism is mobilization of vitamin B_6 to the sites of inflammation, where it may serve as a cofactor in pathways producing metabolites with immune-modulating effects.[15] As with the other vitamins that have been discussed, there is no evidence that providing B vitamins to replete, healthy children has any benefit on immune function.

Trace Elements (see also Chapter 20: Trace Elements)

Iron (see also Chapter 19: Iron)

Iron deficiency is associated with an altered cytokine profile, an increase in cells expressing interferon-alpha, a decrease in the proportion of cells expressing IL-4, reduced lymphocyte proliferation, and impaired delayed-type hypersensitivity responses with relative preservation of humoral immunity.[16] Iron is necessary for myeloperoxidase activity, which is involved in the process of killing bacteria by neutrophils via the formation of highly toxic hydroxyl radicals.[1] A study in France demonstrated that iron supplementation of children of low socioeconomic status who are iron deficient can normalize circulating T-lymphocyte counts and delayed-type hypersensitivity skin responses as well as IL-2 production in vitro, but the clinical consequences are unclear.[17] A more recent supportive study demonstrates changes in several components of humoral and cell-mediated immunity as well as cytokine activity in the context of iron-deficiency anemia in a pediatric population.[18]

Depriving microbial pathogens of iron to inhibit bacterial growth and virulence is a protective feature of the innate immune system; thus, there may be adverse consequences to iron supplementation in parts of the world with a high prevalence of bacterial infections such as malaria and tuberculosis.[16] A small placebo-controlled trial among 6- to 36-month-old children in Togo, West Africa (n=163) found no change in infectious disease incidence after 6 months of iron supplementation.[19] Increased availability of elemental iron in the gut has the potential to promote the growth and survival of pathogenic organisms.[8]

Zinc

Zinc is involved in cytosolic defense against oxidative stress and is an essential cofactor for modulation and proliferation of cytokine release. It supports Th1 response and helps to maintain skin and mucosal membrane integrity.[1] Moderate to severe zinc deficiency can impair both lymphocyte and phagocyte cell function. In developing countries, zinc supplementation has shown therapeutic responses in infectious disease, especially acute diarrhea in children, chronic hepatitis C, shigellosis, leishmaniasis, and the common cold.[20] In a randomized, placebo-controlled trial of more than 1700 cases of acute diarrhea in Nepalese children, zinc supplementation reduced the duration of diarrhea and was not enhanced by or dependent on concomitant vitamin A supplementation.[21] There is no direct evidence that zinc supplementation may benefit zinc-replete children. When given in quantities higher than twice the Recommended Dietary Allowance, zinc may in fact impair immunity,[5] and there is a risk that zinc supplements may also impair copper absorption.[4]

Selenium

Selenium is present in protein-rich foods such as meat, fish, nuts, and seeds. It is essential for optimal functioning of cells comprising both adaptive and innate immunity. It is critical to redox regulation, including the protection against DNA damage, and antioxidant function through glutathione peroxidases.[22] Supranutritional selenium promotes proliferation and favors differentiation of naive CD4+ T lymphocytes toward T helper 1 cells, thus supporting the acute cellular immune response. In contrast, it also directs macrophages toward the M2 phenotype counteracting excessive activation of the immune system and ensuing host tissue damage.[23]

In the presence of selenium deficiency, benign strains of Coxsackie and influenza viruses can mutate to highly pathogenic strains. It has been suggested that dietary supplementation to provide adequate or "supranutritional selenium" may confer health benefits for patients with some viral illnesses, most notably HIV and influenza A viral infections.[23]

Copper

In humans, nutritional or inherited copper deficiency (Menkes syndrome) is associated with multisystem morbidity, including increased susceptibility to bacterial infections. Correspondingly, primary or secondary copper deficiency in animals has been shown to impair the ability of macrophages and neutrophils to generate an oxidative burst and effectively kill phagocytized microbes.[24] Despite the long-standing observations that copper promotes a healthy immune system, the recognition of copper as an integral part of innate immune responses is relatively recent. Many studies have indicated that copper redistribution and mobilization in mammalian tissues and individual cells is a key immune response to bacterial infections.[25]

Nucleotides

Nucleotides and nucleic acids (components of RNA and DNA) constitute approximately 20% of the nonprotein nitrogen content in human milk at concentrations ranging from 70 to 189 μmol/L.[26] Currently, nucleotides are added to several infant formulas in the United States. The mechanism by which dietary nucleotides may modify immune function is unknown,[27] although mouse-model studies indicate they may augment Th1-based immune responses.[28] Most recently, a neonatal pig model of intrauterine growth restriction demonstrated that nucleotide-supplemented formula increased plasma concentrations of IgA, IL-1β, and leukocyte number compared with those receiving unsupplemented formula.[29]

Studies in human infants have reported that adding nucleotides to infant formula increases NK cell activity, IL-2 production by monocytes, serum IgM and IgA concentrations, and serum antibody titers to food antigens.[30] The clinical relevance of these effects is unknown. A systematic review and meta-analysis concluded that nucleotide-supplemented infant formula, compared with human milk or control formula, improved antibody response to several immunizations (influenza, polio, diphtheria) and reduced the number of diarrheal episodes.[31] Such data are promising, but additional studies are needed to understand the mechanism of action, confirm clinical endpoints, and monitor the long-term immune-related effects of adding nucleotides to infant formula.

Long-Chain Polyunsaturated Fatty Acids (see also Chapter 17: Fats and Fatty Acids)

The effects of long-chain polyunsaturated fatty acids (LCPUFAs) on infant immune function are not well understood. Arachidonic acid (ARA) is the precursor for prostaglandins and leukotrienes that regulate normal inflammatory processes.[5] In vivo, docosahexaenoic acid (DHA) supplementation of feeds can inhibit both inflammatory responses and T-lymphocyte signaling in adult humans.[32] Epidemiologic studies suggest an inverse association between human milk DHA content and the development of atopic disease in children with family history of atopic disease. Studies in humans and mice suggest that maternal diet supplementation with DHA during lactation, hence increasing the human milk DHA content, alters infants' immune function and promotes the establishment of oral tolerance in the first year of life. Moreover, preterm infants receiving formula supplemented with ARA and DHA had a higher proportion of memory T lymphocytes and improved cytokine response to immune challenge, compared with unsupplemented formula.[33] Studies are needed to determine whether supplementation or fortification of foods with DHA and ARA have clinically significant in vivo effects on inflammation, immune responses, mucosal immune system development, and long-term immunocompetence in infants and children.

Human Milk (see also Chapter 3: Breastfeeding)

Studies have shown that early nutrition influences the short- and long-term health outcomes of infants. Human milk provides bioactive factors including immunoglobulins, lactoferrin, lysozyme, cytokines, growth factors, hormones, and oligosaccharides that work in concert to fortify mucosal immunity, shape the gut microbiota, and stimulate infant growth.[34,35] The predominant immunoglobulin in human milk is secretory IgA (sIgA). It acts as a first line of defense against foreign antigens by blocking the adhesion of pathogens to intestinal epithelial surfaces and binding bacterial toxins.[36] Its efficacy against *Vibrio cholerae* O antigen and enterotoxin, *Campylobacter*, and enterotoxin-producing *Escherichia coli* has been documented by various investigators.

Lactoferrin is known to have bacteriostatic and bactericidal activity. It was thought that its primary bacteriostatic activity was attributable to its iron scavenging properties; however, specific lactoferrin-binding receptors have been more recently described in several bacterial pathogens.[37] Its

VI

bacterial surface binding causes lipopolysaccharide release from the cell wall and ultimate cell death.[37] Additionally, it stimulates cell proliferation and differentiation, facilitates iron absorption, affects brain development, and has anti-inflammatory activity.[38]

Lysozyme, like lactoferrin, has also been shown to be present in the stool of breastfed infants, has antiviral activity, is capable of degrading the cell membrane of gram-positive bacteria, and has the ability to kill gram-negative bacteria in vitro synergistically with lactoferrin.[39] Beyond being a key energy source, human milk carbohydrates also serve immune-related roles. Oligosaccharides and more complex glycoproteins and glycolipids serve as receptor analogs that interfere with the adherence of pathogens such as pneumococci and *Haemophilus influenzae* and of enterotoxins such as those of *Vibrio cholerae* and *E coli* to epithelial cells.[40]

Similarly, lipids provide essential fatty acids for membrane structures, serving as an important energy source and contributing to the infant's immunologic responses. Free fatty acids and monoglycerides have a lytic effect on several viruses, and fatty acids have an antiprotozoal effect, particularly against *Giardia* species.[41] During the first weeks of life, 2 anti-inflammatory cytokines, IL-10 and transforming growth factor-beta (TGF-β), in human milk contribute to the maturation of mucosal immunity.[42] The TGF-β concentration in human milk correlates with sIgA levels in breastfed infants and a decreased risk for childhood diseases including allergy.[43] TGF-β from human milk also promotes the development of oral tolerance.[43]

Some hormones (cortisol, insulin, thyroxine) and growth factors (epidermal growth factor, nerve growth factor, TGF) found in human milk may influence the growth and development of the gastrointestinal tract as well with potential benefits on host immunoprotection.[44] Colostrum is a potent contributor to immune development and the protective effects of human milk. There are unique nutritional and immunologic differences between human milk at term and preterm,[37] and the short-term benefits of these nutritional-immunologic interactions are clear.

Although the rates of infection are similar among breastfed and non-breastfed infants, the duration and severity of infection are often reduced in breastfed infants. There is strong evidence to support enhanced protection against certain infections many years after the termination of breastfeeding.[45] Some studies suggest that host defense may be actively stimulated by breastfeeding, and this notion is supported by the finding of enhanced vaccine responses in breastfed compared with nonbreastfed infants.[45] The role of breastfeeding in modulating allergy risk remains controversial. Studies have found inconsistent protective effects of breastfeeding on long-term allergic outcomes.[46] The current recommendations of the World Health Organization (WHO) that infants should be exclusively breastfed for 6 months and of the European Academy of Allergy and Clinical Immunology (EACCI) that infants should be exclusively breastfed for 4 to 6 months to prevent development of allergies are not supported by recent study results.[46]

Autoimmunity

Although previous studies have shown the lack of breastfeeding to be a modifiable risk factor for both type 1 and type 2 diabetes mellitus (DM), more recent data suggest no protective association between breastfeeding and the risk of type 1 DM.[47] The use of hydrolyzed formula compared with a conventional formula did not reduce the incidence of DM and may increase the risk of islet autoimmunity in children at risk for type 1 DM.[48] Introduction of gluten before 3 months of age was found to be a risk factor for the development of type 1 DM with associated islet auto-antibodies in children of parents with type 1 DM.[49] Earlier studies suggested breastfeeding at the time of gluten exposure was protective; however, a recent study showed that neither the delayed introduction of gluten nor breastfeeding modified the risk of celiac disease among infants at risk.[50] Therefore, the European Society for Pediatric Gastroenterology, Hepatology and Nutrition (ESPGHAN) recommends that gluten be introduced in the infant's diet anytime between 4 and 12 months of age.[51]

Nutrition and Immunity: the Gut Microbiome

Microbiota

Feeding strategy (breastfeeding vs formula feeding) influences human infant growth by affecting body composition, intestinal maturation, gut microbial succession, and immune responses.[52] A number of factors such as gestational age, mode of delivery, host genetics, antimicrobial medications, lifestyle, and diet, have been shown to potentially influence the acquisition of the infant gastrointestinal microbiome. Which of these factors is most influential in this process is unclear and may vary between individual infants. Human milk possesses an abundance of complex oligosaccharides that are indigestible by infants and instead consumed by microbial populations in the developing intestine.[53,54] These oligosaccharides are believed to be growth factors for bifidobacteria.[55–57] Studies have shown that infants who are exclusively breastfed until weaning tend to have a more stable, less diverse bacterial community with predominant bifidobacterial, compared with formula-fed infants.[58,59] After introduction of solid foods, gut microbiota composition gravitates toward the adult pattern with increasing diversity,[59,60] and increased abundance of anaerobic *Firmicutes*.[61] The characteristics of the gut microbiota of breastfed and formula-fed infants converge gradually, become indistinguishable by approximately 18 months of age,[59] and resemble those of an adult by age 3 years.[62]

It is not fully understood how neonates adapt to the formidable challenges of microbial colonization. The capacity to accept the microbiota can also be explained by the relative immaturity of the intestinal immune system at birth and the tolerogenic environment, as the developing immune system is characterized by blunted inflammatory cytokine production and skewed T and B cell development in favor of regulatory responses.[63] Although this blunted immune response places neonates at high risk for infections, this immunoregulatory environment ensures the establishment of healthy microbial colonization without overt inflammation.[64] Commensal microbiota can profoundly influence the development of the gut mucosal immune system and be crucial in preventing exogenous pathogen intrusion, both by direct interaction with pathogenic bacteria and by beneficial stimulation of the immune system.[64] The gut microbiota interacts with both innate and adaptive immune system components and plays a pivotal role in the induction, development, and ultimate function of the host immune system.[65] This dynamic relationship between the host and its microbiota is important for maintaining immune homeostasis.[66] The immune system is not only controlled by its symbiotic relationship with the microbiota but is also highly sensitive to the nutritional status of the host.

Probiotics

Probiotic organisms as a component of the host microbiome are essential for health and immune system development and are supported by prebiotic dietary nutrients. The following discussion is meant to provide background information on the role of probiotic organisms to place the discussion of prebiotic nutrients in context. The commensal organisms that constitute the intestinal microbiome include several bacterial strains that may provide a health benefit when consumed as a dietary supplement. Although traditionally, probiotics have been consumed orally to promote gastrointestinal tract function, the route of application and target organ effects are expanding.[67] Continuous communication between the intestinal microbiota and components of the intestinal immune system results in an appropriately regulated immune response to luminal bacterial and nutritional antigens. The consumption of probiotics can enhance immune regulation and may even correct immune dysregulation responsible for some immune-mediated disease states. Broadly speaking, probiotic bacteria enhance intestinal health and function through various possible mechanisms. These include, but are not limited to, colonization resistance, promotion of the intestinal mucous layer, enhancement of the intestinal barrier, secretion of antibacterial factors, and positively influencing the intestinal immune system.[68]

Cell surface receptors on epithelial cells and dendritic cells, including toll-like receptors (TLRs), recognize bacterial components and differentiate between beneficial and pathogenic bacteria. This contributes to the process of intestinal colonization and promotes the development of balanced immune responsiveness. Probiotic bacteria have the ability to promote TLR expression and influence receptor localization within the cell. Their interaction with TLRs has also been shown to attenuate the downstream proinflammatory responses associated with TLR activation.[69,70] A specific probiotic strain, *Lactobacillus reuteri*, decreased the lipopolysaccharide (LPS)-activated tumor necrosis factor (TNF) production by immune cells, such as macrophages, of pediatric patients with Crohn disease.[71] Unique immunomodulatory effects on dendritic cells have been shown with the strains contained within a widely available combination probiotic product, which includes lactobacilli, streptococci, and bifidobacteria. These effects include upregulated IL-10 responses and decreased proinflammatory responses, which were most positively influenced by bifidobacteria from the product.[72] These findings support not only the wide immunomodulatory effects of probiotics but also the strain specificity of these effects. Additionally, the induction of regulatory T lymphocytes with probiotics has been described and helps to promote appropriate immune regulation, balancing immune responsiveness and tolerance.[73,74]

Numerous studies have been performed to determine the clinical efficacy of probiotics in the prevention or treatment of infectious or immune-mediated diseases in children. The 2014 The European Society for Pediatric Gastroenterology, Hepatology and Nutrition (ESPGHAN) Working Group for Probiotics and Prebiotics gave a strong recommendation despite low quality of evidence for using *Lactobacillus rhamnosus* GG or *Sachromyces boulardii* in the management of acute infectious diarrhea.[75] A 2010 Cochrane review subgroup analysis concluded that 4 randomized controlled trials (RCTs) have documented *Enterococcus faecium* SF6873 to be effective in reducing the risk of diarrhea lasting ≥4 days.[76,77]

VI

A 2012 meta-analysis of 63 RCTs showed a statistically significant reduction in antibiotic-associated diarrhea (AAD) with probiotics. A subgroup analysis demonstrated that the risk reduction of AAD was associated with the use of *L rhamnosus* GG (95% confidence interval [CI], 0.15–0.6), *S boulardii* (95% CI, 0.07–0.6), or *Bifidobacterium lactis* and *Streptococcus thermophilus* (95% CI, 0.3–0.95).[78] A 2009 systematic review also concluded that probiotics significantly reduced the incidence of pediatric AAD and the incidence of pediatric *Clostridium difficile* infection. A 2013 meta-analysis demonstrated that *S boulardii* (relative risk [RR], 0.43; 95% CI, 0.32–0.60) and *L rhamnosus* GG (RR, = 0.36; 95% CI, 0.19–0.69) are the 2 best-studied strains for this indication. Of note, in most of the reviewed studies, the probiotics were taken concurrently during the antibiotic course.[79–81]

In a 2010 review, McFarland et al[82] concluded that there is comparable evidence for efficacy for *L rhamnosus* GG, *Lactobacillus casei* DN-114001, and *S boulardii* and no efficacy for *Lactobacillus acidophilus* in the management of travelers' diarrhea. The number of studies of probiotics in travelers' diarrhea is relatively limited, which has led to lack of clinical recommendations for this indication, and a recent meta-analysis concluded that probiotics are not effective for travelers' diarrhea.[70,82,83]

Several clinical trials indicate that probiotics generally do not eradicate *Helicobacter pylori* but decrease the density of colonization, maintaining lower levels of this pathogen in the stomach. Many studies show a moderately higher eradication rate (~10%) of *H pylori* when probiotics are added to the antibiotic/acid-suppression regimen. Although *L rhamnosus* GG appears not to improve eradication in a randomized, double-blind, placebo-controlled trial, most probiotic bacteria and yeasts reduce the adverse effects of standard *H pylori* eradication regimens. A 2014 meta-analysis of RCTs of probiotic supplementation of *H pylori* regimen in children showed that probiotics may have beneficial effects on eradication and therapy-related adverse effects, particularly diarrhea.[84–87]

Although some probiotic strains have been shown to objectively improve the intestinal inflammation in milk protein allergy of infancy,[88] a 2014 meta-analysis concluded that there is insufficient evidence to support the beneficial role of probiotics in infants.[89]

Prebiotics
Some components of our diet are not digested but rather are fermented specifically by intestinal bacteria that selectively influence the intestinal microbiome and, in turn, the intestinal health of the host. These dietary

components are referred to as prebiotics, which primarily belong to 1 of 2 distinct categories: inulin-type fructans and galacto-oligosaccharides (GOSs).[90] Several animal model and human studies have demonstrated the various health benefits of prebiotics, which include improvements in intestinal motility, absorption, intestinal barrier function, and intestinal immunity. Additionally, reduction in risk of obesity, metabolic syndrome, colon cancer, enteric infections, and intestinal inflammatory disease has also been described.[91]

A variety of grains, fruits, and vegetables naturally provide inulin-type fructans in the diet,[70] whereas GOSs are derived from lactose. There are qualitative differences in GOSs of cow milk versus human milk, the latter of which is able to promote bifidobacteria populations in the infant intestine. This "bifidogenic effect" of human milk is not observed in infants fed cow milk-based formulas.[92]

The health benefits of prebiotics may be a result of positive influences on the intestinal microbiome or modulating the intestinal immune function more directly via products of their fermentation. These products include defensins and short-chain fatty acids. A reduction of childhood diarrheal illness was demonstrated in a study supplementing healthy infants with fructo-oligosaccharides (FOSs) and in a different study that provided a GOS/FOS-supplemented formula.[93,94] An immunologic response was demonstrated in a group of 8-month-old infants with increased measles IgG levels after measles vaccination when supplemented with inulin-like fructans.[95] Several studies have demonstrated increased sIgA levels after prebiotic supplementation.[90] Prebiotic and probiotic supplementation to modulate immune-related disease risk is an area of great scientific interest and active investigation and will continue to be a rapidly evolving area of nutritional research.

Nutrition and Immunity: Developmental and Acquired Immunodeficiency (HIV)

Developmental Immunodeficiency (Preterm Infants)

For a multitude of unique reasons, infants born preterm or at low birth weight are at risk of a relative immunodeficiency, compared with infants born at term. Some elements of this risk may be influenced by the infant's nutritional sources. Although several immune system components are still developing in the full-term infant, especially those of the adaptive immune system, more marked compromise is present in both innate and adaptive

VI

immunity in the preterm infant.[33,96] Because adaptive immunity requires pathogen and antigen exposure for proper development and these exposures are limited prenatally, adaptive immune responses are particularly immature in all infants.[97] The innate immune system, therefore, is the primary means of defense in the early postnatal period.[98] A compensatory transfer of nutrients and immunoglobulins occurs via the placenta, particularly of maternal IgG.[96] In infants with either low birth weight attributable to placental insufficiency or those delivered preterm, this process of transferred immunity is incomplete. Correspondingly, preterm infants have significantly lower serum IgG concentrations compared with their full-term infant counterparts ($P < .05$).[99] On the other hand, differences in serum IgA and IgM levels have not been noted between term and preterm infants. In addition, CD3+, CD4+, CD8+, and CD19+ T lymphocyte, as well as NK cell, counts are significantly lower in preterm infants than in term infants ($P < .05$). This relative deficiency is less marked as gestational age at birth increases, with statistically significant differences noted even between preterm infants born between 28 and 34 weeks' gestation and those born between 34 and 37 weeks' gestation ($P < .05$).[99] Complement proteins, on the other hand, are not transferred via the placental route and instead are produced endogenously after 20 weeks of gestation.[100] Concurrent with these quantitative differences in immune system components in preterm infants are functional differences as well. Table 35.2 summarizes the various components of immunity and unique characteristics of these components in preterm infants. Clinically, the immature immune status of preterm infants likely plays a role in the development of necrotizing enterocolitis, retinopathy of prematurity, bronchopulmonary dysplasia, and the increased risk of allergy and atopy described in this population.[33]

Postnatally, the continued transfer of several beneficial immune-modulating factors occurs via human milk. These factors, only some of which have been supplemented in preterm infant formulas, provide either protection or maturational influences on the developing intestinal immune system. Preterm infants have different nutritional requirements not only for adequate growth and general development but also specifically to support their immature, developing immunity. When compared human milk of mothers who delivered term infants, human milk of mothers of preterm infants seems to be better suited for host defense, because it contains higher concentrations of sIgA, lactoferrin, lysozyme, and epidermal growth factor.[101] The absolute number of macrophages, neutrophils,

Table 35.2.

Specific Immune Deficiencies in Preterm Infants

Immune System Component	Role and Function	Characteristics in Preterm Infants
Physical Barrier		
Skin	Prevention of pathogen penetration.	The epidermal barrier function fully develops at approximately the 32nd to 24th week of gestation. The skin of very preterm infants is more susceptible to rupture.
Mucous membranes	Mucous and secretory components in the respiratory and GI tracts protect against pathogen entry.	The GI tract is not fully mature in preterm infants with lower gastric acidity. ↓ MHC receptors and secretory components are detectable until 29th week of gestation. ↓ number of antibody producing B cells prior to the first postnatal week.
Innate Immune System		
Complement system proteins	On activation, the complement system (approx 20 proteins) generates different molecules (C3a, C3) that release inflammatory mediators, and stimulate chemotaxis, phagocytosis, and microbial lysis.	↓ amounts of proteins (C1, C4, and factor B) of the complement system before the third trimester of pregnancy. ↓ pathogen-killing abilities and deficiency in the pattern recognition receptor mannose-binding lectin in preterm (PT) vs term infants.

Continued

Abbreviations: ↑, higher; ↓, lower; APC, antigen-presenting cell; APP, antimicrobial proteins and peptide; DC, dendritic cell; GI, gastrointestinal; IFN-g, interferon gamma; Ig, immunoglobulin; IL, interleukin; MHC, major histocompatibility complex; NK, natural killer; OT, oral tolerance; TLR, toll-like receptor; TNF-a, tumor necrosis factor-alpha.

Modified from Lewis, 2017[2] (Originally from Blumer N, Pfefferle PI, Renz H. Development of mucosal immune function in the intrauterine and early postnatal environment. *Curr Opin Gastroenterol. 2007;23(6):655–660;* with permission).

VI

Table 35.2. *Continued*
Specific Immune Deficiencies in Preterm Infants

Immune System Component	Role and Function	Characteristics in Preterm Infants
Innate Immune System Continued		
Monocytes, macrophages, neutrophils, and dendritic cells	Phagocytize microorganisms and intracellular destruction with toxic substances (superoxide anions, hydroxyl radicals, nitric oxide, lysozyme). They are APCs expressing MHC classes I and II that can induce T-cell proliferation through the secretion of cytokines. Leukocytes (neutrophils, macrophages, and lymphocytes) can also release APPs that bind and destroy microorganisms.	↓ capacity at processing/presenting antigens and cytokines production in infants vs adults. ↓ cytokine production (IFN-g and TNF-a) from monocytes in PT vs term infants. ↑ in cytokines and APPs production with gestational age. ↓ neutrophils storage pool before 32nd week of gestation. ↓ amounts of molecules involved in the recruitment of neutrophils to the site of infection (P-selectin, L-selectin, E-selectin, CR3) in PT vs term infants. ↓ capacity of neutrophils to deal with pathogens (ex: ↓ respiratory activity) in PT vs term infants. ↑ with gestational age. Similar number of DCs and level of TLR9 in PT and term infants vs adults. ↓ lower capacity to produce IFN-a on TLR9 challenge in PT vs term infants.
NK cells	Ability to lyse infected cells (tumor and virus-infected cells) but also bacteria, parasites, and fungi.	Similar (or slightly higher) number of NK cells in term infants vs adult. ↓ NK cytotoxic activity (less efficient) in term infants vs adult. ↓ number of NK cells and NK activity in PT vs term infants.

Adaptive Immune System

T cells	Need to be stimulated by APC to get activated and then regulate immune responses by producing cytokines (Th1 and Th2). Also play a role in activating NK cells, monocytes, and B cells.	↓ T cells proliferative response (IL-2), production of Th1 cytokines (IFN-g), and cytolytic activity in infants vs adults. ↓ absolute number of T cells and proliferative capacity in PT vs term infants.
B cells	Activated by T cells. Main producer of Ig antibodies for specific humoral immunity. Igs are involved in oral tolerance	↓ production of Ig antibodies in term infants vs adults ↓ expression of CD40, CD40L, and TNF family receptors needed for B-cell activation and effective antibody response in PT vs term infants.
Passive immune system	Maternal IgG transfer to the fetus through the placenta to compensate for the lack of antibodies produced.	Transfer for IgG starts at approximately the 32nd to 34th week of gestation. ↑ with gestational age.

Abbreviations: ↑, higher; ↓, lower; APC, antigen-presenting cell; APP, antimicrobial proteins and peptide; DC, dendritic cell; GI, gastrointestinal; IFN-g, interferon gamma; Ig, immunoglobulin; IL, interleukin; MHC, major histocompatibility complex; NK, natural killer; OT, oral tolerance; TLR, toll-like receptor; TNF-a, tumor necrosis factor-alpha.

Modified from Lewis, 2017[2] (Originally from Blumer N, Pfefferle PI, Renz H. Development of mucosal immune function in the intrauterine and early postnatal environment. *Curr Opin Gastroenterol.* 2007;23(6):655-660; with permission).

and lymphocytes in human colostrum of mothers who delivered a preterm infant is higher than that in colostrum of mothers who delivered at term.[102] The thorough recent review of this topic by Lewis et al discusses the compositional differences in human milk from mothers who delivered preterm and those who delivered at term, which allows nutritional support specific to an infant's gestational age.[33]

Acquired Immunodeficiency (Human Immunodeficiency Virus Infection)

Although there are many causes of acquired immunodeficiency, this discussion will focus on human immunodeficiency virus (HIV) infection as a primary example of the issues faced in the nutritional support of pediatric patients with acquired immunodeficiency. Although considerable progress has been made toward reducing HIV infection among children as a result of global efforts to expand access to antiretroviral therapy (ART), the global burden of pediatric HIV infection and acquired immune deficiency syndrome (AIDS) remains challenging, particularly in resource-limited countries. The Joint United Nations Programme on HIV/AIDS (UNAIDS) reports that in 2016, there were 36.7 million people living with HIV, and of those, 2.1 million were children younger than 15 years. Worldwide, 160 000 children became newly infected with HIV in 2016.[103] The care of children living with HIV and AIDS is complex and continues to evolve.

HIV Research and Development

Although HIV can negatively affect nutritional status, there is a reciprocal effect, because malnutrition can intensify the immunologic consequences of HIV infection. Nutritional abnormalities including failure to thrive (FTT), malnutrition and obesity, and cardiometabolic problems are potential adverse outcomes of HIV infection in the "highly active antiretroviral therapy" (HAART) era, even as the therapy has contributed to declines in morbidity and mortality.[104] Patients who have nutritional and metabolic disturbances that result in weight loss and wasting may show a chronic inflammatory state secondary to increased viral replication or microbial translocation from the gastrointestinal tract. Furthermore, obesity and its consequences are associated with an inflammatory state, which itself may compromise immune function. Optimal nutritional status can improve an individual's immune function, reduce disease-associated complications, attenuate the progression of HIV infection, improve quality of life, and ultimately, reduce mortality associated with HIV infection.[105] Although many of the nutritional problems in HIV infected children occurred in the pre-HAART era, new nutritional problems such as lipodystrophy, hyperlipidemia, and insulin resistance have appeared since then.[106]

Malnutrition and Wasting

Malnutrition in children with HIV/AIDS may be caused by several mechanisms working independently or synergistically. These causes are summarized in Table 35.3. Insufficient intake of nutrients is one of the most important factors that may lead to undernutrition.

Gastrointestinal tract mucosal abnormalities may lead to compromised macronutrient and micronutrient absorption. These mucosal changes can be attributed to local HIV infection with associated bacterial translocation or secondary enteric infections. Several enteric infections may cause unremitting diarrhea, which predisposes individuals to severe malnutrition and

Table 35.3.

Potential Causes of Malnutrition in HIV-Infected Children

Decreased nutrient intake Primary anorexia Idiopathic aphthous ulcers Dysgeusia (zinc deficiency) Opportunistic infections of the upper GI tract (*Candida*, CMV, HSV) Peptic disease Encephalopathy
Gastrointestinal malabsorption Infectious Inflammatory Disaccharidase deficiency Protein-losing enteropathy Fat malabsorption (pancreatic/hepatobiliary disease)
Increased nutritional requirements or tissue catabolism Protein wasting Increased metabolism secondary to: Fever, infections, sepsis Neoplasms (Kaposi sarcoma, lymphoma) Medications
Psychosocial factors Poverty, food insecurity Illness in biological family members Limited access to health care Substance abuse

GI, gastrointestinal; CMV, cytomegalovirus; HSV, herpes simplex virus; HBV, hepatitis B virus; HCV, hepatitis C virus.

increased mortality, especially in developing nations. Villous atrophy and gastrointestinal tract dysfunction are coincident with a higher HIV-1 viral load in the gut.[107] Gastrointestinal tract bleeding associated with mucosal ulcerations may contribute to loss of nutrients. The effect of opportunistic infections on the hepatobiliary and pancreatic systems can compound a state of malabsorption. Furthermore, HIV encephalopathy may result in the physical inability to consume enough calories to sustain growth.[108] Finally, many medications may result in gastric irritation, nausea, vomiting, and diarrhea.

Growth and Body Composition
Prior to the introduction of HAART, the natural history of somatic growth in HIV-infected infants was characterized by alterations in growth and body composition similar to those produced by acute and chronic malnutrition.[109] In industrialized countries during the pre-HAART era, HIV-infected children showed declines in both weight and length as early as the first 1 to 3 months of life. Follow-up showed that growth of HIV-infected children remained below that of age- and gender-matched uninfected children. Several pediatric studies in the pre-HAART era showed progressive declines in lean body mass over time in children with HIV/AIDS, whereas fat stores remained stable yet low.[110,111] Cytokines may be responsible for some of the growth, metabolic, and immunologic effects associated with HIV infection, and there are positive changes in cytokine patterns after HAART therapy.[112]

Energy Balance
Asymptomatic chronic HIV infections may have some effect on energy utilization and can predispose children to secondary infections, which in turn, can further alter energy utilization patterns. Differences in energy expenditure do not seem to fully explain the variable growth rates of HIV-infected children. Additionally, substandard intake in HIV-infected children contributes to compromised growth, compared with uninfected children.[113] A large prospective study demonstrated this growth difference despite receiving well over the Recommended Dietary Allowance of total calories and protein.[114] Thus, it is generally recommended that stable HIV-infected individuals increase their energy intake by approximately 10% to account for the metabolic needs associated with chronic viral infection.[115]

Gastrointestinal and Hepatobiliary Complications
The evaluation of diarrhea in patients with AIDS yields a specific cause in 50% to 85% of patients, with most being effectively treated.[116] Nonspecific

AIDS enteropathy may be attributable in part to undiagnosed enteric infections or the local inflammatory effects of HIV itself.[117] Impaired absorption of carbohydrate, fat, and protein in children with HIV/AIDS has been described, the extent of which is not always correlated with the degree of malnutrition.[118] Pancreatic and biliary tract disease can also cause vomiting and abdominal pain, leading to poor oral intake or malabsorption. Pancreatic disease has been linked to medications, such as pentamidine isethionate, as well as opportunistic infections (eg, cytomegalovirus, *Cryptosporidium* species, and mycobacterial disease).[119] Biliary tract disease, including sclerosing cholangitis and papillary stenosis, has been linked to *Cryptosporidium*, cytomegalovirus, and *Microsporidia* infections.[119,120]

Nutrition in the HAART Era

The term HAART refers to a combination of antiretroviral agents, generally including a protease inhibitor. Although rates of growth reconstitution in resource-limited settings and industrialized settings in the post-HAART era were comparable or higher in resource-limited settings, children in those settings had continued marked lower growth at 12- and 24-months post-HAART. Earlier age and nutritional supplementation in conjunction with HAART may improve growth outcomes. Despite empiric nutritional supplementation in pediatric ART programs, evidence of the effectiveness of nutritional therapy on growth and morbidity in children receiving ART is lacking.[121]

Symptomatic HIV-1 infection, including associated bacterial infections, still remains an important problem despite HAART utilization. Nevertheless, since the advent of HAART, bacterial infections in HIV-infected children have decreased substantially and predominate in children who have not had a sustained response to HAART.[122] The etiology of HIV-associated wasting in the HAART era continues to be multifactorial, including low socioeconomic status, poor access to care, cultural practices, psychological factors, disease-associated complications, and adverse effects of HAART therapy.[123]

Psychosocial Factors

Psychosocial factors are important contributors to suboptimal growth of HIV-infected children. An unstable home environment and inadequate emotional and social support may affect growth in both HIV-infected and uninfected children.[124] Children with HIV infection are at risk of living with parents who are ill with limited access to social support and adequate nutrition, ongoing drug and substance abuse, and/or psychiatric illness.[125]

Although children perinatally infected with HIV do not appear to be at greater risk of mental health problems than uninfected peers from similar community and home environments, the most prevalent neuropsychiatric disorders in HIV-infected children when they do occur include attention-deficit/hyperactivity disorder (ADHD), oppositional defiant disorder (ODD), anxiety, and major depression.[126,127] For children with comorbid HIV and ADHD, appetite-suppressing stimulants to treat ADHD may exacerbate growth failure and should be used with caution.[128]

Obesity and Cardiometabolic Disease
Obesity is an emerging health problem among adolescents and adults living with HIV/AIDS.[129,130] With the advent of HAART, HIV-infected children can improve their immunologic and disease status, and their eating patterns often become similar to those in healthy children.[131] Coincident with the introduction of HAART, a clinical syndrome of body fat redistribution and metabolic changes, lipodystrophy, was described initially in adults but is now commonly reported among children.[132] The syndrome is characterized by truncal obesity, dorsocervical fat pad, and extremity and facial wasting. Associated complications include diabetes mellitus and premature cardio-vascular disease. Further studies have shown that the majority of children develop fat redistribution within 3 years of initiating a protease inhibitor-containing regimen, and these changes progress over time. The cosmetic effects of lipodystrophy may contribute to poor compliance with drug therapy in children.[133,134]

Cardiometabolic Risk
Atherosclerotic cardiovascular disease (CVD) is a leading comorbidity and cause of mortality among HIV-infected adults.[135] Several studies show that HIV-infected children, compared with healthy peers, have higher rates of CVD risk factors, including dyslipidemia, insulin resistance, obesity, and central adiposity. HIV infection also results in a chronic inflammatory state, thereby further increasing CVD risk.[136,137]

Dyslipidemia
Elevated triglyceride and low-density lipoprotein cholesterol (LDL-C) con-centrations are associated with HIV infection. It has been suggested that proinflammatory cytokines secondary to the chronic viral infection alter lipid pathways, such as lipoprotein lipase activity. After the initiation of protease inhibitor (PI) therapy, several investigators reported a 20% to 50%

increase in serum lipid concentrations of HIV-infected children.[138] Other factors associated with hyperlipidemia include successful viral suppression, better CD4+ T-lymphocyte counts, and demographic factors such as insulin resistance.[139]

Insulin Resistance and Type 2 Diabetes Mellitus

The etiology of insulin resistance is multifactorial and has been linked to both PI and nucleoside/nucleotide reverse transcriptase inhibitors (NNRTI or NRTI), used as monotherapy or in combination. Specific mechanisms have not been well defined. A study by Beregszaszi et al demonstrated that insulin resistance occurs at the level of the adipose tissue, and children with lipodystrophy have more pronounced insulin resistance than those without, suggesting that metabolic changes occur as a result of the central adiposity.[140] A possible mechanism by which HAART causes insulin resistance is by direct inhibition of the transport function of the GLUT4 glucose transporter, which is responsible for insulin-stimulated glucose uptake into muscle and fat.[141] Inflammatory cytokines have been linked to insulin resistance and diminished adiponectin, which affects insulin signaling and glucose homeostasis. Adipose tissue is a major determinant of insulin sensitivity, and changes associated with lipodystrophy can alter the secretion of adiponectin. Although there are fewer studies in children compared with adults, the increased risk of diabetes mellitus in HIV-infected children on HAART is becoming increasingly clear.[142,143]

Bone Mineralization

Several studies have shown that bone mineral density of HIV-infected children is lower than national standards for age and gender and socioeconomically matched cohorts.[144] Tenofovir and other antiretroviral therapies have emerged as contributors to bone density loss in HIV-infected children.[145] Thus, baseline bone density assessments are recommended (typically with dual x-ray absorptiometry), with periodic follow-up. Calcium and vitamin D intake should be optimized with supplements when indicated.

Nutritional Assessment and Interventions

A complete baseline nutritional assessment should be performed on all patients regardless of symptoms as part of the multidisciplinary care plan, with a regular follow-up to achieve care plan goals.[146] This assessment should include a review of the medical and dietary history, analysis of nutrient intake, anthropometric measurements (ie, weight, height, BMI, head

VI

circumference [younger than 3 years], arm muscle circumferences, skin-fold measurements [4 sites]), and measurement of biochemical values (eg, complete blood cell count, albumin, transthyretin, iron, zinc, lipid profile, and absorptive tests, as indicated). When inadequate weight gain or weight loss is identified, aggressive diagnostic evaluation to detect malabsorptive conditions such as opportunistic infections or other inflammatory lesions of the gastrointestinal tract should be pursued. Treatment of underlying infections will likely improve the response to nutritional and medical management. All HIV-infected children and adolescents should be monitored at regular intervals for metabolic concerns. With clinically evident fat redistribution syndrome, a fasting serum glucose and insulin level should be obtained.[147]

The approach to nutrition and nutritional interventions for HIV-infected children and adolescents is summarized in Table 35.4. Multiple strategies to improve nutritional outcomes exist, including HAART, treatment of coinfections, nutritional counseling, pharmacologic agents to stimulate appetite or anabolism, and nutritional supplements. To prevent or delay the development of metabolic syndrome, emphasis should be placed on modifiable lifestyle factors.[148] The dietary plan for infants and children with HIV/AIDS should be individualized on the basis of symptoms and ability to meet nutrient requirements. Dietary management of macronutrient and micronutrient status relevant to disease stage and clinical condition is summarized in Table 35.5. A nutrition support team should be involved to ensure optimal monitoring and care, and this team should optimally include a physician, nurse-specialist, nutritionist, and social worker collaborating with other health care providers as needed. This approach offers the best opportunity to achieve optimal nutritional health for individual patients.

Table 35.4.

Nutritional Interventions for HIV-Infected Children[a]

Healthy with HIV • Combination of antiretroviral drug therapy, adequate dietary intake, and frequent exercise • Nutrition education and counseling • Promote healthy eating habits • Self-monitoring of dietary intake and weight changes • Discourage fad diets, including megavitamins and amino acid supplementation • Psychosocial assessment and appropriate referrals
Poor growth, unintentional weight loss, and lean tissue wasting • Careful monitoring of dietary intake and change in weight and body composition • Assess food and nutrition security, provide appropriate support • Increase calories and protein • Infants: may benefit from increased caloric density of a formula • Certain appetite stimulants may be useful in selected patients • Oral nutritional supplements are preferable • Tube feeding: if optimal food intake and use of oral nutrition supplements cannot achieve sufficient energy supply • Parenteral nutrition: should be used only in patients who are not able to feed enterally
Micronutrient deficiency • Multivitamin/mineral supplementation at DRI levels (high-dose if deficient) • Monitor intake of key nutrients (iron, zinc, calcium, and vitamins A and D) • Drug-nutrient interactions should be considered
Management of symptoms that may affect nutritional status • Nausea, vomiting: small, frequent meals; nutrient-dense beverages between meals • Anorexia: increase nutrient density of foods; small, frequent meals; appetite stimulants • Taste change: use stronger seasonings and salty foods, avoid excessively sweet foods
Diarrhea or malabsorption • Dietary composition adjusted to the degree of gastrointestinal tract dysfunction   o Identify and manage lactose intolerance • Small, frequent feedings • Semi-elemental or elemental formula

Continued

Table 35.4. *Continued*
Nutritional Interventions for HIV-Infected Children[a]

Overweight/obesity and increased cardiovascular risk   • Metabolic complications of HAART should be carefully evaluated and monitored   • Promote weight loss if overweight or obese   • Heart-healthy diet: reduced intake of saturated fat, trans fatty acids, and cholesterol   • Increased fiber intake and limit simple carbohydrates   • Increase consumption of omega-3 fatty acid-rich foods   • Physical activity, counseling, or physical activity program participation
Loss of bone mineral density, osteopenia   • Supplement calcium and vitamin D intakes to DRI levels for age if suboptimal intake   • Regular weight-bearing exercise   • Decrease high-phosphorous carbonated beverage intake

DRI, Dietary Reference Intake.

[a] Adapted from recommendations by the Academy of Nutrition and Dietetics, American Society for Parenteral and Enteral Nutrition, European Society of Parenteral and Enteral Nutrition, and American Heart Association.[146,149-151]

Table 35.5.
Macronutrient and Micronutrient Requirements of HIV-Infected Children

Nutrient	HIV Infection Factors Clinical Situations	Recommendation/Nutrition Intervention
Energy	During adequate growth and no illness	Standard methods of assessing energy needs
	During illness	Energy requirements can increase by up to 20%–30% during infections and recovery[115]
	Recovery phase	Catch-up growth Use equations for estimating catch-up growth requirements for both calories and protein
	Advanced disease	Up to 50%–100% additional energy to recover and regain weight; best achieved through enteral or parenteral (if enteral has failed) feeding
	Overweight or obesity	Weight management: counseling on changing eating habits and patterns Regular exercise: physical activity counseling or physical activity program participation
Protein	During periods of well-being	AMDR[a] can be used to ensure sufficient intake[152]
	Period of catch-up growth	Use equation for estimating catch-up growth requirements

[a] AMDR: acceptable macronutrient distribution ranges is the intake range of a particular energy source that is associated with reduced risk of chronic disease while providing intake of essential nutrients.[152]

Continued

Table 35.5. *Continued*

Macronutrient and Micronutrient Requirements of HIV-Infected Children

Nutrient	HIV Infection Factors Clinical Situations	Recommendation/Nutrition Intervention
Fat	During periods of well-being	Provide anticipatory guidance for all otherwise healthy HIV-infected patients older than 2 years and their families. AMDR: 1–3 years: 30%–40% of total calories 4–18 years: 25%–35% of total calories
	Fat malabsorption in GI enteropathy attributable to HIV or secondary infections Chronic fat malabsorption	In these cases, supplemental medium-chain triglycerides (MCTs) and enteral formulas containing MCTs can be used to supplement caloric intake Supplementation of fat-soluble vitamins is indicated
	Dyslipidemia	Counseling on eating habits and patterns per American Heart Association/American Academy of Pediatrics
Carbohydrate	During periods of well-being	AMDR: 45%–65% of total calories –Added sugars should be <10% of total calories
Fiber		Intake 0.5 g/kg/day to a maximum of 35 g daily
Fluid	The fluid needs of HIV-infected individuals are similar to those of their age-matched peers	Based on weight: 0–10 kg: 100 mL/kg 10–20 kg: 1000 mL + 50 mL/kg over 10 kg >20 kg: 1500 mL + 20 mL/kg over 20 kg –Special clinical circumstances (cardiac disease, renal disease, dehydration) may alter requirements

Vitamins and minerals	Micronutrient deficiencies due to inflammation	Varied diets, fortified foods, and micronutrients when adequate intake cannot be guaranteed by regular foods
	Suboptimal intake	Multivitamin/mineral supplementation
Calcium and vitamin D	Increased risk for low bone mineral density	Optimize intake of calcium and vitamin D; multivitamin use has been associated with better bone mineral density[144]
	Low bone mineral density	Calcium/vitamin D supplementation
Iron	Anemia attributable to a variety of nonnutritional conditions (medications, chronic illness)	Anemia should be evaluated to determine the utility of nutritional intervention, such as dietary iron and supplementation of folate or vitamin B_{12}

a AMDR: acceptable macronutrient distribution ranges is the intake range of a particular energy source that is associated with reduced risk of chronic disease while providing intake of essential nutrients.[152]

VI

References

1. Maggini S, Wintergerst E, Beveridge S, Hornig D. Selected vitamins and trace elements support immune function by strengthening epithelial barriers and cellular and humoral immune responses. *Br J Nutr.* 2007;98(Suppl 1):S29–S35

2. Marcos A, Nova E, Montero A. Changes in the immune system are conditioned by nutrition. *Eur J Clin Nutr.* 2003;57(Suppl 1):S66–S69

3. Imdad A, Mayo-Wilson E, Herzer K, Bhutta ZA. Vitamin A supplementation for preventing morbidity and mortality in children from six months to five years of age. *Cochrane Database Syst Rev.* 2017;(3):CD008524

4. Institute of Medicine. *Dietary Reference Intakes for Vitamin A, Vitamin K, Arsenic, Boron, Chromium, Copper, Iodine, Iron, Manganese, Molybdenum, Nickel, Silicon, Vanadium, and Zinc.* Washington, DC: National Academies Press; 2001

5. Gredel S. *Nutrition and Immunity in Man. ILSI Europe Concise Monograph Series.* 2nd ed. Washington, DC: International Life Sciences Institute; 2011

6. Hart PH, Gorman S, Finlay-Jones JJ. Modulation of the immune system by UV radiation: more than just the effects of vitamin D? *Nature Rev Immunol.* 2011;11(9):584–596

7. Chirumbolo S, Bjørklund G, Sboarina A, Vella A. The role of vitamin D in the immune system as a pro-survival molecule. *Clin Ther.* 2017;39(5):894–916

8. Calder PC. Feeding the immune system. *Proc Nutr Soc.* 2013;72(3):299–309

9. Kutukculer N, Akil T, Egemen A, et al. Adequate immune response to tetanus toxoid and failure of vitamin A and E supplementation to enhance antibody response in healthy children. *Vaccine.* 2000;18(26):2979–2984

10. Muggli R. Vitamin C and phagocytes. In: Cunningham-Rundles S, ed. *Nutrient Modulation of the Immune Response.* New York, NY: Marcel-Dekker Inc; 1993:75–90

11. Johnston CS. The antihistamine action of ascorbic acid. *Subcell Biochem.* 1996;25: 189–213

12. Maggini S, Wenzlaff S, Hornig D. Essential role of vitamin C and zinc in child immunity and health. *J Int Med Res.* 2010;38(2):386–414

13. Douglas RM, Hemilä H. Vitamin C for preventing and treating the common cold. *PLoS Med.* 2005;2(6):e168

14. Specker BL, Black A, Allen L, Morrow F. Vitamin B12: low milk concentrations are related to low serum concentrations in vegetarian women and to methylmalonic aciduria in their infants. *Am J Clin Nutr.* 1990;52(6):1073–1076

15. Ueland PM, McCann A, Midttun Ø, Ulvik A. Inflammation, vitamin B6 and related pathways. *Mol Aspects Med.* 2017;53:10–27

16. Cherayil BJ. Iron and immunity: immunological consequences of iron deficiency and overload. *Arch Immunol Ther Exp.* 2010;58(6):407–415

17. Thibault H, Galan P, Selz F, et al. The immune response in iron-deficient young children: effect of iron supplementation on cell-mediated immunity. *Eur J Pediatr.* 1993;152(2):120–124

18. Ekiz C, Agaoglu L, Karakas Z, Gurel N, Yalcin I. The effect of iron deficiency anemia on the function of the immune system. *Hematol J.* 2005;5(7):579–583

19. Berger J, Dyck JL, Galan P, et al. Effect of daily iron supplementation on iron status, cell-mediated immunity, and incidence of infections in 6–36 month old Togolese children. *Eur J Clin Nutr.* 2000;54(1):29–35

20. Chasapis CT, Loutsidou AC, Spiliopoulou CA, Stefanidou ME. Zinc and human health: an update. *Arch Toxicol.* 2012;86(4):521–534

21. Strand TA, Chandyo RK, Bahl R, et al. Effectiveness and efficacy of zinc for the treatment of acute diarrhea in young children. *Pediatrics.* 2002;109(5):898–903

22. Arthur JR, McKenzie RC, Beckett GJ. Selenium in the immune system. *J Nutr.* 2003;133(5 Suppl 1):1457S–1459S

23. Steinbrenner H, Al-Quraishy S, Dkhil MA, Wunderlich F, Sies H. Dietary selenium in adjuvant therapy of viral and bacterial infections. *Adv Nutr.* 2015;6(1):73–82

24. Neyrolles O, Wolschendorf F, Mitra A, Niederweis M. Mycobacteria, metals, and the macrophage. *Immunol Rev.* 2015;264(1):249–263

25. Hodgkinson V, Petris MJ. Copper homeostasis at the host-pathogen interface. *J Biol Chem.* 2012;287(17):13549–13555

26. Motil KJ. Infant feeding: a critical look at infant formulas. *Curr Opin Pediatr.* 2000;12(5):469–476

27. Grimble GK, Westwood OM. Nucleotides as immunomodulators in clinical nutrition. *Curr Opin Clin Nutr Metab Care.* 2001;4(1):57–64

28. Jyonouchi H, Sun S, Abiru T, Winship T, Kuchan MJ. Dietary nucleotides modulate antigen-specific type 1 and type 2 T-cell responses in young C57Bl/6 mice. *Nutrition.* 2000;16(6):442–446

29. Che L, Hu L, Liu Y, et al. Dietary nucleotides supplementation improves the intestinal development and immune function of neonates with intra-uterine growth restriction in a pig model. *PLoS One.* 2016;11(6):e0157314

30. Navarro J, Maldonado J, Narbona E, et al. Influence of dietary nucleotides on plasma immunoglobulin levels and lymphocyte subsets of preterm infants. *Biofactors.* 1999;10(1):67–76

31. Gutierrez-Castrellon P, Mora-Magana I, Diaz-Garcia L, Jiménez-Gutiérrez C, Ramirez-Mayans J, Solomon-Santibáñez GA. Immune response to nucleotide-supplemented infant formulae: systematic review and meta-analysis. *Br J Nutr.* 2007;98(Suppl 1):S64–S67

32. Calder PC. N-3 polyunsaturated fatty acids, inflammation and immunity: pouring oil on troubled waters or another fishy tale? *Nutr Res.* 2001;21(1-2):309–341

33. Lewis ED, Richard C, Larsen BM, Field CJ. The importance of human milk for immunity in preterm infants. *Clin Perinatol.* 2017;44(1):23–47

34. Hennet T, Borsig L. Breastfed at Tiffany's. *Trends Biochem Sci.* 2016;41(6):508–518

35. Ellison RT, III., Giehl TJ. Killing of Gram-negative bacteria by lactoferrin and lysozyme. *J Clin Invest.* 1991;88(4):1080–1091

VI

36. Cravioto A, Tello A, Villafan H, Ruiz J, del Vedovo S, Neeser JR. Inhibition of localized adhesion of enteropathogenic *Escherichia coli* to Hep-2 cells by immunoglobulin and oligosaccharide fractions of human colostrum and breast milk. *J Infect Dis.* 1991;163(6):1247–1255

37. Xanthou M. Immune protection of human milk. *Biol Neonate.* 1998;74(2):121–133.

38. Lönnerdal B. Nutritional roles of lactoferrin. *Curr Opin Clin Nutr Metab Care.* 2009;12(3):293–297

39. Lönnerdal B. Human milk: bioactive proteins/peptide and functional properties. *Nestle Nutr Inst Workshop Ser.* 2016;86:97–107

40. Newburg DS. Oligosaccharides and glycoconjugates in human milk: their role in host defense. *J Mammary Gland Biol Neoplasia.* 1996;1(3):271–283

41. Palmeira P, Carneiro-Sampaio M. Immunology of breast milk. *Rev Assoc Med Bras.* 2016;62(6):584–593

42. Lalho K, Lampi AM, Hamalainen M, et al. Breast milk fatty acids, eicosanoids, and cytokines in mothers with and without allergic disease. *Pediatr Res.* 2003;53(4):642–647

43. Oddy WH, Rosales F. A systematic review of the importance of milk TGF-beta on immunological outcome in the infant and young child. *Pediatr Allergy Immunol.* 2010;21(1 Pt 1):47–59

44. Sheard NF, Walker WA. The role of breast milk in the development of the gastrointestinal tract. *Nutr Rev.* 1988;46(1):1–8

45. Hanson LA. Breastfeeding provides passive and likely long lasting active immunity. *Ann Allergy Asthma Immunol.* 1998;81(6):523–537

46. Bion V, Lockett GA, Soto-Ramirez N, et al. Evaluating the efficacy of breastfeeding guidelines on long term outcomes for allergic disease. *Allergy.* 2016;71(5):661–670

47. Lund-Blix NA, Dydensborg Sander S, Størdal K, et al. Infant feeding and risk of type I diabetes in two large Scandinavian birth cohorts. *Diabetes Care.* 2017;40(7):920–927

48. Hummel S, Beyeralein A, Tamura R, et al. First infant formula type and risk of islet autoimmunity in the environmental determinants of diabetes in the young (TEDDY) study. *Diabetes Care.* 2017;40(3):398–404

49. Ziegler AG, Schmid S, Huber D, Hummel M, Bonifacio E. Early infant feeding and risk of developing type 1 diabetes-associated autoantibodies. *JAMA.* 2003;290(13):1721–1728

50. Lionetti E, Castellaneta S, Francavilla R, et al. Introduction of gluten, HLA status, and the risk of celiac disease in children. *N Engl J Med.* 2014;371(14):1295–1303

51. Szajewska H, Shamir R, Mearin ML, et al. Gluten introduction and the risk of coeliac disease: a position paper by the European Society for Paediatric Gastroenterology, Hepatology, and Nutrition. *J Pediatr Gastroenterol Nutr.* 2016;62(3):507–513

52. O'Sullivan A, He X, McNiven EM, Haggarty NW, Lönnerdal B, Slupsky CM. Early diet impacts infant Rhesus gut microbiome, immunity and metabolism. *J Proteome Res.* 2012;12(6):2833–2845

53. Chichlowski M, German JB, Lebrilla CB, Mills DA. The influence of milk oligosaccharides on microbiota of infants: opportunities for formulas. *Ann Rev Food Sci Technol.* 2011;2:331–351

54. Ogawa K, Ben RA, Pons S, de Paolo MI, Bustos Fernández L. Volatile fatty acids, lactic acid, and pH on the stools of breast-fed and bottle-fed infants. *J Pediatr Gastroenterol Nutr.* 1992;15(3):248–252

55. LoCascio RG, Ninonuevo M, Kronewitter S, et al. A versatile and scalable strategy for glycoprofiling bifidobacterial consumption of human milk oligosaccharides. *Microb Biotechnol.* 2009;2(3):333–342

56. LoCascio RG, Ninonuevo MR, Freeman SL, et al. Glycoprofiling of bifidobacterial consumption of human milk oligosaccharides demonstrate strain specific, preferential consumption of small chain glycans secreted in early human lactation. *J Agric Food Chem.* 2007;55(22):8914–8919

57. Petschow BW, Talbott RD. Response of bifidobacterium species to growth promoters in human and cow milk. *Pediatr Res.* 1991;29(2):208–213

58. Flint AH, Scott KP, Loius P, Duncan SH. The role of the gut microbiota in nutrition and health. *Nat Rev Gastroenterol Hepatol.* 2012;9(10):577–589

59. Roget LC, McCartney AL. Longitudinal investigation of the faecal microbiota of healthy full term infants using florescence in situ hybridization and denaturing gradient gel electrophoresis. *Microbiology.* 2010;156(Pt 11):3317–3328

60. Favier CF, Vaughan EE, De Vos WM, Akkermans AD. Molecular monitoring of succession of bacterial communities in human neonates. *Appl Environ Microbiol.* 2002;68(1):219–226

61. Fallani M, Amarri S, Uusijarvi A, et al. Determinants of the human infant intestinal microbiota after the introduction of first complementary foods infant samples from five European centres. *Microbiology.* 2011;157(Pt 5):1385–1392

62. Yatsunenko T, Rey FE, Manary MJ, et al. Human gut microbiome viewed across age and geography. *Nature.* 2012;486(7402):222–227

63. PrabhuDas M, Adkins B, Gans H, et al. Challenges in infant immunity: implications for responses to infection and vaccines. *Nat Immunol.* 2011;12(3): 189–194

64. Belkaid Y, Hand T. Role of the microbiota in immunity and inflammation. *Cell.* 2014;157(1):121–141

65. Purchiaroni F, Tortora A, Gabrielli M, et al. The role of intestinal microbiota and the immune system. *Eur Rev Medi Pharmacol Sci.* 2013;17(3):323–333

66. Rooks MG, Garrett WS. Gut microbiota, metabolites and host immunity. *Nat Rev Immunol.* 2016;16(6):341–352

67. Reid G, Abrahamsson T, Bailey M, et al. How do probiotics and prebiotics function at distant sites? *Benef Microbes.* 2017;8(4):1–4

VI

68. Gareau MG, Sherman PM, Walker WA. Probiotics and the gut microbiota in intestinal health and disease. *Nat Rev Gastroenterol Hepatol.* 2010;7(9):503–514

69. Grabig A, Paclik D, Guzy C, et al. *Eschericihia coli* strain Nissle, 1917 ameliorates experimental colitis via toll-like receptor 2- and toll-like receptor 4- dependent pathways. *Infect Immun.* 2006;74(7):4075–4082

70. Trejo F, Sanz Y. Intestinal bacterial and probiotics: effects on the immune system and impacts on human health. In: Calder PC, Yaqoob P, eds. *Diet, Immunity and Inflammation.* Cambridge, United Kingdom: Woodhead Publishing Ltd; 2013:267–291

71. Lin YP, Thibodeaux CH, Pena J, Ferry GD, Versalovic J. Probiotic *Lactobacillus reuteri* suppress proinflammatory cytokines via c-Jun. *Inflamm Bowel Dis.* 2008;14(8):1068–1083

72. Hart AL, Lammers K, Brigidi P, et al. Modulation of human dendritic cell phenotype and function by probiotic bacteria. *Gut.* 2004;53:1602–1609

73. Ho-Keun K, Choong-Gu L, Jae-Seon S, et al. Generation of regulatory dendritic cells and CD4+Foxp3+ T cells by probiotics administration suppresses immune disorders. *Proc Natl Acad Sci USA.* 2010;107(5):2159–2164

74. Smits HH, Engering A, van der Kleij D, et al. Selective probiotic bacteria induce IL-10-producing regulatory T cells in vitro by modulating dendritic cell function through dendritic-cell specific intercellular adhesion molecule 3-grabbing nonintegrin. *J Allergy Clin Immunol.* 2005;115(6):1260–1267

75. Szajewska H, Guarino A, Hojsak I, et al. Use of probiotics for management of acute gastroenteritis: a position paper by the ESPGHAN Working Group for Probiotics and Prebiotics. *J Pediatr Gastroenterol Nutr.* 2014;58(4):531–539

76. Vandenplas Y, Huys G, Daube G. Probiotics: an update. *J Pediatr (Rio J).* 2015;91(1):6–21

77. Lund B, Edlund C. Probiotic Enterococcus faecium strain is a possible recipient of the vanA gene cluster. *Clin Infect Dis.* 2001;32(9):1384–1385.

78. Hempel S, Newberry SJ, Maher AR, et al. Probiotics for the prevention and treatment of antibiotic-associated diarrhea: a systematic review and meta-analysis. *JAMA.* 2012;307(18):1959–1969

79. Tung JM, Dolovich LR, Lee CH. Prevention of *Clostridium difficile* infection with *Saccharomyces boulardii*: a systematic review. *Can J Gastroenterol.* 2009;23(12): 817–821

80. McFarland LV, Goh S. Preventing pediatric antibiotic-associated diarrhea and *Clostridium difficile* infections with probiotics: a meta-analysis. *World J Meta-Anal.* 2013;1(3):102–120

81. Braegger C, Chmielewska A, Decsi T, et al. Supplementation of infant formula with probiotics and/or prebiotics: a systematic review and comment by the ESPGHAN committee on nutrition. *J Pediatr Gastroenterol Nutr.* 2011;52(2): 238–250

82. McFarland LV. Probiotics and diarrhea. *Ann Nutr Metab.* 2010;57(Suppl 1):10–11

83. DuPont HL, Ericsson CD, Farthing MJ, et al. Expert review of the evidence base for prevention of travelers' diarrhea. *J Travel Med.* 2009;16(3):149–160

84. Szajewska H, Albrecht P, Topczewska-Cabanek A. Randomized, double-blind, placebo-controlled trial: effect of lactobacillus GG supplementation on Helicobacter pylori eradication rates and side effects during treatment in children. *J Pediatr Gastroenterol Nutr.* 2009;48(4):431–436

85. Malfertheiner P, Selgrad M, Bornschein J. Helicobacter pylori: clinical management. *Curr Opin Gastroenterol.* 2012;28(6):608–614

86. Wilhelm SM, Johnson JL, Kale-Pradhan PB. Treating bugs with bugs: the role of probiotics as adjunctive therapy for *Helicobacter pylori. Ann Pharmacother.* 2011;45(7-8):960–966

87. Li S, Huang XL, Sui JZ, et al. Meta-analysis of randomized controlled trials on the efficacy of probiotics in *Helicobacter pylori* eradication therapy in children. *Eur J Pediatr.* 2014;173(2):153–161

88. Baldassarre ME, Laforgia N, Fanelli M, Laneve A, Grosso R, Lifschitz C. *Lactobacillus GG* improves recovery in infants with blood in the stools and presumptive allergic colitis compared with extensively hydrolyzed formula alone. *J Pediatr.* 2010;156(3):397–401

89. Kim SO, Ah YM, Yu YM, Choi KH, Shin WG, Lee JY. Effects of probiotics for the treatment of atopic dermatitis: a meta-analysis of randomized controlled trials. *Ann Allergy Asthma Immunol.* 2014;113(2):217–226

90. Guarner F. Impacts of prebiotics on the immune system and inflammation. In: Calder PC, Yaqoob P, eds. *Diet, Immunity and Inflammation.* Cambridge, United Kingdom: Woodhead Publishing Ltd; 2013:292–312

91. Gibson GR, Roberfroid M. *Handbook of Prebiotics.* Boca Raton, FL: CRC Press; 2008

92. Coppa GV, Bruni S, Morelli L, Soldi S, Gabrielli O. The first prebiotics in humans: human milk oligosaccharides. *J Clin Gastroenterol.* 2004;38(6 Suppl):S80–S83

93. Waligora-Dupriet AJ, Campeotto F, Nicolis I, et al. Effect of oligofructose supplementation on gut microflora and well-being in young children attending a day care centre. *Int J Food Microbiol.* 2007;113(1):108–113

94. Bruzzese E, Volpicelli M, Squeglia V, et al. A formula containing galacto- and fructo-oligosaccharides prevents intestinal and extra-intestinal infections: an observational study. *Clin Nutr.* 2009;28(2):156–161

95. Firmansyah A, Pramita G, Fassler AC, Haschke F. Improved humoral immune response to measles vaccine in infants receiving infant cereal with fructooligosaccharides. *J Paediatr Gastroenterol Nutr.* 2001;31:A521

96. Goldman AS. Back to basics: host responses to infection. *Pediatr Rev.* 2000;21(10): 342–349

97. Perez-Cano FJ, Franch A, Castellote C, Castell M. The suckling rat as a model for immunonutrition studies in early life. *Clin Dev Immunol.* 2012;2012:537310

98. Marodi L. Innate cellular immune responses in newborns. *Clin Immunol.* 2006;118(2-3):137–144

VI

99. Li Y, Wei QF, Pan XN, et al. Cellular and humoral immunity in preterm infants of different gestational ages. *Chinese J Contemp Pediatr.* 2014;16(11):1118–1121

100. Goenka A, Kollmann TR. Development of immunity in early life. *J Infect.* 2015;71(Suppl 1):S112–S120

101. Mathur NB, Dwarkadas AM, Sharma VK, Saha K, Jain N. Anti-infective factors in preterm human colostrum. *Acta Paediatr Scand.* 1990;79(11):1039–1044

102. Schlesinger LM, Munoz C, Arevalo M, Arredondo S, Mendez G. Functional capacity of colostral leukocytes from women delivering prematurity. *J Pediatr Gastroenterol Nutr.* 1989;8(1):89–94

103. United Nations Programme on HIV/AIDS. Fact Sheet - latest statistics on the status of the AIDS epidemic. Available at: http://www.unaids.org/en/resources/fact-sheet. Accessed February 11, 2019

104. Ivers LC, Cullen KA, Freedberg KA, Block S, Coates J, Webb P. HIV/AIDS, undernutrition, and food insecurity. *Clin Infect Dis.* 2009;49(7):1096–1102

105. Grobler L, Siegfried N, Visser ME, Mahlungulu SS, Volmink J. Nutritional interventions for reducing morbidity and mortality in people with HIV. *Cochrane Database Syst Rev.* 2013;(2):CD004536

106. Sacilotto LB, Pereira PCM, Manechini JPV, Papini SJ. Body composition and metabolic syndrome components on lipodystrophy different subtypes associated with HIV. *J Nutr Metab.* 2017;2017:8260867

107. Smith PD, Meng G, Salazar-Gonzalez JF, Shaw GM. Macrophage HIV-1 infection and the gastrointestinal tract reservoir. *J Leukoc Biol.* 2003;74(5):642–649

108. Chiriboga CA, Fleishman S, Champion S, Gaye-Robinson L, Abrams EJ. Incidence and prevalence of HIV encephalopathy in children with HIV infection receiving highly active anti-retroviral therapy (HAART). *J Pediatr.* 2005;146(3):402–407

109. Moye J, Jr., Rich KC, Kalish LA, et al. Natural history of somatic growth in infants born to women infected by human immunodeficiency virus. Women and Infants Transmission Study Group. *J Pediatr.* 1996;128(1):58–69

110. Miller TL, Evans SJ, Orav EJ, Morris V, McIntosh K, Winter HS. Growth and body composition in children infected with the human immunodeficiency virus-1. *Am J Clin Nutr.* 1993;57(4):588–592

111. Arpadi SM, Horlick MN, Wang J, Cuff P, Bamji M, Kotler DP. Body composition in prepubertal children with human immunodeficiency virus type 1 infection. *Arch Pediatr Adolesc Med.* 1998;152(7):688–693

112. Theron AJ, Anderson R, Rossouw TM, Steel HC. The role of transforming growth factor beta-1 in the progression of HIV/AIDS and development of non-AIDS-defining fibrotic disorders. *Front Immunol.* 2017;8:1461

113. Johann-Liang R, O'Neill L, Cervia J, et al. Energy balance, viral burden, insulin-like growth factor-1, interleukin-6 and growth impairment in children infected with human immunodeficiency virus. *AIDS.* 2000;14(6):683–690

114. Henderson RA, Talusan K, Hutton N, Yolken RH, Caballero B. Resting energy expenditure and body composition in children with HIV infection. *J Acquir Immune Defic Syndr Hum Retrovirol*. 1998;19(2):150–155

115. World Health Organization. *Guidelines for an Integrated Approach to Nutritional Care of HIV-Infected Children (6 months-14 years)*. Geneva, Switzerland: World Health Organization; 2009

116. Weber R, Ledergerber B, Zbinden R, et al. Enteric infections and diarrhea in human immunodeficiency virus-infected persons: prospective community-based cohort study. *Arch Intern Med*. 1999;159(13):1473–1480

117. Kotler DP. HIV infection and the gastrointestinal tract. *AIDS*. 2005;19(2):107–117

118. Guarino A, Bruzzese E, De Marco G, Buccigrossi V. Management of gastrointestinal disorders in children with HIV infection. *Paediatr Drugs*. 2004;6(6):347–362

119. Miller TL, Winter HS, Luginbuhl LM, Orav EJ, McIntosh K. Pancreatitis in pediatric human immunodeficiency virus infection. *J Pediatr*. 1992;120(2 Pt 1): 223–227

120. Bouche H, Housset C, Dumont JL, et al. AIDS-related cholangitis: diagnostic features and course in 15 patients. *J Hepatol*. 1993;17(1):34–39

121. McGrath CJ, Diener L, Richardson BA, Peacock-Chambers E, John-Stewart GC. Growth reconstitution following antiretroviral therapy and nutritional supplementation: systematic review and meta-analysis. *AIDS*. 2015;29(15): 2009–2023

122. Siberry GK, Abzug MJ, Nachman S, et al. Panel on Opportunistic Infections in HIV-Exposed and HIV-Infected Children. Guidelines for the prevention and treatment of opportunistic infections in HIV-exposed and HIV-infected children: recommendations from the National Institutes of Health, Centers for Disease Control and Prevention, the HIV Medicine Association of the Infectious Diseases Society of America, the Pediatric Infectious Diseases Society, and the American Academy of Pediatrics. *Pediatr Infect Dis J*. 2013;32(Suppl 2):i-KK4

123. Feucht UD, Van Bruwaene L, Becker PJ, Kruger M. Growth in HIV-infected children on long-term antiretroviral therapy. *Trop Med Int Health*. 2016;21(5): 619–629

124. Benki-Nugent S, Wamalwa D, Langat A, et al. Comparison of developmental milestone attainment in early treated HIV-infected infants versus HIV-unexposed infants: a prospective cohort study. *BMC Pediatr*. 2017;17(1):24

125. Steele RG, Nelson TD, Cole BP. Psychosocial functioning of children with AIDS and HIV infection: review of the literature from a socioecological framework. *J Dev Behav Pediatr*. 2007;28(1):58–69

126. Gadow KD, Chernoff M, Williams PL, et al. Co-occuring psychiatric symptoms in children perinatally infected with HIV and peer comparison sample. *J Dev Behav Pediatr*. 2010;31(2):116–128

127. Vreeman RC, McCoy BM, Lee S. Mental health challenges among adolescents living with HIV. *J Int AIDS Soc*. 2017;20(Suppl 3):21497

VI

128. Sirois PA, Montepiedra G, Kapetanovic S, et al. Impact of medications prescribed for treatment of attention-deficit hyperactivity disorder on physical growth in children and adolescents with HIV. *J Dev Behav Pediatr.* 2009;30(5): 403–412

129. Thompson-Paul AM, Wei SC, Mattson CL, et al. Obesity among HIV-infected adults receiving medical care in the United States: data from the cross-sectional medical monitoring project and national health and nutrition examination survey. *Medicine (Baltimore).* 2015;94(27):e1081

130. Crum-Cianflone N, Tejidor R, Medina S, Barahona I, Ganesan A. Obesity among HIV patients: the latest epidemic. *AIDS Patient Care STDS.* 2008;22:925–930

131. Sharma TS, Kinnamon DD, Duggan C, et al. Changes in macronutrient intake among HIV-infected children between 1995 and 2004. *Am J Clin Nutr.* 2008;88(2): 384–391

132. Piloya T, Bakeera-Kitaka S, Kekitiinwa A, Kamya MR. Lipodystrophy among HIV-infected children and adlescents on highly active antiretroviral therapy in Uganda: a cross sectional study. *J Int AIDS Soc.* 2012;15:17427

133. Vigano A, Mora S, Testolin C, et al. Increased lipodystrophy is associated with increased exposure to highly active antiretroviral therapy in HIV-infected children. *J Acquir Immune Defic Syndr.* 2003;32(5):482–489

134. Kumar NS, Shashibhushan J, Malappa, Venugopal K, Vishwanatha H, Menon M. Lipodystrophy in human immunodeficiency virus (HIV) patients on highly active antiretroviral therapy (HAART). *J Clin Diagn Res.* 2015;9:OC05–OC08

135. Grinspoon SK, Grunfeld C, Kotler DP, et al. State of the science conference: Initiative to decrease cardiovascular risk and increase quality of care for patients living with HIV/AIDS: executive summary. *Circulation.* 2008;118(2):198–210

136. Miller TL, Grant YT, Almeida DN, Sharma T, Lipshultz SE. Cardiometabolic disease in human immunodeficiency virus-infected children. *J Cardiometab Syndr.* 2008;3(2):98–105

137. Miller TL, Orav EJ, Lipshultz SE, et al. Risk factors for cardiovascular disease in children infected with human immunodeficiency virus-1. *J Pediatr.* 2008;153(4): 491–497

138. Lainka E, Oezbek S, Falck M, Ndagijimana J, Niehues T. Marked dyslipidemia in human immunodeficiency virus-infected children on protease inhibitor-containing antiretroviral therapy. *Pediatrics.* 2002;110(5):e56

139. Sharma T, Orav E, Weinberg G, et. al. Visceral adiposity and cardiac risk profiles in human immunodeficiency virus-1 infected children. *EPAS.* 2006;59:5523.132

140. Beregszaszi M, Jaquet D, Levine M, et al. Severe insulin resistance contrasting with mild anthropometric changes in the adipose tissue of HIV-infected children with lipohypertrophy. *Int J Obes Metab Disord.* 2003;27(1):25–30

141. Hruz PW. HIV protease inhibitors and insulin resistance: lessons from in vitro, rodent and healthy human volunteer models. *Curr Opin HIV AIDS.* 2008;3: 660–665

142. Araujo S, Bañon S, Machuca I, Moreno A, Pérez-Elías MJ, Casado JL. Prevalence of insulin resistance and risk of diabetes mellitus in HIV-infected patients receiving current antiretroviral drugs. *Eur J Endocrinol.* 2014;171(5):545–554

143. Barlow-Mosha L, Eckard AR, McComsey GA, Musoke PM. Metabolic complications and treatment of perinatally HIV-infected children and adolescents. *J Int AIDS Soc.* 2013;16:18600

144. Jacobson DL, Spiegelman D, Duggan C, et al. Predictors of bone mineral density in human immunodeficiency virus-1 infected children. *J Pediatr Gastroenterol Nutr.* 2005;41(3):339–346

145. Zuccotti G, Vigano A, Gabiano C, et al. Antiretroviral therapy and bone mineral measurements in HIV-infected youths. *Bone.* 2010;46(6):1633–1638

146. Fields-Gardner C, Campa A, American Dietetic Association. Position of the American Dietetic Association: Nutrition Intervention and Human Immunodeficiency Virus Infection. *J Am Diet Assoc.* 2010;110(7):1105–1119

147. Gkrania-Klotsas E, Klotsas AE. HIV and HIV treatment: effects on fats, glucose and lipids. *Br Med Bull.* 2007;84:49–68

148. Kastorini CM, Milionis HJ, Esposito K, Giugliano D, Goudevenos JA, Panagiotakos DB. The effect of Mediterranean diet on metabolic syndrome and its components: a meta-analysis of 50 studies and 534,906 individuals. *J Am Coll Cardiol.* 2011;57(11):1299–1313

149. Krauss RM, Eckel RH, Howard B, et al. AHA Dietary Guidelines: revision 2000: a statement for healthcare professionals from the Nutrition Committee of the American Heart Association. *Stroke.* 2000;31(11):2751–2766

150. Ockenga J, Grimble R, Jonkers-Schuitema C, et al. ESPEN Guidelines on Enteral Nutrition: Wasting in HIV and other chronic infectious diseases. *Clin Nutr.* 2006;25(2):319–329

151. Sabery N, Duggan C. A.S.P.E.N. clinical guidelines: nutrition support of children with human immunodeficiency virus infection. *JPEN J Parenter Enteral Nutr.* 2009;33(6):588–606

152. Institute of Medicine, Food and Nutrition Board. *Dietary Reference Intakes for Energy, Carbohydrate, Fiber, Fat, Fatty Acids, Cholesterol, Protein, and Amino Acids.* Washington, DC: National Academies Press; 2005

VI

Chapter 36

Nutritional Support of Children With Developmental Disabilities

Introduction

Children and adolescents with developmental disabilities encompass a group with a wide spectrum of etiologies and conditions. Over the past several decades, children characterized as having developmental disabilities have been those demonstrating impairment of body structure or body functions that affect their physical, cognitive, academic, and/or emotional and behavioral performance in daily activities and participation. Irrespective of primary etiology, the disabilities may begin early in development and have lifelong impacts.[1] Estimates vary regarding the prevalence of developmental disabilities, but generally, it is reported to be 13% to 15%.[2]

With improved treatments of both primary and secondary causes of disability, more children are surviving into their third decade of life or beyond. Nutrition support has become increasingly recognized as a critical component of those treatments. This aspect of care is best accomplished when integrated into a multidisciplinary, holistic approach to the care of children with disabilities. An excellent overview of this approach was outlined in 2016 by Glader et al.[3] Their framework, based on the components of the International Classification of Function, Disability and Health, underlies the approach provided in this chapter. Because of the many and varied potential barriers that can and do occur, provision of adequate nutrition can be challenging. Families can face medical, psychosocial, cultural, and financial barriers in this regard.

Assessment

Children with developmental disabilities are often at risk of malnutrition and should be screened regularly in primary care. Malnutrition can cause or worsen disability; similarly, malnutrition can result from the disabling condition.[4,5] Subspecialty tertiary-level clinics typically include experienced registered dietitian nutritionists (RDNs) within the interdisciplinary team providing comprehensive care. In the primary medical home setting, care plans may require an RDN as a partner. Outside the medical home, community resources include the Special Supplemental Nutrition Program for Women, Infants, and Children (WIC), Early and Periodic Screening, Diagnostic, and Treatment (EPSDT) benefits under Medicaid, Title V Maternal Child Health Program, early intervention services (0–3 years),

Head Start, the National School Lunch Program, and the benefits specified under the Individuals with Disabilities Education Act (IDEA).[6]

Acute and chronic illness-related malnutrition in children with disabilities can result in loss of lean body mass, muscle weakness, developmental or intellectual delay, delayed wound healing, immune dysfunction, infections, and extended hospitalizations. Chronically malnourished children can appear "proportionate" on weight-for-height standards. Regular nutrition assessments and intervention can reduce health care costs by early identification and intervention.[5] Periodic assessments can be particularly helpful before and after surgeries and/or acute infections. Nutritional assessments are best conducted jointly by the physician and RDN; potential components of nutrition assessments are shown in Table 36.1.

Medical History
Beyond the inherent aspects of the child's developmental disability that directly affect nutritional well-being, there are nutrition-related medical issues that should be considered. A number of these are outlined in Table 36.2.

Growth History/Assessment
The American Academy of Pediatrics (AAP) recommends using the World Health Organization (WHO) growth charts for children younger than 2 years and the Centers for Disease Control and Prevention (CDC) growth charts for children 2 to 20 years of age[7] (see Appendix Q). Current

Table 36.1.
Potential Elements of Nutritional Assessment for the Developmentally Disabled Child

Medical history	Anthropometric measures
Nutrition-focused physical examination	Laboratory data
Complementary/alternative therapies	Food intake pattern
Oral-motor concerns	Bowel patterns
Nutritional/vitamin supplements	Food insecurity
Feeding skills	Environmental factors
Cognitive/social factors	Functional abilities
Social factors	

Table 36.2.

Nutrition-Related Medical Issues Frequently Seen in Children With Developmental Disabilities

Clinical Considerations	Potential Contributing Issues

Altered growth
  Onset; patterns, associated
  clinical issues
	Short stature
	Underweight
	Overweight/obesity

Feeding
  Need for changes in formula,
  volume, rate, additives
  Recent changes in routines
  impacting feeding schedules
  (home, school)
	Feeding route
	Oral
	Enteral
	Parenteral
	Combination of the above

Gastrointestinal Recent or worsening symptoms	Constipation Diarrhea Dumping syndrome Dysmotility Gastroesophageal reflux Malrotation

Orthopedic
  Conditions creating chronic
  pain or anatomical restrictions
  impacting feedings
	Dislocated hips
	Scoliosis
	Contractures
	Osteopenia

Medications Alternative/complementary medicine	Drug-nutrient interactions Medication side effects
Dysphagia Potential for changes with age	Oropharyngeal Esophageal
Effects on energy needs and caloric expenditure	Muscle tone (hypo/hypertonia) Mobility status Medication side effects Underlying diagnosis Degree/level of physical therapy

recommendations are to use the WHO/CDC growth charts and monitor growth velocity of the individual child with serial measurements.[8] Children can have appropriate growth velocity and follow their own curve, even if their measurements are consistently below the 5th percentile. A change in growth velocity of greater than ½ standard deviation should prompt additional monitoring and screening.[9]

Table 36.3.
Selected Sites for Condition-Related Growth Charts

Cerebral Palsy: http://pediatrics.aappublications.org/content/128/2/e299.long
Down Syndrome: http://pediatrics.aappublications.org/content/138/4/e20160541.long
Duchenne Muscular Dystrophy: http://www.sciencedirect.com/science/article/pii/S0022347613009761?via%3Dihub
Prader-Willi Syndrome (non–growth hormone-treated): http://pediatrics.aappublications.org/content/135/1/e126.long
Rett Syndrome: https://www.ncbi.nlm.nih.gov/pmc/articles/PMC3468773/

There are specialty growth charts for some developmental disabilities (eg, Down syndrome) that are useful when growth plotted on the WHO/CDC charts requires additional evaluation.[10] Additional charts are available for other conditions and listed with links in Table 36.3.

Specific measurements by a trained clinician, such as triceps skin fold measurements or mid-upper arm circumference, have been shown to add clinical information about fat stores, malnutrition (in children up to ae 6 years of age), and body composition (see Appendix Q). The reference percentiles for these measurements were generated in children without disabilities, so the measurements derived from a child with a disability should be used serially to detect trends.[5,8,11–13]

Height
Measurements should be to the nearest 0.1 cm. Measuring an accurate length or height in children with developmental disabilities can be challenging because of body habitus, inability to stand, lack of adequate measurement devices, or the child's ability to stand or lie still. Various techniques to measure length have been described including segmental length, recumbent length, knee height, and arm span; training for each is needed for accuracy. Generally, children with cerebral palsy, Down syndrome, cystic fibrosis, Duchenne muscular dystrophy, myelomeningocele, and Prader-Willi syndrome tend to exhibit more diminished linear growth.[10,11,14–17]

Weight
To ensure an accurate weight, scales should be "zeroed" prior to measurement, and individuals should be weighed in light clothing (no shoes, braces,

coats). The weight should be measured to the nearest 0.1 kg. Using the same scale each time ensures the most accurate serial measurements. Although a table, bed, or wheelchair scale are ideal for children unable to stand, these may be available only in specialty facilities. In practice, many physicians weigh both the parent and child together on a standing scale and then subtract the parent's weight to obtain a measurement. Although inaccuracies may occur, consistency allows for some trend analysis. Some diagnoses, particularly those with genetic etiologies such as Down syndrome, have a higher risk of obesity, even if their early weight velocity is similar to typically developing children.[10]

Body Mass Index and Body Composition

Body mass index (BMI) for age is not necessarily the optimal reflection of a child's body habitus, because it is based on muscle and fat distribution in the typically developing population. Children with spina bifida and Prader-Willi syndrome, for example, have higher body fat and lower lean body mass comparatively.[14,18,19]

Family/Social History

The inability to consistently provide adequate amounts of food is a trigger for increased strain and stress in families. The presence of food insecurity is known to be associated with depression, anxiety, and toxic stress, irrespective of social class[20] (see Chapter 49: Community Nutrition Services). When external conditions such as food insecurity are present in the environment of a child with developmental disabilities, there is added risk. Out-of-pocket medical expenses are generally higher among families of children with developmental disabilities. Identification of such added stressors is critical when assessing nutritional concerns in this population. Extensive questionnaires in survey format are available for population research related to food insecurity. Hager et al have shown the value of a simple 2-question inquiry in the clinical setting[21]: *1) Within the past 12 months, we worried whether our food would run out before we got money to buy more (Yes or No); 2. Within the past 12 months, the food we bought just didn't last and we didn't have money to get more (Yes or No).* Affirmative answers should prompt further questions.[21]

Another clinically useful tool to better identify barriers to adequate nutrition related to socioeconomic issues was devised by the National Center for Medical-Legal Partnership using the acronym, IHELLP. This mnemonic assists in remembering barriers that may affect adequate nutrition within the household: **i**ncome; **h**ousing /utilities; **e**ducation; **l**egal status (immigration); **l**iteracy (child and/or parent); **p**ersonal safety (domestic violence,

VI

etc). The AAP has a useful pocket card for the clinician's use at https://www.
aap.org/en-us/Documents/IHELLPPocketCard.pdf. Both of these tools
helps to remind the professional of the tremendous value of a social history
when considering poor nutritional status in a child with developmental
disabilities.

Other resources (see also Chapter 49) available to the clinician and families are the following websites:

- WIC food packages: https://www.fns.usda.gov/wic/links-state-agency-
  wic-approved-food-lists
- Supplemental Nutrition Assistance Program (SNAP) Eligible food
  items: https://www.fns.usda.gov/snap/eligible-food-items
- SNAP-Ed resources: https://snaped.fns.usda.gov/
- National School Lunch and National School Breakfast Programs:
  https://www.fns.usda.gov/school-meals/nutrition-standards-school-
  meals
- Child and Adult Care Food Program (for infants, children, and adults):
  http://www.fns.usda.gov/cacfp/meals-and-snacks
- Summer Food Service Program: https://www.fns.usda.gov/sfsp/
  summer-food-service-program
- USDA Food Distribution Program: https://www.fns.usda.gov/fdd/food-
  distribution-programs
- Modules on training with CSHCN and Nutrition: http://depts.
  washington.edu/chdd/ucedd/ctu_5/pacwestcshcn_5.html

Diet History/Meal Observation
The nutrition assessment should include a diet history and/or 24-hour
food recall. This should include information on the feeding environment,
feeding equipment, feeding abilities, feeding difficulties, length of feedings, preparation of the food, and aspects of feeding (who feeds the child;
which food and drinks are offered, consumed, refused; amount of spillage).[6] Estimations of oral intake by recall can be challenging; in 1 study of
parents of children with cerebral palsy, overestimates of intake ranged as
high as 300%.[22]

Energy
Estimating energy needs in children with developmental disabilities is complicated by altered body composition and variations in mobility/
activity levels. Among some children with developmental disabilities,
weight gain may occur on an intake of 20% to 40% fewer calories than

estimated by prediction equations.[15,19,22,23] In specialty clinics, the Dietary Reference Intakes (DRIs) are used along with a physical activity coefficient[24] to estimate energy needs.

Medications affecting tone, such as trihexyphenidyl and baclofen, can reduce energy expenditure by reducing tone or spasticity; risperidone can increase hunger and energy intake. Gastrostomy tube feedings can result in overfeeding and weight gain in patients with cerebral palsy (CP); close monitoring of weight is essential.[25] Lean body mass, higher levels of mobility, and ambulation increase resting energy expenditure (REE) in CP.[25,26] Enteral feedings have been shown to increase resting energy expenditure (REE) in malnourished children with CP from 70% to 102% of predicted needs.[22]

Protein
Protein needs are calculated using the DRI ratio based on the patient's actual weight. For surgery or wound healing, needs may be increased by 1.5 to 2 g/kg/day.[8,14,23] Additional calories or protein does not necessarily result in increased lean body mass in Duchenne muscular dystrophy or in CP, in which it has been found that increasing energy results in higher fat mass and lower muscle mass.[15,27]

Micronutrients
If a child has an adequate variety and intake of foods, supplementation with a multivitamin/multimineral should not be necessary. The DRI for age for vitamins and minerals provides recommended intake levels. Supplementation is recommended in specific circumstances (eg, when there is low intake of a micronutrients, additional needs based on serum values, surgery, wound healing, underlying diagnosis, drug-nutrient interactions, multiple food allergies).

Fluids
Fluid needs are calculated using the Holliday-Segar equation based on actual body weight and can be further individualized for children as needed. Those estimates are as follows:

Weight	Calculated Estimate
1 – 10 kg	100 mL/kg
10 – 20 kg	1000 mL + 50 mL/kg for each kg >10 kg
≥20 kg	1000 mL + 20 mL/kg for each kg >20 kg

Oral Health Care and Children With Developmental Disabilities
Pathology within the oral pharynx/hypopharynx (anatomic, infectious, gingival, otherwise) can be a direct contributor to suboptimal intake and,

subsequently, malnutrition (see Chapter 48: Nutrition and Oral Health). The AAP published an extensive review of oral health issues that affect children with developmental disabilities.[28] As outlined in the report, a variety of contributors to poor oral health can have direct or secondary effects on nutrition: *oral aversion* (frequently seen in neonatal intensive care graduates who have had noxious experiences to the mouth and/or dysphagia related to their prematurity); *children unable to meet fluid/nutritional needs orally* (those with nonoral feeding have a propensity to a build-up of tartar and gingivitis); *children with severe behavioral problems* (making activities of daily living, such as tooth brushing, difficult/dangerous to caregivers); and *children with craniofacial anomalies* (some of whom may have very limited ability to fully open the mouth for care). These and similar barriers to oral health can affect which and how much food can be provided.

Bone Health

Bone health is a common concern among many categories of developmental disabilities. Risk factors for poor bone health among this cohort of children include: a history of fractures, sustained periods of immobilization (including postsurgical), non–weight-bearing status, feeding difficulties, obesity, diets low in calcium and/or vitamin D, certain medications (proton pump inhibitors, some seizure medications, long-term use of corticosteroids), and limited sun exposure. For those at risk, a systematic plan of monitoring should be devised. For example, the adequate intake of calcium and vitamin D and the monitoring of 25-OH vitamin D blood levels and growth hormone status (when indicated) might be useful.[29–32]

Medication Use

Many youth with developmental disabilities require chronic medications; some require multiple medications daily. As a result, there is potential for medications to negatively affect nutritional interventions; likewise, the child's nutritional status and care plan can affect bioavailability and metabolism of medication. Medications can increase or diminish appetite, with untoward effects that go in either direction. Medications with the adverse effect of nausea or with known associated deficiencies of micronutrients adversely affect growth and well-being.

Physical Examination

Physical findings related to nutrition can range from subtle to blatant among children with developmental disabilities. Monitoring of growth trends based on consistently obtained measurements of height and weight is the first step in physical assessment and is perhaps most important. Other physical changes, compared with prior examinations, need to be considered in the context of the individual child and the underlying diagnosis. Physical findings that suggest malnutrition (decreased subcutaneous tissue, decreased fat stores, edema, oropharyngeal changes such as cheilosis, gingival bleeding, thin and brittle hair, hepato-splenomegaly, or distension) are generally late signs. Evidence of scurvy, although rare, can occur in unusual contexts. Paying attention to the child's demeanor is especially helpful. Irritability, apathy, anxiety, or decreased social interactions may be related to undernutrition. In a child with poor weight trajectory, physical findings of iron deficiency may be absent or quite subtle until anemia occurs.

An examination and description of muscle tone is useful to assess overall energy requirements. A description of hydration status is useful in planning fluid requirements and types of fluids needed. If there have been changes in joint or spine findings, the secondary effects on posture may have functional effect on the feeding process.

It is unlikely that time will permit a formal observation of a feeding during routine examinations. Two avenues to "extend the examination" can be of use: (1) obtaining a 5- to 8-minute video from the family of the child having a typical meal at home; and (2) setting up a clinical feeding evaluation wherein the parent and child join the dietitian and/or feeding therapist for a meal, preferably using food from home and utensils from home. Observation of feeding extends the examination to include information about functional feeding patterns. Close follow-up physical examinations (every 2–3 weeks or every 2–3 months, depending on the situation) are critical to monitor the effectiveness of interventions and assist with decision making when expected outcomes are not being realized.

Diagnostic Studies for Consideration on the Basis of History/Physical Examination

Numerous laboratory and/or imaging studies are available to assist in better describing aspects of nutrition and feeding among children with developmental disabilities. Clearly, the history and physical examination should guide the specific evaluations being ordered and reviewed (see Chapter 24: Nutritional Assessment, for a complete list and description of assessments that might be considered).

Opportunities for Intervention

Patterns and Approaches to Feeding

The "division of responsibility" approach to feeding a young child is based on the trust model that typically developing children can self-regulate food intake with a schedule of meals and snacks. The parents are responsible for what foods are offered at meals and snacks (offering variety and balance), the meal and snack schedule, where the meals take place, and providing a relaxed atmosphere for family meals. Children are responsible for what they eat, whether they eat, and how much they eat.[33] Although all components of this approach are not appropriate for children with disabilities, scheduled meals and snacks, family meals, and reduced pressure to eat at meals can be used at home during meal and snack times. Information and examples for intervention can be found at http://www.ellynsatterinstitute.org/. Feeding difficulties range in severity and determine the need for mealtime assistance, from minimal (setting up tray, cutting food) to maximal (unable to self-feed, totally dependent for feeding). A child who is more dependent for activities of daily living will typically be more dependent for feedings.

Diet Therapy

After a comprehensive evaluation that may include a clinical feeding evaluation and/or videofluoroscopic swallow study, the RDN, speech-language pathologist (SLP), and occupational therapist (OT) work with the families to implement a comprehensive feeding plan. Recommendations should be provided for texture modifications, liquid modifications, feeding environment, positioning, pacing or meals, and behavior modification. Physician orders for school can be implemented into the individualized education program (IEP) or 504 plan.

Intervention for Other Gastrointestinal Conditions

Several gastrointestinal conditions can have direct bearing on feeding and nutrition. Gastroesophageal reflux disease (GERD) is common in children with neurodevelopmental disabilities. Delayed gastric emptying can, in turn, contribute to GERD in children with disabilities such as muscular dystrophy.[15] Medical and/or surgical intervention may be required for management. Appropriately chosen dietary selections can offer clinical improvement among children with GERD (in children receiving enteral feedings, adjustments can be made to the infusion rate, volume per feeding, and formula/additive selections). It should be noted that intestinal bacterial overgrowth related to medications (eg, proton pump inhibitors) and the associated symptoms can negatively affect appetite and nutrient absorption.

Constipation among children with disabilities may be related to their underlying diagnoses, mobility status, medication regimen, and fluid/fiber intake. Constipation can lead to a cycle of reduced appetite, reduced food intake, and weight loss. Constipation can be misattributed; for example, perceived "hip pain" may actually be attributable to increased contractions of the lower abdominal muscles and painful cramping from constipation. Both adequate fluid intake and dietary fiber may mitigate the risks of constipation.

Enteral Feedings (see also Chapter 23: Enteral Nutrition)

Several publications are available to provide guidance on enteral feedings in children with developmental disabilities (also see Chapter 23: Enteral Nutrition).[34–36] Each offers examples of clinical situations in which enteral tube feedings might be considered. General categories for these include inadequate or insufficient oral intake (related to dysphagia, increased metabolic needs, critical illness and sequelae, congenital anomalies), disorders of digestion and/or absorption (short gut syndrome, cystic fibrosis, severe immunodeficiency related to the underlying disability), disorders of gastrointestinal tract motility, growth failure as a result of malnutrition and primary metabolic disorders.

When considering enteral feedings, either complete or as an adjunct to oral feedings, an informed and sensitive approach to the conversation with the child/family is critical. Such decisions necessarily encompass emotional, social, cultural, medical, and financial considerations, at the least. The AAP clinical report provides stepwise guidance in both when to consider use of nonoral feedings *and* the components of shared decision making that should be used.[34] The latter focuses on the context of the decision, the values, and belief systems affecting such a decision and the processes of care by which the child, family, and physician come to a comfortable and confident decision and care plan. An overview can be found at http://pediatrics.aappublications.org/content/early/2014/11/18/peds.2014-2829.

Weight gain is often a measure of success when enteral feedings are initiated in children with developmental disabilities. However, close follow-up over weeks and months or years is needed to ensure that the feeding regimen does not lead to excessive weight gain. Overweight can have its own adverse medical effects and can act as a functional barrier to participation in day-to-day activities of daily living and independence from caregivers.

Vernon-Roberts et al, in a study of gastrostomy tube feeding in children with CP, showed that even those fed with a low-energy, micronutrient-sufficient, high-fiber base formula continued to grow even with energy intakes below 75% of estimated needs.[25] Children with other conditions can require even less. The authors outlined the potential advantages of carefully adjusted feeding regimens to meet individual requirements, which again underscores the importance of close interaction with the pediatric nutritionist trained and familiar with this patient population.

Formula Selection

Polymeric pediatric enteral formulas are available in caloric densities from 0.6 to 2 kcal/mL and are generally appropriate for children 1 to 10 years of age. Adult formulas are available in 0.3 to 2 kcal/mL and are typically recommended for children 10 years or older. However; in clinical practice, a pediatric enteral formula has been used for a longer period of time because of the higher fortification of calcium and vitamin D and to reduce the number of supplements. Depending on volume of formula and age of the child, up to 100% of the DRI for vitamins and minerals may be met. Experts recommend not using adult formulas until the child is at least 8 to 10 years of age.[36] For children with normal gut function, polymeric formulas contain intact nutrients and provide casein-based protein.

Children with disabilities can have primary or secondary conditions that affect absorption and tolerance of various formula components. Thus, formula selection can be particularly important (see Appendix M: Special Enteral Products for Special Indications). Soy formulas do not contain whey, casein, or lactose and are available for vegetarians and those with milk protein allergy. Typically, enteral formulas are gluten free, and many are lactose free or low in lactose. Calorically dense formulas are used for volume intolerance; however, they provide less free water, so it is important to consider total fluid intake when assessing intake. Reduced-calorie formulas provide reduced energy with adequate protein and micronutrients for children who are hypometabolic. Formulas with additional fiber (soy fiber, guar gum, inulin, oligofructose, and fructo-oligosaccharides) can help with bowel function, and high-protein formulas provide additional protein for increased protein needs.

Children with significant malabsorption can be supported on protein hydrolysate-based formulas or those with free amino acids or short-chain peptides and fat provided as medium-chain triglycerides (MCTs).

Commercially prepared, blenderized, "real food" tube feedings and home-blended tube feedings have recently become more popular, although the evidence of benefit is currently limited.[37] Some families prefer the "whole food" blenderized diet to help normalize feeding times, to feed their child like their other children, and to manage costs. The literature has reported reduced gagging and retching, fewer oral aversions, improvement in reflux, constipation, volume tolerance, and support for those who require customized foods for food allergies/sensitivities/vegetarian diets.[38,39]

A combination of blenderized tube feedings with commercial formulas ensures that nutrient needs are met. In a study of pediatric patients on enteral feedings, 90% of patients were given commercial formula for some portion of their daily intake, because not all blenderized feedings are nutritionally complete.[40,41]

If families choose to prepare their own tube feedings at home or use commercially prepared whole food feedings, they should consult with the RDN to ensure adequate nutrient intake and safe handling techniques. Bolus feedings are preferred for administration of these formulas, and they are thick and need to be thinned down to go through and not clog the tubing.

Modular products are used to add additional energy without additional volume in the form of carbohydrate, protein, fat, and fiber. Most modular products provide single nutrients, such as carbohydrate, protein, fat, or fiber. There are modular products that contain 2 types of macronutrients; for example, a product that contains both carbohydrate and fat, and another that contains both fat and protein. The clinician must ensure appropriate nutrient distribution and consider formula displacement when adding modular products.

Feeding Tolerance

Children who are malnourished are at a higher risk of refeeding syndrome (see Chapter 26: Malnutrition, and Chapter 38: Eating Disorders). Recommendations are to provide supplemental potassium, phosphorus, and vitamins in such children. Potassium, phosphate, and magnesium serum levels should be closely monitored when initiating feedings in a child at risk of refeeding syndrome. Children with a BMI <16 kg/m^2; greater than 15% weight loss in the past 3 to 6 months; low levels of potassium, phosphate, and magnesium; and reduced intake for 5 to 10 days are particularly at risk.[36]

The physician and RDN, as part of a multidisciplinary team, should monitor enteral feeding tolerance, growth trends, and when indicated, laboratory values. If a child is also eating by mouth, the combinations of feedings are evaluated to ensure the child is receiving adequate intake of recommended nutrients. Common indicators of intolerance of enteral feedings include diarrhea, nausea, vomiting, bloating, and pulmonary symptoms related to microaspiration from reflux. Management of symptoms by the physician and RDN may include changing formula, infusion volume, rate, feeding schedule, ensuring adequate fluid intake, or medication management.

The Oley Foundation (www.oley.org) and Feeding Tube Awareness Foundation (http://www.feedingtubeawareness.org/) have excellent resources for families and caregivers on enteral feeding management, including how to implement enteral feedings and manage complications.

Summary of Diagnoses and Nutrition-Related Issues

Autism Spectrum Disorder

Characterized by language delays, ritualistic behaviors, and impaired social interactions, many children with autism spectrum disorder (ASD) also have differences in feeding skills and patterns. Limited food repertoires may be seen, with manifestations of limited food variety, rigid rituals around mealtimes, preferences for specific food textures, and resistance in trying new foods.[42,43] Some families follow a gluten-free/casein-free diet in hopes of managing symptoms of ASD. To date, neither approach has been shown to improve symptoms in studies with high levels of evidence. A potential adverse effect of such trials is the potential for micronutrient deficiencies.[44] Medications (eg, antipsychotics, mood stabilizers) can cause appetite changes and resultant significant weight loss or weight gain.

Cerebral Palsy

CP is a disorder of muscle control/coordination. Although considered "nonprogressive," the manifestations clinically can vary over time. Children with CP who do not have feeding difficulties have shown near normal growth.[45] But those with feeding difficulties show slower growth velocity and lower final stature/weight. Excess body weight in nonambulatory children with CP can result and potentially add further medical complications.[46] Similarly, among those with enteral feedings but minimal physical activity, there is higher risk of obesity.

Cystic Fibrosis

Children with cystic fibrosis (CF) tend to be underweight. Guidelines released in 2016 published several recommendations, including the use of enteral tube feedings to help meet needs for growth, as it has been shown that pulmonary function improves when nutritional status improves. Enteral feedings increase the risks of CF-related diabetes, oral aversion, disordered eating, and other behavior issues.[47] These risks should be discussed in the shared decision-making process prior to initiating a regimen of nonoral feedings.[48]

Drug Exposure and Fetal Alcohol Spectrum Disorder

Children exposed to drugs and/or alcohol in utero can demonstrate irreversible delays in neural, mental, and physical growth. Poor nutrition can exacerbate growth deficiency. Although children with fetal alcohol spectrum disorder (FASD) have a higher rate of underweight in early childhood, over time, they are 3 times more likely to become overweight/obese compared with peers; careful monitoring is warranted.[49,50]

Down Syndrome

Children with Down syndrome have higher rates of feeding difficulties in infancy and higher risk for overweight/obesity later in life because of reduced muscle mass, short stature, and mobility problems.[51] The AAP recommends screening children with Down syndrome for symptoms of celiac disease at each preventative care visit if the child consumes gluten.[52]

Muscular Dystrophy

Differences in body composition attributable to the loss of lean body mass and increased fat mass make it difficult to assess energy needs and inaccurate to use BMI for assessment. Steroid therapy for maintaining muscle strength and functional ability often results in weight gain with continuance into adulthood, shorter final height, and lower bone density. Early nutrition intervention with the RDN throughout the lifespan is recommended as part of multidisciplinary care. A significant number of children with Duchenne muscular dystrophy have dysphagia related to oropharyngeal muscle weakness. This carries potential for both poor weight gain and for pulmonary complications; enteral feedings, total or partial, can improve nutritional and respiratory status.[9,15,53]

Genetic/Inherited Metabolic Disorders

Dietitians specially trained in these disorders are critical players, as their skills are necessary working with families to best maintain optimal growth

VI

and development. Children with these conditions require careful monitoring of micronutrient and macronutrient intake throughout the life span.

Orofacial Cleft

Many parents are concerned about feeding their newborn with a cleft. Breastfeeding can be successful in many cases of isolated cleft lip, but direct breastfeeding is rarely successful as the sole means of feeding an infant with cleft palate. Access to a high-quality breast pump is important for mothers who want to provide their infants with all the benefits of human milk. There are a variety of special nipples and assisted-delivery bottles available to facilitate feeding infants with clefts. Because of increased air intake while feeding, infants with a cleft require more frequent burping. Nasal regurgitation is common when there is a palatal opening or dysfunction. Detailed information about feeding methods is available in the Cleft Palate Foundation publication "Feeding Your Baby" (https://cleftline.org/family-resources/feeding-your-baby/).

Prader-Willi Syndrome

Children with Prader-Willi syndrome typically begin with severe hypotonia, sometimes resulting in failure to thrive in infancy because of feeding difficulties. Later, hyperphagia, characterized by food seeking and behavior problems related to food, results in obesity. With this comes an increasing risk for comorbid conditions, such as type 2 diabetes mellitus and metabolic syndrome.[19,54] Monitoring growth patterns, feeding issues, and behavioral issues related to feeding with referral to a dietitian can help maintain appropriate growth velocity. Although care must be taken in its initiation and management, studies have shown that growth hormone treatment improves linear growth and body composition.[6]

Rett Syndrome

Rett syndrome is a neurologic disorder related to a mutation of MECP2 gene and predominantly affects girls. Over time, worsening of feeding difficulties and malnutrition frequently occur. A comprehensive, multidisciplinary approach is required. If oral feedings are not safe, provision of enteral feedings improves respiratory status, nutritional status, growth, and lean body mass and fat stores. With hypotonia and lower physical activity, children with Rett syndrome can have lower lean body mass, higher fat mass, and lower bone density; fracture risk increases by 4 times in children with Rett syndrome.[31,55–58]

Spina Bifida (Myelomeningocele)

Children with spina bifida are shorter than their typically developing peers. The level of the spina bifida lesion is correlated to body fat percentage, and the lower level of lean body mass reduces energy expenditure. Ambulation and active gross motor movement varies widely within the population, making energy expenditure estimates challenging for the team offering advice for growth, wellness, and fitness.

Conclusion

Adequate nutrition is central to growth, comfort, development, behavior, activities of daily living, and quality of life. This is true for all children. For children with developmental disabilities, inadequate nutrition can be obvious to the clinician, or it can be an occult contributor to factors complicating the care of these children. Adding to the challenges for the clinician, the evaluation of nutritional status can be difficult, as many standard measures of nutritional status have not been validated in this population. A keen eye on longitudinal trends and the clinical signs outlined in this chapter offer a reasonable starting point.

Collaboration with other clinicians, the child, and the family has been stressed.[48] This collaboration is particularly the case relative to the pediatric RDN, who ideally is integrated into the care team, whether that is in the primary medical home or the specialty care centers where the children are followed. Finally, as these children grow and "age out" of the pediatric community, close attention to the process of transitioning to adult care is particularly important. Providing an updated care plan and list of resources to the adult medical team can be critical for the young adult.

References

1. Blumberg SJ. Trends in the prevalence of developmental disabilities in U.S. children. National Conference on Health Statistics. 2012. Available at: https://www.cdc.gov/nchs/ppt/nchs2012/ss-22_blumberg.pdf. Accessed March 14, 2019

2. Boyle C, Boulet S, Schieve L, et al. Trends in the prevalence of developmental disabilities in US children, 1997–2008. *Pediatrics.* 2011;127(6):1034–1042

3. Glader L, Plews-Ogan J, Agrawal R. Children with medical complexity: creating a framework for care based on the International Classification of Functioning, Disability and Health. *Dev Med Child Neurol.* 2016;58(11):1116–1123

4. Groce N, Challenger E, Berman-Bieler R, et al. Malnutrition and disability: unexplored opportunities for collaboration. *Paediatr Int Child Health.* 2014;34(4): 308–314

VI

5.   Secker DJ, Jeejeebhoy KN. How to perform subjective global nutritional assessment in children. *J Acad Nutr Diet.* 2012;112(3):424–431

6.   Ptomey LT, Wittenbrook W. Position of the Academy of Nutrition and Dietetics: Nutrition services for individuals with intellectual and developmental disabilities and special health care needs. *J Acad Nutr Diet.* 2015;115(4):593–608

7.   Centers for Disease Control and Prevention, Division of Nutrition, Physical Activity, and Obesity. Growth Chart Training: Using the WHO Growth Charts. Available at: https://www.cdc.gov/nccdphp/dnpao/growthcharts/who/recommendations/development.htm. Accessed March 14, 2019

8.   Wittenbrook W. Nutritional assessment and intervention in cerebral palsy. *Pract Gastroenterol.* 2011;92:16–32

9.   Davidson ZE, Ryan MM, Kornberg AJ, et al. Observations of body mass index in Duchenne muscular dystrophy: a longitudinal study. *Eur J Clin Nutr.* 2014;68(8): 892–897

10. Zemel BS, Pipan M, Stallings VA, et al. Growth charts for children with Down syndrome in the United States. *Pediatrics.* 2015;136(5):e1204–e1211

11. Finbråten AK, Martins C, Andersen GL, et al. Assessment of body composition in children with cerebral palsy: a cross-sectional study in Norway. *Dev Med Child Neurol.* 2015;57(9):858–864

12. Frisancho AR. *Anthropometric Standards: An Interactive Nutritional Reference of Body Size and Body Composition for Children and Adults* 2nd ed. Ann Arbor, MI: University of Michigan Press; 2008

13. Ishizaki M, Kedoin C, Ueyama H, Maeda Y, Yamashita S, Ando Y. Utility of skinfold thickness measurement in non-ambulatory patients with Duchenne muscular dystrophy. *Neuromusc Disord.* 2017;27(1):24–28

14. Wittenbrook W. Best practices in nutrition for children with myelomeningocele. *Infant Child Adolesc Nutr.* 2010;2(4):237–245

15. Davis J, Samuels E, Mullins L. Nutrition considerations in Duchenne muscular dystrophy. *Nutr Clin Pract.* 2015;30(4):511–521

16. Zhang Z, Shoff SM, Lai HJ. Comparing the use of CDC and WHO growth charts in children with cystic fibrosis through two years of age. *J Pediatr.* 2015;167(5): 1089–1095

17. Butler MG, Lee J, Manzardo AM, et al. Growth charts for non-growth hormone treated Prader-Willi syndrome. *Pediatrics.* 2015;135(1):e126–e135

18. Mueske NM. Fat distribution in children and adolescents with myelomeningocele. *Dev Med Child Neurol.* 2015;57(3):273–278

19. Khan MJ. Mechanisms of obesity in Prader–Willi syndrome. *Pediatr Obes.* 2016;13(1). Available at: https://www.researchgate.net/publication/310474357 . Accessed March 14, 2019

20. Schwarzenberg SJ, Kuo AA, Linton JM, Flanagan P, American Academy of Pediatrics, Council on Community Pediatrics. Promoting food security for all children. *Pediatrics.* 2015;136(5):e1431–e1438

21. Hager ER, Quigg AM, Black MM, et al. Development and validity of a 2-item screen to identify families at risk for food insecurity. *Pediatrics.* 2010;126(1): e6–e32

22. Arrowsmith FE. Nutritional rehabilitation increases the resting energy expenditure of malnourished children with severe cerebral palsy. *Dev Med Child Neurol.* 2012;54(2):170–175

23. Quitadamo P, Thapar N, Staiano A, Borrelli O. Gastrointestinal and nutritional problems in neurologically impaired children. *Eur J Paediatr Neurol.* 2016;20(6):810–815

24. Brooks GA, Butte NF, Rand WM, Flatt JP, Caballero B. Chronicle of the Institute of Medicine physical activity recommendation: how a physical activity recommendation came to be among dietary recommendations. *Am J Clin Nutr.* 2004;79(5):921S–930S

25. Vernon-Roberts A, Wells J, Grant H, et al. Gastrostomy feeding in cerebral palsy: enough and no more. *Dev Med Child Neurol.* 2010;52(12):1099–1105

26. Walker JL, Bell KL, Boyd RN, Davies PS. Energy requirements in preschool-age children with cerebral palsy. *Am J Clin Nutr.* 2012;96(6):1309–1315

27. Ohata K, Tsuboyama T, Haruta T, Ichihashi N, Nakamura T. Longitudinal change in muscle and fat thickness in children and adolescents with cerebral palsy. *Dev Med Child Neurol.* 2009;51(12):943–948

28. Norwood KW, Slayton R, American Academy of Pediatrics, Council on Children With Disabilities, Section on Oral Health. Oral health care for children with developmental disabilities. *Pediatrics.* 2013;131(3):614–619

29. Cohen M, Lahat E, Bistritzer T, Livne A, Heyman E, Rachmiel M. Evidence-based review of bone strength in children and youth with cerebral palsy. *J Child Neurol.* 2009;24(8):959–967

30. Kecskemethy HH, Harcke HT. Assessment of bone health in children with disabilities. *J Pediatr Rehabil Med.* 2014;7(2):111–124

31. Jefferson A, Leonard H, Siafarikas A, et al. Clinical guidelines for management of bone health in Rett syndrome based on expert consensus and available evidence. *PLoS One.* 2016;11(2):e0146824

32. Golden NH, Abrams SA, American Academy of Pediatrics, Committee on Nutrition. Optimizing bone health in children and adolescents. *Pediatrics.* 2014;134(4):e1229–e1243

33. Satter E. Eating Competence: Definition and Evidence for the Satter Eating Competence Model. *J Nutr Educ Behav.* 2007;39(5 Suppl):S142–S153

34. Adams RA, Elias E. Nonoral feeding for children and youth with developmental or acquired disabilities. *Pediatrics.* 2014;134(6):e1745–e1762

35. Sisnghai S, Baker SS, Bojczuk GA, Baker RD. Tube feeding in children. *Pediatr Rev.* 2017;38(1):23–33

36. Braegger C, Decsi T, Dias JA, et al. Practical approach to paediatric enteral nutrition: a comment by the ESPGHAN committee on nutrition. *J Pediatr Gastroenterol Nutr.* 2010;51(1):110–122

37. Edwards S, Davis AM, Bruce A, et al. Caring for tube-fed children: a review of management, tube weaning, and emotional considerations. *J Parenter Enteral Nutr.* 2016;40(5):616–622

38. Bobo E. Reemergence of blenderized tube feedings: exploring the evidence. *Nutr Clin Pract.* 2016;31(6):730–735

39. Coad J, Toft A, Lapwood S, et al. Blended foods for tube-fed children: a safe and realistic option? A rapid review of the evidence. *Arch Dis Child.* 2016;102(3): 274–278

40. Epp L, Lammert L, Vallumsetla N, Hurt RT, Mundi MS. Use of blenderized tube feeding in adult and pediatric home enteral nutrition patients. *Nutr Clin Pract.* 2017;32(2):201–205

41. Martin K, Gardner G. Home enteral nutrition: updates, trends, and challenges. *Nutr Clin Pract.* 2017;32(6):712–721

42. Cermak SA, Curtin C, Bandini LG. Food selectivity and sensory sensitivity in children with autism spectrum disorders. *J Am Diet Assoc.* 2010;110(2):238–246

43. Johnson CR, Turner K, Stewart PA, et al. Relationships between feeding problems, behavioral characteristics and nutritional quality in children with ASD. *J Autism Dev Disord.* 2014;44(9):2175–2184

44. Elder JH. The gluten-free, casein-free diet in autism: an overview with clinical implications. *Nutr Clin Pract.* 2008;23(6):583–588

45. Strand KM, Dahlseng MO, Lydersen S, et al. Growth during infancy and early childhood in children with cerebral palsy: a population-based study. *Dev Med Child Neurol.* 2016;58(9):924–930

46. Brooks J, Day S, Shavelle R, Strauss D. Low weight, morbidity, and mortality in children with cerebral palsy: new clinical growth charts. *Pediatrics.* 2011;128(2): e299–e307

47. Schwarzenberg SJ, Hempstead SE, McDonald CM, et al. Enteral tube feeding for individuals with cystic fibrosis: Cystic Fibrosis Foundation evidence-informed guidelines. *J Cystic Fibrosis.* 2016;15(6):724–735

48. Adams RC, Levy SE, American Academy of Pediatrics, Council on Children With Disabilities. Shared decision-making and children with disabilities: pathways to consensus. *Pediatrics.* 2017;139(6):e20170956

49. Fuglestad AJ, Boys CJ, Chang PN, et al. Overweight and obesity among children and adolescents with fetal alcohol spectrum disorders. *Alcohol Clin Exp Res.* 2014;38(9):2502–2508

50. Young JK, Giesbrecht HE, Eskin MN, Aliani M, Suh M. Nutrition implications for fetal alcohol spectrum disorder. *Adv Nutr.* 2014;5(6):675–692

51. Magenis ML, Machado AG, Bongiolo AM, Silva MAD, Castro K, Perry IDS. Dietary practices of children and adolescents with Down syndrome. *J Intellect Disabil.* 2018;22(2):125–134

52. Bull MJ, American Academy of Pediatrics, Committee on Genetics. Health supervision for children with Down syndrome. *Pediatrics.* 2011;128(2):393–406

53. Ramelli GP, Aloysius A, King C, Davis T, Muntoni F. Gastrostomy placement in paediatric patients with neuromuscular disorders: indications and outcome. *Dev Med Child Neurol.* 2007;49(5):367–371

54. May Y, Wu T, Liu Y, et al. Nutritional and metabolic findings in patients with Prader-Willi syndrome diagnosed in early infancy. *J Pediatr Endocrinol Metab.* 2012;25(11-12):1103–1109

55. Leonard H, Ravikumara M, Baikie G, et al. Assessment and management of nutrition and growth in Rett syndrome. *J Pediatr Gastroenterol Nutr.* 2013;57(4): 451–460

56. Motil KJ, Barrish JO, Lane J, et al. Vitamin D deficiency is prevalent in females with Rett syndrome. *J Pediatr Gastroenterol Nutr.* 2011;53(5):569

57. Motil KJ, Ellis KJ, Barrish JO, Caeg E, Glaze DG. Bone mineral content and bone mineral density are lower in older than in younger females with Rett syndrome. *Pediatr Res.* 2008;64(4):435–439

58. Platte P, Jaschke H, Herbert C, Korenke GC. Increased resting metabolic rate in girls with Rett syndrome compared to girls with developmental disabilities. *Neuropediatrics.* 2011;42(5):179–182

VI

Chapter 37

Nutrition of Children Who Are Critically Ill

Introduction

Provision of optimal nutrition therapy is an important aspect of care for critically ill infants and children. The goal of nutrition therapy is to meet energy, macronutrient, and micronutrient requirements and to preserve lean body mass during the catabolic phase of the stress response to illness. The stress of a variety of critical illnesses, such as trauma, sepsis, surgery, or burns, places variable metabolic demands on the patient. Accurate estimation and bedside delivery of nutrient needs is often challenging in the pediatric intensive care unit (PICU) environment. Failure to accurately estimate and meet these demands can result in nutritional deterioration during illness.[1] A proportion of critically ill children have a high incidence of malnutrition on admission to the PICU and low metabolic reserves. Unintended underfeeding for prolonged periods, resulting in cumulative nutrient deficits, might be associated with poor outcomes. On the other hand, hypometabolism, with low resting energy expenditure, has been demonstrated in critically ill patients with a variety of illnesses. The use of inaccurate resting energy expenditure (REE) estimating equations in this setting could result in unintended cumulative overfeeding. Both underfeeding and overfeeding have been documented with deleterious consequences.[2,3] Designing optimal nutritional strategies for critically ill children requires a sound understanding of the metabolic response to critical illness, an awareness of the challenges of bedside nutrient provision, and the associations between nutrient delivery and outcomes. The impact of nutrition therapy on outcomes may be most relevant in patients with underlying nutritional deficiencies.

Malnutrition and Metabolic Reserves

Assessment of nutritional status of PICU patients can be difficult.[4] The routine weighing and measuring of height (and then calculating body mass index) of critically ill children may be inaccurate because of edema resulting from fluid shifts and capillary leak that are inherent to the acute phases of many illnesses. Standard biochemical measures of visceral protein and micronutrient concentrations are also altered during critical illness. Hence, the true incidence of malnutrition in the PICU may be unknown, although reports suggest that more than 25% of children in the PICU are already malnourished at the time of admission.[5,6] Critical illness imposes the risk of further nutritional deterioration, with failure to estimate accurate energy expenditure and to deliver adequate substrate.[6] Following initial resuscitation and stabilization, basic anthropometry may highlight malnourished patients that are at a higher risk of adverse outcomes.[5,7]

The body composition of healthy infants and children differs from that of adults, with limited stores of protein and lipids available during periods of stress.[8,9] The breakdown of protein is a principle feature of the metabolic stress response, providing free amino acids for anti-inflammatory and tissue healing pathways. This adaptive response, while sustaining an individual during acute stress, may cause significant lean body mass depletion during prolonged or chronic stress responses. Thus, infants and children are particularly at risk for the deleterious effects of protein imbalance from protracted catabolic stress. Providing optimal macronutrients to decrease protein turnover is a very important part of caring for the critically ill child.

Protein Metabolism

Critical illness is characterized by high protein turnover, with continuous protein degradation and decreased synthesis.[10] This adaptive response allows a large amount of amino acids to be available in the free amino acid pool. Free amino acids are redistributed away from skeletal muscle for tissue repair, wound healing, and participation in inflammatory response pathways. In addition, the carbon skeleton is conscripted via the gluconeogenetic pathway to provide glucose for various organs. Protein turnover is increased in the acute phase of critical illness, and its contribution to the amino acid pool far outweighs that of dietary protein intake. The reprioritization of amino acids is manifested by a marked increase in the circulation of acute-phase proteins (such as C-reactive protein, fibrinogen, alpha-1-antitrypsin, haptoglobin) and decrease in liver-derived visceral proteins (such as albumin and retinol-binding protein). Overall, protein breakdown during critical illness exceeds protein synthesis and sets the stage for a negative protein (nitrogen) balance. Unlike in starvation, the provision of dietary glucose during critical illness does not suppress the protein breakdown, nor does it decrease endogenous gluconeogenesis, often resulting in hyperglycemia. A protracted response with ongoing protein turnover that is not matched by concomitant adequate protein intake, may result in a steady loss of lean body mass.[11] The likelihood of morbidity increases as muscle loss is not restricted to skeletal muscle but may involve cardiac and diaphragmatic muscles with resultant cardiopulmonary insufficiency. Optimal protein intake might help restore protein balance by enhancing protein synthesis, although it has no effect on protein degradation. Provision of optimal protein intake during critical illness is an important aspect of nutrition therapy in this population. The effect of specific amino acid solutions on outcomes in critically ill children remains investigational at this time.[12] In addition, the role of hormonal and other interventions to reduce the severity of protein degradation during critical illness has not been adequately studied in the general PICU population.[13]

Carbohydrate and Lipid Metabolism

Once protein needs have been determined, the next step in devising the nutrition support plan involves a rational partitioning of carbohydrate and lipids as energy sources. The metabolism of carbohydrates during critical illness is characterized by the increase in glucose production as described previously. Gluconeogenesis ensures that there is an energy source for glucose-dependent organs, such as brain, erythrocytes, and renal medulla. The provision of glucose in the diet does not stop gluconeogenesis, and the concomitant decrease in glucose utilization from insulin insensitivity during critical illness results in hyperglycemia.[14] An association between high serum glucose concentrations and poor outcomes during critical illness has been reported.[15] However, the role of the tight glycemic control (TGC) strategy, aimed at using insulin to prevent hyperglycemia in critically ill children, has not been proven to improve outcomes in large, well-controlled multicenter trials.[16–18] Furthermore, TGC in children may increase the risk of hypoglycemia, which remains the principal hurdle to insulin therapy for TGC.[19] A prudent glycemic control, using a range of acceptable glucose values, is generally practiced at individual centers, although the triggers for insulin use in the PICU remain variable.

The incidence of overfeeding during critical illness might be under-recognized in some critically ill children.[2,20] Inaccurate estimation of the true energy needs, overestimation of the energy demands of the metabolic stress response, and failure to regularly follow weight all contribute to unintended overfeeding in this population. Overfeeding, especially with a predominantly carbohydrate-based diet, results in the excess glucose being synthesized to fat and presents an additional carbon dioxide burden to the individual.[21,22] In critically ill children with respiratory insufficiency, this might increase or prolong the needs for mechanical ventilation. Respiratory quotient, defined as the ratio of carbon dioxide production to oxygen consumption, can be measured by indirect calorimetry and is much higher in cases in which excess glucose is provided with concomitant fat synthesis. On the other hand, excess dietary lipids are stored as triglycerides and do not increase the carbon dioxide burden. Thus, a mixed-fuel system, in which lipids account for 30% to 40% of total energy needs, is commonly employed in the PICU.

Energy Requirement During Critical Illness

Energy needs during critical illness are often related to the nature and severity of the illness. A variety of equations are used to estimate basal energy requirements and prescribe the daily energy allotment for children in the PICU population.[23,24] These equations, based on age, gender, and weight, are derived from healthy population data. Hence, estimates of energy expenditure from these equations are frequently inaccurate in the PICU population.[25] In addition, a variety of stress factors contribute to the equation for the estimated energy requirement, to account for the perceived energy cost of certain conditions, such as fever. Unfortunately, the actual delivery of energy at the bedside may fall far short **or exceed** the prescribed amount. Failure to deliver the prescribed energy over a period results in cumulative energy imbalance with anthropometric deteriorations that eventually result in poor outcomes.[11,26,27]

For some time, the metabolic stress response to critical illness has been associated with a significant energy burden to the patient.[28] Indeed, patients with burn injury exhibit a hypermetabolic response, with energy expenditure that is elevated for several weeks after the initial insult.[29] Underfeeding during this hypermetabolic phase results in nutritional deterioration—in particular, loss of lean body mass—when protein intake is also limited.

In contrast, a variety of factors in critically ill children might decrease total energy expenditure. Lack of physical activity, temperature management in modern PICUs, modern anesthesia and pain-management strategies, and ventilatory support all contribute to the reduction in overall energy expenditure during critical illness. In recent years, newborn infants undergoing uncomplicated major surgery have only a transient 20% increase in energy expenditure that returns to baseline levels within 12 hours.[30] Newborn infants extubated after surgery for closure of large ventricular septal defects or soon after ligation of patent ductus arteriosus have resting energy expenditures that are lower than expected and almost resemble those of healthy infants at baseline.[31,32] Using a stable isotopic technique, the mean energy expenditures of critically ill neonates receiving extracorporeal membrane oxygenation (ECMO) support were similar to age- and diet-matched nonstressed controls.[33] Thus, the muted or transient increase in energy expenditure following a variety of stresses may result in an overestimation of the energy cost using the equations for estimating energy requirements in the critically ill population. As a result, unintended overfeeding is likely prevalent in the PICU and, like underfeeding, poses significant risks.[2,20] If overfeeding is sustained, especially in patients receiving parenteral nutrition with a high percentage of calories from carbohydrates, there is a significant carbon dioxide load on the patient. In children with chronic respiratory insufficiency, this could result in poorer outcomes, including prolonged ventilator dependence and PICU length of stay. Other deleterious effects of overfeeding include increased triglyceride concentrations, hyperglycemia, and hepatotoxicity.

Indirect calorimetry (IC) allows accurate assessment of REE and may be feasible in some centers and select populations.[34,35] The device has been available and utilized for decades and has helped improve understanding of the metabolic state and energy requirements of critically ill children. In centers where IC is not available, cautious use of standard equations to estimate REE must be accompanied by vigilance for unintended cumulative imbalances between required and delivered energy.[25]

Micronutrients

There has been an emphasis on testing the benefits of select micronutrients with antioxidant properties during adult and pediatric critical illness.[36–38] To maintain homeostasis, a complex system of selected enzymes, cofactors (selenium, zinc, iron, and manganese), sulfhydryl group donors (glutathione), and vitamins (E and C) form a defense system that counters the oxidant stress seen in the acute phase of injury or illness. Critically ill patients may have deficiencies of micronutrients in the early phase of illness, as vitamins and trace elements are redistributed from the central circulation to tissues, and fluid losses from wounds, exudates, and third spacing might disturb micronutrient balance.[39] The stores of enzyme cofactors, vitamins, and trace elements decrease rapidly after injury and may remain at subnormal levels for weeks. There is an association between low endogenous antioxidant stores and an increase in free radical generation, augmented systemic inflammatory response, cell injury, and increased morbidity and mortality in critically ill people.[40] There has been increased interest in the role of vitamin D as an antioxidant. Serum concentrations of vitamin D in children with severe burns may be decreased for months after burn injury.[41] The significance of the association of low serum vitamin D concentrations with outcomes, as well as the role of vitamin D supplementation during critical illness, remain to be determined.

The concept of early micronutrient supplementation to prevent the development of acute deficiency, to rectify the oxidant-antioxidant balance, and to reduce oxidative-mediated injuries to organs has been investigated in trials in critically ill adults.[37]

Immunonutrition

In 1997, Bone and colleagues discussed the importance of a fine balance between the inflammatory and compensatory anti-inflammatory responses in an individual challenged with an injury or infection.[42] This highly coordinated biphasic inflammatory response is aimed at mounting an effective defense while keeping the proinflammatory response under control. Hence, it is thought that immunomodulation might play a significant role in the response to an infectious insult and affect outcomes in critically ill children. Immune-enhancing diets (IEDs) have been available for many years. An increasing number of studies in adult patients have examined the effect of IEDs in variety of illnesses, for their role in affecting outcomes. However, adult studies have provided conflicting results because of deficiencies in study design and the heterogeneity of IED formulations used in heterogeneous patient populations.[43] The commercially available diets for adults vary greatly, and the role of individual compounds is impossible to interpret. The immunomodulating effects of individual compounds are dose dependent, and mixtures of different immunomodulating nutrients are likely to have synergistic as well as antagonistic effects. Although no conclusive data on the beneficial effects of IEDs have been established, glutamine, antioxidants, and fish oils were among the nutrients with the promise of beneficial effects in selected patient groups. However, in a recent large multicenter 2-by-2 factorial trial of mechanically ventilated adults with multiple organ failure, a significant increase in hospital and 6-month mortality and a trend toward increased 28-day mortality were seen in the group receiving glutamine.[37] In another trial, no infectious benefits and higher 6-month mortality was recorded in medical patients randomized to receive a formula containing glutamine, omega-3 fatty acids, and antioxidants.[44]

In a comparative effectiveness trial, mechanically ventilated children receiving enteral nutrition were randomly assigned to receive enteral supplementation of a combination of glutamine, zinc, selenium, and metoclopramide, or whey protein. After enrollment of 293 patients, no differences were recorded in PICU length of stay, duration of mechanical ventilation, infections, or mortality between the 2 groups. The study was terminated, but in a subgroup of immunocompromised children, significant reduction in health care-associated infections was noted in the intervention group.[36]

Nutrient Delivery in the PICU: Challenges

The enteral route of feeding is preferred in children with a functioning gastrointestinal tract. The benefits of enteral nutrition include preservation of intestinal mucosal integrity, enhanced mucosal immunity, and reduction in parenteral nutrition use with its associated complications and risk of infections (see Chapter 23: Enteral Nutrition). Patients deprived of enteral nutrients rapidly develop adverse intestinal mucosal changes, including reduced crypt depth and villus height.[45] Overall, enteral nutrition is relatively more physiologic, safer, and more cost-effective compared with parenteral nutrition. However, establishing and maintaining enteral nutrition intake in critically ill children often conflicts with therapeutic and diagnostic interventions in the PICU and is challenging.[46,47] A variety of barriers impede the optimal delivery for enteral nutrition at the bedside in critically ill children. As a result, a large number of patients in the PICU experience interruptions to or delays in initiating enteral nutrition. A majority of these events are related to conflicts with other procedures that require fasting, intolerance of enteral nutrition, or perceived contraindications to enteral nutrition. Prospective audits of nutritional practices suggest that many opportunities to initiate and sustain enteral nutrition are frequently overlooked in the PICU population because of lack of a uniform feeding strategy or myths regarding the safety of enteral nutrition in specific scenarios. Furthermore, some patients do not tolerate enteral nutrition or are at risk of mucosal ischemia or pulmonary aspiration after enteral feeding. The benefits of enteral nutrition must be balanced against the risks in these children. Stepwise algorithms have been shown to facilitate safe delivery of enteral nutrition in the intensive care unit.[48]

Parenteral nutrition has been used to achieve nutritional goals as a supplement to enteral nutrition in children who do not tolerate full enteral

VI

nutrition (see Chapter 22: Parenteral Nutrition). The optimal timing of parenteral nutrition in critically ill children has been recently investigated. In a large controlled trial, critically ill patients in the PICU were randomly assigned to receive early (on day 1 after PICU admission) versus delayed (on day 8 after PICU admission) parenteral nutrition. Clinical outcomes were significantly better in the group receiving delayed parenteral nutrition[49]; similar results have been demonstrated in adult critically ill patients.[50] Therefore, the role of an aggressive, early supplemental parenteral nutrition strategy (within 24 hours of admission) among critically ill children has been questioned. These results have also reemphasized the importance of the enteral route, when feasible, to meet the nutrient needs during acute critical illness.

Summary

Nutrition therapy is an important aspect of critical care. Critically ill children are at risk of nutritional deterioration during acute illness, and careful attention to their metabolic state will allow prescription of optimal macronutrients and micronutrients during their PICU stay. The advantages of enteral nutrition are well documented. Awareness of the many challenges to nutrient delivery in the PICU will allow nutrition goals to be achieved and may improve clinical outcomes in this population. Nutrition therapy in the PICU must be recognized as a clinical and research priority. Because of the heterogeneity of patients in the PICU, an individualized approach to optimal timing, route, and amount of nutrient delivery may be beneficial during critical illness.

References

1.   Hulst J, Joosten K, Zimmermann L, et al. Malnutrition in critically ill children: from admission to 6 months after discharge. *Clin Nutr.* 2004;23(2):223–232

2.   Mehta NM, Bechard LJ, Dolan M, Ariagno K, Jiang H, Duggan C. Energy imbalance and the risk of overfeeding in critically ill children. *Pediatr Crit Care Med.* 2011;12(4):398–405

3.   Mehta NM, Bechard LJ, Leavitt K, Duggan C. Severe weight loss and hypermetabolic paroxysmal dysautonomia following hypoxic ischemic brain injury: the role of indirect calorimetry in the intensive care unit. *JPEN J Parenter Enteral Nutr.* 2008;32(3):281–284

4.   Leite HP, Isatugo MK, Sawaki L, Fisberg M. Anthropometric nutritional assessment of critically ill hospitalized children. *Rev Paul Med.* 1993;111(1):309–313

5. Bechard LJ, Duggan C, Touger-Decker R, et al. Nutritional status based on body mass index is associated with morbidity and mortality in mechanically ventilated critically ill children in the PICU. *Crit Care Med*. 2016;44(8):1530–1537

6. Mehta NM, Duggan CP. Nutritional deficiencies during critical illness. *Pediatr Clin North Am*. 2009;56(5):1143–1160

7. Grippa RB, Silva PS, Barbosa E, Bresolin NL, Mehta NM, Moreno YM. Nutritional status as a predictor of duration of mechanical ventilation in critically ill children. *Nutrition*. 2017;33:91–95

8. Duffy B, Pencharz P. The effects of surgery on the nitrogen metabolism of parenterally fed human neonates. *Pediatr Res*. 1986;20(1):32–35

9. Fomon SJ, Haschke F, Ziegler EE, Nelson SE. Body composition of reference children from birth to age 10 years. *Am J Clin Nutr*. 1982;35(5 Suppl):1169–1175

10. Fullerton BS, Sparks EA, Khan FA, et al. Whole body protein turnover and net protein balance after pediatric thoracic surgery: a noninvasive single-dose 15N glycine stable isotope protocol with end-product enrichment. *JPEN J Parenter Enteral Nutr*. 2018;42(2):361–370

11. Hulst JM, Joosten KF, Tibboel D, van Goudoever JB. Causes and consequences of inadequate substrate supply to pediatric ICU patients. *Curr Opin Clin Nutr Metab Care*. 2006;9(3):297–303

12. Hauschild DB, Ventura JC, Mehta NM, Moreno YMF. Impact of the structure and dose of protein intake on clinical and metabolic outcomes in critically ill children: a systematic review. *Nutrition*. 2017;41:97–106

13. Herndon DN, Hart DW, Wolf SE, Chinkes DL, Wolfe RR. Reversal of catabolism by beta-blockade after severe burns. *N Engl J Med*. 2001;345(17):1223–1229

14. Long CL, Kinney JM, Geiger JW. Nonsuppressability of gluconeogenesis by glucose in septic patients. *Metabolism*. 1976;25(2):193–201.

15. Branco RG, Garcia PC, Piva JP, Casartelli CH, Seibel V, Tasker RC. Glucose level and risk of mortality in pediatric septic shock. *Pediatr Crit Care Med*. 2005;6(4):470–472

16. Agus MS, Asaro LA, Steil GM, et al. Tight glycemic control after pediatric cardiac surgery in high-risk patient populations: a secondary analysis of the safe pediatric euglycemia after cardiac surgery trial. *Circulation*. 2014;129(22): 2297–2304

17. Agus MS, Hirshberg E, Srinivasan V, et al. Design and rationale of Heart and Lung Failure - Pediatric INsulin Titration Trial (HALF-PINT): a randomized clinical trial of tight glycemic control in hyperglycemic critically ill children. *Contemp Clin Trials*. 2017;53:178–187

18. Macrae D, Grieve R, Allen E, et al. A randomized trial of hyperglycemic control in pediatric intensive care. *N Engl J Med*. 2014;370(2):107–118

19. Selig PM, Popek V, Peebles KM. Minimizing hypoglycemia in the wake of a tight glycemic control protocol in hospitalized patients. *J Nurs Care Qual*. 2010;25(3):255–260.

VI

20. Chwals WJ. Overfeeding the critically ill child: fact or fantasy? *New Horiz.* 1994;2(2):147–155

21. Askanazi J, Rosenbaum SH, Hyman AI, Silverberg PA, Milic-Emili J, Kinney JM. Respiratory changes induced by the large glucose loads of total parenteral nutrition. *JAMA.* 1980;243(14):1444–1447

22. Alaedeen DI, Walsh MC, Chwals WJ. Total parenteral nutrition-associated hyperglycemia correlates with prolonged mechanical ventilation and hospital stay in septic infants. *J Pediatr Surg.* 2006;41(1):239–244

23. Human energy requirements: report of a joint FAO/ WHO/UNU Expert Consultation. *Food Nutr Bull.* 2005;26(1):166

24. Schofield WN. Predicting basal metabolic rate, new standards and review of previous work. *Hum Nutr Clin Nutr.* 1985;39(Suppl 1):5–41

25. Smallwood CD, Mehta NM. Estimating energy expenditure in critically ill children: still shooting in the dark? *J Pediatr.* 2017;184:10–12

26. Mehta NM, Bechard LJ, Cahill N, et al. Nutritional practices and their relationship to clinical outcomes in critically ill children—an international multicenter cohort study. *Crit Care Med.* 2012;40(7):2204–2211

27. Mehta NM, Bechard LJ, Zurakowski D, Duggan CP, Heyland DK. Adequate enteral protein intake is inversely associated with 60-d mortality in critically ill children: a multicenter, prospective, cohort study. *Am J Clin Nutr.* 2015;102(1):199–206

28. Cuthbertson D. Intensive-care-metabolic response to injury. *Br J Surg.* 1970;57(10):718–721

29. Suman OE, Mlcak RP, Chinkes DL, Herndon DN. Resting energy expenditure in severely burned children: analysis of agreement between indirect calorimetry and prediction equations using the Bland-Altman method. *Burns.* 2006;32(3):335–342

30. Jones MO, Pierro A, Hammond P, Lloyd DA. The metabolic response to operative stress in infants. *J Pediatr Surg.* 1993;28(10):1258–1262

31. Shew SB, Beckett PR, Keshen TH, Jahoor F, Jaksic T. Validation of a [13C] bicarbonate tracer technique to measure neonatal energy expenditure. *Pediatr Res.* 2000;47(6):787–791

32. Shew SB, Keshen TH, Glass NL, Jahoor F, Jaksic T. Ligation of a patent ductus arteriosus under fentanyl anesthesia improves protein metabolism in premature neonates. *J Pediatr Surg.* 2000;35(9):1277–1281

33. Shew SB, Keshen TH, Jahoor F, Jaksic T. The determinants of protein catabolism in neonates on extracorporeal membrane oxygenation. *J Pediatr Surg.* 1999;34(7):1086–1090

34. Mehta NM, Bechard LJ, Leavitt K, Duggan C. Cumulative energy imbalance in the pediatric intensive care unit: role of targeted indirect calorimetry. *JPEN J Parenter Enteral Nutr.* 2009;33(3):336–344

35. Mehta NM, Smallwood CD, Graham RJ. Current applications of metabolic monitoring in the pediatric intensive care unit. *Nutr Clin Pract.* 2014;29(3): 338–347

36. Carcillo JA, Dean JM, Holubkov R, et al. The randomized comparative pediatric critical illness stress-induced immune suppression (CRISIS) prevention trial. *Pediatr Crit Care Med.* 2012;13(2):165–173

37. Heyland D, Muscedere J, Wischmeyer PE, et al. A randomized trial of glutamine and antioxidants in critically ill patients. *N Engl J Med.* 2013;368(16):1489–1497

38. Heyland DK, Dhaliwal R, Day AG, et al. REducing Deaths due to OXidative Stress (The REDOXS Study): rationale and study design for a randomized trial of glutamine and antioxidant supplementation in critically-ill patients. *Proc Nutr Soc.* 2006;65(3):250–263

39. Galloway P, McMillan DC, Sattar N. Effect of the inflammatory response on trace element and vitamin status. *Ann Clin Biochem.* 2000;37(Pt 3):289–297

40. Goode HF, Cowley HC, Walker BE, Howdle PD, Webster NR. Decreased antioxidant status and increased lipid peroxidation in patients with septic shock and secondary organ dysfunction. *Crit Care Med.* 1995;23(4):646–651

41. Gottschlich MM, Mayes T, Khoury J, Warden GD. Hypovitaminosis D in acutely injured pediatric burn patients. *J Am Diet Assoc.* 2004;104(6):931–941

42. Bone RC, Grodzin CJ, Balk RA. Sepsis: a new hypothesis for pathogenesis of the disease process. *Chest.* 1997;112(1):235–243

43. Heyland DK, Samis A. Does immunonutrition in patients with sepsis do more harm than good? *Intensive Care Med.* 2003;29(5):669–671

44. van Zanten AR, Sztark F, Kaisers UX, et al. High-protein enteral nutrition enriched with immune-modulating nutrients vs standard high-protein enteral nutrition and nosocomial infections in the ICU: a randomized clinical trial. *JAMA.* 2014;312(5):514–524

45. Hernandez G, Velasco N, Wainstein C, et al. Gut mucosal atrophy after a short enteral fasting period in critically ill patients. *J Crit Care.* 1999;14(2):73–77

46. Mehta NM, McAleer D, Hamilton S, et al. Challenges to optimal enteral nutrition in a multidisciplinary pediatric intensive care unit. *JPEN J Parenter Enteral Nutr.* 2010;34(1):38–45

47. Rogers EJ, Gilbertson HR, Heine RG, Henning R. Barriers to adequate nutrition in critically ill children. *Nutrition.* 2003;19(10):865–868

48. Hamilton S, McAleer DM, Ariagno K, et al. A stepwise enteral nutrition algorithm for critically ill children helps achieve nutrient delivery goals. *Pediatr Crit Care Med.* 2014;15(7):583–589

49. Fivez T, Kerklaan D, Mesotten D, et al. Early versus Late Parenteral Nutrition in Critically Ill Children. *N Engl J Med.* 2016;374(12):1111–1122

50. Casaer MP, Hermans G, Wilmer A, Van den Berghe G. Impact of early parenteral nutrition completing enteral nutrition in adult critically ill patients (EPaNIC trial): a study protocol and statistical analysis plan for a randomized controlled trial. *Trials.* 2011;12:21

VI

Chapter 38

Eating Disorders in Children and Adolescents

Introduction

Eating disorders are complex biopsychosocial disorders defined by behavioral, cognitive, emotional, and physical criteria. They usually have their onset during adolescence and are associated with significant medical and psychiatric morbidity. The estimated lifetime prevalence of an eating disorder is 5.7% for adolescent girls and 1.2% for adolescent boys.[1] The hallmarks of an eating disorder are severe disturbances in eating behavior and body image that are associated with psychological distress, functional impairment, and often, physical symptoms. Medical complications develop either as a result of adaptive responses to malnutrition or secondary to unhealthy weight control practices such as self-induced vomiting or the use of laxatives, diuretics, or diet pills.

The *Diagnostic and Statistical Manual of Mental Disorders, Fifth Edition (DSM-5)*[2] includes several changes from previous editions that improve the clinical utility of the diagnostic categories for feeding and eating disorders. The eating disorder diagnostic categories most frequently encountered clinically in children and adolescents include anorexia nervosa (AN), bulimia nervosa (BN), binge eating disorder (BED), avoidant restrictive food intake disorder (ARFID), and atypical anorexia nervosa. Although eating disorders most often occur in females, approximately 10% to 15% of patients with AN or BN are male, with a higher proportion of males in the younger age groups.[3-6] The prevalence of eating disorders may be increasing in male, minority, and younger populations.[7] Often, eating disorder symptoms first appear in childhood or early adolescence, and frank disorders typically have their onset in middle or late adolescence or early adulthood. Lifetime prevalence estimates of eating disorders in individuals of all ages range from approximately 1% for AN to 1% to 4% for BN[8,9]; one recent epidemiologic study of adolescents reported lifetime prevalence rates of 0.3% for AN, 0.9% for BN, and 1.6% for BED.[9] The reported prevalence rates may be underestimates, because eating disorders often go unrecognized, and individuals may be reluctant to acknowledge symptoms or seek treatment because of shame and fear of stigmatization. Early detection and intervention are critical and can lead to improved outcomes.[7]

Clinical research has focused on AN and BN, but children and adolescents, in particular, often do not meet full criteria for AN or BN, because they may present with failure to gain weight adequately rather than marked weight loss, or they may minimize or deny body image dissatisfaction or overvaluation of weight/shape. Because of the potential long-term effects of eating disorders on physical and emotional growth, clinicians should lower the threshold for intervention in children and adolescents. Early recognition is associated with improved prognosis,[10] so it is crucial that pediatricians identify these disorders as soon as possible.

The goals of this chapter are to provide clinicians working with children and adolescents with practical information regarding the assessment and treatment of eating disorders and, in particular, the assessment and treatment of the common problems that occur related to nutrition and health in these complex disorders.

Clinical Features

Anorexia Nervosa

Diagnostic Criteria

The key features of AN are persistent low body weight, marked fear of weight gain, and disturbance in the way that body image is experienced (eg, believing one is fat even though underweight). Peak age of diagnosis is 13 to 15 years, with a range of 10 to 25 years. In the *DSM-5*, the amenorrhea criterion was eliminated and the specific low weight cutoff for "low body weight" was removed but guidance provided that a body weight associated with a BMI for age less than the 5th percentile suggests a low body weight. When working with children and adolescents, clinicians should review growth charts to ascertain historical growth trajectory to determine whether weight and height have "fallen off" the expected curve for the individual patient.

Individuals with AN achieve low weight through dietary restriction and often engage in excessive physical activity and manifest strict food rules. Although all individuals with AN are restricting intake to below nutritional needs, a subset periodically engage in binge eating and/or purging. *DSM-5* specifies 2 subtypes of AN: restricting type and binge-eating/purging type (Table 38.1). Whereas individuals with the restricting type may appear constricted in affect and personality, those with the binge-eating/purging type may be more likely to have comorbid impulsivity, including substance use disorders, cluster B personality disorders, mood lability, and suicidality. Additionally, those with binge/purge type AN may develop more severe medical complications, such as electrolyte disturbances.

Table 38.1.

Diagnostic Criteria for Anorexia Nervosa

A. Restriction of energy intake relative to requirements, leading to a significantly low body weight in the context of age, sex, development trajectory, and physical health. Significantly low weight is defined as a weight that is less than minimally normal or, for children and adolescents, less than that minimally expected.

B. Intense fear of gaining weight or of becoming fat, or persistent behavior that interferes with weight gain, even though at a significantly low weight.

C. Disturbance in the way in which one's body weight or shape is experienced, undue influence of body weight or shape on self-evaluation, or persistent lack of recognition of the seriousness of the current low body weight.

Restricting type: During the last 3 months, the individual has not engaged in recurrent episodes of binge-eating or purging behavior (ie, self-induced vomiting or the misuse laxatives, diuretics, or enemas). This subtype describes presentations in which weight loss is accomplished primarily through dieting, fasting, and/or excessive exercise.

Binge-eating/purging type: During the last 3 months, the individual has engaged in recurrent episodes of binge-eating or purging behavior (ie, self-induced vomiting or the misuse of laxatives, diuretics, or enemas).

VI

Associated Signs and Medical Complications

Psychologically, individuals with AN often present with severe body image distortion; preoccupation with weight, shape, and eating; restricted or negative affect; and limited insight into the illness. They may be perfectionistic, obsessive, interpersonally insecure, and unsure of their own identity. Further, they often experience intrapersonal conflict around maturation, sexual development, separation, and individuation. Notably, AN has the highest mortality rate for any mental disorder; suicide and cardiac complications are the leading causes of death.

In individuals with AN, most systems are affected as weight loss becomes pronounced (Table 38.2). Physical signs include bradycardia, hypotension, orthostasis (defined as an increase in pulse rate by >20 beats on standing or a drop in systolic blood pressure by >20 mm Hg on standing), lanugo, alopecia, and edema. Those who self-induce vomiting may exhibit dental erosion, parotid hypertrophy, and calluses on the dorsum of the hand

Table 38.2.
Associated Signs and Medical Complications of Anorexia Nervosa

System	Features
Cardiac	Bradycardia, orthostatic hypotension, arrhythmia, mitral valve prolapse/murmur, decreased left ventricular forces, prolonged QT interval corrected for heart rate, increased vagal tone, pericardial effusion, congestive heart failure
Endocrine and metabolic	Amenorrhea, hypothyroidism, delayed puberty, arrested growth, hypothermia, reduced bone mineral density, sick euthyroid syndrome, electrolyte disturbances, decreased serum testosterone or estradiol, hypercholesterolemia, hypercortisolism
Skeletal	Low bone mineral density, fractures
Breasts	Breast atrophy
Dermatologic	Cheilosis, acrocyanosis, hypercarotenemia, alopecia, xerosis, acne, lanugo, pallor
Oral/dental	Enamel erosion and gum recession; swelling of the parotid gland; salivary gland hypertrophy; elevated serum amylase levels; halitosis
Gastrointestinal	Palpable stool secondary to constipation, rectal prolapse, scaphoid abdomen; esophagitis; chest pain, dyspepsia; gastroesophageal reflux disease; esophageal rupture; hiatal hernias; irritable bowel syndrome; melanosis coli; atonic or cathartic colon
Pulmonary	Pneumothorax or aspiration secondary to vomiting, pulmonary edema during refeeding
Neurologic and mental status	Neurocognitive deficit, diminished muscle strength, peripheral neuropathy, movement disorder
Hematologic	Anemia, leukopenia, thrombocytopenia
Renal	Increased blood urea nitrogen, calculi

(Russell sign). Laboratory findings could include electrolyte abnormalities, in particular hypokalemia, hypophosphatemia, hypomagnesemia, and hyponatremia. Gastrointestinal complications, such as constipation, delayed gastric motility, and delayed gastric emptying, are common. Elevated transaminases occur in approximately 40% of adolescents hospitalized with anorexia nervosa.[11] High concentrations of blood urea nitrogen may reflect renal abnormalities resulting from dehydration. Polyuria related to an abnormality in vasopressin secretion may also develop. Approximately 20% of patients experience peripheral edema, usually during refeeding. Mild anemia, leukopenia, and thrombocytopenia are often observed[12] but typically reverse with refeeding. Neurologic abnormalities may include reduced gray matter volumes and increased sulcal cerebrospinal fluid volumes that are partially reversible with recovery.

Electrocardiographic abnormalities (eg, low voltage, bradycardia, T-wave inversions, ST segment depression, and arrhythmias) are common and often normalize with refeeding. Some cardiac problems, including prolonged corrected QT intervals, myocardial damage, and arrhythmias secondary to electrolyte imbalances, may be fatal. Amenorrhea secondary to starvation-induced suppression of the hypothalamic-pituitary-gonadal axis, is common in adolescent girls with AN and may precede significant weight loss in up to 20% of patients.[13] Other endocrine complications include the "sick euthyroid" or "low T3 syndrome," relative growth hormone resistance with low insulin-like growth factor-1 levels,[14,15] and decreased serum leptin concentrations.[12] The likelihood of these complications increases in those who are more severely malnourished (as determined by absolute BMI or percent of median BMI). Although many medical complications resolve with weight restoration, deficits in bone mineral density (BMD) may persist,[16] leading to increased fracture risk.[17-20] Although estrogen deficiency is an important cause of low BMD, administration of estrogen as an oral estrogen-progesterone combination pill is not effective in increasing BMD in women or girls with AN.[21-23] In contrast, physiologic estrogen administration as replacement doses with transdermal estrogen or as small incremental doses of oral estrogen to mimic the early pubertal rise in estrogen does increase BMD in adolescent girls with AN when compared with placebo.[24] However, bone accrual rates remain lower than in normal-weight controls, likely because other hormonal deficits are not addressed by estrogen replacement alone in the absence of weight restoration.[24]

In low-weight female athletes, the constellation of low energy availability, with or without an eating disorder, hypothalamic amenorrhea, and low

BMD for age, has been termed the "female athlete triad."[25] Energy availability refers to dietary energy intake minus exercise energy expenditure. Energy availability is the amount of dietary energy remaining for other bodily functions. Some athletes resort to abnormal eating patterns, including dietary restriction, fasting, binge eating, and purging, or may use diet pills, laxatives, diuretics, or enemas and, thus, have low energy availability. The female athlete triad is more common in adolescent athletes who participate in sports in which leanness is emphasized.

Bulimia Nervosa

Diagnostic Criteria

In the *DSM-5*, BN is characterized by a regular pattern of binge eating and compensatory behaviors and an overvaluation of weight and shape (see Table 38.3). Binge eating and compensatory behaviors occur at a threshold frequency of once a week for at least 3 months. A binge episode is defined as the consumption of an objectively large amount of food accompanied by a subjective feeling of being out of control during the eating episode. Often, individuals with BN alternate between binge eating and strict dieting. Binge eating typically occurs alone, involves consumption of calorie-dense foods, and is associated with abdominal discomfort and feelings of guilt, disgust,

Table 38.3.
Diagnostic Criteria for Bulimia Nervosa

A. Recurrent episodes of binge eating. An episode of binge eating is characterized by both of the following:
   1. Eating, in a discrete period of time (eg, within any 2-hour period), an amount of food that is definitely larger than what most individuals would eat in a similar period of time under similar circumstances.
   2. A sense of lack of control over eating during the episode (eg, a feeling that one cannot stop eating or control what or how much one is eating).
B. Recurrent inappropriate compensatory behaviors in order to prevent weight gain, such as self-induced vomiting; misuse of laxatives, diuretics, or other medications; fasting; or excessive exercise.
C. The binge-eating and inappropriate compensatory behaviors both occur, on average, at least once a week for 3 months.
D. Self-evaluation is unduly influenced by body shape and weight.
E. The disturbance does not occur exclusively during episodes of anorexia nervosa.

Table 38.4.

Associated Signs and Medical Complications of Bulimia Nervosa

System	Features
Cardiovascular	Arrhythmia, mitral valve prolapse, murmur, cardiomyopathy
Musculoskeletal	Tetany, skeletal muscle myopathy
Gastrointestinal	Gastric dilation, abdominal fullness, esophagitis, gastroesophageal reflux disease or rupture, hiatal hernias, Barrett esophagus, irritable bowel syndrome, melanosis coli, atonic or cathartic colon
Oral/dental	Mouth sores, palatal scratches, dental caries, enamel erosion and gum recession, swelling of the parotid gland, submandibular adenopathy, elevated serum amylase levels
Skin	Periorbital petechiae, Russell sign (calluses over the knuckles due to induction of emesis, swelling of hands and feet, dryness, lack of hair sheen
Metabolic	Pitting edema, poor skin turgor, Chvostek signs, Trousseau sign, hypokalemia, metabolic acidosis or alkalosis secondary to purging by vomiting and/or use of diuretics and laxatives
Neurologic	Cognitive impairment, irritability

VI

and depression. Individuals with BN engage in compensatory behaviors, including purging (self-induced vomiting, laxative, diuretic, or enema abuse) and nonpurging behaviors (excessive exercise or fasting) in efforts to counteract the effects of the binge and prevent weight gain. Clinical features of BN are listed in Table 38.4.

Associated Signs and Medical Complications
Patients with BN may complain of bloating, weakness, fatigue, dyspepsia, chest pain, and dry mouth. Physical signs may include facial swelling, sialadenosis (parotid gland hypertrophy, bilateral and nontender) or excoriations on the dorsal aspect of the hand and fingers (Russell sign). Oral findings may include dental caries, absence of a gag reflex, petechiae of the posterior pharyngeal wall, and bleeding gums. Additional signs include peripheral edema, petechiae in the skin surrounding the eyes, subconjunctival hemorrhages (resulting from increased pressure from vomiting), or

angular cheilitis. Angular cheilitis may be secondary to vomiting or vitamin (often B complex) deficiencies.

Laboratory findings are not diagnostic but can be helpful in assessing medical complications. Depending on the method of purging, there can be alterations in serum electrolyte concentrations. Hypokalemia, hypochloremia, hypophosphatemia, hypomagnesemia, and hyponatremia (associated with excess water ingestion) are commonly seen. The serum pH can be increased from purging. There may be an elevated serum amylase. Because of electrolyte disturbances, purging may lead to weakness, tetany, and arrhythmias; diuretic overuse may cause Pseudo-Barter syndrome (hypokalemia secondary to diuretic or laxative misuse). Further complications include renal failure and electrolyte imbalances, leading to seizures. Albumin concentrations are typically normal in patients with eating disorders; if they are low, clinicians should investigate a comorbid or alternative diagnosis, such as inflammatory bowel disease.

Medical complications of BN are varied, often occult, and carry significant risk of morbidity and mortality. Gastrointestinal tract complications are often secondary to self-induced vomiting and include esophagitis, dyspepsia, gastroesophageal reflux disease, hiatal hernias, and gastric dilatation. In severe cases, self-induced vomiting may lead to Mallory-Weiss tears, aspiration pneumonia, esophageal or gastric rupture, or a pneumothorax. More commonly, delayed gastric emptying and elevated intestinal transit time lead to presenting complaints of bloating, postprandial fullness, and constipation.

It is very important to inquire about laxative abuse, because this leads to depletion of potassium bicarbonate and a resultant metabolic acidosis. Laxative and diuretic abuse or chronic dehydration may lead to renal stones. Laboratory abnormalities seen with laxative abuse include metabolic acidosis, hyperuricemia, elevated blood urea nitrogen concentration, hypocalcemia, and hypomagnesemia. Laxative abuse may lead to irritable bowel syndrome, melanosis coli, an atonic or cathartic colon, or rectal prolapse. Cessation of chronic laxative abuse may cause rapid increase in weight because of fluid retention and edema. Other times, cessation of laxative abuse leads to constipation and may be managed with increased fluid and fiber intake.

Patients with BN should undergo electrocardiography (ECG), and abnormal results should prompt consideration of hospitalization. Self-induced vomiting and laxative and diuretic abuse may lead to electrolyte and acid base disturbances, and resultant cardiac complications may ensue. Cardiac arrhythmias and prolonged QTc intervals can lead to sudden death in purging patients. T-wave changes may also be noted on ECG. Although no longer commercially available, ipecac abuse is associated with distinct, potentially life-threatening cardiac complications. Ipecac contains emetine, which can cause a skeletal muscle myopathy, diffuse myositis, and cardiomyopathy (which could lead to irreversible myocardial damage and cardiac failure). The development of pericardial pain, dyspnea, weakness, hypotension, or tachycardia or abnormalities detected on ECG may suggest ipecac ingestion and require urgent medical attention.

Many endocrine abnormalities are associated with BN. Thyroid function tests may show the sick euthyroid syndrome marked by low triiodothyronine (T_3), elevated reverse T_3, and low to normal thyroxine (T_4) and thyroid-stimulating hormone (TSH). Cortisol and growth hormone may be increased. Vasopressin depression often leads to polyuria. Patients may have irregular or absent menstruation; this may be seen in normal-weight or even overweight adolescents with BN.

Certain complaints suggest acute complications of BN. Volume depletion may lead to hypotension, dizziness, and syncope. In the case of severe abdominal pain, it is necessary to rule out gastric dilatation (perhaps requiring urgent medical intervention). Because ipecac use is associated with cardiomyopathy, any complaints of chest pain, dyspnea, hypotension, or tachycardia or abnormalities detected on ECG require urgent medical attention. In addition, hematemesis or rectal bleeding may require emergent care. Other clinical signs that suggest hospitalization may be necessary include serum potassium concentration less than 3.5 mmol/L, serum chloride concentration less than 88 mmol/L, hematemesis, cardiac arrhythmias (ie, prolonged QTc), or hypothermia. Hypokalemia must be carefully corrected in a hospital setting with careful observation for cardiac instability.

Binge Eating Disorder, Avoidant Restrictive Food Intake Disorder, and Atypical Anorexia Nervosa

BED describes those individuals who binge-eat but do not purge or compensate in any other way. Individuals with BED are usually overweight or obese. Avoidant restrictive food intake disorder (ARFID), a new diagnostic category in *DSM-5*, describes patients who avoid certain foods because of color, texture, or fear of choking or vomiting. There is no distortion in body image and no fear of gaining weight, but eating behaviors interfere with normal growth and development. Such patients account for approximately

12% to 14% of children and adolescents referred to specialized eating disorder programs.[10,26,27] ARFID is more common in males than either AN or BN.[10,26] Body weight is usually low. Atypical anorexia nervosa describes patients who have lost a large amount of weight, have the cognitions associated with classic AN, but are of normal weight. Such patients have severe body image dissatisfaction and share the same medical and psychological complications as those with AN. They are often missed by pediatricians, because weight loss in these patients is typically seen as beneficial and because of their normal appearance. However, they engage in unhealthy weight control practices that can lead to medical instability.[28-30] The proportion of such patients presenting to 1 tertiary care inpatient service increased fivefold over a period of 5 years.[29] The American Academy of Pediatrics recommends carefully monitoring weight loss and vital signs in an adolescent who is trying to lose weight. The pediatrician should inquire about the methods used to lose weight, and if an eating disorder is suspected, the patient should be referred for evaluation of a possible eating disorder.[31]

Etiology of AN and BN

The etiology of eating disorders is multifactorial and dependent on sociocultural, psychological, biological, and familial factors. Both AN and BN typically have onset during adolescence, although patients frequently have a history of body image concerns and disordered eating that precede the onset of the illness.

Sociocultural factors that may increase risk for eating disorders include the Western emphasis on a thin ideal for women and a muscular ideal for men. Dieting is a behavior that increases risk for eating disorders. Further, certain populations may be at heightened risk of eating disorders. For example, sports such as ballet, gymnastics, long-distance running, ice skating, and wrestling or activities such as modeling or acting all value a slender body shape and may promote thinness and weight loss. In addition, patients with diabetes mellitus represent an at-risk group; patients with type 1 (or insulin-dependent) diabetes mellitus must adhere to strict diet plans and may underdose insulin to cause intentional weight loss. Diabetic patients with eating disorders more frequently present with ketoacidosis and vascular complications associated with poor glycemic control. Gay males may also be at increased risk. Environmental factors, including transitions from middle school to high school, the experience of a loss, and physical or sexual abuse, may also precipitate maladaptive coping responses, including eating disorders.

Psychological characteristics such as personality or temperament as well as comorbid psychopathology may also play a role in the development of eating disorders. Perfectionism, low self-esteem, and difficulty in regulating affect or managing emotions are personality characteristics that may be present in individuals with eating disorders. Patients with BN frequently demonstrate other impulsive behaviors, such as substance abuse, promiscuity, and self-destructive/injurious behaviors that may require their own medical intervention and monitoring. Anxiety and mood disorders often co-occur with eating disorders; although anxiety disorders most often have onset before eating disorders, mood disorders may be more likely to develop at the same time as or following the eating disorder onset.

Research in the past decade has begun to explore the genetics and heritability of eating disorders. Family and twin studies demonstrate that the risk of AN and/or BN is significantly increased in first-degree relatives of those with eating disorders, with one study indicating the relative risk of eating disorders in female relatives to be 11.3.[32,33] Further, there is growing evidence that specific symptoms, such as binge eating and self-induced vomiting, may also be heritable. Biological factors, such as obesity, may increase vulnerability to eating disorders.[31] Neurobiological research has also demonstrated alterations in hormonal and neurohormonal systems among individuals with eating disorders. Impaired serotonergic regulation has been implicated in obesity and overeating; studies have shown patients with BN to have dysregulated serotonin function as well as lower cerebrospinal 5-HT1A levels. Ghrelin, a hormone that acts on the hypothalamus to stimulate appetite, has been shown to have an abnormal response to normal-sized meals in patients with BN.[34] Because patients with BN often have an abnormal satiety following normal-sized meals, ghrelin may play a role in the pathogenesis in the lack of satiety that characterizes a binge episode. Yet, the degree to which these neurochemical and hormonal alterations are premorbid risks rather than secondary effects of eating disorders is unclear.

Within a biopsychosocial model, the family environment may also reinforce socioculturally based thin ideal expectations. This influence may occur through modeling of healthful or unhealthful attitudes or behaviors or through direct encouragement of children or adolescents to adopt disordered eating patterns.

VI

Assessment

The medical provider plays an important role in the diagnosis and management of eating disorders in children and adolescents.[7,35] Given that eating disorders often involve private behaviors or secret thoughts that may not be apparent from the outside, a careful medical, nutritional, and psychological assessment is critical. It is often pediatricians who are on the front line of screening for eating disorders in children and adolescents. Although eating disorder symptoms may be distressing to patients and often leave them feeling ashamed, lonely, or remorseful, many are ambivalent about seeking treatment and may not readily disclose their symptoms. Further, children and adolescents with eating disorders deny or minimize symptoms, either unconsciously because of a distorted perception of their behavior/ attitudes or consciously to keep clinicians from recognizing the extent of their symptoms. A strong alliance with a trusted health care professional is crucial in the success of treating the ambivalent patient. Inquiring in a direct yet caring and nonjudgmental/non-shaming manner can help many patients who are unsure how to disclose their symptoms. Data have shown that patients are more likely disclose their symptoms to a professional when directly asked.[36] With adolescents, it is important for the clinician to meet with the adolescent alone as well as with his or her parents to obtain a more complete perspective on the referral; the family may cite concerns about the child's diet changes, eating alone, skipping meals, and mood changes.

Obtaining a weight history (highest, lowest, current, and desired weight) can shed light on body image concerns and weight fluctuations. Evaluation will include inquiry about the amount of time spent thinking about food, calories, and weight, as patients will often report that these topics consume their thoughts and may also interfere with their ability to attend to or enjoy other activities. A detailed 24-hour nutritional history is important to obtain to allow providers to estimate energy, macronutrient, and micronutrient intake. Are patients restricting or avoiding certain foods or food groups (eg, fats)? Direct assessment of pattern of eating and frequency of meals consumed provides information about whether some meals/snacks are more challenging than others and whether there may be large gaps between eating episodes. It is important to ascertain whether there are periods of time when the patient eats an unusually large amount of food in an uncontrolled way. If present, gather more details about the episodes (the length of time, feeling during episode, kinds of food eaten). Assessment should include inquiry about all compensatory behaviors, because each is associated with specific medical complications (eg, ipecac abuse and cardiomyopathy), and many patients engage in more than one compensatory behavior. Ask about vomiting, emetic drugs, laxatives, enemas, "recreational" drugs, insulin underdosing, exercise, and skipping meals. Inquiring about all compensatory measures (regardless of whether patient endorses this behavior) provides an opportunity for psychoeducation about the risks associated with each behavior (ie, after asking about ipecac use, explain risk of cardiac death). Further, it can be important to ask about unusual behaviors, such as hoarding food, chewing food and spitting it out, eating in secret, and limiting fluid consumption.

The initial laboratory evaluation should include a urinalysis, complete blood cell count with sedimentation rate, electrolytes (including sodium, potassium, chloride, phosphorus, magnesium, and calcium), amylase, thyroid-function studies, and a urine pregnancy test for females. If there are concerns about celiac disease, an immunoglobulin (Ig) A and serum anti-tissue transglutaminase determination are helpful. A baseline ECG is recommended. Amenorrhea can be further evaluated with determinations of follicle-stimulating hormone, luteinizing hormone, prolactin, and estradiol.

Differential Diagnosis
Assessment of eating disorders should include carefully ruling out underlying medical causes of changes in weight or eating behavior. Although medical disorders may co-occur with eating disorders, if the eating disorder symptoms are better accounted for by the medical condition, an eating disorder diagnosis may not be appropriate. One should consider gastrointestinal tract disorders (such as celiac disease, inflammatory bowel disease, achalasia, or ulcers) and endocrine disorders (such as diabetes mellitus, Addison disease, or pituitary or thyroid dysfunction) as well as pregnancy. The clinician should consider malignancies (eg, lymphoma, central nervous system tumor) or neurologic disorders (eg, Kluver-Bucy syndrome) that may impair appetite regulation. The differential diagnosis should also include depression, substance abuse, and the illicit use of diet pills. Further, conversion disorders, schizophrenia, and mood disorders are among the psychiatric disorders that may manifest weight loss and binge/purge behavior.

Psychiatric Comorbidity
Screening for co-occurring psychiatric disorders is important. Among individuals with eating disorders, lifetime prevalence estimates of affective disorders range from 50% to 80%, and those of anxiety disorders, including obsessive compulsive disorder, generalized anxiety disorder,

and social phobia, are also high, ranging from 30% to 65%.[37] Substance use disorders co-occur, particularly among individuals with bulimic symptoms, and alcohol use disorder is the strongest predictor of premature death in individuals with AN.[38] Further, screening for amphetamine misuse and other use of over-the-counter and prescribed drugs used for weight loss is indicated. Although the most commonly recognized abused substance in patients with BN is alcohol, many patients with eating disorders also use caffeine and tobacco to control appetite.[39,40] A toxicology screening is useful in assessment and ongoing monitoring for substance abuse. Personality disorders also frequently co-occur with eating disorders; avoidant or obsessive compulsive personality disorder may occur among those with AN, and borderline personality disorder has been associated with BN. Personality styles, irrespective of eating disorder diagnosis, including perfectionism, interpersonal avoidance/constriction/restraint, and affective/behavioral dysregulation, may also be important to assess, because they can be useful in informing treatment approach. For all patients with eating disorders, assessment of suicidal ideation, intent, and behavior is imperative.

Treatment

Eating disorders are complex illnesses that require multimodal treatments. They are best managed by a multidisciplinary team, with the medical provider an essential member.[41] In addition to medical management, a comprehensive team comprises psychiatric/psychological care and nutrition management. Depending on the severity of illness, care may be delivered with variable intensity, ranging from outpatient management to higher levels of care, including intensive outpatient (evening treatment programs), partial hospitalization, residential care, and inpatient treatment. Most patients can be treated as outpatients, but those with severe malnutrition, electrolyte disturbances, or vital sign instability may require medical hospitalization. Indications supporting hospitalization in an adolescent with an eating disorder are listed in Table 38.5.[35]

Psychiatric Treatment

Psychotherapy

Family-based treatment (FBT), also known as the Maudsley method because of its initial development at the Maudsley Hospital in London, is an outpatient treatment in which parents are recognized as key resources who are integral participants in the recovery process. The treatment takes an agnostic approach to the etiology of eating disorders and empowers parents

Table 38.5.

Indications Supporting Hospitalization in an Adolescent With an Eating Disorder

One or more of the following justify hospitalization:
1. ≤75% median BMI for age and sex
2. Dehydration
3. Electrolyte disturbance (hypokalemia, hyponatremia, hypophosphatemia)
4. EKG abnormalities (eg, prolonged QTc or severe bradycardia)
5. Physiological instability
   a. Severe bradycardia (heart rate <50 beats/minute daytime; <45 beats/minute at night)
   b. Hypotension (<90/45 mm Hg)
   c. Hypothermia (body temperature <96°F [35.6°C])
   d. Orthostatic increase in pulse (>20 beats per minute) or decrease in blood pressure (>20 mm Hg systolic or >10 mm Hg diastolic)
6. Arrested growth and development
7. Failure of outpatient treatment
8. Acute food refusal
9. Uncontrollable binging and purging
10. Acute medical complications of malnutrition (eg, syncope, seizures, cardiac failure, pancreatitis, etc)
11. Comorbid psychiatric or medical condition that prohibits or limits appropriate outpatient treatment (eg, severe depression, obsessive compulsive disorder, type 1 diabetes mellitus)

VI

to initially take more control over the child's eating to restore health; as eating disorder symptoms come under better control, the parents step back. Thus, treatment proceeds through 3 phases determined by the patient's progress, beginning with weight restoration/nutritional rehabilitation, which is managed by the parents, moving to careful return of food/eating control to the adolescent, and ending with focus on issues associated with healthy adolescent development. A number of studies have demonstrated the benefits of using FBT for adolescents with AN[42] and more recently for adolescents with BN[43]; preliminary work also suggests FBT may be useful in treating children, adolescents, and young adults with a wider range of eating disorders.[44]

Psychotherapy is an integral component of care for the child or adolescent with an eating disorder. Individual and/or family therapy or parent training can be used to support the medical and nutritional recommendations of the team, which can be challenging for the patient or family to enact. Therapy also helps the child or adolescent identify and address underlying or associated issues that may include separation-individuation, identity development, comorbidities (such as anxiety or depression), and perfectionism, for example. When individual psychotherapy is recommended for the adolescent, meetings with the patient's family must be part of the treatment as well. The goals of individual therapy will include improving nutritional health, modifying unhealthy eating attitudes and behaviors, improving self-esteem and quality of life, and treating coexisting conditions, such as depression and anxiety disorders.

Psychopharmacology
Limited data are available on the efficacy of psychiatric medications in adolescents with eating disorders. Among low-weight patients, the mainstay of treatment is nutritional rehabilitation and weight restoration; psychiatric medications have generally not been shown to improve eating disorder outcomes, and the efficacy of these medications is likely diminished as a result of malnutrition. They should not be the first line of treatment.[45] However, psychiatric medications are often used to treat comorbid conditions, such as depression and anxiety, and are frequently prescribed, even for underweight patients.[46] More recently, there is some evidence that atypical neuroleptics, such as olanzapine, may improve distorted body image and may assist with weight gain, although clinicians should be aware that many patients with AN will be resistant to taking a medication associated with weight gain[47]; in addition, atypical neuroleptics have been associated with long-term complications, including diabetes mellitus and dyslipidemia.

Better evidence exists for the use of psychopharmacologic interventions in adult BN. Serotonergic medications, such as selective serotonin reuptake inhibitors (SSRIs) and serotonin-norepinephrine reuptake inhibitors (SNRIs), and tricyclic antidepressants have been shown to decrease binge/purge behaviors.[48] Fluoxetine is the best-studied SSRI and the only medication approved by the Food and Drug Administration for the treatment of BN in adults.[49]

Nutrition Management
The nutritional management for AN begins with the focus on weight restoration; in BN, although weight restoration may be important as well, the treatment focus is on interrupting and arresting the binge/purge cycle by establishing a regular pattern of eating. The help of a licensed nutritionist with expertise in eating disorders is invaluable.

Determining Treatment Goal Weight

Nutritional management of an eating disorder begins with establishment of a treatment goal weight. However, in children and adolescents, because of ongoing growth and development, treatment goal weight should be reassessed every 3 to 6 months.[35] Height and weight should be measured and BMI calculated and plotted on the Centers for Disease Control and Prevention (CDC) growth charts (www.cdc.gov/growthcharts) (see Appendix Q). A 2-step process is recommended[35,41]:

   a. Determine the degree of malnutrition compared with the reference population by calculating the percent of median BMI (current BMI/50th percentile BMI for age and sex x 100)
   b. Determine a healthy weight range for that individual, taking into account previous height, weight, and BMI as well as pubertal stage and growth trajectory. The weight associated with median BMI can be calculated using the following formula:

Height (m²) × the 50th percentile body mass index (BMI) for age and gender

BMI information is available on the CDC Web site for girls (http://www.cdc.gov/growthcharts/data/set1clinical/cj41l024.pdf) and for boys (http://www.cdc.gov/growthcharts/data/set1clinical/cj41l023.pdf).

Treatment goal weight is not necessarily the same as the weight associated with median BMI. For example, for the adolescent who had always tracked at the 25th percentile BMI curve, it is possible that returning to the 25th percentile would be an appropriate and justifiable goal. In females, weight associated with resumption of menses is one biological indicator of a healthy weight for that individual. Resolution of the cognitive distortions and focus on body shape and weight is another important indicator of recovery.

Calculating Nutrition Requirements

Estimating caloric needs for eating disorders varies on the basis of physical state (eg, percent of median BMI), patient's recent energy intake, and risk of refeeding syndrome. Nutrition requirements will change throughout treatment and must be reevaluated frequently on the basis of rate of weight gain, laboratory levels, goal weight, and stage of treatment (inpatient versus outpatient). Overall, many factors such as age, weight, activity level, and overall state of illness can affect calorie needs for weight gain. Indirect calorimetry is the most accurate method to determine energy needs; however, cost and availability make its use difficult.[50] The constant change of metabolic rate during weight restoration in underweight patients would result in requiring indirect calorimetry more frequently than is feasible to maintain accuracy.

The patient should be followed carefully by a team for continued monitoring and reevaluation during both inpatient and outpatient treatment. If the patient has severe abnormalities on laboratory tests or is very low weight, an inpatient setting for refeeding is the safest option. A 24-hour dietary recall can provide an estimate of dietary intake, but it should be noted that patients with AN frequently overestimate intake in a dietary recall.[51]

For inpatients with AN, older regimens started patients on 1000 to 1200 kcal/day to prevent development of the refeeding syndrome. However, refeeding hypophosphatemia, the hallmark biochemical feature of the refeeding syndrome, is correlated with the degree of malnutrition rather than the rate of refeeding.[52-54] Current research supports a higher initial caloric prescription (1400 to 2000 kcal/day) with close medical monitoring. Such practices reduce hospital length of stay and increase the rate of weight gain without increasing rates of refeeding syndrome.[53,55-57] At the time of admission to the hospital, patients with AN are initially hypometabolic, but during inpatient nutritional rehabilitation, both basal and postprandial energy expenditure increase, contributing to greater energy needs.[58] Prescribed caloric intake should, therefore, be increased every 24 to 48 hours. A weight gain of 0.5 lb daily or 2 to 3 lb per week is appropriate.[50] The patient's rate of weight gain should be followed, and energy intake should be adjusted accordingly. In an inpatient setting, females often peak around 3000 to 3500 kcal/day, and males often peak around 4000 kcal/day.

For patients with AN being treated on an outpatient basis, initial caloric prescription should be 200 to 400 kcal above estimated intake, and energy intake is usually advanced at a slower pace. An increase of 500 kcal weekly is usually the maximum of what can be tolerated for energy intake advancement. A gain of 1 to 2 lb weekly is appropriate. Once children and adolescents achieve a healthy weight, an increased energy prescription may be needed to support future growth and development.[50]

It may be difficult to determine energy intake in patients with BN, given variability with binge/purge behaviors. Generally, 50% of kcal consumed in a binge/purge cycle should be added to total calorie count.[59] To determine energy intake for normal or overweight patients with BN, the resting energy expenditure equation (REE) covers basal needs and assumes sedentary activity levels and should prevent excessive weight gain in children.

REE (kcals):
Males 3–10 years of age: (22.7 x wt (kg)) + 495
Females 3–10 years of age: (22.5 x wt (kg)) + 499

Males 10–18 years of age: (17.5 x wt (kg)) + 651
Females 10–18 years of age (12.2 x wt (kg)) + 746

Weight loss calorie goals should be avoided regardless of overweight/ obesity until an eating pattern is stabilized, because caloric restriction may trigger binging.[60] Patients with BN or those with a history of BN may be hypometabolic, requiring less energy intake than typically estimated for a patient of similar weight and height.

Notably, patients with BN are most often treated on an outpatient basis; higher level of care may be recommended at times for interrupting the binge/purge cycle or managing medical complications of BN.

Meal Planning

Snacks and/or supplements are helpful to increase energy and protein intake while keeping meals manageable in size. Increasing calorie-dense foods as well as providing fluids with calories may be helpful to avoid excessive fullness after eating. In addition, low-lactose foods or providing lactase supplements may decrease abdominal discomfort from nutritionally mediated lactase deficiency. Frequently, behavioral interventions are necessary to facilitate patients meeting energy intake and weight goals.[7] An eating protocol that provides clear criteria for expected energy intake, weight gain, activity, and behavior and that outlines expectations for the patients, family members, and treatment providers is a valuable tool to help patients to meet goals. The exchange list created by the American Diabetes Association in collaboration with the Academy of Nutrition and Dietetics is a helpful tool to plan meals, but not all programs use the exchange system. The exchange system groups foods into starch, protein, fruit, vegetable, milk, and fat categories and within each category indicates specific portion sizes, which provide similar nutrition content (eg, 1 serving of starch can be fulfilled by 1 slice of bread or 1/3 cup of pasta) (https://www.nhlbi.nih.gov/health/ educational/lose_wt/eat/fd_exch.htm). Meals are planned by prescribing a number of exchanges from each food group. This decreases focus on calories and fat and increases emphasis on the inclusion of a variety of foods and food groups.[50] In some cases, allowing patients to make food choices can be empowering and help them to feel in control; yet for other patients, this level of control may feel overwhelming. Patients with AN may find food

VI

choices difficult despite the method of meal planning or the protocols, and there are no longitudinal outcome data to support one method of meal planning over another.[59] In families participating in FBT, the parents are responsible for making the meal choices. For normal-weight patients with BN, encouraging 3 meals and snacks daily promotes normal eating and helps the patient break the cycle of restriction and binge/purge behaviors.[61]

Nutrition Support

Oral feedings are the preferred method of restoring nutrition. The decision to start nutrition support should consider both the patient's immediate physical health and psychological health. The indications for tube feedings include refusing any oral intake, rapid weight loss despite improved oral intake, and inability to meet nutritional needs orally.[7] If enteral nutrition via tube feedings is necessary, starting at 25% of the estimated goal and increasing to the initial goal over 3 to 5 days is recommended by some.[62] Some patients may need to have both tube feedings and oral nutrition to achieve nutrition and weight gain goals. Bolus feedings or nocturnal feedings are useful to provide uneaten calories or supplement intake. However, continuous feedings are less likely to result in dumping syndrome or purging. If tube feedings are initiated, typically a polymeric isotonic, fiber-containing, enteral feeding will be sufficient. Formulas with high glucose content should be avoided. If absorption or digestion is impaired, an elemental or peptide-based formula may be indicated. Parenteral nutrition should be used rarely and with caution, because it leads to the continued loss of hunger cues and increases risk of refeeding syndrome.[60,62]

Refeeding Syndrome

When starved or severely malnourished patients begin nutrition repletion, they are at risk of refeeding syndrome, a potentially life-threatening constellation of clinical and metabolic changes that occur on nutritional rehabilitation. As the metabolism shifts from catabolism to anabolism, it may result in fluid and electrolyte shifts that can cause cardiac, pulmonary, neurologic, and hematologic complications, including sudden death.

As patients are refed, metabolic disturbances may occur, including hypophosphatemia, hypokalemia, and hypomagnesemia. Hypophosphatemia may result from the intracellular shift of serum phosphorus needed for the generation of adenosine triphosphate (ATP) in the cellular anabolic processes. Low serum concentrations of phosphorus are associated with cardiac and neuromuscular dysfunction as well as blood cell dysfunction. Hypokalemia and hypomagnesemia may increase risk of cardiac arrhythmias and gastrointestinal and neuromuscular complications. During refeeding, extracellular expansion is common, causing peripheral edema; in extreme cases, congestive heart failure may occur. In a recent systematic review of hospitalized adolescents with AN, the average incidence of hypophosphatemia was found to be 18%.[54] Hypophosphatemia is believed to be a biochemical hallmark of the refeeding syndrome and, contrary to earlier beliefs, has been correlated more with the degree of malnutrition than with the rate of refeeding.[52] Hypophosphatemia and other electrolyte disturbances can be carefully corrected in the inpatient setting in order to prevent the refeeding syndrome. Frequent physical examinations as well as determinations of serum phosphorus, magnesium, and potassium concentrations are needed. In addition, there should be careful monitoring of the patient's vital signs, daily weights, fluid intake, and urine output.

Macronutrients, Fiber, and Fluids

No optimal macronutrient intake regimen has been found to be more beneficial for patients with eating disorders; however, a standard recommendation of 25% to 30% fat, 15% to 20% protein, and 50% to 55% carbohydrate may be helpful to provide a balance of macronutrients.[50,59] In patients at risk of developing refeeding syndrome, a slightly higher intake of fat and protein calories may be somewhat protective, because carbohydrate metabolism drives refeeding syndrome. Initially, when prescribing a meal plan or tube feedings, 150 to 200 g/day of carbohydrate should not be exceeded, and the protein goal should be approximately 1.2 to 1.5 g/kg of ideal body weight to preserve lean body mass while feeding hypocalorically. Patient access to simple sugars and sodium should be limited to avoid the risk of refeeding syndrome. The patient's previous intake of fiber should guide how much fiber is prescribed. Excessive fiber may result in discomfort or gastrointestinal distress, and insufficient fiber may contribute to constipation. Adequate hydration should be provided as needed to prevent dehydration or fluid retention.

Micronutrients

Vitamin deficiencies are frequently seen in patients with AN and BN. Eating disorders usually begin during adolescence, the critical period for bone mineral accretion, and adolescents with eating disorders are at risk for both vitamin D deficiency and increased bone fragility. They should be screened for vitamin D deficiency by obtaining a serum 25 hydroxyvitamin D level.[63] Most studies show that approximately 30% of patients with AN who have not previously been supplemented with vitamin D have 25 hydroxyvitamin

VI

D levels below 20 ng/mL, indicating deficiency.[64-66] Such patients should be treated with 50 000 IU of vitamin D_2 or D_3 once a week for 6 to 8 weeks or 2000 IU of vitamin D_2 or D_3 daily for 6 to 8 weeks, followed by a maintenance dose of 600 to 1000 IU/day.[63] The 6- to 8-week course of high-dose vitamin D treatment is necessary to replete diminished vitamin D stores, but this high dose needs to be followed by the lower maintenance dose. Increased dietary intake of calcium and vitamin D-containing foods and beverages should be encouraged, but it is common practice to supplement the patient with a multivitamin and calcium supplement during treatment.[59] The current recommendation for adolescent females is 1300 mg/day of calcium and 600 IU/day of vitamin D.[63,67]

Longitudinal Outcome

The course and outcome of eating disorders is variable; adolescents with a shorter duration of illness have a more favorable outcome compared with adults or those with a longer duration of illness, underscoring the importance of early detection and intervention.

A recent meta-analysis of 36 quantitative studies of individuals with eating disorders found significantly elevated mortality rates,[68] and AN is associated with the highest risk of mortality among all psychiatric disorders.[69] Among adults with AN, longitudinal studies suggest the rate of mortality is 0.56% per year, which is more than 12 times higher than that for young women in the general population.[38,69] Further, the rate of suicide is also elevated, with 1 study demonstrating a 57-fold increase in death by suicide among adult women with AN.[38] Yet, the longitudinal course and prognosis is better for adolescents. One recent analysis of multiple outcome studies for adolescent-onset AN found that 57% recovered, 26% more had improved substantially, 17% went on to have a chronic course of AN, and 2% had died.[70]

Patients with BN generally have a more favorable course. Longitudinal research suggests that approximately 50% of adult women with BN achieve full recovery from their eating disorder at 5 to 12 years of follow-up, although approximately one third of these will go on to relapse.[71] In contrast to the high mortality rates in patients with AN, mortality does not appear to be significantly increased in those with BN.[38,72] One review of 88 studies demonstrated a crude mortality rate of 0.3% during longitudinal follow-up, although the authors cautioned that this may have been an underestimate because of variable lengths of follow-up (6 months to 10 years) and low ascertainment across follow-up.[73]

Conclusions

Eating disorders are prevalent problems among adolescents, and to a lesser extent, among children. These illnesses carry the risk of severe medical and psychosocial consequences and poor long-term outcome. As such, early detection and intervention involving a multidisciplinary team consisting of a pediatrician or primary medical provider, a nutritionist, and a mental health provider is required.

References

1. Smink FR, van Hoeken D, Oldehinkel AJ, Hoek HW. Prevalence and severity of DSM-5 eating disorders in a community cohort of adolescents. *Int J Eat Disord.* 2014;47(6):610–619

2. American Psychiatric Association. *Diagnostic and Statistical Manual of Mental Disorders, 5th Edition.* Washington, DC: American Psychiatric Association; 2013

3. Pinhas L, Morris A, Crosby RD, Katzman DK. Incidence and age-specific presentation of restrictive eating disorders in children: a Canadian Paediatric Surveillance Program study. *Arch Pediatr Adolesc Med.* 2011;165(10):895–899

4. Nicholls DE, Lynn R, Viner RM. Childhood eating disorders: British national surveillance study. *Br J Psychiatry.* 2011;198(4):295–301

5. Madden S, Morris A, Zurynski YA, Kohn M, Elliot EJ. Burden of eating disorders in 5-13-year-old children in Australia. *Med J Austr.* 2009;190(8):410–414

6. Peebles R, Wilson JL, Lock JD. How do children with eating disorders differ from adolescents with eating disorders at initial evaluation? *J Adolesc Health.* 2006;39(6):800–805.

7. Rosen DS. Identification and management of eating disorders in children and adolescents. *Pediatrics.* 2010;126(6):1240–1253

8. Hudson JI, Hiripi E, Pope HG, Jr., Kessler RC. The prevalence and correlates of eating disorders in the National Comorbidity Survey Replication. *Biol Psychiatry.* 2007;61(3):348–358

9. Swanson SA, Crow SJ, Le Grange D, Swendsen J, Merikangas KR. Prevalence and correlates of eating disorders in adolescents. Results from the national comorbidity survey replication adolescent supplement. *Arch Gen Psychiatry.* 2011;68(7):714–723

10. Forman SF, McKenzie N, Hehn R, et al. Predictors of outcome at 1 year in adolescents with DSM-5 restrictive eating disorders: report of the national eating disorders quality improvement collaborative. *J Adolesc Health.* 2014;55(6):750–756

11. Nagata JM, Park KT, Colditz K, Golden NH. Associations of elevated liver enzymes among hospitalized adolescents with anorexia nervosa. *J Pediatr.* 2015;166(2):439–443.e431

12. Misra M, Aggarwal A, Miller KK, et al. Effects of anorexia nervosa on clinical, hematologic, biochemical, and bone density parameters in community-dwelling adolescent girls. *Pediatrics.* 2004;114(6):1574–1583

13. Golden NH, Jacobson MS, Schebendach J, Solanto MV, Hertz SM, Shenker IR. Resumption of menses in anorexia nervosa. *Arch Pediatr Adolesc Med.* 1997;151(1):16–21

14. Golden NH, Kreitzer P, Jacobson MS, et al. Disturbances in growth hormone secretion and action in adolescents with anorexia nervosa. *J Pediatr.* 1994;125(4):655–660

15. Misra M, Miller KK, Bjornson J, et al. Alterations in growth hormone secretory dynamics in adolescent girls with anorexia nervosa and effects on bone metabolism. *J Clin Endocrinol Metab.* 2003;88(12):5615–5623

16. Misra M, Golden NH, Katzman DK. State of the art systematic review of bone disease in anorexia nervosa. *Int J Eat Disord.* 2016;49(3):276–292

17. Lucas AR, Melton LJ III, Crowson CS, O'Fallon WM. Long-term fracture risk among women with anorexia nervosa: a population-based cohort study. *Mayo Clin Proc.* 1999;74(10):972–977

18. Vestergaard P, Emborg C, Stoving RK, Hagen C, Mosekilde L, Brixen K. Fractures in patients with anorexia nervosa, bulimia nervosa, and other eating disorders—a nationwide register study. *Int J Eat Disord.* 2002;32(3):301–308

19. Faje AT, Fazeli PK, Miller KK, et al. Fracture risk and areal bone mineral density in adolescent females with anorexia nervosa. *Int J Eat Disord.* 2014;47(5):458–466

20. Nagata JM, Golden NH, Leonard MB, Copelovitch L, Denburg MR. Assessment of sex differences in fracture risk among patients with anorexia nervosa: a population-based cohort study using the health improvement network. *J Bone Miner Res.* 2017;32(5):1082–1089

21. Golden NH, Lanzkowsky L, Schebendach J, Palestro CJ, Jacobson MS, Shenker IR. The effect of estrogen-progestin treatment on bone mineral density in anorexia nervosa. *J Pediatr Adolesc Gynecol.* 2002;15(3):135–143

22. Klibanski A, Biller BM, Schoenfeld DA, Herzog DB, Saxe VC. The effects of estrogen administration on trabecular bone loss in young women with anorexia nervosa. *J Clin Endocrinol Metab.* 1995;80(3):898–904

23. Strokosch GR, Friedman AJ, Wu SC, Kamin M. Effects of an oral contraceptive (norgestimate/ethinyl estradiol) on bone mineral density in adolescent females with anorexia nervosa: a double-blind, placebo-controlled study. *J Adolesc Health.* 2006;39(6):819–827

24. Misra M, Katzman D, Miller KK, et al. Physiologic estrogen replacement increases bone density in adolescent girls with anorexia nervosa. *J Bone Miner Res.* 2011;26(10):2430–2438

25. Nattiv A, Loucks AB, Manore MM, Sanborn CF, Sundgot-Borgen J, Warren MP. American College of Sports Medicine position stand. The female athlete triad. *Med Sci Sports Exerc.* 2007;39(10):1867–1882

26. Fisher MM, Rosen DS, Ornstein RM, et al. Characteristics of avoidant/restrictive food intake disorder in children and adolescents: a "new disorder" in DSM-5. *J Adolesc Health*. 2014;55(1):49–52

27. Ornstein RM, Rosen DS, Mammel KA, et al. Distribution of eating disorders in children and adolescents using the proposed DSM-5 criteria for feeding and eating disorders. *J Adolesc Health*. 2013;53(2):303–305

28. Lebow J, Sim LA, Kransdorf LN. Prevalence of a history of overweight and obesity in adolescents with restrictive eating disorders. *J Adolesc Health*. 2015;56(1):19–24

29. Whitelaw M, Gilbertson H, Lee KJ, Sawyer SM. Restrictive eating disorders among adolescent inpatients. *Pediatrics*. 2014;134(3):e758–e764

30. Sim LA, Lebow J, Billings M. Eating disorders in adolescents with a history of obesity. *Pediatrics*. Oct 2013;132(4):e1026–1030

31. Golden NH, Schneider M, Wood C, American Academy of Pediatrics, Committee on Nutrition, Committee on Adolescence, Section on Obesity. Preventing obesity and eating disorders in adolescents. *Pediatrics*. 2016;138(3):e20161649

32. Strober M, Freeman R, Lampert C, Diamond J, Kaye W. Controlled family study of anorexia nervosa and bulimia nervosa: evidence of shared liability and transmission of partial syndromes. *Am J Psychiatry*. 2000;157(3):393–401

33. Bulik CM, Breen G. The genetics of eating disorders. In: Brownell KD, Walsh BT, eds. *Eating Disorders and Obesity: A Comprehensive Handbook*. 3rd ed. New York, NY: Guilford Press; 2017:249–253

34. Monteleone P, Martiadis V, Rigamonti AE, et al. Investigation of peptide YY and ghrelin responses to a test meal in bulimia nervosa. *Biol Psychiatry*. 2005;57(8): 926–931

35. Golden NH, Katzman DK, Sawyer SM, et al. Update on the medical management of eating disorders in adolescents. *J Adolesc Health*. 2015;56(4): 370–375

36. Becker AE, Thomas JJ, Franko DL, Herzog DB. Disclosure patterns of eating and weight concerns to clinicians, educational professionals, family, and peers. *Int J Eat Disord*. 2005;38(1):18–23

37. Herzog DB. Psychiatric comorbidity in eating disorders. In: Wonderlich S, Mitchell, J.E., de Zwaan, M., Steiger H., ed. *Annual Review of Eating Disorders*. Oxford, United Kingdom: Radcliff Publishing Ltd; 2007:35–50

38. Keel PK, Dorer DJ, Eddy KT, Franko D, Charatan DL, Herzog DB. Predictors of mortality in eating disorders. *Arch Gen Psychiatry*. 2003;60(2):179–183

39. Burgalassi A, Ramacciotti CE, Bianchi M, et al. Caffeine consumption among eating disorder patients: epidemiology, motivations, and potential of abuse. *Eat Weight Disord*. 2009;14(4):e212–e218

40. Krug I, Treasure J, Anderluh M, et al. Present and lifetime comorbidity of tobacco, alcohol and drug use in eating disorders: a European multicenter study. *Drug Alcohol Depend*. 2008;97(1-2):169–179

VI

41. Society for Adolescent Health and Medicine, Golden NH, Katzman DK, et al. Position Paper of the Society for Adolescent Health and Medicine: medical management of restrictive eating disorders in adolescents and young adults. *J Adolesc Health*. 2015;56(1):121–125

42. Lock J, Le Grange D, Agras WS, Moye A, Bryson SW, Jo B. Randomized clinical trial comparing family-based treatment with adolescent-focused individual therapy for adolescents with anorexia nervosa. *Arch Gen Psychiatry*. 2010;67(10): 1025–1032

43. le Grange D, Crosby RD, Rathouz PJ, Leventhal BL. A randomized controlled comparison of family-based treatment and supportive psychotherapy for adolescent bulimia nervosa. *Arch Gen Psychiatry*. 2007;64(9):1049–1056

44. Loeb KL, le Grange D. Family-Based Treatment for Adolescent Eating Disorders: Current Status, New Applications and Future Directions. *Int J Child Adolesc health*. 2009;2(2):243–254

45. Golden NH, Attia E. Psychopharmacology of eating disorders in children and adolescents. *Pediatr Clin North Am*. 2011;58(1):121–138

46. Monge MC, Forman SF, McKenzie NM, et al. Use of Psychopharmacologic Medications in Adolescents With Restrictive Eating Disorders: Analysis of Data From the National Eating Disorder Quality Improvement Collaborative. *J Adolesc Health*. 2015;57(1):66–72

47. Bissada H, Tasca GA, Barber AM, Bradwejn J. Olanzapine in the treatment of low body weight and obsessive thinking in women with anorexia nervosa: a randomized, double-blind, placebo-controlled trial. *Am J Psychiatry*. 2008;165(10):1281–1288

48. Broft A, Berner, L.A., Walsh, B.T.,. Pharmacotherapy for bulimia nervosa. In: Grilo CM, Mitchell J.E., ed. *The treatment of eating disorders*. New York: Guilford Press; 2010:388–401

49. Fluoxetine in the treatment of bulimia nervosa. A multicenter, placebo-controlled, double-blind trial. Fluoxetine Bulimia Nervosa Collaborative Study Group. *Arch Gen Psychiatry*. 1992;49(2):139–147

50. Reiter CS, Graves L. Nutrition therapy for eating disorders. *Nutr Clin Pract*. 2010;25(2):122–136

51. Schebendach JE, Porter KJ, Wolper C, Walsh BT, Mayer LE. Accuracy of self-reported energy intake in weight-restored patients with anorexia nervosa compared with obese and normal weight individuals. *Int J Eat Disord*. 2012;45(4): 570–574

52. Katzman DK, Garber, A.K., Kohn, M., Golden, N.H. Refeeding hypophosphatemia in hospitalized adolescents with anorexia nervosa. *J Adolesc Health*. 2014;55(3):455–457

53. Golden NH, Keane-Miller C, Sainani KL, Kapphahn CJ. Higher caloric intake in hospitalized adolescents with anorexia nervosa is associated with reduced length of stay and no increased rate of refeeding syndrome. *J Adolesc Health*. 2013;53(5):573–578

54. O'Connor G, Nicholls D. Refeeding hypophosphatemia in adolescents with anorexia nervosa: a systematic review. *Nutr Clin Pract.* 2013;28(3):358–364

55. Garber AK, Mauldin K, Michihata N, Buckelew SM, Shafer MA, Moscicki AB. Higher calorie diets increase rate of weight gain and shorten hospital stay in hospitalized adolescents with anorexia nervosa. *J Adolesc Health.* 2013;53(5): 579–584

56. Garber AK, Sawyer SM, Golden NH, et al. A systematic review of approaches to refeeding in patients with anorexia nervosa. *Int J Eat Disord.* 2016;49(3):293–310

57. Madden S, Miskovic-Wheatley J, Clarke S, Touyz S, Hay P, Kohn MR. Outcomes of a rapid refeeding protocol in adolescent anorexia nervosa. *J Eat Disord.* 2015;3:8

58. Schebendach JE, Golden NH, Jacobson MS, Hertz S, Shenker IR. The metabolic responses to starvation and refeeding in adolescents with anorexia nervosa. *Ann N Y Acad Sci.* 1997;817:110–119

59. Schebendach JE. Nutrition in eating disorders. In: Mahan LK, Escott-Stump S, ed. *Krauses's Food and Nutrition Therapy.* 12th ed. St. Louis, MO: Saunders/ Elsevier; 2005:563–586

60. Fitzgerald C. Eating disorders. In: Corkins MR, ed. *Pediatric Nutrition Core Support Curriculum.* Silver Spring, MD: American Society for Parenteral and Enteral Nutrition (A.S.P.E.N); 2010:204–212

61. Ozier AD, Henry BW, American Dietetic Association. Position of the American Dietetic Association: nutrition intervention in the treatment of eating disorders. *J Am Diet Assoc.* 2011;111(8):1236–1241

62. Kraft MD, Btaiche IF, Sacks GS. Review of the refeeding syndrome. *Nutr Clin Pract.* 2005;20(6):625–633

63. Golden NH, Abrams SA, Committee on Nutrition; Committee on Adolescence; Section on Obesity. Optimizing bone health in children and adolescents. *Pediatrics.* 2014;134(4):e1229–e1243

64. Modan-Moses D, Levy-Shraga Y, Pinhas-Hamiel O, et al. High prevalence of vitamin D deficiency and insufficiency in adolescent inpatients diagnosed with eating disorders. *Int J Eat Disord.* 2015;48(6):607–614

65. Gatti D, El Ghoch M, Viapiana O, et al. Strong relationship between vitamin D status and bone mineral density in anorexia nervosa. *Bone.* 2015;78:212–215

66. Veronese N, Solmi M, Rizza W, et al. Vitamin D status in anorexia nervosa: a meta-analysis. *Int J Eat Disord.* 2015;48(7):803–813

67. Institute of Medicine. *2011 Dietary Reference Intakes for Calcium and Vitamin D.* Washington DC: The National Academies Press; 2011

68. Arcelus J, Mitchell AJ, Wales J, Nielsen S. Mortality rates in patients with anorexia nervosa and other eating disorders. A meta-analysis of 36 studies. *Arch Gen Psychiatry.* 2011;68(7):724–731

69. Sullivan PF. Mortality in anorexia nervosa. *Am J Psychiatry.* 1995;152(7):1073–1074

VI

70. Steinhausen HC. Outcome of eating disorders. *Child Adolesc Psychiatr Clin North Am.* 2009;18(1):225–242

71. Herzog DB, Dorer DJ, Keel PK, et al. Recovery and relapse in anorexia and bulimia nervosa: a 7.5-year follow-up study. *J Am Acad Child Adolesc Psychiatry.* 1999;38(7):829–837

72. Nielsen S, Moller-Madsen S, Isager T, Jorgensen J, Pagsberg K, Theander S. Standardized mortality in eating disorders—a quantitative summary of previously published and new evidence. *J Psychosom Res.* 1998;44(3-4):413–434

73. Keel PK, Mitchell JE. Outcome in bulimia nervosa. *Am J Psychiatry.* 1997;154(3):313–321

Nutrition for Children With Sickle Cell Disease and Thalassemia

Introduction

Hemoglobin synthesis disorders are among the most common genetic disorders worldwide. Approximately 5.2% of the worldwide population are carriers for a hemoglobinopathy trait, and the global incidence of a significant hemoglobinopathy is 2.6 in 1000 live births.[1,2]

Thalassemia (thal) is a term describing a heterogeneous group of disorders with inadequate or inappropriate production of the alpha or beta globin chains of hemoglobin, which leads to clinical conditions characterized by varying degrees of ineffective hematopoiesis with chronic anemia, intermittent hemolysis, and iron overload. Thal has a high prevalence in Mediterranean and Asian populations, with carrier rates as high as 60% in some regions of southeast Asia, and has been increasing in incidence in the United States because of migration patterns.

There are 4 alpha thal states—silent carrier, trait, hemoglobin H, and hydrops fetalis—determined by the number (1 to 4) of alpha genes deleted, respectively. Mutations may occur in the alpha globin gene, but alpha thal is more likely related to deletions than mutations. In contrast, mutations in the 2 beta globin genes are the etiology of beta thal. Regardless of genotype, patients with thalassemia major are, by definition, transfusion dependent. Transfusion is generally initiated in the first year of life and continued chronically. Patients with thal intermedia do not currently require chronic transfusions but may in the future. Unaffected carriers have thal minor or thal trait. This chapter focuses on nutritional complications in patients with thal major but may also be relevant to those affected by more severe thal intermedia.

Sickle cell disease (SCD) defines a group of hemoglobinopathies in which the abnormal hemoglobin variant S, sickle hemoglobin, is produced because of a mutation in the beta globin gene and is found in conjunction with a second S mutation or a mutation resulting in another hemoglobin variant such as C, D, or E, leading to a clinical condition marked by anemia, vaso-occlusive events, and inflammation with tissue injury. The S in conjunction with a beta thal zero mutation (no normal A hemoglobin) or a beta thal plus mutation (reduced A production) manifests similarly because of the abnormal sickle-shaped red blood cells, which are less deformable than normal.

VI

Sickle cell (SS) anemia is the most common type of SCD. An estimated 1 in every 8 African American people carries at least 1 S gene, and the prevalence of SS anemia in African American newborn infants is approximately 1 in 375. Hemoglobin SCD occurs approximately 1 in 835 African American live births, and S beta-thalassemia occurs in about 1 in 1700 African American live births. Thus, SCD, with an autosomal-recessive inheritance pattern, is the most common medically significant genetic condition in African American children but also occurs in children with a Mediterranean, East Indian, Middle Eastern, Caribbean, or South and Central American ancestry.

The discussion of nutrition and diet in the hemoglobinopathies that follows relates primarily to people affected by thal major, SS anemia, and sickle beta-zero thal, because they are the most severe conditions and the best studied. However, even for people affected by those conditions, the literature is primarily limited to small, single-institutional, nonrandomized, non–placebo-controlled studies, and the findings may reflect local nutritional status. Accordingly, the National Heart, Lung, and Blood Institute (NHLBI) of the National Institutes of Health has suggested there is a need for adequately powered clinical studies to effectively evaluate nutritional status and potential interventions for people with hemoglobinopathies.

Macronutrient Intake, Requirements, and Energy Expenditure

Growth retardation, delayed pubertal development, and poor nutritional status are frequently observed in both thal major and SCD. The pattern of poor growth and abnormal body composition has not been completely established, but it is generally recognized to be multifactorial, and nutritional factors likely play a role.

In thal major, growth failure has been reported with an incidence ranging from 25% to 75% depending on the thal syndrome and severity of disease. Linear growth, expressed as height z-score, tends to decrease with age and is commonly associated with pubertal delays. Contributing factors to growth failure in thal major include chronic anemia, chelation toxicity, and iron-associated endocrinopathies, such as hypogonadism, hypothyroidism, and growth hormone deficiency.

However, recent reports of studies conducted mostly outside the United States suggest that nutritional inadequacy also plays a major role in growth failure and pubertal development in thal major. Several small studies have demonstrated that nutritional supplementation in toddlers with thal improves markers of immune function and growth.[3,4] Children with thal major have similar dietary intake when compared with age- and gender-matched controls, despite marked growth and body fat deficits. In a randomized controlled trial, increasing energy intake by 30% to 50% over an 8-week period resulted in significant improvements in weight, fat stores, and albumin and insulin-like growth factor 1 (IGF-1) levels, compared with a nonsupplemented thal major group.[5] The improvement in IGF-1 following nutritional therapy supports the notion that a component of the growth failure is related to global nutritional deficiency.

One explanation for the reduced growth rates in thal, despite seemingly adequate energy intake, could be increased energy expenditure. Increased energy expenditure is possible, given the existence of hyperactive bone marrow and increased cardiac output attributable to chronic anemia. In one study, energy expenditure in chronically transfused adults with thal major was 12% higher than expected before transfusion (at the nadir of hemoglobin concentration) and decreased to near-normal levels after transfusion.[6]

Poor nutritional intake may also contribute to growth deficiencies. The Thalassemia Clinical Research Network conducted a cross-sectional analysis of dietary intake in 221 adult and pediatric patients with a variety of thal syndromes.[7] The results suggest that patients with thal generally have adequate and sometimes excess intakes of macronutrients (fat and protein); however, they have inadequate intake of some vitamins and micronutrients.

Growth retardation, delayed pubertal development, and poor nutritional status are also seen in some children with SCD.[8] Physical findings in these children include decreased body weight, height/length, arm circumference, skin fold thicknesses, and bone age. Direct measures of body composition by several research methods have shown lower total body fat.[9,10] Episodic acute illnesses in children with SCD further aggravate growth and nutritional status.[11]

Patients with SCD have increased energy requirements because of chronic hemolysis and increased, erythropoiesis, cardiac output, protein turnover, and proinflammatory cytokines.[12–17] Several studies have documented increased resting energy expenditure in children and adults with SCD in the United States and other countries.[18–20] The increase is generally 10% to 20% above the predicted energy expenditure of healthy control children. Unfortunately, children with SCD do not necessarily increase energy intake to compensate for increased energy needs. The increased

VI

resting energy expenditure has been correlated with low hemoglobin concentrations.[21,22]

Although acute vaso-occlusive events in children with SCD do not appear to increase resting energy expenditure, the events are associated with decreased energy intake.[22,23] Some of the new treatments for SCD, such as oral glutamine supplementation and hydroxyurea therapy, may decrease resting energy expenditure.[24,25]

Dietary intake of many nutrients may be inadequate in children with SCD. A large cohort study of 97 children and adolescents with SCD evaluated dietary intake longitudinally over 4 annual visits using 24-hour recall data.[8] Children receiving chronic transfusions and hydroxyurea were excluded from this study. Although the median estimated energy intake was equal to the estimated energy requirements for children with a low-active physical activity level, overall growth was suboptimal (mean height z-score, −0.5 ± 1.0; weight z-score, −0.8 ± 1.2), and intake of many specific micronutrients was found to be low. Specifically, intake of vitamins D and E, folate, calcium, and fiber was inadequate, with 63% to 85% of the children falling below the estimated average requirement. Additionally, like what is observed in thal, there was a general decline in adequacy of dietary intake as the children aged, with decreased intakes of protein, vitamins A, B_{12}, C; and riboflavin, and magnesium and phosphorus. In a recent study from Italy, data on 29 children with 24-hour recall diary showed that their total caloric, carbohydrate, and lipid intakes were moderately less than daily requirements.[26] Total calorie intake did not correlate with clinical outcome or laboratory data. Protein and lipid intakes showed a negative correlation with the days of hospitalization. Lipid and carbohydrate intakes were negatively associated with fetal hemoglobin levels.

Another factor contributing to inadequate nutrient intake in children with SCD may be the emphasis placed on encouraging fluid intake to maintain hydration to help prevent vaso-occlusive events; children with SCD have increased fluid needs resulting from hyposthenuria, the inability of the kidneys to appropriately concentrate urine.[27] This may lead to inadequate intake of other dietary nutrients. In addition, suboptimal intakes during periods of illness at home or in the hospital may contribute to the pattern of decreased dietary intake and poor growth, particularly in patients with severe SCD disease.

The amino acids glutamine and L-arginine may be deficient in patients with SCD, especially adults, related to long-standing increased hemolysis.[28]

Glutamine and L-arginine deficiency have been associated with increased hemolysis, acute chest syndrome, and pulmonary hypertension in SCD.[29-31] A randomized trial of arginine administration for treatment of vaso-occlusive crisis and another for treatment of ulcers in SCD have been promising.[32,33]

Specific Micronutrient Deficiencies

In addition to the potential increased requirement for total kilocalories, there are specific essential micronutrients for which patients with SCD and thal may be at risk of deficiency (Table 39.1).

Water-Soluble Vitamins

Folate is an essential nutrient required for normal erythropoietic activity and theoretically may be deficient in thal and SCD because of increased red blood cell turnover and a hyperactive bone marrow. In one study, children with SCD remained folate deficient despite supplementation with 1 mg/day of folate, supporting the hypothesis that folate requirements are significantly increased.[34] In contrast, a Canadian study reported normal folate levels in children receiving folate supplementation as part of routine care.[35] However, a recent Cochrane review suggested that there were not enough data to routinely recommend folate supplementation for SCD.[36] Folate is readily catabolized by ferritin; therefore, in patients with thal major or SCD and transfusional iron overload, folate requirements are increased and supplementation is indicated.

Vitamin B_6 deficiency has been reported in thal and SCD. Vitamin B_{12} is reportedly normal in thal, but there are mixed reports in SCD.[37] Vitamin B status is of particular interest in SCD, because folate and plasma homocysteine levels may be associated with increased risk of stroke in children with SCD.[38-40] In SCD, it was shown that supplementation with folate, vitamin B_6, and vitamin B_{12} decreased plasma homocysteine levels, but no studies have demonstrated an associated reduction in the incidence of stroke.[41] In another study of children with SCD, vitamin B_6 status correlated positively with weight and body mass index but was negatively correlated with the reticulocyte count.[42]

Vitamin C is an antioxidant that is often deficient in children with thal major and SCD, and deficiency has been associated with ineffective chelation.[26,43-45] It has been known for decades that vitamin C is important both in nonheme iron absorption as well as in the mobilization of iron from

VI

Table 39.1.
Nutrients of Concern in Sickle Cell Disease and Thalassemia

Nutrient	Sickle Cell Disease	Thalassemia	Possible Signs
Macronutrients: Kilocalories	Poor dietary quality/ nutrient density	Poor dietary quality/ nutrient density	Growth failure
Micronutrients: Fat-soluble vitamins	Amino acids[a]		Increased oxidative stress
	Vitamin A		Increased vaso-occlusive crises
	Vitamin D	Vitamin D	Reduced bone mineral density
	Vitamin E	Vitamin E	Increased oxidative damage
Water-soluble vitamins	Vitamin C	Vitamin C	Increased oxidative damage, decreased chelator efficacy
	Folate and vitamin B$_{12}$	Folate	Ineffective erythropoiesis; increased homocysteine (SCD)
	Vitamin B$_6$		Increased reticulocyte count
Minerals	Zinc	Zinc	Increased vaso-occlusive crises and infection (SCD), poor growth, reduced bone density (thal)
	Calcium	Calcium	Reduced bone mineral density

[a]There may be increased requirements for certain amino acids (glutamine, arginine).

tissues.[46] Vitamin C supplementation in iron-overloaded children with thal major augments the efficacy of the iron chelators, especially deferoxamine.[47] Although vitamin C supplementation has been demonstrated to reduce the percentage of irreversibly sickled cells, it also increased hemolysis.[48]

Fat-Soluble Vitamins

Fat-soluble vitamin deficiency appears to be of concern in children with hemoglobinopathies. Vitamin D deficiency has received much attention in the scientific literature with the revised dietary guidelines for vitamin D intake from the Institute of Medicine (now National Academy of Medicine).[49] Vitamin D has many unique hormonal functions; its active form, calcitriol (1,25-dihydroxyvitamin D), has been shown to affect bone and is associated with improved cardiovascular health and immune function. However, the literature related to hemoglobinopathies is primarily based upon the inactive, 25-OH vitamin D concentrations, which complicates interpretation of the impact of vitamin D.

The prevalence of vitamin D deficiency (25-hydroxy vitamin D <50 nmol/L) in children with thal in North American and Europe is 40% to 60%.[50] International reports have found the same.[51–55] Vitamin D deficiency may occur in thal major because of one or more of the following: impaired 25-hydroxylation of vitamin D in the liver, decreased production in the skin, or intestinal malabsorption. The relationship of vitamin D to bone mineral density is unclear in SCD. In a survey of participants from the Thalassemia Clinical Research Network, those with vitamin D deficiency had lower bone mineral density.[56] However, 2 studies have found no association between 25-hydroxyvitamin D (25-OH-D) levels and either bone mass or bone density in children with SCD.[57,58]

There are a few reports exploring the association between vitamin D levels and cardiovascular health in thal major. Wood et al found a weak although significant correlation between 25-OH-D levels and left ventricular ejection fraction in patients with thal ($r^2 = 0.35$); all 4 subjects with dysfunctional ejection fractions (<57%) also had low levels of vitamin D.[59] In a recent study of 34 children with thal major, vitamin D levels significantly correlated with left ventricular ejection fraction, shortening fraction and N-terminal prohormone B-type natriuretic peptide (NT-proBNP) levels.[60]

Children with SCD are also at risk of vitamin D deficiency, in part because they commonly have dark skin color. However, children with SCD have decreased serum 25-OH-D concentrations and decreased vitamin D and calcium intakes, even compared with healthy age-matched African

VI

American controls.[61] In a study of 65 children with SCD, 93% of the subjects had low serum 25-OH-D concentrations, defined as 25-OH-D <30 ng/mL (75 nmol/L). After adjustments were made for seasonal effects and age, the risk of a low serum 25-OH-D in patients with SCD was 5 times greater than in healthy African American controls. When considering treatment of children with SCD, who commonly are African Amercan, it is important to appreciate that both levels of total 25-OH-D and vitamin D-binding protein are lower in African American individuals than in white individuals, resulting in similar concentrations of estimated bioavailable 25-OH-D.[62]

Despite the contradictory literature, on the basis of the high prevalence of low vitamin D concentrations and the potential for comorbidities in both thal and SCD patients, some guidelines suggest that vitamin D status be monitored every 6 months. People who reside in Northern latitudes, are dark skinned, who customarily shroud themselves, or who have limited exposure to sunlight and have limited dietary intake of vitamin D are particularly at risk. Given that vitamin D is a fat-soluble vitamin and stored in fat tissue, it can be provided in large, infrequent doses to improve compliance. For subjects who regularly receive transfusion therapy and who have low vitamin D concentrations (<20 ng/mL [50 nmol/L]), a 50 000-IU vitamin D oral dose at time of transfusion has been used successfully to improve vitamin D status.[63]

Vitamins A and E, essential nutrients with antioxidant effects, are frequently reported to be deficient in children and adolescents with SCD.[64-69] This is particularly important in SCD, which is a disorder marked by increased oxidative stress resulting from chronic hemolysis. In one study of young children with SCD, vitamin A status was found to be suboptimal in two thirds of the studied children and was associated with poor growth and lower hematocrit, increased episodes of pain and fever, and a 10-fold increased frequency of hospitalizations.[70] However, vitamin A supplementation at the dose recommended for healthy children did not improve retinol levels or change the frequency of vaso-occlusive events, fever, or hospitalization rates in children with SCD.[71]

Vitamin E has been shown to help stabilize the red blood cell membrane, whereas vitamin E deficiency enhances red blood cell susceptibility to peroxidative damage.[72,73] Chronic red blood cell transfusions may increase oxidative stress because of iron overload.[74] Accordingly, supplementation with 400 to 600 IU of vitamin E for 3 months in patients with either thal intermedia or E-beta thal has been found to reduce oxidative stress.[75] In a study of 39 children with β thalassemia major who were iron overloaded and receiving a chelating agent, treatment with vitamins containing A, C, and E for 1 year translated to significantly higher vitamin levels and lower liver iron content as compared with the 21 children in the placebo group.[47]

A study of adults with SCD found that 60% were deficient in vitamin C, 70% were deficient in vitamin E, and 45% were deficient in both vitamins. With treatment, all adults achieved normal vitamin C levels and 90% achieved normal vitamin E levels, but hemolytic markers increased. Treatment did not change the baseline hemoglobin or rate of vaso-occlusive events.[48]

Trace Minerals

Zinc is an essential trace mineral required for cell division and differentiation and gene expression. It is critical for the function of more than 300 enzymes regulating development and maintenance of the immune system, bone health, vitamin A metabolism, and the actions of insulin, testosterone, thyroid, and growth hormones.

Zinc deficiency has been documented in nontransfusion-dependent and chronically transfused patients with thal.[76] Proximal renal tubular damage can increase urinary zinc concentration by as much as fourfold compared with controls. Increases in urinary zinc may also be related to the presence of diabetes, a comorbidity associated with iron overload. Zinc is similar in size and charge to iron, so it has the potential to be depleted by chelation.[77] Zinc supplementation for regularly transfused but nonchelated patients with thal was shown to improve growth velocity.[78]

Zinc deficiency may play a role in the pathology of osteoporosis, because osteoblasts need zinc for bone formation, and osteoclastic bone resorption is inhibited by zinc. In thal, bone mineral density (BMD) z-scores are lower in males and females with severe zinc deficiency compared with those with normal serum zinc levels.[79] In iron-overloaded patients with thal major, deficient serum zinc levels are also associated with lower insulin concentrations.[80]

Zinc deficiency has been recognized in children with SCD for several decades.[81] There is evidence that patients with SCD have increased urinary zinc losses and likely have increased needs because of chronic hemolysis and increased protein turnover.[82] A zinc supplement taken for 1 year has been shown to improve linear growth and weight gain in prepubertal children with SCD, even in those with normal plasma zinc levels before supplementation.[83] A benefit to zinc supplementation has also been demonstrated with regard to sexual maturation and decreased infections and hospitalizations.[84,85]

Unique Nutritional Situations

Pica and SCD

Pica is the consumption and/or craving of nonfood substances, such as paper, fabric, dirt, foam, ice, or powder. The most commonly linked nutritional deficiencies include the trace elements iron and zinc. Pica is highly prevalent in children with SCD; it is reported that 32% to 56% of children have pica.[86,87] Pica has been associated with younger age and lower hemoglobin levels. Although generally benign, there is a potential for serious medical complications, including dental injury, constipation, intestinal obstruction, lead poisoning, malabsorption of essential nutrients, and poor growth.

Iron Overload in Thalassemia: The Dogma and the Dilemma

Given the relationship between iron overload and organ dysfunction in thal major, counseling to consume a diet low in iron has been part of the standards of care for decades. Typically, a diet that is low in iron-rich foods, such as red and organ meats and fortified breakfast cereals, is recommended. However, there is debate regarding the effectiveness of reducing dietary iron consumption for the transfused subject. Typical daily iron accumulation from transfusion-related iron is approximately 20 mg/day (2 transfusion units every 3 weeks), compared with daily iron accumulation from an iron-rich diet of approximately 4 mg (assuming 30% absorption). A low-iron diet may decrease the quality of life in some transfusion-dependent patients and/or create a false sense of security—that is, if they decrease their dietary iron intake, they may need to be less diligent about chelator adherence.

For the child with thal who is not transfusion dependent, reducing iron in the diet is an important part of nutritional counseling, to compensate for over absorption of iron from the intestinal track. Ingestion of tea is suggested for all children, because it reduces iron absorption.[88]

Nutrition and Bone Health

Bone health is an important nutritional consideration for both children with SCD and thal. Bone marrow hyperplasia in response to increased red blood cell turnover expands the marrow medullary space in long bones, thinning the cortical bone compartment. Cortical thinning likely results in increased bone fragility and increased lifelong risk of fracture.

Elevations in protein and energy metabolism are also associated with increased bone turnover in SCD. Increased protein turnover and decreased lean body mass may be significant when considering the concept of the bone-muscle unit. Forces produced by muscle contractions influence the restructuring of bone, and changes in muscle mass affect bone mass, size, and strength and may be relevant to SCD.

Bone mineral content deficits may occur in children with SCD, even when adjusting for age, height, pubertal status, and lean body mass. A study from France found a slightly decreased bone mineral density when they evaluated 53 children with SCD with a mean age of 12.8 ± 2.4 years. Multiple factors likely contribute to poor bone health, including decreased vitamin D and calcium intake.[89]

A study from Iran evaluated 140 transfusion-dependent children with thal between 8 and 18 years of age. The authors noted lower bone density in the lumbar spine in 82% of the children and found better nutritional status was associated with higher bone mineral density.[55]

Nutritional Guidelines for SCD and Thalassemia

For children with SCD and thal, routine, longitudinal growth and nutritional status assessments are suggested. The data obtained from these assessments should inform nutritional interventions to prevent growth failure or malnutrition. The biological parents' heights should be obtained, recorded on the patient's growth chart, and used to assess the pattern of linear growth. It is important to remember that short stature is not a part of the genetic expression of either hemoglobinopathy, and with optimal nutritional intake, most children will be able to grow to their genetic potential for height. An accurate longitudinal growth (length, height, weight, head circumference) and body composition (fat stores measurements) record is essential to monitoring nutritional status and evaluating the results of nutrition intervention efforts. Pubertal progression should be evaluated and documented.

As to SCD, a 2004 statement from the NHLBI stressed the importance of nutritional counseling but made no specific recommendations for monitoring or intervention.[90] The only routine nutritional supplement recommended by the NHLBI is folate, but a recent Cochrane review did not support routine folic acid supplementation for children with SCD.[36]

Guidelines for the nutritional management of children with thal receiving chronic transfusions are available.[91,92] The Thalassemia International

VI

Federation recommends a high-calorie diet in growing children. All children should have a diet high in calcium (ie, milk, cheese, and oily fish) and take vitamin D at 2000 IU daily. Vitamin D levels are to be checked every 6 months, given the seasonal variability in vitamin D concentrations. A diet rich in vitamin E (ie, eggs, vegetable oils, nuts, and cereals) is recommended, and supplementation with 400 IU/day may be helpful. Zinc levels are to be monitored every 6 months, especially if iron chelators are prescribed. Zinc sulfate, 220 mg, 3 times daily, is recommended. Vitamin C is potentially toxic as it increases iron absorption, so is to be given only with a chelator to increase iron excretion.[91] If children are infrequently being transfused red blood cells or not at all, folic acid, 1 mg/day, is recommended. The Northern California Comprehensive Thalassemia Center also has published a set of nutritional monitoring recommendations that may provide a useful guide for clinicians.[92]

Conclusions

Deficient concentrations of key fat- and water-soluble vitamins, as well as important essential minerals, have been reported in children patients with thal and SCD. There is increasing evidence that children with both disorders have increased requirements for some nutrients because of poor nutrient absorption and/or elevated losses and/or increased nutrient turnover. It is suggested that affected children receive nutritional counseling, are monitored for deficiencies, and are treated as indicated. Large, multicenter, randomized, placebo-controlled research trials are indicated to better determine the nutritional needs and determine effective interventions to improve the quality of life for children with thal and SCD.

References

1. Weatherall DJ, Clegg JB. Inherited hemoglobin disorders: an increasing global health problem. *Bull World Health Organ.* 2001;79(8):704–712

2. Modell B, Darlison M. Global epidemiology of haemoglobin disorders and derived service indicators. *Bull World Health Organ.* 2008;86(6):480–487

3. Tienboon P. Effect of nutrition support on immunity in paediatric patients with beta-thalassaemia major. *Asia Pacific J Clin Nutr.* 2003;12:61–65

4. Fuchs GJ, Tienboon P, Linpisarn S, et al. Nutritional factors and thalassemia major. *Arch Dis Child.* 1996;74(3):224–227

5. Soliman AT, El-Matary W, Fattah M, Nasr IS, El Alaily RK, Thabet MA. The effect of a high calorie diet on nutritional parameters of children with beta-thalassemia major. *Clin Nutr.* 2004;23(5):1153–1158

6. Vaisman N, Akivis A, Sthoeger D, Barak Y, Matitau A, Wolach B. Resting energy expenditure in patients with thalassemia major. *Am J Clin Nutr.* 1995;61(3): 582–584

7. Fung EB, Xu Y, Trachtenberg F, et al. Thalassemia Clinical Research Network. Inadequate dietary intake in patients with thalassemia. *J Acad Nutr Diet.* 2012;112(7):980–990

8. Kawchak DA, Schall JI, Zemel BS, Ohene-Frempong K, Stallings VA. Adequacy of dietary intake declines with age in children with sickle cell disease. *J Am Diet Assoc.* 2007;107(5):846–848

9. Barden EM, Kawchak DA, Ohene-Frempong K, Stallings VA, Zemel BS. Body composition in children with sickle cell disease. *Am J Clin Nutr.* 2002;76(1): 218–225

10. VanderJagt DJ, Harmatz P, Scott-Emuakpor AB, Vichinsky E, Glew RH. Bioelectrical impedance analysis of the body composition of children and adolescents with sickle cell disease. *J Pediatr.* 2002;140(6):681–687

11. Malinauskas BM, Gropper SS, Kawchak DA, Zemel BS, Ohene-Frempong K, Stallings VA. Impact of acute illness on nutritional status of infants and young children with sickle cell disease. *J Am Diet Assoc.* 2000;100(3):330–334

12. Modebe O, Ifenu SA. Growth retardation in homozygous sickle cell disease: role of calorie intake and possible gender-related differences. *Am J Hematol.* 1993;44(3):149–154

13. Gray NT, Bartlett JM, Kolasa KM, Marcuard SP, Holbrook CT, Horner RD. Nutritional status and dietary intake of children with sickle cell anemia. *Am J Pediatr Hematol Oncol.* 1992;14(1):57–61

14. Salman EK, Haymond MW, Bayne E, et al. Protein and energy metabolism in prepubertal children with sickle cell anemia. *Pediatr Res.* 1996;40(1):34–40

15. Singhal A, Thomas P, Cook R, Wierenga K, Serjeant G. Delayed adolescent growth in homozygous sickle cell disease. *Arch Dis Child.* 1994;71(5):404–408

16. Singhal A, Davies P, Wierenga KJ, Ghomas P, Serjeant G. Is there an energy deficiency in homozygous sickle cell disease? *Am J Clin Nutr.* 1997;66(2):386–390

17. Buchowski MS, Townsend KM, Williams R, Chen KY. Patterns and energy expenditure of free-living physical activity in adolescents with sickle cell anemia. *J Pediatr.* 2002;140(1):86–92

18. Borel MJ, Muchowski MS, Turner EA, Peeler BB, Goldstein RE, Flakoll PJ. Alterations in basal nutrient metabolism increase resting energy expenditure in sickle cell disease. *Am J Physiol.* 1998;274(2 Pt 1):e357–e364

19. Badaloo A, Jackson AA, Jahoor F. Whole body protein turnover and resting metabolic rate in homozygous sickle cell disease. *Clin Sci.* 1989;77(1):93–97

20. Singhal A, Davies P, Sahota A, Thomas PW, Serjeant GR. Resting metabolic rate in homozygous sickle cell disease. *Am J Clin Nutr.* 1993;57(1):32–34

21. Barden EM, Zemel BS, Kawchak DA, Goran MI, Ohene-Frempong K, Stallings VA. Total and resting energy expenditure in children with sickle cell disease. *J Pediatr.* 2000;136(1):73–79

VI

22. Williams R, Olivi S, Mackert P, Fletcher L, Tian GL, Wang W. Comparison of energy prediction equations with measured resting energy expenditure in children with sickle cell anemia. *J Am Diet Assoc.* 2002;102(7):956–961

23. Fung EB, Malinauskis BM, Kawchak DA, et al. Energy expenditure and intake in children with sickle cell disease during acute illness. *Clin Nutr.* 2001;20(2):131–138

24. Williams R, Olivi S, Li CS, et al. Oral glutamine supplementation decreases resting energy expenditure in children and adolescents with sickle cell anemia. *J Pediatr Hematol Oncol.* 2004;26(10):619–625

25. Fung EB, Barden EM, Kawchak DA, Zemel BS, Ohene-Frempong K, Stallings VA. Effect of hydroxyurea therapy on resting energy expenditure in children with sickle cell disease. *J Pediatr Hematol Oncol.* 2001;23(9):604–608

26. Mandese V, Marotti F, Bedetti L, Bigi E, Palazzi G, Iughetti L. Effects of nutritional intake on disease severity in children with sickle cell disease. *Nutr J.* 2016;15(1):46

27. Smith JA, Wethers DL. Health care maintenance. In: Embury SH, Hebbel RP, Mohandas N, Steinberg MH, eds. *Sickle Cell Disease.* New York, NY: Raven Press; 1994:739–744

28. Morris CR, Suh JH, Hagar W, et al. Erythrocyte glutamine depletion, altered redox environment, and pulmonary hypertension in sickle cell disease. *Blood.* 2008;111(1):402–410

29. Morris CR, Kuypers FA, Larkin S, Vichinsky EP, Styles LA. Patterns of arginine and nitric oxide in patients with sickle cell disease with vasoocclusive crisis and acute chest syndrome. *J Pediatr Hematol Oncol.* 2000;22(6):515–520

30. Morris CR, Kato GJ, Poljakovic M, et al. Dysregulated arginine metabolism, hemolysis-associated pulmonary hypertension, and mortality in sickle cell disease. *JAMA.* 2005;294(1):81–90

31. Sullivan KJ, Kissoon N, Sandler E, et al. Effect of oral arginine supplementation on exhaled nitric oxide concentration in sickle cell anemia and acute chest syndrome. *J Pediatr Hematol Oncol.* 2010;32(7):e249–e258

32. Morris CR, Kuypers FA, Lavrisha L, et al. A randomized placebo-controlled trial of arginine therapy for the treatment of children with sickle cell disease hospitalized with vaso-occlusive pain episodes. *Haematologica.* 2013;98(9): 1375–1382

33. Morris CR, Morris SM, Jr., Hagar W, et al. Arginine therapy: a new treatment for pulmonary hypertension in sickle cell disease? *Am J Respir Crit Care.* 2003;168(1): 63–69

34. Kennedy TS, Fung EB, Kawchak DA, Zemel BS, Ohene-Frempong K, Stallings VA. Red blood cell folate and serum vitamin B12 status in children with sickle cell disease. *J Pediatr Hematol Oncol.* 2001;23(3):165–169

35. Martyres DJ, Vijenthira A, Barrowman N, Harris-Janz S, Chretien C, Klassen RJ. Nutrient insufficiencies/deficiencies in children with sickle cell disease and its association with increased disease severity. *Pediatr Blood Cancer.* 2016;63(6): 1060–1064

36. Dixit R, Nettem S, Madan SS, et al. Folate supplementation in people with sickle cell disease. *Cochrane Database Syst Rev.* 2016;(2):CD011130

37. Ajayi O, Bwayo-Weaver S, Chirla S, et al. Cobalamin status in sickle cell disease. *Int J Hematol.* 2013;35(1):31–37

38. van der Dijs FP, Schnog JJ, Brouwer DA, et al. Elevated homocysteine levels indicate suboptimal folate status in pediatric sickle cell patients. *Am J Hematol.* 1998;59(3):192–198

39. Segal JB, Miller ER, Brereton NH, Resar LM. Concentrations of B vitamins and homocysteine in children with sickle cell anemia. *South Med J.* 2004;97(2):149–155

40. Houston PE, Rana S, Sekhsaria S, Perlin E, Kim KS, Castro OL. Homocysteine in sickle in sickle cell disease: relationship to stroke. *Am J Med.* 1997;103(3):192–196

41. van der Dijs FP, Fokkema MR, Dijck-Brouwer DA, et al. Optimization of folic acid, vitamin B12, and vitamin B6 supplements in pediatric patients with sickle cell disease. *Am J Hematol.* 2002;69(4):239–246

42. Nelson MC, Zemel BS, Kawchak DA, et al. Vitamin B6 status of children with sickle cell disease. *J Pediatr Hematol Oncol.* 2002;24(6):463–469

43. Wapnick AA, Lynch SR, Charlton RW, Seftel HC, Bothwell TH. The effect of ascorbic acid deficiency on desferrioxamine induced urinary iron excretion. *Br J Haematol.* 1969;17(6):563–568

44. Chapman RW, Hussain MA, Gorman A, et al. Effect of ascorbic acid deficiency on serum ferritin concentration in patients with B-thalassemia major and iron overload. *J Clin Pathol.* 1982;35(5):487–491

45. Claster S, Wood JC, Noetzli L, et al. Nutritional deficiencies in iron overloaded patients with hemoglobinopathies. *Am J Hematol.* 2009;84(6):344–348

46. Fung EB, Xu Y, Trachtenberg F, et al. Inadequate dietary intake in patients with thalassemia. *J Acad Nutr Diet.* 2012;112(7):980–990

47. Elalfy MS, Saber MM, Adly AA, et al. Role of vitamin C as an adjuvant therapy to different iron chelators in young β-thalassemia major patients: efficacy and safety in relation to tissue iron overload. *Eur J Haematol.* 2016;96(3):318–326

48. Arruda MM, Mecabo G, Rodrigues CA, Matsuda SS, Rabelo IB, Figueiredo MS. Antioxidant vitamins C and E supplementation increases markers of haemolysis in sickle cell anaemia patients: a randomized, double-blind, placebo-controlled trial. *Br J Haematol.* 2013;160(5):688–700

49. Institute of Medicine, Food and Nutrition Board. *Dietary Reference Intakes for Calcium and Vitamin D.* Washington, DC: National Academies Press; 2011

50. Giusti A, Pinto V, Forni GL, Pilotto A. Management of beta-thalassemia-associated osteoporosis. *Ann N Y Acad Sci.* 2016;1368(1):73–81

51. Napoli N, Carmina E, Bucchieri S, Sferrazza C, Rini GB, Di Fede G. Low serum levels of 25-hydroxy vitamin D in adults affected by thalassemia major or intermedia. *Bone.* 2006;38(6):888–892

VI

52. Soliman A, Adel A, Wagdy M, Al Ali M, El Mulla N. Calcium homeostasis in 40 adolescents with beta-thalassemia major: a case control study of the effects of intramuscular injection of a megadose of cholecalciferol. *Pediatr Endocrinol Rev.* 2008;6(Suppl 1):149–154

53. Nakavachara P, Viprahasit V. Children with hemoglobin E/β-thalassemia have a high risk of being vitamin D deficient even if they get abundant sun exposure: a study from Thailand. *Pediatr Blood Cancer.* 2013;60(10):1683–1688

54. Pirinccioglu AG, Akpolat V, Koksal O, Haspolat K, Soker M. Bone mineral density in children with beta-thalassemia major in Diyarbakir. *Bone.* 2011;49(4): 819–823

55. Mirhosseini NZ, Shahar S, Ghayour-Mobarhan M, et al. Bone-related complications of transfusion-dependent beta thalassemia among children and adolescents. *J Bone Miner Metab.* 2013;31(4):468–476

56. Vogiatzi MG, Macklin EA, Trachtenberg FL, et al. Differences in the prevalence of growth, endocrine and vitamin D abnormalities among the various thalassemia syndromes in North America. *Br J Haematol.* 2009;146(5):546–556

57. Tzoulis P, Ang AL, Shah FT, et al. Prevalence of low bone mass and vitamin D deficiency in b-thalassemia major. *38.* 2014;3(173–178)

58. Rovner A, Stallings VA, Kawchak DA, Schall JI, Ohene-Frempong K, Zemel BS. High risk of vitamin D deficiency in children with sickle cell disease. *J Am Diet Assoc.* 2008;108(9):1512–1516

59. Wood JC, Claster S, Carson S, et al. Vitamin D deficiency, cardiac iron and cardiac function in thalassemia major. *Br J Haematol.* 2008;141(6):891–894

60. Ambarwati L, Rahayuningsih SE, Setiabudiawan B. Association between vitamin D levels and left ventricular function and NT-proBNP among thalassemia major children with iron overload. *Ann Pediatr Cardiol.* 2016;9(2):126–131

61. Buison AM, Kawchak DA, Schall JI, Ohene-Frempong K, Stallings VA, Zemel BS. Low vitamin D status in children with sickle cell disease. *J Pediatr.* 2004;145(5): 622–627

62. Powe CE, Evans MK, Wenger J, et al. Vitamin D-binding protein and vitamin D status of black Americans and white Americans. *N Engl J Med.* 2013;369(21): 1991–2000

63. Fung EB, Aguilar C, Micaily I, Foote D, Lal A. Treatment of vitamin D deficiency in transfusion-dependent thalassemia. *Am J Hematol.* 2011;86(10):871–873

64. Marwah SS, Wheelwright D, Blann AD, et al. Vitamin E correlates inversely with non-transferrin-bound iron in sickle cell disease. *Br J Haematol.* 2001;114(4): 917–919

65. Nur E, Biemond BJ, Otten HM, Brandjes DP, Schnog JJ. Oxidative stress in sickle cell disease; pathophysiology and potential implications for disease management. *Am J Hematol.* 2011;86(6):484–489

66. Ray D, Deshmukh P, Goswami K, Garg N. Antioxidant vitamin levels in sickle cell disorders. *Natl Med J India.* 2007;20(1):11–13

67. Ren H, Ghebremeskel K, Okpala I, Lee A, Ibegbulam O, Crawford M. Patients with sickle cell disease have reduced blood antioxidant protection. *Int J Vitam Nutr Res.* 2008;78(3):139–147

68. Marwah SS, Blann AD, Rea C, Phillips JD, Wright J, Bareford D. Reduced vitamin E antioxidant capacity in sickle cell disease is related to transfusion status but not to sickle crisis. *Am J Hematol.* 2002;69(2):144–146

69. Hasanato R. Zinc and antioxidant vitamin deficiency in patients with severe sickle cell anemia. *Ann Saudi Med.* 2006;26(1):17–21

70. Schall JI, Zemel BS, Kawchak DA, Ohene-Frempong K, Stallings VA. Vitamin A status, hospitalizations, and other outcomes in young children with sickle cell disease. *J Pediatr.* 2004;145(1):99–106

71. Dougherty KA, Schall JI, Kawchak DA, et al. No improvement in suboptimal vitamin A status with a randomized, double-blind, placebo-controlled trial of vitamin A supplementation in children with sickle cell disease. *Am J Clin Nutr.* 2012;96(4):932–940

72. Chiu D, Vichinsky E, Yee M, Kleman K, Lubin B. Peroxidation, vitamin E and sickle cell anemia. *Ann N Y Acad Sci.* 1982;393:323–335

73. Pfeifer WP, Degasperi GR, Almeida MT, Vercesi AE, Costa FF, Saad ST. Vitamin E supplementation reduces oxidative stress in beta thalassemia intermedia. *Acta Haematol.* 2008;10(4):225–231

74. Walter PB, Fung EB, Killilea DW, et al. Oxidative stress and inflammation in iron-overloaded patients with beta-thalassaemia or sickle cell disease. *Br J Haematol.* 2006;135(2):254–263

75. Tesoriere L, D'Arpa D, Butera D, et al. Oral supplements of vitamin E improve measures of oxidative stress in plasma and reduce oxidative damage to LDL and erythrocytes in beta-thalassemia intermedia patients. *Free Radic Res.* 2001;34(5):529–540

76. Kajanchumpol S, Tatu T, Sasanakul W, Chuansumrit A, Hathirat P. Zinc and copper status of thalassemic children. *Southeast Asian J Trop Med Public Health.* 1997;28(4):877–880

77. Uysal Z, Akar N, Kemahli S, Dincer N, Arcasoy A. Desferrioxamine and urinary zinc excretion in b-thalassemia major. *Pediatr Hematol Oncol.* 1993;10(3):257–260

78. Arcasoy A, Cavdar A, Cin S, et al. Effects of zinc supplementation on linear growth in beta thalassemia (a new approach). *Am J Hematol.* 1987;24(2):127–136

79. Shamshirsaz AA, Bekheirnia MR, Kamgar M, et al. Bone mineral density in Iranian adolescents and young adults with beta-thalassemia major. *Pediatr Hematol Oncol.* 2007;24(7):469–479

80. Dehshal MH, Hooghooghi AH, Kebryaeezadeh A, et al. Zinc deficiency aggravates abnormal glucose metabolism in thalassemia major patients. *Med Sci Monit.* 2007;13(5):CR235–CR239

81. Prasad AS, Schoomaker EB, Ortega J, Brewer GJ, Oberleas D, Oelshlegel FJ. Zinc deficiency in sickle cell disease. *Clin Chem.* 1975;21(4):582–587

VI

82. Prasad AS. Zinc deficiency in patients with sickle cell disease. *Am J Clin Nutr.* 2002;75(2):181–182

83. Zemel BS, Kawchak DA, Fung EB, Ohene-Frempong K, Stallings V. Effect of zinc supplementation on growth and body composition in children with sickle cell disease. *Am J Clin Nutr.* 2002;75(2):300–307

84. Prasad AS, Abbasi AA, Rabbani P, DuMouchelle E. Effect of zinc supplementation on serum testosterone level in adult male sickle cell anemia subjects. *Am J Hematol.* 1981;10(2):119–127

85. Prasad AS, Beck F, Kaplan J, et al. Effect of zinc supplementation on incidence of infections and hospital admissions in sickle cell disease. *Am J Hematol.* 1999;61(3):194–202

86. Aloni MN, Lecerf P, Lê PQ, et al. Is pica under-reported in children with sickle cell disease? A pilot study in a Belgian cohort. *Hematology.* 2015;20(7):429–432

87. Ivascu NS, Sarnaik S, McCrae J, Whitten-Shurney W, Thomas R, Bond S. Characterization of pica prevalence among patients with sickle cell disease. *Arch Pediatr Adolesc Med.* 2001;155(11):1243–1247

88. Badiee MS, Nili-Ahmadabadi H, Zeinvand-Lorestani H. Green tea consumption improves the therapeutic efficacy of deferoxamine on iron overload in patients with beta-thalassemia major: a randomized clinical study. *Biol Forum.* 2015;7(2): 383–387

89. Buison AM, Kawchak DA, Schall JI, et al. Bone area and bone mineral content deficits in children with sickle cell disease. *Pediatrics.* 2005;116(4):943–949

90. National Heart, Lung, and Blood Institute. *The Management of Sickle Cell Disease.* Washington, DC: National Institutes of Health; 2004

91. Cappellini MD, Cohen A, Eleftheriou A, et al. Guidelines for the Management of Transfusion Dependent Thalassemia. Nicosia, Cyprus: Thalassemia International Federation; 2014: Available at: https://www.ncbi.nlm.nih.gov/books/NBK269382/. Accessed April 10, 2019

92. Northern California Comprehensive Thalassemia Center. Nutrition. *Standard-of-Care Clinical Practice Guidelines.* Oakland, CA: Northern California Comprehensive Thalassemia Center; 2012: Available at: http://hemonc.cho.org/thalassemia/treatment-guidelines-16.aspx. Accessed March 18, 2019

Chapter 40

Nutrition in Renal Disease

Introduction

Children with normal renal function have great latitude in day-to day nutritional intake, but those who have renal disease often require significant nutritional guidance to support their nutrient needs. Nutritional management of infants and children with renal disease requires an understanding not only of the primary renal disease but also evaluation of the family dynamic surrounding daily eating patterns. Nutritional management of such children is best accomplished as a collaborative effort of a skilled pediatric renal dietitian and other members of the pediatric nephrology team.

The dietary prescription for a patient with renal disease is not static and changes in parallel with gradual loss in glomerular filtration rate (GFR) and corresponding filtration capacity or urine production. With the diverse array of renal disease in children, there is no universal nutritional prescription that can be comprehensively recommended—that is, a singular "renal diet" does not exist. Rather, nutrition in pediatric renal disease must be tailored to the underlying disease, the stage of renal function, and the underlying glomerular and tubular physiology. And unlike adults with renal disease, more than half of children with renal disease have excess fluid loss attributable to abnormal tubular function; these children may need far more fluid than children with normal renal function to maintain an appropriate fluid balance for euvolemia.

Lastly, the effects of neurodevelopmental status (including oro-motor skills), uremia-associated dysgeusia and anorexia, and potential socioeconomic limitations to adequate nutritional sources must also be taken into consideration when developing a dietary prescription for patients with complex needs. In fact, nutrition is often the most challenging aspect of these diseases for families to manage. The entire family is often focused on getting adequate calories and fluids into a small child who simply cannot or will not take what is required by mouth or without emesis.

This chapter reviews nutritional considerations for patients with nephrolithiasis, hypertension, nephrotic syndrome, acute glomerulonephritis, acute kidney injury, and chronic kidney disease. Special populations, including end-stage renal disease requiring dialysis and transplant, are also reviewed briefly.

The Food and Nutrition Board of the Institute of Medicine (now National Academy of Medicine) has presented nutritional standards in the form of Dietary Reference Intakes (DRIs). Previously, this information was presented as Recommended Dietary Allowances (RDAs). For the nutrients to be discussed in this chapter, the term RDA is used when describing experimental results performed using RDAs as standards, and the term DRI is used when noting current standard values. Whenever possible, evidence-based recommendations for nutritional support are provided, and controlled studies are cited. Unfortunately, critical studies in children are often lacking; therefore, studies performed in adults are referenced.

Nutritional Assessment and Needs in Renal Disease

Accurate nutritional assessment in the pediatric renal patient requires longitudinal attention to laboratory and growth measures by a multidisciplinary medical team including physician, nursing, and dietitian/nutrition staff. Key markers of growth include height (or length in children younger than 2 years or those unable to stand without assistance), head circumference (in children younger than 3 years), and weight. These measurements should be plotted on standardized growth charts for age and/or preexisting condition (eg, preterm infant status and various syndromes) and followed serially for growth trends.

Comprehensive growth evaluation requires an understanding of the patient's ideal or estimated "dry weight." Dry weight represents a target, stable weight that the medical team could expect in a euvolemic person with normal renal function. Dry weight is most critical in a patient receiving dialysis but can be challenging in others with renal disease. In establishing a dry weight, the team must allow for interval weekly growth in the youngest of patients receiving dialysis; thus, close communication between the dialysis nursing and dietitian teams with physician staff is necessary to provide adequate fluid and calories for growth.

Routine laboratory studies are key components for assessing nutritional adequacy in renal disease. Serum albumin is most often used as a surrogate for nutritional protein status. Hypoalbuminemia may also be noted in urinary protein losing disease-states such as nephrotic syndrome or during episodes of peritonitis for those on peritoneal dialysis; in these conditions, serum albumin concentration may be a difficult measure of nutritional status. Blood urea nitrogen (BUN) concentration can also be used to understand protein intake status. A low BUN concentration together with elevated creatinine (eg, progressive renal disease) is suggestive of inadequate protein intake and/or significant malnutrition.

Enteral Nutrition and Fluid Provision

Individuals with normal renal function have great latitude in the quantity (and quality) of the nutrients they can ingest. Those with kidney disease have less flexibility in their nutritional choices because of decreased renal excretion and/or increased renal tubular losses. Nutritional renal prescriptions can be complex, and it is often necessary to increase the intake of some nutrients (for example, higher protein-energy needs; see Table 40.1). Conversely, some electrolytes may be restricted while others are supplemented to support cellular homeostasis and growth. Oral aversion and decreased appetite are frequently reported symptoms in advanced chronic kidney disease (CKD).[1,2] For young children and infants, supplemental enteral nutrition may be required to meet nutritional goals if energy intakes are otherwise inadequate to prevent further growth delays.[3,4] Energy requirements for children with CKD should be targeted to 100% of the estimated energy requirement for age with adjustment as appropriate for body size and response in rate of weight gain or loss.[5] In many cases, placement of a gastrostomy tube is necessary given the long-term nutritional and fluid requirements of this population, even following transplantation. A variety of specialized formulas exists for infants, children, and young adults with renal disease and should be used with the assistance of an experienced renal dietitian (see Table 40.2).

Fluid needs may be variable depending on the underlying renal disease. In the case of nonoliguric CKD, fluid needs may be significantly greater than typically estimated for age/size given the lack of tubular concentrating ability. Infants and young children with nonoliguric CKD may require substantial water intake to compensate for urinary losses, and this can hinder the ability to meet complete calorie goals by mouth and reinforcing the need for a gastrostomy tube in these children.

Nutritional Considerations in Specific Renal Conditions

Nephrolithiasis

The incidence of nephrolithiasis in pediatric patients has increased in the past 20 years with some speculation that this increase is related to the increased prevalence of obesity, hypertension, and diabetes in the pediatric population.[6,7] Most renal stones are formed of calcium and oxalate; less commonly, cystine or uric acid are the primary constituents of renal stones in pediatric patients.

VI

Table 40.1.
Recommended Energy and Protein Intakes in Children With Chronic Kidney Disease and End-Stage Renal Disease[5,74]

Age	Predialysis		Hemodialysis		Peritoneal Dialysis	
	Energy[a]	Protein[b]	Energy[a]	Protein[b,c]	Energy[a,d]	Protein[b,e]
0–6 mo	100–110	2.2	100–110	2.6	100–110	3
6–12 mo	95–105	1.5	95–105	2	95–105	2.4
1–3 y	90	1.1	90	1.6	90	2.0
4–10 y	70	0.95	70	1.6	70	1.8–2.0
11–14 y (boys)	55	0.95	55	1.4	55	1.8
11–14 y (girls)	47	0.95	47	1.4	47	1.8
15–18 y (boys)	45	0.85	45	1.3	45	1.5
15–18 y (girls)	40	0.85	40	1.2	40	1.5

[a] kcal/kg/day.

[b] g/kg/day.

[c] Protein intakes increased by approximately 0.4 g/kg/day to account for hemodialysis losses.

[d] Note: up to 10% of the total caloric intake (10 kcal/kg/day) can be absorbed as dextrose via the dialysate. Obesity may become a concern for some children and adolescents on peritoneal dialysis.

[e] Protein requirements on peritoneal dialysis reflect the significant loss of proteins through the dialysis fluid.

Table 40.2.

Nutrient Content of Selected Renal Formulas[a]

| Content per 100 mL | gm/100 mL | | | mg (mEq)/100 mL | | | |
	CHO	Fat	Pro	Na	K	Ca	P
Standard formula	7.2	3.8	1.4	16 (0.7)	71 (1.8)	53 (2.6)	28
Similac PM 60/40	6.9	3.8	1.5	16 (0.7)	54 (1.4)	38 (1.9)	19
Calcilo	52.3	28.7	11.4	125 (5.4)	420 (10.7)	<50 mg	128
Suplena[b]	20	9.6	4.5	80 (3.5)	114 (2.9)	105 (5.3)	72
Nepro[b]	16	9.6	8.1	106 (4.6)	106 (2.7)	106 (5.3)	72

Ca indicates calcium; CHO, carbohydrate; K, potassium; Na, sodium; P, phosphorous; Pro, protein. Carbohydrate, fat, and protein calories in g/100 mL. Electrolyte composition in mg (mEq)/100 mL.

[a] Content value from individual formulas can be compared to percent daily recommended intake needs for patient age and gender as seen on Table 40.1.

[b] Denotes a formula often used in adult dialysis populations but can be utilized in the pediatric setting as indicated by nutritional needs.

Renal sodium reabsorption is linked to the reabsorption of urine calcium. Sodium-restricted diets should be advised, because high sodium intakes lead to increased sodium excretion with subsequent increases in excretion of elements such as calcium. Thus, a high-water, low-sodium diet (defined as less than 1000–1500 mg sodium for children weighing less than 20 kg and less than 2000–2500 mg for children weighing more than 20 kg) is recommended as first-line therapy. When a high-fluid, low-sodium diet is insufficient to improve urinary calcium excretion and stone formation continues, a distal tubule (thiazide) diuretic may be required. There is *no role for dietary calcium restriction*, and conversely, dietary calcium should be provided at the level of the DRI (see Table 40.3). Furthermore, children experiencing nephrolithiasis are more likely to have hypocitraturia and may also benefit from urinary alkalinization in addition to increased fluid volume intakes.[8]

Hyperoxaluria can be divided into primary (hereditary) and secondary (enteric/dietary) forms. In primary hyperoxaluria, there is no indication to limit dietary oxalate. In secondary hyperoxaluria and/or hypercalciuria with

Table 40.3.
Select Dietary Reference Intakes (DRIs) for Healthy Individual Infants, Children, and Adolescents[74]

	Protein (g/d)	Protein g/kg/d	Sodium g/d	Phosphorous mg/d	Calcium mg/d	Potassium g/d
Infants						
0–6 mo	9.1	1.5	0.12	100	210	0.4
7–12 mo	**11**	**1.5**	0.37	275	270	0.7
Children						
1–3 y	**13**	**1.1**	1	**460**	500	3
4–8 y	**19**	**0.95**	1.2	**500**	800	3.8
Males						
9–13 y	**34**	**0.95**	1.5	**1250**	1300	4.5
14–18 y	**52**	**0.85**	1.5	**1250**	1300	4.7
Females						
9–13 y	**34**	**0.95**	1.5	1250	1300	4.5
14–18 y	**46**	**0.85**	1.5	1250	1300	4.7

Unbolded values are adequate intake (AI) the recommended average daily intake level based on observed or experimentally determined approximations or estimates of nutrient intake by a group (or groups) of apparently healthy people that are assumed to be adequate—used when an DRI cannot be determined.

Values in **bold** typeface are listed as the DRI – adequate for 97.5% of the population.

Table 40.4.
Foods With High Oxalate Content[75]

Spinach
Rhubarb
Beets
Nuts
Chocolate
Tea
Wheat bran
Strawberries

mild hyperoxaluria, it is advisable to avoid high-oxalate food (see Table 40.4) if the patient has experienced symptomatic oxalate stone formation.[9,10] Dietary calcium should be optimized, because any inadvertent restriction can augment oxalate absorption in secondary hyperoxaluria.[11] Excessive vitamin C intake (more than 100 mg/day) should be discouraged as vitamin C can be converted to oxalate in alkaline urine.

Although there are many conditions that predispose children to renal stones, common therapeutic interventions exist. In all cases, a high fluid intake is the primary intervention. Specifically, the volume of fluid intake should be adjusted to maintain urine volume greater than 750 mL/day for infants, greater than 1000 mL/day for children younger than 5 years, greater than 1500 mL/day for children between 5 and 10 years, and more than 2000 mL/day for children older than 10 years.[12] To avoid excess calorie intake from increased fluid needs, the primary fluid should come from water and/or low-calorie flavored water (expert opinion-based recommendation). Children should meet their daily nutritional goal for protein intake without specific restriction or excess. Sources of fresh fruit and vegetables should be encouraged as the citrate and potassium found in these foods serve as urinary stone inhibitors.

Hypertension

Data continue to support a strong association between childhood obesity and risk for hypertension.[13] Body weights track from childhood through adulthood, and there is evidence that obesity (also characterized by increased body mass index [BMI]) is related to development of essential hypertension in children.[14–16] Dietary modification aimed at weight stabilization (or gradual weight loss in the older adolescent) to normalize BMI is appropriate.[17] Specific nutritional modifications for reduction in blood pressure are aligned with the "DASH" (Dietary Approaches to Stop Hypertension) eating plan. The DASH diet is a low-fat, high-potassium dietary strategy that has been associated with modest weight loss and significant decreases in blood pressure in pediatric and adult cohorts.[18,19] See Table 40.5 for a description of the DASH eating plan. In adults, lowering sodium intake has an additive effect on the decrease in blood pressure seen with the DASH diet.[20,21] Data from the National Health and Nutrition Examination Survey (NHANES) IV revealed that more than 90% of adolescents and adults in the United States consume sodium in excess of the DRI.[22] The Institute of Medicine, through its Food and Nutrition Board, recommended an upper limit for sodium intake of approximately 1.5 to 2 g/day in otherwise healthy children beginning at around 3 years of age (Table 40.3).[23] A meta-analysis of trials conducted in children suggested that

Table 40.5.

Description of the Dietary Approach to Stop Hypertension (DASH) Eating Plan[76]

The DASH plan is often considered flexible and balanced – it requires no special foods. Participants are encouraged to choose foods that are rich in potassium, calcium, magnesium, fiber and protein but low in sodium, low in fat.

Food Group	Servings per Day (based on a 2000 calorie per day diet)
Grains	6–8
Meat, poultry, fish	6 or less
Vegetables	4–5
Fruit	4–5
Low-fat, fat-free dairy	2–3
Fats and oils	2–3
Sodium	2300 mg (1500 mg intake lowers blood pressure to a greater extent than 2300 milligram DASH diet)
	Servings per Week
Nuts, seeds, peas, dry beans	4–5
Sweets	Less than 5

sodium reduction can lower mean systolic and diastolic blood pressure by 1.2 and 1.3 mm Hg, respectively.[24] Depending on the child's usual sodium intake, limiting sodium intake to 2 to 3 g/day may be a reasonable starting point if sodium intake is excessive at baseline. Encouraging a diet high in fruits and vegetables is appropriate as a means of increasing dietary potassium intake and is safe in individuals with normal renal function. However, in people with significant renal impairment, potassium intake should be carefully monitored and/or modified.

Nephrotic Syndrome

Nephrotic syndrome is defined clinically by the presence of proteinuria, hypoalbuminemia, edema, and hypercholesterolemia. The mainstay of dietary therapy for children with nephrotic syndrome is sodium restriction, which serves to palliate symptomatic edema. Although no studies have defined the optimal level to which sodium should be restricted in these children, reasonable strategies and daily dietary sodium estimates are noted in Table 40.6. This level of sodium restriction requires lifestyle adjustment for patients and their families—specifically, limiting processed foods and eliminating salted snack foods. A limited sodium diet is important during times when the patient is nephrotic (to help limit edema formation) and while the patient is on steroids (to limit possible hypertension). The majority of pediatric patients respond to corticosteroids and can be weaned from them within 3 to 6 months. Unfortunately, most will relapse and require the reinstitution of steroid therapy. A minority of children will require the use of additional/other medications to limit proteinuria and keep them edema free. Additional therapy may include angiotensin-converting enzyme (ACE) inhibitors or angiotensin receptor blockers, either of which may lead to hyperkalemia, in which case, dietary potassium restriction may be indicated.

Because of the risk for relapse of nephrotic syndrome, it is reasonable practice to counsel families to adopt a low-sodium lifestyle even with remission of nephrotic syndrome. However, many families may have a misconception about the role of sodium intake, so it is helpful for them to understand that sodium intake does not cause relapse nor remission.

Children with severe edema may sometimes need to be hospitalized for aggressive fluid removal. One common error is the simultaneous provision of intravenous "maintenance" or "partial maintenance" fluids in the patient with severe hypoalbuminemia. In the absence of intravascular volume depletion, there is no need to provide intravenous fluids, and unnecessary

Table 40.6.
Reasonable Starting Points for Dietary Modification in Renal Disease

Overview	Evaluating patient and family lifestyle eating patterns may reveal areas that can be improved without limiting all sources of the nutrient in question. Ongoing nutritional follow-up is important to monitor nutrient intake and assess adequacy
	Obtain a detailed diet history to determine current food and beverage intake. All diet changes are based on evaluation of this current intake. Focus on decreasing the amount of frequently-consumed high sources of elevated nutrients.
	Resist the temptation to restrict nutrients until there is a need demonstrated.
	The word "low" in front of a nutrient ("low sodium," "low potassium") is not a diet order. Be specific (suggestions below). "Renal diet" is not a diet order.
	Selective micronutrient restrictions may result in the patient refusing to consume adequate amounts of macronutrients (calories, protein, and fat). Follow-up is important to ensure adequacy of intake to meet growth needs.
	Limit as few nutrients as possible to optimize intake.

Nutrient	Possible Diet Order	Description	Recommended Starting Points			Comment
			Weight	Outpatient	Inpatient	
Sodium	3–4 g sodium (formerly No Added Salt)	Food is cooked with some salt; high sources such as pizza, hot dogs, and chips are limited or avoided	<20 kg	Begin with 2 g/day	1 g/day	A sodium restriction will automatically decrease fat intake in most children

	Restriction level	Food preparation / sources	Pediatric recommendation	Notes
	2 g sodium	Food is prepared with no salt; high sources are eliminated.	Begin with 3 g/day; >20 kg: 2 g/day	
	1 g sodium	Food is prepared with no salt; low-sodium products are used exclusively		
Potassium	Limit food sources with high potassium content	Foods high in potassium include citrus, bananas, potatoes.	Limit only high sources of potassium child is currently eating/drinking	Correct acidosis, bleeding, and other potential causes of elevated potassium. Potassium binding agents may be required.
Phosphorus	800 mg/day	High sources are limited to 8 ounces of milk/day or the phosphorus equivalent of cheese, yogurt, ice cream, beans, nuts	Start with 800 mg/day, smaller children will consume less because of smaller portion sizes	Infants require higher serum phosphorus levels for adequate bone mineralization. Start phosphorus binders with meals as necessary. A phosphorus limitation will automatically limit protein and potassium intake.
Protein	Regular diet	Highest sources include meat, poultry, fish, egg, dairy products	Start with a diet history to determine need for supplementation.	Children with rising blood urea nitrogen (BUN) levels rarely consume more than the DRI due to poor appetite and phosphorus restriction. Ensure adequate calorie intake for protein-sparing; otherwise BUN may be elevated because of protein catabolism. Protein needs are elevated in dialysis.

VI

salt and water administration should be avoided. When using diuretic therapy to reestablish euvolemia in the nephrotic patient, the family should be given a daily fluid goal/limit to ensure that the child is receiving adequate enteral hydration while avoiding an excess that might cause rebound edema and weight gain.

Hypercholesterolemia is common in patients with nephrotic syndrome, both as a component of the nephrotic syndrome itself and as an adverse effect of steroid administration. The medical and dietary approach to children with persistent nephrotic syndrome and resultant hyperlipidemia remains a dilemma. Although there is evidence that use of statin-based therapy lowers total cholesterol and low-density lipoprotein concentrations, there is currently no consensus as to the best approach to the treatment of hyperlipidemia in the young child with nephrotic syndrome. Prolonged hyperlipidemia is a recognized cardiovascular risk factor; however, it does not appear that the transient hypercholesterolemia seen in children who have recovered from the nephrotic syndrome has any negative effect on cardiovascular mortality later in life.[25] Given that the outcome of nephrotic syndrome (with coincident steroid use) for an individual child is difficult to predict, attention to dietary lipid content is prudent, and care may involve restriction of dietary fat to 30% of daily energy intake (see Chapter 17: Fats and Fatty Acids). Treatment with a statin is typically not necessary.

Given the association between steroid use and both weight gain and hypertension, all patients can benefit from nutritional counseling with initial clinical assessment at the time of presentation. This counseling should include warnings about the risk for steroid-associated obesity, strategies to avoid rapid weight gain, and careful weight monitoring throughout the course of steroids.

Glomerulonephritis

Clinically, glomerulonephritis (GN) is characterized by the presence of both hematuria and proteinuria. The care of children with GN is dependent on whether the condition is acute or chronic as well as on the presence of associated findings, such as hypertension or nephrotic syndrome.

In the case of acute GN (such as acute postinfectious GN), there is a risk for rapid loss of GFR over the first few days that may lead to hypertension (from salt and water overload) and hyperkalemia. These children may benefit from limitation of sodium and potassium in their diets, whether they are to be managed as inpatients or outpatients. They should usually be allowed to drink fluids according to their thirst, as "pushing fluids" will not improve outcome and excess limitation of oral fluids may contribute to loss of GFR.

The nutritional management of GN depends on maintenance or loss of renal function; electrolytes should be monitored closely. If nephrosis is also present, hyperlipidemia is likely as mentioned previously, but will likely not need to be addressed acutely.

Nutrition as Therapy for Acute Kidney Injury

Acute kidney injury (AKI) describes a spectrum ranging from mild injury to major renal impairment potentially requiring dialysis. Causes of AKI are broad—for example: prerenal hypoperfusion injury, intrinsic (tubular) nephrotoxin exposure, and obstructive (postrenal) lesions preventing urinary outflow. AKI is increasingly recognized as a common medical complication in both critically ill and noncritically ill pediatric patients,[26] occurring in up to 3.9/1000 at-risk hospitalized pediatric patients in the United States.[27] For the critically ill and medically complex pediatric patient, acute and chronic malnutrition are very unfortunate and common phenomena in pediatric AKI, with data suggesting a significant lag in adequate provision of dietary energy and/or protein in a substantial percentage of these patients.[28] Underfeeding carries significant risk for morbidity and mortality with worse wound healing outcomes and higher risk of infection.[29,30] Nutritional goals in individuals with AKI include maintaining appropriate hydration and electrolyte balance, providing adequate energy intake, optimizing nitrogen balance, and providing appropriate vitamin and mineral supplementation.[31,32] With the widespread availability of pediatric dialysis in most major medical centers, it is now possible to provide adequate nutritional intake for the majority of infants and children with AKI in combination with appropriately used dialysis therapy. Indeed, the need to provide nutrition serves as an important indication for starting renal replacement therapies.

AKI may either be associated with low levels of urinary water output (oliguria/anuria) or with normal or even increased urine volumes (nonoliguria). In general, patients with AKI cannot adjust urine output effectively, and the physician will be called on to manage fluid intakes to prevent either volume overload or depletion. Furthermore, the patient with AKI is often unable to control the excretion of metabolic wastes, such as urea, sodium, potassium, phosphorus, and acids/bases. Specific dietary requirements will depend on the clinical circumstances. Individuals with oligoanuria who are not clinically volume overloaded should receive daily fluid intakes equivalent to their urine output plus estimated insensible water loss.

Electrolyte requirements may change on a day-to-day basis in AKI and require careful attention with individual prescription. Potassium and phosphate intakes are often restricted, with allowable intakes based on the clinical setting. If oral restriction of potassium and/or phosphorus (especially in the chronic setting) does not provide adequate improvement in laboratory status, the use of "binding agents" may be necessary. Typical enteral binding agents include sodium polystyrene sulfonate (potassium binding), calcium carbonate, and/or sevelamer hydrochloride (phosphorus binding). Of note, aggressive polystyrene sulfonate administration may result in hypomagnesemia and hypocalcemia; furthermore, caution should be exercised in rectal use of polystyrene sulfonate in the acute postoperative period following bowel surgeries, for patients with neutropenia, and those at risk for necrotizing enterocolitis.

Protein and Carbohydrate Metabolism in Acute Kidney Injury

AKI is associated with activation of net protein catabolism with excessive release of amino acids from skeletal muscle, leading to a sustained negative nitrogen balance.[33] Furthermore, the tubular brush border of the kidney plays a key role in peptide and protein clearance. With AKI, diminished clearance of these protein molecules may lead to increased tubular inflammation and may further drive the AKI process.

Varying recommendations exist regarding minimal protein intake in pediatric AKI; however, a **minimum protein intake** (typically 1–2 g/kg/day) to meet the child's basal needs is suggested to minimize protein catabolism.[34–36] Additional factors that may be important in slowing excessive protein catabolism include stabilization of endocrine abnormalities (specifically hyperglycemia and providing insulin when applicable) and correcting metabolic acidosis to avoid additional muscle protein breakdown and oxidation.[37,38]

Hyperglycemia is a common phenomenon in critically ill children. The odds of AKI increase 12% for every peak in glycemia by 10 mg/dL,[39] likely because of hyperglycemia-driven oxidative damage at the renal mitochondrial level. As such, insulin may be warranted in multimodal care for the patient with AKI.

Use of Enteral and Parenteral Nutrition in Acute Kidney Injury

For pediatric patients with AKI hospitalized in the general pediatric unit, it may be reasonable to expect that they will maintain oral intake without supplemental nutritional support. However, children with AKI who are more ill appearing and remain hospitalized in the general pediatric unit (eg, young children with fever, sepsis, postsurgical pain) may require supplemental nutrition to meet basal metabolic needs to prevent excessive catabolism, as outlined previously. Whenever possible, enteral nutrition should be used, but depending on the child's age and ability to tolerate enteral nutrition or to ingest solid foods, parenteral nutrition may be necessary.

A variety of "renal-friendly formulas" exist (see Table 40.2) that have both high energy and protein content but typically lower phosphorus and/or potassium content. In the case of inadequate oral intake, the family should be counseled about placement of a temporary nasogastric tube to facilitate provision of adequate nutrition. Existing data suggest that advancement of enteral nutrition in AKI may be associated with higher gastric residual volumes; therefore, enteral nutrition should be initiated at slow rates to observe for tolerance.[40] Prokinetic and/or antiemetic agents may be required.

When providing parenteral nutrition for the child with AKI, the solution used must be complete and must contain all essential micronutrients, specifically water-soluble vitamins and selenium. As noted, there is aberrant glucose tolerance in AKI, and parenteral nutrition should be prescribed to ensure euglycemia, as outlined previously.

Nutritional Losses With RRT

Dialysis therapies may be required in severe AKI—for example, hemodialysis, peritoneal dialysis, and continuous renal replacement therapy. A key indication for dialysis in pediatric patients is the inability to provide adequate nutrition because of the presence of fluid overload. With the increasingly widespread availability of pediatric dialysis modalities, it is now possible to provide appropriate nutritional intake for the majority of infants and children with AKI while addressing concerns of fluid overload with provision of full nutrition.

All patients requiring dialysis for any appreciable period of time should receive a water-soluble vitamin supplement, especially if there is any concern for preexisting inadequacy in nutritional status, because of the risk for acute water-soluble vitamin depletion.[5] Filtration-based modalities of dialysis (eg, hemodialysis and continuous renal replacement therapy) carry higher risk for acute thiamine depletion compared with peritoneal dialysis in patients who have poor nutritional status. In either case, water-soluble vitamin supplementation is indicated.

VI

Nutrition in Advanced Chronic Kidney Disease

Current terminology divides CKD into 5 categories (Table 40.7). When renal function declines to a GFR of <60 mL/min/1.73 m² (stage 3 CKD), changes in blood chemistries become apparent and growth failure becomes more likely. In young children, changes in growth rate may be seen as early as stage 2 CKD (GFR 60–89 mL/min/1.73 m²). The National Kidney Foundation Kidney Disease Outcomes Quality Initiative has published consensus nutrition guidelines for the care of children with CKD. These data are presented broadly here, but the recommendations themselves are beyond the scope of this chapter.[5]

Intensive nutritional intervention and assessment is required for this population, particularly in the smallest of patients, when rapid growth and development occurring within the first 2 years of life are very nutrition dependent.[3] After 1 to 2 years of age, growth retardation associated with CKD is usually amenable to use of growth hormone therapy, but nutrition still needs to be optimized to achieve that benefit. In counseling parents of older children with CKD, it is important to note that food frequency data suggest that dietary sources of energy, protein, and sodium intake in this population are heavily driven by consumption of milk and fast foods.[41] For

Table 40.7.

National Kidney Foundation Kidney Disease Outcomes Quality Initiative Classification of the Stages of Chronic Kidney Disease (CKD)[77]

Stage	GFR (mL/min/ 1.73 m²)	Description	Action Plan
1	≥90	Kidney damage with normal or increased GFR	Treat primary and comorbid conditions Slow CKD progression, CVD risk reduction
2	60–89	Kidney damage with mild reduction of GFR	Estimate rate of progression of CKD
3	30–59	Moderate reduction of GFR	Evaluate and treat complications
4	15–29	Severe reduction of GFR	Prepare for kidney replacement therapy
5	<5	Kidney failure	Kidney replacement therapy

GFR indicates glomerular filtration rate; CVD, cardiovascular disease.

a subset of patients, frequency of eating from fast-food options raises the long-term risk for obesity-associated progression of CKD[42] and potential for complications such as metabolic syndrome into adulthood.

Protein Energy and Calorie Needs

Spontaneous food (and therefore energy) intake declines with progression of CKD so that significant undernutrition and lean body mass wasting are often seen in advanced renal disease.[43,44] Energy intake should, therefore, be supplemented to provide approximately 100% of the daily estimated energy expenditure for chronologic age, activity level, and body size.[5] Protein intake should be at least 100% of the DRI (see Table 40.3) for age and body size in CKD, with some patients with advanced CKD requiring up to 140% of the DRI for protein (see Table 40.1). In pediatric patients, there is no evidence that restricting protein intake is effective at delaying progression of renal disease or time to dialysis initiation.[45-47] With the progression of CKD to more severe stages, the use of dietary enteral feeding in combination with protein powder supplementation may be required for children who are unable to meet recommended daily goals for age with spontaneous food or enteral/fluid intake, and tube feeding may be necessary to provide full nutrition for growth.

Acidosis

Maintenance of normal serum bicarbonate concentrations is vital for growth in pediatric patients with CKD. The National Kidney Foundation Kidney Disease Outcomes Quality Initiative recommends that serum bicarbonate concentrations be maintained at 22 mmol/L or greater.[5] Acidosis is believed to contribute to protein energy wasting[48] with additional deleterious effects on bone and statural growth and to have a possible role in hastening the progression of CKD.[49] Physiologic bicarbonate supplementation appears to slow the progression of CKD and improves nutritional status.[50] Acidosis should be treated with enteral sodium bicarbonate or sodium citrate solutions.

Bone Mineral Status

Calcium and phosphorus homeostasis is a complex interplay between calcium, phosphate, vitamin D, parathyroid hormone, and the phosphate-controlling hormone fibroblast growth factor 23 (FGF-23; see also Chapter 18: Calcium, Phosphorous, and Magnesium). At baseline, nearly 30% of children with mild to moderate CKD have 25-hydroxyvitamin D (25-OH-D) deficiency (<20 ng/mL) that is associated with potentially modifiable dietary risk factors such as low daily milk intake and low nutritional vitamin D supplementation.[51] Vitamin D concentrations should be maintained in the normal range (>20 ng/mL) by supplementation of vitamin D_2 or vitamin D_3. Hypocalcemia is a primary feature of untreated, late CKD secondary to decreased hydroxylation of 25-OH-D to active 1,25-dihydroxyvitamin D (1,25-OH-$_2$D) within the renal tubular cells. Most patients with stage 3 through 5 CKD will achieve better bone health with supplementation of enteral calcitriol (1,25-OH-$_2$D).

Phosphorus excretion is dependent on native GFR and tubular function; therefore, urinary phosphorus excretion decreases with progressive CKD.[52] When serum phosphate concentrations are elevated, restriction to 80% of the DRI is suggested (Table 40.3). In practice, patients with CKD stages 4 and 5 may require an enteral phosphorus binding agent to decrease the total amount of dietary phosphorus absorbed and prevent hyperphosphatemia. Examples of phosphate binders include sevelamer and various calcium carbonate preparations. Table 40.6 reviews dietary mechanisms of phosphorus reduction. Poor control of serum calcium and phosphorus concentrations is associated with hyperparathyroidism, the development of metabolic bone disease, and an increased risk of systemic cardiovascular calcifications.[53,54] FGF-23 is a key hormone involved in bone-mineral homeostasis via modulation of renal phosphate handling, regulation of parathyroid hormone concentrations, and calcitriol production. In patients with CKD, FGF-23 levels increase with declining renal function. Adult data suggest that higher FGF-23 levels are linked to accelerated atherosclerosis rates[55] as well as aberrancy in dynamic measurements of vascular function—specifically, arterial stiffness and endothelial dysfunction.[56]

Sodium Supplementation

One subset of children with chronic renal failure requires special mention—infants and toddlers with nonoliguric (polyuric) CKD, usually as a result of severe congenital hydronephrosis, posterior urethral valves, or renal dysplasia. These children may not be able to conserve sodium or bicarbonate because of impaired nephrogenesis/tubular maturation acquired prenatally. They often require significant sodium chloride and alkali supplementation for growth.[57] Animal data demonstrate substantial gains in growth following provision of a sodium replete diet (in contrast to a sodium-deficient diet) in early life.[58] Signs of sodium depletion are often subtle and include failure to gain weight despite adequate caloric intake, hyperkalemia, and mild hypochloremia. In these children, it is reasonable to initiate supplementation with approximately 2 to 3 mEq/kg/day of sodium chloride.

Substantially greater amounts of sodium may be necessary to ensure optimal growth. Sodium bicarbonate cannot substitute for sodium chloride to restore intravascular volume, and underlying severe acidosis may not be apparent until the infants receive sufficient (replete) sodium chloride. Supplementation should be slowed/stopped if the serum sodium concentration is greater than 140 mEq/L or the infant develops either hypertension or volume overload.

Special Populations

End-Stage Renal Disease Requiring Dialysis

There are 2 common forms of maintenance dialysis for children with end-stage renal disease—peritoneal dialysis and hemodialysis. The National Kidney Foundation Kidney Disease Outcomes Quality Initiative workgroup has separated its recommendations for these 2 dialysis types on the basis of available existing data.[5]

To date, there have been no randomized controlled trials examining the intake and/or needs of vitamins and trace elements in pediatric patients with CKD or end-stage renal disease. This lack of research leads to an absence of data on ideal vitamin and trace element intakes in infants and children with advanced renal disease, in contrast to well-defined standards for healthy children. It is suggested that pediatric dialysis patients receive a water-soluble vitamin supplement such that the combination of enteral nutrition and supplemental vitamin provision meet age- and gender-based values for DRIs in the general pediatric population (see Table 40.8) to reduce risk for development of adverse health-related conditions associated with vitamin deficiency.[5,59]

With the exception of vitamin D, there is no evidence to indicate that supplementation of fat-soluble vitamins is necessary in advanced renal disease. Vitamin D has a special role in the care of these children. Recent estimates suggest a marked increase in the diagnosis of 25-OH-D deficiency (<20 ng/mL) in the general pediatric population since the year 2000.[60] In contrast to the general pediatric population, the consequence of untreated vitamin D deficiency in CKD and end-stage renal disease is secondary hyperparathyroidism; therefore, current guidelines for the care of patients with advanced renal disease suggest the routine measurement of 25-OH-D concentrations and appropriate **supplementation to achieve a serum 25-OH-D concentration of ≥20 ng/mL.**[61] Vitamin A supplements should be specifically avoided, because vitamin A can accumulate in children with

VI

Table 40.8.

Suggested Dietary Allowance and Adequate Intake for Water-Soluble Vitamins and Trace Elements in the General Pediatric Population[5]

	Infants 0-6 mo	Infants 7-12 mo	Children 1-3 y	Children 4-8 y	Males 9-13 y	Males 14-18 y	Females 9-13 y	Females 14-18 y
Vitamin A (μg/d)	400	500	**300**	**400**	**600**	**900**	**600**	**700**
Vitamin C (mg/d)	40	50	**15**	**25**	**45**	**75**	**45**	**65**
Vitamin E (mg/d)	4	5	**6**	**7**	**11**	**15**	**11**	**15**
Vitamin K (μg/d)	2.0	2.5	30	55	60	75	60	75
Thiamin (mg/d)	0.2	0.3	**0.5**	**0.6**	**0.9**	**1.2**	**0.9**	**1.0**
Riboflavin (mg/d)	0.3	0.4	**0.5**	**0.6**	**0.9**	**1.3**	**0.9**	**1.0**
Niacin (mg/d; NE)	2*	4	**6**	**8**	**12**	**16**	**12**	**14**
Vitamin B$_6$ (mg/d)	0.1	0.3	**0.5**	**0.6**	**1.0**	**1.3**	**1.0**	**1.2**
Folate (μg/d)	65	80	**150**	**200**	**300**	**400**	**300**	**400**
Vitamin B$_{12}$ (μg/d)	0.4	0.5	**0.9**	**1.2**	**1.8**	**2.4**	**1.8**	**2.4**
Pantothenic acid (mg/d)	1.7	1.8	2	3	4	5	4	5
Biotin (μg/d)	5	6	8	12	20	25	20	25
Copper (μg/d)	200	220	**340**	**440**	**700**	**890**	**700**	**890**
Selenium (μg/d)	15	20	**20**	**30**	**40**	**55**	**40**	**55**
Zinc (mg/d)	2	3	**3**	**5**	**8**	**11**	**8**	**9**

Note: Recommended Dietary Allowances (RDAs) are in bold with adequate intakes in standard font (see also Appendix E).

CKD resulting in vitamin A toxicity.[62] Vitamin E is not necessary as a standard nutritional supplement.

Some pediatric dialysis patients who meet daily caloric goals through a combination of general diet and/or enteral formula supplements could actually meet or exceed the recommended 100% DRI for individual vitamins and trace elements through the use of adult multivitamin preparations occasionally given to children on dialysis because of the paucity of commercially available, dialysis-specific multivitamin supplement options available for pediatric use.[63,64] **Care should be taken not to greatly exceed 100% of the DRI for vitamin and trace element intake** (Table 40.8) because of the potential for toxicity with oversupplementation of vitamins for patients receiving dialysis. Table 40.9 highlights the vitamin and trace element content of commonly used enteral formulas in pediatric patients receiving dialysis.

Particular attention should be paid to folate, because folate depletion can limit the effectiveness of administered erythropoietin.

Hyperhomocysteinemia has been shown to be an independent predictor of heart disease. Although supplementation with vitamin B_6, folate, and vitamin B_{12} appears to lower homocysteine concentrations in patients with CKD including those having undergone transplantation, adult data do not support a long-term reduction in cardiovascular morbidity or mortality with resolution of hyperhomocysteinemia.[65]

Carnitine, a transporter of fatty acids, may be deficient in CKD, and carnitine supplementation has been suggested as a treatment for both anemia and hyperlipidemia.[66,67] Studies involving carnitine supplementation are difficult to interpret, in part because of the variability in dosing and delivery methods. There is little pediatric evidence available to support carnitine supplementation in pediatric patients, and routine supplementation is not recommended.[5,68,69]

Trace elements such as zinc and selenium are mineral substances that constitute less than 0.01% of the total human body weight. Daily requirements in adults are in the range of 1 to 100 mg/day.[59] Intact renal function is required for trace mineral homeostasis. Existing adult data suggest that for most individuals with renal disease, trace mineral supplements are not required. In individual clinical situations, it may be prudent to assess serum concentrations, particularly of selenium and zinc, as an approximation of body stores so that supplements can be provided as necessary.

Renal Transplant
Current immunosuppressive regimens for children after a renal transplant most often include the use of some combination of corticosteroids,

Table 40.9.
Vitamin and Trace Element Content of Commonly Used Enteral Formulas in Pediatric Dialysis Patients[a]

Content per 100 mL	Thiamine (B₁)	Pyridoxine (B₆)	Folate (B₉)	Vitamin C	Zinc	Selenium
Similac Standard	0.07 mg	0.04 mg	10.7 µg	6 mg	0.5 mg	1.67 µg
Gerber GoodStart Gentle	0.07 mg	0.05 mg	10 µg	6.7 mg	0.5 mg	2 µg
Similac PM 60/40	0.07 mg	0.04 mg	10 µg	6 mg	0.5 mg	1.2 µg
Calcilo	0.07 mg	0.04 mg	10 µg	6 mg	0.5 mg	1.67 µg
Suplena[b]	0.23 mg	0.8 mg	104 µg	10.4 mg	4.2 mg	12 µg
Nepro[b]	0.23 mg	0.8 mg	104 µg	10.4 mg	4.2 mg	12 µg

[a] Content value from individual formulas can be compared to percent daily recommended intake needs for patient age and gender as seen in Table 40.1.

[b] Denotes a formula often used in adult dialysis populations but can be utilized in the pediatric setting as indicated by nutritional needs.

calcineurin inhibitors, and/or mTOR inhibitors. Consequences of these therapies include increased risk for obesity, type 2 diabetes mellitus, hyperlipidemia, and hypertension after transplantation.[70] In the initial post-transplant period, the focus of medical nutrition therapy should be on limitation of sodium (2-3 g/day), weight control, and adequate fluid intake, especially for smaller children who receive adult-size kidneys. Long-term goals include achieving or maintaining age-and gender-appropriate BMI, regular physical activity, and eating a variety of foods, including fruits and vegetables, with moderate consumption of high-fat and high-sodium foods. Lipids should be monitored after transplantation.[71,72] There are currently no agreed on recommendations for use of either omega-3 fatty acids or statin-based therapy, although single-center data suggest use in pediatric solid organ recipients to be safe[73]; conversely, opinion-based recommendations largely defer to lifestyle modification and dietary changes.

Conclusion

Nutritional assessment and provision for the pediatric patient with kidney disease requires regular attention to critical growth and development parameters in conjunction with fluid, electrolyte, acid-base, vitamin, and mineral status. Partnership with a knowledgeable dietitian is a key factor for success in the care of the renal patient population. The objectives for optimal nutrition may vary widely depending on renal disease state, although a uniting focus is to understand the very significant challenges for the patient and family around all aspects of optimizing nutrition in the collaborative effort to achieve optimal outcomes.

References

1. Ayestaran FW, Schneider MF, Kaskel FJ, et al. Perceived appetite and clinical outcomes in children with chronic kidney disease. *Pediatr Nephrol.* 2016;31(7): 1121–1127

2. Warady BA, Kriley M, Belden B, Hellerstein S, Alan U. Nutritional and behavioral-aspects of nasogastric tube-feeding in infants receiving chronic peritoneal-dialysis. *Adv Perit D.* 1990;6:265–268

3. Rees L, Jones H. Nutritional management and growth in children with chronic kidney disease. *Pediatr Nephrol.* 2013;28(4):527–536

4. Rees L, Shaw V. Nutrition in children with CRF and on dialysis. *Pediatr Nephrol.* 2007;22(10):1689–1702

5. National Kidney Fountation. KDOQI clinical practice guideline for nutrition in children with CKD: 2008 update. *Am J Kidney Dis.* 2009; 53(3): S1–123

6. Rendina D, De Filippo G, D'Elia L, Strazzullo P. Metabolic syndrome and nephrolithiasis: a systematic review and meta-analysis of the scientific evidence. *J Nephrol.* 2014;27(4):371–376

7. Tiwari R, Campfield T, Wittcopp C, et al. Metabolic syndrome in obese adolescents is associated with risk for nephrolithiasis. *J Pediatr.* 2012;160(4): 615–620 e612

8. Cambareri GM, Kovacevic L, Bayne AP, et al. National multi-institutional cooperative on urolithiasis in children: age is a significant predictor of urine abnormalities. *J Pediatr Urol.* 2015;11(4):218–223

9. Krishnamurthy MS, Hruska KA, Chandhoke PS. The urinary response to an oral oxalate load in recurrent calcium stone formers. *J Urol.* Jun 2003;169(6): 2030–2033

10. Penniston KL, Nakada SY. Effect of dietary changes on urinary oxalate excretion and calcium oxalate supersaturation in patients with hyperoxaluric stone formation. *Urology.* 2009;73(3):484–489

11. Curhan GC, Willett WC, Rimm EB, Stampfer MJ. A prospective study of dietary calcium and other nutrients and the risk of symptomatic kidney stones. *N Engl J Med.* 1993;328(12):833–838

12. Edvardsson VO, Goldfarb DS, Lieske JC, et al. Hereditary causes of kidney stones and chronic kidney disease. *Pediatr Nephrol.* 2013;28(10):1923–1942

13. Sorof JM, Lai D, Turner J, Poffenbarger T, Portman RJ. Overweight, ethnicity, and the prevalence of hypertension in school-aged children. *Pediatrics.* 2004;113 (3 Pt 1):475–482

14. Lambert M, Delvin EE, Levy E, et al. Prevalence of cardiometabolic risk factors by weight status in a population-based sample of Quebec children and adolescents. *Can J Cardiol.* 2008;24(7):575–583

15. Kuwahara E, Asakura K, Nishiwaki Y, et al. Steeper increases in body mass index during childhood correlate with blood pressure elevation in adolescence: a long-term follow-up study in a Japanese community. *Hypertens Res.* 2014;37(2):179–184

16. Graf C, Rost SV, Koch B, et al. Data from the StEP TWO programme showing the effect on blood pressure and different parameters for obesity in overweight and obese primary school children. *Cardiol Young.* 2005;15(3):291–298

17. Morrison KM, Damanhoury S, Buchholz A, et al. The CANadian Pediatric Weight management Registry (CANPWR): study protocol. *BMC Pediatr.* 2014;14:161

18. Couch SC, Saelens BE, Levin L, Dart K, Falciglia G, Daniels SR. The efficacy of a clinic-based behavioral nutrition intervention emphasizing a DASH-type diet for adolescents with elevated blood pressure. *J Pediatr.* 2008;152(4):494–501

19. Harsha DW, Lin PH, Obarzanek E, Karanja NM, Moore TJ, Caballero B. Dietary Approaches to Stop Hypertension: a summary of study results. DASH Collaborative Research Group. *J Am Diet Assoc.* 1999;99(8 Suppl):S35–39

20. Sacks FM, Svetkey LP, Vollmer WM, et al. Effects on blood pressure of reduced dietary sodium and the Dietary Approaches to Stop Hypertension (DASH) diet. DASH-Sodium Collaborative Research Group. *N Engl J Med.* 2001;344(1):3–10

21. Vollmer WM, Sacks FM, Ard J, et al. Effects of diet and sodium intake on blood pressure: subgroup analysis of the DASH-sodium trial. *Ann Intern Med.* 2001;135(12):1019–1028

22. Centers for Disease Control and Prevention. Trends in the prevalence of excess dietary sodium intake - United States. *MMWR Morb Mortal Wkly Rep.* 2013;62(50):1021–1025

23. Institute of Medicine, Food and Nutrition Board. *Dietary Reference Intakes: Electrolytes and Water.* Washington, DC: The National Academies Press; 2004

24. He FJ, MacGregor GA. Importance of salt in determining blood pressure in children: meta-analysis of controlled trials. *Hypertension.* 2006;48(5):861–869

25. Lechner BL, Bockenhauer D, Iragorri S, Kennedy TL, Siegel NJ. The risk of cardiovascular disease in adults who have had childhood nephrotic syndrome. *Pediatr Nephrol.* 2004;19(7):744–748

26. Holmes J, Roberts G, May K, et al. The incidence of pediatric acute kidney injury is increased when identified by a change in a creatinine-based electronic alert. *Kidney Int.* 2017;92(2):432–439

27. Sutherland SM, Ji J, Sheikhi FH, et al. AKI in hospitalized children: epidemiology and clinical associations in a national cohort. *Clin J Am Soc Nephrol.* 2013;8(10):1661–1669

28. Kyle UG, Akcan-Arikan A, Orellana RA, Coss-Bu JA. Nutrition support among critically ill children with AKI. *Clin J Am Soc Nephrol.* 2013;8(4):568–574

29. Cano NJ, Aparicio M, Brunori G, et al. ESPEN Guidelines on Parenteral Nutrition: adult renal failure. *Clin Nutr.* 2009;28(4):401–414

30. Fiaccadori E, Cremaschi E, Regolisti G. Nutritional assessment and delivery in renal replacement therapy patients. *Semin Dial.* 2011;24(2):169–175

31. Abitbol CL, Warady BA, Massie MD, et al. Linear growth and anthropometric and nutritional measurements in children with mild to moderate renal insufficiency: a report of the Growth Failure in Children with Renal Diseases Study. *J Pediatr.* 1990;116(2):S46–54

32. Sethi SK, Maxvold N, Bunchman T, Jha P, Kher V, Raina R. Nutritional management in the critically ill child with acute kidney injury: a review. *Pediatr Nephrol.* 2017;32(4):589–601

33. Flugel-Link RM, Salusky IB, Jones MR, Kopple JD. Protein and amino acid metabolism in posterior hemicorpus of acutely uremic rats. *Am J Physiol.* 1983;244(6):E615–623

34. Briassoulis G, Tsorva A, Zavras N, Hatzis T. Influence of an aggressive early enteral nutrition protocol on nitrogen balance in critically ill children. *J Nutr Biochem.* 2002;13(9):560

35. Mehta NM, McAleer D, Hamilton S, et al. Challenges to optimal enteral nutrition in a multidisciplinary pediatric intensive care unit. *JPEN J Parenter Enteral Nutr.* 2010;34(1):38–45

36. Kyle UG, Jaimon N, Coss-Bu JA. Nutrition support in critically ill children: underdelivery of energy and protein compared with current recommendations. *J Acad Nutr Diet.* 2012;112(12):1987–1992

VI

37. Bailey JL, Mitch WE. Twice-told tales of metabolic acidosis, glucocorticoids, and protein wasting: what do results from rats tell us about patients with kidney disease? *Semin Dial.* 2000;13(4):227–231

38. Bailey JL. Metabolic acidosis and protein catabolism: mechanisms and clinical implications. *Miner Electrolyte Metab.* 1998;24(1):13–19

39. Gordillo R, Ahluwalia T, Woroniecki R. Hyperglycemia and acute kidney injury in critically ill children. *Int J Nephrol Renovasc Dis.* 2016;9:201–204

40. Fiaccadori E, Maggiore U, Giacosa R, et al. Enteral nutrition in patients with acute renal failure. *Kidney Int.* 2004;65(3):999–1008

41. Chen W, Ducharme-Smith K, Davis L, et al. Dietary sources of energy and nutrient intake among children and adolescents with chronic kidney disease. *Pediatr Nephrol.* 2017;32(7):1233–1241

42. Kramer H. Dietary patterns, calories, and kidney disease. *Adv Chronic Kidney Dis.* 2013;20(2):135–140

43. Foreman JW, Abitbol CL, Trachtman H, et al. Nutritional intake in children with renal insufficiency: a report of the growth failure in children with renal diseases study. *J Am Coll Nutr.* 1996;15(6):579–585

44. Rees L, Mak RH. Nutrition and growth in children with chronic kidney disease. *Nat Rev Nephrol.* 2011;7(11):615–623

45. Wingen AM, Fabian-Bach C, Schaefer F, Mehls O. Randomised multicentre study of a low-protein diet on the progression of chronic renal failure in children. European Study Group of Nutritional Treatment of Chronic Renal Failure in Childhood. *Lancet.* 1997;349(9059):1117–1123

46. Kopple JD, Levey AS, Greene T, et al. Effect of dietary protein restriction on nutritional status in the Modification of Diet in Renal Disease Study. *Kidney Int.* 1997;52(3):778–791

47. Chaturvedi S, Jones C. Protein restriction for children with chronic renal failure. *Cochrane Database Syst Rev.* 2007;(4):CD006863

48. Verove C, Maisonneuve N, El Azouzi A, Boldron A, Azar R. Effect of the correction of metabolic acidosis on nutritional status in elderly patients with chronic renal failure. *J Renal Nutr.* 2002;12(4):224–228

49. Mitch WE. Influence of metabolic acidosis on nutrition. *Am J Kidney Dis.* 1997;29(5):R46–R48

50. de Brito-Ashurst I, Varagunam M, Raftery MJ, Yaqoob MM. Bicarbonate supplementation slows progression of CKD and improves nutritional status. *J Am Soc Nephrol.* 2009;20(9):2075–2084

51. Kumar J, McDermott K, Abraham AG, et al. Prevalence and correlates of 25–hydroxyvitamin D deficiency in the Chronic Kidney Disease in Children (CKiD) cohort. *Pediatr Nephrol.* 2016;31(1):121–129

52. Hong YA, Lim JH, Kim MY, et al. Assessment of tubular reabsorption of phosphate as a surrogate marker for phosphate regulation in chronic kidney disease. *Clin Exp Nephrol.* 2015;19(2):208–215

53. Cozzolino M, Gallieni M, Brancaccio D. The mechanisms of hyperphosphatemia-induced vascular calcification. *Int J Artif Organs.* 2008;31(12): 1002–1003

54. Hruska KA, Choi ET, Memon I, Davis TK, Mathew S. Cardiovascular risk in chronic kidney disease (CKD): the CKD-mineral bone disorder (CKD-MBD). *Pediatr Nephrol.* 2010;25(4):769–778

55. Mirza MAI, Hansen T, Johansson L, et al. Relationship between circulating FGF23 and total body atherosclerosis in the community. *Nephrol Dial Transpl.* 2009;24(10):3125–3131

56. Mirza MA, Larsson A, Lind L, Larsson TE. Circulating fibroblast growth factor-23 is associated with vascular dysfunction in the community. *Atherosclerosis.* 2009;205(2):385–390

57. Parekh RS, Flynn JT, Smoyer WE, et al. Improved growth in young children with severe chronic renal insufficiency who use specified nutritional therapy. *J Am Soc Nephrol.* 2001;12(11):2418–2426

58. Wassner SJ. The effect of sodium repletion on growth and protein turnover in sodium-depleted rats. *Pediatr Nephrol.* 1991;5(4):501–504

59. Kleinman RE, Greer FR. Trace Elements. *Pediatric Nutrition.* 7th ed. Elk Grove Village: American Academy of Pediatrics; 2013

60. Basatemur E, Horsfall L, Marston L, Rait G, Sutcliffe A. Trends in the Diagnosis of Vitamin D Deficiency. *Pediatrics.* 2017;139(3)

61. Inker LA, Astor BC, Fox CH, et al. KDOQI US commentary on the 2012 KDIGO clinical practice guideline for the evaluation and management of CKD. *Am J Kidney Dis.* 2014;63(5):713–735

62. Yatzidis H, Digenis P, Fountas P. Hypervitaminosis A accompanying advanced chronic renal failure. *Br Med J.* 1975;3(5979):352–353

63. Kriley M, Warady BA. Vitamin status of pediatric patients receiving long-term peritoneal dialysis. *Am J Clin Nutr.* 1991;53(6):1476–1479

64. Warady BA, Kriley M, Alon U, Hellerstein S. Vitamin status of infants receiving long-term peritoneal dialysis. *Pediatr Nephrol.* 1994;8(3):354–356

65. Jamison RL, Hartigan P, Kaufman JS, et al. Effect of homocysteine lowering on mortality and vascular disease in advanced chronic kidney disease and end-stage renal disease: a randomized controlled trial. *JAMA.* 2007;298(10):1163–1170

66. Huang HH, Song LJ, Zhang H, Zhang HB, Zhang JP, Zhao WC. Influence of L-carnitine supplementation on serum lipid profile in hemodialysis patients: a systematic review and meta-analysis. *Kidney Blood Press R.* 2013;38(1):31–41

67. Aoun B, Berard E, Vitkevic R, Dehee A, Bensman A, Ulinski T. L-carnitine supplementation and EPO requirement in children on chronic hemodialysis. *Pediatr Nephrol.* 2010;25(3):557–560

68. Steinman TI. L-carnitine supplementation in dialysis patients: does the evidence justify its use? *Semin Dialysis.* 2005;18(1):1–2

VI

69. Schroder CH, Dialysi EPP. The management of anemia in pediatric peritoneal dialysis patients - Guidelines by an ad hoc European committee. *Pediatr Nephrol.* 2003;18(8):805–809

70. Bonthuis M, van Stralen KJ, Verrina E, et al. Underweight, overweight and obesity in paediatric dialysis and renal transplant patients. *Nephrol Dial Transpl.* 2013;28:195–204

71. Habbig S, Volland R, Krupka K, et al. Dyslipidemia after pediatric renal transplantation-The impact of immunosuppressive regimens. *Pediatr Transplant.* 2017;21(3). doi: 10.1111/petr.12914

72. Filler G. Challenges in pediatric transplantation: the impact of chronic kidney disease and cardiovascular risk factors on long-term outcomes and recommended management strategies. *Pediatr Transplant.* 2011;15(1):25–31

73. Argent E, Kainer G, Aitken M, Rosenberg AR, Mackie FE. Atorvastatin treatment for hyperlipidemia in pediatric renal transplant recipients. *Pediatr Transplant.* 2003;7(1):38–42

74. Otten JJ, Hellwij JP, Meyers LD. *Dietary Reference Intakes: The Essential Guide to Nutrient Requirements.* Washington, DC: National Academies; 2006

75. Massey LK, Sutton RA. Modification of dietary oxalate and calcium reduces urinary oxalate in hyperoxaluric patients with kidney stones. *J Am Diet Assoc.* 1993;93(11):1305–1307

76. National Heart, Lung, and Blood Institute. Description of the DASH Eating Plan. 2015; https://www.nhlbi.nih.gov/health/health-topics/topics/dash. Accessed June 30, 2017

77. Hogg RJ, Furth S, Lemley KV, et al. National Kidney Foundation's Kidney Disease Outcomes Quality Initiative clinical practice guidelines for chronic kidney disease in children and adolescents: evaluation, classification, and stratification. *Pediatrics.* 2003;111(6 Pt 1):1416–1421

78. Minister of Public Works and Government Services. Dietary reference intake: recommended dietary allowance and adequate intake. 2010; https://www.canada.ca/en/health-canada/services/food-nutrition/healthy-eating/dietary-reference-intakes/tables.html. Accessed May 10, 2017.

Chapter 41

Nutritional Management of Children With Cancer

Background

Nutrition-related pathologies are well described and can add to both the morbidity and mortality in pediatric oncology. Children and adolescents with cancer who are malnourished (both under- and overnutrition) experience increased infections, reduced quality of life, poor neurodevelopmental and growth outcomes, and poorer cancer outcomes.[1] The clinical risks associated with malnutrition are more threatening to children with cancer. Epidemiologic data reveal that children from low- and middle-income countries (LMICs) often have overt undernutrition at the time of cancer diagnosis.[2] After controlling for stage of disease, these studies have found that poor nutritional status correlates with reduced survival and adherence to therapy in children and adolescents.[2] Remediation of malnutrition in both LMIC and high-income countries has been one of many strategies leading to improved survival rates for children with cancer.[3,4] These studies underscore the importance of directing attention and resources toward preventing undernutrition and optimizing nutritional status for children with cancer to ensure maintenance of adequate growth and development, improve well-being, minimize associated treatment toxicities, and provide children with the best odds for survival.

The prevalence of malnutrition in pediatric cancer patients has been well-documented in the medical literature; however, the degree of poor nutrition (mild to severe) and pattern (at diagnosis or developing over the course of therapy) will largely depend on the diagnosis, stage of disease, intensity of the treatment regimen, socioeconomic status, nutritional status at diagnosis, and other comorbidities.[1,5] The severity of either under- or overnutrition has been associated with the pathologic type of the malignancy and the degree of tumor involvement. Undernutrition frequently develops over the course of therapy because of treatment-related adverse effects and complications.[6] However, overnutrition is becoming an increasingly important clinical challenge in pediatric oncology. Because of the consistently poorer outcomes observed among this patient group, effective interventions aimed at maintaining a healthy weight during and after treatment is a research priority of the Nutrition Committee of the Children's Oncology Group (COG), the largest clinical trials and basic science consortium in pediatric oncology funded by the National Institutes of Health, National Cancer Institute.[7]

The importance of nutritional status in pediatric oncology is best exemplified by several recent studies that have been performed in homogenous patient populations with moderately large sample sizes, have addressed some of the weaknesses of earlier studies. Although most of the studies were retrospective reviews, significant relationships between nutritional status and toxicity and/or survival have been consistently reported. A recent meta-analysis consisting of nearly 5000 children with leukemia found a significant association between nutritional status and outcome.[8] In children with acute lymphoblastic leukemia (ALL), the most common childhood cancer, reduced survival was observed in children with a higher body mass index (BMI; relative risk [RR], 1.35; 95% confidence interval [CI], 1.20–1.51) compared with those at a lower BMI, as was a nonstatistically significant trend toward greater risk of relapse (RR, 1.17; 95% CI, 0.99–1.38) with a higher versus lower BMI. In children with acute myelogenous leukemia (AML), a higher BMI was also significantly associated with poorer survival (RR, 1.56; 95% CI 1.32–1.86) compared with a lower BMI.[8] The observed survival effect has been postulated to be equal to the advances in the survival of children with AML over the past 10 years.[9] The association of poor nutritional status in children with solid tumors is less well-described largely because of the heterogeneity of studies and the rarity of the disease itself, thereby limiting the sample size of existing studies.[10-16]

Remediation of malnutrition reduces the risk of toxicity and improves survival. A retrospective study exploring the effect of nutritional status at diagnosis and throughout therapy in children with high-risk ALL found that those who remained malnourished for the majority of treatment experienced increased toxicity and had reduced survival rates.[4] Similar observations have been reported in children residing in Central America.[3] These studies underscore the importance of timely and effective nutritional interventions. Enhanced supportive care strategies, including nutritional therapy, have an integral role during and after treatment for a pediatric malignancy.

Nutrition Assessment

This topic is comprehensively discussed in Chapter 24: Assessment of Nutritional Status. Evaluation of nutritional status is necessary throughout the continuum of cancer care to ensure normal growth and development and optimize clinical outcomes. Nutrition assessment should commence at diagnosis and be conducted longitudinally during treatment as well as into survivorship. As in most aspects of clinical medicine, the importance of history and physical assessment cannot be underestimated. Dietary assessment studies have found that dietary intake of specified micronutrients may be associated with increased toxicities during treatment for ALL.[17,18] Baseline evaluation should include dietary history to ascertain intake of macro- and micronutrients and identify known food aversions, allergies, or intolerances (see also Chapter 34: Food Allergy). Clinical evaluation includes appropriate anthropometric measurements and biochemical measurements.

Weight and height are the anthropometric measurements most frequently documented in pediatric patients with cancer, as they are used to ascertain body surface area in order to determine the dosage of chemotherapy. Body mass index (BMI) is calculated as a proxy for body fat and lean body mass compared to weight alone, however, it is not without limitations.[19,20] Nutritional assessments based on weight alone can be misleading, especially in the acutely ill cancer patient when fluid balance may be disturbed, particularly in the presence of edema, disease mass, or limb-sparing interventions. Mid upper-arm circumference and triceps skinfolds provide the best estimate of lean body mass and adipose tissue. Recent studies performed in children with ALL have found both an increase in fat mass and a reduction in lean mass during and after treatment.[19,20] The clinical implications of body composition in pediatric oncology remains unknown and is an important area of current research.

Many children with cancer undergo treatment for several years.[21] Anthropometric percentiles should be compared with those prediagnosis and should be monitored longitudinally. However, the presence of subclinical malignancy may have influenced the child's growth pattern for some period prior to diagnosis, so it may be necessary to go back further in time. Longitudinal assessments are critical for children at high risk for nutritional depletion (Table 41.1) resulting from the treatment itself or as an expected adverse effect of treatment, each of which may require specialized forms of nutritional intervention. Nutritional assessment of hospitalized patients is usually performed by an inpatient dietitian or nutritionist. For outpatients, the maintenance of a diary of food and supplement intakes can be used to construct a 24-hour dietary recall over several nonsequential days, or a 3- to 5-day food record. These are valuable aids for the dietitian to ascertain if the patient is meeting daily nutrient requirements.

Biochemical laboratory assessments that may be altered because of cancer therapy and concurrent infection may be misleading in the

VI

Table 41.1.

Patients at High Risk for Malnutrition

- Patients with malnutrition or evidence of cachexia present at diagnosis
- Patients expected to receive highly emetogenic regimens
- Patients treated with regimens associated with severe gastrointestinal complications such as constipation, diarrhea, loss of appetite, mucositis, enterocolitis
- Patients with relapsed disease
- Patients who are <2 months old
- Patients who are expected to receive radiation to the oropharynx/esophagus or abdomen
- Patients on chemotherapy treatment protocols with high occurrence of gastrointestinal or appetite-depressing effects such as those for Burkitt lymphoma, osteogenic sarcoma, and central nervous system tumors
- Patients with postsurgical complications such as prolonged ileus or short gut syndrome
- Patients receiving a hematopoietic stem cell transplant
- Patients with inadequate availability of nutrients because of low socioeconomic status

assessment of nutritional status. Any condition that can alter the rate of protein synthesis, degradation, or excretion and/or alter the inflammatory status may alter serum protein concentrations. Transthyretin (prealbumin) is a better indicator than albumin of the acute nutritional state because of its shorter half-life. Biochemical nutritional assessment should include the monitoring of liver and renal function as well as serum lipids and glucose to determine whether dietary modifications are required. For example, in patients with ALL, a very low-fat diet (<10 g of fat per day) may be indicated in children with hypertriglyceridemia because of coadministration of corticosteroids and L-asparaginase. Glucose concentrations should be monitored in patients receiving high-dose steroids and L-asparaginase. Furthermore, the pediatric cancer patient is at an increased risk for episodes of sepsis, usually because of immunosuppression, which may be further increased by a catabolic state and nutritional deficiency.

In both the inpatient and outpatient setting, a complete assessment of nutritional status should include a full evaluation of the dietary intake of micronutrients.[22,23] Ongoing cytotoxic therapy may also deplete the body of micronutrients. Decreased intake of micronutrients has been reported following chemotherapy and may be associated with the development of some therapeutic-related toxicities. For example, reduced intake of B vitamins may be associated with the development of neuropathy.[24,25] Zinc is important to immune function, mucosal integrity, and wound healing and has been associated with increased infection and changes in taste. Reduced intake of antioxidant nutrients may also be associated with infection and increased hospital stay.[17] Reduced intake of bone-related nutrients, specifically vitamin D and calcium, may increase the risk of bone morbidities among children with ALL.[26] Thus, a thorough analysis of dietary intake should accompany anthropometric and biochemical measurements to assess micronutrient status. The routine use of micronutrient supplements is controversial, because some oncologists are concerned about the theoretical effect on chemotherapy cytotoxic action. For example, folate supplementation may interfere with the effects of methotrexate, an anti-folate chemotherapeutic agent. Concerns have also arisen regarding nutritional supplements containing high-dose antioxidants. However, in the depleted patient, micronutrient supplementation within the recommended intakes set forth by the Institute of Medicine (now the National Academy of Medicine) in the Dietary Reference Intakes (DRIs) is generally regarded as safe (see also Appendix E: Dietary Reference Intakes).[27,28]

Nutritional Intervention

Nutritional interventions are challenging for the child with cancer because of the multiple factors concurrently impacting appetite and dietary intake (Figure 41.1). The primary goal for nutritional intervention in the child with cancer is to sustain and promote normal growth and development while the patient is receiving the necessary anticancer therapy. Historically, clinicians were primarily concerned with maintaining optimal weight and preventing nutritional deficiencies. However, the increasing prevalence of obesity has caused most clinicians to balance both ends of the nutritional spectrum, under- and overnutrition. Nutritional intervention should be proactive so as to prevent the development of undernutrition in patients at high risk of becoming nutritionally depleted rather than being reactive and targeting reversal of undernutrition only when it becomes apparent. The most appropriate intervention must be able to meet nutritional requirements resulting from the treatment of malignancy. Typical adverse effects of cancer treatment that can alter dietary intake are oral, esophageal, and bowel mucositis, severe nausea/vomiting, gastrointestinal tract obstruction, constipation, and diarrhea. A family-based approach to nutritional support is generally

VI

Figure 41.1.

Factors Affecting Nutritional Status of the Child with Cancer

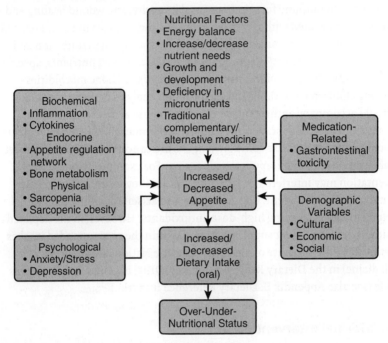

regarded as optimal, because parents or guardians are essential to providing appropriate nutrition to the infant or child throughout the course of therapy. An awareness of culturally driven food choices is essential for providing effective advice among a diverse patient population. In addition, the socioeconomic status of the parents can affect their ability to sustain adequate nutritional needs when at home and must be taken into consideration. Reliance on a dietitian to provide the support and education to staff, families, and patients is a crucial component of optimal nutritional care.

Dietary Counseling

Nutrition counseling should begin with strategies to ensure that the child is meeting the energy and nutrient requirements as set forth by the DRIs while also considering the planned cancer therapy for the child. Oral dietary intake may be difficult for many children and adolescents undergoing treatment but may be offered as an initial strategy prior to advancing to enteral tube feeding (ETF) or parenteral nutrition (PN).[5] For children undergoing highly intensive therapy, proactive ETF should be used to prevent the development of undernutrition. Children treated for ALL and others receiving chronic steroid medications, such as children with glioblastoma multiforme, are at increased risk for weight gain during therapy. Dietary strategies aimed at weight maintenance are a priority in developing dietary plans for these children. Dietary plans aimed at minimizing added sugar intake may have a role in cancer therapy.[29–31] Parents frequently request advice on special diets, such as the ketogenic diet, that are promoted in the lay literature. There is little evidence available about most of these diets for children with cancer, and therefore, evidence-based recommendations are not available at this time.

Dietary counseling should emphasize nutrient-dense foods in children who have difficulty with oral intake. This may include nutritionally fortified drinks or shakes to enhance caloric and protein intake. Table 41.2 provides a list of some commercially available supplements typically used in pediatric oncology patients. Other formulations that maintain electrolyte balance, such as coconut water or Pedialyte, may be necessary, particularly in patients receiving highly emetic chemotherapy medications. Medium-chain triglyceride oil may be another complement to feeding strategies to increase total calories in a readily absorbable formulation.

Appetite stimulants may augment dietary intake, although their efficacy has not been consistently demonstrated. Although corticosteroids increase appetite in many patients, they are not routinely used as appetite stimulants because of their immunosuppressive effects. A small pilot study found that megestrol acetate, a progestin with antiandrogen activity, stimulated dietary intake but was also associated with a disproportionate increase in fat mass.[32] Other investigators have evaluated the role of cyproheptadine hydrochloride, an anti-seratonin agent, for weight gain attributable to the lack of adrenal suppression.[33] Additional research, particularly looking at the effect of all appetite stimulants on body composition, is needed prior to their routine inclusion into clinical care.[34]

Children undergoing hematopoietic stem cell transplantation (HSCT) or receiving highly intensive therapies often experience severe immunosuppression for prolonged periods of time. When the absolute neutrophil count falls below 500 cells/μL, a neutropenic diet or low-microbial diet is often prescribed to minimize the introduction of pathogenic organisms into the gastrointestinal tract.[35,36] Adherence to these diets is difficult and provides

Table 41.2.
Commonly Used Commercial Nutrition Supplements

Oral
Ensure
Boost
Pediasure (with and without fiber)[a]
Boost Kid Essentials
Carnation Breakfast Essentials
Orgain
Bright Beginnings (Kosher)
Ensure Clear

High-Calorie Oral
Ensure Plus
Boost Plus
Pediasure 1.5[a]
Boost Kid Essentials 1.5 (with and without fiber)
Enu

Enteral
Osmolite 1.0, 1.2, 1.5
Jevity 1.0, 1.2, 1.5
Pediasure Peptide 1.0, 1.5 (with and without fiber)
Nutren 1.0, 1.5, 2.0 (1.0 with and without fiber)
Nutren Jr. (with and without fiber)
Compleat
Compleat Pediatric
Peptamen
Peptamen Jr 1.0, 1.5 (1.0 with and without fiber)
Liquid Hope
Nourish

[a] May also be used for enteral feeding.

further constraints on the individual's dietary intake. Most importantly, clinical trials have not found these diets to be effective in the prevention of infection over and above that of a diet provided using standard food safety guidelines.[35–37] Counseling and education on food safety guidelines are important components of nutritional counseling. A summary of food safety guidelines may be found on the US Food and Drug Administration's website (https://www.fda.gov/food/resourcesforyou/consumers/ucm255180.htm) (see also Chapter 51: Food Safety: Infectious Disease).

An emerging area of research in the field of pediatric oncology is the importance of maintaining a healthy microbiome during cancer therapy.

Several clinical studies in oncology have found that cancer therapy has an adverse effect on the composition of the microbiome.[38] Concomitant exposure to prophylactic antibiotic therapy provides further insult to the microbiome. Probiotic administration may be associated with reduced acute gastrointestinal graft-versus-host disease (GvHD) in HSCT.[39-41] However, the existing literature is not sufficiently robust to recommend routine supplementation with probiotics at this time.

Enteral Tube Feeding

Because of a variety of influences (Figure 41.1), oral intake frequently becomes inadequate to support growth or meet nutritional requirements in a child with cancer. When oral supplementation is unsuccessful in maintaining adequate nutrition and there are no contraindications for enteral intake, ETF may be considered and is the preferred route versus total parenteral nutrition (PN). ETF has numerous advantages over PN, which include the maintenance of gastrointestinal tract mucosal function and microbial communities, low cost, and avoidance of the known complications associated with PN (see also Chapter 22: Parenteral Nutrition, and Chapter 23: Enteral Nutrition). ETF eases the burden of administering oral medications, a significant benefit for children with cancer who are often required to consume multiple medicines daily.

There continues to be hesitation and reluctance in the provision of ETF within the pediatric oncology community. The presentation of ETF is often coercive and perceived as a punishment for not eating. Therefore, it is important to present ETF as a positive and not punitive intervention.[22] There may be concern on behalf of the parent or child because of the inconvenience, discomfort, and poor body image associated with the placement of the ETF tube. These concerns are especially noteworthy among adolescents with cancer. To optimize acceptance of ETF, it should be proposed as a positive intervention measure that is part of a comprehensive supportive care plan so as to optimize clinical outcomes.

Several studies have demonstrated that ETF is successful in maintaining adequate nutritional status and in reversing malnutrition in pediatric oncology patients.[42,43] ETF has been found to be feasible and safe in patients with mucositis, severe neutropenia, and thrombocytopenia.[44] Most children tolerate ETF without significant vomiting or diarrhea, even if they have thrombocytopenia. A noteworthy finding among several studies has been the cost efficiency associated with ETF compared with PN. Proactive ETFs have been found to improve and avert the use of PN. A small pilot study

VI

reported an increased risk of infection with EN[43]; however, this was not confirmed in a larger systematic review.[45]

Considerations in determining feeding schedules and formulas may be found in Chapter 23: Enteral Nutrition. Continuous feeding schedules are generally better tolerated than intermittent bolus feedings and are the preferred schedule in patients at high risk for nausea and vomiting, constipation, or diarrhea. If frequent vomiting persists, postpyloric tube feedings may help improve tolerance.[5] Daytime continuous feeds may be initiated on days that children are unable to consume adequate intake or cannot tolerate any oral intake. The use of ETF has potential risks such as aspiration and vomiting. Attention to guidelines of tube insertion is important to reduce the risk of aspiration.

The choice of formula will depend on the clinical condition of the patient. In most oncology patients, a standard milk-based formula with or without fiber may be used to initiate tube feedings (Table 41.2). Formulas that have a lower osmolarity are better tolerated and should preferably be used for ETF. In patients with lactose intolerance, a soy-based or lactose-free formula should be the preferred formula. Elemental or extensively hydrolyzed protein-based (small peptide) formulas are suited for patients with significant gastrointestinal tract inflammation or malabsorption conditions. Modification of any selected formula provided to the patient may be necessary if intolerance develops with symptoms such as persistent constipation, diarrhea, or abdominal pain.

In children with uncontrolled or severe vomiting, placement of postpyloric tubes often will minimize the risk of repeated reinsertions of the tube. Considering formulas with fiber or low osmolarity may minimize the duration and severity of diarrhea. Lactose intolerance can develop over the course of treatment, especially among children undergoing HSCT and may be a contributing factor in children unable to tolerate ETFs.

Indications for placement of a percutaneous endoscopic gastrostomy (PEG) tube include significant dysphagia and/or risk of aspiration; intractable vomiting; esophageal strictures; cancer of the head and neck; radiation to the head, neck, or chest; or anticipated long-term need for enteral nutritional support. Placement of a PEG tube needs to be coordinated with the timing of chemotherapy or radiation to avoid an endoscopic or surgical procedure during periods of severe immunosuppression. Adequate gastrointestinal tract function is also necessary for PEG tube insertion. Infection at the local insertion site can occur, and careful hygiene is required.

Parenteral Nutrition

PN may be required when all attempts for sufficient enteral feeding have failed or are contraindicated. A well-designed systematic review of PN found limited evidence that PN is not more effective than EN in promoting weight gain or maintaining nutritional status.[45,46] Despite the limited evidence, there are clinical conditions in which PN is essential. These include neutropenic enterocolitis, ileus, chylous ascites after surgery, and gastrointestinal GvHD after HSCT. Maintaining some EN is beneficial in an effort to preserve gut integrity and function. Short-term PN supplementation is rarely of benefit because of PN risks in the immunocompromised patient and should only be considered in those temporally unable to tolerate any enteral feeding. Determining PN requirements and administration are discussed in Chapter 22: Parenteral Nutrition.

Most pediatric patients with cancer have a central line placed to receive intravenous (IV) chemotherapy because of the inconvenience, pain, and difficulty with frequent peripheral IV access. Thus, the central line may also be used for administration of PN. PN is associated with mechanical complications of the central line, such as increased risk of thrombosis and line occlusion, which are morbidities that add considerable risk to the cancer patient (see Chapter 22: Parenteral Nutrition). Children with cancer receiving PN are more vulnerable to develop hepatotoxicity because of hepatic dysfunction secondary to hepatotoxic chemotherapeutic agents and infections attributable to immunosuppression. The transition back to enteral feeding requires a careful weaning approach and is dependent on gastrointestinal function. For the patient who has had a prolonged period of no oral intake, the clinician should be aware of the refeeding syndrome (see also Chapter 38: Eating Disorders in Children and Adolescents). Special consideration should be given to taste, smell, and food intolerance, as these often change or develop over the course of therapy and after PN.

Common Gastrointestinal Tract Complications in Pediatric Oncology

Neutropenic Enterocolitis

Neutropenic enterocolitis, sometimes called typhlitis (related to the caecum), is a severe complication of intensive chemotherapy and often preceded by chemotherapy-induced gut mucositis. It is seen in prolonged neutropenia presenting with fever, severe abdominal pain, and sometimes

VI

diarrhea. In severe cases, it may lead to sepsis, associated with gram-negative, gram-positive, and anaerobic bacteria, shock, and bowel perforation. Radiologic imaging often reveals the diagnosis and may show bowel wall thickening, thumb printing, air in the bowel wall, or free air in the abdomen. Urgent administration of intravenous broad-spectrum antibiotics including coverage for anaerobes is required in addition to cessation of all enteral feeds. Early surgical consultation is recommended. Dietary management initially involves complete bowel rest, during which PN may be required.

Bowel Perforation and/or Obstruction

Non-Hodgkin lymphoma with invasion of the bowel (especially Burkitt lymphoma) can present with bowel perforation or intussusception. Intussusception presenting after 2 years of age may be caused by a lymphoma. The early commencement of chemotherapy can resolve the invasion of the bowel wall, but intussusceptions may require surgery and additional chemotherapy.

Some solid tumors of the abdomen can present with bowel obstruction, such as Wilms tumor and neuroblastoma. The obstruction is often attributable to extrinsic pressure causing occlusion of the bowel. This bowel obstruction is treated by initial surgical removal followed by chemotherapy and sometimes radiation therapy. Nutritional intervention maybe required if the response to therapy does not resolve the problem.

Mucositis

Mucositis is a common adverse effect of intensive chemotherapy, most frequently seen within several days after the administration of anthracyclines, high-dose methotrexate, or radiation involving the head and neck or abdomen. Gastrointestinal tract mucosa contains rapidly dividing cells, which are affected by the chemotherapy used to stop the cell cycle of cancer cells. Mucositis may be limited to the mouth and esophagus but sometimes may extend into the entire length of the bowel. Mucositis is associated with significant pain with impairment of swallowing and, thus, diminished oral nutritional intake. It is a definite portal of entry for bacteria and other gut microorganisms and, therefore, increases the risk for sepsis in severely affected patients, especially in children who are also neutropenic. Nutritional interventions for mucositis include avoiding acidic, spicy, or hot foods and drinks, because they may cause further irritation to the mucosa and usually cause significant pain when consumed. In severe cases, placement of a nasogastric tube may be indicated to ensure adequate nutritional intake.

Chemotherapy-Induced Nausea and Vomiting

At some point in therapy, most children will experience nausea and vomiting (NV), which may not be always be adequately managed with antiemetic agents.[47] The emetic potential of most chemotherapy drugs has been classified into 3 categories: anticipatory NV (before chemotherapy administration), acute NV (during chemotherapy), and delayed NV (immediately or several hours after chemotherapy). Unfortunately, the prevention and treatment of NV is not always successful and often results in diminished nutritional intake. Other factors that may also contribute to NV include infections, bowel obstruction or inflammation, disorders of the central nervous system, and psychological conditions. Most recently, an evidence-based clinical guideline on antiemetic agents has been developed for the diagnosis and management of NV for practicing clinicians.[47] Dietary management of NV should involve consultation with a registered dietitian and includes routine monitoring of anthropometrics.

Gastrointestinal Tract Hemorrhage

Gastrointestinal tract hemorrhage is a severe and potentially life-threatening adverse effect of cancer therapy. It may occur as a result of bowel infections, enterocolitis, ulcers, primary bowel tumors, GvHD, complications of thrombocytopenia, and coagulation defects. The presentation is varied and can include abdominal pain and distension, hematemesis, and melena, as well as signs and symptoms associated with acute blood loss. The bleeding may be diffuse or localized and require endoscopy and radiologic imaging to ascertain the source. Supportive care with appropriate blood products and possible surgical intervention is required. Enteral feeding is contraindicated until cessation of bleeding and active bowel motility is present.

Pancreatitis

Pancreatitis is a serious complication that most often occurs following administration of L-asparaginase and cytarabine but has also been associated with HSCT and chronic use of PN. Its presentation includes severe abdominal pain, frequently radiating to the back, and elevated pancreatic enzymes (lipase and amylase). Changes to the pancreas itself may also be observed with abdominal ultrasonography or an abdominal computed tomography (CT) scan. Management is supportive and may require changes

VI

to nutritional, fluid, and drug management. Short-term PN may be indicated if oral feeds cannot be tolerated.

Hematopoietic Stem Cell Transplantation

HSCT is the most intensive form of therapy for the treatment of pediatric and adolescent malignancies. It is most commonly used for children with very high-risk leukemias or leukemia that relapses after standard front-line chemotherapy. It is also used in some high-risk advanced solid tumors such as neuroblastoma. Allogeneic HSCTs infuse related or nonrelated donor stem cells, and autologous HSCTs infuse the patient's own stem cells that are harvested once the patient is in remission. Stem cells can be obtained from the bone marrow or collected from the peripheral blood using a pheresis machine. The underlying concept of HSCT is that by using very high-dose chemotherapy, with or without radiation, the malignancy can be eradicated. Because this preparative regimen could damage the normal bone marrow beyond recovery, the marrow can be rescued by replacing hematopoietic stem cells. This modality of therapy has been used since the 1970s with ever-improving disease-free survival. Unfortunately, it is associated with a very high risk of treatment-related morbidity and mortality.

From a nutritional perspective, the gut is often profoundly damaged by the preparative chemotherapy/radiation regimen. In the case of allogenic HSCT, this may be further exacerbated by the child's risk of acute or chronic GvHD. Approximately 30% of acute GvHD affects the gastrointestinal tract, which affects the ability to consume oral nutrition and may complicate the delivery of nutritional support.[48] ETF is the preferred modality in delivery, particularly because of its ability to preserve the beneficial bacterial composition of the gut and prevent bacterial translocation. Provision of nutritional support is often necessary for 100 days or longer after HSCT because of prolonged effects of therapy or GvHD.

Nutrition and Survivorship

Survivors of childhood and adolescent cancers are at risk of multiple long-term morbidities because of their previous disease and the treatment of those cancers. Up to 40% of long-term survivors have one or more long-term effect(s) from their disease and/or treatment, many of which are nutrition-related conditions such as obesity, metabolic syndrome, heart disease, osteopenia/osteoporosis, and mechanical issues that can make eating difficult, such as reduced salivary function.[49–51] The increased risk of each of these nutrition-related conditions underscores the continued need for medical providers to ensure patients are receiving adequate nutrition assessment and counseling.

It is well recognized that pediatric and adolescent cancer survivors are at increased risk of second malignancies. This risk is increased for patients who have received alkylating chemotherapy drugs such as cyclophosphamide and/or radiation therapy. The use of lifestyle education programs has been found to be successful in promoting long-term behavior change among adult survivors of cancer.[52] The effect of these programs is unknown among survivors of childhood cancer, but studies are being conducted. Current clinical practice in the follow-up of survivors of childhood and adolescent cancer should incorporate all aspects of lifestyle intervention and provide the opportunity for survivors to receive continual access to nutrition information designed for survivors of cancer.

References

1. Brinksma A, Huizinga G, Sulkers E, Kamps W, Roodbol P, Tissing W. Malnutrition in childhood cancer patients: a review on its prevalence and possible causes. *Crit Rev Oncol Hematol.* 2012;83(2):249–275

2. Sala A, Rossi E, Antillon F, et al. Nutritional status at diagnosis is related to clinical outcomes in children and adolescents with cancer: a perspective from Central America. *Eur J Cancer.* 2012;48(2):243–252

3. Antillon F, Rossi E, Molina AL, et al. Nutritional status of children during treatment for acute lymphoblastic leukemia in Guatemala. *Pediatr Blood Cancer.* 2012;60(6):911–915

4. Orgel E, Sposto R, Malvar J, et al. Impact on survival and toxicity by duration of weight extremes during treatment for pediatric acute lymphoblastic leukemia: a report from the Children's Oncology Group. *J Clin Oncol.* 2014;32(13):1331–1337

5. Ladas EJ, Sacks N, Meacham L, et al. A multidisciplinary review of nutrition considerations in the pediatric oncology population: a perspective from children's oncology group. *Nutr Clin Pract.* 2005;20(4):377–393

6. Sala A, Pencharz P, Barr RD. Children, cancer, and nutrition—a dynamic triangle in review. *Cancer.* 2004;100(4):677–687

7. Sung L, Zaoutis T, Ullrich NJ, Johnston D, Dupuis L, Ladas E. Children's Oncology Group's 2013 blueprint for research: cancer control and supportive care. *Pediatr Blood Cancer.* 2013;60(6):1027–1030

8. Orgel E, Genkinger JM, Aggarwal D, Sung L, Nieder M, Ladas EJ. Association of body mass index and survival in pediatric leukemia: a meta-analysis. *Am J Clin Nutr.* 2016;103(3):808–817

9. Lange BJ, Gerbing RB, Feusner J, et al. Mortality in overweight and underweight children with acute myeloid leukemia. *JAMA.* 2005;293(2):203–211

VI

10. Small AG, Thwe le M, Byrne JA, et al. Neuroblastoma, body mass index, and survival: a retrospective analysis. *Medicine*. 2015;94(14):e713

11. Rodeberg DA, Stoner JA, Garcia-Henriquez N, et al. Tumor volume and patient weight as predictors of outcome in children with intermediate risk rhabdomyosarcoma: a report from the Children's Oncology Group. *Cancer*. 2011;117(11):2541–2550

12. Hingorani P, Seidel K, Krailo M, et al. Body mass index (BMI) at diagnosis is associated with surgical wound complications in patients with localized osteosarcoma: a report from the Children's Oncology Group. *Pediatr Blood Cancer*. 2011;57(6):939–942

13. Goldstein G, Shemesh E, Frenkel T, Jacobson JM, Toren A. Abnormal body mass index at diagnosis in patients with Ewing sarcoma is associated with inferior tumor necrosis. *Pediatr Blood Cancer*. 2015;62(11):1892–1896

14. Fernandez CV, Anderson J, Breslow NE, et al. Anthropomorphic measurements and event-free survival in patients with favorable histology Wilms tumor: a report from the Children's Oncology Group. *Pediatric Blood Cancer*. 2009;52(2):254–258

15. Brown TR, Vijarnsorn C, Potts J, Milner R, Sandor GG, Fryer C. Anthracycline induced cardiac toxicity in pediatric Ewing sarcoma: a longitudinal study. *Pediatr Blood Cancer*. 2013;60(5):842–848

16. Altaf S, Enders F, Jeavons E, et al. High-BMI at diagnosis is associated with inferior survival in patients with osteosarcoma: a report from the Children's Oncology Group. *Pediatr Blood Cancer*. 2013;60(12):2042–2046

17. Kennedy DD, Tucker KL, Ladas EJ, Blumberg J, Rheingold SR, Kelly KM. Low antioxidant vitamin intakes are associated with increases in adverse effects of chemotherapy in children with acute lymphoblastic leukemia. *Am J Clin Nutr*. 2004;79(6):1029–1036

18. Kennedy DD, Ladas EJ, Rheingold SR, Blumberg J, Kelly KM. Antioxidant status decreases in children with acute lymphoblastic leukemia during the first six months of chemotherapy treatment. *Pediatr Blood Cancer*. 2004;44(4):378–385

19. Barr R, Collins L, Nayiager T, et al. Nutritional status at diagnosis in children with cancer. 2. An assessment by arm anthropometry. *J Pediatr Hematol Oncol*. 2011;33(3):e101–e104

20. Orgel E, Mueske NM, Sposto R, Gilsanz V, Freyer DR, Mittelman SD. Limitations of body mass index to assess body composition due to sarcopenic obesity during leukemia therapy. *Leuk Lymphoma*. 2016;59(1):138–145

21. Pizzo PA. *Principles and Practice of Pediatric Oncology*. 6th ed. Philadelphia, PA: Lippincott Williams & Wilkins; 2011

22. Ladas EJ, Sacks N, Brophy P, Rodgers PC. Standards of nutritional care in pediatric oncology: results from a nationwide survey on the standards of practice in pediatric oncology. A Children's Oncology Group Study. *Pediatric Blood Cancer*. 2005;46(3):377–393

23. Ladas EJ, Orjuela M, Stevenson K, et al. Dietary intake and childhood leukemia: the Diet and Acute Lymphoblastic Leukemia Treatment (DALLT) cohort study. *Nutrition*. 2016;32(10):1103–1109.e1

24. Ozyurek H, Turker H, Akbalik M, Bayrak AO, Ince H, Duru F. Pyridoxine and pyridostigmine treatment in vincristine-induced neuropathy. *Pediatr Hematol Oncol.* 2007;24(6):447–452

25. Youssef S, Hachem R, Chemaly RF, et al. The role of vitamin B6 in the prevention of haematological toxic effects of linezolid in patients with cancer. *J Antimicrob Chemother.* 2008;61(2):421–424

26. Tylavsky FA, Smith K, Surprise H, et al. Nutritional intake of long-term survivors of childhood acute lymphoblastic leukemia: evidence for bone health interventional opportunities. *Pediatr Blood Cancer.* 2010;55(7):1362–1369

27. Institute of Medicine. *Dietary Reference Intakes for Energy, Carbohydrate, Fiber, Fat, Fatty Acids, Cholesterol, Protein, and Amino Acids (Macronutrients).* Washington, DC: National Academies Press; 2002

28. Institute of Medicine. Panel on Dietary A, Related C. *Dietary Reference Intakes for Vitamin C, Vitamin E, Selenium, and Carotenoids.* Washington DC: National Academies Press; 2000

29. Young PC, West SA, Ortiz K, Carlson J. A pilot study to determine the feasibility of the low glycemic index diet as a treatment for overweight children in primary care practice. *Ambul Pediatr.* 2004;4(1):28–33

30. Ebbeling CB, Leidig MM, Sinclair KB, Hangen JP, Ludwig DS. A reduced-glycemic load diet in the treatment of adolescent obesity. *Arch Pediatr Adolesc Med.* 2003;157(8):773–779

31. Spieth LE, Harnish JD, Lenders CM, et al. A low-glycemic index diet in the treatment of pediatric obesity. *Arch Pediatr Adolesc Med.* 2000;154(9):947–951

32. Cuvelier GD, Baker TJ, Peddie EF, et al. A randomized, double-blind, placebo-controlled clinical trial of megestrol acetate as an appetite stimulant in children with weight loss due to cancer and/or cancer therapy. *Pediatr Blood Cancer.* 2014;61(4):672–679

33. Couluris M, Mayer JL, Freyer DR, Sandler E, Xu P, Krischer JP. The effect of cyproheptadine hydrochloride (periactin) and megestrol acetate (megace) on weight in children with cancer/treatment-related cachexia. *J Pediatr Hematol Oncol.* 2008;30(11):791–797

34. Ladas EJ. Future directions in evaluating cancer-associated cachexia. *J Pediatr Hematol Oncol.* 2009;31(1):1–2

35. Tramsen L, Salzmann-Manrique E, Bochennek K, et al. Lack of effectiveness of neutropenic diet and social restrictions as anti-infective measures in children with acute myeloid leukemia: an analysis of the AML-BFM 2004 trial. *J Clin Oncol.* 2016;34(23):2776–2783

36. Moody KM, Baker RA, Santizo RO, et al. A randomized trial of the effectiveness of the neutropenic diet versus food safety guidelines on infection rate in pediatric oncology patients. *Pediatr Blood Cancer.* 2018;65(1). doi: 10.1002/pbc.26711.

37. Maia JE, da Cruz LB, Gregianin LJ. Microbiological profile and nutritional quality of a regular diet compared to a neutropenic diet in a pediatric oncology unit. *Pediatr Blood Cancer.* 2018;65(3). doi: 10.1002/pbc.26828

VI

38. Docampo MD, Auletta JJ, Jenq RR. Emerging influence of the intestinal microbiota during allogeneic hematopoietic cell transplantation: control the gut and the body will follow. *Biol Blood Marrow Transplant.* 2015;21(8):1360–1366

39. Jenq RR, Taur Y, Devlin SM, et al. Intestinal Blautia is associated with reduced death from graft-versus-host disease. *Biol Blood Marrow transplant.* 2015;21(8): 1373–1383

40. Jenq RR, Ubeda C, Taur Y, et al. Regulation of intestinal inflammation by microbiota following allogeneic bone marrow transplantation. *J Exp Med.* 2012;209(5):903–911

41. Ladas EJ, Bhatia M, Chen L, et al. The safety and feasibility of probiotics in children and adolescents undergoing hematopoietic cell transplantation. *Bone Marrow Transplant.* 2016;51(2):262–266

42. Deswarte-Wallace J, Firouzbakhsh S, Finklestein JZ. Using research to change practice: enteral feedings for pediatric oncology patients. *J Pediatr Oncol Nurs.* 2001;18(5):217–223

43. Sacks N, Hwang WT, Lange BJ, et al. Proactive enteral tube feeding in pediatric patients undergoing chemotherapy. *Pediatr Blood Cancer.* 2014;61(2):281–285

44. Trimpe K, Shaw MR, Wilson M, Haberman MR. Review of the effectiveness of enteral feeding in pediatric oncology patients. *J Pediatr Oncol Nurs.* 2017;34(6): 439–445

45. Chow R, Bruera E, Chiu L, et al. Enteral and parenteral nutrition in cancer patients: a systematic review and meta-analysis. *Ann Palliat Med.* 2016;5(1):30–41

46. Ward EJ, Henry LM, Friend AJ, Wilkins S, Phillips RS. Nutritional support in children and young people with cancer undergoing chemotherapy. *Cochrane Database Syst Rev.* 2015(8):CD003298

47. Dupuis LL, Sung L, Molassiotis A, Orsey AD, Tissing W, van de Wetering M. 2016 updated MASCC/ESMO consensus recommendations: prevention of acute chemotherapy-induced nausea and vomiting in children. *Support Care Cancer.* 2017;25(1):323–331

48. Jacobsohn DA, Vogelsang GB. Acute graft versus host disease. *Orphanet J Rare Dis.* 2007;2:35

49. Oeffinger KC, Hudson MM. Long-term complications following childhood and adolescent cancer: foundations for providing risk-based health care for survivors. *CA Cancer J Clin.* 2004;54(4):208–236

50. Oeffinger KC, Mertens AC, Sklar CA, et al. Chronic health conditions in adult survivors of childhood cancer. *New Engl J Med.* 2006;355(15):1572–1582

51. Oeffinger KC, Mertens AC, Sklar CA, et al. Obesity in adult survivors of childhood acute lymphoblastic leukemia: a report from the Childhood Cancer Survivor Study. *J Clin Oncol.* 2003;21(7):1359–1365

52. Mosher CE, Lipkus I, Sloane R, Snyder DC, Lobach DF, Demark-Wahnefried W. Long-term outcomes of the FRESH START trial: exploring the role of self-efficacy in cancer survivors' maintenance of dietary practices and physical activity. *Psychooncology.* 2013;22(4):876–885

Chapter 42

Nutrition in the Management of Chronic Autoimmune Inflammatory Bowel Diseases in Children

Introduction

The incidence of chronic gastrointestinal inflammatory diseases, such as inflammatory bowel disease (IBD) and celiac disease, is increasing globally. IBD and celiac disease commonly develop in childhood and share similar presentations, often exhibiting both gastrointestinal and extraintestinal manifestations. Both IBD and celiac disease have a prevalence that varies according to ethnicity and geography. In addition, Crohn disease, one of the two major forms of IBD, and celiac disease affect nutrient and vitamin absorption given their common distribution in the small intestine. Thus, in both IBD and celiac disease, children are at risk for malnutrition and growth failure/delay states. This chapter highlights the problems, approaches, and challenges to managing nutrition in patients with IBD and gluten-related disorders like celiac disease.

Inflammatory Bowel Disease

IBD, most typically classified as either Crohn disease or ulcerative colitis, develops during childhood or adolescence in as many as 25% of patients.[1] Although the incidence and prevalence of IBD varies by ethnicity and geography, recent reports suggest that the incidence, currently estimated to be approximately 7 to 20/100 000 children, is increasing globally.[2] Although IBD incidence in westernized countries has recently stabilized, the most rapid increases in incidence have occurred in newly industrialized nations such as those in Africa, Asia, and South America, where IBD was rarely seen before,[3] highlighting the role of environmental risk factors that accompany industrialization, such as pollution and changes in diet, in the pathogenesis of IBD.[4] Diet is increasingly believed to play an important part in IBD pathogenesis, likely, in part, through diet-induced changes in the intestinal microbiota and metabolome. Specifically, diets high in fiber, fruits, and vegetables and omega-3 fatty acids have been shown to protect against the development of IBD, and diets high in total and omega-6 fatty acids appear to increase IBD risk.[5]

Crohn disease and ulcerative colitis are chronic, relapsing, and remitting bowel diseases that are manifest by abdominal pain, diarrhea (often with blood), and often fever, fatigue, and anemia. Extraintestinal manifestations, such as arthritis and/or arthralgia, uveitis, hepatobiliary diseases, and dermatologic disorders such as erythema nodosum and psoriasis, may accompany gastrointestinal tract-related symptoms. Although ulcerative colitis affects only the mucosa of the large intestine, Crohn disease can affect any region of the gastrointestinal tract, and the inflammation can extend deeper into and, at times, through the intestinal wall, increasing risk for the phenotypic hallmarks of Crohn disease, such as strictures and fistulae.[6]

Because Crohn disease is more likely to affect macro- and micronutrient absorption, given that its distribution often involves the small intestine, many children affected with Crohn disease suffer from malnutrition and growth failure/delay. However, impaired linear growth and malnutrition can also occur in ulcerative colitis.

Growth Failure

Prevalence

Growth failure is common in children with IBD, particularly in children in whom the disease is diagnosed before or during the early stages of puberty, and is far more common in Crohn disease than in ulcerative colitis. The prevalence of growth impairment in children with Crohn disease varies with the definition of growth impairment and with the interval between symptom onset and diagnosis but has been reported to be as high as 40% and is more common in boys than in girls.[7] It is important to recognize that impairment of linear growth in IBD can occur before any overt gastrointestinal symptoms.[8] Growth failure is often accompanied by delayed puberty and skeletal maturation. Despite advances in treatment, linear growth impairment persists in some children with IBD and can lead to a deficit in final adult height.[9]

Pathophysiology

Several interrelated factors contribute to growth impairment in children with Crohn disease. Chronic undernutrition, attributable to decreased calorie intake, nutrient malabsorption, and increased caloric requirements, certainly contributes, as does the use of corticosteroids as a treatment modality. However, more recently, the direct growth-inhibiting effects of proinflammatory cytokines released in the setting of acute and chronic inflammation are now well described.[7] This is supported by the consistent observation that linear growth in Crohn disease improves with therapy that effectively reduces inflammation and that these improvements can occur independent of weight gain or corticosteroid reduction.[10] Thus, enhancement of linear growth may be best achieved through provision of adequate nutrition in addition to control of intestinal inflammation.

Role of Cytokines and Endocrine Mediators in Growth Impairment

Insulin-like growth factor-1 (IGF-1), produced by the liver in response to growth hormone (GH) stimulation, normally mediates GH effects on the growth plate of bones. The association between impaired linear growth in Crohn disease and low IGF-1 levels is well recognized. Several interrelated factors may decrease IGF-1 levels, including malnutrition, direct cytokine effects (such as interleukin-6 [IL-6]), and suppression by chronic daily corticosteroid therapy.[11]

Animal studies support a direct role for IL-6 in growth impairment in IBD, likely via inhibition of growth hormone signal transduction in hepatocytes and reduction of IGF-1 levels. Transgenic mice that overexpress IL-6 have reduced levels of IGF-1 production and impaired growth, and rats with chemical-induced colitis and poor growth have high levels of IL-6 and low levels of circulating IGF-1 and show improved growth with inhibition of IL-6.[12,13] In children with IBD, serum and tissue IL-6 levels are increased and correlate with mucosal inflammation, which may help explain the high rates of growth impairment at diagnosis.[14,15]

Linear growth, in addition to nutritional status and pubertal development, needs to be frequently monitored in children with IBD, with the goal of achieving maximum adult height potential.

Monitoring of Nutritional Status

Assessment of nutritional status includes a dietary history and a physical examination and a laboratory assessment for signs of micro- and/or macronutrient deficiencies when indicated. A thorough dietary history should be obtained with assistance from a registered dietitian, who can perform a 24-hour dietary intake history and/or analyze a 3- to 5-day dietary diary to assess calorie and micro- and macronutrient intake and compare with estimated needs. Documentation of medication intake, including corticosteroids and other immune suppressants, as well as use of nutritional supplements, including vitamins and minerals, is also important. Symptoms associated with the underlying illness that might affect nutrient requirements, such as difficulty swallowing, chronic nausea and/or vomiting, or

VI

diarrhea, should be documented. A review of social factors should include the home environment, economic status, issues of food security, and access to appropriate medications or other therapies.

Physical examination includes anthropometric assessment of body habitus, including weight, height, and BMI; all measurements should be recorded on appropriate standardized charts at each clinic visit. Sexual maturation should be documented by Tanner staging. Physical signs of generalized undernutrition (eg, protein-calorie malnutrition) or specific nutrient deficiencies, including skin rashes, hair changes, oral lesions, hepatomegaly, clubbing of the nail beds, and edema, should be documented.

Laboratory determination of serum albumin may be helpful for nutritional assessment, although albumin correlates better with inflammation of the intestinal tract than with nutritional status in patients with IBD. Serum prealbumin (transthyretin) has a much shorter half-life (2 days) than does albumin (18–20 days) and has been used to assess the efficacy of nutrition support. Additional nutritional laboratory assessment should include periodic assessment for anemia and iron deficiency, folate and vitamin B_{12} deficiency (particularly if there is ileal involvement of Crohn disease), zinc deficiency, and 25-hydroxyvitamin D (25-OH-D).[16]

Although bone density scanning with dual x-ray absorptiometry (DXA) has not yet been recommended for all children with IBD, it should be considered for patients with growth impairment, pubertal delay, persistent disease activity, and frequent corticosteroid use.[16] DXA should be analyzed with pediatric specific standards and reported as a z-score to help prevent underestimation of bone mineral density (BMD). BMD of children with delayed skeletal age/delayed puberty needs to be further adjusted for skeletal age as opposed to chronologic age.

Selected Nutrient Requirements and Nutrient Deficiencies

Daily nutrient requirements may be increased above the dietary reference intakes (DRIs) because of the metabolic cost of chronic disease and inflammation, malabsorption, and diarrhea. Children with Crohn disease generally have greater nutrient needs for their age, gender, and weight than do children with ulcerative colitis. During disease exacerbation, energy consumption in children with Crohn disease is often less than the Recommended Dietary Allowance (RDA) because of gastrointestinal symptoms such as nausea, vomiting, and abdominal pain, which limit adequate intake. The diet of pediatric patients with IBD should be well balanced, based on the US Department of Agriculture's ChooseMyPlate campaign[17] and the DRIs. Dietary restrictions should be avoided unless intestinal obstruction or specific abnormalities of digestion exist. Dietary supplementation of selected nutrients (eg, vitamin D, folate, and elemental iron) may be warranted.

Energy

There is inconsistent evidence supporting higher energy requirements in children with IBD. Although some studies have shown that resting energy expenditure (REE [kcal/day]) is higher in children with Crohn disease, it appears that this difference may be a result of factors other than body composition, such as inflammation.[18] Most pediatric studies assessing the influence of disease activity on REE have not shown an increase in REE in children with active versus inactive IBD.[19,20] One study in well-nourished children who underwent ileocolonic resection for stricture or medically refractory Crohn disease showed a decrease in REE of only about 5% after accounting for the energy expended by the resected gut.[21] Furthermore, studies have found no differences in REE before and after tumor necrosis factor (TNF)-inhibitor treatment in children.[22,23] Thus, REE does not appear to be significantly higher in children with IBD compared with controls when corrected for body composition, and disease activity appears to have little effect on REE in children with established IBD.

Protein

Whole-body protein turnover has been shown to be increased in children with acute and chronic disease activity, and can be reduced following induction of remission with either corticosteroid therapy or consumption of an elemental diet.[24] Proteolysis and protein synthesis may also be reduced following infliximab therapy and surgical resection in children.[21,22] These findings have led some groups to recommend increasing protein intake above typical goals during disease exacerbation when the inflammatory burden is high.[25] Dietary protein deficiency is generally uncommon in Western diets; nevertheless, the metabolic costs of inflammation and growth on protein nutrition in children with Crohn disease need more elucidation, and no specific recommendations for quantitative and qualitative protein and/or amino acid needs can be made at this time.

Vitamins, Minerals, and Trace Elements

Deficiencies for virtually every vitamin, mineral, and trace element have been reported in children with Crohn disease. During disease exacerbation, dietary intakes of iron, zinc, copper, folic acid, and vitamin C may

VI

decrease, on average, 20% to 50% below their recommended dietary allow-ance.[26] Altered serum or plasma concentrations often are used to define the deficiency state; however, these values may reflect inflammation rather than body tissue stores or functional deficits.[27] With severe, extensive inflam-mation or after resection of the terminal ileum, parenteral vitamin B_{12} supplementation may be necessary. Many patients require oral or occasional parenteral iron supplementation to replace chronic and ongoing losses attributable to bleeding and dietary malabsorption.

Vitamin D

Vitamin D is known to play important role in calcium and phosphate regula-tion and bone mineralization but is also thought to have an expanding role in immune regulation and, perhaps, in IBD course and response to treat-ment. Serum concentrations of 25-OH-D >20 ng/mL are considered suf-ficient for healthy children in the United States, although this cutoff was set mostly to help prevent rickets in early childhood. and the true level of suf-ficiency in IBD is not known. Vitamin D deficiency (25-OH-D ≤15 ng/mL) is common in children and young adults with IBD, with a prevalence as high as 35%.[28] Reduced dietary intake, decreased sun exposure, and reduced absorption attributable to intestinal inflammation may contribute to higher rates of vitamin D deficiency in children with IBD. Consistent risk factors for vitamin D deficiency include winter season, darker skin, and upper gastrointestinal tract involvement. Disease activity has not been consistently shown to correlate with vitamin D status in pediatric IBD.[28,29] In addition, it is not clear whether BMD correlates with serum vitamin D status.[29] The optimal dose for vitamin D supplementation to correct defi-ciency is not known. A randomized controlled trial (RCT) showed that doses of 50 000 IU of vitamin D_2/week and 2000 IU of vitamin D_3/day for 6 weeks were more effective at correcting deficiency (25-OH-D <20 ng/mL) than 2000 IU per day of vitamin D_2 in children with IBD.[30] Interestingly, 2000 IU of vitamin D_2/day was not sufficient to maintain levels >32 ng/mL throughout a calendar year, pointing to a potential need for even higher maintenance doses.[31] More recently, a retrospective single-center study showed that a single treatment with high-dose oral cholecalciferol (200 000–800 000 IU) sustained vitamin D sufficiency (25-OH-D >20 ng/mL) for children with IBD for 6 months.[32] The effect of vitamin D supplementation on BMD and fracture risk in children with IBD is not clear.

Bone mineralization is an important consideration in the care of the growing child with IBD. The World Health Organization defines osteopenia as the loss of bone mineral and matrix z-scores >1 standard deviation (SD) and osteoporosis as matrix z-scores >2 SDs below the mean for male and female populations. High rates of osteopenia and osteoporosis are reported in children with IBD.[33,34] Vertebral compression fracture has been reported as a presenting manifestation of the disease, and the rate of bone fracture is increased in children after corticosteroid treatment.

Gender and pubertal staging are important considerations in understanding reported rates of osteopenia and osteoporosis. In most studies, a greater proportion of adolescent boys exhibit osteoporosis. However, when osteoporosis occurs in girls with Crohn disease, it tends to persist. Because bone density is heavily influenced by growth and puberty, correction for height for age, bone age, or BMI reduces the apparent prevalence of osteoporosis. An independent risk factor for low bone density may be genetic predisposition. Patient groupings can be further subdivided by disease classification (Crohn disease vs ulcerative colitis), treatment with corticosteroids, or previous surgery. Patients with Crohn disease have far greater impairment of bone density than do patients with ulcerative colitis. Bone mineral density has consistently been reported to be low at diagnosis in pediatric patients with Crohn disease, after 2 years of treatment, and in adults with longstanding disease.[35–37]

Corticosteroids reduce calcium absorption, down-regulate calcitriol synthesis, decrease gene expression of calcium-binding protein, inhibit osteoblast proliferation, and stimulate osteoclastic bone resorption. Corticosteroid use at >7.5 mg/day, 5 g lifetime cumulative dose, or >12 months of lifetime exposure are risk factors for a low bone mineral density z-score.[38,39]

Patients with newly diagnosed Crohn disease often exhibit hypercalciuria, indicating negative calcium balance, because of the effects of systemic inflammation. Serum from pediatric patients with Crohn disease inhibits osteoblastic activity in bone cell culture, potentially attributable to the effects of IL-6, TNF-alpha, and other cytokines.[40] In states of systemic inflammation, products of activated T lymphocytes, such as the proinflammatory cytokines IL-6 and TNF-alpha, appear to directly and indirectly affect bone cells and cause a disruption in bone turnover.[41] Thus, inflammation itself appears to directly contribute to decreased BMD in IBD.

Treatment of Bone Disease

Effective therapy of the underlying disease by reducing the inflammatory burden is the most powerful treatment for osteoporosis and an appropriate

BMD for age and gender should be regarded as an important clinical end-point. Provision of adequate calcium and vitamin D is also essential. Recent guidelines have increased recommended intakes of calcium and vitamin D in healthy growing adolescents (age 9-18 years) to 1300 mg/day and 600 IU/day, respectively,[42] but goals are really to maintain sufficiency. Ensuring adequate calcium and vitamin D intake is important in patients with lactose intolerance (may have low dairy intake), dietary restrictions, decreased intake, and malabsorption. Patients may be monitored by bone density assessment correlated to height for age, bone age, or BMI.

Patients with IBD are at greater risk of physical inactivity, an independent risk factor for osteoporosis. Immobilization and bed rest compound other risk factors in patients with acute illness. Maintaining activity, encouraging full participation in sports, and minimizing bed rest are important factors. Smoking exacerbates Crohn disease and should be particularly discouraged in adolescents.[43]

The use of calcitonin to treat low BMD has not been widely studied in children. A double-blind, placebo-controlled trial testing the efficacy and safety of intranasal calcitonin on bone mineral density in pediatric patients with IBD did not show any sustained efficacy.[44] Bisphosphonates inhibit osteoclasts and have been used to prevent osteoporosis and prevent the risk of fracture in adults. A Cochrane meta-analysis of 13 trials involving 842 patients showed that the use of bisphosphonates is effective in preventing and treating bone loss in patients treated with chronic corticosteroids.[45] Increasing bone strength is a separate consideration from increasing bone density. No published data support use of bisphosphonates in children with IBD. The early implementation of nutritional or immunosuppressive therapies as an alternative to chronic corticosteroid treatment may reduce the prevalence of osteoporosis in children with IBD. Recent reports of improved bone formation and bone mineral content with infliximab suggest that treatment of the underlying inflammatory state may be sufficient to improve bone health in these patients.[46,47] Increases in IGF-1 may predict bone accrual following anti-TNFα therapy in pediatric Crohn disease.[48]

Zinc
Zinc functions as a cofactor in more than 200 metalloenzymes that are vital to RNA and DNA synthesis and immune functions including lymphocyte proliferation, cytokine production, free radical activity, and wound healing. Zinc deficiency can result in growth retardation, anorexia, impaired

cell-mediated immunity, diarrhea, alopecia, and acrodermatitis, all of which have been documented in patients with IBD.

Dietary zinc is absorbed along the length of the small intestine. Reduced serum zinc concentrations have been reported in patients with IBD compared with controls and particularly in patients with Crohn disease. As many as 40% of children with newly diagnosed IBD have been found to have low serum zinc concentrations, which may influenced by decreased dietary intake and by poor absorption and increased fecal excretion.[49] The role of zinc deficiency in IBD is poorly understood, and serum zinc concentration is not a reliable marker of total body zinc status, because much of zinc is intracellular. Despite this, the current recommendation is to assess zinc status in children with prolonged IBD flares and to correct zinc deficiency if found, with a 2- to 4-week course of oral zinc replacement.[25] There has been investigation into the use of supraphysiologic doses of zinc as adjunctive treatment for IBD, but there is no current evidence to support its use.

Iron

Iron deficiency and iron-deficiency anemia are common in patients with IBD, are correlated with disease activity, and have a higher prevalence in children than in adults.[50] Iron deficiency is influenced by inadequate dietary intake, malabsorption, and chronic gastrointestinal blood loss. In addition, there appears to be a direct effect of inflammatory cytokines on the hepcidin-ferroportin axis, leading to reduced absorption of dietary iron.[51] Anemia and iron status should be assessed periodically in patients with IBD. Iron status is most accurately measured by serum ferritin. However, ferritin is an acute phase reactant and its value is affected by active inflammation. Thus, low serum ferritin levels have been defined as <30 ng/mL in patients with normal C-reactive protein (CRP) values and <100 ng/mL in patients with elevated CRP levels.

Optimal iron replacement in children with IBD has not been established. The oral method, with compounds such as ferrous sulfate or gluconate, is most common but may be limited by poor absorption in children with active disease and by intolerance, including abdominal pain and constipation. Intravenous iron replacement is being increasingly used in children with IBD, is well tolerated, and appears effective at improving iron deficiency and anemia.[52,53] Newer intravenous iron preparations like iron sucrose and ferric-carboxymaltose appear safer than prior preparations, and there may be significant advantage of intravenous over oral iron replacement in patients with active inflammation.

Folate

Studies investigating folate status in children with IBD have shown mixed results, with some studies showing low serum folate levels but more recent studies showing normal or even elevated folate levels compared with controls, despite lower folate intake.[49,54] Despite this uncertainty, current guidelines from the European Society for Paediatric Gastroenterology, Hepatology and Nutrition (ESPGHAN) recommend annual assessment of serum folic acid or assessment if macrocytosis is present in the absence of thiopurine use.[25] If folate deficiency is confirmed, replacement with 1 mg daily by mouth for 2 to 3 weeks appears adequate, although the optimal replacement has not been determined. Importantly, folate supplementation is recommended for all IBD patients receiving medications that may interfere with folate metabolism, such as sulfasalazine and methotrexate.

Vitamin B_{12} (Cobalamin)

Vitamin B_{12} is a water-soluble vitamin with absorption limited to the distal ileum. Therefore, patients with Crohn disease with active ileal inflammation and those who have had extensive ileal resections (>20 cm) appear to be at highest risk for vitamin B_{12} deficiency. Patients with ulcerative colitis who have undergone a restorative proctocolectomy also appear to be at higher risk. There are very limited data on the prevalence of vitamin B_{12} deficiency in children. Prevalence in adults varies depending on measurement technique (serum vitamin B_{12} level vs serum methylmalonic acid). ESPGHAN guidelines recommend annual measurement of vitamin B_{12} status in children with active ileal Crohn disease, those who have had >20 cm of ileum removed, and patients with ulcerative colitis following ileal pouch anal anastomosis.[25] The optimal replacement strategy in children has not been determined, but one group suggests that children with clinical signs of B_{12} deficiency receive intramuscular B_{12} replacement with 1000 µg every other day for 1 week and then weekly until clinical resolution and normalization of levels.[25]

Nutritional Therapy for IBD

Dietary Therapy

Specific dietary therapies including "exclusion" diets are being increasingly used and studied as primary therapy in children with IBD. Although many such diets exist, only those that have been specifically studied in children will be discussed. These include exclusive enteral nutrition (EEN), partial enteral nutrition (PEN), and the specific carbohydrate diet (SCD). As with any diet that, by definition, limits intake of specific foods or food groups, patients using dietary therapy should be followed regularly by an experienced dietitian to ensure that macro- and micronutrient goals are being met to avoid iatrogenic nutritional deficiencies. Although the mechanism of these dietary therapies is incompletely understood, they likely exert their effect by manipulation of the gut microbiota and microbial products that are implicated in the pathogenesis of IBD, as opposed to targeting the immune system as many traditional IBD medications do.

Exclusive Enteral Nutrition

EEN is a formula-based treatment in which all solid food is excluded so that 100% of calories are taken in liquid form by mouth or nasogastric tube. Different formula preparations have been used, including those containing intact protein as well as semi-elemental and elemental formulas. The typical length of treatment ranges from 6 to 12 weeks, and it is generally well tolerated without many adverse effects. EEN is the best studied nutritional therapy in children with IBD and is used frequently as primary therapy in children with newly diagnosed Crohn disease in Europe, Canada, and other parts of the world. Historically, it has been used much less frequently in the United States, although use here is increasing. EEN, as monotherapy, has been repeatedly shown to improve clinical and biochemical outcomes, linear growth, and nutritional status in children with Crohn disease and can induce mucosal healing.[55] Meta-analyses have generally shown EEN to be as effective as corticosteroids at inducing clinical remission in children with Crohn disease.[56] A small Italian study showed EEN to be superior to systemic corticosteroids in inducing mucosal healing in children with active luminal Crohn disease.[55] More recently, a multicenter prospective study showed similar clinical response and remission rates in children with Crohn disease treated with EEN and those treated with anti-TNF therapy.[57] This evidence has led to the recommendation that EEN be strongly considered as first-line therapy for induction of remission in children with active luminal Crohn disease in both Europe and North America.[58,59] The role of EEN in ulcerative colitis appears limited.

Elemental Versus Polymeric Diets

The mechanism by which EEN improves clinical and biochemical outcomes is not clear but is thought to involve its effect on the fecal and intestinal mucosa-associated microbiome and metabolome. Both elemental and polymeric diets are associated with improved disease activity scores, histologic healing, and down-regulation of proinflammatory cytokines.[15,60,61] A meta-analysis considered results from 9 clinical trials that included a total of approximately 300 patient treated with elemental and nonelemental diets.[62] No differences were observed between the groups, although the study was limited in that several different types of formula diets were included in the nonelemental group. A more recent meta-analysis that incorporated more trials also found no difference in outcomes between patients using polymeric versus elemental or semi-elemental formula for EEN.[63]

Specific formula contents have been a target of investigation to better elucidate mechanism of action. Specifically, formulas with various concentrations of amino acids like glutamine and fat and fatty acid compositions have been compared with minimal differences in efficacy found, if any.[61,64,65] Because there appears to be no significant clinical difference between formulas, cow milk based, polymeric formulas are often recommended because they are more palatable and less expensive than more specialized formulas. Symptoms generally improve within the first week of EEN treatment. Although physical adverse effects with EEN are rare, refeeding syndrome is possible in malnourished patients who begin EEN and should be monitored for (see below). In addition, nausea, vomiting, and diarrhea have been reported. Some patients may have issues with social adjustment with family and peers, and this should also be assessed and addressed. There is little evidence to support the use of EEN as a maintenance therapy.

Partial Enteral Nutrition

PEN can be defined as receiving less than 80% to 100% of caloric needs from formula. PEN has been clearly shown to be inferior to EEN in the induction of clinical and biochemical remission in children with Crohn disease.[57] However, PEN, when combined with a regular diet, does appear to be more effective than an all-food diet at preventing Crohn disease relapse.[66] Additionally, although PEN is not effective at inducing remission when used alone, it may augment the benefits of more traditional medical therapy or other specific dietary therapy/exclusion diets.[67]

Specific Carbohydrate Diet

The SCD is a whole food exclusion diet that has been used to treat IBD for decades but is increasing in popularity. First developed as a diet for celiac disease, the diet excludes all grains, sweeteners apart from honey, processed foods, and all cow milk products except hard cheeses and yogurt that is fermented for >24 hours. There have been 2 prospective trials evaluating the efficacy of the SCD in pediatric IBD. Neither study contained a control group, and subjects and providers were not blinded to treatment. In the first open-label study, 9 of 10 patients completed the 12-week trial and 7 of 10 continued the SCD for 52 weeks. There were improvements in both clinical symptoms and mucosal inflammation (assessed by video capsule endoscopy) for many patients.[68] In the second study, 8 of 12 children with IBD were in clinical remission 12 weeks following the initiation of the SCD.[69] In addition, there was significant improvement in mean CRP value before and after treatment. Finally, in addition to clinical and biochemical improvement, there were significant changes in the stool microbiome following diet change. Although these studies are very small and uncontrolled, the encouraging results support the need for more intensive and larger interventional diet studies.

Although the SCD is a whole food diet, a small study showed that the majority of children on the diet had intakes of vitamins B_1 and B_9, vitamin D, and calcium less than the RDA.[70] This finding underscores the importance of regular follow-up with an experienced pediatric dietitian who can evaluate the need for nutrient supplementation and to ensure nutritional adequacy.

Finally, it appears that a "modified" SCD with inclusion of some "illegal" foods like rice or other grains is not as effective as the SCD. In a small single-center, retrospective study, patients on a modified SCD did not show improvement in mucosal inflammation after diet initiation.[71]

Despite a paucity of data, limited information on mechanism of action, and the cautions noted previously, there is enthusiasm among some about the potential role for the SCD or other similar anti-inflammatory and specific exclusion diets in the management of IBD. However, before such diets can be recommended, more and higher-quality studies assessing efficacy and safety are needed.

Total Parenteral Nutrition in IBD

There are limited data to support the use of total parenteral nutrition (TPN) as primary therapy in children with IBD, because enteral nutrition, when tolerated, is generally effective and safer than TPN. In certain circumstances in which enteral nutrition is contraindicated, such as intestinal obstruction or ischemia, hemodynamic instability, or high-output fistula, TPN can be used in the short-term to ensure adequate nutritional intake until enteral nutrition can be tolerated.

TPN can be effective in the preoperative setting in patients with IBD. Preoperative parenteral nutrition has been shown to be efficacious in reducing postoperative complications when therapy is administered for at least 5 days to patients with IBD who are severely undernourished.[72,73] Short bowel syndrome (SBS) can be a morbid outcome in patients with Crohn disease and repeated small bowel resections. These patients often require longer courses of TPN, although teduglutide, a glucagon-like peptide-2 analogue, has shown early promise in reducing the need for TPN in these patients.[74]

Fish Oil

Attention has recently been directed at the immunomodulatory role of polyunsaturated fatty acids. Omega-3 fatty acids have been shown to down-regulate the inflammatory response in both human and rodent models. Thus, their role for maintaining remission in patients with IBD has been recently investigated. Unfortunately, although it appears safe and showed early promise in clinical trials, oral fish oil therapy does not appear to be effective in maintaining remission in adults with Crohn disease or ulcerative colitis.[75,76]

Curcumin

Curcumin, a natural phytochemical derived from turmeric, has anti-inflammatory and antioxidative qualities in vitro and improves murine colitis. Recently, curcumin has shown to be more effective than placebo in inducing remission in adults with mild to moderate ulcerative colitis who were not responding to mesalamine.[77] In one small pediatric study, curcumin was well tolerated as adjunctive therapy in children with IBD.[78] Although more study is needed, curcumin shows early promise as adjunctive treatment in IBD.

Psychosocial Impact of Nutritional Interventions in the Care of Children With IBD

IBD represents a major, lifelong health threat that challenges the psychological resources of both the affected child and his or her family. Acute, active disease may necessitate hospital admission, causing major disruptions in children's academic, social, and family life. Many children with IBD experience considerable worry, distress, and concern about their disease and its effects on school absences, academic achievement, and participation in family and social activities away from home.

Well-conducted studies regarding the effects of nutrition support on psychosocial functioning in children with IBD are lacking. Treatment interventions can have both direct and indirect effects on psychosocial functioning. For example, although EEN is not associated with the potential adverse effects of corticosteroids and other IBD treatments, it does have drawbacks, particularly social concerns. Nasogastric tube feeding is often needed, particularly when elemental formulas are used. EEN support requires high patient and family motivation. Social factors, including support from family and friends, as well as peer pressure at school, are recognized as important influences on tolerance of EEN.[79]

During EEN treatment, patients endure prolonged periods of oral food deprivation and can experience frustration because of disruption of social and family activities during meals. EEN can be difficult for children who eat their meals at school, particularly if they are already embarrassed about the disease. Use of tube feedings and special liquid diets can also exacerbate feelings of being different and, thus, further contribute to a sense of alienation.[80] An additional consideration is that use of the feeding tube and pump apparatus makes the disease more visible, both to patients and to those around them. This can accentuate feelings of self-consciousness and heighten embarrassment in social situations. In addition, patients initially experience the insertion of a nasogastric tube as intrusive. The psychological meanings that patients attribute to treatment procedures as well as emotional reactions such as anxiety, fear, and depression may well be more influential than physical status in determining adherence to treatment and the success of nutritional therapies.[81]

Gluten-Related Disorders

Gluten-related disorders include celiac disease and nonceliac gluten sensitivity.[82–86] The prevalence of celiac disease approximates 1%. Nonceliac gluten sensitivity has been described infrequently in pediatric patients, and the prevalence is unknown, but it is estimated that up to 7.4% of children in the United States may avoid gluten.[83,84,86] There are no diagnostic biomarkers for nonceliac gluten sensitivity, and biomarkers for celiac disease are absent. The pathophysiology is unknown, and whether or not gluten is the cause of symptoms has yet to be confirmed. A diagnosis of nonceliac gluten sensitivity is commonly made in a patient who reports gastrointestinal or extraintestinal symptoms following gluten ingestion, with resolution after elimination of gluten from the diet.[85,87] Patients with nonceliac gluten sensitivity follow a gluten-free diet and, therefore, benefit from similar clinical assessment and nutrient supplementation.[85]

VI

Celiac disease is an autoimmune enteropathy that occurs in genetically predisposed individuals in response to ingestion of gluten, found in wheat, rye, and barley.[83] When individuals with celiac disease ingest gluten, the result is damage to the mucosa of the small intestine and subsequent malabsorption. Although celiac disease can develop at any age, common symptoms of celiac disease in childhood include gastrointestinal symptoms such as diarrhea, abdominal pain, or constipation.[83] Extraintestinal manifestations in children include growth failure, which may result in short stature, anemia, bone fractures, and dental enamel hypoplasia.[88] Children may also have clinically silent disease.[83] Serum antibodies such as anti-tissue transglutaminase (anti-tTG) are useful to screen individuals at risk for or suspected of having celiac disease. However, a small-intestinal biopsy must be obtained to confirm the diagnosis.[88] Because gluten-containing grains are the known environmental trigger for patients with celiac disease, removal of gluten from the diet leads to symptom improvement and resolution of histologic abnormalities in the small intestine. Rarely in pediatric patients, there may be a lack of response to the gluten-free diet. This lack of response may be confirmed by a small intestinal biopsy that fails to show mucosal recovery despite adherence to the gluten-free diet.[89] Children with untreated celiac disease are at risk for complications often seen at the time of presentation, such as iron-deficiency anemia, vitamin deficiencies, and stunted growth.[90] Further research must be conducted to establish whether these complications also occur in pediatric patients who fail to respond to the gluten-free diet. Compliance with a gluten-free diet is challenging and therefore supervision and nutritional counseling by a dietitian is essential to a patients' success.

The Gluten-Free Diet

The only known and available treatment for celiac disease is a gluten-free diet. Gluten is the general name for the prolamins found in wheat (gliadin), rye (secalin), barley (hordein), and oats (avenin).[91] Any food product that contains rye, barley, or malt (a partial hydrolysate of barley) has prolamins that are considered harmful.[91] The oat prolamin is thought not to elicit the same immune response as gliadin and is generally safe for 99% of patients with celiac disease to ingest. However, the majority of oats in the United States are contaminated with wheat because oats are often crop-rotated, harvested, and milled with wheat. For this reason, patients are instructed to use only labeled gluten-free oats in their diet. Recent studies have evaluated the addition of oats into the diet of patients with celiac disease, and these studies have confirmed the safety of oats that are labeled gluten free.[92,93] The education of the person with a new diagnosis of celiac disease should consist of a team approach between the patient (and guardians), the gastro-enterologist, the primary care physician, the dietitian, and local branches of support groups. After the gastroenterologist confirms the diagnosis with a small intestinal biopsy, the patient should be immediately referred to a knowledgeable dietitian for medical nutritional therapy.[94] Physicians and dietitians should encourage the patient to join support organizations, which can aid in finding local resources for gluten-free foods, such as supermarkets, food manufacturers, and restaurants.

Lifelong compliance with the gluten-free diet, although necessary, is challenging. Numerous barriers face those following a strict gluten-free diet, including availability of gluten-free foods, taste and quality of the safe foods, and the high cost of gluten-free items. On average, products may be up to 240% more expensive than their gluten-containing counterparts.[95] Maintaining a strict gluten-free diet can be difficult because of inadvertent cross-contamination during food processing and preparation and confusing food labeling (see Chapter 50.II: Federal Regulation of Food Labeling). For patients with celiac disease, even 1/100th of a slice of bread is enough to stimulate the immune system and cause intestinal damage.[91] Yet even patients maintaining a gluten-free diet may be inadvertently exposed to up to 2 g of gluten per day.[96,97] In children, poor availability of gluten-free items and cost are the most significant barriers to adherence.[98] Studies using questionnaires to assess dietary adherence report compliance rates in children of approximately 59%, whereas adherence in adults ranges from 42% to 91%.[99,100]

Changes in labeling practices have made it easier and faster for patients with celiac disease and gluten-related disorders to choose foods that are gluten free. The Food Allergen Labeling and Consumer Protection Act (FALCPA) was signed into law in August 2004.[101] It requires food labels to clearly state if a product contains any of the top 8 food allergens: milk, eggs, fish, crustacean shellfish, tree nuts, peanuts, soybeans, and wheat. All food products manufactured and sold in the United States after January 1, 2006, are required to have updated labels declaring the presence of any of the top 8 food allergens in the product. FALCPA was primarily passed to benefit individuals with food allergies.[101] However, it is also of tremendous value to those with celiac disease and nonceliac gluten sensitivity, because wheat is often hidden on ingredient labels as "modified food starch," "flavorings,"

VI

"seasonings," or "dextrin." Wheat is often used as a flavoring in candy, sauces, seasonings, soups, and salad dressings.[91,102] Because wheat is the most commonly used grain in the United States, by clarifying the source of ingredients and identifying "wheat," approximately 90% of labeling concerns are resolved for patients with celiac disease and nonceliac gluten sensitivity.[103] In the United States, the US Food and Drug Administration (FDA) rule establishing the definition of "gluten-free" for food labels was passed and enacted as of August 2013. The rule establishes a standard to increase consumer confidence in the safety of products labeled gluten free (see Chapter 50.II.) A summary of the FDA gluten-free label rules includes:

- A food labeled gluten free:
  - Must be inherently gluten free (raw vegetables, water, 100% juice)
  - Must not contain an ingredient that is gluten containing such as wheat, rye, or barley
  - Must not contain an ingredient derived from gluten that has not been processed to remove the gluten
  - May contain an ingredient derived from a gluten-containing grain that has been processed to remove gluten (wheat starch) as long as the food does not contain more than 20 parts per million (ppm) gluten
  - Must contain less than 20 ppm of gluten

These rules apply only to foods that are regulated by the FDA and not to toiletries, art supplies, and other products that contain gluten. Patients with celiac disease and nonceliac gluten sensitivity should be mindful of non-FDA regulated dietary supplements, which are not regulated by this act and may contain undocumented gluten.

Management of Patients With Gluten-Related Disorders

An excellent resource for patients and families beginning the gluten-free diet is available from the North American Society for Pediatric Gastroenterology, Hepatology and Nutrition at https://www.gikids.org/files/documents/resources/Gluten-FreeDietGuideWeb.pdf. For physicians, current guidelines for the management of pediatric celiac disease state that patients' growth parameters should be monitored closely, patients should have access to a dietitian, and a serum IgA anti-tissue transglutaminase (tTG) should be determined after a patient is on a gluten-free diet for 6 months as a surrogate marker of dietary adherence and mucosal recovery.[104] However, research confirms that celiac serology does not predict patients' adherence to the gluten-free diet or whether a patient has attained mucosal recovery.[89,105] Therefore, the only clinically available objective marker to confirm dietary compliance and small intestinal mucosal recovery is endoscopy with a repeat small intestinal biopsy. However, repeating the endoscopy to confirm mucosal recovery is not the current standard of care for pediatric patients with celiac disease.

Monitoring of Nutritional Status

Screening and assessing the nutrition of children with celiac disease is essential to complete medical care. Symptoms associated with celiac disease should be assessed. As for children with IBD, screening includes weight for age, height for age, and calculation of the BMI followed longitudinally on appropriate growth charts.[104] Social factors should be assessed, including the home environment for the possibility of cross contamination, and economic factors that may impact food security. Assessment of nutritional status also includes history, physical examination, and repeat laboratory testing of any abnormal labs.[104] A thorough dietary history including all medications and supplements taken should be obtained by a registered dietitian who can assess the dietary intake and identify any minute gluten contamination. In the first year after the diagnosis of celiac disease is made, patients should meet with a dietitian to review their diet and any supplements. After 1 year on a gluten-free diet, if signs and symptoms suggest mucosal recovery, patients should meet with a gastroenterologist and registered dietitian annually to review the history, physical examination, growth, and diet. Specific nutrient and micronutrient deficiencies are common in children with celiac disease and should be considered in the nutritional assessment.

Selected Nutrient Requirements and Nutrient Deficiencies

Children with active celiac disease should consume a well-balanced diet. Up to 28% of children with celiac disease have a deficiency of nutrients such as iron, folate (14%), vitamin B_{12} (1%), or vitamin D (27%) at diagnosis.[106] Low bone mineral density is common in children with newly diagnosed celiac disease.[107] In most cases, these nutrient deficiencies will resolve within 1 year of adopting the gluten-free diet regardless of whether dietary supplements are used.[106,107] Unlike fortified processed foods made with gluten-containing grains, gluten-free foods are not fortified with folate and B vitamins, and therefore, patients should work with a dietitian to ensure they are meeting recommended daily requirements. Additionally, patients with celiac disease should be counseled on appropriate intake of foods containing calcium and vitamin D, and supplementation should be suggested when

VI

necessary.[104] Recommended intakes of calcium and vitamin D are the same as those for children with Crohn disease, discussed earlier in this chapter.

Although historically, pediatric patients with celiac disease had poor weight gain and were malnourished at diagnosis, today, studies suggest that up to 40% of patients may be overweight at the time of diagnosis.[108] Manufacturers of gluten-free foods often improve palatability by increasing fat, sugar, and calorie content.[109] Therefore, children may gain weight because of the high calorie content of these foods as well as to the resolution of malabsorption of ingested calories. For this reason, patients should be counseled on the use of gluten-free whole grains, fruits, vegetables, dairy, and lean meats in preference to gluten-free processed foods in their diets.

Patients with celiac disease may suffer from other complications related to their underlying disease or adoption of the gluten-free diet. Patients should be counseled about the possibility of a temporary secondary lactase deficiency because of the loss of the lactase enzyme located on the blunted small intestinal villous tip.[110] Decreases in fiber intake and subsequent constipation commonly occur when patients transition to a gluten-free diet.[111] Therefore, patients should pay attention to their overall fiber intake.

Psychosocial Impact of Nutritional Therapy in the Care of Children With Gluten-Related Disorders

Celiac disease requires a lifelong dietary change. For patients with celiac disease and nonceliac gluten sensitivity, the challenges associated with following a gluten-free diet, some of which have previously been mentioned, include cost and ease of availability, difficulty reading labels, poor palatability, traveling and the challenges of eating at restaurants, and feeling socially isolated.[112] Adolescents following a gluten-free diet must learn how to navigate social events such as restaurants, parties, and camp attendance. Studies suggest that a diagnosis of celiac disease negatively affects the quality of life in children, but adherence to the gluten-free diet is associated with a decrease in reported depression symptoms and improve organizational skills.[113,114] Poor adherence has been associated with poor food palatability, frequent eating out at restaurants, increasing age, and the absence of acute symptoms following ingestion of gluten. Although many find a strict gluten-free diet extremely difficult to maintain,[112] adherence to a gluten-free diet in patients with celiac disease has been shown to improve physical outcomes as well as improve the quality of life.

Summary

Important clinical practices can enhance the growth and nutritional status of children and adolescents with celiac disease and IBD. These include but are not limited to:

1. Screen and assess pediatric patients with celiac disease and IBD for malnutrition and growth failure. At a minimum, this includes:
   - Height, weight, and BMI followed serially and plotted on standardized reference growth charts; and
   - Biochemical tests of nutrient and micronutrient status and, in patients at high risk of bone disease, medical imaging for bone mineral content and density.
2. Provide a diet based on the DRIs and the Dietary Guidelines for Americans for all pediatric patients. Dietary supplementation of selected nutrients may be warranted on the basis of a nutritional assessment of the individual patient.
3. Provide adequate calcium and vitamin D intake for all children with celiac disease and IBD. Patients at greatest risk of osteopenia and osteoporosis may be monitored by bone mineral density assessment. Maintaining full physical activity and minimizing bed rest are important to reduce the risk of bone disease.
4. Exclusive enteral nutrition is effective in inducing remission for active Crohn disease; enteral nutrition should be considered before parenteral nutrition, because it is safer and less costly.
5. Total parenteral nutrition is considered for nutrition support in children with IBD when enteral nutrition is contraindicated or inadequate.
6. Psychosocial dysfunction is common in children with celiac disease and active IBD. Adherence to a strict gluten-free diet in celiac disease and to exclusion diets in IBD may also have negative effects on social and psychological functioning. For such children, ongoing support of a mental health professional who is experienced in helping children develop coping strategies to deal with the effects of chronic illness and the treatments used for celiac disease and IBD is a critical component of the child's therapy.

VI

References

1.   Kelsen J, Baldassano RN. Inflammatory bowel disease: the difference between children and adults. *Inflamm Bowel Dis.* 2008;14(Suppl 2):S9-S11

2.   Benchimol EI, Fortinsky KJ, Gozdyra P, Van den Heuvel M, Van Limbergen J, Griffiths AM. Epidemiology of pediatric inflammatory bowel disease: a systemic review of international trends. *Inflamm Bowel Dis.* 2011;17(1):423–439

3.   Ng SC, Shi HY, Hamidi N, et al. Worldwide incidence and prevalence of inflammatory bowel disease in the 21st century: a systematic review of population-based studies. *Lancet.* 2017;390(10114):2769–2778

4.   Ananthakrishnan AN, Bernstein CN, Iliopoulos D, et al. Environmental triggers in IBD: a review of progress and evidence. *Nat Rev Gastroenterol Hepatol.* 2018;15(1):39–49

5.   Lee D, Albenberg L, Compher C, et al. Diet in the pathogenesis and treatment of inflammatory bowel diseases. *Gastroenterology.* 2015;148(6):1087–1096

6.   Van Limbergen J, Russell RK, Drummond HE, et al. Definition of phenotypic characteristics of childhood-onset inflammatory bowel disease. *Gastroenterology.* 2008;135(4):1114–1122

7.   Sanderson IR. Growth problems in children with IBD. *Nat Rev Gastroenterol Hepatol.* 2014;11(10):601–610

8.   Kanof ME, Lake AM, Bayless TM. Decreased height velocity in children and adolescents before the diagnosis of Crohn's disease. *Gastroenterology.* 1988;95(6):1523–1527

9.   Lee JJ, Escher JC, Shuman MJ, et al. Final adult height of children with inflammatory bowel disease is predicted by parental height and patient minimum height Z-score. *Inflamm Bowel Dis.* 2010;16(10):1669–1677

10. Malik S, Wong SC, Bishop J, et al. Improvement in growth of children with Crohn disease following anti-TNF-α therapy can be independent of pubertal progress and glucocorticoid reduction. *J Pediatr Gastroenterol Nutr.* 2011;52(1): 31–37

11. Gupta N, Lustig RH, Kohn MA, McCracken M, Vittinghoff E. Sex differences in statural growth impairment in Crohn. *Inflamm Bowel Dis.* 2011;17(11):2318–2325

12. De Benedetti F, Alonzi T, Moretta A, et al. Interleukin 6 causes growth impairment in transgenic mice through a decrease in insulin-like growth factor-I. A model for stunted growth in children with chronic inflammation. *J Clin Invest.* 1997;99(4):643–650

13. Sawczenko A, Azooz O, Paraszczuk J, et al. Intestinal inflammation-induced growth retardation acts through IL-6 in rats and depends on the -174 IL-6 G/C polymorphism in children. *Proc Natl Acad Sci U S A.* 2005;102(37):13260–13265

14. Brown KA, Back SJ, Ruchelli ED, et al. Lamina propria and circulating IL-6 in newly diagnosed pediatric inflammatory bowel disease patients. *Am J Gastroenterol.* 2002;97(10):2603–2608

15. Carey R, Jurickova I, Ballard E, et al. Activation of an IL-6: STAT3-dependent transcriptome in pediatric-onset inflammatory bowel disease. *Inflamm Bowel Dis.* 2008;14(4):446–457

16. Rufo PA, Denson LA, Sylvester FA, et al. Health supervision in the management of children and adolescents with IBD: NASPGHAN recommendations. *J Pediatr Gastroenterol Nutr.* 2012;55(1):93–108

17. US Department of Agriculture. ChooseMyPlate. Available at: http://www.choosemyplate.gov/. Accessed March 18, 2019

18. Azcue M, Rashid M, Griffiths A, Pencharz PB. Energy expenditure and body composition in children with Crohn's disease: effect of enteral nutrition and treatment with prednisolone. *Gut.* 1997;41(2):203–208

19. Wiskin AE, Wooten SA, Cornelius VR, Afzal NA, Elia M, Beattie RM. No relation between disease activity measured by multiple methods and REE in childhood Crohn disease. *54.* 2012;2(271–276)

20. Wiskin AE, Wootton SA, Culliford DJ, Afzal NA, Jackson A, Beattie RM. Impact of disease activity on resting energy expenditure in children with inflammatory bowel disease. *28.* 2009;6(652–656)

21. Varille V, Cézard JP, de Lagausie P, et al. Resting energy expenditure before and after surgical resection of gut lesions in pediatric Crohn's disease. *J Pediatr Gastroenterol Nutr.* 1996;23(1):13–19

22. Steiner SJ, Pfefferkorn MD, Fitzgerald JF, Denne SC. Protein and energy metabolism response to the initial dose of infliximab in children with Crohn's disease. *Inflamm Bowel Dis.* 2007;13(6):737–744

23. Steiner SJ, Pfefferkorn MD, Fitzgerald JF, Denne SC. Carbohydrate and lipid metabolism following infliximab therapy in pediatric Crohn's disease. *Pediatr Res.* 2008;64(6):673–676

24. Thomas AG, Miller V, Taylor F, Maycock P, Scrimgeour CM, Rennie MJ. Whole body protein turnover in childhood Crohn's disease. *Gut.* 1992;33(5):675–677

25. Miele E, Shamir R, Aloi M, et al. Nutrition in pediatric inflammatory bowel disease: a position paper on behalf of the Porto Inflammatory Bowel Disease Group of the European Society of Pediatric Gastroenterology, Hepatology and Nutrition. *J Pediatr Gastroenterol Nutr.* 2018;66(4):687–708

26. Thomas AG, Taylor F, Miller V. Dietary intake and nutritional treatment in childhood Crohn's disease. *J Pediatr Gastroenterol Nutr.* 1993;17(1):75–81

27. Ainley C, Cason J, Slavin BM, Wolstencroft RA, Thompson RP. The influence of zinc status and malnutrition on immunological function in Crohn's disease. *Gastroenterology.* 1991;100(6):1616–1625

28. Pappa HM, Gordon CM, Saslowsky TM, et al. Vitamin D status in children and young adults with inflammatory bowel disease. *Pediatrics.* 2006;118(5):1950–1961

29. El-Matary W, Sikora S, Spady D. Bone mineral density, vitamin D, and disease activity in children newly diagnosed with inflammatory bowel disease. *Dig Dis Sci.* 2011;56(3):825–829

VI

30. Pappa HM, Mitchell PD, Jiang H, et al. Treatment of vitamin D insufficiency in children and adolescents with inflammatory bowel disease: a randomized clinical trial comparing three regimens. *J Clin Endocrinol Metab.* 2012;97(6): 2134–2142

31. Pappa HM, Mitchell PD, Jiang H, et al. Maintenance of optimal vitamin D status in children and adolescents with inflammatory bowel disease: a randomized clinical trial comparing two regimens. *J Clin Endocrinol Metab.* 2014;99(9): 3408–3417

32. Shepherd D, Day AS, Leach ST, et al. Single high-dose oral vitamin D3 therapy (Stoss): a solution to vitamin D deficiency in children with inflammatory bowel disease? *J Pediatr Gastroenterol Nutr.* 2015;61(4):411–414

33. Gokhale R, Favus MJ, Karrison T, Sutton MM, Rich B, Kirschner BS. Bone mineral density assessment in children with inflammatory bowel disease. *Gastroenterology.* 1998;114(5):902–911

34. Issenman RM, Atkinson SA, Radoja C, Fraher L. Longitudinal assessment of growth, mineral metabolism, and bone mass in pediatric Crohn's disease. *J Pediatr Gastroenterol Nutr.* 1993;17(4):401–406

35. Andreassen H, Hylander E, Rix M. Gender, age, and body weight are the major predictive factors for bone mineral density in Crohn's disease: a case—control cross-sectional study of 113 patients. *Am J Gastroenterol.* 1999;94(3):824–828

36. Herzog D, Bishop N, Glorieux F, Seidman EG. Interpretation of bone mineral density values in pediatric Crohn's disease. *Inflamm Bowel Dis.* 1998;4(4):261–267

37. Warner JT, Cowan FJ, Dunstan FD, Evans WD, Webb DK, Gregory JW. Measured and predicted bone mineral content in healthy boys and girls aged 6–18 years: adjustment for body size and puberty. *Acta Paediatr.* 1998;87(3):244–249

38. Lopes LH, Sdepanian VL, Szejnfeld VL, de Morais MB, Fagundes Neto U. Risk factors for low bone mineral density in children and adolescents with inflammatory bowel disease. *Dig Dis Sci.* 2008;53(10):2746–2753

39. Semeao EJ, Jawad AF, Stouffer NO, Zemel BS, Piccoli DA, Stallings VA. Risk factors for low bone mineral density in children and young adults with Crohn's disease. *J Pediatr* 1999;135(5):593–600

40. Hyams JS, Wyzga N, Kreutzer DL, Justinich CJ, Gronowicz GA. Alterations in bone metabolism in children with inflammatory bowel disease: an in vitro study. *J Pediatr Gastroenterol Nutr.* 1997;24(3):289–295

41. Pappa H, Thayu M, Sylvester F, Leonard M, Zemel B, Gordon C. Skeletal health of children and adolescents with inflammatory bowel disease. *J Pediatr Gastroenterol Nutr.* 2011;53(1):11–25

42. Institute of Medicine, Food and Nutrition Board. *Dietary Reference Intakes for Calcium and Vitamin D.* Washington, DC: National Academies Press; 2010

43. Rubin DT, Hanauer SB. Smoking and inflammatory bowel disease. *Eur J Gastroenterol Hepatol.* 2000;12(8):855–862

44. Pappa HM, Saslowsky TM, Filip-Dhima R, et al. Efficacy and harms of nasal calcitonin in improving bone density in young patients with inflammatory bowel disease: a randomized, placebo-controlled, double-blind trial. *Am J Gastroenterol.* 2011;106(8):1527–1543

45. Homik J, Cranney A, Shea B, et al. Bisphosphonates for steroid induced osteoporosis. *Cochrane Database Syst Rev.* 2000(2):CD001347

46. Griffin LM, Thayu M, Baldassano RN, et al. Improvements in bone density and structure during anti-TNF-α therapy in pediatric Crohn's disease. *J Clin Endocrinol Metab.* 2015;100(7):2630–2639

47. Abreu MT, Geller JL, Vasiliauskas EA, et al. Treatment with infliximab is associated with increased markers of bone formation in patients with Crohn's disease. *J Clin Gastroenterol.* 2006;40(1):55–63

48. DeBoer MD, Lee AM, Herbert K, et al. Increases in IGF-1 after anti-TNF-α therapy are associated with bone and muscle accrual in pediatric Crohn disease. *J Clin Endocrinol Metab.* 2018;103(3):936–945

49. Alkhouri RH, Hashmi H, Baker RD, Gelfond D, Baker SS. Vitamin and mineral status in patients with inflammatory bowel disease. *J Pediatr Gastroenterol Nutr.* 2013;56(1):89–92

50. Goodhand JR, Kamperidis N, Rao A, et al. Prevalence and management of anemia in children, adolescents, and adults with inflammatory bowel disease. *Inflamm Bowel Dis.* 2012;18(3):513–519

51. Martinelli M, Strisciuglio C, Alessandrella A, et al. Serum hepcidin and iron absorption in paediatric inflammatory bowel disease. *J Crohns Colitis.* 2016;10(5):566–574

52. Danko I, Weidkamp M. Correction of iron deficiency anemia with intravenous iron sucrose in children with inflammatory bowel disease. *J Pediatr Gastroenterol Nutr.* 2016;63(5):e107–e111

53. Stein RE, Plantz K, Maxwell EC, Mamula P, Baldassano RN. Intravenous iron sucrose for treatment of iron deficiency anemia in pediatric inflammatory bowel disease. 66. 2018;2(e51–e55)

54. Heyman MB, Garnett EA, Shaikh N, et al. Folate concentrations in pediatric patients with newly diagnosed inflammatory bowel disease. *Am J Clin Nutr.* 2009;89(2):545–550

55. Borrelli O, Cordischi L, Cirulli M, et al. Polymeric diet alone versus corticosteroids in the treatment of active pediatric Crohn's disease: a randomized controlled open-label trial. *Clin Gastroenterol Hepatol.* 2006;4(6):744–753

56. Dziechciarz P, Horvath A, Shamir R, Szajewska H. Meta-analysis: enteral nutrition in active Crohn's disease in children. *Aliment Pharmacol Ther.* 2007;26(6):795–806

57. Lee D, Baldassano RN, Otley AR, et al. Comparative effectiveness of nutritional and biological therapy in North American children with active Crohn's disease. *Inflamm Bowel Dis.* 2015;21(8):1786–1793

VI

58. Critch J, Day AS, Otley A, King-Moore C, Teitelbaum JE, Shashidhar H. NASPGHAN IBD Committee. Use of enteral nutrition for the control of intestinal inflammation in pediatric Crohn disease. *J Pediatr Gastroenterol Nutr.* 2012;54(2):298–305

59. Ruemmele FM, Veres G, Kolho KL, et al. European Crohn's and Colitis Organisation, European Society of Pediatric Gastroenterology, Hepatology and Nutrition. Consensus guidelines of ECCO/ESPGHAN on the medical management of pediatric Crohn's disease. *J Crohns Colitis.* 2014;8(10):1179–1207

60. Teahon K, Smethurst P, MacPherson A, Levi J, Menzies IS, Bjarnason I. Intestinal permeability in Crohn's disease and its relation to disease activity and relapse following treatment with elemental diet. *Eur J Gastroenterol Hepatol.* 1993;5(2):79–84

61. Leiper K, Woolner J, Mullan MM, et al. A randomised controlled trial of high versus low long chain triglyceride whole protein feed in active Crohn's disease. *Gut.* 2001;49(6):790–794

62. Zachos M, Tondeur M, Griffiths AM. Enteral nutritional therapy for inducing remission of Crohn's disease. *Cochrane Database Syst Rev.* 2001(3):CD000542

63. Narula N, Dhillon A, Zhang D, Sherlock ME, Tondeur M, Zachos M. Enteral nutritional therapy for induction of remission in Crohn's disease. *Cochrane Database Syst Rev.* 2018(4):CD000542

64. Sakurai T, Matsui T, Yao T, et al. Short-term efficacy of enteral nutrition in the treatment of active Crohn's disease: a randomized, controlled trial comparing nutrient formulas. *JPEN J Parenter Enteral Nutr.* 2002;26(2):98–103

65. Gassull MA, Fernandez-Banares F, Cabre E, et al. Eurpoean Group on Enteral Nutrition in Crohn's Disease. Fat composition may be a clue to explain the primary therapeutic effect of enteral nutrition in Crohn's disease: results of a double blind randomized multicentre European trial. *Gut.* 2002;51(2):164–168

66. Takagi S, Utsunomiya K, Kuriyama S, et al. Effectiveness of an 'half elemental diet' as maintenance therapy for Crohn's disease: a randomized-controlled trial. *Aliment Pharmacol Ther.* 2006;24(9):1333–1340

67. Sigall-Boneh R, Pfeffer-Gik T, Segal I, Zangen T, Boaz M, Levine A. Partial enteral nutrition with a Crohn's disease exclusion diet is effective for induction of remission in children and young adults with Crohn's disease. *Inflamm Bowel Dis.* 2014;20(8):1353–1360

68. Cohen SA, Gold BD, Oliva S, et al. Clinical and mucosal improvement with specific carbohydrate diet in pediatric Crohn disease. *J Pediatr Gastroenterol Nutr.* 2014;59(4):516–521

69. Suskind DL, Cohen SA, Brittnacher MJ, et al. Clinical and fecal microbial changes with diet therapy in active inflammatory bowel disease. *J Clin Gastroenterol.* 2018;52(2):155–163

70. Braly K, Williamson N, Shaffer ML, et al. Nutritional adequacy of the specific carbohydrate diet in pediatric inflammatory bowel disease. *J Pediatr Gastroenterol Nutr.* 2017;65(5):533–538

71. Wahbeh GT, Ward BT, Lee DY, Giefer MJ, Suskind DL. Lack of mucosal healing from modified specific carbohydrate diet in pediatric patients with Crohn disease. *J Pediatr Gastroenterol Nutr.* 2017;65(3):289–292

72. Han PD, Burke A, Baldassano RN, Rombeau JL, Lichtenstein GR. Nutrition and inflammatory bowel disease. *Gastroenterol Clin North Am.* 1999;28(2):423–443

73. Gouma DJ, von Meyenfeldt MF, Rouflart M, Soeters PB. Preoperative total parenteral nutrition (TPN) in severe Crohn's disease. *Surgery.* 1988;103(6): 648–652

74. Kochar B, Long MD, Shelton E, et al. Safety and efficacy of teduglutide (Gattex) in patients with Crohn's disease and need for parenteral support due to short bowel syndrome-associated intestinal failure. *J Clin Gastroenterol.* 2017;51(6): 508–511

75. Turner D, Steinhart AH, Griffiths AM. Omega 3 fatty acids (fish oil) for maintenance of remission in ulcerative colitis. *Cochrane Database Syst Rev.* 2007(3):CD006443

76. Turner D, Zlotkin SH, Shah PS, Griffiths AM. Omega 3 fatty acids (fish oil) for maintenance of remission in Crohn's disease. *Cochrane Database Syst Rev.* 2009(1):CD006320

77. Lang A, Salomon N, Wu JC, et al. Curcumin in combination with mesalamine induces remission in patients with mild-to-moderate ulcerative colitis in a randomized controlled trial. *Clin Gastroenterol Hepatol.* 2015;13(8):1444–1449

78. Suskind DL, Wahbeh G, Burpee T, Cohen M, Christie D, Weber W. Tolerability of curcumin in pediatric inflammatory bowel disease: a forced-dose titration study. *J Pediatr Gastroenterol Nutr.* 2013;56(3):277–279

79. Seidman EG. Nutritional therapy for Crohn's disease: lessons from the Ste-Justine Hospital experience. *Inflamm Bowel Dis.* 1997;3(1):S43–S45

80. Allison SP. Some psychological and physiological aspects of enteral nutrition. *Gut.* 1986;27(Suppl 1):18–24

81. Gray WN, Denson LA, Baldassano RN, Hommel KA. Treatment adherence in adolescents with inflammatory bowel disease: the Collective Impact of Barriers to Adherence and Anxiety/Depressive Symptoms. *J Pediatr Psychol.* 2012;37(3):282–291

82. Sapone A, Bai JC, Ciacci C, et al. Spectrum of gluten-related disorders: consensus on new nomenclature and classification. *BMC Med.* 2012;10:13

83. Fasano A, Berti I, Gerarduzzi T, et al. Prevalence of celiac disease in at-risk and not-at-risk groups in the United States: a large multicenter study. *Arch Intern Med.* 2003;163(3):286–292

84. Tanpowpong P, Broder-Fingert S, Katz AJ, Camargo CA, Jr. Predictors of gluten avoidance and implementation of a gluten-free diet in children and adolescents without confirmed celiac disease. *J Pediatr.* 2012;161(3):471–475

85. Fasano A, Sapone A, Zevallos V, Schuppan D. Nonceliac gluten sensitivity. *Gastroenterology.* 2015;148(6):1195–1204

VI

86. Francavilla R, Cristofori F, Castellaneta S, et al. Clinical, serologic, and histologic features of gluten sensitivity in children. *J Pediatr.* 2014;164(3):463–467.e461

87. Leonard MM, Sapone A, Catassi C, Fasano A. Celiac disease and nonceliac gluten sensitivity: a review. *JAMA.* 2017;318(7):647–656

88. Hill ID, Dirks MH, Liptak GS, et al. Guideline for the diagnosis and treatment of celiac disease in children: recommendations of the North American Society for Pediatric Gastroenterology, Hepatology and Nutrition. *J Pediatr Gastroenterol Nutr.* 2005;40(1):1–19

89. Leonard MM, Weir DC, DeGroote M, et al. Value of IgA tTG in predicting mucosal recovery in children with celiac disease on a gluten-free diet. *J Pediatr Gastroenterol Nutr.* 2017;64(2):286–291

90. Fasano A. Clinical presentation of celiac disease in the pediatric population. *Gastroenterology.* 2005;128(4 Suppl):S68–S73

91. Case S. *The Gluten-Free Diet: A Comprehensive Resource Guide.* Saskatchewan, Canada: Centax Books; 2001

92. Pinto-Sanchez MI, Causada-Calo N, Bercik P, et al. Safety of adding oats to a gluten-free diet for patients with celiac disease: systematic review and meta-analysis of clinical and observational studies. *Gastroenterology.* 2017;153(2): 395–409.e393

93. Lionetti E, Gatti S, Galeazzi T, et al. Safety of oats in children with celiac disease: a double-blind, randomized, placebo-controlled trial. *J Pediatr.* 2018;194: 116–122.e112

94. Pietzak MM. Follow-up of patients with celiac disease: achieving compliance with treatment. *Gastroenterology.* 2005;128(4 Suppl 1):S135–S141

95. Stevens L, Rashid M. Gluten-free and regular foods: a cost comparison. *Can J Diet Pract Res.* 2008;69(3):147–150

96. Leffler DA, Edwards-George J, Dennis M, et al. Factors that influence adherence to a gluten-free diet in adults with celiac disease. *Dig Dis Sci.* 2008;53(6): 1573–1581

97. Gibert A, Espadaler M, Angel Canela M, Sanchez A, Vaque C, Rafecas M. Consumption of gluten-free products: should the threshold value for trace amounts of gluten be at 20, 100 or 200 p.p.m.? *Eur J Gastroenterol Hepatol.* 2006;18(11):1187–1195

98. MacCulloch K, Rashid M. Factors affecting adherence to a gluten-free diet in children with celiac disease. *Paediatr Child Health.* 2014;19(6):305–309

99. Jadresin O, Misak Z, Sanja K, Sonicki Z, Zizic V. Compliance with gluten-free diet in children with coeliac disease. *J Pediatr Gastroenterol Nutr.* 2008;47(3): 344–348

100. Hall NJ, Rubin G, Charnock A. Systematic review: adherence to a gluten-free diet in adult patients with coeliac disease. *Aliment Pharmacol Ther.* 2009;30(4): 315–330

101. Food Allergen Labeling and Consumer Protection Act of 2004. Pub L No. 108–282

102. Crowe JP, Falini NP. Gluten in pharmaceutical products. *Am J Health Syst Pharm.* 2001;58(5):396–401

103. Thompson T, Kane RR, Hager MH. Food Allergen Labeling and Consumer Protection Act of 2004 in effect. *J Am Diet Assoc.* 2006;106(11):1742–1744

104. Snyder J, Butzner JD, DeFelice AR, et al. Evidence-informed expert recommendations for the management of celiac disease in children. *Pediatrics.* 2016;138(3):e20153147

105. Silvester JA, Kurada S, Szwajcer A, Kelly CP, Leffler DA, Duerksen DR. Tests for serum transglutaminase and endomysial antibodies do not detect most patients with celiac disease and persistent villous atrophy on gluten-free diets: a meta-analysis. *Gastroenterology.* 2017;153(3):689–701.e681

106. Wessels MM, van V I, Vriezinga SL, Putter H, Rings EH, Mearin ML. Complementary serologic investigations in children with celiac disease is unnecessary during follow-up. *J Pediatr.* 2016;169:55–60

107. Kalayci AG, Kansu A, Girgin N, Kucuk O, Aras G. Bone mineral density and importance of a gluten-free diet in patients with celiac disease in childhood. *Pediatrics.* 2001;108(5):e89

108. Dickey W, Kearney N. Overweight in celiac disease: prevalence, clinical characteristics, and effect of a gluten-free diet. *Am J Gastroenterol.* 2006;101(10):2356–2359

109. Saturni L, Ferretti G, Bacchetti T. The gluten-free diet: safety and nutritional quality. *Nutrients.* 2010;2(1):16–34

110. Heyman MB, American Academy of Pediatrics, Committee on Nutrition. Lactose intolerance in infants, children, and adolescents. *Pediatrics.* 2006;118(3): 1279–1286

111. Theethira TG, Dennis M. Celiac disease and the gluten-free diet: consequences and recommendations for improvement. *Dig Dis.* 2015;33(2):175–182

112. White LE, Bannerman E, Gillett PM. Coeliac disease and the gluten-free diet: a review of the burdens; factors associated with adherence and impact on health-related quality of life, with specific focus on adolescence. *J Hum Nutr Diet.* 2016;29(5):593–606

113. Simsek S, Baysoy G, Gencoglan S, Uluca U. Effects of gluten-free diet on quality of life and depression in children with celiac disease. *J Pediatr Gastroenterol Nutr.* 2015;61(3):303–306

114. Sevinc E, Cetin FH, Coskun BD. Psychopathology, quality of life, and related factors in children with celiac disease. *J Pediatr (Rio J).* 2017;93(3):267–273

VI

Chapter 43

Liver Disease

Introduction

The liver is the major site for (1) the synthesis of serum proteins, such as albumin and coagulation factors; (2) urea synthesis for nitrogen metabolism and ammonia clearance; (3) glucose production for maintaining euglycemia; and (4) lipid metabolism including the generation of lipoproteins and ketone bodies. These metabolic functions consume approximately 20% of resting energy requirements, although the liver constitutes only 2% of body weight. Patients who have significant liver disease demonstrate impaired hepatic metabolic function as well as extrahepatic alterations in glucose (hypoglycemia is most likely in infants, but insulin resistance and impaired glucose tolerance also occur, particularly in older children), lipid (increased lipolytic rates), and protein (decreased protein synthesis and increased amino acid oxidation rates) metabolism.

Nutritional support of an infant or child with liver disease is dependent on the type of liver disease. Needs vary depending on whether the disease is acute or chronic, the degree of cholestasis and hepatic dysfunction, and the age of the patient. These categories are useful for developing nutritional protocols but may overlap in any one child; a careful assessment of each child is necessary to understand the factors that increase nutritional risk. This chapter focuses on the nutritional support of the child with *chronic liver disease with hepatic impairment or cirrhosis*. The common causes of such disease in childhood include drug-induced hepatitis, chronic viral hepatitis, metabolic liver disease, nonalcoholic fatty liver disease, biliary atresia, and autoimmune hepatitis, although many other diagnoses are possible. *Acute liver disease*, such as acute viral hepatitis or drug-induced liver disease, may cause vomiting and diarrhea and may result in weight loss. Chronic malnutrition, however, is uncommon. Because these acute diseases are brief, they may require no special nutritional therapy unless encephalopathy ensues. Various *inborn errors of metabolism* that cause liver disease (ie, galactosemia, tyrosinemia, hereditary fructose intolerance, Wilson disease) have specific nutritional requirements and dietary restrictions. The disease-specific diets of these children are generally managed by the hepatologist or metabolic physician, but if the disease progresses to hepatic insufficiency or cirrhosis, the principles described in this chapter apply. Note that children may have chronic liver disease, such as chronic hepatitis B infection, without impairment of hepatic function; these forms of liver disease generally do not impair nutrition.

VI

Advanced chronic liver disease commonly causes protein-energy malnutrition for several reasons. Decreased nutrient intake occurs because of anorexia and nausea. The presence of tense ascites, especially in an infant, makes food intake much more difficult as a result of the intra-abdominal pressure on the stomach. Diminished food intake may result from depression caused by hospitalization, encephalopathy, or the unpalatable nature of many restricted diets. Malabsorption of fat and fat-soluble vitamins frequently complicates childhood chronic cholestatic liver disease. Fat and fat-soluble vitamins require a critical concentration of intraluminal bile acids for micellar solubilization. Cholestasis, with diminished bile flow, results in reduced biliary secretion of bile acids and consequent fat and fat-soluble vitamin malabsorption. Supplementation with the fat-soluble vitamins A, D, E, and K is required to avoid potential deficiencies of these vitamins. Cirrhosis and portal hypertension may lead to hypermetabolism, protein oxidation, enteropathy, and malabsorption secondary to increased mesenteric venous system pressure and villous atrophy from malnutrition. Some liver diseases may be associated with extrahepatic organ dysfunction, such as pancreatic insufficiency (eg, cystic fibrosis), inflammatory bowel disease (primary sclerosing cholangitis), or kidney failure (eg, polycystic kidney disease associated with congenital hepatic fibrosis), which may aggravate the malabsorption and/or increase nutritional needs, increasing the risk of malnutrition.

Recognizing and managing the nutritional challenges of chronic liver disease improves childhood growth and development, and allows the child to lead as normal a life as possible. Children with chronic liver disease and severe compromise of hepatic function may eventually be considered for liver transplantation, a very successful form of organ transplant, with the ability to effect a long-term cure of the primary disease.[1] The success of pediatric liver transplantation is optimized in the child with appropriate pretransplant nutritional support.[2]

Nutritional Assessment of the Child With Liver Disease

It is imperative that any child with chronic liver disease undergo a thorough nutritional assessment to determine the risk factors for malnutrition and the existing degree of malnutrition, if present, and to tailor the nutritional intervention. The severity of malnutrition may not correlate with the degree of vitamin or trace mineral deficiency or the degree of hepatic dysfunction.

A number of obstacles complicate the accurate assessment of the nutritional status of a child with liver disease.

Body weight may be deceptive, because organomegaly from an enlarged liver or spleen, edema, or ascites can mask weight loss or increase the weight. Height (or length in infants and young children) is a better indicator of malnutrition in these children and can be a reliable tool to determine chronic malnutrition. A decrease in height/length for age percentile may be indicative of prolonged malnutrition.

In addition to weight and height/length measurements, triceps skinfold and arm circumference measurements provide a sensitive indicator of nutritional status in children with chronic liver disease.[3] Lower extremities are more prone to peripheral edema and fluid retention than upper extremities; thus, upper extremity measurements are a better indicator of body fat stores and muscle mass. In children, early reduction in fat and muscle stores reflects the preferential utilization of fat stores to conserve protein stores for energy in the malnourished state. To optimize the accuracy of anthropometric measurements, it is best to use a single observer using a standard technique with serial measurements.

Measurement of plasma proteins, including albumin, transferrin, prealbumin, and retinol-binding protein, which are synthesized by the liver, has been used to determine visceral protein nutriture. However, diminished serum concentrations of these proteins may not accurately reflect the body's visceral protein status. The serum concentrations of these proteins more closely correlate with the severity of liver injury rather than the degree of malnutrition as assessed by anthropometric measurements. Hypoalbuminemia in chronic liver disease patients often results from third spacing of fluid and protein in ascites or the extravascular compartment. Further, increased catabolism of albumin without a compensatory increase in albumin synthesis because of inadequate reserves and malabsorption of amino acids and peptides often makes albumin an inaccurate measure of nutritional status. Poor oral intake may further contribute to the hypoalbuminemia.

Nitrogen balance studies are difficult to evaluate in children with chronic liver disease. Impairment of hepatic urea synthesis leads to underestimation of urinary nitrogen losses. In addition, ammonia accumulates in the intra- and extracellular compartments instead of being excreted by the kidneys. The creatinine-height index is a good indicator of lean body mass

VI

if renal function is unimpaired. When using the creatinine-height index, dietary protein intake, trauma, and infection must be considered, because they all can alter creatinine excretion.

Immune status is sometimes used as an indirect measure of nutritional status. However, because liver disease and, in particular, hypersplenism can result in lymphopenia, abnormal skin test results for delayed hypersensitivity, or decreased concentrations of complement irrespective of nutritional status, these immunologic markers are of limited usefulness in children with liver disease.

Another problem with using biochemical measurements to determine nutritional status in children with liver disease is that many of the drugs used to treat children with liver disease may alter blood concentrations of vitamins. For example, cholestyramine and colestipol, bile acid binding resins, may deplete enteral bile acids and interfere with fat-soluble vitamin absorption from the intestines. Diphenylhydantoin and phenobarbital increase the hepatic metabolism of vitamin D and, thus, decrease cholecalciferol concentrations in plasma.

A well-prepared 24-hour diet diary can be invaluable in assessing the usual caloric intake and should always account for use of dietary supplements or any dietary restrictions that have been imposed. Problems such as nausea, vomiting, diarrhea, or anorexia should be recorded, because these may contribute to poor intake. A careful and thorough physical examination can determine the degree of muscle wasting, depletion of subcutaneous fat, and any evidence of vitamin or mineral deficiencies.

Malabsorption in Chronic Liver Disease

Calories

Ensuring normal growth pattern is important in children with liver disease. Although children with early liver disease may have normal growth with ordinary calorie intake for age, as children approach end-stage liver disease, calorie needs increase and may reach as high as 130% to 150% of the Recommended Dietary Allowance (RDA). Infants with liver disease are at particular risk.[4] Increased frequency of monitoring is important. As liver disease advances, anorexia and vomiting may limit oral intake. Many children with severe liver disease require nasogastric or nasojejunal feedings to achieve appropriate growth and weight gain. Such interventions should be performed early in the course of liver disease. Portal hypertension and esophageal varices are not a contraindication to nasogastric feedings.[4]

Protein

Studies in adults have shown muscle mass is an independent risk factor for poor outcomes in cirrhosis and death on the liver transplantation wait list.[5,6] Protein restriction is not recommended for children with liver disease unless they have severe hepatic encephalopathy. Families should be encouraged to provide high-bioavailable protein to their children with liver disease.

Fat

Steatorrhea (fat malabsorption) is frequently observed in patients with cirrhosis and/or chronic cholestasis, although the degree of biliary obstruction correlates poorly with the amount of fat excreted in the stools. Even in the absence of biliary obstruction, intraluminal bile salt concentrations may be below the critical micellar concentration such that intraluminal products of lipolysis cannot form micellar solutions.[7] Typically, the prothrombin time or international normalized ratio (INR) is prolonged. A trial of parenteral vitamin K administration daily will often correct the prothrombin time or INR and suggests poor fat-soluble vitamin absorption. Failure of parenteral vitamin K to correct the INR suggests poor hepatic synthesis of vitamin K-dependent proteins, and, thus, worse hepatic function.

Treatment with a low-fat diet supplemented with medium-chain triglyceride (MCT [C8-C12 fatty acids]) helps to decrease the degree of steatorrhea and may help to improve the nutritional status of the infant by providing more calories. MCTs do not require intraluminal bile salts for micellar formation to be absorbed in the intestinal lumen. MCTs are relatively water soluble and directly absorbed into the portal circulation. For infants, breastfeeding with MCT supplementation is the preferred feeding; mothers of children with liver disease should be encouraged to breastfeed. If human milk is not available, appropriate MCT-containing formulas are hydrolyzed (eg, Pregestimil [Mead Johnson, approximately 55% of fat as MCT], Alimentum [Ross, approximately 33% fat as MCT]). It should be noted that elemental formulas are not necessary in these infants; the hydrolyzed formulas are used because they contain high percentages of MCT. For older children, MCT oil may be prescribed and added to foods.[4] However, when hepatic decompensation ensues, although steatorrhea may be diminished with MCT dietary supplementation, growth failure may progress.

Essential Fatty Acids

The malabsorption of fat, especially long-chain triglycerides (LCTs), and inadequate intake can lead to essential fatty acid (EFA) deficiency. EFAs

are fatty acids that cannot be synthesized by desaturation or elongation of shorter fatty acids. Linoleic acid and linolenic acid are the 2 EFAs
in humans. Deficiency of EFAs may result in growth impairment, a dry
scaly rash, thrombocytopenia, and impaired immune function.[8] LCTs
are poorly absorbed if cholestasis is present. Infants have a small store of
linoleic acid and cholestasis places them at an increased EFA deficiency
risk.[7] Pregestimil and Alimentum provide only 14% to 16% of calories as
linoleic acid. To prevent EFA deficiency, at least 3% to 4% of calories should
be linoleic acid. If cholestasis is severe enough to allow 30% to 40% of
dietary fat to be malabsorbed, then EFA deficiency may ensue.[9] Portagen
or Enfaport (Mead Johnson), containing 87% MCTs and <7% EFAs, are not
recommended for use in children with cholestatic liver disease, because
EFA deficiency may occur if supplementation is not provided.[10] Corn oil or
safflower oil containing linoleic acid can be added to foods, or a lipid emulsion (Microlipid [Novartis]) can be added to formula to provide additional
linoleic acid.

Fat-Soluble Vitamins *(see also Chapter 21.I: Fat-Soluble Vitamins)*
Bile acids in the intestinal lumen are not only important for fat absorption from the lumen but also for fat-soluble vitamin absorption. Vitamins
A, D, E, and K are all dependent on intraluminal bile acid concentration
for absorption. When the intraluminal bile acid concentration falls below
a critical micellar concentration (1.5–2.0 mM), malabsorption of fat-
soluble vitamins ensues. Cholestyramine and colestipol, bile acid-binding
resins, are sometimes used to relieve cholestatic itching, but may deplete
enteral bile acids and interfere with fat-soluble vitamin absorption from
the intestine. Vitamin A and vitamin E require hydrolysis by an intestinal
esterase that is bile acid dependent before intestinal absorption. In infants,
cholestasis leads to rapid depletion of body stores of fat-soluble vitamins
with evidence of both biochemical and clinical features of deficiency unless
adequate supplementation is provided. Evaluation for fat-soluble vitamin
deficiency, supplementation, and follow-up monitoring are critical for
infants and children with cholestasis.

At the time of diagnosis of chronic liver disease or cholestasis, serum
vitamin A, 25-hydroxyvitamin D (25-OH-D), and vitamin E concentrations generally are measured to assess for fat-soluble vitamin sufficiency.
As a surrogate for direct vitamin K measurement, prothrombin time and/
or INR can be used. In the child with cholestasis, or if deficiency is found,
follow-up monitoring of fat-soluble vitamin levels is crucial. Achieving

adequate supplementation without toxicity is difficult and may require both preparations containing several fat-soluble vitamins in water-miscible form and individual water-miscible forms of the fat-soluble vitamins.[11] Yearly monitoring may be adequate in mild-moderate, slowly progressive disease. More frequent monitoring should be considered in children with more progressive disease. After initiating supplementation or changing the dose of supplementation, repeat measurement should be performed in 2 to 3 months. This repeat measurement ensures adequate replacement of the vitamin and reduces risk of excessive doses of these vitamins. Specifics of measurement will be noted for each vitamin in the sections to follow.

Initial therapy to alleviate the malabsorption of fat-soluble vitamins in chronic liver disease can be a double daily dose of an aqueous preparation of vitamins A, D, E, and K. In some cases, only a single vitamin will be deficient and can be supplemented individually. However, as liver disease progresses, it frequently becomes necessary to prescribe water-soluble forms of the fat-soluble vitamins to achieve appropriate serum concentrations. Some preparations of individual fat-soluble vitamins are available in water-soluble form (for example, Liqui-E, d-α-tocopherol polyethylene glycol succinate [vitamin E]), but most often, more than one deficiency exists and use of a multivitamin designed for individuals with fat malabsorption is appropriate. Many of these vitamins were originally designed for use by individuals with cystic fibrosis and contain all 4 fat-soluble vitamins in water-miscible forms. Varying forms are available for children of different ages.

A major concern for all supplementation is the cost of the water-miscible products necessary to achieve adequate fat-soluble vitamin levels in children with cholestasis and chronic liver disease. These products are much more expensive than standard supplemental vitamins and are generally not covered by insurance. If children do not achieve the response to supplementation expected, questions regarding both compliance and financial issues are important.

Each fat-soluble vitamin will be discussed individually, because evaluation, supplementation, and monitoring differ.

Vitamin A
Vitamin A refers to retinol and its derivatives having similar biologic activities. The principal vitamin A compounds include retinol, retinal (retinaldehyde), retinoic acid, and retinyl esters that differ in the terminal group at the end of the side chain. Dietary vitamin A predominantly is derived from animal sources (liver, fish liver oils, dairy products, kidney, eggs) and

carotenoids (provitamin A, beta carotene) in darkly colored vegetables, oily fruits, and red palm oil. The Adequate Intake for vitamin A for infants is 400 to 500 µg/day. The RDA of vitamin A for children 1 to 3 years of age is 300 µg/day, for 4 to 8 years of age is 400 µg/day, and for older children and adults is 600 to 1000 µg/day.[12]

As a fat-soluble vitamin, vitamin A absorption can be adversely affected by cholestasis. Determinations of serum retinol and/or retinol-binding protein are routinely used to screen for vitamin A nutritional status in children with chronic liver disease. Vitamin A deficiency is reported in 35% to 69% of children with cholestatic liver disease. In general, serum concentrations of retinol and/or retinol-binding protein are used to monitor vitamin A concentrations, although they may not accurately reflect vitamin A sufficiency or deficiency states, particularly in cholestatic liver disease, because vitamin A is stored in the liver.

Detecting vitamin A deficiency is important, because vitamin A deficiency may lead to xeropthalmia, keratomalacia and irreversible damage to the cornea of the eye, night blindness, and pigmentary retinopathy. Although these ocular findings are rare in cholestatic children, the potential for eye damage and visual disturbance is real.

Oral supplementation of vitamin A in children with liver disease ranges from 5000 to 25 000 IU/day of water-miscible vitamin A. Oral water-miscible vitamin A, as an individual vitamin, is not readily available for use in infants. Vitamin A capsules (8000 U/capsule, 10 000 U/capsule, 15 000 U/capsule, or 25 000 U/capsule, generic) are available. AquADEKs Pediatric Liquid (Axcan Pharma) contains 5751 IU/mL of vitamin A (www.axcan.com) in a water-miscible form; other preparations are available. Vitamin A parenteral (Aquasol A Parenteral, Mayne Pharma, 50 000 U/mL-15 mg retinol) may be used for vitamin A replacement therapy intramuscularly.

Monitoring during vitamin A supplementation is obligatory, both to ensure adequate levels of vitamin A and to prevent toxicity. Vitamin A toxicity may cause fatigue; malaise; anorexia; vomiting; increased intracranial pressure; painful bone lesions, including osteopenia and higher risk of fractures; hypercalcemia; and a massive desquamation dermatitis.[13] Vitamin A hepatotoxicity is associated with elevated retinyl esters, which can be assayed.[14] Recent studies suggest that relatively little excess vitamin A can lead to toxicity, so close monitoring of vitamin A status and of any supplementation is warranted.[15]

Vitamin D

Vitamin D (calciferol) includes vitamin D_2 (ergocalciferol) and vitamin D_3 (cholecalciferol). Vitamin D_2 is found in plants and fungi. Vitamin D_3 is found naturally in very few foods, an exception being saltwater fish. It is added to milk in the United States and is in most supplemental vitamins. Although there is some evidence that vitamin D_3 as a dietary supplement may be more effective than vitamin D_2, in treating patients requiring large amounts of vitamin D, vitamin D_2 is more economical. Vitamin D_3 is photosynthesized in the skin of vertebrates by the action of ultraviolet B radiation. Vitamin D is biologically inert and requires hydroxylation to form its biologically active hormone 1,25-dihydroxyvitamin-D (1,25-OH-2D). Hydroxylation at the 1 position occurs in the kidney, and 25-hydroxylation occurs in the liver. A major biologic function of vitamin D in humans is to maintain serum calcium and phosphorus concentrations within the normal range by enhancing the efficiency of the small intestine to absorb these minerals from the diet. The adequate intake for vitamin D is 10 µg/day (400 IU) for infants and 15 µg/day (600 IU) for children and adults.[16]

Vitamin D deficiency is demonstrated by its effect on calcium metabolism, resulting in hypocalcemia, hypophosphatemia, tetany, osteomalacia, and rickets. Children with chronic liver disease may develop hepatic osteodystrophy manifested by rickets, bone demineralization (osteopenia), or pathologic fractures.[17] These findings are in part the result of fat malabsorption attributable to diminished bile outflow, leading to steatorrhea and associated calcium and vitamin D malabsorption. Hypocalcemia and vitamin D insufficiency result in secondary hyperparathyroidism and increased bone resorption. Despite vitamin D repletion by supplementation to normal values, some patients continue to have low bone mass, implying that vitamin D status alone does not account for hepatic osteodystrophy.[18] Magnesium deficiency has been proposed to play a role in the development of this bone disease.[19] Liver transplantation has demonstrated remarkable improvement in bone mineral density of these children.[20]

Assessment of bone health is complex. Children with liver disease who are being monitored ahead of bone disease may require few laboratory studies while children with existing or suspected osteomalacia, osteopenia, and rickets may require extensive laboratory and radiographic studies. Children with liver disease should have vitamin D measured as serum concentration of 25-OH-D. If the child is being treated with large amounts

VI

of vitamin D_2, the most economical form of supplementation, the total 25-OH-D concentration may be underestimated in some assays. It is important to use an assay that accurately measures both 25-OH-D_2 and 25-OH-D_3. The AAP and the IOM recommend a target for serum 25-OH-D concentration $\geq$50 nmol/L (20 ng/mL) (see Chapter 21.I). Measurement of 1,25-OH-$_2$D is only necessary when there is kidney disease in addition to liver disease. Additional useful information may include serum concentrations of calcium, phosphorous, magnesium, alkaline phosphatase, albumin, and parathyroid hormone. When indicated, bone mineral content is assessed by dual-energy x-ray absorptiometry. Dietary calcium and phosphorus intake can also be assessed using a trained nutritionist.

Periodic assessment of total serum 25-OH-D concentration, adequate sunlight exposure, and adequate dietary intake of calcium and phosphorous is recommended for cholestatic children. Vitamin D insufficiency can be treated with oral vitamin D supplementation, usually at a dose range of 600 to 2000 IU/day. Serum 25-OH-D concentrations must be closely monitored along with calcium and phosphorus concentrations during supplementation to ensure repletion of vitamin D. Vitamin D deficiency and hypocalcemia attributable to dietary calcium deficiency or malabsorption can lead to rickets and osteopenia on bone radiographs. Large doses of vitamin D supplements (5000–20 000 IU/day) may be required to correct this condition.

Parenteral vitamin D preparations are available in some counties but are generally unavailable in the United States. They are painful injections and should be used only if patients fail to respond to oral therapy because of increased costs and risks for toxicity. If available, careful monitoring for vitamin D intoxication should be performed using urine calcium-to-creatinine ratio, serum calcium and phosphorus, and serum 25-OH-D concentrations. Vitamin D toxicity may include hypercalcemia causing central nervous system depression, ectopic calcifications, hypercalciuria resulting in nephrocalcinosis, and nephrolithiasis. Bisphosphonates are not recommended for use for children with chronic liver disease.[21]

Vitamin E

Vitamin E refers to a group of 8 compounds including the tocopherols and the tocotrienols. The 4 major forms of vitamin E (alpha, beta, gamma, and delta) differ by the position and number of methyl group substitutions and their bioactivity. Alpha-tocopherol is the predominant form found in food and has the highest biologic activity. The RDA for adequate vitamin E is

4 mg/day in infants 0 to 6 months of age, 5 mg/day in infants 7 to 12 months of age, 6 mg/day in children 1 to 3 years of age, 7 mg/day in children 4 to 8 years of age, 11 mg/day in children 9 to 13 years of age, and 15 mg/day in adolescents 14 to 18 years of age. Oral vitamin E requires solubilization by bile acids to mixed micelles and esterase hydrolysis by pancreatic or intestinal esterases that are bile acid dependent before absorption by the intestinal enterocyte. In blood, vitamin E is transported in low-density and high-density lipoprotein.[22]

In infants and children with cholestasis, impaired secretion of bile acids results in malabsorption of vitamin E.[23] Vitamin E is the most hydrophobic of the fat-soluble vitamins and has the greatest need for bile acids intra-luminally for absorption. Vitamin E absorption, as determined by an oral vitamin E tolerance test, is profoundly diminished in cholestatic children who are vitamin E deficient and can be improved by coadministration of bile acids.[23] Vitamin E is necessary to maintain the structure and function of the nervous system and muscular system. Peripheral neuropathy, ataxia, ophthalmoplegia, and muscle weakness characterize vitamin E deficiency in children with cholestasis.[24] Reversal of these findings may be accomplished before permanent injury occurs if supplementation and normalization of serum vitamin E concentrations is accomplished before 3 years of age.[25] The best predictor of vitamin E status in cholestatic children is the ratio of serum vitamin E to total serum lipids (the sum of the serum cholesterol and triglycerides, and phospholipids), because vitamin E partitions into the plasma lipoproteins that may be increased in cholestasis.[26] The serum vitamin E level may be increased into the normal range as a result of its partitioning into the plasma lipoproteins. The ratio of serum vitamin E to lipid compensates for this phenomenon. Biochemical vitamin E deficiency in older children and adults is <0.8 mg total tocopherol/g total lipid and for infants younger than 1 year is <0.6 mg/g. The target vitamin E-to-lipid ratio for correction of vitamin E deficiency is 0.8 to 1.0 mg/g. Other measure-ments of vitamin E, including measurement of vitamin E in adipose tissue, red blood cell (RBC) hydrogen peroxide hemolysis, the RBC malondialde-hyde release test,[27,28] and breath ethane and pentane measurements[29] are rarely available or impractical.

To prevent vitamin E deficiency in cholestatic infants and children, vitamin E supplementation as a water-miscible product is indicated. In infants, 50 to 100 IU/day of vitamin E (alpha-tocopherol [Aqua-E, Yasoo Health], 20 IU/mL; Liqui-E, TPGS-d-alpha-tocopheryl poly-ethylene

VI

glycol 1000 succinate, 400 IU/15 mL, Twinlabs) may be prescribed. In older children with vitamin E deficiency, 15 to 25 IU/kg/day of vitamin E therapy is initiated. Vitamin E is also included in the products designed for patients with cystic fibrosis. Vitamin E should not be administered with medications that might hamper its intestinal absorption (ie, cholestyramine) and may benefit from morning administration, when bile flow may be maximal after an overnight fast. Monitoring by vitamin E-to-lipid ratio and neurologic examination will help determine the need to increase vitamin E dosing if normalization does not occur within several weeks of therapy. Vitamin E toxicity is rare and may present as bleeding in children taking anticoagulants or sepsis in neonates.

Vitamin K

Vitamin K is a member of the naphthoquinone family and has 3 forms.[30] Phylloquinone (vitamin K_1) is found in leafy vegetables, soybean oil, fruits, seeds, and cow milk. Menaquinone (vitamin K_2) is produced by intestinal bacteria. Menadione (vitamin K_3) is a synthesized form of vitamin K and has better water solubility. Because of the lack of data to estimate an average requirement, a recommended adequate intake is based on representative dietary intake data from healthy individuals. The Adequate Intake for vitamin K is 2.0 µg/day for infants 0 to 6 months of age, 2.5 µg/day for infants 7 to 12 months of age, 30 µg/day for children 1 to 3 years of age, 55 µg/day for children 4 to 8 years of age, 60 µg/day for children 9 to 13 years of age, and 75 µg/day for children 14 to 18 years of age. The Adequate Intake for men and women is 120 and 90 µg/day, respectively. No adverse effect has been reported for individuals consuming higher amounts of vitamin K.[31]

Absorption of vitamin K_1 requires bile and pancreatic secretions that are impaired by cholestasis. Intestinal absorption of vitamin K_1 is an active process, while vitamin K_2 absorption is by passive diffusion. Absorbed vitamin K is incorporated into chylomicrons and is transported to the blood via the lymph. Little vitamin K is stored in the liver.

Vitamin K functions as a coenzyme during the synthesis of the biologically active form of a number of proteins involved in blood coagulation and bone metabolism. The vitamin K-dependent coagulation proteins include factors II, VII, IX, and X; protein C; and protein S.[32] Another family of vitamin K-dependent proteins includes the gla proteins. Osteocalcin is one of these proteins involved in bone mineralization.[33] Vitamin K deficiency in infancy can cause a coagulopathy resulting in intracranial bleeding.[34] In cholestatic children, malabsorption of vitamin K accompanied by antibiotic suppression of intestinal flora vitamin K production predisposes to vitamin K deficiency.[35]

Vitamin K status is frequently measured by using the prothrombin time/INR, which is dependent on vitamin K-dependent clotting factors. If the prothrombin time/INR is prolonged in comparison with the partial thromboplastin time, then vitamin K deficiency is likely. Liver disease may prolong the prothrombin time/INR because of impaired synthesis of clotting factors active in the intrinsic coagulation pathway. Vitamin K deficiency in liver disease may be underestimated by as much as 50% by the use of prothrombin time/INR as a surrogate marker.[36] However, other measures of vitamin K are not widely available or are impractical. Vitamin K status can be more sensitively ascertained by the plasma protein-induced in vitamin K absence (PIVKA)-II assay (enzyme-linked immunosorbent assay). Plasma PIVKA-II values greater than 3 ng/mL are indicative of vitamin K deficiency. Plasma-conjugated bilirubin, total bile acids, and severity of liver disease all have positively correlated with plasma PIVKA-II concentrations. However, some have suggested that this test is not clinically useful, because abnormal concentrations may also be found in healthy patients. Measurement of vitamin K-dependent clotting factors is costly and offers no advantage over monitoring prothrombin time for assessing vitamin K deficiency.

Vitamin K deficiency in children with cholestasis should be avoided; supplementation should begin prior to demonstration of elevated INR, to prevent vitamin K-deficient bleeding. Supplementation with oral vitamin K should be provided (Mephyton, Aton Pharma Inc [vitamin K1], 5-mg tablets) in a daily or twice-weekly dose of 2.5 to 10 mg, depending on response to therapy. There is also a water miscible form in vitamin preparations for patients with cystic fibrosis (Table 43.1). Failure to respond to oral vitamin K supplementation may require subcutaneous or intravenous vitamin K administration (AquaMephyton, Merck and Co, [vitamin K₁], 2 mg/mL or 10 mg/mL). If administered intravenously, it should be administered slowly, not to exceed 1 mg/minute, to avoid anaphylaxis. To attempt correction of coagulopathy, vitamin K may be administered subcutaneously or intravenously for 3 days consecutively. Failure to respond to this regimen suggests significant hepatic dysfunction.

VI

Table 43.1.
Vitamin Supplementation in Children With Cholestasis

Vitamin	Recommended Dose	Preparation	Dose Provided
Vitamin A	Oral supplementation of vitamin A ranges from 5000–25 000 IU/day of water-miscible vitamin A	Water-miscible form of fat soluble vitamins ("cystic fibrosis vitamin")[a]	3170–16 000 IU/mL or capsule, beta carotene or retinol palmitate, depending on product
		Vitamin A capsules (**not** water-miscible)	10 000 U/capsule or 25 000 U/capsule, generic
		Vitamin A parenteral (Aquasol A Parenteral, Mayne Pharma)	50 000 U/mL–15 mg retinol
Vitamin D	600–2000 IU/day[b]	Oral vitamin D supplementation	Ergocalciferol (D_2) oral solution, tablets or capsules OR Cholecalciferol (D_3) oral solution, tablets or capsules
		Water-miscible form of fat soluble vitamins ("cystic fibrosis vitamin")	400–3000 IU/mL or capsule, depending on product

Vitamin E	In infants, 50–200 IU/kg/day In older children with vitamin E deficiency, 15–25 IU/kg/day	Liqui-E (TPGS-d-alpha-tocopheryl polyethylene glycol 1000 succinate, Twinlabs)[a]	400 IU/15 mL
		A-tocopherol, Aqua-E (Yasoo Health)	20 IU/mL
		Water-miscible form of fat soluble vitamins ("cystic fibrosis vitamin")	50–200 IU/mL or capsule, depending on product
Vitamin K	Daily or twice weekly dose of 2.5–10 mg, dependent on response to therapy	Mephyton, Anton Pharma (vitamin K_1)	5-mg tablets
		Water-miscible form of fat soluble vitamins ("Cystic Fibrosis vitamin")	300–1000 mcg/mL or capsule, depending on product
	Subcutaneous or intravenous vitamin K administration (1–5 mg, dependent on size)	AquaMephyton, Merck and Co (vitamin K_1)	2 mg/mL or 10 mg/mL

[a] Preferred form for supplementation in cholestasis.

[b] Starting dose for maintenance. For deficient children or those with rickets, see Hogler et al.[21]

Water-Soluble Vitamins *(see also Chapter 21.II: Water-Soluble Vitamins)*

Although in theory, decreased intake and malabsorption secondary to enteropathy are risk factors for deficiencies of water-soluble vitamins in children with chronic liver diseases, no systematic deficiencies of these vitamins in these conditions have been reported. Deficiencies of water-soluble vitamins in children with chronic liver disease are likely to be uncommon, because infant and enteral formulas used to feed children with chronic liver disease are supplemented with these vitamins.

Trace Elements *(see also Chapter 20: Trace Elements)*

Zinc

Although children with chronic liver disease are often considered at risk of trace element deficiencies, no systematic studies of these deficiencies have been reported. Zinc is an important trace metal that is essential for normal cellular growth and differentiation, immune function, wound healing, and protein synthesis. Zinc deficiency is associated with acrodermatitis, diarrhea, and poor growth. Zinc metabolism is altered in children and adults with chronic liver disease. Infants and children with biliary atresia have been observed to have lower plasma zinc concentrations compared with controls.[37] Plasma zinc concentrations do not correlate with age, episodes of cholangitis, or repeated surgical procedures. Inappropriate urinary zinc excretion has been documented in children with chronic liver disease and hypozincemia and may be the pathogenesis for the observed deficiency in chronic liver disease.[38] Other potential causes of zinc deficiency in patients with chronic liver disease include decreased intestinal absorption, decreased dietary intake, and reduced portal-venous extraction secondary to portosystemic shunting. After liver transplantation, abnormal zinc homeostasis can rapidly improve and biochemical zinc deficiency reverses.[39] Serum zinc concentrations may not reflect total body zinc status. For example decreased zinc levels are associated with food intake and stress and increased zinc levels occur with muscle catabolism. Identification of subclinical zinc deficiency is difficult, although occasionally a low concentration of alkaline phosphatase, a zinc-dependent enzyme, can indicate a zinc deficiency state. If clinical signs of zinc deficiency are suspected (acrodermatitis, diarrhea, and poor growth), an empiric trial of zinc supplementation is warranted. The standard dose of zinc for supplementation is 1 to 2 mg/kg/day of elemental zinc.

Copper

Copper is an essential trace element and functions as a cofactor for several important enzymes, such as lysyl oxidase, elastase, monoamine oxidase, cytochrome oxidase, ceruloplasmin, and superoxide dismutase. Deficiency of copper may be expressed by impaired activity of these enzymes. Signs of copper deficiency include neutropenia, microcytic anemia nonresponsive to iron supplementation, bone abnormalities, skin disorders, and depigmentation of hair and skin. The immune system is affected, resulting in diminished phagocytic activity of neutrophils and impaired cellular immunity. The anemia is the result of low concentrations of ceruloplasmin or ferroxidase. This enzyme is required for the incorporation of iron into hemoglobin.

Wilson disease is an autosomal-recessive disorder of copper metabolism that results in toxic effects of copper. In patients with Wilson disease, excess copper is stored in the body, especially in the liver and brain. Clinically, patients develop cirrhosis, eye lesions (Kayser-Fleisher rings), kidney abnormalities, and neurologic disease. Despite high concentrations of copper in the liver, serum concentrations of copper and ceruloplasmin are often low. Treatment includes chelation therapy with d-penicillamine or triethylenetetramine (trientine) and oral zinc therapy to reduce intestinal copper absorption. Avoidance of high-copper foods (for example, organ meats, shellfish, dried beans) is necessary.

Copper is excreted into the intestinal tract via the biliary route. Thus, copper deficiency is unlikely to occur in children with cholestasis. However, when cholestatic children receive parenteral nutrition, copper concentrations should be monitored carefully to avoid excessive accumulation of systemic copper. Presumptively removing copper from parenteral nutrition trace elements in the absence of elevated copper concentrations is not recommended, because it can increase risk for copper deficiency, which can lead to anemia, leukopenia, and bone fractures. Copper deficiency in children receiving parenteral nutrition appears to be more common than toxicity.[40]

Chromium

Chromium functions as a cofactor for insulin. Chromium deficiency is associated with poor growth and impaired glucose, lipid, and protein metabolism. Although peripheral insulin resistance and glucose intolerance occur in liver disease and chromium deficiency in adults, studies of the utility of chromium supplementation in adults or children with chronic liver disease are nonexistent. Chromium deficiency in infants is probably rare and

VI

only associated with protein-calorie malnutrition or prolonged parenteral nutrition without supplementation. Other than occasional development of glucose intolerance and hyperglycemia, the only indicator of chromium deficiency is the demonstration of a beneficial effect to chromium supplementation.

Manganese

Manganese is a cofactor for enzymes such as arginase, glutamate-ammonia ligase, manganese superoxide dismutase, and pyruvate carboxylase. Deficiency of manganese has not been reported in infants and children. Toxic effects of manganese accumulation in the basal ganglia are reported in adults with cirrhosis and liver disease and may cause lack of coordination and balance, mental confusion, and muscle cramps and may contribute to hepatic encephalopathy. Extrapyramidal effects may resemble Parkinson disease. Because manganese is excreted in bile, children with cholestatic liver disease may develop elevated plasma concentrations.[41] Children with cholestatic liver disease who receive parenteral nutrition should have manganese eliminated or reduced in trace mineral supplementation in parenteral nutrition solutions.

Selenium

Selenium deficiency has been demonstrated in children receiving long-term parenteral nutrition without supplementation. Selenium deficiency results in macrocytosis and loss of hair and skin pigmentation.[42] Selenium is a required part of several proteins, such as selenium-dependent glutathione peroxidase, selenoprotein P, and deiodinase. Serum selenium concentration may be decreased in adults with liver disease. Selenium should be measured in children with end-stage liver disease and can be supplemented at 1 to 2 µg/kg/day to achieve repletion.[4]

Calcium

In end-stage liver disease, hypoalbuminemia may lead to low serum calcium concentrations. In such situations, it is recommended that ionized calcium should be measured to accurately determine concentrations. Calcium supplementation may be required in liver disease, particularly in children receiving very high levels of vitamin D to avoid "hungry bone" syndrome.[43]

Ascites Management

Ascites development in chronic liver disease usually signifies advanced disease with portal hypertension. Only the nutritional issues related to ascites management are considered here. Although sodium and fluid restriction were recommended in the past for management of ascites, it has been found that severe restriction may lead to poor nutrient intake and malnutrition.[44] A diet that is sodium free or severely sodium restricted may be unpalatable for a child. Although the diet should restrict excess sodium (sodium intake >2–3 mEq/kg body weight/day), management with diuretics and paracentesis is used before severe sodium restriction. During hospitalization for severe ascites, all sources of sodium intake, whether dietary, in intravenous fluids, medications, etc, must be counted.

Liver Failure

Children with acute liver failure may develop hepatic encephalopathy (hepatic coma). Ammonia, the result of protein metabolism, is considered to be a contributing factor in the development and progression of encephalopathy. Thus, protein restriction is recommended for children with severe hepatic encephalopathy, and for children in deep coma, a completely protein-free diet may be warranted. However, to regenerate new liver tissue, some protein is advisable (1 g/kg/day) in children who can tolerate small amounts so that anabolism, and not catabolism, of protein stores occurs. Some studies suggested administration of branched-chain amino acid (BCAA)-enriched formulas might improve encephalopathy; a Cochrane review found BCAA supplementation improved hepatic encephalopathy in adults without affecting mortality.[45] Formulas containing high levels of BCAA are expensive, and their role for children with liver failure has not been defined.

Parenteral Nutrition-Associated Liver Disease

Parenteral nutrition-associated liver disease results from prolonged use of parenteral nutrition. It is especially prevalent among neonates with short bowel, recurrent sepsis, surgical procedures, or prematurity (see Chapter 22: Parenteral Nutrition). Infants and older children sustaining severe liver toxicity that leads to cirrhosis and irreversible liver injury may require liver with or without small intestinal transplantation as a life-saving measure. Parenteral nutrition-associated liver disease may be prevented or treated by advancement of enteral nutrition; however, some children cannot tolerate adequate enteral feeds to avoid hepatic injury. Both restriction of parenteral lipid emulsions[46] and provision of lipid emulsions containing fish oil with a high content of long-chain polyunsaturated fatty acids[47] may be effective at preventing and treating parenteral nutrition-associated liver disease. Soybean/medium-chain triglyceride/olive/fish oil emulsion (SMOF) is now available as an option for lipids in children requiring parenteral nutrition.[48-50] Further investigations are ongoing to determine efficacy of these treatments.

Nonalcoholic Fatty Liver Disease

Nonalcoholic fatty liver disease (NAFLD) is associated with obesity and is the most common form of liver disease in children. The estimated prevalence in the United States is 9.6% for children 2 to 19 years old; however, it is estimated to be present in 38% of obese children.[51] Untreated NAFLD may progress to cirrhosis and end-stage liver disease, even in adolescents. In adults, lifestyle modification leading to at least 5% to 10% weight loss improves liver histology and reverses fibrosis.[52,53] For children with NAFLD related to obesity, lifestyle modification with weight loss is recommended; however, no studies in children have been performed that allow recommendation of any specific weight-loss diet.[54] Trials have been conducted on various medications in children with NAFLD; these trials are complicated by differing outcome measures (liver enzymes vs hepatic ultrasonography vs liver biopsy), small sample sizes, and extent of randomization. Some experts recommend vitamin E supplementation (400 IU twice daily in children >6 years old) on the basis of available data; however, although vitamin E reduced hepatocellular ballooning and hepatic enzymes, it had no effect on steatosis, inflammation, or fibrosis.[55] More studies of specific lifestyle alterations is crucial to determining the optimal management of this important liver disease.

Liver Transplantation

Liver transplantation is a life-saving intervention in children with end-stage liver disease or life-threatening acute liver disease or metabolic liver disease. The child's nutritional status has an effect on survival after transplantation as well as wait-list mortality.[2,56] Thus, particular attention must be paid to the nutrition of the child on the liver transplantation wait list. After transplantation, it should be recognized that hepatic osteodystrophy may take 1 to 2 years to resolve and may be prolonged by steroid use in the immunosuppression regimen. Children who have undergone liver transplantation may be at increased risk of obesity. Obesity can lead to metabolic syndrome but may also risk damage to the transplanted organ.[57] Increased risk is associated with Hispanic ethnicity, steroid use in the postoperative period, and pretransplant overweight or obesity.[58]

References

1. Tanpowpong P, Broder-Fingert S, Katz AJ, Camargo CA, Jr. Predictors of gluten avoidance and implementation of a gluten-free diet in children and adolescents without confirmed celiac disease. *J Pediatr.* 2012;161(3):471–475

2. Utterson EC, Shepherd RW, Sokol RJ, et al. Biliary atresia: clinical profiles, risk factors, and outcomes of 755 patients listed for liver transplantation. *J Pediatr.* 2005;147(2):180–185

3. Sundaram SS, Mack CL, Feldman AG, Sokol RJ. Biliary atresia: Indications and timing of liver transplantation and optimization of pretransplant care. *Liver Transpl.* 2017;23(1):96–109

4. Young S, Kwarta E, Azzam R, Sentongo T. Nutrition assessment and support in children with end-stage liver disease. *Nutr Clin Pract.* 2013;28(3):317–329

5. Hanai T, Shiraki M, Nishimura K, et al. Sarcopenia impairs prognosis of patients with liver cirrhosis. *Nutrition.* 2015;31(1):193–199

6. Montano-Loza AJ. Muscle wasting: a nutritional criterion to prioritize patients for liver transplantation. *Curr Opin Clin Nutr Metab Care.* 2014;17(3):219–225

7. Badley BW, Murphy GM, Bouchier IA, Sherlock S. Diminished micellar phase lipid in patients with chronic nonalcoholic liver disease and steatorrhea. *Gastroenterology.* 1970;58(6):781–789

8. Wene JD, Connor WE, DenBesten L. The development of essential fatty acid deficiency in healthy men fed fat-free diets intravenously and orally. *J Clin Invest.* 1975;56(1):127–134

9. Pettei MJ, Daftary S, Levine JJ. Essential fatty acid deficiency associated with the use of a medium-chain-triglyceride infant formula in pediatric hepatobiliary disease. *Am J Clin Nutr.* 1991;53(5):1217–1221

10. Kaufman SS, Scrivner DJ, Murray ND, Vanderhoof JA, Hart MH, Antonson DL. Influence of portagen and pregestimil on essential fatty acid status in infantile liver disease. *Pediatrics.* 1992;89(1):151–154

11. Shneider BL, Magee JC, Bezerra JA, et al. Efficacy of fat-soluble vitamin supplementation in infants with biliary atresia. *Pediatrics.* 2012;130(3):e607–e614

12. Ross AC. Vitamin A. In: Ross AC, Caballero B, Cousins RJ, Tucker KL, Ziegler TR, eds. *Modern Nutrition in Health and Disease.* Eleventh ed. Baltimore: Wolters Kluwer/Lippincott Williams & Wilkins; 2014:260–277

13. Lippe B, Hensen L, Mendoza G, Finerman M, Welch M. Chronic vitamin A intoxication. A multisystem disease that could reach epidemic proportions. *Am J Dis Child.* 1981;135(7):634–636

VI

14. Smith FR, Goodman DS. Vitamin A transport in human vitamin A toxicity. *N Engl J Med.* 1976;294(15):805–808

15. Penniston KL, Tanumihardjo SA. The acute and chronic toxic effects of vitamin A. *Am J Clin Nutr.* 2006;83(2):191–201

16. Jones G. Vitamin D. In: Ross AC, Caballero B, Cousins RJ, Tucker KL, Ziegler TR, eds. *Modern Nutrition in Health and Disease.* 11th ed. Baltimore: Wolters Kluwer/ Lippincott Williams & Wilkins; 2014:278–292

17. Heubi JE, Hollis BW, Specker B, Tsang RC. Bone disease in chronic childhood cholestasis. I. Vitamin D absorption and metabolism. *Hepatology.* 1989;9(2): 258–264

18. Bucuvalas JC, Heubi JE, Specker BL, Gregg DJ, Yergey AL, Vieira NE. Calcium absorption in bone disease associated with chronic cholestasis during childhood. *Hepatology.* 1990;12(5):1200–1205

19. Heubi JE, Higgins JV, Argao EA, Sierra RI, Specker BL. The role of magnesium in the pathogenesis of bone disease in childhood cholestatic liver disease: a preliminary report. *J Pediatr Gastroenterol Nutr.* 1997;25(3):301–306

20. Argao EA, Balistreri WF, Hollis BW, Ryckman FC, Heubi JE. Effect of orthotopic liver transplantation on bone mineral content and serum vitamin D metabolites in infants and children with chronic cholestasis. *Hepatology.* 1994;20(3):598–603

21. Hogler W, Baumann U, Kelly D. Endocrine and bone metabolic complications in chronic liver disease and after liver transplantation in children. *J Pediatr Gastroenterol Nutr.* 2012;54(3):313–321

22. Traber MG. Vitamin E. In: Ross AC, Caballero B, Cousins RJ, Tucker KL, Ziegler TR, eds. *Modern Nutrition in Health and Disease.* 11th ed. Baltimore: Wolters Kluwer/Lippincott Williams & Wilkins; 2014:293–304

23. Sokol RJ, Heubi JE, Iannaccone S, Bove KE, Balistreri WF. Mechanism causing vitamin E deficiency during chronic childhood cholestasis. *Gastroenterology.* 1983;85(5):1172–1182

24. Guggenheim MA, Jackson V, Lilly J, Silverman A. Vitamin E deficiency and neurologic disease in children with cholestasis: a prospective study. *J Pediatr.* 1983;102(4):577–579

25. Sokol RJ, Guggenheim MA, Iannaccone ST, et al. Improved neurologic function after long-term correction of vitamin E deficiency in children with chronic cholestasis. *N Engl J Med.* 1985;313(25):1580–1586

26. Sokol RJ, Heubi JE, Iannaccone ST, Bove KE, Balistreri WF. Vitamin E deficiency with normal serum vitamin E concentrations in children with chronic cholestasis. *N Engl J Med.* 1984;310(19):1209–1212

27. Cynamon HA, Isenberg JN, Nguyen CH. Erythrocyte malondialdehyde release in vitro: a functional measure of vitamin E status. *Clin Chim Acta.* 1985;151(2): 169–176

28. Gordon HH, Nitowsky HM, Cornblath M. Studies of tocopherol deficiency in infants and children. I. Hemolysis of erythrocytes in hydrogen peroxide. *Am J Dis Child.* 1955;90(6):669–681

29. Refat M, Moore TJ, Kazui M, Risby TH, Perman JA, Schwarz KB. Utility of breath ethane as a noninvasive biomarker of vitamin E status in children. *Pediatr Res.* 1991;30(5):396–403

30. Olson RE. The function and metabolism of vitamin K. *Annu Rev Nutr.* 1984;4: 281–337

31. Suttie JW. Vitamin K. In: Ross AC, Caballero B, Cousins RJ, Tucker KL, Ziegler TR, eds. *Modern Nutrition in Health and Disease.* 11th ed. Baltimore: Wolters Kluwer/Lippincott Williams & Wilkins; 2014:305–316

32. Shah DV, Suttie JW. The vitamin K dependent, in vitro production of prothrombin. *Biochem Biophys Res Commun.* 1974;60(4):1397–1402

33. Price PA, Parthemore JG, Deftos LJ. New biochemical marker for bone metabolism. Measurement by radioimmunoassay of bone GLA protein in the plasma of normal subjects and patients with bone disease. *J Clin Invest.* 1980;66(5):878–883

34. Bancroft J, Cohen MB. Intracranial hemorrhage due to vitamin K deficiency in breast-fed infants with cholestasis. *J Pediatr Gastroenterol Nutr.* 1993;16(1):78–80

35. Yanofsky RA, Jackson VG, Lilly JR, Stellin G, Klingensmith WC, 3rd, Hathaway WE. The multiple coagulopathies of biliary atresia. *Am J Hematol.* 1984;16(2): 171–180

36. Strople J, Lovell G, Heubi J. Prevalence of subclinical vitamin K deficiency in cholestatic liver disease. *J Pediatr Gastroenterol Nutr.* 2009;49(1):78–84

37. Goksu N, Ozsoylu S. Hepatic and serum levels of zinc, copper, and magnesium in childhood cirrhosis. *J Pediatr Gastroenterol Nutr.* 1986;5(3):459–462

38. Hambidge KM, Krebs NF, Lilly JR, Zerbe GO. Plasma and urine zinc in infants and children with extrahepatic biliary atresia. *J Pediatr Gastroenterol Nutr.* 1987;6(6):872–877

39. Narkewicz MR, Krebs N, Karrer F, Orban-Eller K, Sokol RJ. Correction of hypozincemia following liver transplantation in children is associated with reduced urinary zinc loss. *Hepatology.* 1999;29(3):830–833

40. MacKay M, Mulroy CW, Street J, et al. Assessing copper status in pediatric patients receiving parenteral nutrition. *Nutr Clin Pract.* 2015;30(1):117–121

41. Bayliss EA, Hambidge KM, Sokol RJ, Stewart B, Lilly JR. Hepatic concentrations of zinc, copper and manganese in infants with extrahepatic biliary atresia. *J Trace Elem Med Biol.* 1995;9(1):40–43

42. Vinton NE, Dahlstrom KA, Strobel CT, Ament ME. Macrocytosis and pseudoalbinism: manifestations of selenium deficiency. *J Pediatr.* 1987;111(5): 711–717

43. Misra M, Pacaud D, Petryk A, et al. Vitamin D deficiency in children and its management: review of current knowledge and recommendations. *Pediatrics.* 2008;122(2):398–417

44. Shepherd RW. Chronic liver disease, cirrhosis, and complications. In: Murray KF, Horslen S, eds. *Diseases of the Liver in Children.* New York, NY: Springer Science+Business Media; 2014:483–495

VI

45. Gluud LL, Dam G, Les I, et al. Branched-chain amino acids for people with hepatic encephalopathy. *Cochrane Database Syst Rev.* 2015(2):CD001939

46. Sanchez SE, Braun LP, Mercer LD, Sherrill M, Stevens J, Javid PJ. The effect of lipid restriction on the prevention of parenteral nutrition-associated cholestasis in surgical infants. *J Pediatr Surg.* 2013;48(3):573–578

47. Premkumar MH, Carter BA, Hawthorne KM, King K, Abrams SA. Fish oil-based lipid emulsions in the treatment of parenteral nutrition-associated liver disease: an ongoing positive experience. *Adv Nutr.* 2014;5(1):65–70

48. Pichler J, Simchowitz V, Macdonald S, Hill S. Comparison of liver function with two new/mixed intravenous lipid emulsions in children with intestinal failure. *Eur J Clin Nutr.* 2014;68(10):1161–1167

49. Dai YJ, Sun LL, Li MY, et al. Comparison of Formulas Based on Lipid Emulsions of Olive Oil, Soybean Oil, or Several Oils for Parenteral Nutrition: A Systematic Review and Meta-Analysis. *Adv Nutr.* 2016;7(2):279–286

50. Diamond IR, Grant RC, Pencharz PB, et al. Preventing the progression of intestinal failure-associated liver disease in infants using a composite lipid emulsion: a pilot randomized controlled trial of SMOFlipid. *JPEN J Parenter Enteral Nutr.* 2017;41(5):866–877

51. Schwimmer JB, Deutsch R, Kahen T, Lavine JE, Stanley C, Behling C. Prevalence of fatty liver in children and adolescents. *Pediatrics.* 2006;118(4):1388–1393

52. Promrat K, Kleiner DE, Niemeier HM, et al. Randomized controlled trial testing the effects of weight loss on nonalcoholic steatohepatitis. *Hepatology.* 2010;51(1):121–129

53. Vilar-Gomez E, Martinez-Perez Y, Calzadilla-Bertot L, et al. Weight Loss Through Lifestyle Modification Significantly Reduces Features of Nonalcoholic Steatohepatitis. *Gastroenterology.* 2015;149(2):367–378 e365

54. Nobili V, Alisi A, Newton KP, Schwimmer JB. Comparison of the phenotype and approach to pediatric vs adult patients with nonalcoholic fatty liver disease. *Gastroenterology.* 2016;150(8):1798–1810

55. Lavine JE, Schwimmer JB, Van Natta ML, et al. Effect of vitamin E or metformin for treatment of nonalcoholic fatty liver disease in children and adolescents: the TONIC randomized controlled trial. *JAMA.* 2011;305(16):1659–1668

56. Malenicka S, Ericzon B-G, Jørgensen MH, et al. Impaired intention-to-treat survival after listing for liver transplantation in children with biliary atresia compared to other chronic liver diseases: 20 years' experience from the Nordic countries. *Pediatr Transplant.* 2017 Mar;21(2). doi: 10.1111/petr.12851

57. Nobili V, de Ville de Goyet J. Pediatric post-transplant metabolic syndrome: new clouds on the horizon. *Pediatr Transplant.* 2013;17(3):216–223

58. Sundaram SS, Alonso EM, Zeitler P, Yin W, Anand R, SPLIT Research Group. Obesity after pediatric liver transplantation: prevalence and risk factors. *J Pediatr Gastroenterol Nutr.* 2012;55(6):657–662

Chapter 44

Cardiac Disease

Introduction

Malnutrition, impaired growth, and growth failure are prevalent in children with congenital heart disease (CHD) but result from undernutrition. Technically speaking, malnutrition can refer to undernutrition as well as overnutrition. For the purposes of this chapter, malnutrition and undernutrition will be used interchangeably as synonyms. There are generally 3 categories that describe undernutrition: inadequate intake, inefficient absorption and utilization, and/or increased energy needs, and children with CHD can be affected by all of these. Growth failure in heart disease has a multifactorial etiology and follows a pattern identical to acute and chronic protein-calorie undernutrition with wasting of body mass acutely and stunting of linear growth chronically. Hypoxemia (which commonly presents as cyanosis), congestive heart failure (CHF), and pulmonary hypertension are the sentinel features of CHD-associated with growth failure. Growth failure attributable to a congenital heart malformation may begin before birth. Many newborn infants with CHD carry the prenatal diagnosis of intrauterine growth restriction. Infants with most forms of cardiac malformations (transposition of the great arteries [TGA] being a notable exception) have a lower than normal birth weight.[1-3] Not only do children who have CHD have difficulty growing (short- and long-term), but that difficulty is compounded by the presence of concomitant chromosomal abnormalities, hypoxemia, prematurity, or other congenital syndromes and malformations (eg, trisomy 21, trisomy 18, Turner syndrome, VACTER association [vertebral defects, anal atresia, cardiac malformations, tracheo-esophageal fistula, renal abnormalities and limb abnormalities], CHARGE syndrome [coloboma, heart malformations, choanae atresia, retarded growth and development, genital abnormalities, ear abnormalities]), which are frequently associated with CHD.[4-6]

Acute undernutrition, defined as reduced weight relative to the median weight predicted by length (wasting), and chronic undernutrition, based on reduced length relative to the median length predicted for age (stunting), are more prevalent among hospitalized patients with CHD. Approximately 40% to 50% of patients with CHD meet criteria for some category of undernutrition, either acute or chronic,[7,8] although some older studies have found that number to be closer to 60% to 70%.[9] One newer study reported the prevalence of undernutrition at only 15%, but the power of this study was perhaps limited by its retrospective nature and small sample size of

VI

125 patients.[10] In the current age of successful single-ventricle palliative surgeries, it has been noted that infants who undergo the stage 1 Norwood palliation are at increased risk for undernutrition before surgery and that this risk continues during the postoperative period.[11–13] Even patients with atrial septal defect (ASD), not typically associated with growth failure in the minds of most physicians, can experience undernutrition associated with the hemodynamic impact of the lesion. In one study, the authors found that in patients with secundum ASD and body mass index (BMI) <5th percentile, there was improved growth after transcatheter closure.[14] Nearly all types of congenital heart defects can contribute to growth failure. Delay in skeletal maturation as assessed by bone age is related to severity of hypoxemia in cyanotic heart disease but also is observed in CHF.[15] Conversely, acyanotic lesions in which no significant intracardiac shunting is present (eg, aortic stenosis, coarctation, and pulmonary stenosis) without congestive heart failure or pulmonary hypertension may not be associated with undernutrition.

Undernutrition in CHD

Undernutrition occurs when metabolic demands for protein or energy (expenditure) combined with nutrient losses (regurgitation or malabsorption) exceed energy and protein nutrient intake. Delayed gastric emptying[16] and gastroesophageal reflux[17] in children with CHD as well as oral aversion may be significant features that reduce voluntary intake and compromise nutrition. There may be early satiety induced by gastroparesis and gut hypomotility related to edema or hypoxia as well as by distention from hepatomegaly associated with CHF. Investigators have attempted to study each of these components of nutrient balance, and as will be demonstrated below, measuring each of these components in seriously ill children with CHD is rife with challenges. In addition to deficits in these macronutrients affecting growth and body composition, clinically important deficiency in certain micronutrients may also occur.

Energy Expenditure

A number of studies have confirmed that total daily energy expenditure (TDEE), including components of physical activity, such as cardiorespiratory work associated with movement and dietary thermogenesis—the energy required to assimilate and metabolize nutrients—is increased significantly in children with CHD. TDEE comprises resting energy expenditure (REE), energy expended during physical activity, and dietary-induced thermogenesis. Energy intake must exceed TDEE to permit normal growth. The degree to which the increased TDEE observed in children with CHD is attributable to increases in REE is difficult to quantify. In patients with CHD who are already undernourished, 3 typical predictive REE models (Schofield,[18] World Health Organization,[19] and White et al[20]) yielded statistically significant different values than REE measured by indirect calorimetry.[21] Predictive models for REE, when used for properly selected patients, are a good "rough guide" to help guide the nutrition prescription. There are other predictive equations for calculating resting energy expenditure, but they either have not been tested in CHD, or literature suggests their utility in patients with congenital heart disease is limited. Some studies have demonstrated insignificant increases in REE relative to lean body mass.[22–26] Nydegger et al showed that infants with CHD have increased REE compared with healthy controls (247 kJ/kg/day vs 210 kJ/kg/day), which then normalizes 1 week after surgery,[27] while Farrell et al found that although measured REE was higher in infants with CHF compared with controls, it was not statistically significant.[28] More recently, Trabulsi et al could not demonstrate a statistically significant difference in TDEE when comparing healthy infants versus those with CHD.[29] After adjusting for fat-free mass, the 36.4 kcal/day increase in TDEE observed in infants with CHD versus healthy infants was not statistically significant ($P = .37$).[29] Together, these studies show the difficulty in quantifying what is readily observed at the bedside. Infants with CHD have higher energy requirements than their healthy counterparts.

Nutrient Losses

Some patients with CHD have abnormalities of gastrointestinal tract function or renal losses that may affect nutrition. Urinary losses of energy as glycosuria and proteinuria may be significant in certain patients with renal disease or glucose intolerance. Approximately 8% of infants with CHD have associated major gastrointestinal tract malformations, such as tracheoesophageal fistula and esophageal atresia, malrotation, or diaphragmatic hernia that generally will limit intake and cause losses of nutrients.[30] Fecal losses of energy in subclinical steatorrhea or of protein in protein-losing enteropathy may be more significant and prevalent than expected, affecting up to 50% of patients with a variety of congenital heart lesions. In one study, protein-losing enteropathy was found in 8 of 21 infants with severe CHD[31] and is a major complication common in patients who undergo the Fontan procedure or have severe right-sided CHF. Steatorrhea, indicative of disturbed digestion or absorption, was found in 5 of 21 infants with CHD (1 of 8 patients with CHF and 4 of 12 cyanotic patients). Mucosal small-bowel biopsies were normal, and mean resting oxygen consumption was higher in infants with CHF than in those with cyanotic heart disease.[31]

No significant malabsorption of energy or fat in stools was observed in the study of children receiving diuretics by Vaisman et al.[32] However, total body water and extracellular water excess were measured and correlated directly with fat losses and inversely with energy intake, suggesting a relationship to the degree of CHF and diuretic efficacy. Therefore, infants with increased total body water (ie, not effectively diuresed) had more malabsorption than did euvolemic diuresed patients. Van der Kuip et al noted that infants with CHD who were not effectively diuresed had increased total body water and a concomitant increase in TDEE. Those who were diuresed showed an attenuation in the increase of measured TDEE.[33] The same paper noted that infants with growth retardation and CHD experienced a 12% loss of ingested energy attributable to vomiting.

Yahav et al studied malabsorption relative to energy requirements in 14 infants with CHD 2 to 36 months of age (mean age, 10.4 months).[34] Ten infants with CHF and 4 with cyanosis were studied in 3 periods of 3 to 7 days each, comparing baseline oral intake, supplemented oral intake, and nasogastric feedings of a high-caloric density formula. Nasogastric feedings of a high-caloric density formula (1.5 kcal/mL or 45 kcal/oz) were administered to 11 patients. Consistent weight gain averaging 13 g/day was observed only in patients receiving >170 kcal/kg/day, with only 50% of the children gaining weight on 149 kcal/kg/day. Increased cardiac and respiratory rates were observed in patients after feeding and were attributed to dietary thermogenesis but did not appear to be clinically significant. Minor intestinal losses of fat were observed in 3 patients, and protein-losing enteropathy in zero patients, and these were not considered to be significant limiting factors in weight gain.[34]

Energy Intake

Several studies have examined energy/nutrient intake requirements of infants and young children with CHD (Table 44.1). Approximately 140 to 150 kcal/kg/day is required to effect linear growth and increase subcutaneous fat and muscle in infants with CHD and CHF. In one study of 19 infants randomly assigned to 3 groups, only the group receiving continuous 24-hour nasogastric feedings over a 5-month study period was able to achieve intakes >140 kcal/kg/day (mean, 147 kcal/kg/day).[35] Only this group

Table 44.1.

Protein Load in Relation to Energy Provided in Selected Formulas

Formula	Protein g/dL (% kcal)	kcal/mL	kcal/g Protein	kcal/kg @ 3.5 g/kg Protein	Protein g/kg @ 140 kcal/kg/day
Human milk	0.9 (5)	0.69	77	269	1.83
Enfamil/Similac	1.4 (8)	0.67	48	168	2.9
Pediasure/KidEssential/Nutren Jr	3 (12)	1	33	116	4.25
Portagen	2.4 (14)	0.67	28	98	5
Nutramigen/Pregestimil	1.9 (11)	0.67	35	123	4
Peptamen Jr/Peptide	3 (12)	1	33	116	4.25
Neocate/Elecare	2 (12)	0.67	35	123	4
Vivonex Ped	2.4 (12)	0.8	33	116	4.2
Enfaport	3.6 (14)	1	28	98	5
Vital HN	4.2 (16.7)	1	24	84	5.8
Monogen	3 (12)	1	33	117	4.2
Perative	6.6 (20.5)	1.3	20	70	7
Tolerex	2.1 (8)	1	44	154	3.18

VI

of patients was able to demonstrate improved nutritional status manifested as increased weight, length, and anthropometric measures of fat and muscle stores. The groups that received either 12-hour supplemental nocturnal infusions or oral feedings alone failed to achieve such intakes and growth responses. The 12-hour oral plus infusion group received only 122 kcal/kg, well below the threshold for growth. Fatigue during oral feedings was considered a limiting factor in both groups. In addition, in the 12-hour infusion group, daytime oral intake (52 kcal/kg) actually dropped to approximately 50% of the prestudy mean calorie intake (98 kcal/kg). The investigators concluded that only 24-hour continuous enteral feeding by nasogastric tube of a 1-kcal/mL formula was able to provide >140 kcal/kg/day and improve nutritional status.[35]

Two studies have concluded that children with CHD who fail to grow consume insufficient calories, because they reliably respond to nutritional supplementation, supporting the proposition that failure to gain weight can be simply a matter of inadequate intake, not intrinsic genetic or cardiac factors. These studies found that the type of cardiac defect did not necessarily predict or limit the response to dietary counseling and oral supplementation.[36,37] More recent studies have confirmed this in patients with CHD that has been repaired or palliated.[11,38-40]

Hemodynamic Factors

Congestive Heart Failure

Growth failure in children with CHF is common, although the pathogenesis is not always clear and is likely multifactorial. CHF causes increased energy requirements because of increased myocardial and respiratory work and increased catecholamines. There is reduced net nutrient intake as a result of intestinal malabsorption, anorexia, vomiting, and fatigability during feedings and even iatrogenic fluid restriction and diuresis.[35,41] Elevated right atrial pressures may cause intestinal protein losses and fat malabsorption and/or anorexia because of splanchnic and mesenteric venous and lymphatic congestion.[42,43] The increased right atrial pressure can transmit to the liver, causing hepatomegaly and, in some cases, decreased gastric capacity.[44,45] Oxygen consumption and basal metabolic rate are increased in infants with CHF when compared with healthy children or children with cyanotic CHD.[31,46-49] Traditionally, growth failure has been most common in infants with CHF attributable to pulmonary over circulation from large left-to-right shunts, such as a ventricular septal defect (VSD) or atrioventricular septal defect. This has been most evident in children with a VSD and large left-to-right shunt and pulmonary hypertension.[37,50,51]

Cyanotic Heart Disease

The role of hypoxemia as a primary cause of growth retardation in children is unclear. Cyanotic CHD (eg, tetralogy of Fallot, tricuspid atresia) with chronic hypoxemia is frequently associated with undernutrition and linear growth retardation, especially if prolonged and if complicated by CHF (TGA or single ventricle). Isolated hypoxemia or desaturation does not necessarily result in tissue hypoxia, because tissue aerobic metabolism may not be impaired until arterial oxygen partial pressure falls below 30 mmHg, a threshold also affected by such factors as oxygen-carrying capacity determined by hemoglobin concentration and tissue perfusion. Therefore, the added complication of CHF with decreased cardiac output probably contributes to chronic tissue hypoxia limiting growth. In addition to oxygen desaturation and CHF, anemia has been identified as an important factor predicting undernutrition in CHD.[7,52]

Some studies have demonstrated significant differences in growth between children with and without cyanotic heart disease, whereas others have failed to do so.[15] More recently, Costello et al found some correlation between presence of cyanosis ($P < .15$), presence of feeding difficulty ($P < .15$) and growth restriction in children 0 to 3 months of age presenting for surgery.[53] Children with cyanosis without pulmonary hypertension or CHF can demonstrate a normal nutritional state with stunting of growth being more common than poor weight gain.[54] Part of the perception that children with cyanosis grow better than children with other types of CHD may stem from the commonly observed "fat tet" infants. These children are fed frequently, perhaps overfed in some cases, to provide soothing and stave off a hypercyanotic spell. The more we learn, it seems that the specific cardiac lesion and the presence or absence of heart failure are 2 of the most important factors in determining risk for undernutrition.

Systemic to Pulmonary Shunts

Extracardiac shunting from the systemic circulation to the pulmonary circulation is a special circumstance that is perhaps the most frequently encountered hemodynamically significant systemic to pulmonary shunt among pediatric practitioners. Persistence of the ductus arteriosus, commonly known as patent ductus arteriosus (PDA), is found in 57 of 100 000 live births.[55] In very low birth weight (VLBW) infants, 1 in 3 will have a PDA.[56] In the extremely low birth weight (ELBW) population, the prevalence of symptomatic PDA requiring treatment has been reported to be as high as 55%.[57,58] Neonates with persistence of the ductus arteriosus have decreased intestinal blood flow compared to age-matched controls.[59] This has implications in terms of increased risk for necrotizing enterocolitis (NEC) and malnutrition.[60] Several studies have shown that treating the PDA, whether medically or surgically, especially in ELBW neonates, reduces the risk of developing NEC.[61]

Certain patients with single ventricle defect are offered palliative surgery that involves placing a type of surgical extracardiac systemic to pulmonary shunt, the Blalock-Taussig shunt. This procedure is used to supply pulmonary circulation and can be thought of as similar to the ductus arteriosus in vivo. It turns out that infants with surgical systemic to pulmonary artery shunts have many similarities to preterm neonates with persistence of the ductus arteriosus. The Pediatric Heart Network Investigators have looked at weight-for-age z scores in this population and found that the largest decline in weight-for-age z scores occurred between birth and hospital discharge after Norwood stage 1 procedure (when the Blalock-Taussig shunt is placed).[62] The challenge with these particular patients is that the systemic to pulmonary shunt is necessary for survival until the next stage surgery can be completed (typically around 4 months), so medical or surgical closure is out of the question. Providing adequate nutrition is vital, and it has been shown that adequate weight gain between Norwood stage 1 and stage 2 (average 2.5 kg) is associated with interstage survival.[63]

Management

Surgery

Significant protein-calorie undernutrition may delay surgical correction and impair postoperative recovery and growth. Radman et al found an association between malnutrition and decreased myocardial function.[64] Children demonstrate improvement in growth following corrective or palliative repair of a congenital heart lesion, and available data support the use of early surgical correction of major cardiac malformations to optimize growth.[24,65]

Within 1 week of surgery in infants with heart disease, energy expenditure decreases sharply to reach levels significantly below preoperative levels. As soon as 3 months after corrective surgery, weight, body composition, resting energy expenditure, TDEE, or energy expended during physical activity are similar to those of healthy children without CHD.[21,66,67] Studies have demonstrated a reversal of decreased growth velocity in infants who have undergone repair of VSD, tetralogy of Fallot, and TGA in the first year of life.[68] There are conflicting data regarding somatic growth in patients who have undergone the Fontan procedure. Some studies have demonstrated improvement in growth parameters, so much so that the reported incidence of obesity in adults who underwent the Fontan procedure as children is 14% to 39%.[69-71] Other studies have shown persistent growth failure, especially before 20 years of age.[71,72] These differences may relate to many factors, including different malformations (eg, systemic right ventricle versus systemic left ventricle), timing for surgery, etc. Catch-up linear growth is more likely with corrective than palliative surgery and with early repair. Residual, although reduced, CHF or shunt may still prevent normal nutritional recovery.[68,73]

It should be noted that although corrective and palliative surgery generally result in improvement in overall hemodynamic balance and improved growth, patients with severe CHD associated with high right heart pressures and disturbances to mesenteric venous drainage (eg, patients with hypoplastic left heart syndrome having undergone the Fontan procedure) remain at increased risk for protein-losing enteropathy.[42] Although the precise mechanism by which protein-losing enteropathy occurs is incompletely understood, initial clinical reports have shown some improvement in patients treated with oral budesonide.[74-76]

Chylothorax may complicate up to 6.5% of corrective surgeries. Biewer et al reported that most cases (71%) will resolve on a medium-chain triglyceride (MCT)-based diet administered for at least 10 days, after which customary feedings can be resumed gradually without recurrence.[77]

Vocal cord dysfunction, especially after congenital heart surgery, is an important contributor to feeding problems in this population. Incidence of vocal cord dysfunction ranges from 1.7% in 1 large retrospective study that reviewed 2255 patients undergoing heart surgery[78] to 38% in neonates undergoing coarctation or hypoplastic aortic arch repair.[79] In cases in which vocal cord dysfunction is suspected or confirmed, feeding by nasogastric tube may be required for several months until the dysfunction resolves.

Current literature suggests that in general, early enteral feeding after congenital heart surgery, whether by mouth or via gavage tube, expedites catch-up growth and reduces ventilator time, length of stay (both hospital and intensive care unit), and mortality.[40,63,80] In patients undergoing the Norwood stage I palliation for univentricular heart disease, gavage feeding was associated with a longer hospital stay, more medications at time of discharge, and lower weight-for-age z-score.[81] Patients requiring Norwood palliation appear to be at the greatest risk for undernutrition and its associated morbidities. These 2 studies highlight that although enteral feeding is important, reasonable efforts toward encouraging oral feeding should be made, especially in patients at highest risk for morbidity. Early integration of enteral nutrition with parenteral nutrition may be more beneficial rather than using enteral nutrition alone. Using enteral nutrition as the sole route for nutrition support in critically ill children may result in a prolonged period of underfeeding because of the patient's inability to tolerate adequate volumes to achieve anabolism. In high-risk patients (ie, after aortic arch repair or with preoperative shock), gradual escalation of enteral nutrition in conjunction with weaning of parenteral nutrition is recommended.[82] Because of the obvious negative consequences of chronic fluid (and, thus, calorie) restriction in children, fluid restriction is now only sparingly used in patients who are either awaiting some type of intervention (eg, surgery or heart transplantation) or recovering from some type of acute process (eg, surgery, acute decompensation, pleural effusions, etc) and is not recommended as a general principle of management.

Nutritional Assessment

A complete nutritional history includes feeding pattern and schedule, including frequency, duration, and volume of feedings. The volume of each feeding may be inversely related to the duration of feeding as the child fatigues. Diaphoresis with feedings reflects autonomic stimulation effects. Gastrointestinal tract function should be assessed to identify reflux and vomiting losses, irritability attributable to esophagitis or cramping, diarrhea or constipation, and early satiety, which may respond to acid-control and motility medications or may be signs of associated anomalies. The physical examination must include accurate nude weight, length, or height and head circumference plotted on a growth curve. Consider changes in rate of growth or growth velocity as well as the relation of actual body weight to the ideal body weight predicted by height or length for age and sex. Specialized appropriate charts should still be used for children who were born preterm or with Turner syndrome, trisomy 21, or trisomy 18. Of note, new growth charts for US children with trisomy 21 were published in 2015 after a few years' hiatus while new data were being collected.[83] Assessment of subcutaneous fat and muscle mass may be helpful, if measured by a skilled dietitian with calipers, although dehydration or edema may affect validity (see Chapter 24: Assessment of Nutritional Status). Signs of CHF, pulmonary hypertension, clubbing, cyanosis, and hepatomegaly connote increased risk of nutritional failure.

Laboratory evaluation initially should include hemoglobin, oxygen saturation, albumin, and prealbumin. Protein-losing enteropathy as a cause of hypoalbuminemia can be confirmed by fecal alpha-1 antitrypsin assay and is encountered in conditions of systemic venous hypertension, which occur with right-sided CHF, constrictive pericardial disease, or restrictive cardiac disease or after Fontan operation. A low alkaline phosphatase or cholesterol concentration may signify zinc deficiency, which may affect taste and linear growth.

Nutritional Support

The goals of nutritional intervention are to (1) achieve nutritional balance by providing sufficient energy to stop catabolism of lean body mass and sufficient protein to match nitrogen losses; (2) provide additional nutrients to restore deficits and allow growth, thus, normalizing weight for height and promoting linear growth; (3) provide enteral feedings to replace parenteral nutrition, as tolerated by the gastrointestinal tract; and (4) develop and maintain oral feeding competence to enable voluntary independent feeding.

Nutrient Prescription

The optimal nutritional support should provide sufficient energy and protein not only to prevent catabolism of protein and maintain body composition and weight but also to restore deficits and permit growth toward genetic potential. Electrolyte losses with diuretics and deficiencies in micronutrients, such as the trace minerals iron and zinc or vitamins, may be limiting factors. As a general principle, for any given level of nitrogen (or protein) provided in the diet, increasing the energy (calories) will improve nitrogen balance and protein synthesis or accretion. Similarly, for a given level of energy intake, increasing the protein intake will improve the nitrogen balance or protein accretion. If energy provided by carbohydrate and fat in the diet is below the patient's requirements, protein will be catabolized as an energy source and not used in synthesis of lean body mass. Even if sufficient calories are provided to stop gluconeogenesis and restore body glycogen and fat stores, enough protein must be provided as a nitrogen source to allow accretion of lean body protein mass and effective growth.

A marginal or negative electrolyte balance, such as low net sodium or potassium intake in the setting of fluid restriction and diuretic use, required for some patients in CHF, may impair growth independent of energy and protein sufficiency. Zinc deficiency has been implicated in cases of failure to thrive, with improved growth demonstrated after supplementation.[84,85]

Energy Requirement

Additional energy above the Recommended Dietary Allowance for age is required to permit normal growth rates, with even greater amounts required to restore nutritional deficits in "catch-up" or accelerated growth (rapid increase in weight, length, and head circumference, which continues until the normal individual growth pattern is resumed) in patients with CHF, especially in the perioperative period. A portion of this incremental energy requirement may be explained by simply calculating needs based on the patient's ideal or median body weight predicted from body length or even head circumference. This calculation assumes that metabolic needs for energy and protein are determined by the relatively preserved brain and visceral and lean body mass with a minimal contribution from the adipose or fat mass that is depleted with undernutrition. In undernutrition, the ratio of metabolically active lean body mass to total weight is increased. For example, 150 kcal/kg of actual body weight in the typical lean child with CHD, who may be 80% of the expected or "ideal" weight for length, corresponds to 120 kcal/kg for a healthy robust infant of the same length but at ideal body weight because of increased fat mass. Therefore, energy requirements may be more reliably based on the child's "ideal" body weight for length or height. An alternative calculation of a reference weight (kg) for predicting energy requirements is the 50th percentile body mass index (BMI) for age multiplied by the patient's length in meters squared.

Increased cardiac and respiratory work in the child with CHF, shunt, or cyanosis undoubtedly adds to the energy requirement. Increased catecholamines in CHF will increase energy expenditure, as will the demands of increased respiratory rate and hematopoiesis in cyanotic heart disease. The myocardium itself is a significant consumer of energy, with demands increased with pulmonary hypertension, hypertrophy, shunting, and CHF. Barton et al estimated the energy requirement for growth of an infant with CHD.[22] The energy cost of normal tissue deposition is 21 kJ/g (5 kcal/g).[86] This energy cost is 30% less than the 31 kJ/g (7.4 kcal/g) estimated in infants with CHD receiving high-energy feedings.[87] In a very real sense, feeding can be considered "exercise" for an infant with significant CHD. Assuming 75% of the energy cost of growth is stored in this new tissue and the remainder is used during synthesis (part of TDEE), an intake of 600 kJ/kg/day (143 kcal/kg/day) is required to allow average weight gain during the first 3 months of life.[22] The parenteral requirements for energy will be approximately 70% to 80% of enteral estimates.

Feeding Complications

One must also consider the metabolic load imposed by feeding. Cardiac output is determined by tissue metabolic demand. As additional nutrients are provided, cardiac output must increase to oxygenate these tissues, and ventilatory demands on the lungs increase to eliminate the carbon dioxide generated by metabolic activity. This phenomenon of increased energy demands of nutrition support known as dietary thermogenesis, the thermic effect of food, varies for different nutrients, being minimal for fat metabolism and quite significant—up to 5% of calories—for carbohydrate. Carbohydrates are used for fat synthesis when carbohydrates or equivalent glucose amounts are administered at a rate exceeding 8 mg/kg/minute. This endothermic process requires energy and oxygen and liberates carbon dioxide, which must be expired. For this reason, the energy provided should be distributed between fat and carbohydrate, with fat providing at least 30% of the total caloric intake. At least 6% of fat should be long-chain triglycerides (linoleic acid, as in corn, soy, safflower oils) and some linolenic acid to provide essential fatty acids. The value and safety of additional omega-3 fatty acids beyond essential fatty acid requirements is the subject of ongoing research.

Overfeeding or overly rapid increments in nutrition support can precipitate or worsen CHF. A refeeding syndrome has been described in which overzealous nutritional support has caused complications, not only with cardiac failure, but also with conduction disturbances and dysrhythmias related to electrolyte and mineral shifts with anabolism (see Chapter 38: Eating Disorders in Children and Adolescents). Provision of glucose leads to an insulin-mediated influx of potassium, and intermediary metabolism demands for phosphorus (phosphorylated intermediate metabolites and production of adenosine triphosphate) lead to an intracellular shift, causing profound hypokalemia, hypophosphatemia, hypomagnesemia, and hypocalcemia. Prolongation of QT_c interval may be observed. Sudden death suspected to be related to lethal arrhythmias, such as torsade de pointes, has been attributed to the rapid refeeding of patients accommodated to the undernourished state.

In neonates with CHD, especially the preterm infant, there is a higher incidence of necrotizing enterocolitis. In those with ductal-dependent systemic circulation (eg, hypoplastic left heart syndrome), the prevalence of NEC is approximately 7% to 13%.[88,89] Diastolic flow reversal in the superior mesenteric artery is common before and immediately after the stage 1 Norwood palliation and is likely one of the prime movers behind the observed increased incidence of NEC. The flow reversal is attributable to the diastolic runoff, preoperatively through the patent ductus arteriosus, and postoperatively through the Blalock-Taussig shunt, which may deprive the intestines of adequate perfusion during diastole.[90] As convincing as the diastolic runoff theory may sound, the issue is more complex, and there are other factors at play. For example, Miller et al showed that infants with hypoplastic left heart syndrome who developed NEC had a lower abdominal aorta pulsatility index compared with those without NEC on both preoperative and postoperative echocardiograms, despite similar ventricular function and operative risk, suggesting a role for some intrinsic vascular abnormality.[91]

There remains wide variance among centers when it comes to enteral feeds in the preterm or term infant with congenital heart disease,[11,92] with some centers still advocating a strict "nothing by mouth" policy in patients with ductal dependent systemic circulation. In a large cohort study, Becker et al demonstrated no increased risk of NEC in infants with ductal-dependent circulation receiving enteral feeds,[93] and others have found that enteral feeding prior to cardiac surgery, if administered judiciously, may actually reduce the risk of NEC.[94] For those on parenteral nutrition, trophic feedings of approximately 10 to 20 mL/kg, preferably expressed human milk, for enteral and enterohepatic stimulation is beneficial.[92] Evidence is mounting that standardized feeding protocols, focused on judicious advancement of feeding in the newborn period and monitoring tolerance in terms of abdominal distention, accumulating gastric residual volume, and hematochezia, might reduce the incidence of NEC.

Protein Intake
There is little discussion in the literature about nitrogen balance or protein intake in children with CHD. In general, if sufficient nonprotein energy is provided to prevent gluconeogenesis from catabolism of dietary amino

acids, provision of more protein (up to specific limits) leads to greater incorporation of protein and its nitrogen in lean body mass. Protein generally constitutes 5% to 12% of total calories, reflected in the composition of human milk and infant formulas that model human milk. Fomon and Ziegler suggested a formula calorie composition of 9% protein, 60% carbohydrate, and 31% fat provided in a density of 1 kcal/mL for infants with CHD.[95] The ratio of energy to protein in infant formulas is 30 to 50 kcal/g of protein (corresponding to nonprotein calorie-to-nitrogen ratios of 287:140). Thus, a child receiving 140 kcal/kg/day of energy would receive 2.9 to 4.25 g/kg of protein, if derived from standard or concentrated formula, with protein constituting 8% to 12% of total calories. To avoid excessive hepatic protein metabolic and renal solute load, assuming a limit of 3.5 g/kg/day of protein, the additional energy required above 120 kcal/kg based on ideal body weight for length should be provided by either glucose polymers (Polycose or starch) or by fat (Microlipid or oils) added to the formula, unless using a standard infant formula or human milk (Table 44.1). These formulas are low enough in protein content that their high calorie-to-protein ratio allows concentration of the formula to achieve a higher calorie intake without exceeding the threshold for protein tolerance. Once the child approaches 1 year of age, an intact protein-based 1-kcal/mL formula (eg, Pediasure, Kids Essential, Nutren Jr), a protein-hydrolysate (eg, Peptamen Jr), or an amino acid-based (eg, Neocate Jr, Elecare, Nutramigen AA Vivonex Pediatric) formula should be substituted for infant formula.

Protein-losing enteropathy is diagnosed by identification of hypoalbuminemia, lack of proteinuria, and positive fecal alpha-1-antitrypsin assay. Typically, protein-losing enteropathy is encountered in patients with Fontan anatomy, constrictive pericarditis, or other lesions that cause right heart failure. Additional protein is probably necessary, and the fat provided should be predominantly MCTs, which are transported via portal circulation, to reduce mesenteric lymphatic flow and pressures contributing to the protein loss. A similar rationale leads to the use of MCTs in patients with chylothorax or chylous ascites. Formulas with predominant MCTs as the fat source can be found in Appendix M. Human milk cannot support these protein needs without supplementation and is very high in long-chain triglycerides, which are absorbed via the lymphatic system. Essential fatty acid deficiency can occur with MCT-dominant feeding and should be monitored. Providing 2% to 4% of the total calories as essential fatty acids should prevent deficiency. When addressing the nutritional needs of a patient with chylothorax, it is important to:

1. Limit dietary long-chain triglycerides for up to 6 weeks after surgery by offering very high-MCT formula for infants or a diet very low (<10 g/day) in total fat for toddlers and children. Human milk can be skimmed using a centrifuge and then fortified with high-MCT formula or oil.
2. Ensure that 2% to 4% of calories are from long-chain fat to prevent essential fatty acid deficiency.
3. According to age and need, ensure adequate protein, electrolyte, and vitamin intake requirements are being met, keeping in mind that nutrients are lost in the chyle that is drained via chest tube. In refractory cases, parenteral nutrition may be required to meet nutritional needs in the intermediate term but should not be considered first-line therapy.[77,79]

Electrolytes, Minerals, and Micronutrients

Disturbances in electrolyte and mineral homeostasis accompany diuretic therapy or refeeding. Hypokalemia or hypocalcemia may cause changes in myocardial conduction and contractility. Diuretic therapy is irrational if sodium intake is not controlled. Concentrated formulas provide an increased electrolyte and mineral load without accompanying free water, challenging renal regulation, especially in the patient receiving diuretic therapy for congestive heart failure. This is one of the main arguments for limiting the calorie concentration of formulas to 24 kcal/oz and providing additional calorie requirements by fat emulsion or glucose polymer additives. Potassium and chloride depletion commonly occur and may require supplementation. Calcium, magnesium, and zinc may also be depleted. Calciuria may be diminished by using chlorothiazide instead of furosemide. Calcium absorption from the gut is limited in magnesium deficiency (magnesium-dependent adenosine triphosphatase). Potassium may be spared by addition of spironolactone in selected cases.

Current recommendations for vitamin D according to the "Global Consensus Recommendations of Prevention and Management of Ricketts" (2016) are daily supplementation of 400 IU of vitamin D in infants from birth to 12 months of age and 600 IU for children 12 months through adulthood. The daily intake of each child may include other dietary sources of vitamin D, such as fortified food.[96] Human milk does not contain sufficient vitamin D and, therefore, must be supplemented with exogenous vitamin D. This makes it more likely for infants to be deficient in vitamin D. Infant formula, on the other hand, is fortified to provide approximately 400 IU of vitamin D per L.[97] A study by McNally and colleagues determined vitamin

D status in children undergoing congenital heart surgery, found that 42% of patients were vitamin D deficient preoperatively and 86% of the same patients were deficient postoperatively.[98] This study might suggest the current recommendations are too low, especially for postoperative critically ill patients. Regular monitoring of vitamin D in children with CHD seems prudent in the light of current data.

Loop and thiazide diuretics, commonly used in children with CHD, cause increased urinary magnesium excretion.[40] Magnesium is a known antiarrhythmic and plays a role in myocardial contractility through intracellular potassium regulation. Patients who are prone to arrhythmias may benefit from magnesium supplementation.[99]

Zinc depletion may manifest as a low alkaline phosphatase activity and low cholesterol concentration (zinc-dependent enzymatic products). Iron needs are increased in cyanotic heart disease to maintain the increased erythroid mass demanded by hypoxemia. Anemia contributes to tissue hypoxia in patients with ventricular pressure overload, volume overload, CHF, or hypoxemia/cyanosis. In aortic valve stenosis, anemia may contribute to subendocardial ischemia, causing angina or arrhythmia. In patients with a large VSD, anemia causes decreased blood viscosity and pulmonary vascular resistance, which allows increased left-to-right shunting and increased CHF and pulmonary blood flow. Selenium and carnitine deficiency may occur in unsupplemented parenteral nutrition and may manifest as cardiomyopathy.

Thiamine (vitamin B_1) deficiency may present as the syndrome of wet beriberi with varying severity of CHF attributable to impaired myocardial function and impaired autonomic regulation of circulation. Clinical manifestations include edema, fatigue, dyspnea, and tachycardia with signs of CHF. Shoshin is a severe form of beriberi that may affect infants with pulmonary edema and CHF. Thiamine depletion may occur in settings of high carbohydrate intake without thiamine, as in a nursing mother on an inadequate diet or consuming alcohol or in settings of prolonged parenteral nutrition or glucose administration without a multivitamin supplement. Thiamine requirements are increased with the stress of surgery and critical illness, and losses of thiamine increase with loop diuretics such as furosemide, putting patients with CHD at risk of deficiency. Shamir et al identified thiamine deficiency in 4 of 22 children with CHD before surgery, 3 of whom had adequate thiamine intake.[100] Six of the 22 also had thiamine deficiency after surgery. However, no relationship to the level of undernutrition, thiamine intake, or furosemide use could be proven.[100]

VI

Fluids

Many patients, especially those with CHF, are restricted in fluid intake with or without diuretic treatment. Providing adequate calories in the setting of fluid restriction is challenging and requires a concentrated formula, often requiring continuous administration via nasogastric or transpyloric tube (see earlier section on Energy Intake). The use of fat emulsions, such as Microlipid 4.5 kcal/mL, provides an energy-dense supplement to boost formula caloric density without increasing volume or osmolarity as well as avoiding the protein and electrolyte load incurred by concentrating formula.

Feeding Strategies

Oral or enteral feedings are preferred, and there need be no restriction in volume of formula in infants with CHF or cyanosis if they feed voluntarily. However, many patients with CHD have voluntary oral intake insufficient to supply nutrient requirements to maintain growth. The increased cardiopulmonary demands of eating or associated problems, such as gastrointestinal tract dysmotility, prematurity, and airway or pulmonary disease, may prevent adequate intake. Volume may also be restricted, especially in patients with lesions associated with CHF or pulmonary hypertension requiring diuretic therapy, fluid, and sodium restriction. Reparative or palliative surgery may be safer if performed after achieving a target weight. Formula concentration is frequently increased to provide more energy and protein in a restricted volume. If volume is the limiting factor, a more concentrated formula will be necessary to provide up to 3.5 g/kg/day of protein, above which additional calories may be added with carbohydrates (Polycose powder or liquid) or fats (Microlipid emulsion). Concentrating a formula leads to increased protein and solute load, osmolarity, or tonicity and decreased free water, but a study of postoperative infants showed that advancement to a high-concentration formula within 2 days rather than 5 days safely improved energy intake and weight gain and decreased length of stay.[38] Overall, providing a more concentrated feed (fortified human milk or concentrated formula to higher calorie) is recommended when volume is compromised.

Supplemental enteral nutrition is frequently instituted to achieve nutritional goals via nasogastric or gastrostomy tube. Consequences of coercive oral feeding efforts or nasopharyngeal tube placement and feeding include a high incidence of oral aversion, which may prove quite refractory long after the cardiac issues have improved. Patients who are considered likely to require chronic nasogastric tube feedings for longer than 6 months should be considered early for gastrostomy tube placement. Given the possibility that gastrostomy feeding may alter gastroduodenal motility and increase gastroesophageal reflux, evidence of airway penetration, impaired airway protective reflexes such as absent gag or cough, or lower respiratory tract disease may mandate protective antireflux surgery (Nissen fundoplication). If airway protective reflexes are intact (eg, no vocal cord dysfunction or recurrent laryngeal nerve palsy) and there is no evidence of respiratory compromise, such as reactive airway disease, laryngospasm/stridor, or aspiration pneumonia, then percutaneous gastrostomy without antireflux surgery is a safe and effective option.[101] The need for fundoplication has been associated with increased morbidity and mortality in infants with congenital heart disease, perhaps because of the additional comorbidities present in patients requiring both gastrostomy and Nissen procedures.[102] The anatomy of the upper gastrointestinal tract should be evaluated using contrast studies to exclude associated anomalies of tracheoesophageal fistula; vascular ring; gross airway penetration, directly or with reflux; and intestinal rotational anomalies. For patients with aspiration risks who are not considered safe candidates for antireflux fundoplication surgery, transpyloric feeding with a nasojejunal or percutaneous gastrojejunal tube or direct-feeding jejunostomy are alternatives. Although transpyloric duodenal or jejunal feeding may prevent formula entry into the stomach, gastroduodenal motility may be inhibited, and duodenogastric reflux of bile or gastroesophageal reflux of acid and/or bile may still occur.

The breastfed infant may require manual or pump expression of milk if there is fatigue or problems suckling either because of inability to latch on, excessive respiratory effort, and/or tachypnea competing with sucking and swallowing. Tube feeding either fortified human milk or a high-caloric density formula continuously to augment a marginal nursing intake will be required for sufficient calories.

Parenteral nutrition is reserved for patients who cannot be fed effectively or safely by the enteral routes described previously. Examples would be patients with associated gastrointestinal tract disease, such as necrotizing enterocolitis or at risk of aspiration because of tachypnea or gastroesophageal reflux. Because cardiac output is determined by the demands of peripheral tissue metabolism, advancement of feedings, whether parenteral or enteral, in the patient accommodated to chronic malnutrition, should be gradual and monitored for refeeding complications. Peripheral capillary vasodilation in response to tissue anabolism can lead to high-output cardiac failure, and excessive volume administration can provoke CHF and anasarca. Glucose uptake and metabolism will cause intracellular influx of potassium, magnesium, calcium, and most dramatically, phosphate. Dysrhythmias, particularly atrial arrhythmias related to changes in venous return, and ventricular arrhythmias related to conduction disturbances may be associated with electrolyte fluxes (hypokalemia, hypocalcemia, hypophosphatemia) and can manifest in changes in the corrected QT interval on electrocardiogram. Other cardiac complications of parenteral nutritional support include volume overload, increased viscosity and pulmonary artery pressures with high lipid infusions (exceeding 0.15 g/kg/hour or 3.5 g/kg/day), increased tissue metabolic demand for cardiac output, arrhythmias, and endocarditis/sepsis related to the central venous catheter.

Monitoring Outcome

Precise weights and lengths (or standing heights for patients older than 3 years) should be obtained at each encounter and plotted on the appropriate growth curve. There are separate growth curves for several genetic syndromes and for preterm infants. In theory, the same dietitian should obtain measurements of mid-upper arm circumference and triceps skinfold thickness to help assess muscle and fat stores, understanding that fluid status and edema may affect the measures (see Chapter 24: Assessment of Nutritional Status). Review of diet is important. The current formula and methods for mixing and adding supplements should be reviewed to eliminate errors in formulation. The family should be instructed to bring a 3- or 5-day diet record to the clinic visit for evaluation by the dietitian for nutrient analysis. Attention should be paid to total calorie intake, proportion of fat and carbohydrate intake, protein intake, and adequacy of micronutrients, including iron, zinc, and vitamins. Fluid volume intake, urinary frequency, and hydration status in the context of diuretic therapy should be assessed. More sophisticated measures of body composition, including bone mineral status, may be obtained in certain groups or research settings, if the technology such as dual energy x-ray absorptiometry or bioelectrical impedance analysis is available. Indirect calorimetry can assess resting energy expenditure and respiratory quotient to assess energy requirements and avoid overfeeding in patients in the intensive care unit. In the absence of direct measures of lean body mass or energy requirements, the surrogate parameter of weight expected for length for age or ideal body weight for length, can be helpful in estimating energy and protein requirements for the very lean or obese child (see Table 44.1). However, serial measurement of changes in weight, length, and other measures of anthropometry are the best indicators of nutrient adequacy.

References

1. Levy RJ, Rosenthal A, Castaneda AR, Nadas AS. Growth after surgical repair of simple D-transposition of the great arteries. *Ann Thorac Surg.* 1978;25(3):225–230

2. Kramer HH, Tramisch HJ, Rammos S, Giese A. Birth weight of children with congenital heart disease. *Eur J Pediatr.* 1990;149(11):752–757

3. Archer JM, Yeager SB, Kenny MJ, Soll RF, Horbar JD. Distribution of and mortality from serious congenital heart disease in very low birth weight infants. *Pediatrics.* 2011;127(2):293–299

4. Patel A, Costello JM, Backer CL, et al. Prevalence of noncardiac and genetic abnormalities in neonates undergoing cardiac operations: analysis of the The Society of Thoracic Surgeons Congenital Heart Database. *Ann Thorac Surg.* 2016;102(5):1607–1614

5. Steurer MA, Baer RJ, Keller RL, et al. Gestational age and outcomes in critical congenital heart disease. *Pediatrics.* 2017;140(4):E20170999

6. Rosenthal GL, Wilson PD, Permutt T, Boughman JA, Ferencz C. Birth weight and cardiovascular malformations: a population-based study. The Baltimore-Washington Infant Study. *Am J Epidemiol.* 1991;133(12):1273–1281

7. Batte A, Lwabi P, Lubega S, et al. Wasting, underweight and stunting among children with congenital heart disease presenting at Mulago hospital, Uganda. *BMC Pediatr.* 2017;17(1):10

8. Toole BJ, Toole LE, Kyle UG, Cabrera AG, Orellana RA, Coss-Bu JA. Perioperative nutritional support and malnutrition in infants and children with congenital heart disease. *Congenit Heart Dis.* 2014;9(1):15–25

9. Cameron JW, Rosenthal A, Olson AD. Malnutrition in hospitalized children with congenital heart disease. *Arch Pediatr Adolesc Med.* 1995;149(10):1098–1102

10. Blasquez A, Clouzeau H, Fayon M, et al. Evaluation of nutritional status and support in children with congenital heart disease. *Eur J Clin Nutr.* 2016;70 (528–531)

11. McCrary AW, Clabby ML, Mahle WT. Patient and practice factors affecting growth of infants with systemic-to-pulmonary shunt. *Cardiol Young.* 2013;23(4): 499–506

12. Kelleher DK, Laussen P, Teixeira-Pinto A, Duggan C. Growth and correlates of nutritional status among infants with hypoplastic left heart syndrome (HLHS) after stage 1 Norwood procedure. *Nutrition.* 2006;22(3):237–244

13. Medoff-Cooper B, Naim M, Torowicz D, Mott A. Feeding, growth, and nutrition in children with congenitally malformed hearts. *Cardiol Young.* 2010;20(Suppl 3): 149–153

14. Chlebowski MM, Dai H, Kaine SF. The effect on somatic growth of surgical and catheter treatment of secundum atrial septal defects. *Pediatr Cardiol.* 2017;38(7): 1410–1414

15. Leitch CA. Growth, nutrition and energy expenditure in pediatric heart failure. *Progr Pediatr Cardiol.* 2000;11(3):195–202

16. Cavell B. Gastric emptying in infants with congenital heart disease. *Acta Paediatr Scand.* 1981;70(5):517–520

17. Forchielli ML, McColl R, Walker WA, Lo C. Children with congenital heart disease: a nutrition challenge. *Nutr Rev.* 1994;52(10):348–353

18. Schofield WN. Predicting basal metabolic rate, new standards and review of previous work. *Hum Nutr Clin Nutr.* 1985;39(Suppl 1):5–41

19. Food and Agriculture Organization of the United Nations, World Health Organization, United Nations University. Human Energy Requirements: Report of a Joint FAO/WHO/UNU Expert Consultation. Rome, Italy: Food and Agriculture Organization of the United Nations, World Health Organization, United Nations University; 2001: Available at: ftp://ftp.fao.org/docrep/fao/007/y5686e/y5686e00.pdf. Accessed March 21, 2019

20. White MS, Shepherd RW, McEniery JA. Energy expenditure in 100 ventilated, critically ill children: improving the accuracy of predictive equations. *Crit Care Med.* 2000;28(7):2307–2312

21. De Wit B, Meyer R, Desai A, Macrae D, Pathan N. Challenge of predicting resting energy expenditure in children undergoing surgery for congenital heart disease. *Pediatr Crit Care Med.* 2010;11(4):496–501

22. Barton JS, Hindmarsh PC, Scrimgeour CM, Rennie MJ, Preece MA. Energy expenditure in congenital heart disease. *Arch Dis Child.* 1994;70(1):5-9

23. Leitch CA, Karn CA, Peppard RJ, et al. Increased energy expenditure in infants with cyanotic congenital heart disease. *J Pediatr.* 1998;133(6):755–760

24. Mitchell IM, Davies PS, Day JM, Pollock JC, Jamieson MP. Energy expenditure in children with congenital heart disease, before and after cardiac surgery. *J Thorac Cardiovasc Surg.* 1994;107(2):374–380

25. Huse DM, Feldt RH, Nelson RA, Novak LP. Infants with congenital heart disease. Food intake, body weight, and energy metabolism. *1975.* 1975;129(1):65–69

26. Menon G, Poskitt EM. Why does congenital heart disease cause failure to thrive? *Arch Dis Child.* 1985;60(12):1134–1139

27. Nydegger A, Walsh A, Penny DJ, Henning R, Bines JE. Changes in resting energy expenditure in children with congenital heart disease. *Eur J Clin Nutr.* 2009;63(3):392–397

28. Farrell AG, Schamberger MS, Olson IL, Leitch CA. Large left-to-right shunts and congestive heart failure increase total energy expenditure in infants with ventricular septal defect. *Am J Cardiol.* 2001;87(9):1128–1131

29. Trabulsi JC, Irving SY, Papas MA, et al. Total Energy Expenditure of Infants with Congenital Heart Disease Who Have Undergone Surgical Intervention. *Pediatr Cardiol.* 2015;36(8):1670–1679

30. Rosenthal A. Congenital cardiac anomalies and gastrointestinal malformations. In: Pierpont M, Moller J, eds. *Genetics of Cardiovascular Disease.* Boston, MA: Martinus Nijhoff; 1986:113–126

31. Sondheimer JM, Hamilton JR. Intestinal function in infants with severe congenital heart disease. *J Pediatr.* 1978;92(4):572–578

32. Vaisman N, Leigh T, Voet H, Westerterp K, Abraham M, Duchan R. Malabsorption in infants with congenital heart disease under diuretic treatment. *Pediatr Res.* 1994;36(4):545–549

33. van der Kuip M, Hoos MB, Forget PP, Westerterp KR, Gemke RJ, de Meer K. Energy expenditure in infants with congenital heart disease, including a meta-analysis. *Acta Paediatr* 2003;92(8):921–927

34. Yahav J, Avigad S, Frand M, et al. Assessment of intestinal and cardiorespiratory function in children with congenital heart disease on high-caloric formulas. *J Pediatr Gastroenterol Nutr.* 1985;4(5):778–785

35. Schwarz SM, Gewitz MH, See CC, et al. Enteral nutrition in infants with congenital heart disease and growth failure. *Pediatrics.* 1990;86(3):368–373

36. Unger R, DeKleermaeker M, Gidding SS, Christoffel KK. Calories count. Improved weight gain with dietary intervention in congenital heart disease. *Am J Dis Child.* 1992;146(9):1078–1084

37. Salzer HR, Haschke F, Wimmer M, Heil M, Schilling R. Growth and nutritional intake of infants with congenital heart disease. *Pediatr Cardiol.* 1989;10(1):17–23

38. Pillo-Blocka F, Adatia I, Sharieff W, McCrindle BW, Zlotkin S. Rapid advancement to more concentrated formula in infants after surgery for congenital heart disease reduces duration of hospital stay: a randomized clinical trial. *J Pediatr.* 2004;145(6):761–766

39. Nicholson GT, Clabby ML, Kanter KR, Mahle WT. Caloric intake during the perioperative period and growth failure in infants with congenital heart disease. *Pediatr Cardiol.* 2013;34(2):316–321

40. Lewis KD, Conway J, Cunningham C, Larsen BMK. Optimizing nutrition in pediatric heart failure: the crisis is over and now it's time to feed. *Nutr Clin Pract.* 2018;33(3):397–403

41. Weintraub RG, Menahem S. Growth and congenital heart disease. *J Paediatr Child Health.* 1993;29(2):95–98

42. Roche SL, Redington AN. The failing right ventricle in congenital heart disease. *Canadian J Cardiol.* 2013;29(7):768–778

43. Kay JD, Colan SD, Graham TP. Congestive heart failure in pediatric patients. *Am Heart J.* 2001;142(5):923–928

44. Kantor PF, Lougheed J, Dancea A, et al. The Children's Heart Failure Study Group. Presentation, diagnosis, and medical management of heart failure in children: Canadian Cardiovascular Society Guidelines. *Can J Cardiol.* 2013;29(12):1535–1552

45. Gervasio MR, Buchanan CN. Malnutrition in the pediatric cardiology patient. *CCQ.* 1985;8(3):49–56

46. Sinclair JC, Thorlund K, Walter SD. Longitudinal measurements of oxygen consumption in growing infants during the first weeks after birth: old data revisited. *Neonatology.* 2013;103:223–231

47. Seckeler MD, Hirsh R, Beekman III RH, Goldstein BH. A new predictive equation for oxygen consumption in children and adults with congenital and acquired heart disease. *Heart.* 2015;101(7):517–524

VI

48. Krauss AN, Auld PA. Metabolic rate of neonates with congenital heart disease. *Arch Dis Child.* 1975;50(7):539–541

49. Stocker FP, Wilkoff W, Miettinen OS, Nadas AS. Oxygen consumption in infants with heart disease. Relationship to severity of congestive failure, relative weight, and caloric intake. *80.* 1972;1(43–51)

50. Vaidyanathan B, Roth SJ, Gauvreau K, Shivaprakasha K, Rao SG, Kumar RK. Somatic growth after ventricular septal defect in malnourished infants. *J Pediatr.* 2006;149(2):205–209

51. Manso PH, Carmona F, Jácomo AD, Bettiol H, Barbieri MA, Carlotti AP. Growth after ventricular septal defect repair: does defect size matter? A 10-year experience. *Acta Paediatr.* 2010;99(9):1356–1360

52. Okoromah CAN, Ekure EN, Lesi FEA, Okunowo WO, Tijani BO, Okeiyi JC. Prevalence, profile and predictors of malnutrition in children with congenital heart defects: a case-control observational study. *Arch Dis Child.* 2011;96(4): 354–360

53. Costello CL, Gellatly M, Daniel J, Justo RN, Weir K. Growth restriction in infants and young children with congenital heart disease. *10.* 2015;5(447–456)

54. Varan B, Tokel K, Yilmaz G. Malnutrition and growth failure in cyanotic and acyanotic congenital heart disease with and without pulmonary hypertension. *Arch Dis Child.* 1999;81(1):49–52

55. Hoffman JI, Kaplan S. The incidence of congenital heart disease. *J Am Coll Cardiol.* 2002;29(12):1890–1900

56. Investigators of the Vermont Oxford Trials Network. Very low birth weight outcomes for 1990. *Pediatrics.* 1993;91(3):540–545

57. Koch J, Hensley G, Roy L, Brown S, Ramaciotti C, Rosenfeld CR. Prevalence of spontaneous closure of the ductus arteriosus in neonates at a birth weight of 1000 grams or less. *Pediatrics.* 2006;117(4):1113–1121

58. Richards J, Johnson A, Fox G, Campbell M. A second course of ibuprofen is effective in the closure of a clinically significant PDA in ELBW infants. *Pediatrics.* 2009;124(2):e287–e293

59. Shimada S, Kasai T, Hoshi A, Mrata A, Chida S. Cardiocirculatory effects of patent ductus arteriosus in extremely low-birth-weight infants with respiratory distress syndrome. *Pediatr Int.* 2003;45(3):255–262

60. Westin V, Stoltz-Sjöström E, Ahlsson F, Domellöf M, Norman M. Perioperative nutrition in extremely preterm infants undergoing surgical treatment for patent ductus arteriosus is suboptimal. *Acta Paediatr.* 2014;103(3):282–288

61. Clyman RI, Chorne N. Patent ductus arteriosus: evidence for and against treatment. *J Pediatr.* 2007;150(3):216–219

62. Burch PT, Gerstenberger E, Ravishankar C, et al. Pediatric Heart Network Investigators. Longitudinal assessment of growth in hypoplastic left heart syndrome: results from the single ventricle reconstruction trial. *J Am Heart Assoc.* 2014;3(3):e000079

63. Evans CF, Sorkin JK, Abraham DS, Wehman B, Kaushal S, Rosenthal GL. Interstage weight gain is associated with survival after first-stage single-ventricle palliation. *Ann Thorac Surg.* 2017;104(2):674–680

64. Radman M, Mack R, Barnoya J, et al. The effect of preoperative nutritional status on postoperative outcomes in children undergoing surgery for congenital heart defects in San Francisco (UCSF) and Guatemala City (UNICAR). *J Thorac Cardiovasc Surg.* 2014;147(1):442–450

65. Leitch CA, Karn CA, Ensing GJ, Denne SC. Energy expenditure after surgical repair in children with cyanotic congenital heart disease. *J Pediatr.* 2000;137(3): 381–385

66. Irving SY, Medoff-Cooper B, Stouffer NO, et al. Resting energy expenditure at 3 months of age following neonatal surgery for congenital heart disease. 80. 2013;4(343–351)

67. Ackerman IL, Karn CA, Denne SC, Ensing GJ, Leitch CA. Total but not resting energy expenditure is increased in infants with ventricular septal defects. *Pediatrics.* 1998;102(5):1172–1177

68. Sholler GF, Celermajer JM. Cardiac surgery in the first year of life: the effect on weight gains of infants with congenital heart disease. *Aust Paediatr J.* 1986;22(4): 305–308

69. Chung ST, Hong B, Patterson L, Petit CJ, Ham JN. High overweight and obesity in Fontan patients: a 20 year history. *Pediatr Cardiol.* 2016;37(1):192–200

70. Stenbog EV, Hjortdal VE, Ravn HB, Skjaerbaek C, Sorensen KE, Hansen OK. Improvement in growth, and levels of insulin-like growth factor-I in the serum, after cavopulmonary connections. *Cardiol Young.* 2000;10(5):440–446

71. Freud LR, Webster G, Costello JM, et al. Growth and obesity among older single ventricle patients presenting for Fontan conversion. *World J Pediatr Congenit Heart Surg.* 2015;6(4):514–520

72. Cohen MI, Bush DM, Ferry RJ, Jr., et al. Somatic growth failure after the Fontan operation. *Cardiol Young.* 2000;10(5):447–457

73. Baum D, Beck RQ, Haskell WL. Growth and tissue abnormalities in young people with cyanotic congenital heart disease receiving systemic-pulmonary artery shunts. *Am J Cardiol.* 1983;52(3):349–352

74. John AS, Johnson JA, Khan M, Driscoll DJ, Warnes CA, Cetta F. Clinical outcomes and improved survival in patients with protein-losing enteropathy after the Fontan operation. *J Am Coll Cardiol.* 2014;64(1):54–62

75. John AS, Driscoll DJ, Warnes CA, Phillips SD, Cetta F. The use of oral budesonide in adolescents and adult patients with protein-losing enteropathy after the Fontan operation. *Ann Thorac Surg.* 2011;92(4):1451–1456

76. Gursu HA, Erdogan I, Varan B, et al. Oral budesonide as a therapy for protein-losing enteropathy in children after the Fontan operation. *J Cardiol Surg.* 2014;29(5):712–716

VI

77. Biewer ES, Zurn C, Arnold R, et al. Chylothorax after surgery on congenital heart disease in newborns and infants—risk factors and efficacy of MCT-diet. *J Cardiothoracic Surg.* 2010;5:127–134

78. Sachdeva R, Hussain E, Moss MM, et al. Vocal cord dysfunction and feeding difficulties after pediatric cardiovascular surgery. *J Pediatr.* 2007;151(3):312–315

79. Mery CM, Guzmán-Pruneda FA, Carberry KE, et al. Aortic arch advancement for aortic coarctation and hypoplastic aortic arch in neonates and infants. *Ann Thorac Surg.* 2014;98(2):625–633

80. Manoj KS, Singal A, Menon R, et al. Early enteral nutrition therapy in congenital cardiac repair postoperatively: a randomized controlled pilot study. *Ann Cardiol Anaesth.* 2016;19(4):653–661

81. Lambert LM, Pike NA, Medoff-Cooper B, et al. Pediatric Heart Network Investigators. Variation in feeding practices following the Norwood procedure. *J Pediatr.* 2014;164(2):237–242

82. Cabrera AG, Prodhan P, Bhutta AT. Nutritional challenges and outcomes after surgery for congenital heart disease. *Curr Opin Cardiol.* 2010;25(2):88–94

83. Zemel BS, Pipan M, Stallings VA, et al. Growth charts for children with Down syndrome in the United States. *Pediatrics.* 2015;136(5):e1204–e1211

84. Brown KH, Peerson JM, Allen LHBND-. Effect of zinc supplementation on children's growth: a meta-analysis of intervention trials. *Bibl Nutr Dieta.* 1998(54):76–83

85. Walravens PA, Hambidge KM, Koepfer DM. Zinc supplementation in infants with a nutritional pattern of failure to thrive: a double-blind controlled study. *Pediatrics.* 1989;83(4):522–528

86. Payne PR, Waterlow JC. Relative energy requirements for maintenance, growth, and physical activity. *Lancet.* 1971;2(7717):210–211

87. Jackson M, Poskitt EM. The effects of high-energy feeding on energy balance and growth in infants with congenital heart disease and failure to thrive. *Br J Nutr.* 1991;65(2):131–143

88. Niemarkt HJ, de Meij TG, van de Velde ME, et al. Necrotizing enterocolitis: a clinical review on diagnostic biomarkers and the role of the intestinal microbiota. *Inflamm Bowel Dis.* 2015;21(2):436–444

89. Jeffries HE, Wells WJ, Starnes VA, Wetzel RC, Moromisato DY. Gastrointestinal morbidity after Norwood palliation for hypoplastic left heart syndrome. *Ann Thorac Surg.* 2006;81(3):982–987

90. Sharma R, Tepas JJ, III. Microecology, intestinal epithelial barrier and necrotizing enterocolitis. *Pediatr Surg Int.* 2010;26(1):11–21

91. Miller TA, Minich LL, Lamber LM, Joss-Moore L, Puchalski MD. Abnormal abdominal aorta hemodynamics are associated with necrotizing enterocolitis in infants with hypoplastic left heart syndrome. *Pediatr Cardiol.* 2014;35(4):616–621

92. Karpen HE. Nutrition in the cardiac newborns. Evidence-based nutrition guidelines for cardiac newborns. *Clin Perinatol.* 2016;43(1):131–145

93. Becker KC, Hornik CP, Cotton CM, et al. Necrotizing enterocolitis in infants with ductal dependent congenital heart disease. *Am J Perinatol.* 2015;32(7): 633–638

94. Scahill CJ, Graham EM, Atz AM, Bradley SM, Kavarana MN, Zyblewski SC. Preoperative feeding neonates with cardiac disease: Is the necrotizing enterocolitis fear justified? *World J Pediatr Congenit Heart Surg.* 2017;8(1):62–68

95. Fomon SJ, Ziegler EE. Nutritional management of infants with congenital heart disease. *Am Heart J.* 1972;83(5):581–588

96. Munns CF, Shaw N, Kiely M, et al. Global consensus recommendations on prevention and management of nutritional rickets. *J Clin Endocrinol Metab.* 2016;101(2):394–415

97. Ahrens KA, Rossen LM, Simon AE. Adherence to vitamin D recommendations among US infants aged 0-11 months, NHANES, 2009 to 2012. *Clin Pediatr (Phila).* 2016;55(6):555–556

98. McNally JD, Menon K. Vitamin D deficiency in surgical congenital heart disease: prevalence and relevance. *Transl Pediatr.* 2013;2(3):99–111

99. Dittrich S, Germanakis J, Dähnert I, et al. Randomised trial on the influence of continuous magnesium infusion on arrhythmias following cardiopulmonary bypass surgery for congenital heart disease. *Intensive Care Med.* 2003;29(7): 1141–1144

100. Shamir R, Dagan O, Abramovitch D, Abramovitch T, Vidne BA, Dinari G. Thiamine deficiency in children with congenital heart disease before and after corrective surgery. *JPEN J Parenter Enteral Nutr.* 2000;24(3):154–158

101. Ciotti G, Holzer R, Pozzi M, Dalzell M. Nutritional support via percutaneous endoscopic gastrostomy in children with cardiac disease experiencing difficulties with feeding. *Cardiol Young.* 2002;12(6):537–541

102. Short HL, Travers C, McCracken C, Wulkan ML, Clifton MS, Raval MV. Increased morbidity and mortality in cardiac patients undergoing fundoplication. *Pediatr Surg Int.* 2017;33(4):559–567

VI

Chapter 45

Nutrition in Children With Short Bowel Syndrome

Background

Short bowel syndrome (SBS) is a complex disorder that is characterized as a malabsorptive state in the setting of a reduced length of small bowel. The complexity of this disorder stems from the nutritional, metabolic, and infectious complications that often occur as a consequence of altered anatomy and physiology. In pediatrics, SBS typically results from congenital anomalies, such as intestinal atresia, gastroschisis, midgut volvulus, and acquired causes, the most common of which is necrotizing enterocolitis (NEC; see Table 45.1). Although the actual incidence and prevalence of SBS in the United States are not precisely known, advances in neonatal intensive care and surgical techniques has likely increased the frequency with which pediatricians will encounter such patients.

There is a wide spectrum of functionality associated with SBS, but a number of patients will develop intestinal failure, defined as an inability of the small intestine to maintain adequate fluid, nutrient, and electrolyte absorption to support normal growth and development. Such patients are dependent on parenteral nutrition. Although parenteral nutrition can serve as a life-saving treatment for patients who otherwise would not survive, its use does not come without risk. Central catheter-associated bloodstream infections, mechanical catheter-associated complications (breakage and/or thrombosis), and parenteral nutrition-associated liver disease (PNALD) are the main contributors to the morbidity and mortality associated with chronic use of parenteral nutrition. A study of infants with intestinal failure from 2000–2004 showed an overall mortality rate of 25% (primarily attributable to liver disease, multisystem organ failure, sepsis, and need for

Table 45.1.
Etiology of Short Bowel Syndrome in Infants and Children

Intestinal atresia
Necrotizing enterocolitis
Gastroschisis
Midgut volvulus
Total intestinal aganglionosis
Congenital short bowel
Ischemic injury
Tumor
Radiation enteritis

Table 45.2.
Factors Affecting Prognosis of SBS

Length of residual bowel
Presence or absence of ileocecal valve
Type of enteral feeds used
Early introduction of enteral feeds
Adaptive potential of residual bowel
Frequency of infections
Health of other organs (ie, stomach, pancreas, liver, colon)

intestinal transplantation).[1] Encouragingly, more recent advances regarding treatment of catheter-related complications and PNALD plus the development of multidisciplinary programs specializing in the care of short bowel syndrome have improved survival to >90%.[2-5]

A number of factors have been identified that are thought to influence the prognosis of SBS (see Table 45.2).[6-8] Loss of bowel length is the most significant, because this results in reduced surface area for absorption, decreased exposure of nutrients to brush-border digestive enzymes, and decreased exposure to pancreatic and biliary secretions. It has been estimated that 10 to 30 cm of small bowel with a preserved ileocecal valve or 30 to 50 cm of small bowel without an ileocecal valve is required for successful weaning from parenteral nutrition.[9] However, because residual length is only one of several factors involved in the prognosis of these patients, there are considerable exceptions to these estimations. Recognizing the importance of these various factors can help guide the management of these patients and ultimately facilitate the process of weaning from parenteral nutrition.

The optimal outcome for patients with SBS is to become independent from parenteral nutrition or attain what is referred to as enteral autonomy. Although there is still much to learn in this field, experience and data have been emerging to help us better understand how to achieve such an outcome through a physiologic mechanism known as intestinal adaptation. The act of promoting intestinal adaptation through nutritional, medical, and surgical therapies has been increasingly recognized and is now more commonly referred to as intestinal rehabilitation.

Intestinal Adaptation

Intestinal adaptation is a complex process that ensues following bowel resection. Throughout this process, the bowel undergoes both structural and functional changes in an attempt to compensate for the loss of absorptive surface area (see Table 45.3). Structurally, the villi lengthen and the

Table 45.3.

Changes Associated With Intestinal Adaptation

Increased villus height
Increased crypt depth
Increased bowel length
Increased bowel circumference
Increased bowel wall thickness
Increased enterocyte proliferation

bowel lengthens and dilates, all of which serve to increase the intestinal absorptive surface area.[10-13] Functionally, the bowel undergoes changes in nutrient transport, enzyme activity, and intestinal transit. Because of the innate ability of the maturing intestine to grow, infants may have an advantage for achieving better intestinal adaptation compared with older children or adults.[14-16] Small bowel length is estimated to be approximately 125 cm at 20 weeks' gestation, 200 cm at 30 weeks' gestation, and 275 cm at term.[16] An accelerated increase in bowel length during the last trimester of gestation could provide a theoretical advantage for bowel lengthening for the newborn infant.[14-16] Linear growth proceeds at a relatively rapid rate during the first year of life and continues for the next several years, although at a slower velocity.

A number of factors have been identified that influence the adaptive process, including enteral nutrition, hormones, and growth factors.[17] Enteral nutrients are an important stimulant for mucosal hyperplasia.[18] Complex nutrients, such as disaccharides and intact proteins have more of a stimulatory effect compared with monosaccharides and protein hydrolysates.[19,20] However, the use of intact nutrients must be carefully weighed against the possibility that they will be malabsorbed. The role of hormones and growth factors have been investigated, and currently, glucagon-like peptide 2 (GLP-2) is considered one of the more important hormones involved in intestinal adaptation (see "Medical Therapies").

Intestinal Physiology

The distinct functions of the proximal versus distal small intestine have a significant effect on the management of patients with SBS. Because different segments of the small intestine may be compromised, each patient has a unique anatomy and physiology. Treatment for these patients is based on their underlying disease, which segments have been resected, which segments are retained, and the functional capacity of retained remaining bowel. To determine the optimal nutritional therapy for each patient, it is

VI

important to appreciate the various functions of each area of small intestine and the consequences of its resection (Fig 45.1).

The duodenum is rarely affected in patients with SBS, perhaps because of its separate vascular supply. It is primarily responsible for the ongoing

Fig 45.1.
Gastrointestinal Manifestations of Intestinal Failure.

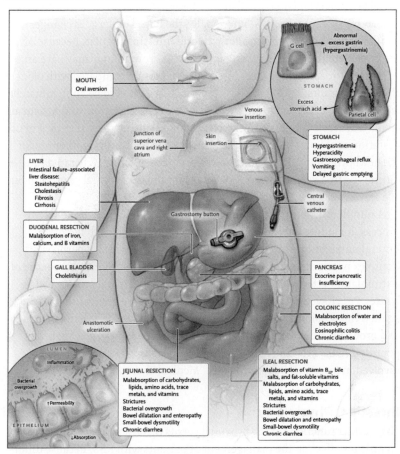

After intestinal resection, malabsorption of several classes of nutrients ensues (depending on the site of resection) and numerous inflammatory complications (e.g., bacterial overgrowth, colitis, anastomotic ulcerations, peptic disease with hypergastrinemia, and increased intestinal permeability) occur. Water and electrolyte losses are also commonly observed. Intestinal failure–associated liver disease has multiple manifestations. Reprinted with permission from: Duggan CP, Jaksic T. Pediatric intestinal failure. *N Engl J Med.* 2017;377(7):666–675 digestion of chyme (the semifluid mass of food released from the stomach) and is the preferred site of iron and folate absorption. When chyme is expelled from the stomach, the hormones secretin and cholecystokinin are released. Secretin stimulates pancreatic secretion of bicarbonate-rich fluid and of mucus-rich alkaline secretions from Brunner glands. The net effect is to neutralize the acidic chyme, establishing a pH favorable to the action of digestive enzymes. Cholecystokinin (CCK) is secreted in response to the presence of fat and protein. CCK stimulates biliary and pancreatic secretions, which promote further digestion of chyme.

The jejunum has long villi, a large absorptive surface area, and a high concentration of enzymes and transport carrier proteins. It is the primary absorptive site for most nutrients. Loss of jejunum is associated with decreased absorption attributable to loss of surface area, impaired digestion resulting from loss of brush-border enzymes, and decreased secretin and CCK with resultant compromise in pancreatic and biliary secretions. Following resection of the jejunum, however, through the process of intestinal adaptation over time, these functions of the jejunum may be acquired by the remaining bowel.

The ileum is characterized by shorter villi, more lymphoid tissue, and less absorptive capacity compared with the jejunum. Unlike the jejunum, however, 2 unique functions of the ileum cannot be acquired by other sites in the intestine following resection. The first is absorption of bile acids and vitamin B_{12}. Resections involving the ileum, therefore, can result in steatorrhea, cholelithiasis, and vitamin B_{12} deficiency. The second is the production of hormones that regulate intestinal motility. Normally, motility is more rapid in the proximal small bowel and slows in the distal ileum. Consequently, resection of the ileum may have more of an adverse effect on transit time compared with a proximal resection.

The ileocecal valve (ICV) controls the amount and rate of passage of ileal contents into the colon. Absence of the ICV shortens transit time and can lead to increased losses of fluid and nutrients. The ICV also serves to prevent reflux of colonic bacterial back into the small intestine. Reflux of colonic bacteria into the small intestine can cause mucosal inflammation and small intestine bacterial overgrowth, which can then lead to malabsorption.

Nutritional Assessment

The primary goals in the treatment of SBS patients are (1) to provide adequate nutrition to achieve normal growth and development; (2) to promote intestinal adaptation; and (3) to avoid complications associated with intestinal resection and use of parenteral nutrition. The first steps in assessing a child with SBS are to identify the underlying disease leading to a shortened gut, assess the residual anatomy, and anticipate the individual physiology of the patient on the basis of this information. Patients with intestinal atresias may not have developed a normal length of bowel in utero and, despite undergoing relatively limited resections, may be left with a significantly compromised length of bowel. Patients with gastroschisis are often compromised by a dilated, dysfunctional bowel and motility disorders, despite having a residual length that should otherwise be adequate for adaptation. NEC occurs predominantly in preterm infants and most commonly affects the terminal ileum and proximal colon. For such infants, the ICV is more likely to be resected and can contribute to more rapid transit and the development of small bowel bacterial overgrowth. The ischemic and inflammatory reactions associated with the pathogenesis of NEC can also contribute to the development of strictures.

Once the underlying diagnosis and anticipated physiology is determined, the focus becomes the assessment of the patient's nutritional status. Accurate measurements of weight, length/height, and head circumference obtained serially are essential. Fluid shifts, changes in stool and ostomy output, and the presence of ascites may affect the accuracy of weight measurements. In such cases, assessment of mid-upper arm circumference and triceps skinfold thickness may provide a better representation of nutritional status.

Nutritional Management

Parenteral Nutrition
In the early postoperative stage, parenteral nutrition is used to stabilize fluid and electrolyte status. Once a postoperative ileus resolves, large fluid volume and electrolyte losses may occur, along with hypergastrinemia and a need for acid suppression. Achieving adequate fluid and electrolyte balance can often pose a significant challenge. Because these losses can vary from day to day, it is advantageous to use a standard parenteral nutrition solution that meets basic fluid, electrolyte, and macro- and micronutrient requirements. Excessive fluid losses from ostomy output and stool losses can then be replaced based on the volume and electrolyte content of these secretions. It is preferable to measure the volume of these secretions and replace them using a separate fluid and electrolyte solution. Adjustment of parenteral

nutrition should be based on daily weights; strict measurements of urine, stool, ostomy output, serum electrolytes, and triglycerides; and a liver panel (inclusive of aspartate transaminase, alanine transaminase, alkaline phosphatase, gamma glutamyl transpeptidase, total bilirubin, direct bilirubin, and albumin [see Chapter 22: Parenteral Nutrition]).

Enteral Nutrition

A slow introduction of enteral feeding should be started as soon as possible after surgery. The role of early enteral feedings is important, because the process of intestinal adaptation begins as soon as 12 to 24 hours after surgical resection. Enteral nutrients stimulate the adaptive process by providing direct contact with the epithelial cells, thereby inducing villous hyperplasia and by stimulating the secretion of trophic gastrointestinal tract hormones. The use of enteral feedings is also important in the prevention of PNALD (see "Complications").

Mothers of newborn infants with SBS should be encouraged to continue with their production of human milk, because it offers several beneficial effects. In addition to the immunologic and anti-infective properties, human milk also contains growth factors, nucleotides, glutamine, and other amino acids thought to be important in the process of intestinal adaptation.[21] Human milk from mothers of preterm infants may require fortification to increase the caloric density as well as protein concentration. Donated human milk is also preferable to enteral formula.

When human milk is unavailable, the optimal enteral formula has not been clearly established. Some animal studies suggest that complex nutrients stimulate the intestinal adaptive process more effectively, but human data are limited.[20,22,23] However, because of potentially compromised digestive capabilities and limited absorptive surface area, the use of a standard infant formula can lead to malabsorption, resulting in fluid, electrolyte, and metabolic imbalance. Therefore, it has become customary to use either a protein hydrolysate or amino acid-based formula (see Chapter 4: Formula Feeding of Term Infants, for web links to manufacturers for product composition and other information]). These formulas contain glucose, glucose polymers, medium-chain triglycerides (MCTs), and hydrolyzed proteins, which may add significantly to the osmolality of the formula. Observations of a higher incidence of gastrointestinal allergies in SBS and the association with successful weaning from total parenteral nutrition have also supported the use of amino acid-based formulas.[8,24]

VI

Although fats tend to be poorly absorbed in patients with SBS, they are an important source of calories and are necessary for the prevention of essential fatty acid deficiency. MCTs are more water soluble than long-chain triglycerides and are more readily absorbed, particularly in the settings of bile acid malabsorption, liver disease, or pancreatic insufficiency. However, MCTs have slightly lower caloric density and a higher osmotic load, which can aggravate diarrhea. Long-chain triglycerides have a greater trophic effect on the small intestine and are, therefore, thought to be beneficial in stimulating intestinal adaptation. Ultimately, a combination of MCTs to maximize absorption and long-chain triglycerides to stimulate adaptation is recommended.

Carbohydrates may be difficult to tolerate, because they are rapidly metabolized to small molecules that can produce an increased osmotic load in the small intestine, resulting in high-volume stool or ostomy output. An increase in stool reducing substances and/or a low stool pH may indicate carbohydrate malabsorption.

The use of soluble dietary fiber, such as pectin or guar gum, has potentially beneficial effects on colonic adaptation but there have been case reports however of late onset necrotizing enterocolitis with the use of gum-containing thickening agents.[25] Fiber can slow transit and is also fermented by bacteria in the colon to produce short-chain fatty acids. In adults, the provision of fiber and the resultant short-chain fatty acids can provide as much as 500 to 1000 calories per day. In addition, butyrate (a short-chain fatty acid) has been shown to enhance sodium and water absorption via up-regulation of sodium-hydrogen exchanges. This up-regulation, however, may be delayed initially, causing stool output to worsen before it improves.[26,27] The dilution of formula to lower caloric density may allow improved tolerance by reducing malabsorption, maldigestion and lowering the osmotic load.

How to Feed

Once the appropriate source of enteral nutrition has been established, the next step is to determine the appropriate method of feeding. Continuous enteral feedings via a nasogastric or gastrostomy tube are generally preferred. Continuous enteral feeding allows for constant saturation of transport carrier proteins, thereby maximally utilizing the available absorptive surface area. Controlling the rate of feeds in this fashion may also help to reduce emesis and allow for more consistent advancement. Enteral feedings are slowly advanced by increasing either concentration or volume, depending on their tolerance. With this regimented approach to feeding, it is also important to introduce some oral feedings, even at nonnutritive volumes, so as to stimulate the normal development of oromotor skills. Missing this window of developmental opportunity often results in significant oral aversion later in life. As an infant is advancing his or her enteral feeds, 1 hour's worth of volume may be given by mouth, during which time tube feedings should be paused (Fig 45.2).

Fig 45.2.
Suggested Guidelines for Starting Enteral Feeds

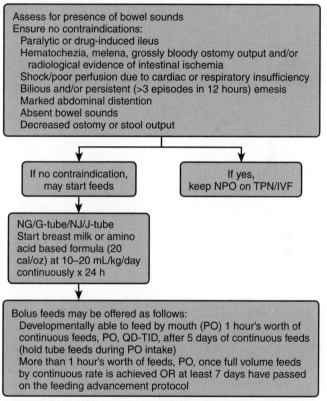

NPO, nil per os (nothing by mouth); TPN/IVF, total parenteral nutrition/intravenous fluids; NG/G, nasogastric/gastrostomy; NJ/J, nasojejunal/jejunostomy; QD-TID, every day to 3 times/ day; PO, oral.

Adapted from Sonneville K, Duggan C, ed. *Manual of Pediatric Nutrition*. 5th ed. Shelton, CT: People's Medical Publishing house; 2014.

The rate at which enteral feedings are advanced is determined by a number of factors including stool or ostomy output, and signs of malabsorption (Table 45.4). Carbohydrate malabsorption can be assessed by stool pH and reducing substances and can be an important and easily measurable factor to help in determining readiness for advancement. If feeding intolerance occurs after an increase in rate or concentration, a decrease to the previously tolerated rate or concentration should be made. Once tolerance is again established, another attempt at advancement may be made. Frequent setbacks are not uncommon. The development of diarrhea is inevitable in most patients and does not necessarily serve as a rate-limiting factor to advancing enteral feedings. As long as there is adequate weight gain, positive electrolyte and fluid balance, and lack of significant carbohydrate malabsorption, as reflected by stool pH and reducing substances, advancement should continue. Once a patient achieves his or her target for enteral feedings, a gradual transition to oral/bolus feedings should be pursued. This is generally accomplished by compressing a set volume of feeds over a shorter period of time. For example, if the patient is tolerating a rate of 40 mL/hour, one could compress the feedings to be given as 48 mL/hour for 2.5 hours with 30 minutes off, then 60 mL/hour for 2 hours with 1 hour off, etc.

Medical Therapies

The therapeutic effect of gastrointestinal hormones to promote intestinal adaptation has shown promise as a specific medical therapy for SBS. Glucagon-like peptide-2 (GLP-2) is a hormone secreted in response to ingestion of nutrients, has inhibitory effects on motility, decreases gastric acid secretion, and stimulates expansion of the intestinal mucosa, and its secretion has been found to be impaired in patients without a terminal ileum or colon.

The induction of intestinal epithelial proliferation by GLP-2 was first demonstrated in animal models in the mid-1990s. Since that time, a synthetic GLP-2 analogue (Teduglutide) has been studied and now is approved by the US Food and Drug Administration for the indication of short bowel syndrome in adult patients.[28–30] A recently published randomized, open-label, 12-week trial in pediatric patients showed a trend toward reduction in need for parenteral nutrition.[31] A 24-week trial to determine efficacy at higher doses is currently being conducted.

Table 45.4.
Suggested Guidelines for Advancing Enteral Feeds

Measure	Advance Rate by 10–20 mL/kg/day	No Change	Reduce Rate or Hold Feeds x 8 h, Then Restart at ¾ Previous Rate
Ostomy output (g)	<2 g/kg/h	2–3 g/kg/h	>3 g/kg/h
Stool output (g)	<10 g/kg/day or <10 stools/day	10–20 g/kg/day or 10–12 stools/day	>20 g/kg/day or >12 stools/day
Gastric residuals (mL)	<4 times previous hour's infusion		>4 times previous hour's infusion
Signs of malabsorption			
Stool-reducing substances	<1%	1%	>1%
Dehydration	Absent		Present
Weight loss	Absent		Present

Advancement Principles: Quantify feeding intolerance per stool or ostomy output; assess tolerance no more than twice per 24 hours; advance no more than once per 24 hours; goals: 150–200 mL/kg/day and 100–140 kcal/kg/day; as feedings are advanced, PN should be reduced while maintaining weight gain velocity.

Adapted from Sonneville K, Duggan C, eds. *Manual of Pediatric Nutrition*. 5th ed. Shelton, CT: People's Medical Publishing house; 2014

Surgical Therapies

As mentioned previously, one of the developments associated with intestinal adaptation is an increase in intestinal circumference or dilation of the bowel. Although this results in an increased absorptive surface area, such dilation can lead to compromised motility and stasis of intestinal contents, which often predisposes to the development of bacterial overgrowth. To optimize the absorptive surface area and address these adverse effects, surgical techniques to reconfigure the bowel have been pursued. For a longitudinal lengthening procedure, a dilated segment of intestine is divided along its longitudinal axis into 2 tubes, and the ends are then anastomosed in an isoperistaltic fashion (Fig 45.3). Unfortunately, this procedure is technically challenging, because it requires meticulous dissection of the mesenteric blood supply, is often complicated by the development of anatomic strictures, and ultimately has not been demonstrated to be of any significant benefit in weaning patients with SBS from total parenteral nutrition.[32]

The serial transverse enteroplasty (STEP) was introduced in 2003 as a novel surgical technique for patients with SBS.[33] In contrast to the longitudinal intestinal lengthening and tailoring (LILT) procedure, the STEP procedure involves applying a surgical stapler perpendicular to the bowel axis from alternating sides. This creates a more normal caliber, longer lumen

Fig 45.3.
Longitudinal Intestinal Lengthening Procedure

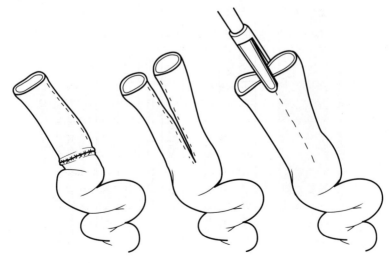

Fig 45.4.
Serial Transverse Enteroplasty Procedure

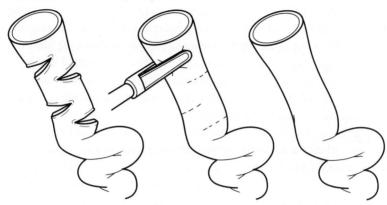

through which enteral contents can pass (Fig 45.4). Advantages to this technique include preservation of the vascular supply and avoiding the creation of new anastomotic sties. A study of nutritional and clinical outcomes with this procedure demonstrated both improved enteral tolerance and catch-up growth.[34] Data from the International STEP Registry have shown that after an initial STEP procedure, 66% had improved enteral tolerance and 47% were able to fully wean off parental nutrition.[35] In contrast to the LILT, a STEP procedure may be repeated.[36]

VI

Complications

As mentioned earlier, the use of parenteral nutrition offers a life-saving therapy for patients with SBS but does not come without risk. The 2 most significant complications associated with the long-term use of parenteral nutrition include catheter-related complications and the development of PNALD. Central venous catheter complications include catheter breakage, central venous thrombosis, loss of access, and most commonly, catheter-related blood stream infections. The risk of infection, particularly with gram-negative organisms, may be increased in patients with SBS because of the presence of an ostomy as well as increased stool output. Patients with intestinal pathology are significantly more likely to have life-threatening catheter-associated infections than other patients with indwelling lines (ie, for medication administration).[37] The propensity for bacteria to form a biofilm of bacterial colonies adherent to the wall of the catheters can contribute to repeated line infections. Preventive measures include diligent sterile technique when manipulating catheters as well as the use of lock therapy. With lock therapy, either ethanol or an antibiotic, such as vancomycin, is instilled into the central venous catheter and left to dwell for varying durations of time in an attempt to prevent and/or breakdown the film and kill the bacteria. A systematic review supports the use of ethanol instillation into central venous catheters to significantly decrease the rate of central catheter-associated bloodstream infections in patients receiving total parenteral nutrition.[38] A recent study incorporating ethanol lock therapy into a standardized protocol for central catheter care demonstrated a decrease in central catheter-associated bloodstream infections from 6.99 per 1000 catheter days to 0.42 per 1000 catheter days.[39] Although there were no significant adverse events in this study, there have been reports of structural changes, elution of molecules from catheter polymers (predominantly in polyurethane-based catheters, less so in silicone catheters), and increased risk of thrombosis with the use of ethanol; therefore, appropriate patient selection remains important[40,41] (see also Chapter 22: Parenteral Nutrition).

PNALD is most commonly identified by a serum direct bilirubin concentration >2 mg/dL with no other cause for liver disease. Histologic changes associated with PNALD include cholestasis, steatosis, steatohepatitis, fibrosis, and cirrhosis. It is estimated that two thirds of patients with intestinal failure will develop PNALD with 25% advancing to end-stage liver disease.[42] Multiple hypotheses regarding the pathogenesis of PNALD have been proposed including altered gut hormones, bacterial overgrowth-related cholangitis, intestinal stasis-associated hepatotoxic bile acids, and deficiencies of or toxic components in the total parenteral nutrition itself.[43–47] Risk factors for the development of PNALD include preterm birth, low birth weight, prolonged duration of PN, enteral nutrition intolerance, disrupted enterohepatic circulation of bile acids, intestinal stasis with bacterial overgrowth, catheter-related sepsis, excess glucose intake leading to steatosis, micronutrient deficiency, and high parenteral protein, fat, and/or energy intake.[48]

The mainstay of therapy for PNALD is the elimination of parenteral nutrition and parenteral lipids with advancement to full enteral nutrition. For those who are unable to wean from parenteral nutrition, alternative strategies for lipid administration are implemented and include lipid restriction and lipid replacement. A comparison of reduced dosing (1 g/kg/day, twice a week) versus standard dosing (3 g/kg/day) have shown a significantly higher rate of resolution of cholestasis in the reduced dosing group.[49,50] However, although lipid restriction may be effective in treatment of PNALD, the consequences for brain development are unknown, so this must be considered carefully. Essential fatty acid deficiency may occur at restricted doses; therefore, regular clinical and biochemical monitoring is required for those receiving lowered dosing.

With regard to lipid replacement, there are currently 2 main intravenous lipid emulsions approved for use in the United States: Intralipid and Smoflipid (FDA approved for adults; under investigation in pediatrics). An additional fish oil-based intravenous lipid emulsion (Omegaven) has been used in clinical trials that showed a decreased incidence of cholestasis and reduced mortality rates among infants with SBS.[51,52] It has been proposed that the increased amounts of omega-3 fatty acids and the decreased amounts of hepatotoxic phytosterols and proinflammatory omega-6 fatty acids in fish oil-based emulsions account for the beneficial effects of these alternative lipid emulsions.[53–56] The abundance of omega-6 fatty acids and relative paucity of antioxidants found in soybean-based emulsions may also potentiate inflammation and liver injury.[57,58] A recent multicenter blinded randomized trial comparing Smoflipid and Intralipid resulted in lower conjugated bilirubin concentrations, suggesting less liver disease.[59] Administration of ursodeoxycholic acid may alter bile composition, enhance bile flow, reduce gallbladder stasis, and provide cytoprotective, membrane stabilizing, and immunomodulatory effects.[60]

Aside from complications associated with the use of long-term parenteral nutrition, patients with SBS are at risk of developing complications inherent to their altered anatomy and physiology (Table 45.5). These include micronutrient deficiency, gastric acid hypersecretion, cholelithiasis, nephrolithiasis, bacterial overgrowth, and D-lactic acidosis.[61]

Periodic surveillance of micronutrient status is recommended as part of the nutritional assessment (Table 45.6) of patients with SBS. For patients at risk of fat malabsorption attributable to ileal resection and/or associated liver or pancreatic disease, routine monitoring of fat-soluble vitamins is recommended. In addition, as a consequence of fat malabsorption, long-chain fatty acids can form calcium and magnesium soaps, resulting in a deficiency of these minerals.[62] Zinc and copper deficiencies are common in patients with SBS, particularly those with an ostomy.[63]

Gastric acid hypersecretion results from loss of CCK and secretin, both of which regulate gastrin secretion. Without this negative feedback control,

VI

Table 45.5.

Complications Associated With SBS

Central venous catheter related
    Loss of venous access
    Thrombosis of veins
    Line infections/sepsis
Parenteral nutrition-associated liver disease
    Cholestasis
    Steatosis
    Steatohepatitis
    Fibrosis
    Cirrhosis
    Liver failure
    Cholelithiasis
    Cholecystitis
Metabolic complications
    Fluid and electrolyte imbalance
    Micronutrient deficiency/toxicity
Metabolic bone disease
    Osteopenia
    Osteoporosis
Renal complications
    Nephrolithiasis
    Hyperoxaluria
Bacterial overgrowth
D-lactic acidosis
Gastric acid hypersecretion
    Peptic injury
    Maldigestion
    Malabsorption

gastrin concentrations in the stomach are elevated, resulting in increased acid production. This can result in caustic injury to the proximal small bowel, adversely affecting its absorptive capacity. Also, because pancreatic enzymes and bile salts function optimally at a pH of 7 to 8, such hyperacidity can impair carbohydrate and protein digestion, micelle formation, and lipolysis of fat, resulting in malabsorption. The suppression of acid with either H_2 blockers or proton pump inhibitors can help to improve absorption.[64] There has been evidence suggesting the use of acid blockade increases the risk of respiratory and gastrointestinal tract infections; therefore, it is important to carefully weigh the risks and benefits of their use.[65]

Compromised enterohepatic circulation of bile or bile acid malabsorption related to ileal resection may allow for cholesterol to precipitate more readily in bile because of a low concentration of bile salts. Independent of

Table 45.6.

Micronutrient Monitoring

Micronutrient	Mechanism for Deficiency
Fat-soluble vitamins	
A<D<E<K	Fat malabsorption, cholestasis
Water-soluble vitamins	
B_{12}	Gastric or ileal resection
Folate	Proximal small bowel malabsorption
Minerals and trace elements	
Calcium	Fat malabsorption
Magnesium	Fat malabsorption
Zinc	Diarrhea, ostomy losses
Iron	Proximal small bowel malabsorption, omission from total parenteral nutrition
Copper	Diarrhea, ostomy losses, inadequate repletion in total parenteral nutrition
Selenium	Inadequate repletion in total parenteral nutrition

ileal resection, the chronic use of parenteral nutrition, in and of itself, has been associated with the development of biliary sludge and cholelithiasis as well.[66]

As mentioned previously, long-chain fatty acids are able to combine with calcium and magnesium, leading to deficiency of these minerals. When this occurs, calcium becomes less available to bind to oxalate that is normally excreted in the stool in the form of calcium-oxalate. Oxalate is then reabsorbed through the colon, the permeability of which is increased when bile salts are not adequately taken up in the ileum and are, thus, present in the colon. These factors increase enteric oxalate absorption that, in turn, increases the risk of developing oxalate renal stones. This is a complication that can affect patients with SBS long after they have achieved intestinal adaptation. Often, such patients will need to maintain a low-oxalate diet to prevent recurrent nephrolithiasis.[67]

Bacterial overgrowth is a common complication associated with SBS. Adverse effects include deconjugation of bile acids with resultant steatorrhea, competitive metabolism, competition for enteral nutrients, synthesis of toxic metabolites including D-lactic acid, and translocation resulting in bacteremia and potentially in sepsis.[68] Factors that can predispose to the development of bacterial overgrowth include dysmotility, stasis of intestinal contents in a dilated lumen, and absence of an ileal cecal valve allowing reflux of colonic contents into the small intestine. The organisms associated with bacterial overgrowth are usually anaerobes or gram-negative bacteria. Such bacteria can deconjugate bile salts, cause steatorrhea, and lead to mucosal inflammation, which then compromises intestinal absorption. Bacterial overgrowth should be suspected in patients who lose weight or plateau or require increasingly higher amounts of calories.[69] An added complication of bacterial overgrowth is the development of D-lactic acidosis. D-lactic acidosis is a rare occurrence in humans and results when unabsorbed carbohydrates are metabolized by colonic bacteria. The bacteria produce the D-isomer of lactic acid, which is unable to be metabolized by the human form of lactate dehydrogenase and can cross the blood-brain barrier. Therefore, this condition should be suspected when there is unexplained acidosis or unexplained neurologic changes, including headache, drowsiness, confusion, behavioral changes, altered mental status, slurred speech, and ataxia. Therapy is directed toward treatment and prevention of small intestinal bacterial overgrowth as well as limitation of dietary carbohydrates.[70,71]

Summary

SBS is a complex condition because of the nutritional, metabolic, and infectious complications that can occur from having an altered anatomy and physiology. The primary goals in the treatment of SBS are to provide adequate nutrition to achieve normal growth and development, promote intestinal adaptation, and avoid complications associated with intestinal resection and use of parenteral nutrition. These goals are best achieved by the advancement of enteral feedings, weaning from parenteral nutrition, and monitoring closely for the development of potential complications.

References

1.   Squires RH, Duggan C, Teitelbaum DH, et al. Natural history of pediatric intestinal failure: initial report from the Pediatric Intestinal Failure Consortium. *J Pediatr.* 2012;161(4):723–728

2.   Javid PJ, Malone FR, Bittner R, Healey PJ, Horslen SP. The optimal timing of referral to an intestinal failure program: the relationship between hyperbilirubinemia and mortality. *J Pediatr Surg.* 2011;46(6):1052–1056

3. Fullerton BS, Sparks EA, Hall AM, Duggan C, Jaksic T, Modi BP. Enteral autonomy, cirrhosis, and long term transplant-free survival in pediatric intestinal failure patients. *J Pediatr Surg.* 2016;51(1):96–100

4. Stanger JD, Oliveira C, Blackmore C, Avitzur Y, Wales PW. The impact of multi-disciplinary intestinal rehabilitation programs on the outcom of pediatric patients with intestinal failure: a systematic review and meta-analysis. *J Pediatr Surg.* 2013;48(5):983–992

5. Hess RA, Welch KB, Brown PI, Teitelbaum DH. Survival outcomes of pediatric intestinal failure patients: analysis of factors contributing to improved survival over the past two decades. *J Surg Res.* 2011;170(1):27–31

6. Sondheimer JM, Cadnapaphornchai M, Sontag M, Zerbe GO. Predicting the duration of dependence on parenteral nutrition after neonatal intestinal resection. *J Pediatr.* 1998;132(1):80–84

7. Kaufman SS, Loseke CA, Lupo JV, et al. Influence of bacterial overgrowth and intestinal inflammation on duration of parenteral nutrition in children with short bowel syndrome. *J Pediatr.* 1997;131(3):356–361

8. Andorsky DJ, Lund DP, Lillehei CW, et al. Nutritional and other postoperative management of neonates with short bowel syndrome correlates with clinical outcomes. *J Pediatr.* 2001;139(1):27–33

9. Kurkchubasche AG, Rowe MI, Smith SD. Adaptation in short-bowel syndrome: reassessing old limits. *J Pediatr Surg.* 1993;28(8):1069–1071

10. Dowling RH, Booth CC. Structural and functional changes following small intestinal resection in the rat. *Clin Sci.* 1967;32(1):139–149

11. Hanson WR, Osborne JW, Sharp JG. Compensation by the residual intestine after intestinal resection in the rat. II. influence of postoperative time interval. *Gastroenterology.* 1977;72(4 Pt 1):701–705

12. Sacks AI, Warwick GJ, Barnard JA. Early proliferative events following intestinal resection in the rat. *J Pediatr Gastroenterol Nutr.* 1995;21(2):158–164

13. Williamson RC. Intestinal adaptation (first of two parts). structural, functional and cytokinetic changes. *N Engl J Med.* 1978;298(25):1393–1402

14. Siebert JR. Small-intestine length in infants and children. *Am J Dis Child.* 1980;134(6):593–595

15. Weaver LT, Austin S, Cole TJ. Small intestinal length: a factor essential for gut adaptation. *Gut.* 1991;32(11):1321–1323

16. Touloukian RJ, Smith GJ. Normal intestinal length in preterm infants. *J Pediatr Surg.* 1983;18(6):720–723

17. Tappenden KA. Intestinal adaptation following resection. *JPEN J Parenter Enteral Nutr.* 2014;38(Suppl):23S–31S

18. DiBaise JK, Young RJ, Vanderhoof JA. Intestinal rehabilitation and the short bowel syndrome: part 1. *Am J Gastroenterol.* 2004;99(7):1386–1395

19. Vanderhoof JA, Grandjean CJ, Burkley KT, Antonson DL. Effect of casein versus casein hydrolysate on mucosal adaptation following massive bowel resection in infant rats. *J Pediatr Gastroenterol Nutr.* 1984;3(2):262–267

VI

20. Weser E, Babbitt J, Hoban M, Vandeventer A. Intestinal adaptation. different growth responses to disaccharides compared with monosaccharides in rat small bowel. *Gastroenterology.* 1986;91(6):1521–1527

21. Pereira-Fantini PM, Thomas SL, Taylor RG, et al. Colostrum supplementation restores insulin-like growth factor-1 levels and alters muscle morphology following massive small bowel resection. *JPEN J Parenter Enteral Nutr.* 2008;32(3): 266–275

22. Clarke RM. "Luminal nutrition" versus "functional work-load" as controllers of mucosal morphology and epithelial replacement in the rat small intestine. *Digestion.* 1977;15(5):411–424

23. Vanderhoof JA, Grandjean CJ, Kaufman SS, Burkley KT, Antonson DL. Effect of high percentage medium-chain triglyceride diet on mucosal adaptation following massive bowel resection in rats. *JPEN J Parenter Enteral Nutr.* 1984;8(6): 685–689

24. Bines J, Francis D, Hill D. Reducing parenteral requirement in children with short bowel syndrome: Impact of an amino acid-based complete infant formula. *J Pediatr Gastroenterol Nutr.* 1998;26(2):123–128

25. Beal J, Silverman B, Young T, Klontz K. Late onset necrotizing enterocolitis in infants following use of a xanthan gum-containing thickening agent. *J Pediatr.* 2012;161:354–356

26. Musch MW, Bookstein C, Xie Y, Sellin JH, Chang EB. SCFA increase intestinal na absorption by induction of NHE3 in rat colon and human intestinal C2/bbe cells. *Am J Physiol Gastrointest Liver Physiol.* 2001;280(4):G687–G693

27. Matarese LE, O'Keefe SJ, Kandil HM, Bond G, Costa G, Abu-Elmagd K. Short bowel syndrome: Clinical guidelines for nutrition management. *Nutr Clin Pract.* 2005;20(5):493–502

28. Jeppesen PB, Gilroy R, Pertkiewicz M, Allard JP, Messing B, O'Keefe SJ. Randomised placebo-controlled trial of teduglutide in reducing parenteral nutrition and/or intravenous fluid requirements in patients with short bowel syndrome. *Gut.* 2011;60(7):902–914

29. Schwartz LK, O'Keefe S, Fujioka K, et al. Long term Teduglutide for the treatment of patients with intestinal failure associated with short bowel syndrome. *Clin Transl Gastroenterol.* 2016;7:e142

30. Iyer KR, Kunecki M, Boullata JI, et al. Independence from parenteral nutrition and intravenous fluid support during treatment with teduglutide among patients with intestinal failure associated with short bowel syndrome. *J Parenter Enteral Nutr.* 2017;41(6):946–951

31. Carter BA, Cohran VC, Cole CR, et al. Outcomes from a 12-week, open-label, multicenter clinical trial of Teduglutide in pediatric short bowel syndrome. *J Pediatr.* 2017;181:102–111

32. Thompson JS, Pinch LW, Young R, Vanderhoof JA. Long-term outcome of intestinal lengthening. *Transpl Proc.* 2000;32(6):1242–1243

33. Kim HB, Fauza D, Garza J, Oh JT, Nurko S, Jaksic T. Serial transverse enteroplasty (STEP): A novel bowel lengthening procedure. *J Pediatr Surg.* 2003;38(3):425–429

34. Ching YA, Fitzgibbons S, Valim C, et al. Long-term nutritional and clinical outcomes after serial transverse enteroplasty at a single institution. *J Pediatr Surg.* 2009;44(5):939–943

35. Jones BA, Hull MA, Potanos KM, et al. Report of 111 consecutive patients enrolled in the International Serial Transverse Enteroplasty (STEP) Data Registry: a retrospective observational study. *J Am Coll Surg.* 2013;216(3):438–446

36. Mercer SF, Hobson BD, Gerhardt BK, et al. Serial transverse enteroplasty allows children with short bowel to wean from parenteral nutrition. *J Pediatr.* 2014;164(1):93–98

37. Dahan M, O'Donnell S, Hebert J, et al. CLABSI Risk Factors in the NICU: Potential for Prevention: A PICNIC Study. *Infect Control Hosp Epidemiol.* 2016;37(12):1446–1452

38. Oliveira C, Nasr A, Brindle M, Wales PW. Ethanol Locks to Prevent Catheter-Related Bloodstream Infections in Parenteral Nutrition: A Meta-Analysis. *Pediatrics.* 2012;129(2):318–329

39. Ardura MI, Lewis J, Tansmore JL, Harp PL, Dienhart MC, Balint JC. Central catheter-associated bloodstream infection reduction with ethanol lock prophylaxis in pediatric intestinal failure: broadening quality improvement initiatives from hospital to home. *JAMA Pediatr.* 2015;169(4):324–331

40. Wong T, Clifford V, McCallum Z, et al. Central venous catheter thrombosis associated with 70% ethanol locks in pediatric intestinal failure patients on home parenteral nutrition: a case series. *J Parenter Enteral Nutr.* 2012;36(3):358–360

41. Mermel LA, Alang N. Adverse effects associated with ethanol lock solutions: a systematic review. *J Antimicrob Chemother.* 2014;69(10):2611–2619

42. Wales PW, Allen N, Worthington P, George D, Compher C, American Society for Parenteral and Enteral Nutrition. ASPEN Clinical Guidelines: support of pediatric patients with intestinal failure at risk of parenteral-nutrition associated liver disease. *JPEN J Parenter Enteral Nutr.* 2014;38(5):538–557

43. Beath SV, Davies P, Papadopoulou A, et al. Parenteral nutrition-related cholestasis in postsurgical neonates: multivariate analysis of risk factors. *J Pediatr Surg.* 1996;31(4):604–606

44. Colomb V, Jobert-Giraud A, Lacaille F, Goulet O, Fournet JC, Ricour C. Role of lipid emulsions in cholestasis associated with long-term parenteral nutrition in children. *JPEN J Parenter Enteral Nutr.* 2000;24(6):345–350

45. Greenberg GR, Wolman SL, Christofides ND, Bloom SR, Jeejeebhoy KN. Effect of total parenteral nutrition on gut hormone release in humans. *Gastroenterology.* 1981;80(5 Pt 1):988–993

VI

46. Cooper A, Ross AJ, O'Neill JA, Bishop HC, Templeton JM, Ziegler MM. Resolution of intractable cholestasis associated with total parenteral nutrition following biliary irrigation. *J Pediatr Surg.* 1985;20(6):772–774

47. Kubota A, Yonekura T, Hoki M, et al. Total parenteral nutrition-associated intrahepatic cholestasis in infants: 25 years' experience. *J Pediatr Surg.* 2000;35(7):1049–1051

48. Peyret B, Collardeau S, Touzet S, et al. Prevalence of liver complications in children receiving long-term parenteral nutrition. *Eur J Clin Nutr.* 2011;65(6): 743–749

49. Cober MP, Killu G, Brattain A, et al. Intravenous fat emulsions reduction for patients with parenteral nutrition-associated liver disease. *J Pediatr.* 2012;160(3): 421–427

50. Rollins MD, Ward RM, Jackson WD, et al. Effect of decreased parenteral soybean lipid emulsion on hepatic function in infants at risk for parenteral nutrition-associated liver disease: a pilot study. *J Pediatr Surg.* 2013;48(6):1348–1356

51. Puder M, Valim C, Meisel JA, et al. Parenteral fish oil improves outcomes in patients with parenteral nutrition-associated liver injury. *Ann Surg.* 2009;250(395–402)

52. Nandivada P, Fell GL, Gura KM, Puder M. Am J Clin Nutr. 103. 2016;2 (629S–634S)

53. Buchman A. Total parenteral nutrition-associated liver disease. *JPEN J Parenter Enteral Nutr.* 2002;26(5 Suppl):S43–S48

54. Kurvinen A, Nissinen MJ, Gylling H, et al. Effects of long-term parenteral nutrition on serum lipids, plant sterols, cholesterol metabolism, and liver histology in pediatric intestinal failure. *J Pediatr Gastroenterol Nutr.* 2011;53(4): 440–446

55. El Kasmi KC, Anderson AL, Devereaux MW, et al. Phytosterols promote liver injury and Kupffer cell activation in parental nutrition associated liver disease. *Sci Transl Med.* 2013;5(206):206ra137

56. Clayton PT, Whitfield P, Iyer K. The role of phytosterols in the pathogenesis of liver complications of pediatric parenteral nutrition. *Nutrition.* 1998;14(1): 158–164

57. Chen WY, Lin SY, Pan HC, et al. Beneficial effect of docosahexaenoic acid on cholestatic liver injury in rats. *J Nutr Biochem.* 2012;23(3):252–264

58. Yeh SL, Chang KY, Huang PC, Chen WJ. Effects of n-3 and n-6 fatty acids on plasma eicosanoids and liver antioxidant enzymes in rats receiving total parenteral nutrition. *Nutrition.* 1997;13:32–36

59. Diamond IR, Grant RC, Pencharz PB, et al. Preventing the progression of intestinal failure-associated liver disease in infants using a composite lipid emulsion:a pilot randomized controlled trial of SMOFlipid. *JPEN J Parenter Enteral Nutr.* 2017;41(5):866–877

60. San Luis VA, Btaich IF. Ursodiol in patients with parenteral nutrition-associated cholestasis. *Ann Pharmacother.* 2007;41(11):1867–1872

61. Nightingale J. The medical management of intestinal failure: methods to reduce the severity. *Proc Nutr Soc.* 2003;62(3):703–710

62. Haderslev KV, Jeppesen PB, Mortensen PB, Staun M. Absorption of calcium and magnesium in patients with intestinal resections treated with medium chain fatty acids. *Gut.* 2000;46(6):819–823

63. Balay KS, Hawthorne KM, Hicks PD, Chen Z, Griffin IJ, Abrams SA. Low zinc status and absorption exist in infants with jejunostomies or ileostomies which persists after intestinal repair. *Nutrients.* 2012;4(9):1273–1281

64. Cortot A, Fleming CR, Malagelada JR. Improved nutrient absorption after cimetidine in short-bowel syndrome with gastric hypersecretion. *N Engl J Med.* 1979;300(2):79–80

65. Canani RB, Cirillo P, Rogerro P, et al. Therapy with gastric acidity inhibitors increases the risk of acute gastroenteritis and community-acquired pneumonia in children. *Pediatrics.* 2006;117(5):e817–e820

66. Murray FE, Hawkey CJ. Therapeutic approaches to the problem of biliary sludge and gallstone formation during total parenteral nutrition. *Clin Nutr.* 1992;11(10):12–17

67. American Gastroenterological Association. Medical position statement: short bowel syndrome and intestinal transplantation. *Gastroenterology.* 2003;124(4):1105–1110

68. Cole CR, Frem JC, Schmotzer B, et al. The rate of bloodstream infection is high in infants with short bowel syndrome: relationship with small bowel bacterial overgrowth, enteral feeding, and inflammatory and immune responses. *J Pediatr.* 2010;156(6):941–947

69. Vanderhoof JA. Short bowel syndrome. In: Walker WA, Watkins JB, Duggan C, eds. *Nutrition in Pediatrics.* Hamilton, Ontario: BC Decker Inc; 2003:771–789

70. Perlmutter DH, Boyle JT, Campos JM, Egler JM, Watkins JB. D-lactic acidosis in children: an unusual metabolic complication of small bowel resection. *J Pediatr.* 1983;102(2):234–238

71. Mayne AJ, Handy DJ, Preece MA, George RH, Booth IW. Dietary management of D-lactic acidosis in short bowel syndrome. *Arch Dis Child.* 1990;65(2):229–231

VI

Chapter 46

Nutrition in Cystic Fibrosis

Introduction

Cystic fibrosis (CF) is a life-shortening, autosomal-recessive disorder that affects the sweat glands and digestive, respiratory, and reproductive systems. It is caused by mutations in the cystic fibrosis transmembrane conductance regulator (CFTR) gene, a 250 kb gene found on the long arm of chromosome 7 that encodes a chloride transport protein.[1,2] More than 2000 mutations of the CFTR gene have been reported (http://www.genet.sickkids.on.ca/cftr/app), and more are still being discovered; however, most occur infrequently, and approximately 10% are common enough to be well characterized (http://www.cftr2.org). Among these gene mutations, some are disease causing, some are sequence variations that do not cause CF, some are associated with single or milder organ system involvement than typically seen in CF (sometimes called "CFTR-associated disorders" or "CFTR-related metabolic syndrome"), and some have variable or unknown consequences.[3] The most common is the first mutation discovered, F508del, which is a 3-base pair deletion at codon 508 that leads to loss of a phenylalanine residue that, in turn, causes a protein-folding defect and a failure in processing through the cytoplasm to the epithelial surface of affected cells.[1] Approximately half of patients with CF are homozygous for F508del, and nearly 40% more have at least 1 such mutation; however, in the latter circumstance, it is the second mutation that determines genotype-phenotype implications.[4-6]

The strongest relation between the genotype and the phenotype is observed for the exocrine pancreas.[4-6] The majority of people with CF have pancreatic insufficiency (PI) at birth or develop PI by 1 year of age. Most patients with the PI phenotype present with signs and symptoms of malabsorption and/or failure to thrive at an early age, although some may appear normal. Approximately 10% to 15% of children with CF have evidence of pancreatic dysfunction but retain sufficient residual pancreatic function to permit considerable digestion without the need for exogenous pancreatic enzyme supplements with meals. The term pancreatic sufficiency (PS) is used to describe patients with this phenotype who tend to have a milder form of CF disease.[2] Analyses of large patient cohorts have revealed that different mutations in the CFTR gene confer either the PI or the PS phenotypes.[2,4]

The lungs of infants with CF are structurally and functionally normal at birth, but there is often evidence of airway obstruction and structural

VI

changes within the first few months of life.[7,8] The lungs of patients with CF are highly susceptible to infection, especially with the gram-negative bacterium *Pseudomonas aeruginosa*.[9] Intermittent, then chronic, pulmonary infection occurs over the course of months to years, leading to bronchiectasis and, ultimately, respiratory failure. Infection increases caloric requirements because of the increased work of breathing and ultimately causes premature death in 90% of affected individuals.

In the United States, most cases of CF in children are diagnosed in early infancy through newborn screening. Early screening and identification has allowed early aggressive intervention to maintain growth and preserve lung function. Up to 20% of newborn infants with the PI phenotype of CF present with meconium ileus.[10] The spectrum of meconium ileus ranges from neonatal bowel obstruction attributable to thick meconium to intrauterine intestinal perforation with intra-abdominal calcifications. Treatment depends on the degree of obstruction and injury to the colon. Microcolon frequently results from the prolonged intrauterine intestinal obstruction. Studies suggest children with CF who have meconium ileus have reduced fat mass, bone mineral density, and lung function compared with those who do not have meconium ileus.[11] The need for surgical intervention to relieve obstruction (as opposed to relief of the obstruction by enemas) increases the risk of poor growth.[12]

Role of the Pediatrician

In the United States, children with CF generally receive CF-focused medical care through a Cystic Fibrosis Center; these are developed, funded, and monitored by the Cystic Fibrosis Foundation (CFF). Contact with the center may be made by the pediatrician in the first days of life, when the newborn screening result positive for CF. Although it may seem that the comprehensive care provided by the CF center reduces the importance of the pediatrician, nothing could be further from the truth. Children with CF, similarly to all children, need regular pediatric care for good health. Indeed, providing a "typical child" medical experience may benefit both parents and child. Importantly, the pediatrician providing primary care to the child with CF may be best able to observe depression in the parent or child, and issues with feeding and compliance. For families living at a distance from their CF center, the pediatrician has a crucial role in supporting and monitoring recommendations of the center. The CF center and the pediatrician are a critical team in the management of growth and nutrition in the child with CF, and changes made by one partner should be communicated to the other for consistent management.

Importance of Nutrition in CF

Many lines of evidence demonstrate that people with CF who have normal growth and development have better pulmonary function than those with deficient growth. A prospective observational study using data from the Cystic Fibrosis Foundation Registry identified 3142 children with CF from 1989–1992 and stratified them by peak weight-for-age percentile at 4 to 5 years of age.[13] They found that individuals with CF who had weight for age >50th percentile at 4 years of age reached a much higher height for age early in life and maintained this advantage into adulthood. In addition, pulmonary function, measured as percent forced expiratory volume in 1 second (FEV1) of the total forced vital capacity (FVC), was much lower in people with CF with weight for age <10th percentile at 4 years of age. This trend tracked through 18 years of age. Finally, weight for age at 4 years of age predicted survival at 18 years of age, with higher weight for age at 4 years of age predicting higher survival. This study has been supported by several other lines of evidence, including a single center study showing that infants with CF who recovered a weight z score comparable to that at birth within 2 years of diagnosis had better lung function and fewer symptoms of pulmonary disease than nonresponders.[14] A study of 6805 children from the Cystic Fibrosis Foundation Registry showed that children followed from age 2 to 7 years whose weight-for-length and body mass index (BMI) percentiles increased by >10 percentile points by 6 years of age had FEV1 significantly higher than those whose weight for length and BMI was <50th percentile and stable or decreased >10 percentile points. Achieving weight for length BMI >50th percentile and maintaining this level was associated with significantly higher FEV1 at 6 to 7 years of age.[15] In summary, maintaining optimal nutritional status at all times is crucial in prolonging survival in CF. Optimal survival requires close monitoring and aggressive attention to poor growth or weight loss. Pediatricians can significantly affect survival in their patients with CF by supporting aggressive nutritional management of CF with families and alerting the CF team if they note lagging growth or weight loss.

VI

Pathogenesis of Poor Weight Gain in Cystic Fibrosis

Children with CF have increased energy needs, but complications associated with CF impede intake or increase malabsorption of nutrients. Several lines of evidence show that children with CF have increased resting energy expenditure,[16–18] which is generally attributed to increased work of breathing, chronic inflammation (both pulmonary and intestinal[19,20]), and chronic infection but may also be a direct effect of the defective CFTR.

At the same time, children with CF may have impaired intake of nutrients. The appetite of a child with CF may be diminished by poor sense of smell associated with sinusitis,[21] or the child may experience anorexia associated with medications. Abdominal pain associated with gastroesophageal reflux, small bowel bacterial overgrowth, constipation, distal intestinal obstruction syndrome, or other gastrointestinal complications of CF,[22] may limit intake of food. At every stage of life, children with CF are at risk of disordered eating behaviors. Initially, this may be associated with intense focus by parents on intake, driven by their fear of their child being underweight, but later, depression may cause reduced intake in the older child.

Calories ingested may not be digested adequately as a result of pancreatic insufficiency or poor adherence to pancreatic enzyme replacement therapy (PERT). Intestinal bile acids are essential for production of mixed micelles and absorption of fat.[23] Children with CF may have reduced intestinal bile acid content because of cystic fibrosis related liver disease and because the relatively acidic intestinal environment leads to precipitation of bile salts. Low intestinal pH resulting from the lack of pancreatic bicarbonate secretion[24] may prevent the enteric coating on the PERT beads from dissolving at the optimal site in the intestine. Children with meconium ileus in infancy may have residual short bowel or dysmotility of the bowel, leading to poorer absorption.[11] CF-related diabetes occurs in about 2% of young children, 20% of adolescents, and about 40% of adults.[25] Untreated, it is associated with diminished body mass index and decreased survival. Energy loss through glycosuria is one mechanism of this impact.

Overview of Therapy

Without therapeutic interventions, CF is usually fatal within the first decade of life. Current treatment is multifaceted and requires close monitoring by an expert multidisciplinary care team. This care includes, at minimum, quarterly evaluation, counseling, and intervention by expert physicians, nurses, dietitians, respiratory and/or physical therapists, and social workers. Genetic counselors, psychologists, and exercise physiologists are also important resources. A key goal is to support nutrition to promote normal growth and development. In addition, high priority is given to effective disease education so that the family can understand and be equipped to manage this complex chronic disorder.

The core objectives of treatment for children with CF treatment are to prevent malnutrition, control respiratory infections, and promote mucus clearance.[7] The CFF has published evidence-informed guidelines on many aspects of CF care including diagnosis[3] and pulmonary management.[26] For the purposes of this review, guidelines for nutritional management for patients with CF were first published in 1992[27] and revised in 2002[28] and 2008[29] to incorporate more evidence-based recommendations. Since this time, key updates to nutritional guidelines were published with the age-specific guidelines for infants[7,8] and for children 2 to 5 years of age[30] with CF. All CFF-endorsed guidelines are available at www.cff.org. The European Cystic Fibrosis society recently published guidelines for nutritional care of infants, children, and adults with CF.[31]

Nutritional Care

Goals

The goal of nutritional care in children with CF is to achieve normal growth and optimize nutritional status. A review of Cystic Fibrosis Foundation Registry data from 1994 to 2003 led the CFF to recommend a goal for BMI of $\geq$50th percentile for all children with CF, and an adult goal for BMI of $\geq$22 for women and $\geq$23 men. This is an aggressive goal, but the data showed better lung function with a higher BMI percentile.[29] Major interventions include: (1) PERT to reduce malabsorption caused by PI; (2) a high-energy, nutrient-dense diet to compensate for nutrient losses, increased energy requirement, and decreased dietary intake; and (3) vitamin/mineral supplementation to prevent micronutrient deficiencies.

Pancreatic Enzyme Replacement Therapy

Diagnosis of Pancreatic Insufficiency

Exocrine pancreatic function should be assessed in the following situations: (1) at or shortly after diagnosis to provide objective evaluation of pancreatic status before enzyme therapy is initiated; and (2) to monitor patients with previous studies demonstrating PS for evidence of developing fat maldigestion, particularly when frequent bulky bowel movements or unexplained weight loss occur. The preferred test for assessment of pancreatic functional status is fecal elastase-1 concentration.[8] Fecal elastase-1 concentration is not diagnostic by itself but aids in defining PS (>200 µg/g) or PI (<100 µg/g). This test does not quantitate the degree of malabsorption. Because the fecal elastase-1 test measures human elastase, it is not affected by the ingestion of porcine-derived PERT, nor can it be used to assess adherence to PERT.

PERT Regimen

Because of the strong association between genotype and pancreatic phenotype, PERT should be initiated if the patient is known to have 2 CFTR mutations associated with PI or objective evidence of PI.[8] PERT should not be initiated in infants with a CFTR mutation known to be associated with PS, unless there are unequivocal signs or symptoms of malabsorption. In some infants with CF diagnosed through newborn screening, PI is not present at the time of diagnosis but develops later in infancy or even early childhood. Therefore, it is important to repeat fecal elastase-1 measurement in infants who initially have PS, especially when gastrointestinal tract symptoms appear or poor weight gain occurs. Children with CF who have laboratory evidence of PI should be started on PERT, even in the absence of signs or symptoms of fat malabsorption.

Pancreatic enzymes are extracts of porcine origin containing amylase, proteases, and lipase. Enzyme dosing is based on lipase content, and commercial products are sold in capsules with varying lipase activity, ranging from 4200 to 24 000 lipase units/capsule. The majority of US Food and Drug Administration (FDA)-approved PERT agents are enteric-coated enzymes that are protected from stomach acid and released in the intestine at neutral pH. There is a single nonenteric coated enzyme, Viokase. It is not suitable for ordinary management of children with CF. Only FDA-approved pancreatic enzymes are appropriate for children with CF. "Organic" or "natural" or generic enzyme preparations sold in supermarkets, online, and at "health food" stores are ineffective at preventing maldigestion and malnutrition in patients with pancreatic insufficiency and should not be used by children with CF.

The enteric-coated forms of pancreatic enzymes vary considerably in their biochemical coating, biophysical dissolution properties, and size of microspheres or microtablets.[32–34] There are few carefully performed clinical studies comparing the different formulations,[35] and few in vivo data are available that demonstrate the superiority of a single product. In fact, all currently available enzyme products fail to completely correct nutrient malabsorption in all patients with CF; fat absorption is estimated at 85% to 90% of that of children with normal pancreatic function.[23] The reasons are multiple, are likely to vary from patient to patient, and in some cases, may be attributable to factors unrelated to failed pancreatic digestion.[36] The enteric coating of enzyme microspheres or microtablets requires a pH >5.2 to 6.0 for dissolution to occur in the proximal intestine, and the intestinal milieu is acidic in the patient with CF because of loss of pancreatic bicarbonate secretion and impaired intestinal bicarbonate secretion.[24] Histamine (H_2) antagonists or proton-pump inhibitors may be used to suppress gastric acid production and increase intestinal pH, but there are no direct studies to confirm the effectiveness of this strategy to improve digestion.[37,38] Intestinal dysbiosis, dysmotility, and mucosal inflammation may also impair absorption.[39] Nevertheless, enzymes do improve nutrient digestion and absorption in patients with CF, but the caregiver must be aware of the less-than-ideal efficacy of these products in individual patients.

Dosing Guidelines

Dosing of PERT is based on consensus recommendations established by the CFF and the FDA.[8,29,30,40] These include: 500 to 2500 U of lipase/kg of body weight/meal OR 2000 to 4000 U of lipase/g of dietary fat/day AND a total of <10 000 U of lipase/kg/day. These guidelines were established when it was recognized that many CF centers were giving excessive doses of enzymes, which is strongly associated with a severe intestinal complication termed fibrosing colonopathy.[40] Total doses of PERT >10 000 lipase units/kg/day may occur for short periods in infants because of high caloric needs in the first months of life. No direct studies of this have been performed, but it has not appeared to be harmful over this limited period.[41]

Enzyme Administration

There are no convincing data concerning timing of enzyme dosing with meals, but for practical reasons, it is recommended that enzymes be taken in 2 to 3 divided doses before and during meals.[42] Theoretically, this will result in more even mixing and gastric emptying of enzymes, although this has not been clinically proven. Enzymes are not required with foods containing only simple carbohydrates (eg, hard candy, popsicles, fruit juice, carbonated beverages, gelatins) but are needed for foods containing fat, protein, and/or starch (rice, potatoes, etc).

Diet: Nutritional Requirements

Energy and Macronutrients

Patients with CF are at high risk of energy deficiency as a result of their increased requirement and decreased consumption. The consequence of energy deficiency leads to impaired growth in children with CF. Weight retardation and linear growth failure are particularly prevalent during times of rapid growth (ie, infancy and adolescence) as well as in patients before diagnosis of CF.[43,44]

Recommended energy intake for children with CF is from 110% to 120% of estimated intake for a similarly aged child without CF.[28] To obtain adequate energy intake and compensate for fat malabsorption, it is recommended that patients with CF increase their ingestion of fat from 30% to 35% to 40% of their total daily calories.[28] Because fat is the most energy-dense macronutrient, fat restriction is not recommended as a means to alleviate symptoms of malabsorption. Instead, a high-fat diet combined with adequate PERT should be prescribed. This diet is difficult for some children; studies show that most children with CF fail to achieve the recommended calorie intake.[45–47] Despite energy intake recommendations, the amount of energy a child with CF should ingest is the amount that leads to normal growth and achievement of goals of age-appropriate weight gain and height growth. Intake must be individualized to meet goals.

With regard to macronutrients, it was believed that protein digestion and absorption posed less of a problem than fat in the CF population. Although low concentrations of serum proteins (eg, albumin, prealbumin, and retinol-binding protein), are commonly found in infants at the time of diagnosis of CF, normalization of serum albumin concentration often occurs following comprehensive nutrition therapy.[48,49] Recent data have suggested that while most children with CF meet their target protein intake, energy intake from protein is a predictor of height for age z score.[47] Thus, focusing on adequate protein intake, particularly early in life, is important

Essential Fatty Acids

Although essential fatty acid deficiency (EFAD) occurs in children with CF with both PI and PS,[50,51] overt symptoms (alopecia, skin rashes, etc) are rare. Serum linoleic acid is a convenient biomarker for deficiency.[52] Recent studies demonstrated that achieving normal growth in the first 2 years of life depends not only on sufficient energy intake but also normal essential fatty acid status.[53] However, at present there is believed to be insufficient evidence to recommend supplementation of children with CF with essential fatty acids unless it is the suspected cause of growth failure.[7,8]

Vitamin and Mineral Supplementation

Fat-Soluble Vitamins

Deficiencies of fat-soluble vitamins in untreated CF are common.[54,55] As many as 45% of children with CF may have one or more fat-soluble vitamin deficiency, most commonly vitamin D.[55] These deficiencies have clinical consequences. Vitamin D insufficiency is directly linked to poor bone mineralization.[56] Vitamin E deficiency can lead to hemolytic anemia.[57] In addition, early, prolonged vitamin E deficiency has been shown to be associated with cognitive dysfunction later in life.[58]

The CFF recommends monitoring of fat-soluble vitamins (serum vitamin A, E, and D and international normalized ratio [INR] as a surrogate for vitamin K) (Table 46.1). Vitamin supplementation is necessary to treat and

Table 46.1.
Vitamin Supplementation Guidelines for Pancreatic-Insufficient Children With CF

Vitamin	Supplementation[a]
Vitamin A	Retinol: Infants 1500 IU/d Children and adolescents 5000–10 000 IU/d
Vitamin D	D3 (cholecalciferol) : Infants 400–500 IU/d, increased to achieve levels of at least 30 ng/mL with a maximum of 800–1000 IU/d Children and adolescents: 800–1000 IU/d, increased to achieve levels of at least 30 ng/mL with a maximum of 2000 IU/d
Vitamin E (tocopherols)	A-tocopherol : Infant–1 year 50 IU/day >1 year 100–400 IU/day
Vitamin K	Infants 0.3–1.0 mg/day Older children 1–10 mg/day
Vitamin B$_{12}$[b]	100 μg/month, intramuscularly

[a] In all cases, initiate supplementation and monitor levels to allow appropriate dose modification to achieve normal levels. Infants should have levels measured 2 months after initiating supplementation. For all others, monitor vitamin A, E, D, and international normalized ratio (INR) annually and 3–6 months after a dosing change.

[b] Monitor yearly after ileal resection and initiate supplementation when deficiency detected.

Sources: Cystic Fibrosis Foundation, Turck et al, and Tangpricha et al.[7,31,56]

prevent deficiencies. Even children with normal fat-soluble vitamin concentrations and/or those with PS are recommended to start supplementation at the time of diagnosis. This is most commonly accomplished using an age-appropriate dose of a water-miscible form of the fat soluble vitamins (eg, AquaDEKs, MVW Complete, etc). Deficiencies found at monitoring should be corrected. As a general rule, children with CF do not have deficiencies of water-soluble vitamins, but most water-miscible forms of fat-soluble vitamins also contain variable amounts of water-soluble vitamins.

Minerals and Electrolytes

For patients with CF, sodium is of great concern, because they lose large amounts of sodium in their sweat; marginal or low body sodium may limit the growth of children with CF.[59] The CFF recommends infants with CF should receive salt supplementation. Current guidelines recommend a daily dose of ⅛ teaspoon of table salt, which contains 12.5 mEq of sodium, for infants younger than 6 months.[8] For infants 6 to 12 months of age, ¼ teaspoon per day, but not to exceed 4 mEq/kg/day, is recommended.[8] In older children and adolescents with CF, it is recommended to add additional salt at meals and snacks, particularly during warmer weather.[29,30]

Studies with stable isotopes have reported increased fecal zinc losses and decreased zinc absorption in infants and children with CF.[60,61] Zinc deficiency affects growth and vitamin A status but is difficult to diagnose, because serum zinc concentration is not an adequate measure of zinc status. Therefore, current CFF guidelines recommend a trial of zinc supplementation, 1 mg/kg/day of elemental zinc for 6 months, for children with CF experiencing poor growth despite adequate caloric intake and pancreatic enzyme supplementation.[8]

Anemia in patients with CF has been reported with varying prevalence as high as 33%, with iron deficiency proposed to be the main cause.[62] Current CFF recommendations are for yearly monitoring of hemoglobin and hematocrit.[28]

Nutritional Assessment and Monitoring

Frequent assessment and monitoring of nutritional status for patients with CF is essential to ensure early detection of any deterioration and prompt initiation of intervention. This comprehensive assessment is generally performed by the CF dietitian in the CF center. Assessment of nutritional status for children with CF must include anthropometric, biochemical, clinical, and dietary assessments. Current recommendations for these assessments are summarized in the CFF guidelines.[8,29,30]

Anthropometric Assessment

Anthropometric assessment, with an emphasis on physical growth, is the most important component of nutritional assessment in children with CF. Accurate and sequential measurements of head circumference (0–3 years), recumbent length (0–2 years), height (2–20 years), weight (0–20 years), weight for length (0–2 years), and BMI (2–20 years) should be obtained at each clinic visit using standardized techniques. These measurements should be plotted on the 2000 CDC growth charts and/or the 2009 World Health Organization growth charts (0–2 years) to determine sex- and age-specific percentiles (see Appendix Q).

In addition to weight and length/height percentiles, weight gain velocity and length/height velocity are more sensitive indicators of growth and should be evaluated when growth faltering is observed.[8,28,30] Other anthropometric assessments, such as measurements of skinfold thickness (eg, mid-upper arm circumference, triceps skinfold thickness, etc), provide additional information on body composition (ie, lean body mass and subcutaneous fat stores). However, skinfold thickness measurements are prone to measurement errors, and reference standards are not available for all ages of children (see Chapter 24, Table 24.3).

Biochemical Assessment

Monitoring biochemical indices of nutritional status was described earlier in the chapter. Briefly, current guidelines recommend yearly measurements of serum protein (albumin), vitamin A (retinol), vitamin D (25-OH-D), and vitamin E (alpha-tocopherol) concentrations, and measurement of hemoglobin and hematocrit to detect anemia[8,28,30] (see Chapter 24, Table 24.5).

Clinical Assessment

Clinical assessment of nutritional status in children with CF focuses on evaluation of the severity of maldigestion and malabsorption caused by PI. The clinical signs and symptoms of PI include abdominal discomfort (bloating, flatus, pain) and steatorrhea (frequent, malodorous, greasy stools), although some children with PI have no symptoms. Attention should be paid to confounders of nutrition, including previous intestinal resection (note that even small intestinal resections confound good nutrition in CF), gastrointestinal tract symptoms, liver disease, cystic fibrosis-related diabetes mellitus, and frequent pulmonary exacerbations. The psychosocial environment of the child is crucially important to the achievement of nutritional goals and should be assessed at each visit.

Dietary Assessment

Assessments of energy requirements and dietary intake are important ways of determining whether the patient is in negative energy balance. Evaluation of dietary intake is best performed by dietitians specializing in the care of patients with CF. For patients with good nutritional status, the dietitian may assess dietary habits and the quality of dietary intake using a 24-hour dietary recall. However, for patients with suboptimal nutritional status, a 3- to 7-day prospective food record is the best way to obtain quantitative estimates of energy and nutrient intakes. This assessment can then be used as the basis for initiating appropriate nutritional intervention.

Patient and Parent Education

Education of patients and their caregivers is a vital and routine component of the multidisciplinary care of patients with CF. A solid grounding in the special nutritional needs of a patient with CF should be established at diagnosis. This should include an explanation of the role of the pancreas and how enzyme replacement therapy helps to improve maldigestion. Parents should be given specific instructions on how to provide an appetizing, high-energy, nutritionally balanced diet, particularly with a liberal use of fat to provide extra calories. It is important to communicate the expectation that most children with CF are able to grow and gain weight normally. Patients and their parents require education about the importance of fat-soluble vitamins. Details on when to administer enzymes and vitamins must be reviewed on several occasions. For older children, the pediatrician should ensure that there is adequate understanding of the nature of the disease process, and concerns about adherence should be emphasized and assessed at each follow-up visit.

Age-Specific Guidelines for Nutritional Management

Infants and Young Children (Through 2 Years of Age) With CF

Initial Visits and Coordination With Primary Care Physician

The majority of young infants with CF diagnosed through newborn screening appear to be totally healthy to the parents, and the diagnosis of CF is largely unexpected. Therefore, the psychosocial impact on the family must be carefully addressed at the initial visits.[8] Infants with newly diagnosed CF should be seen at an accredited CF center, ideally within 24 to 72 hours of diagnosis; however, they are usually seen by their primary care provider for referral. Thus, although the CF center may ultimately provide diagnosis and comprehensive education and counseling, the initial disbelief, anger, and anxiety about the new diagnosis may fall on the primary care physician. Parents may also express these emotions in subsequent routine primary care visits, so primary care physicians should familiarize themselves with some of the recommendations for care of an infant with CF. Basic information should be provided in the clearest of terms, and information should be conveyed in a sensitive, empathetic, and positive manner. A variety of formats should be used to provide information, including verbal, written, and audiovisual. Information should be repeated or understanding should be assessed at subsequent visits.

The pivotal role that both parents and primary care provider play as part of the CF team should be emphasized at the early visits.[8] Coordination between the primary care physician and the CF center is essential, because families will be making numerous visits to their primary care provider and CF center during the first 2 years of life. Therefore, regular and open trilateral communications among the family, the primary care physician, and the CF center should be established. Communication between the primary care physician and the CF center is critical to ensure that parents do not get conflicting messages, because many CF care goals are different from those of standard pediatric care (eg, an emphasis on the need for the CF child to be "chubby" versus concerns about obesity in the general pediatric population).

Types of Feeding

Special attention to growth and nutrition early in life is essential, because it is a time of extraordinary growth. The first months of life represent a unique window of opportunity to promote optimal growth, whereas poor growth during this critical period may be irreversible.[14] The CFF recommends that children reach a weight-for-length status of the 50th percentile by 2 years of age, with an emphasis on achieving this goal early in infancy.[8,29] However, optimal nutritional care to achieve this goal has not been defined.

HUMAN MILK VERSUS INFANT FORMULA

The basic principles of infant feeding for healthy term infants apply to feeding infants with CF. However, optimal feeding (ie, human milk, infant formula, or combination) to meet the increased nutritional requirement for infants with CF is unknown. The most recent 2009 CFF infant care guidelines[8,29] recommend human milk as the initial type of feeding for infants with CF on the basis of studies demonstrating equivalent growth between breastfed and formula fed infants with CF.[63-66] A study from Wisconsin revealed that exclusive breastfeeding for less than 2 months was associated

VI

with adequate growth and protected against *Pseudomonas aeruginosa* infections during the first 2 years of life.[66] On the other hand, exclusive breast-feeding longer than 2 months was associated with attenuated growth without additional reduction in respiratory infections. Attention to weight gain is important in the first months of life, regardless of feeding type, to ensure appropriate growth. More studies are needed to evaluate the long-term risks on growth faltering associated with prolonged exclusive breastfeeding in patients with cystic fibrosis, including potential benefits of human milk fortification.

STANDARD FORMULA VERSUS SPECIAL FORMULA

There is limited evidence to address whether formula-fed infants with CF and PI should consume special formula (eg, predigested formula containing protein hydrolysates and/or MCTs). Similar nutritional status was found between infants with CF fed hydrolyzed and standard formulas in 1 study,[67] while another showed better anthropometric measures in infants fed hydrolysate-based formulas.[68] The CFF concluded that there was insufficient evidence to recommend a special formula for formula-fed infants with CF.[8] It should be noted that the presence of confounding factors, such as intestinal resection in infancy, may affect formula recommendations.

It is also unclear whether human milk and standard formula should be fortified routinely to increase caloric and nutrient densities for feeding infants with CF who are growing adequately, for the purpose of sustaining normal growth or preventing growth faltering. This is a nutritional issue recommended by the CFF for research.[8]

COMPLEMENTARY FOODS

Infants with CF should be introduced to complementary solid foods at the same age as healthy infants (ie, at about 6 months of life or when developmentally ready), according to recommendations from the American Academy of Pediatrics. Nutrient- and calorie-dense foods, such as meat, that will enhance weight gain and provide a good source of iron and zinc,[69] are ideal as first foods for infants with CF. Human milk or formula should continue to be fed through the first year of life. Thereafter, in a thriving child, whole cow milk is recommended, to maximize calorie intake.

As infants are introduced to table foods, it is important that families and primary care physicians understand that most children with CF need a balanced diet that is moderately high in fat to meet their nutritional requirement, which is different from the usual nutritional education given to families with healthy children for overweight and obesity prevention. For example, families should buy whole milk for the child with CF and lower-fat milk for other children. During the second year of life, children establish self-feeding skills, food preferences, and dietary habits. Dietitians caring for children with CF should inquire about feeding behaviors to promote positive interactions and to prevent negative behaviors.

Enzyme Dose and Administration

PERT should be given with human milk and formulas, including elemental and MCT-containing formulas, and all foods. An initial dose of 2000 to 4000 U of lipase for each 120-mL feeding is recommended.[8] As the infant grows and the volume of intake increases, the dose is adjusted to up to 2500 U lipase/kg/feeding, not to exceed a maximal daily dose of 10 000 U lipase/kg/day.[8] Enzyme dose in relation to calorie/fat intake and weight gain should be evaluated at each visit. The goal is to prescribe enzyme doses that are sufficient but not excessive to support optimal weight gain while minimizing the risk of fibrosing colonopathy. Nevertheless, caution to avoid fibrosing colonopathy may lead to excessive conservatism in enzyme dosing, and brief periods of enzyme dosing slightly above the recommended levels may occur in early infancy.[41]

In infants with CF, PERT should be offered before feeding, mixed with 2 to 3 mL (½ teaspoon) applesauce, and given by spoon.[8] Other strained fruit can be tried if applesauce is not accepted, but parents should be encouraged to use only one type of food to avoid problems with potential food refusal if many different types of food are used as the vehicle for enzyme delivery.

After 1 year of age, children can be offered enteric-coated products, mixed with 1 type of food. Swallowing of capsules is encouraged as soon as parents consider the child is ready. This varies considerably from patient to patient but occurs usually around 4 to 5 years of age. If children continue to experience difficulties swallowing capsules, parents should open the capsule and sprinkle the beads in the mouth to be ingested by drinking a liquid. Children should be discouraged from chewing the capsules, as this will destroy the protective coating of the enzymes within.

Nutrient Supplementation

All infants with CF should receive standard, age-appropriate water-soluble vitamins plus fat-soluble vitamins A, D, E, and K, as recommended by the CFF guidelines. Because of increased risk of hyponatremia, sodium supplementation is especially important for infants with CF, particularly in those fed human milk, which contains very low amount of sodium. Older infants receiving solid foods are also likely to have low sodium intake, because

VI

infant foods contain no added salt. Infants younger than 6 months with CF should receive a daily dose of 1/8 teaspoon of table salt; this amount should be increased to ¼ teaspoon for infants 6 to 12 months of age.[8]

Young Children With CF (Age 2–5 Years)

The CFF has published guidelines for the management of children 2 to 5 years of age with CF.[30] Critical issues include appropriate development of normal feeding behaviors and early intervention for children not achieving goals of weight and height.

Children in this age group are developing food preferences and dietary habits. Food intake and physical activity vary from day to day. For these reasons, close monitoring of dietary habits, energy intake, and growth are important. Routinely adding calories to table foods may help with maintaining optimal growth at this stage. The importance of serving calorie-dense foods (such as providing whole milk and avoiding low-fat foods) should be emphasized.

Studies have demonstrated that toddlers with CF have longer meal times than do their peers without CF, yet still do not meet the CFF's dietary recommendations for increased energy intake.[70] As the duration of meal times increases, challenging behaviors also occur more frequently.[71] Therefore, dietary counseling should include assessment of eating behaviors. One strategy to address behavioral problems is to limit mealtimes to 15 minutes for toddlers and use snack times as mini-meals. Another strategy is to teach parents alternative ways of responding to their child who eats slowly or negotiates what he or she will eat. The importance of establishing positive mealtime interactions should be emphasized.

School Age (5–10 Years)

Children in this age group are at risk of declining growth for various reasons. They typically participate in a variety of activities, leading to limited time for meals and snacks. They also begin to be exposed to peer pressure and may begin self-managing their disease. These life changes may affect compliance with prescribed therapies, such as pancreatic enzymes and fat-soluble vitamins. In addition, acceptance and understanding by teachers and fellow students may be lacking, further compounding stress for a child with CF. Encouraging children to help in meal planning and preparation maybe helpful in improving food intake.

Preadolescence and Adolescence (10–18 Years)

This stage represents another vulnerable period for developing malnutrition because of increased nutritional requirements associated with accelerated growth, puberty, and high levels of physical activity. In addition, pulmonary disease often becomes more severe in this period, increasing energy requirement. This is also the age when other complications, such as CF-related diabetes mellitus (see comorbid conditions below), begin to occur more frequently, which further increases the risk of poor growth and malnutrition.

Puberty is often delayed in adolescents with CF. It usually is related to growth failure and poor nutritional status rather than to a primary endocrine disorder. Assessment of puberty should be performed annually beginning at 9 years of age in girls and 10 years of age in boys (see Chapter 8). Nutritional counseling should be directed toward the patient rather than the parents. Teenagers may be more receptive to efforts to improve muscular strength and body image as a justification for better nutrition than emphasis on weight gain and improved disease status.

Overweight and Obesity in Children With CF

Several centers report an increase in children with CF who have overweight or obesity. In 1 center, the prevalence increased from 7% in 1985 to 18% in 2011.[72] In general, children with CF who are overweight or obese have milder CFTR mutations and often have PS. Although there is a small benefit to increased BMI with respect to pulmonary function,[72,73] recent data suggest that obese individuals with CF are at risk for dyslipidemia.[74] Although rapid weight loss diets are not recommended in CF, appropriate intervention in these individuals has not been determined.

Nutrition Intervention for Poor Growth and Malnutrition

If poor weight gain is observed or the child is failing to exhibit catch-up growth, careful assessment of energy intake and malabsorption is needed. Careful assessment for underlying pulmonary exacerbation also should be conducted, because inadequate control of respiratory infections is still a common basis of growth faltering. In addition, evaluation of confounders of nutrition in CF[36] (gastrointestinal disease,[22] liver disease,[75] psychosocial problems,[76,77] or cystic fibrosis-related diabetes[25]) should be considered. It is beyond the scope of this chapter to review each of these issues. In general, because of the profound implications of prolonged poor growth in CF, children should be referred to their CF center or to the appropriate specialist with knowledge of CF as soon as weight faltering is noticed.

Dietary Interventions

Oral Supplementation

For infants experiencing inadequate weight gain, increasing caloric density of the feedings is the first step. This can be achieved by fortifying human milk or by concentrating formula. For infants who are eating solids, additional calories can be added to infant cereal with the addition of carbohydrate polymers (eg, Polycose) and/or fats (eg, vegetable oil, MCT oil, or Microlipid).

Dietary modification should begin by adding high-calorie foods to the child's regular diet without dramatically increasing the amount of food consumed. For example, margarine or butter may be added to many foods, and half and half can be used in place of milk or water when preparing canned soup. If dietary modification is ineffective, use of an energy supplement may be introduced. However, it is important to ensure that the energy supplement is not used as a substitute for normal food intake.

Enteral Feedings

For children with growth deficits that do not improve with oral supplementation, enteral feeding should be initiated. The CFF has published guidelines on the use of enteral feedings in people with CF.[78] The goals of enteral feeding should be explained to the patient and family (ie, as a supportive therapy to improve quality of life and outcome), and their acceptance and commitment to this intervention should be realistically assessed.

Enteral feeding can be delivered via nasogastric tubes, gastrostomy tubes, or jejunostomy tubes. The choice of feeding tube and technique for its placement should be based on the expertise of the CF center. Nasogastric tubes are appropriate for short-term nutritional support in highly motivated patients. Gastrostomy tubes are more appropriate for patients who need long-term enteral nutrition. Jejunostomy tubes may be indicated in patients with severe gastroesophageal reflux; use of predigested or elemental formula may be needed with jejunostomy feeding.

Standard enteral feeding formulas (complete protein, long-chain fat) are typically well tolerated.[78] Calorically dense formulas (1.5–2.0 kcal/mL) are usually required to provide adequate energy. Nocturnal infusion is encouraged to promote normal eating patterns during the day. Initially, 30% to 50% of estimated energy requirement may be provided overnight. Pancreatic enzymes should be given with enteral feedings; however, the optimal dosing regimen is unclear with overnight feeding.

Behavioral Intervention

To increase dietary intakes, caregivers of young children with CF may engage in ineffective feeding practices, such as coaxing, commanding, physical prompts, and parental feeding. Adolescents with CF may intentionally skip pancreatic enzymes to achieve a certain body image. An in-depth assessment of eating behavior, feeding patterns, and family interactions at mealtimes should be performed in patients with CF at risk of experiencing malnutrition. If negative behaviors are present, behavioral intervention should be used in conjunction with dietary intervention to improve intake. Behavioral modification techniques have demonstrated significant and prolonged improvement in nutritional intake and weight gain in toddlers with CF.[79] Referral for more in-depth behavioral therapy is also encouraged.

Conclusions

The clear associations between nutritional status and clinical outcomes in CF mandate careful nutritional assessment, management, and monitoring of all patients with CF. In recent years, with new knowledge arising from newborn screening research, there has been a shift away from the idea that malnutrition is inevitable for most patients with CF toward the more optimistic view that normal nutrition and growth are possible if early diagnosis and aggressive nutritional monitoring and therapy are accomplished for each patient. This task is best accomplished by involving a multidisciplinary team that includes the primary care physician in the care and management of patients with CF. In this way, the goals of normal growth and prevention of malnutrition can be attained, which will improve the prognosis and quality of life for patients with CF.

References

1. Kerem B, Rommens JM, Buchanan JA, et al. Identification of the cystic fibrosis gene: genetic analysis. *Science*. 1989;245(4922):1073–1080
2. Kerem E, Corey M, Kerem BS, et al. The relation between genotype and phenotype in cystic fibrosis—analysis of the most common mutation (delta F508). *N Engl J Med*. 1990;323(22):1517–1522

3. Farrell PM, White TB, Ren CL, et al. Diagnosis of cystic fibrosis: consensus guidelines from the Cystic Fibrosis Foundation. *J Pediatr.* 2017;181S:S4–S15 e11

4. Castellani C, Cuppens H, Macek M, Jr., et al. Consensus on the use and interpretation of cystic fibrosis mutation analysis in clinical practice. *J Cyst Fibros.* 2008;7(3):179–196

5. Kristidis P, Bozon D, Corey M, et al. Genetic determination of exocrine pancreatic function in cystic fibrosis. *Am J Hum Genet.* 1992;50(6):1178–1184

6. Sosnay PR, Raraigh KS, Gibson RL. Molecular genetics of cystic fibrosis transmembrane conductance regulator: genotype and phenotype. *Pediatr Clin North Am.* 2016;63(4):585–598

7. Cystic Fibrosis Foundation, Borowitz D, Parad RB, et al. Cystic Fibrosis Foundation practice guidelines for the management of infants with cystic fibrosis transmembrane conductance regulator-related metabolic syndrome during the first two years of life and beyond. *J Pediatr.* 2009;155(6 Suppl):S106–116

8. Cystic Fibrosis Foundation, Borowitz D, Robinson KA, et al. Cystic Fibrosis Foundation evidence-based guidelines for management of infants with cystic fibrosis. *J Pediatr.* 2009;155(6 Suppl):S73–93

9. Li Z, Kosorok MR, Farrell PM, et al. Longitudinal development of mucoid Pseudomonas aeruginosa infection and lung disease progression in children with cystic fibrosis. *JAMA.* 2005;293(5):581–588

10. Carlyle BE, Borowitz DS, Glick PL. A review of pathophysiology and management of fetuses and neonates with meconium ileus for the pediatric surgeon. *J Pediatr Surg.* 2012;47(4):772–781

11. Doulgeraki A, Petrocheilou A, Petrocheilou G, Chrousos G, Doudounakis SE, Kaditis AG. Body composition and lung function in children with cystic fibrosis and meconium ileus. *Eur J Pediatr.* 2017;176(6):737–743

12. Lai HC, Kosorok MR, Laxova A, Davis LA, FitzSimmon SC, Farrell PM. Nutritional status of patients with cystic fibrosis with meconium ileus: a comparison with patients without meconium ileus and diagnosed early through neonatal screening. *Pediatrics.* 2000;105(1 Pt 1):53–61

13. Yen EH, Quinton H, Borowitz D. Better nutritional status in early childhood is associated with improved clinical outcomes and survival in patients with cystic fibrosis. *J Pediatr.* 2013;162(3):530–535 e531

14. Lai HJ, Shoff SM, Farrell PM, Wisconsin Cystic Fibrosis Neonatal Screening G. Recovery of birth weight z score within 2 years of diagnosis is positively associated with pulmonary status at 6 years of age in children with cystic fibrosis. *Pediatrics.* 2009;123(2):714–722

15. Sanders DB, Fink A, Mayer-Hamblett N, et al. Early life growth trajectories in cystic fibrosis are associated with pulmonary function at age 6 years. *J Pediatr.* 2015;167(5):1081–1088 e1081

16. Davies PSW, Erskine JM, Hambidge KM, Accurso FJ. Longitudinal investigation of energy expenditure in infants with cystic fibrosis. *Eur J Clin Nutr.* 2002;56(10): 940–946

17. Moudiou T, Galli-Tsinopoulou A, Vamvakoudis E, Nousia-Arvanitakis S. Resting energy expenditure in cystic fibrosis as an indicator of disease severity. *J Cyst Fibros.* 2007;6(2):131–136

18. Thomson MA, Wilmott RW, Wainwright C, Masters B, Francis PJ, Shepherd RW. Resting energy expenditure, pulmonary inflammation, and genotype in the early course of cystic fibrosis. *J Pediatr.* 1996;129(3):367–373

19. Munck A. Cystic fibrosis: evidence for gut inflammation. *Int J Biochem Cell Biol.* 2014;52:180–183

20. Nichols DP, Chmiel JF. Inflammation and its genesis in cystic fibrosis. *Pediatr Pulmonol.* 2015;50 Suppl 40:S39–56

21. Lindig J, Steger C, Beiersdorf N, et al. Smell in cystic fibrosis. *Eur Arch Otorhinolaryngol.* 2013;270(3):915–921

22. Gelfond D, Borowitz D. Gastrointestinal complications of cystic fibrosis. *Clin Gastroenterol Hepatol.* 2013;11(4):333–342

23. Wouthuyzen-Bakker M, Bodewes FAJA, Verkade HJ. Persistent fat malabsorption in cystic fibrosis; lessons from patients and mice. *J Cyst Fibros.* 2011;10(3):150–158

24. Gelfond D, Ma C, Semler J, Borowitz D. Intestinal pH and gastrointestinal transit profiles in cystic fibrosis patients measured by wireless motility capsule. *Dig Dis Sci.* 2013;58(8):2275–2281

25. Moran A, Brunzell C, Cohen RC, et al. Clinical care guidelines for cystic fibrosis-related diabetes: a position statement of the American Diabetes Association and a clinical practice guideline of the Cystic Fibrosis Foundation, endorsed by the Pediatric Endocrine Society. *Diabetes Care.* 2010;33(12):2697–2708

26. Mogayzel PJ, Jr., Naureckas ET, Robinson KA, et al. Cystic Fibrosis Foundation pulmonary guideline. pharmacologic approaches to prevention and eradication of initial *Pseudomonas aeruginosa* infection. *Ann Am Thorac Soc.* 2014;11(10): 1640–1650

27. Ramsey BW, Farrell PM, Pencharz P. Nutritional assessment and management in cystic fibrosis: a consensus report. The Consensus Committee. *Am J Clin Nutr.* 1992;55(1):108–116

28. Borowitz D, Baker RD, Stallings V. Consensus report on nutrition for pediatric patients with cystic fibrosis. *J Pediatr Gastroenterol Nutr.* 2002;35(3):246–259

29. Stallings VA, Stark LJ, Robinson KA, et al. Evidence-based practice recommendations for nutrition-related management of children and adults with cystic fibrosis and pancreatic insufficiency: results of a systematic review. *J Am Diet Assoc.* 2008;108(5):832–839

30. Lahiri T, Hempstead SE, Brady C, et al. Clinical practice guidelines from the Cystic Fibrosis Foundation for preschoolers with cystic fibrosis. *Pediatrics.* 2016;137(4):e2015178

31. Turck D, Braegger CP, Colombo C, et al. ESPEN-ESPGHAN-ECFS guidelines on nutrition care for infants, children, and adults with cystic fibrosis. *Clin Nutr.* 2016;35(3):557–577

VI

32. Carroccio A, Pardo F, Montalto G, et al. Effectiveness of enteric-coated preparations on nutritional parameters in cystic fibrosis. A long-term study. *Digestion.* 1988;41(4):201–206

33. Durie P, Kalnins D, Ellis L. Uses and abuses of enzyme therapy in cystic fibrosis. *J R Soc Med.* 1998;91 Suppl 34:2–13

34. Somaraju UR, Solis-Moya A. Pancreatic enzyme replacement therapy for people with cystic fibrosis. *Cochrane Database Syst Rev.* 2016;(11):CD008227

35. Taylor CJ, Thieroff-Ekerdt R, Shiff S, Magnus L, Fleming R, Gommoll C. Comparison of two pancreatic enzyme products for exocrine insufficiency in patients with cystic fibrosis. *J Cyst Fibros.* 2016;15(5):675-680

36. Borowitz D, Durie PR, Clarke LL, et al. Gastrointestinal outcomes and confounders in cystic fibrosis. *J Pediatr Gastroenterol Nutr.* 2005;41(3):273–285

37. Heijerman HG, Lamers CB, Bakker W. Omeprazole enhances the efficacy of pancreatin (pancrease) in cystic fibrosis. *Ann Intern Med.* 1991;114(3):200–201

38. Sander-Struckmeier S, Beckmann K, Janssen-van Solingen G, Pollack P. Retrospective analysis to investigate the effect of concomitant use of gastric acid-suppressing drugs on the efficacy and safety of pancrelipase/pancreatin (CREON®) in patients with pancreatic exocrine insufficiency. *Pancreas.* 2013;42(6):983-989

39. De Lisle RC, Borowitz D. The Cystic fibrosis intestine. *Cold Spring Harb Perspect Med.* 2013;3(9):a009753

40. Borowitz DS, Grand RJ, Durie PR. Use of pancreatic enzyme supplements for patients with cystic fibrosis in the context of fibrosing colonopathy. Consensus Committee. *J Pediatr.* 1995;127(5):681–684

41. Borowitz D, Gelfond D, Maguiness K, Heubi JE, Ramsey B. Maximal daily dose of pancreatic enzyme replacement therapy in infants with cystic fibrosis: a reconsideration. *J Cyst Fibros.* 2013;12(6):784–785

42. Brady MS, Rickard K, Yu PL, Eigen H. Effectiveness of enteric coated pancreatic enzymes given before meals in reducing steatorrhea in children with cystic fibrosis. *J Am Diet Assoc.* 1992;92(7):813–817

43. Lai HC, Corey M, FitzSimmons S, Kosorok MR, Farrell PM. Comparison of growth status of patients with cystic fibrosis between the United States and Canada. *Am J Clin Nutr.* 1999;69(3):531–538

44. Lai HC, Kosorok MR, Sondel SA, et al. Growth status in children with cystic fibrosis based on the National Cystic Fibrosis Patient Registry data: evaluation of various criteria used to identify malnutrition. *J Pediatr.* 1998;132(3 Pt 1): 478–485

45. White H, Morton AM, Peckham DG, Conway SP. Dietary intakes in adult patients with cystic fibrosis—do they achieve guidelines? *J Cyst Fibros.* 2004;3(1):1–7

46. Woestenenk JW, Castelijns SJ, van der Ent CK, Houwen RH. Dietary intake in children and adolescents with cystic fibrosis. *Clin Nutr.* 2014;33(3):528–532

47. Filigno SS, Robson SM, Szczesniak RD, et al. Macronutrient intake in preschoolers with cystic fibrosis and the relationship between macronutrients and growth. *J Cyst Fibros.* 2017;16(4):519-524

48. Benabdeslam H, Garcia I, Bellon G, Gilly R, Revol A. Biochemical assessment of the nutritional status of cystic fibrosis patients treated with pancreatic enzyme extracts. *Am J Clin Nutr.* 1998;67(5):912–918

49. Marcus MS, Sondel SA, Farrell PM, et al. Nutritional status of infants with cystic fibrosis associated with early diagnosis and intervention. *Am J Clin Nutr.* 1991;54(3):578–585

50. Christophe AB, Warwick WJ, Holman RT. Serum fatty acid profiles in cystic fibrosis patients and their parents. *Lipids.* 1994;29(8):569–575

51. Strandvik B. Fatty acid metabolism in cystic fibrosis. *Prostaglandins Leukot Essent Fatty Acids.* 2010;83(3):121–129

52. Maqbool A, Schall JI, Garcia-Espana JF, Zemel BS, Strandvik B, Stallings VA. Serum linoleic acid status as a clinical indicator of essential fatty acid status in children with cystic fibrosis. *J Pediatr Gastroenterol Nutr.* 2008;47(5):635–644

53. Shoff SM, Ahn HY, Davis L, Lai H, Wisconsin CFNSG. Temporal associations among energy intake, plasma linoleic acid, and growth improvement in response to treatment initiation after diagnosis of cystic fibrosis. *Pediatrics.* 2006;117(2):391–400

54. Feranchak AP, Sontag MK, Wagener JS, Hammond KB, Accurso FJ, Sokol RJ. Prospective, long-term study of fat-soluble vitamin status in children with cystic fibrosis identified by newborn screen. *J Pediatr.* 1999;135(5):601–610

55. Rana M, Wong-See D, Katz T, et al. Fat-soluble vitamin deficiency in children and adolescents with cystic fibrosis. *J Clin Pathol.* 2014;67(7):605–608

56. Tangpricha V, Kelly A, Stephenson A, et al. An update on the screening, diagnosis, management, and treatment of vitamin D deficiency in individuals with cystic fibrosis: evidence-based recommendations from the Cystic Fibrosis Foundation. *J Clin Endocrinol Metab.* 2012;97(4):1082–1093

57. Wilfond BS, Farrell PM, Laxova A, Mischler E. Severe hemolytic anemia associated with vitamin E deficiency in infants with cystic fibrosis. Implications for neonatal screening. *Clin Pediatr (Phila).* 1994;33(1):2–7

58. Koscik RL, Farrell PM, Kosorok MR, et al. Cognitive function of children with cystic fibrosis: deleterious effect of early malnutrition. *Pediatrics.* 2004;113(6):1549–1558

59. Ozcelik U, Gocmen A, Kiper N, Coskun T, Yilmaz E, Ozguc M. Sodium chloride deficiency in cystic fibrosis patients. *Eur J Pediatr.* 1994;153(11):829–831

60. Krebs NF, Sontag M, Accurso FJ, Hambidge KM. Low plasma zinc concentrations in young infants with cystic fibrosis. *J Pediatr.* 1998;133(6):761–764

61. Krebs NF, Westcott JE, Arnold TD, et al. Abnormalities in zinc homeostasis in young infants with cystic fibrosis. *Pediatr Res.* 2000;48(2):256–261

VI

62. von Drygalski A, Biller J. Anemia in cystic fibrosis: incidence, mechanisms, and association with pulmonary function and vitamin deficiency. *Nutr Clin Pract.* 2008;23(5):557–563

63. Bronstein MN, Sokol RJ, Abman SH, et al. Pancreatic insufficiency, growth, and nutrition in infants identified by newborn screening as having cystic fibrosis. *J Pediatr.* 1992;120(4 Pt 1):533–540

64. Colombo C, Costantini D, Zazzeron L, et al. Benefits of breastfeeding in cystic fibrosis: a single-centre follow-up survey. *Acta Paediatr.* 2007;96(8):1228–1232

65. Parker EM, O'Sullivan BP, Shea JC, Regan MM, Freedman SD. Survey of breast-feeding practices and outcomes in the cystic fibrosis population. *Pediatr Pulmonol.* 2004;37(4):362–367

66. Jadin SA, Wu GS, Zhang Z, et al. Growth and pulmonary outcomes during the first 2 y of life of breastfed and formula-fed infants diagnosed with cystic fibrosis through the Wisconsin Routine Newborn Screening Program. *Am J Clin Nutr.* 2011;93(5):1038–1047

67. Ellis L, Kalnins D, Corey M, Brennan J, Pencharz P, Durie P. Do infants with cystic fibrosis need a protein hydrolysate formula? A prospective, randomized, comparative study. *J Pediatr.* 1998;132(2):270–276

68. Farrell PM, Mischler EH, Sondel SA, Palta M. Predigested formula for infants with cystic fibrosis. *J Am Diet Assoc.* 1987;87(10):1353–1356

69. Baker RD, Greer FR, Committee on Nutrition American Academy of P. Diagnosis and prevention of iron deficiency and iron-deficiency anemia in infants and young children (0-3 years of age). *Pediatrics.* 2010;126(5):1040–1050

70. Powers SW, Patton SR, Byars KC, et al. Caloric intake and eating behavior in infants and toddlers with cystic fibrosis. *Pediatrics.* 2002;109(5):E75–75

71. Stark LJ, Opipari-Arrigan L, Quittner AL, Bean J, Powers SW. The effects of an intensive behavior and nutrition intervention compared to standard of care on weight outcomes in CF. *Pediatr Pulmonol.* 2011;46(1):31–35

72. Stephenson AL, Mannik LA, Walsh S, et al. Longitudinal trends in nutritional status and the relation between lung function and BMI in cystic fibrosis: a population-based cohort study. *Am J Clin Nutr.* 2013;97(4):872–877

73. Kastner-Cole D, Palmer CN, Ogston SA, Mehta A, Mukhopadhyay S. Overweight and obesity in deltaF508 homozygous cystic fibrosis. *J Pediatr.* 2005;147(3):402–404

74. Rhodes B, Nash EF, Tullis E, et al. Prevalence of dyslipidemia in adults with cystic fibrosis. *J Cyst Fibros.* 2010;9(1):24–28

75. Flass T, Narkewicz MR. Cirrhosis and other liver disease in cystic fibrosis. *J Cyst Fibros.* 2013;12(2):116-124

76. Barker DH, Quittner AL. Parental depression and pancreatic enzymes adherence in children with cystic fibrosis. *Pediatrics.* 2016;137(2):e20152296

77. Quittner AL, Saez-Flores E, Barton JD. The psychological burden of cystic fibrosis. *Curr Opin Pulm Med.* 2016;22(2):187–191

78. Schwarzenberg SJ, Hempstead SE, McDonald CM, et al. Enteral tube feeding for individuals with cystic fibrosis: Cystic Fibrosis Foundation evidence-informed guidelines. *J Cyst Fibros.* 2016;15(6):724–735

79. Powers SW, Stark LJ, Chamberlin LA, et al. Behavioral and nutritional treatment for preschool-aged children with cystic fibrosis: a randomized clinical trial. *JAMA Pediatr.* 2015;169(5):e150636

VI

Chapter 47

The Ketogenic Diet

Introduction

The ketogenic diet is a high-fat, low-carbohydrate, and minimal-protein diet designed to mimic the fasting state. It is used most commonly to treat intractable epilepsy but is also a primary therapy for some metabolic defects involving glucose transport and metabolism. The diet increases the body's reliance on fatty acids rather than on glucose for energy. This chapter reviews the history, physiology, mechanism of action, indications, efficacy, and contraindications of the ketogenic diet. The emphasis is on implementing and maintaining the classic ketogenic diet while preventing and managing its complications. Alternative dietary therapies for epilepsy, including the medium-chain triglyceride (MCT) oil version of the ketogenic diet, the low-glycemic index treatment, and the modified Atkins diet, are also described.

History

The benefits of fasting for seizure control have been known for ages.[1] Although the first scientific report did not appear until 1911 in France, fasting for seizure therapy was used by Hippocrates and was described in the Bible (Mark 9:14–29). In the United States, the first report of fasting as a treatment for epilepsy was presented to the American Medical Association in 1921 by endocrinologist H. R. Geyelin (New York Presbyterian Hospital) based on his observation of patients treated by the osteopath H. W. Conklin (Battle Creek, Michigan), who believed that epilepsy could be caused by toxic secretions from intestinal Peyer patches. Because fasting is not a practical long-term treatment, R. M. Wilder (Mayo Clinic) described a high-fat, low-carbohydrate, "ketogenic" diet to mimic fasting. The first efficacy studies of this ketogenic diet by M. G. Peterman (1925, Mayo Clinic) and F. B. Talbot (1926, Massachusetts General Hospital) showed remarkable efficacy, with 50% to 60% of patients becoming seizure free.[2] Interest in the diet waned after the introduction of phenytoin in 1938, but a resurgence of interest in the diet occurred in the 1990s, in part because of the advocacy of the Charlie Foundation (http://www.charliefoundation.org) and in part because of the media attention surrounding the 1997 movie *First Do No Harm*.[1] The diet is currently administered at major medical centers around the United States as well as in at least 41 other countries.[3] A list of dietary centers following patients on the ketogenic diet can be found on the Charlie Foundation website (Document8https://charliefoundation.org/find-a-hospital/).

Physiologic Basis

The basis of the ketogenic diet is to simulate a fasting state. During fasting, the brain is able to obtain 30% to 60% of its energy from serum ketone bodies derived from β-oxidation of fatty acids (Fig 47.1).[4-8] Fasting lowers serum glucose concentration, resulting in a low insulin-to-glucagon ratio. The decrease in this ratio and changes in other hormones, such as epinephrine, stimulate lipolysis in adipocytes. The free fatty acids released into the blood cannot cross the blood-brain barrier and, therefore, cannot be used directly to sustain brain metabolism. Instead, fatty acids are converted by the liver to ketone bodies that cross the blood-brain barrier and serve as a

Fig 47.1.
Summary of ketogenesis

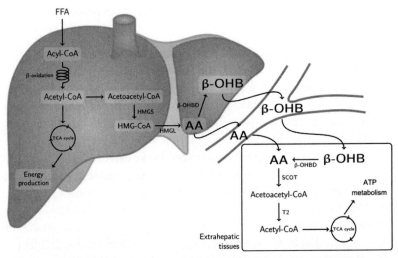

In the liver, free fatty acids are first converted into acyl-CoA. This compound then undergoes β-oxidation and is converted into acetyl-CoA. Acetyl-CoA then either enters the TCA cycle to generate energy, or it is converted into ketone bodies, specifically acetoacetate (AA), β-hydroxybutyrate (β-OHB), and acetone. Hydroxymethylglutaryl-lyase (HMG), and β-OHB dehydrogenase (β-OHBD) facilitate this process. Ketone bodies are then transported to extrahepatic tissues in the blood. In brain, heart or muscle, ketone bodies are converted back into acetyl-CoA. This process depends on β-OHBD, succinyl-CoA: 3-ketoacid CoA transferase (SCOT), and thiolase (T2). Acetyl-CoA is then available to enter the TCA cycle for energy production.
Reprinted with permission from Branco et al.[70]

major energy source for the brain. Similar to a fasting state, with the ketogenic diet, serum glucose concentrations are lower, resulting in decreased glycolysis and increased mitochondrial oxidation. With fatty acids serving as the primary available fuel, metabolism is driven away from gluconeogenesis and toward of β-oxidation, resulting in the formation of 3 primary ketone bodies: β-hydroxybutyrate, acetoacetate, and acetone. These ketones replace glucose as the primary fuel source for the brain.[9,10]

Fatty acids from lipolysis undergo β-oxidation to acetyl coenzyme A (acetyl CoA) in the mitochondria of liver, cardiac muscle, and skeletal muscle cells. Typically, acetyl CoA condenses with oxaloacetate to enter the tricarboxylic acid cycle (TCA cycle or Krebs cycle). However, liver oxaloacetate is low during fasting (or with the ketogenic diet) because it is used to synthesize glucose. The liver, therefore, converts excess acetyl CoA to acetoacetate, some of which is then converted to β-hydroxybutyrate. These 2 ketones are released into the bloodstream and cross the blood-brain barrier.

In the brain, as in other tissues, β-hydroxybutyrate and acetoacetate are converted back to acetyl CoA and enter the TCA cycle, yielding biosynthetic carbon compounds and energy (in the form of reduced nicotinamide adenine dinucleotide [NADH] and reduced flavin adenine dinucleotide [FADH$_2$]). The mitochondrial electron transport chain then oxidizes NADH and FADH$_2$ to yield adenosine triphosphate (ATP).

Mechanisms of Action in Epilepsy

The therapeutic mechanisms of action of the ketogenic diet in epilepsy remain incompletely understood. Several mechanisms are likely contributing, including disruption of glutamatergic synaptic transmission, activation of ATP-sensitive potassium channels (K$_{ATP}$), and inhibition of glycolysis.[9] The direct anticonvulsant effect of ketone bodies has long been questioned, and in human studies, it has been shown that increased serum ketone levels correlate with seizure reduction.[9,11–13] One hypothesis is that acetoacetate may mediate this effect by decreasing glutamate transport into synaptic vesicles, resulting in a decrease in the release of glutamate, an excitatory neurotransmitter. Additionally, it has also been proposed that the ketogenic diet may result in increased production of gamma aminobutyric acid (GABA), an inhibitory neurotransmitter.[9,14] In animal models, ketone bodies increase neuronal K$_{ATP}$ channel activity and reduce the firing rates of neurons in the substantia nigra pars reticulata.[9,15] These neurons are thought to be important in the modulation of seizure threshold.[9,16]

VI

Beyond the direct effects of ketone bodies, it is also possible that the anticonvulsant mechanisms of the ketogenic diet may be secondary to altered glucose metabolism.[9] This theory is supported by the observation that modified versions of the diet are effective even in the absence of a sustained ketosis.[9,17] In animal models, in addition to the possible direct effect of ketones, reduced glucose oxidation has also been shown to lead to activation of K_{ATP} channels, potentially conferring reduced neuronal excitability and seizure resistance.[9,18] The impact of decreased glycolysis has also been studied using the glucose analog, 2-deoxyglucose. By limiting glucose uptake, this compound inhibits glycolysis and has been shown to slow seizure progression through a mechanism of decreased expression of brain-derived neurotrophic factor in experimental models.[9,19] Finally, the ketogenic diet has been shown to augment metabolic mechanisms against oxidative stress, reducing reactive oxygen species.[9,20–23] These metabolic shifts are likely to be neuroprotective but may also decrease neuronal excitability.[9,24] Despite the many hypotheses that have been proposed, none have been universally accepted. The ketogenic diet likely has multiple mechanisms of action, given the complex nature of the metabolic changes involved.

Indications

Intractable Epilepsy

Historically, the ketogenic diet has been most commonly used in the treatment of intractable epilepsy. It effectively treats multiple seizure types (including generalized seizures and focal-onset seizures[25,26]) and epilepsy syndromes (including Lennox-Gastaut syndrome,[27–30] Landau Kleffner syndrome [acquired epileptic aphasia],[31] Dravet syndrome [severe myoclonic epilepsy of infancy],[27,32–34] Doose syndrome [myoclonic-astatic epilepsy of early childhood],[35,36] and West syndrome [infantile spasms],[37–40]), as well as childhood and juvenile absence epilepsy.[41] It is also effective for seizures caused by tuberous sclerosis complex[42–44] and other inherited disorders. There are case reports of efficacy in febrile infection-related epilepsy syndrome (FIRES), a likely immune-mediated epileptic encephalopathy.[45] Efficacy has also been reported in a few cases of infants in the neonatal intensive care unit with drug-resistant epilepsy.[46] In recent years, there has been increasing interest of the efficacy of the ketogenic diet for the treatment of super-refractory status epilepticus for both children and adults.[47–52]

Traditionally, the ketogenic diet has been considered too difficult for use as a first-line agent and has been treated as a last resort. However, the majority of the 2009 expert consensus panel felt that the ketogenic diet should be strongly considered after a patient has failed 2 antiepileptic drugs.[53]

The ketogenic diet is indicated for patients of all ages. In most studies, efficacy is similar across age groups,[54–56] although some studies suggest slightly lower tolerability in older patients.[26] A ketogenic formula can also be effectively administered to formula-fed infants and gastrostomy tube-fed children or adults (see "Calculation of the Ketogenic Diet").[57–59]

Inborn Metabolic Disorders

The ketogenic diet is the preferred treatment for 2 congenital disorders affecting glucose metabolism and transport: pyruvate dehydrogenase complex (PDHc) deficiency[60,61] and glucose transporter type 1 (GLUT-1) deficiency.[62,63] Pyruvate dehydrogenase converts pyruvate (from glycolysis) to acetyl CoA, which then enters the TCA cycle. GLUT-1 is responsible for the facilitated transport of glucose across the blood-brain barrier. In both disorders, mutations limit the availability of glucose to serve as the primary energy substrate for the brain. The ketogenic diet should be considered soon after diagnosis of these metabolic disorders.

Experimental Uses

The ketogenic diet has been explored in a broad spectrum of neurologic and psychiatric disorders including Alzheimer disease, amyotrophic lateral sclerosis, autism spectrum disorder, bipolar disorder, depression, hypoxic/ischemic brain injury, migraine, narcolepsy, Parkinson disease, and traumatic brain injury.[64–66] Beyond PDHc and GLUT-1 deficiencies, the ketogenic diet has been trialed in other metabolic disorders including glycogen storage disease type III, glycogen storage disease type V (McArdle disease), and phosphofructokinase deficiency.[64,67] Several systemic illnesses have also been studied, including type 2 diabetes mellitus, polycystic ovary syndrome, obesity, and cardiac ischemia.[64,68,69] Efficacy and safety have not been fully established for any of these indications and treatment remains experimental.

Malignancy

In recent years, there has been increasing interest in a possible therapeutic role of the ketogenic diet as part of cancer treatment. Malignant cells are highly dependent on glucose for growth, proliferation, and transformation.[70] The theory behind treatment with the ketogenic diet is to reduce glucose availability to tumor cells, which are often dependent on glycolysis.[70] The tumor cell may then undergo "selective starvation" as they are often unable to perform ketone metabolism secondary to metabolic inflexibility, genomic instability, and mitochondrial abnormalities.[70,71] Preclinical studies have shown that the of ketogenic diet may reduce tumor growth and improve survival in animal models of malignant glioma, prostate cancer, colon cancer, and gastrointestinal cancer.[72] There are currently several open clinical trials investigating the ketogenic diet as adjuvant therapy in the treatment of glioblastoma.[70]

Efficacy in Epilepsy

For patients with refractory epilepsy who are treated with the ketogenic diet, typically about one third of patients achieve seizure control and another one third show meaningful but incomplete reduction in seizure frequency. In a 2016 Cochrane review, 7 randomized controlled trials (RTCs) of the classic ketogenic diet and modified versions were reviewed.[25,73–80] These studies included a total of 427 children and adolescents.[80] Authors described "promising, although limited, evidence for the use of the ketogenic diet in epilepsy."[80] There have been 2 additional RTCs published since this review.[81,82] Across these studies, at 3 months of ketogenic diet treatment, 38% to 75% of the cohorts showed greater than 50% seizure reduction and 7% to 60% showed greater than 90% seizure reduction or seizure-freedom.[25,73,75,77,82]

In general, efficacy does not vary significantly based on age, sex, seizure type, or etiology.[83,84] The ketogenic diet has been reported to be effective in the treatment of both generalized and focal epilepsy syndromes. The classic formulations provide a ratio of 3:1 or 4:1 of fat to combined protein and carbohydrate. One RCT has shown that the 4:1 ratio may be slightly more effective compared with the 3:1 ratio.[75] In this study, however, for the majority of cases, individuals who became seizure free while on the 4:1 treatment, remained seizure free through a transition to 3:1 treatment. Further, the 3:1 diet was better tolerated with lower rates of gastrointestinal symptoms.[75,80] Finally, one trial found no significant difference in seizure freedom between the fasting-onset versus gradual-onset ketogenic diet protocols and reported a higher rate of seizure reduction in the gradual-onset cohort.[73,80]

Clinically, it is often reported that individuals with epilepsy treated with the ketogenic diet show improvements in learning and attention. Two prospective studies and 1 RCT have shown significant improvements in neurobehavioral and cognitive functioning associated with ketogenic diet treatment in children with epilepsy.[85–87]

Contraindications

The ketogenic diet is contraindicated for patients with the following diseases: fatty acid oxidation defects (including defects involving fatty acid transportation, enzymes of β-oxidation, and ketone body production), primary carnitine deficiency or other carnitine cycle defects, pyruvate carboxylase deficiency, or porphryia.[53] Candidates for the ketogenic diet should be screened for metabolic disorders, including a comprehensive metabolic blood panel, prior to diet initiation. Although high-fat diets can exacerbate ketotic hypoglycemia, the ketogenic diet is not strictly contraindicated in this condition; however, it does require careful monitoring.[88]

Cotherapy with some medications may increase the risk of certain adverse events, but there are no treatments that are absolutely contraindicated with the ketogenic diet. Because cotherapy may provide optimal seizure control for some patients, the risks and benefits must be weighed. Furthermore, all medications must be reviewed for carbohydrate content (see "Concurrent Medications and Occult Carbohydrates"). In a study of cotherapy, it was shown that serum concentrations trended down for carbamazepine, lamotrigine, levetiracetam, topiramate and valproate, and phenobarbital slightly increased. However, valproate was the only medication that showed a statistically significant change with the ketogenic diet.[89]

Patients using the ketogenic diet and carbonic anhydrase inhibitors (including acetazolamide, topiramate, and zonisamide) may be at increased risk of metabolic acidosis and renal stones.[90,91] However, with adequate hydration and appropriate prophylaxis with a buffering agent, such as potassium citrate, as well as careful monitoring of urine calcium, creatinine, citrate, pH, specific gravity, occult hematuria, and serum bicarbonate, carbonic anhydrase inhibitors and the ketogenic diet can often be safely coadministered.

There have been rare reports of adverse events associated with valproate and the ketogenic diet including acute pancreatitis and hepatic failure.[92] In one such case, hepatic dysfunction seemed to be trigged by a concomitant respiratory viral infection.[92] In general, cotherapy has not been shown to significantly increase the risk of adverse events.[93,94] Long-term use of valproate can induce carnitine deficiency, and it has been suggested that cotherapy may induce hepatotoxicity by a carnitine-related mechanism.[95,96] For patients undergoing treatment with both valproate and the ketogenic diet, liver function, pancreatic amylase, and carnitine levels should be monitored carefully. In the case above, with an identified viral infection, hepatotoxic effects reversed following discontinuation of valproate alone, allowing for ongoing ketogenic diet treatment.[92]

Adverse Effects

Common short-term adverse effects of the ketogenic diet include dehydration, hypoglycemia, acidosis, vomiting, diarrhea, constipation, and loss of appetite.[94,97] These complications are generally treated symptomatically. Younger children may be at increased risk of adverse effects during initiation.[97] The risks of dehydration, hypoglycemia, and acidosis are mitigated with revised initiation protocols and prophylactic potassium citrate (see "Initiation Protocol"). Constipation is very common and is typically managed with medication, such as polyethylene glycol (MiraLax) or through dietary modification, such as increasing fluid and fiber intake, adding MCT oil, or supplementing with carnitine.

Common longer-term adverse effects include renal stones, hypertriglyceridemia, decreased bone density, decreased linear growth, increased bruising, irritability, and lethargy. Some patients on the ketogenic diet may be more susceptible to infection, but the attribution of this adverse effect is not well understood.[98,99]

Rare but serious adverse events have been reported with the ketogenic diet, including acute (possibly hypertriglyceridemia-induced) pancreatitis,[100] cardiomyopathy associated with prolonged QT_c interval,[101] iron-deficiency anemia,[94] hepatotoxicity, and Fanconi renal tubular acidosis.[93,96] In a review of 45 studies, severe adverse effects occurred in less than 0.5% of children on the ketogenic diet.[99]

Growth

There have been several reports demonstrating decreased growth for children on the ketogenic diet.[102-105] The mechanism of this is not fully understood. The ketogenic diet does not appear to change an individual's resting energy expenditure; however, the respiratory quotient does decrease with this treatment.[99,106,107] Changes in weight-for-age percentile appear to be most notable within the first several months on the diet, whereas the most significant changes in height-for-age percentile occur after 6 months of treatment. Younger children who are on the diet for longer periods of time may be at greatest risk for decreased growth. In a literature review of the ketogenic diet and growth, the lowest reported mean z score for height was −1.39 across treatment cohorts.[99,108] In a retrospective study, patients were stratified into groups of satisfactory or poor linear growth. There was an association between decreased linear growth and a total protein or caloric intake of <80% of the recommended daily intake and with a protein-to-energy ratio of 1.4 g protein/100 kcal or less. Given these results, a protein-to-energy ratio of 1.5 g protein/100 kcal is recommended to help support optimal linear growth.[109] In a study of the long-term effects of the ketogenic diet, growth appeared to improve after discontinuation of the diet; however, 40% of the subjects were still <10th percentile height for age after the diet was discontinued.[110] The risk of decreased linear growth, especially with long-term treatment, should be considered when weighing the risks and benefits of the ketogenic diet. Height and weight should be monitored closely (at least every 3 months) and protein and total kilocalories should be adjusted for patients with suboptimal growth.

Renal Stones
Although older studies have indicated that renal calculi occur in approximately 3% to 10% of children treated with the ketogenic diet,[111,112] a recent review of 45 prospective studies reported a rate of 1.4%.[99] This improvement is likely secondary to changes to the diet initiation and maintenance protocols, including the elimination of fluid restriction and preinitiation fasting, as well as prophylactic use of potassium citrate or other buffering agents.[91,113] Cotherapy with carbonic anhydrase inhibitors (including acetazolamide, topiramate, and zonisamide) may increase the risk of calculi.[90,91] Calculi can be composed of uric acid, calcium oxalate, or calcium phosphate. Patients with hematuria (gross or microscopic), crystalluria, abdominal pain, or flank pain should be evaluated for possible nephrolithiasis. Analgesia and hydration are appropriate for acute episodes, and lithotripsy, and/or medical or surgical extraction may be indicated in some cases. Recurrent calculi may be prevented by liberalization of fluids and further alkalinization of the urine with potassium citrate or other buffering agents.

Lipid Profiles
Studies monitoring lipid profiles for patients on the ketogenic diet have found that there is an associated increase in plasma cholesterol, low-density lipoprotein, very low-density lipoprotein, triglycerides, and total apolipoprotein B levels, as well as a decrease in the high-density lipoprotein.[99,114,115]

Reported rates of these changes as adverse events among patients on the ketogenic diet are as follows: hyperlipidemia, 4.6%; hypercholesterolemia, 3.8%; hypertriglyceridemia, 3.2%; gallstones, 0.1%; and fatty liver, 0.1%.[99] Individuals on a formula-based diet are at lower risk of hypercholesterolemia compared with those who are eating solid foods.[114] With the discontinuation of the diet, the lipid profile normalizes. The ketogenic diet has not been associated with changes in vascular function such as carotid intima-media thickness, carotid stiffness, or aortic dispensability.[99,116,117]

Bone Mineral Content

As with antiepileptic drugs, long-term use of the ketogenic diet may increase risk of osteopenia, osteoporosis, and bone fractures.[94,103,108] Although all patients on the ketogenic diet are supplemented with vitamin D and calcium, this may not be sufficient to prevent decreased bone density.[118] Therefore, periodic dual energy x-ray absorptiometry (DEXA) screening for bone health should be considered for patients who are treated with the ketogenic diet long-term.[53]

The Keto Team

The ketogenic diet requires a multidisciplinary team approach. The primary members of the "keto team" are the patient and his or her family, a neurologist, a dietitian, a pediatrician, and a nurse. The inpatient pediatric house staff, a pharmacist, a gastroenterologist, the hospital foodservice staff, a social worker, and other specialists are typically involved as well.[119] Implementing the ketogenic diet is very time intensive for families and for clinicians. Close coordination and communication among the team is critical.

Calculation of the Ketogenic Diet

The ketogenic diet is traditionally calculated at a 4:1 ketogenic ratio (4 g of fat for every 1 g of protein and carbohydrate), although this ratio may be modified to suit the needs of individual patients. Lower ratios may be necessary to meet some patients' protein requirements or to improve tolerability. During follow-up, the diet may be recalculated with an increased or decreased ketogenic ratio. The ratio may be increased for improved seizure control or it may be decreased to allow for more protein to optimize growth.

The energy requirements of children with intractable epilepsy, especially those with impaired mobility, often differ substantially from other children.

In preinitiation consultation, the dietitian collects and analyzes a 3-day food record, measures height and weight, and assesses activity level. Using these variables, a goal for total daily caloric intake while on the ketogenic diet is formulated.

The calculation of macronutrient requirements for the ketogenic diet is outlined in Table 47.1. Menus should be calculated by, or in consultation with, a registered dietitian with experience using the ketogenic diet. These calculations can be made by hand, but the process is greatly facilitated by ketogenic diet software (eg, KetoCalculator, Nutricia North America). Many families rely exclusively on menus calculated by the dietitian; however, some parents learn to calculate menus independently. There are now smart phone applications as well that automate the computations of the ketogenic diet using linear algebra modeling.[120] Meals and recipes are calculated to the nearest gram, and individual foods are weighed to the nearest tenth of a gram.

Developing menus that satisfy the daily allotment of macronutrients as well as the necessary fat requirements (from heavy cream, butter or margarine, oils, mayonnaise, and other sources) takes several steps. Heavy cream

Table 47.1.

Ketogenic Diet Macronutrient Calculations

1. Calculate calories needed per day
   (Example: 15 kg child × 68 kcal/kg/day = 1000 kcal per day)
2. Calculate number of dietary units needed per day[a]
   (For example, on a 4:1 diet, each dietary unit (4 g fat + 1 g protein or carbohydrate) = 40 kcal (1000 kcal/day)/(40 kcal/unit) = 25 units/day)
3. Calculate the number of g of fat required per day
   (Fat: 25 units/day × 4 g/unit = 100 g per day)
4. Calculate the remainder of units/kcal, allotted to protein and carbohydrate
   (Protein and carbohydrate: 25 units/day × 1 g/unit = 25 g/day)
5. Maintain at least the minimum protein requirement (1 g/kg/day)
   (Protein: 1 g/kg/day × 15 kg = 15 g/day of protein)
6. Calculate remainder, allotted to carbohydrate
   (Carbohydrate: 25 g/day − 15 g/day protein = 10 g/day carbohydrate)
7. Divide the allotments into the number of meals per day

[a] The calories per dietary unit vary with the ratio of the ketogenic diet as follows: for a 2:1 diet, 22 kcal per dietary unit; for a 3:1 diet, 31 kcal per dietary unit; for a 4:1 diet, 40 kcal per dietary unit; and for a 5:1 diet, 49 kcal per dietary unit.

VI

(36% fat) is a good source of fat. Patients may drink it as is or add water, and it may be whipped or flavored and frozen as ice cream. Consistent use of the same brand of heavy cream and careful calculations using nutritional tables[121] or standard software is typically step 1. Once fat is allotted, protein sources (eg, meat, fish, poultry, eggs, and cheese) are added, taking into account the protein already present in cream or an alternative fat source. Carbohydrate-containing foods (eg, fruits and vegetables) are added last, taking into account the carbohydrates already present in cream, protein sources, and medications. Small quantities of certain "free foods" (eg, a lettuce leaf, 2 macadamia nuts, or 2 olives) may be added to increase dietary flexibility and palatability.

Ketogenic formulas are available for gastrostomy tube-fed children and formula-fed infants. These formulas can also be used as meal replacements for patients eating by mouth. Ross Carbohydrate Free soy-based formula (RCF), combined with a glucose polymer (Polycose, Ross) and emulsified safflower oil (Microlipid, Novartis Nutrition) to yield the desired ketogenic ratio, is primarily used for tube feedings. There are also a milk-based formulas (KetoCal, Nutricia North America and KetoVie) available in both powdered or ready-to-consume formulations.

Micronutrient Supplementation

The ketogenic diet is deficient in several vitamins (including vitamin D and B vitamins) and minerals (including magnesium, potassium, and calcium) necessitating supplementation. Parents must understand that these supplements are not elective. Prior to the clinical recognition of these vitamin requirements in the 1920s and 1930s, patients developed serious complications of vitamin and mineral deficiencies. Patients should receive an age-appropriate low-carbohydrate multivitamin every day, as well as a carbohydrate-free calcium supplement with vitamin D.[53] Recommendations from the Institute of Medicine for vitamin D intake include 400 IU/day for infants up to 1 year of age and 600 IU/day for children 1 to 18 years of age (Chapter 21.I: Fat-Soluble Vitamins). Because carnitine is important for fatty acid transport, carnitine concentrations should be routinely monitored and supplemented as needed.[95]

Initiation Protocol

Prior to scheduling diet initiation, patents and parents typically meet with the ketogenic dietitian. In addition to assessing the patient's anthropometric and nutritional status, the dietitian educates the family about the ketogenic diet and the initiation protocol, as well as psychosocial issues associated with the ketogenic diet. Laboratory studies (complete blood cell count, complete metabolic panel, lipid profile, pancreatic functions, electrolytes, uric acid, magnesium, phosphorus, carnitine, ß-hydroxybutyrate, and urinalysis) are performed to screen for any possible contraindications and to establish baseline levels. The family should commit to the diet under close supervision for at least 3 months if possible.

Traditionally, the ketogenic diet was initiated with a 24- to 48-hour fast, followed by the introduction of ketogenic meals once the patient was in ketosis (large ketones on urine dipstick). In recent years, this approach has been called into question; many medical centers have introduced modified initiation protocols that do not involve fasting. Although some evidence suggests that fasting leads to a quicker onset of ketosis and seizure control,[122] other studies do not support this claim and show that nonfasting protocols may be more tolerable and reduce the risk of some adverse effects (symptomatic acidosis, hypoglycemia, and electrolyte imbalances).[73,123,124]

Whether fasting or not, standard practice is to initiate the ketogenic diet on an inpatient basis. However, two retrospective studies have shown that it is possible to successfully initiate the ketogenic diet in an outpatient setting.[124,125] Hospital admission has many benefits, however, as it allows for closer monitoring for adverse events, symptomatic treatment, and adjustment of medications. Furthermore, it provides an opportunity for the keto team to meet with the patient and family and provide additional education and support.

If a classic fasting protocol is used, the patient is asked to fast after dinner the night prior to the admission. After 48 hours of fasting, ketogenic meals are introduced, first at one third of goal calculated calories for 24 hours, then at two thirds goal calculated calories for 24 hours, then at full strength.[121] Alternatively, with a nonfasting protocol, full-strength ketogenic meals may be given from day 1. Under an alternative nonfasting protocol, full-calorie meals are given from day 1 at a 1:1 ketogenic ratio. The ratio is then increased daily to 2:1, 3:1, and finally 4:1.[73]

During the course of the hospital admission, blood glucose concentration is typically monitored every 6 hours, more often if hypoglycemia is detected, until the child is in ketosis and tolerating the full ketogenic diet. Once eating the diet and in ketosis, the child is monitored clinically and blood glucose measurements are performed only if there are symptoms of hypoglycemia. Unless the child is symptomatic, blood glucose concentrations as low as 25 mg/dL are not treated. Urine ketone dipsticks are typically checked every void. Serum bicarbonate is checked every 24 hours, and the prescribed potassium citrate dose is adjusted accordingly.

The traditional ketogenic diet involved restricted fluid intake on the basis of the observation that urine ketones may decrease with increased hydration. However, fluid intake generally does not affect serum ß-hydroxybutyrate, which is a more reliable indicator of ketosis than urine ketones.[12] To reduce the risk of dehydration and nephrolithiasis, the majority of practitioners do not recommend fluid restriction with the ketogenic diet.[112,123] Liberalization of fluid intake does not decrease efficacy.

During initiation, all children are supplemented with a multivitamin, calcium, and vitamin D. To reduce the risk of renal stones, children may also be prophylactically supplemented with potassium citrate.[90,113]

Maintenance and Follow-Up

A child on the ketogenic diet requires close supervision by his or her pediatric neurologist/epileptologist, dietitian, and pediatrician. Following initiation, ketogenic diet clinic follow-up visits typically occur at 2 weeks, 1 month, 3 months, and every 3 months thereafter. More frequent visits may be necessary for infants to ensure adequate nutrition and growth.[104] At these visits, height and weight are measured, and routine laboratory studies are performed, as during the preinitiation consult. The child's parents or caregivers should provide records of seizure frequency, food diaries, and records of urine dipsticks for ketones to the neurologist and the dietitian. The majority of the 2009 expert consensus panel suggested routine urine ketosis evaluation by parents several times per week.[53] Clinicians should ask about common adverse effects. The diet may be adjusted at these visits to optimize growth and seizure control.

Minor viral illnesses and more serious infections typically make it difficult to maintain ketosis and may increase metabolic acidosis. During intercurrent illnesses, breakthrough seizures can often be managed with a benzodiazepine pulse (eg, lorazepam or diazepam).

It is relatively safe for patients on the ketogenic diet to undergo anesthesia. In a recent study, 3 or 24 children who underwent surgery had reports of minor complications, 2 of whom had increased seizure frequency postoperatively and one had metabolic acidosis.[126] Of course, within this population, it is very difficult to attribute a cause for seizure exacerbation following surgery given the high risk at baseline, with or without the ketogenic diet.

Concurrent Medications and Occult Carbohydrates

Most oral drug formulations and almost all syrups contain carbohydrates in the form of sugars, starches, or reduced carbohydrates such as glycerin. Parents and caregivers should be instructed to check with the dietitian before giving any new prescription or over-the-counter medications to children on the ketogenic diet. They should also be made aware that some toothpastes, lotions (including sunscreen), and shampoos contain carbohydrates, such as sorbitol, which can be absorbed transdermally. Hidden sources of carbohydrates should be considered if seizure exacerbations occur.

Likewise, physicians who care for children on the ketogenic diet should consult with the dietitian and with appropriate references when prescribing medications.[127,128] A compounding pharmacy should be identified that can prepare carbohydrate-free drug formulations, and the hospital pharmacist may be contacted for inpatient hospitalization. Any added carbohydrates in medication formulations must be included in diet calculations. During inpatient hospital stays, physicians, pharmacists, and nursing staff should be reminded to avoid intravenous fluids containing dextrose. In general, normal saline is the preferred intravenous fluid option compared with lactated Ringer solution; however, normal saline can increase the risk of metabolic acidosis so patients need to be monitored carefully.[126]

Adjusting the Diet for Optimal Seizure Control

The experienced pediatric neurologist and dietitian adjust the ketogenic diet like an antiepileptic drug. Breakthrough seizures may occur at times of day when ketosis is suboptimal; in these cases, the diet may be adjusted to optimize seizure control. For example, breakthrough seizures on waking in the morning might be treated with a small, high-fat snack at bedtime (eg, olives) to help sustain ketosis overnight.

Discontinuation of the Ketogenic Diet

Discontinuation of the diet should be considered for patients who have been seizure free for 2 years or who have not had an effective treatment response after 3 months.[53] Some children with severe epilepsy may need to continue dietary treatment for many years, and for patients with GLUT-1 or PDHc deficiencies, treatment is lifelong.[53,103]

Weaning by reducing the ketogenic ratio should occur gradually over several months for patients who have been on long-term therapy. If seizures recur during the weaning process, the diet can be immediately increased back to the original ratio without necessitating hospital admission. In a retrospective study of 557 children, 80% of individuals who were seizure free on the ketogenic diet remained so after the diet was discontinued.[129] The risk of recurrence was highest for children with abnormal electroencephalograms, structural brain abnormalities, and tuberous sclerosis complex. However, the majority of patients who experienced a recurrence of seizures with discontinuation were able to regain seizure control with reinitiation of the ketogenic diet or adjustment of anticonvulsants.[129]

Alternative Dietary Therapy

Although the ketogenic diet is highly effective, some patients are not able to tolerate it for a variety of reasons. As a result, serval modified versions of this diet have been developed.

In the 1970s, Huttenlocher introduced the MCT oil version of the ketogenic diet.[130] Because MCT oil is, gram-for-gram, more ketogenic than other fats, the MCT diet allows liberalized quantities of protein and carbohydrate. An RCT found no difference in efficacy and tolerability between the MCT oil diet and classic ketogenic diet.[76] However, the MCT oil diet tends to have increased adverse effects of bloating, nausea, and vomiting.

In 2002, the low-glycemic index treatment (LGIT) was developed at Massachusetts General Hospital as a liberalized alternative to the traditional ketogenic diet.[17] This approach permits greater total intake of carbohydrate (40–60 g/day) than the traditional ketogenic diet but limits foods to those with a glycemic index of <50 relative to glucose (ie, foods that produce a relatively low increase in blood glucose per g of carbohydrate). In 4 retrospective studies (total n=169), the efficacy of LGIT approached that of the ketogenic diet but with fewer adverse effects.[131–134] Across these studies, at variable follow-up time points (2 months–14 months), 53% to 78% of the cohorts showed greater than 50% seizure reduction, and 6% to 40% showed greater than 90% seizure reduction or seizure freedom.[131–134]

LGIT has been shown to effectively treat epilepsy associated with tuberous sclerosis complex and Angelman syndrome. In a retrospective study of LGIT in 15 patients with tuberous sclerosis complex, 47% experienced a >50% reduction in seizure frequency after 6 months.[135] In a prospective study of LGIT in 6 children with Angelman syndrome, 67% experienced a >90% reduction in seizure frequency after 4 months.[136] In a larger retrospective study of LGIT in 23 patients with Angelmen syndrome, 22% were seizure free, and an additional 30% were seizure free with the exception of few breakthrough seizures with systemic illnesses.[137]

In 2003, the modified Atkins diet was developed at Johns Hopkins Hospital as another alternative to the classic ketogenic diet.[138] This approach initially restricts carbohydrates to 10 g/day in children and 15 g/day in adults during the first month of treatment and then gradually increases daily carbohydrate intake by 5 g/month to an upper limit of 30 g/day. Once implementation is complete, most patients are on a ketogenic ratio ranging from 1:1 to 2:1.[139]

In a review of 30 retrospective and prospective studies, at 3 to 6 months, 48% of the individuals showed greater than 50% seizure reduction, and 39% showed greater than 90% seizure reduction or seizure freedom.[140] There have been 4 RCTs investigating the efficacy of the modified Atkins diet.[74,78,79,82] In 2 of these studies, at 3 months, 10% to 60% of the cohorts showed greater than 50% seizure reduction, and 0 to 30% showed greater than 90% seizure reduction or seizure freedom.[74,78] In one of these trials, it was shown that initiating the modified Atkins diet with a 10-g/day carbohydrate limit is more effective than a 20-g/day limit.[78] Two trials have compared the modified Atkins diet with the ketogenic diet. In the first, the ketogenic diet group showed higher efficacy; among the ketogenic diet cohort, a reduction in seizure frequency was seen in 100% of patients with a mean decrease of 58% at 3 months and 71% at 6 months. The modified Atkins diet group showed a reduction in seizure frequency in 40% of patients at 3 months (mean decrease of 7%), and 62% of patients at 6 months (mean decrease of 28%).[79] Similarly, in the second trial, seizure freedom rates were higher among the ketogenic diet cohort (53%) compared with the modified Atkins cohort (20%) however, the modified Atkins diet was better tolerated and there were fewer reported adverse effects.[82]

Conclusions

The ketogenic diet is the most effective treatment for intractable epilepsy available. An expert ketogenic team is required to guide patients and families through diet initiation and maintenance to optimize this powerful therapy and to ameliorate risks of adverse effects.

References

1. Bailey EE, Pfeifer HH, Thiele EA. The use of diet in the treatment of epilepsy. *Epilepsy Behav.* 2005;6(1):4–8

2. Wheless JW. History and origin of the ketogenic diet. In: Stafstrom CE, Rho JM, eds. *Epilepsy and the Ketogenic Diet.* Totowa, NJ: Humana Press; 2004:31–50

3. Kossoff EH, McGrogan JR. Worldwide use of the ketogenic diet. *Epilepsia.* 2005;46(2):280–289

4. Cullingford TE. Molecular regulation of ketogenesis. In: Stafstrom CE, Rho JM, eds. *Epilepsy and the Ketogenic Diet.* Totowa, NJ: Humana Press; 2004:201–215

5. Nordli DR, DeVivo DC. Effects of the ketogenic diet on cerebral energy metabolism. In: Stafstrom CE, Rho JM, eds. *Epilepsy and the Ketogenic Diet.* 2004:179–184

6. Mitchell GA, Fukao T. Inborn errors of ketone body metabolism. In: Scriver CR, Beaudet AL, Sly WS, Valle D, eds. *The Metabolic and Molecular Bases of Inherited Disease.* New York, NY: McGraw-Hill Co; 2001:2327–2356

7. Sankar R, Sotero de Menezes M. Metabolic and endocrine aspects of the ketogenic diet. *Epilepsy Res.* 1999;37(3):191–201

8. Williamson DH. Ketone body metabolism during development. *Fed Proc.* 1985;44(7):2342–2346

9. Lutas A, Yellen G. The ketogenic diet: metabolic influences on brain excitability and epilepsy. *Trends Neurosci.* 2013;36(1):32–40

10. DeVivo DC, Leckie MP, Ferrendelli JS, McDougal DB. Chronic ketosis and cerebral metabolism. *Ann Neurol.* 1978;3(4):331–337

11. Wilder RM. The effects of ketonemia on the course of epilepsy. *Mayo Clin Bull.* 1921;2:307–308

12. Gilbert DL, Pyzik PL, Freeman JM. The ketogenic diet: seizure control correlates better with serum beta-hydroxybutyrate than with urine ketones. *J Child Neurol.* 2000;15(12):787–790

13. van Delft R, Lambrechts D, Verschuure P, Hulsman J, Majoie M. Blood beta-hydroxybutyrate correlates better with seizure reduction due to ketogenic diet than do ketones in the urine. *Seizure.* 2010;19(1):36–39

14. Yudkoff M, Daikhin Y, Melø TM, Nissim I, Sonnewald U, Nissim I. The ketogenic diet and brain metabolism of amino acids: relationship to the anticonvulsant effect. *Annu Rev Nutr.* 2007;27:415–430

15. Ma W, Berg J, Yellen G. Ketogenic diet metabolites reduce firing in central neurons by opening K(ATP) channels. *J Neurosci.* 2007;27(14):3618–3625

16. Depaulis A, Vergnes M, Marescaux C. Endogenous control of epilepsy: the nigral inhibitory system. *Prog Neurobiol.* 1994;42(1):33–52

17. Pfeifer HH, Thiele EA. Low glycemic index treatment: a liberalized ketogenic diet for treatment of intractable epilepsy. 2005. 2005;65(11):1810–1812

18. Giménez-Cassina A, Martínez-François JR, Fisher JK, et al. BAD-dependent regulation of fuel metabolism and K(ATP) channel activity confers resistance to epileptic seizures. *Neuron.* 2012;74(4):719–730

19. Garriga-Canut M, Schoenike B, Qazi R, et al. 2-Deoxy-D-glucose reduces epilepsy progression by NRSF-CtBP-dependent metabolic regulation of chromatin structure. *Nat Neurosci.* 2006;9(11):1382–1387

20. Kim DY, Davis LM, Sullivan PG, et al. Ketone bodies are protective against oxidative stress in neocortical neurons. *J Neurochem.* 2007;101(5):1316–1326

21. Maalouf M, Sullivan PG, Davis L, Kim DY, Rho JM. Ketones inhibit mitochondrial production of reactive oxygen species production following glutamate excitotoxicity by increasing NADH oxidation. *Neuroscience.* 2007;145(1):256–264

22. Jarrett SG, Milder JB, Liang LP, Patel M. The ketogenic diet increases mitochondrial glutathione levels. *J Neurochem.* 2008;106(3):1044–1051

23. Kim DY, Vallejo J, Rho JM. Ketones prevent synaptic dysfunction induced by mitochondrial respiratory complex inhibitors. *J Neurochem.* 2010;114(1):130–141

24. Stringer JL, Xu K. Possible mechanisms for the anticonvulsant activity of fructose-1,6-diphosphate. *Epilepsia.* 2008;49(Suppl 8):101–103

25. Neal EG, Chaffe H, Schwartz RH, et al. The ketogenic diet for the treatment of childhood epilepsy: a randomised controlled trial. *Lancet Neurol.* 2008;7(6): 500–506

26. Maydell BV, Wyllie E, Akhtar N, et al. Efficacy of the ketogenic diet in focal versus generalized seizures. *Pediatr Neurol.* 2001;25(3):208–212

27. Dressler A, Stöcklin B, Reithofer E, et al. Long-term outcome and tolerability of the ketogenic diet in drug-resistant childhood epilepsy—the Austrian experience. *Seizure.* 2010;19(7):404–408

28. Trevathan E. Infantile spasms and Lennox-Gastaut syndrome. *J Child Neurol.* 2002;17(Suppl 2):2S9–2S22

29. Lemmon ME, Terao NN, Ng YT, Reisig W, Rubenstein JE, Kosso EH. Efficacy of the ketogenic diet in Lennox-Gastaut syndrome: a retrospective review of one institution's experience and summary of the literature. *Dev Med Child Neurol.* 2012;54(5):464–468

30. Caraballo RH, Fortini S, Fresler S, et al. Ketogenic diet in patients with Lennox-Gastaut syndrome. *Seizure.* 2014;23(9):751–755

31. Bergqvist AG, Chee CM, Lutchka LM, Brooks-Kayal AR. Treatment of acquired epileptic aphasia with the ketogenic diet. *J Child Neurol.* 1999;14(11):696–701

32. Korff C, Laux L, Kelley K, Goldstein J, Koh S, Nordli DR. Dravet syndrome (severe myoclonic epilepsy in infancy): a retrospective study of 16 patients. *J Child Neurol.* 2007;22(2):185–194

33. Caraballo RH, Cersosimo RO, Sakr D, Cresta A, Escobal N, Fejerman N. Ketogenic diet in patients with Dravet syndrome. *Epilepsia.* 2005;46(9): 1539–1544

34. Dressler A, Trimmel-Schwahofer P, Reithofer E, et al. Efficacy and tolerability of the ketogenic diet in Dravet syndrome - comparison with various standard antiepileptic drug regimen. *Epilepsy Res.* 2015;109:81–89

VI

35. Kilaru S, Bergqvist AG. Current treatment of myoclonic astatic epilepsy: clinical experience at the Children's Hospital of Philadelphia. *Epilepsia.* 2007;48(9): 1703–1707

36. Caraballo RH, Cerosimo RO, Sakr D, Cresta A, Escobal N, Fejerman N. Ketogenic diet in patients with myoclonic-astatic epilepsy. *Epileptic Disord.* 2006;8(2): 151–155

37. Numis AL, Yellen MB, Chu-Shore CJ, Pfeifer HH, Thiele EA. The relationship of ketosis and growth to the efficacy of the ketogenic diet in infantile spasms. *Epilepsy Res.* 2011;96(1-2):172–175

38. Hong AM, Turner Z, Hamdy RF, Kossoff EH. Infantile spasms treated with the ketogenic diet: prospective single-center experience in 104 consecutive infants. *Epilepsia.* 2010;51(8):1403–1407

39. Kossoff EH, Hedderick EF, Turner Z, Freeman JM. A case-control evaluation of the ketogenic diet versus ACTH for new-onset infantile spasms. *49.* 2008;9(1504–1509)

40. Prezioso G, Carlone G, Zaccara G, Verrotti A. Efficacy of ketogenic diet for infantile spasms: a systematic review. *Acta Neurol Scand.* 2018;137(1):4–11

41. Groomes LB, Pyzik PL, Turner Z, Dorward JL, Goode VH, Kossoff EH. Do patients with absence epilepsy respond to ketogenic diets? *J Child Neurol.* 2011;26(2):160–165

42. Coppola G, Klepper J, Ammendola E, et al. The effects of the ketogenic diet in refractory partial seizures with reference to tuberous sclerosis. *Eur J Pediatr Neurol.* 2006;10(3):148–151

43. Kossoff EG, Thiele EA, Pfeifer HH, McGrogan JR, Freeman JM. Tuberous sclerosis complex and the ketogenic diet. *Epilepsia.* 2005;46(10):1684–1686

44. Park S, Lee EJ, Eom S, Kang HC, Lee JS, Kim HD. Ketogenic diet for the management of epilepsy associated with tuberous sclerosis complex in children. *J Epilepsy Res.* 2017;7(1):45–49

45. Millichap JJ, Millichap JG. Ketogenic diet as preferred treatment of FIRES. *Pediatr Neurol Briefs.* 2015;29(1):3

46. Thompson L, Fecske E, Salim M, Hall A. Use of the ketogenic diet in the neonatal intensive care unit - safety and tolerability. *Epilepsia.* 2017;58(2):e36–e39

47. Lin JJ, Lin KL, Chan OW, Hsia SH, Wang HS, CHEESE Study Group. Intravenous ketogenic diet therapy for treatment of the acute stage of super-refractory status epilepticus in a pediatric patient. *Pediatr Neurol.* 2015;52(4):442–445

48. Appavu B, Vanatta L, Condie J, Kerrigan JF, Jarrar R. Ketogenic diet treatment for pediatric super-refractory status epilepticus. *Seizure.* 2016;41:62–65

49. Farias-Moeller R, Bartolini L, Pasupuleti A, Brittany Cines RD, Kao A, Carpenter JL. A practical approach to ketogenic diet in the pediatric intensive care unit for super-refractory status epilepticus. *Neurocrit Care.* 2017;26(2):267–272

50. Cervenka MC, Hocker S, Koenig M, et al. Phase I/II multicenter ketogenic diet study for adult superrefractory status epilepticus. *Neurology.* 2017;88(10): 938–943

51. Kossoff EH, Nabbout R. Use of dietary therapy for status epilepticus. *J Child Neurol.* 2013;28(8):1049–1051

52. Smith G, Press CA. Ketogenic diet in super-refractory status epilepticus. *Pediatr Neurol Briefs.* 2017;31(3):8

53. Kossoff EH, Zupec-Kania BA, Amark PE, et al. Charlie Foundation, Practice Committee of the Child Neurology Society; Practice Committee of the Child Neurology Society; International Ketogenic Diet Study Group. Optimal clinical management of children receiving the ketogenic diet: recommendations of the International Ketogenic Diet Study Group. *Epilepsia.* 2009;50(2):304–317

54. Sperling MR, Nei M. The ketogenic diet in adults. In: Stafstrom CE, Rho JM, eds. *Epilepsy and the Ketogenic Diet.* Totowa, NJ: Humana Press; 2004:103–109

55. Mady MA, Kossoff EH, McGregor AL, Wheless JW, Pyzik PL, Freeman JM. The ketogenic diet: adolescents can do it, too. *Epilepsia.* 2003;44(6):847–851

56. Sirven J, Whedon B, Caplan D, et al. The ketogenic diet for intractable epilepsy in adults: preliminary results. *Epilepsia.* 1999;40(12):1721–1726

57. Hosain SA, La Vega-Talbott M, Solomon GE. Ketogenic diet in pediatric epilepsy patients with gastrostomy feeding. *Pediatr Neurol.* 2005;32(2):81–83

58. Kossoff EH, McGrogan JR, Freeman JM. Benefits of an all-liquid ketogenic diet. *Epilepsia.* 2004;45(9):1163

59. Nordli DR, Kuroda MM, Carroll J, et al. Experience with the ketogenic diet in infants. *Pediatrics.* 2001;108(1):129–133

60. Weber TA, M.R. A, Stacpoole PW. Caveats when considering ketogenic diets for the treatment of pyruvate dehydrogenase complex deficiency. *J Pediatr.* 2001;138(3):390–395

61. Wexler ID, Hemalatha SG, McConnell J, et al. Outcome of pyruvate dehydrogenase deficiency treated with ketogenic diets. Studies in patients with identical mutations. *Neurology.* 1997;49(6):1655–1661

62. Leen WG, Klepper J, Verbeek MM, et al. Glucose transporter-1 deficiency syndrome: the expanding clinical and genetic spectrum of a treatable disorder. *Brain.* 2010;133(Pt 3):655–670

63. Klepper J. Glucose transporter deficiency syndrome (GLUT1DS) and the ketogenic diet. *Epilepsia.* 2008;49(Suppl 8):46–49

64. Barañano KW, Hartman AL. The ketogenic diet: uses in epilepsy and other neurologic illnesses. *Curr Treat Options Neurol.* 2008;10(6):410–419

65. Yaroslavsky Y, Stahl Z, Belmaker RH. Ketogenic diet in bipolar illness. *Bipolar Disord.* 2002;4(1):75

66. Barbanti P, Fofi L, Aurilia C, Egeo G, Caprio M. Ketogenic diet in migraine: rationale, findings and perspectives. *Neurol Sci.* 2017;38:111–115

67. Scholl-Bürgi S, Höller A, Pichler K, Michel M, Haberlandt E, Karall D. Ketogenic diets in patients with inherited metabolic disorders. *J Inherit Metab Dis.* 2015;38(4):765–773

68. Yancy WS, Foy M, Chalecki AM, Vernon MC, Westman EC. A low-carbohydrate, ketogenic diet to treat type 2 diabetes. *Nutr Metab (Lond).* 2005;2:34

VI

69. Moreno B, Bellido D, Sajoux I, et al. Comparison of a very low-calorie-ketogenic diet with a standard low-calorie diet in the treatment of obesity. *Endocrine.* 2014;47(3):793–805

70. Branco AF, Ferreira A, Simões RF, et al. Ketogenic diets: from cancer to mitochondrial diseases and beyond. *Eur J Clin Invest.* 2016;46(3):285–298

71. Seyfried TN, Kiebish MA, Marsh J, Shelton LM, Huysentruyt LC, Mukherjee P. Metabolic management of brain cancer. *Biochim Biophys Acta.* 2011;1807(6): 577–594

72. Chung H, Y., Park YK. Rationale, feasibility and acceptability of ketogenic diet for cancer treatment. *J Cancer Prev.* 2017;22(3):127–134

73. Bergqvist AG, Schall JI, Gallagher PR, Cnaan A, Stallings VA. Fasting versus gradual initiation of the ketogenic diet: a prospective, randomized clinical trial of efficacy. *Epilepsia.* 2005;46(11):1810–1819

74. Kossoff EH, Turner Z, Bluml RM, Pyzik PL, Vining EPG. A randomized, crossover comparison of daily carbohydrate limits using the modified Atkins diet. *Epilepsy Behav.* 2007;10(3):432–436

75. Seo JH, Lee YM, Lee JS, Kang HC, Kim HC. Efficacy and tolerability of the ketogenic diet according to lipid: nonlipid ratios—comparison of 3:1 with 4:1 diet. *Epilepsia.* 2007;48(4):801–805

76. Neal EG, Chaffe H, Schwartz RH, et al. A randomized trial of classical and medium-chain triglyceride ketogenic diets in the treatment of childhood epilepsy. *Epilepsia.* 2009;50(5):1109–1117

77. Raju KN, Gulati S, Kabra M, et al. Efficacy of 4:1 (classic) versus 2.5:1 ketogenic ratio diets in refractory epilepsy in young children: a randomized open labeled study. *Epilepsy Res.* 2011;96(1-2):96–100

78. Sharma S, Sankhyan N, Gulati S, Agarwala A. Use of the modified Atkins diet for treatment of refractory childhood epilepsy: a randomized controlled trial. *Epilepsia.* 2013;54(3):481–486

79. El-Rashidy OF, Nassar MF, Abdel-Hamid IA, et al. Modified Atkins diet vs classic ketogenic formula in intractable epilepsy. *Acta Neurol Scand.* 2013;128(6):402–408

80. Martin K, Jackson CF, Levy RG, Cooper PN. Ketogenic diet and other dietary treatments for epilepsy. *Cochrane Database Syst Rev.* 2016(2):CD001903

81. Lambrechts DA, de Kinderen RJ, Vles JS, de Louw AJ, Aldenkamp AP, Majoie HJ. A randomized controlled trial of the ketogenic diet in refractory childhood epilepsy. *Acta Neurol Scand.* 2017;135(2):231–239

82. Kim JA, Yoon JR, Lee EJ, et al. Efficacy of the classic ketogenic and the modified Atkins diets in refractory childhood epilepsy. *Epilepsia.* 2016;57(1):51–58

83. Hallböök T, Sjölander A, Åmark P, Miranda M, Bjurulf B, Dahlin M. Effectiveness of the ketogenic diet used to treat resistant childhood epilepsy in Scandinavia. *Eur J Paediatr Neurol.* 2015;19(1):29–36

84. Vehmeijer FO, van der Louw EJ, Arts WF, Catsman-Berrevoets CE, Neuteboom RF. Can we predict efficacy of the ketogenic diet in children with refractory epilepsy? *Eur J Paediatr Neurol.* 2015;19(6):701–705

85. Pulsifer MB, Gordon JM, Brandt J, Vining EPG, Freeman JM. Effects of ketogenic diet on development and behavior: preliminary report of a prospective study. *Dev Med Child Neurol.* 2001;43(5):301–306

86. Zhu D, Wang M, Wang J, et al. Ketogenic diet effects on neurobehavioral development of children with intractable epilepsy: a prospective study. *Epilepsy Behav.* 2016;55:87–91

87. IJff DM, Postulart D, Lambrechts DAJE, et al. Cognitive and behavioral impact of the ketogenic diet in children and adolescents with refractory epilepsy: a randomized controlled trial. *Epilepsy Behav.* 2016;60:153–157

88. DeVivo DC, Pagliara AS, Prensky AL. Ketotic hypoglycemia and the ketogenic diet. *Neurology.* 1973;23(6):640–649

89. Heo G, Kim SH, Chang MJ. Effect of ketogenic diet and other dietary therapies on anti-epileptic drug concentrations in patients with epilepsy. *J Clin Pharm Ther.* 2017;42(6):758–764

90. Paul E, Conant KD, Dunne IE, et al. Urolithiasis on the ketogenic diet with concurrent topiramate or zonisamide therapy. *Epilepsy Res.* 2010;90(1-2):151–156

91. Takeoka M, Riviello JJ, Pfeifer H, Thiele EA. Concomitant treatment with topiramate and ketogenic diet in pediatric epilepsy. *Epilepsia.* 2002;43(9):1072–1075

92. Stevens CE, Turner Z, Kossoff EH. Hepatic dysfunction as a complication of combined valproate and ketogenic diet. *Pediatr Neurol.* 2016;54:82–84

93. Lyczkowski DA, Pfeifer HH, Ghosh S, Thiele EA. Safety and tolerability of the ketogenic diet in pediatric epilepsy: effects of valproate combination therapy. *Epilepsia.* 2005;46(9):1533–1538

94. Kang HC, Cheung DE, Kim DW, Kim HD. Early- and late-onset complications of the ketogenic diet for intractable epilepsy. *Epilepsia.* 2004;45(9):1116–1123

95. De Vivo DC, Bohan TP, Coulter DL, et al. L-carnitine supplementation in childhood epilepsy: current perspectives. *Epilepsia.* 1998;39(11):1216–1225

96. Ballaban-Gil K, Callahan C, O'Dell C, Pappo M, Moshé S, Shinnar S. Complications of the ketogenic diet. *Epilepsia.* 1998;39(7):744–748

97. Lin A, Turner Z, Doerrer SC, Stanfield A, Kossoff EH. Complications during ketogenic diet initiation: prevalence, treatment, and influence on seizure outcomes. *Pediatr Neurol.* 2017;68:35–39

98. Woody RC, Steele RW, Knapple WL, Pilkington NS. Impaired neutrophil function in children with seizures treated with the ketogenic diet. *J Pediatr.* 1989;115(3):427–430

99. Cai QY, Zhou ZJ, Luo R, et al. Safety and tolerability of the ketogenic diet used for the treatment of refractory childhood epilepsy: a systematic review of published prospective studies. *World J Pediatr.* 2017;13(6):528–536

100. Stewart WA, Gordon K, Camfield P. Acute pancreatitis causing death in a child on the ketogenic diet. *J Child Neurol.* 2001;16(9):682

101. Best TH, Franz DN, Gilbert DL, Nelson DP, Epstein MR. Cardiac complications in patients on the ketogenic diet. *Neurology.* 2000;4(12):2328–2330

VI

102. Neal EG, Chaffe HM, Edwards N, Lawson MS, Schwartz RH, Cross JH. Growth of children on classical and medium-chain triglyceride ketogenic diets. *Pediatrics*. 2008;122(2):e334–e340

103. Groesbeck DK, Bluml RM, Kossoff EH. Long-term use of the ketogenic diet in the treatment of epilepsy. *Dev Med Child Neurol*. 2006;48(12):978–981

104. Vining EP, Pyzik P, McGrogan J, et al. Growth of children on the ketogenic diet. *Dev Med Child Neurol*. 2002;44(12):796–802

105. Williams S, Basualdo-Hammond C, Curtis R, Schuller R. Growth retardation in children with epilepsy on the ketogenic diet: a retrospective chart review. *J Am Diet Assoc*. 2002;102(3):405–407

106. Tagliabue A, Bertoli S, Trentani C, Borrelli P, Veggiotti P. Effects of the ketogenic diet on nutritional status, resting energy expenditure, and substrate oxidation in patients with medically refractory epilepsy: a 6-month prospective observational study. *Clin Nutr*. 2012;31(2):246–249

107. Groleau V, Schall JI, Stallings VA, Bergqvist CA. Long-term impact of the ketogenic diet on growth and resting energy expenditure in children with intractable epilepsy. *Dev Med Child Neurol*. 2014;56:898–904

108. Bergqvist AC, Schall JI, Stallings VA, Zemel BS. Progressive bone mineral content loss in children with intractable epilepsy treated with the ketogenic diet. *Am J Clin Nutr*. 2008;88(6):1678–1684

109. Nation J, Humphrey M, MacKay M, Boneh A. Linear growth of children on a ketogenic diet: does the protein-to-energy ratio matter? *J Child Neurol*. 2014;29(11):1496–1501

110. Patel A, Pyzik PL, Turner Z, Rubenstein JE, Kossoff EH. Long-term outcomes of children treated with the ketogenic diet in the past. *Epilepsia*. 2010;51(7):1277–1282

111. Furth SL, Casey JC, Pyzik PL, et al. Risk factors for urolithiasis in children on the ketogenic diet. *Pediatr Neurol*. 2000;15(1-2):125–128

112. Kielb S, Koo HP, Bloom DA, Gaerber GJ. Nephrolithiasis associated with the ketogenic diet. *J Urol*. 2000;164(2):464–466

113. McNally MA, Pyzik PL, Rubenstein JE, Hamdy RF, Kossoff EH. Empiric use of potassium citrate reduces kidney-stone incidence with the ketogenic diet. *Pediatrics*. 2009;124(2):e300–e304

114. Nizamuddin J, Turner Z, Rubenstein JE, Pyzik PL, Kossoff EH. Management and risk factors for dyslipidemia with the ketogenic diet. *J Child Neurol*. 2008;23(7):758–761

115. Kwiterovich PO, Vining EP, Pyzik P, Skolasky R, Freeman JM. Effect of a high-fat ketogenic diet on plasma levels of lipids, lipoproteins, and apolipoproteins in children. *JAMA*. 2003;290:912–920

116. Kapetanakis M, Liuba P, Odermarsky M, Lundgren J, Hallböök T. Effects of ketogenic diet on vascular function. *Eur J Paediatr Neurol*. 2014;18(4):489–494

117. Doksöz Ö, Güzel O, Yılmaz Ü, et al. The short-term effect of ketogenic diet on carotid intima-media thickness and elastic properties of the carotid artery and the aorta in epileptic children. *J Child Neurol.* 2015;30(12):1646–1650

118. Simm PJ, Bicknell-Royle J, Lawrie J, et al. The effect of the ketogenic diet on the developing skeleton. *Epilepsy Res.* 2017;136:62–66

119. Jung DE, Joshi SM, Berg AT. How do you keto? Survey of North American pediatric ketogenic diet centers. *J Child Neurol.* 2015;30(7):868–873

120. Li H, Jauregui JL, Fenton C, Chee CM, Bergqvist AGC. Epilepsy treatment simplified through mobile ketogenic diet planning. *J Mob Technol Med.* 2014;3(2): 11–15

121. Freeman JM, Kossoff EH, Freeman JB, Kelly MT. *The Ketogenic Diet: A Treatment for Children and Others with Epilepsy.* 4th ed. New York, NY: Demos Medical Publishing; 2007

122. Kossoff EH, Laux LC, Blackford R. When do seizures usually improve with the ketogenic diet? *Epilepsia.* 2008;49(2):329–333

123. Kim DW, Kang HC, Park JC, Kim HD. Benefits of the nonfasting ketogenic diet compared with the initial fasting ketogenic diet. *Pediatrics.* 2004;114(6): 1627–1630

124. Wirrell EC, Darwish HZ, Williams-Dyjur C, Blackman M, Lange V. Is a fast necessary when initiating the ketogenic diet? *J Child Neurol.* 2002;17(3):179–182

125. Vaisleib II, Buchhalter JR, Zupanc ML. Ketogenic diet; outpatient initiation, without fluid, or caloric restrictions. *Pediatr Neurol.* 2004;31(3):198–202

126. Soysal E, Gries H, Wray C. Pediatric patients on ketogenic diet undergoing general anesthesia-a medical record review. *J Clin Anesth.* 2016;35:170–175

127. Karvelas G, Lebel D, Carmant L. The carbohydrate and caloric content of drugs [Appendix]. In: Stafstrom CE, Rho JM, eds. *Epilepsy and the Ketogenic Diet.* Totowa, NJ: Humana Press; 2004:311–344

128. McGhee B, Katyal N. Avoid unnecessary drug-related carbohydrates for patients consuming the ketogenic diet. *J Am Diet Assoc.* 2001;101(1):87–101

129. Martinez CC, Pyzik PL, Kossoff EH. Discontinuing the ketogenic diet in seizure-free children: recurrence and risk factors. *Epilepsia.* 2007;48(1):187–190

130. Huttenlocher PR, Wilbourn AJ, Signore JM. Medium-chain triglycerides as a therapy for intractable childhood epilepsy. *Neurology.* 1971;21(11):1097–1103

131. Muzykewicz DA, Lyczkowski DA, Memon N, Conant KD, Pfeifer HH, Thiele EA. Efficacy, safety, and tolerability of the low glycemic index treatment in pediatric epilepsy. *Epilepsia.* 2009;50(5):1118–1126

132. Coppola G, D'Aniello A, Messana T, et al. Low glycemic index diet in children and young adults with refractory epilepsy: first Italian experience. *Seizure.* 2011;20(7):526–528

133. Karimzadeh P, Sedighi M, Beheshti M, Azargashb E, Ghofrani M, Abdollahe-Gorgi F. Low glycemic index treatment in pediatric refractory epilepsy: the first Middle East report. *Seizure.* 2014;23(7):570–572

VI

134. Kim SH, Kang HC, Lee EJ, Lee JS, Kim HD. Low glycemic index treatment in patients with drug-resistant epilepsy. *Brain Dev.* 2017;39(8):687–692

135. Larson AM, Pfeifer HH, Thiele EA. Low glycemic index treatment for epilepsy in tuberous sclerosis complex. *Epilepsy Res.* 2012;99(1-2):180–182

136. Thibert RL, Pfeifer HH, Larson AM, et al. Low glycemic index treatment for seizures in Angelman syndrome. *Epilepsia.* 2012;53(9):1498–1502

137. Grocott OR, Herrington KS, Pfeifer HH, Thiele EA, Thibert RL. Low glycemic index treatment for seizure control in Angelman syndrome: A case series from the Center for Dietary Therapy of Epilepsy at the Massachusetts General Hospital. *Epilepsy Behav.* 2017;68:45–50

138. Kossoff EH, Krauss GL, McGrogan JR, Freeman JM. Efficacy of the Atkins diet as therapy for intractable epilepsy. 61. 2003;12(1789–1791)

139. Kossoff EH, Dorward JL. The modified Atkins diet. *Epilepsia.* 2008;49(Suppl 8): 37–41

140. Kossoff EH, Cervenka MC, Henry BJ, Haney CA, Turner Z. A decade of the modified Atkins diet (2003–2013): results, insights, and future directions. *Epilepsy Behav.* 2013;29(3):437–442

Chapter 48

Diet, Nutrition, and Oral Health

Introduction

Nutrition plays an important role in the development, progression, management, and treatment of oral and dental diseases. Inadequate or inappropriate dietary intake of certain nutritional components can have a direct effect on the hard and soft tissues of the oral cavity, such as in the development and structure of the teeth or the health of the oral mucosa (eg, vitamin B_{12} deficiency causing angular cheilitis and aphthous ulcers). Poor nutrition can also facilitate the development of disease directly, as in dental erosion, or indirectly, as in dental caries. By understanding the role that nutrition plays in oral health and disease, pediatricians can not only be better prepared to prevent and manage dental disease, but also help children and their families manage their own oral health. The first section of this chapter reviews how malnutrition affects dental development and how the teeth of malnourished children are at risk for disease. The second section of this chapter reviews how micronutrient deficiency manifests itself in the mouth and also highlights specific disease states with important oral manifestations. The third and final section reviews the impact that nutrition has on dental caries, the most common chronic disease of childhood[1] and also highlights breastfeeding and obesity in the context of dental caries.

Influence of Protein-Energy Malnutrition on Dental Development and Disease

Protein-energy malnutrition results from inadequate dietary energy (calories) and protein. Protein-energy malnutrition can be primary, when intake of proteins and energy sources is insufficient to support metabolic needs (found mostly in developing countries), or secondary, when associated with serious diseases like AIDS, chronic diarrhea, cancer, chronic kidney failure, Crohn disease, or ulcerative colitis. When protein-energy malnutrition occurs in early childhood, it may have detrimental effects on dental and oral development and is a risk factor for dental caries in the primary and permanent dentition.

The literature regarding the impact of protein-energy malnutrition on the timing of eruption of permanent teeth is limited and inconclusive. Alvarez and colleagues detected accelerated eruption of permanent molars and incisors in their most malnourished children, the wasted and stunted group.[2] Elamin and Liversidge studied the timing of tooth eruption in 2115 subjects aged 2 to 22 years in Khartoum, Sudan.[3] They found no statistical difference in timing of tooth formation between malnourished children and those of normal nutritional status using the World Health Organization z-scores for body mass index for age and height for age. A third study conducted in Haiti noted delayed exfoliation of primary teeth and delayed eruption of permanent teeth in adolescents with early childhood protein-energy malnutrition and current stunting.[4]

Alvarez and colleagues conducted 2 cross-sectional studies as well as a longitudinal study that examined the influence of past and current nutritional status on tooth eruption, exfoliation, and presence of dental caries.[5-7] Their studies confirmed delayed as well as more severe dental caries in the primary dentition, especially in the settings of either acute (wasting) or chronic (stunting) malnutrition. They identified delayed eruption of the primary dentition as the reason for delayed timing of peak caries activity in their malnourished subjects.

Enamel defects are prevalent in children exposed to malnutrition. Sweeney and colleagues examined the maxillary primary incisors of 104 Guatemalan children ages 2 to 7 years recovering in the hospital from third-degree malnutrition.[9] They noted the presence of linear enamel hypoplasia in 73% of the subjects, a finding consistent with protein-energy malnutrition around the time of birth. Caufield et al further described linear enamel hypoplasia and other forms of developmental defects of enamel as markers of perinatal and postnatal stresses on the child, including malnutrition, infections, low birth weight, and other antecedents.[10] Takaoka and others noted that preterm subjects that were small for gestational age, a surrogate for malnourishment, were 7.8 times more likely to have enamel defects compared with other children who were born preterm.[8]

The presence of enamel defects in malnourished children and others are clinically significant. Numerous studies, including a 2017 systematic review and meta-analysis by Costa and colleagues, have shown that enamel defects increase the dental caries risk in the primary dentition and are associated with severe early childhood caries.[10-16] The presence of malnutrition in early childhood should raise the clinician's suspicion that enamel defects could be present and the child's caries risk is elevated (see Chapter 10: Pediatric Global Nutrition, and Chapter 26: Malnutrition, Failure to Thrive).

Reduced salivary flow in malnourished children may predispose them to dental caries. Psoter and colleagues reported significantly reduced unstimulated and stimulated salivary flow among 1017 Haitian adolescents

(11–19 years) with a history of protein-energy malnutrition before 6 years of age or with chronic nutritional impairment leading to growth stunting; however, salivary pH did not differ statistically among normal and malnourished groups.[17] Johansson et al studied the salivary flow and dental caries among 68 8- to 12-year-old children in Madras, India.[18] They found that the secretory rate for stimulated saliva decreased as malnutrition was classified as more severe. The number of decayed primary and permanent tooth surfaces was statistically increased in subjects with severe malnutrition as compared with controls and children with less severe stunting.

Dental and Oral Manifestations of Micronutrient Deficiency

In recent years, interest in the relationship between malnutrition and severe early childhood caries (S-ECC) has increased as society's dietary habits have changed. Many children with S-ECC are malnourished when anthropometric data is investigated. Furthermore, micronutrients including iron and vitamin D maybe depleted in these children. Nonetheless, few studies in North America have specifically examined malnutrition and micronutrient deficiency in children with S-ECC.

In 2006, Clarke and colleagues examined the nutritional status of 46 Canadian children (median age, 3.8 years) with S-ECC when they presented to hospital for comprehensive dental surgery under general anesthesia.[19] The team, using body weight percentiles, identified 17% of the children as malnourished. Twenty-four percent of the subjects had low (less than 10th percentile) body fat as well. The subjects' serum chemistries were especially notable, including low serum albumin (16%) and low serum ferritin (80%) concentrations. Eleven percent of the children with S-ECC had iron-deficiency anemia. This finding was confirmed in a 2013 study by Schroth and colleagues who conducted a case-control study comparing the iron status of 144 children with S-ECC to a group of 122 caries-free, healthy children in Winnipeg, Canada.[20] Children with S-ECC were found to have lower mean hemoglobin levels ($P <.001$), low ferritin ($P = .033$), and a significantly greater likelihood of having iron-deficiency anemia (adjusted odds ratio [OR], 6.58; 95% confidence interval [CI], 1.01–2.76; $P <.0001$). Low levels of vitamin D and calcium with elevated serum parathyroid hormone have also been observed in children with S-ECC as compared with a control group.[21]

Vitamins A and D have been also identified as important nutrients for normal tooth development (ie, without enamel hypoplasia).[22,23] Schroth et al examined the relationship between 25-hydroxyvitamin D (25-OH-D) levels in pregnant mothers and subsequent S-ECC and enamel hypoplasia in aboriginal Canadian infants at 1 year of age.[24] Enamel hypoplasia and S-ECC were detected in 22% and 36% of the infants, respectively. Mothers of infants with S-ECC had significantly lower prenatal 25-OH-D levels (41 ± 20 vs 52 ± 27 nmol/L; $P = .05$) than those with caries-free infants. Enamel hypoplasia ($P < .001$) and lower prenatal 25-OH-D levels ($P = .02$) were significantly associated with S-ECC in logistic regression analyses.

The relationship between 25-OH-D levels in children and dental caries has been examined in several recent investigations. Hujoel conducted a systematic review of controlled clinical trials to determine the role of vitamin D on prevention of dental caries.[25] This review included 2827 children compiled from 24 controlled clinical trials found reduced (OR, 0.53; 95% CI, 0.43–0.65) relative rate estimates of caries when supplemental vitamin D was used. Other studies using Canadian and US nationally representative samples have produced mixed results. Using data obtained from the 2007 to 2009 Canadian Health Measures Survey, Schroth and colleagues studied the interaction between measured levels of 25-OH-D and caries detected on dentist-conducted dental examination in 1017 children between the ages of 6 and 11 years.[26] Dental caries were present in 56% of the children. Children with 25-OH-D concentrations of ≥75 nmol/L and between 50 nmol/L but less than 75 nmol/L had lower odds of having dental caries, a 47% and 39% decrease, respectively. In contrast, 2005–2006 National Health and Nutrition Examination Survey data failed to show an association between serum 25-OH-D levels and dental caries in 5- to 12-year-old United States school children.[27]

The soft tissues of the oral cavity and perioral tissues are also sensitive to vitamin and mineral deficiency secondary to inadequate dietary intake or malabsorption. Angular cheilitis, mucosal atrophy, and glossitis are associated findings in the setting of nutrient deficiency.[28] In adults, taste disturbances and oral burning mouth sensitivity have been reported in cases of vitamin B_1, vitamin B_6, and zinc deficiency.[28, 29] In the pediatric population, inadequate iron, folate, zinc, magnesium, vitamin C, and vitamins B_1, B_2, B_6, and B_{12} should be explored when recurrent oral ulcerations are noted on history or physical examination.[30, 31] Vitamin C deficiency presenting clinically as scurvy should be considered when gingival bleeding, gingival overgrowth, and gingivitis are noted in children with concurrent musculoskeletal pain and weakness.[32–34] For patients with cobalamin (B_{12}) deficiency, the use of nitrous oxide—oxygen inhalation analgesia, is contraindicated because it may exacerbate the methionine synthase dysfunction.[35,36]

Oral Manifestations in Celiac Disease

Celiac disease, an immune-mediated, gluten-induced enteropathy, produces diet-modified effects to developing teeth and the oral mucosa (see Chapter 27: Chronic Diarrheal Disease). Aine reported that patients with celiac disease developed symmetric, specific types of developmental defects of enamel in all 4 quadrants of the dentition that are associated with exposure to dietary gluten.[37] Numerous studies have corroborated these findings and have shown that later developing primary teeth (ie, second primary molars) and earlier developing permanent teeth (ie, permanent incisors) have a higher prevalence of developmental defects of enamel, likely because of dietary gluten exposure.[38-42]

Developmental defects of enamel have been shown to be less common, or present in reduced severity, in later-developing permanent teeth if celiac disease is diagnosed and a strict gluten-free diet is established.[39,42] The etiology of developmental defects of enamel seen in celiac disease is unknown. Preliminary studies have explored the impact of abnormal calcium malabsorption and the cross-reactivity of celiac disease antibodies (eg, anti-gliadin immunoglobulin G) with enamel proteins during amelogenesis.[39,42,43] Despite widespread developmental defects of enamel and reports of reduced salivary flow in patients with celiac disease, the prevalence and severity of dental caries is reduced compared with matched control populations.[39,40]

Recurrent oral aphthous ulcerations are also seen more frequently in children with celiac disease. A 2008 study by Campisi and colleagues compared 269 children with serologically and histologically confirmed celiac disease to 575 clinical healthy subjects for the presence of positive history of aphthous ulcerations.[44] Twenty-three percent of celiac disease subjects had aphthous like ulcerations as compared with 7.1% in the control group. Among the celiac disease group with aphthous like ulcerations, roughly 80% saw improvement or complete resolution of their ulcerations after 1 year of strict adherence to a gluten-free diet. Several other investigators have reported recurrent aphthous stomatitis to resolve in the setting of a gluten-free diet.[38,45]

In light of these findings, it is important for pediatricians to examine the dentition of patients with celiac disease for signs and symptoms of developmental defects of enamel and recurrent aphthous stomatitis. In some cases, referral to a dentist may even lead to the diagnosis of celiac disease and the introduction of a strict gluten-free diet.

VI

Children Fed Exclusively Via Gastrostomy Tube

Children fed exclusively via gastrostomy tube because of oral-motor dysfunction and neurologic abnormalities that make oral feeding unsafe highlight the importance of route of nutrition on oral microflora and the development of dental caries. These children are generally unlikely to have dental caries because they do not have oral exposure to fermentable carbohydrates, a necessary component of the dental caries process. Two landmark studies by Littleton and colleagues found that the dental plaque of people nourished by stomach tube was less acidogenic, responded with minimal pH decline after sucrose, glucose, or fructose exposure, and was colonized by fewer acid-producing streptococci and lactobacilli, the primary bacteria responsible for dental caries.[46,47] The decline in pH noted in these plaque samples did not reach the critical pH of 5.5 needing for acid dissolution of tooth structure. Furthermore, they concluded that the amount of food entering the mouth via emesis after exclusive tube feeding was inadequate to change the acidogenic properties of the dental plaque.[46,47] In contrast, patients transitioned from stomach tube to oral feeding regained acidogenic plaque as quickly as 1 week after introducing frequent oral fermentable carbohydrate exposures.[46] More recently, Hidas and coworkers found similar results when studying 12 gastrostomy tube fed children as compared with 17 healthy children and 16 children with disabilities fed orally.[48] They reported that children fed via gastrostomy tube were all free of dental caries and had significantly reduced levels of *Streptococci mutans* and lactobacilli as compared with the control groups.

In clinical practice, children fed exclusively by gastrostomy tube differ in their risk for dental caries when compared with children who utilize a feeding tube supportively. In this more common approach to enteral nutrition, regular oral intake of patient tolerated fermentable carbohydrates is encouraged for oral-motor development, taste stimulation, and patient comfort but is supplemented by tube feedings to ensure adequate nutritional intake. Published studies on the influence of supportive tube feeding on dental caries are currently unavailable. Empirically, children with supportive tube feeding behaviors can develop dental caries, especially when development defects of enamel are present, oral hygiene is poor, and fermentable carbohydrates that adhere to teeth are introduced with regularity with prolonged oral clearance times.

Children With End-Stage Renal Disease

Another clinical example of diet intersecting with chronic systemic disease is the child with chronic renal failure (see Chapter 40: Renal Disease). These children commonly present with enamel hypoplasia, poor oral hygiene, increased dental plaque accumulations, and gingivitis.[49–51] The need for a protein-sparing diet compensated calorically with refined carbohydrates and sugar-sweetened beverages can cause rapid development of dental caries in these children. Multiple studies, however, have reported low rates of dental caries in this population attributable to high salivary pH from elevated salivary urea nitrogen concentrations, a by-product of systemic uremia.[49, 51, 52] In these children, sugar exposure reduces salivary pH in comparable magnitude to healthy children, but the more alkaline baseline pH prevents the dental plaque and saliva from reaching pH 5.5, the critical pH needed for development and progression of dental caries.[53]

As kidney function returns to normal and uremia resolves after transplant, salivary pH normalizes as well.[54] As a result, the risk of dental caries increases substantially after transplant because of the interaction of well-established cariogenic dietary habits, poor oral hygiene behaviors, and presence of teeth weakened by enamel hypoplasia. It is, therefore, important that patients with chronic renal failure are followed closely by their dentists in anticipation of these changes in oral health status and to reinforce appropriate dietary and oral hygiene behaviors before, during, and after kidney transplant.

Nutritional Influences on Dental Caries

Dental caries (commonly referred to as tooth decay) is a multifactorial, diet-dependent, fluoride mediated, transmissible infectious disease. It is the most common chronic disease of childhood.[1] Approximately 23% of US children 2 to 5 years of age, 21% of those 6 to 11 years of age, and 58% of those 12 to 18 years of age experienced caries in 2011–2012.[55] Dental caries occurs when cariogenic bacteria in the dental biofilm (plaque) metabolize fermentable carbohydrates and produce organic acids. These acids dissolve the mineral structure of the tooth enamel and can lead ultimately to cavitation in the tooth enamel.

Dietary sugar consumption is the main driver of dental caries. The primary dietary sugars associated with dental caries are monosaccharides (glucose, galactose, fructose) and disaccharides (sucrose, maltose, lactose). Sugars naturally present in grains, whole fruits, vegetables, and milk are less likely to be associated with dental caries compared with those sugars added to foods and those present in honey, syrups, and fruit juices/concentrates.[56]

When sugars are introduced to the cariogenic bacteria in the biofilm (plaque), the acids produced begin to lower the normally neutral pH of the biofilm, almost immediately. The acids then diffuse through the mineral structure of the tooth and, when the acid reaches a susceptible site in the mineral crystal structure (hydroxyapatite), calcium and phosphate are dissolved. As long as there is sugar available, the demineralization will continue. Once sugar is unavailable to the bacteria, the pH can return to normal with the help of the buffering capacity of saliva. As the pH returns to its normal neutral level, calcium and phosphate, from saliva and within the biofilm, diffuse into the tooth and remineralize the tooth. When fluoride is present during this process, a new crystal structure is formed, fluorapatite, that is much more resistant to demineralization (see below).

The type of sugar is not the only factor that is important for the development of dental caries. The amount ingested and the frequency of ingestion are also important in the development and progression of dental caries.[56,57] As described above, demineralization and remineralization occur in the crystal structure of the tooth, during and between meals that contain sugars.[58] The longer sugars are retained in the mouth and oral clearance is delayed, the longer the periods of acid production and demineralization and the shorter the periods of remineralization. For example, frequent sipping of sugary drinks via a bottle or a sippy cup and sucking on a hard candy or lollipop will decrease the time for remineralization and increase decay. Thus, the frequency of intake of sugars is especially important.[59] Similarly, sweet foods that are sticky like fruit roll ups or starch-sugar combinations like cookies, cakes, and crackers can prolong the exposure of the sugar substrate to the acid-producing bacteria, increasing demineralization and worsening the disease process.

Pediatricians can play an important role in the prevention and management of dental caries by addressing nutritional issues.[60] Pediatricians should advise against the introduction of fruit juice before 12 months of age. When introduced, it should be limited to, at most, 4 oz/day in toddlers 1 through 3 years of age, and 4 to 6 oz/day for children 4 through 6 years of age.[61] For children 7 to 18 years of age, juice intake should be limited to 8 oz or 1 cup of the recommended 2 to 2.5 cups of fruit servings per day. Similarly, pediatricians should discourage routine ingestion of carbohydrate-containing sports drinks by children and adolescents.[62] Pediatricians can also advocate for the reduction in schools and school meals of added sugars in nutrient-poor foods like soft drinks, sugar, and sweets.[63]

It is also important to recognize that some populations of children have poor access to healthy foods, and this puts them at risk for dental caries. Children in low-income families may face challenges in obtaining high-quality, nutritious foods and may suffer from food insecurity.[64, 65] Fifty-four percent of American Indian/Alaska Native children between 1 and 5 years of age have experienced tooth decay.[66] Opportunities exist to promote improvement in the availability of healthy foods to native communities and education to decrease the frequent consumption of sugar-containing drinks and sugary snacks.[67]

Breastfeeding and Dental Caries

The American Academy of Pediatrics recommends exclusive breastfeeding for 4 to 6 months, followed by continued breastfeeding as complementary foods are introduced, with continuation of breastfeeding for 1 year or longer as mutually desired by mother and infant.[68] One cup of human milk has 17 g of sugar, the primary sugar being lactose. An important question, then, is whether breastfeeding is associated with dental caries. The literature has been very contradictory on this question, depending on the duration, timing, and exclusivity of breastfeeding as well as the population studied, methods of breastfeeding assessment, and the intake of complementary foods (see Chapter 3: Breastfeeding).

A meta-analysis of cross-sectional studies showed that breastfed children were less affected by dental caries than formula-fed children.[69] Another systematic review found that children exposed to longer versus shorter duration of breastfeeding—up to age 12 months—had a reduced risk of caries, although children breastfed more than 12 months had an increased risk of caries compared with children breastfed less than 12 months.[70] Among children breastfed >12 months, those fed during the night or more frequently had a further increased caries risk. A longitudinal study from the US found that children who were breastfed less than 6 months were more likely to have dental caries in their first molars than children breastfed at least 6 months. This difference diminished with age.[71] A study from Brazil found that breastfeeding for up to 24 months was associated with elevated risk of dental caries at 38 months compared with breastfeeding for less than 6 months.[72] A study from Japan found that infants who had been breastfed for at least 6 or 7 months, both exclusively and partially, were at elevated risk of dental caries at the age of 30 months compared with those who had been exclusively fed with formula.[73] Most recently, a cohort study from Thailand found that that children who were fully breastfed for 6 to 11 months had a significantly lower risk for dental caries than those who were fully breastfed for less than 6 months.[74]

Despite the variability in the study results mentioned here, it is important to restate the importance of and the support that organizations like the American Academy of Pediatrics, World Health Organization, and others place on exclusive breastfeeding up to 6 months of age.[68] Pediatric health care providers should encourage parents and other caregivers to start proper oral hygiene with children as soon as the first tooth erupts, breastfeeding children included.

Fluoride and Dental Caries

Fluoride is the ionic form of the element fluorine. Fluoride has been shown to reduce dental decay by 3 specific mechanisms: (1) it reduces the solubility of enamel; (2) it reduces the bacteria's ability to produce acid; and (3) it promotes remineralization.[76,77] It is most often found in the diet as sodium fluoride and in the body as calcium fluoride. The most common dietary sources of fluoride in children are fluoridated water and water-based beverages, although it is important to note that many, if not most, foods have some level of natural fluoride in them.[78] Other sources of fluoride include fluoridated toothpaste, fluoride supplements, and topically applied fluorides, like fluoride varnish and gels. When incorporated into the structure of enamel during the remineralization process, fluoride ions adsorb to the crystal surface of the tooth, attracting calcium ions. These then attract phosphate ions and begin to rebuild a fluorapatite crystal surface that is much more resistant to the bacteria-produced acids than the original crystal structure.

In many communities across the United States, public water systems are fluoridated. In 2014, 74.4% of the US population received fluoridated water through their community water systems. This ranged from 99.9% in Kentucky to 11.7% in Hawaii.[79] Community water fluoridation is an effective way to prevent and control dental caries. The current recommended level of fluoride in community water systems is 0.7 ppm.[80] Although the main effect of fluoride is topical, community water fluoridation helps to maintain a low concentration of fluoride in saliva and the biofilm. Pediatricians can advocate for water fluoridation in the local community and can maximize the preventive value of fluoride by assessing a child's exposure to fluoride and determine the need for topical or systemic supplements.[81]

Dental Erosion

Dental erosion is the loss of dental hard tissue and occurs when acids are in direct, sustained contact with the tooth surface. The prevalence of dental erosion in children has been estimated to be between 2% and 80%.[82–84] What makes dental erosion different from the acid-induced dissolving of the crystal structure of the tooth is that the acids are nonbacterial. The acids can come from both extrinsic and intrinsic sources.

In children, acids from external sources come primarily from carbonated soft drinks, fruit juices, sports drinks, and some foods such as fruits. These acids tend to be phosphoric acid and citric acid. The pH of certain beverages can vary from 2.3 to 3.2 in carbonated sodas, 2.7 to 3.0 in sports drinks, to 2.9 to 3.3 in grapefruit juice.[85, 86] The most acidic beverages include some lemon and cranberry fruit juices, certain colas, and sports drinks.[86] Intrinsic acids are also associated with erosion, usually hydrochloric acid from gastric juices. Children who frequently consume carbonated drinks or natural fruit juices have increased odds for tooth erosion.[82] Children who consume acidic snacks or sweets also have higher odds of tooth erosion.[82]

Children with gastroesophageal reflux disease (GERD), bulimia, and asthma are at risk for enamel erosion.[87–89] Erosion in children with GERD and bulimia is caused by exposure to acidic stomach contents. In asthma, erosion is attributable to the reduction in salivary flow caused by prolonged beta-2 agonist use and GERD that can accompany asthma.[87] Children who have decreased salivary flow, decreasing the ability to buffer acids in the mouth, whether induced by medication (ie anticholinergics, antihistamines, tricyclic antidepressants, etc), radiation (cancer therapy) or chronic disease (ie, diabetes, cystic fibrosis, ectodermal dysplasia, Sjogren disease), are also at increased risk for dental erosion.[83, 90, 91] Pediatricians can play a role in the prevention of dental erosion by educating families to limit the frequency of intake of low pH beverages including those with high sugar content, carbonated sodas, and sports energy drinks.[61–63] In addition, pediatricians can be diligent about monitoring for dental erosion in patients with GERD and patients with bulimia.[92,93]

Obesity and Dental Caries

Obesity and dental caries share a key common risk factor—the volume and frequency of intake of sugar-sweetened food and drink. By decreasing both the volume and frequency of sugar intake, it might be possible to decrease the prevalence of each of these diseases. Thus, it is important to understand whether there is an association between obesity and dental caries (see Chapter 33: Pediatric Obesity).

Systematic reviews of the literature on the association between childhood obesity and dental caries have been mixed. An early review found inconclusive evidence of an association between obesity and dental caries and recommended further well-designed studies.[94] A more recent systematic review focused solely on children's BMI and dental caries and found mixed results: 48% of studies reviewed found no association between dental caries and BMI; 35% found a positive association and 19% found an inverse association.[95] The authors suggested there is a nonlinear (U-shaped) association between BMI and dental caries with associations greater at both low and high BMIs. A systematic review and meta-analysis found a small association between obesity and caries in the permanent teeth but no association between obesity and caries in the primary dentition.[96] Finally, a recent systematic review of longitudinal studies concluded that consensus has not been reached on the association between obesity (or any anthropometric measures) and dental caries.[97]

Pediatricians have an important role to play in preventing and addressing childhood obesity and, by doing so, may concurrently have an important impact on preventing dental caries. Pediatricians can encourage caregivers to make healthy foods accessible, encourage the drinking of water, and limit the availability of sweetened beverages and other foods containing refined carbohydrates.[98,99] Also, as mentioned previously, they can advocate for healthy foods and drinks in school and at out-of-school events.[62,63]

References

1. National Institutes of Dental and Craniofacial Research, National Institutes of Health. Oral Health in America: A Report of the Surgeon General. Rockville, MD: U.S. Department of Health and Human Services; 2000

2. Alvarez JO. Nutrition, tooth development, and dental caries. *Am J Clin Nutr.* 1995;61(2):410S–416S

3. Elamin F, Liversidge HM. Malnutrition has no effect on the timing of human tooth formation. *PLoS One.* 2013;8(8):e72274

4. Psoter W, Gebrian B, Prophete S, Reid B, Katz R. Effect of early childhood malnutrition on tooth eruption in Haitian adolescents. *Community Dent Oral Epidemiol.* 2008;36(2):179–189

5. Alvarez JO, Caceda J, Woolley TW, Carley KW, Baiocchi N, Caravedo L, et al. A longitudinal study of dental caries in the primary teeth of children who suffered from infant malnutrition. *J Dent Res.* 1993;72(12):1573–1576

6. Alvarez JO, Eguren JC, Caceda J, Navia JM. The effect of nutritional status on the age distribution of dental caries in the primary teeth. *J Dent Res.* 1990;69(9): 1564–1566

7. Alvarez JO, Lewis CA, Saman C, Caceda J, Montalvo J, Figueroa ML, et al. Chronic malnutrition, dental caries, and tooth exfoliation in Peruvian children aged 3-9 years. *Am J Clin Nutr.* 1988;48(2):368–372

8. Takaoka LA, Goulart AL, Kopelman BI, Weiler RM. Enamel defects in the complete primary dentition of children born at term and preterm. *Pediatr Dent.* 2011;33(2):171–176

9. Sweeney EA, Saffir AJ, De Leon R. Linear hypoplasia of deciduous incisor teeth in malnourished children. *Am J Clin Nutr.* 1971;24(1):29–31

10. Caufield PW, Li Y, Bromage TG. Hypoplasia-associated severe early childhood caries—a proposed definition. *J Dent Res.* 2012;91(6):544–550

11. Costa FS, Silveira ER, Pinto GS, Nascimento GG, Thomson WM, Demarco FF. Developmental defects of enamel and dental caries in the primary dentition: A systematic review and meta-analysis. *J Dent.* 2017;60:1–7

12. American Academy of Pediatric Dentistry. Guideline on caries-risk assessment and management for infants, children, and adolescents. In: *Reference Manual.* 2016–2017. p. 142–149

13. Hong L, Levy SM, Warren JJ, Broffitt B. Association between enamel hypoplasia and dental caries in primary second molars: a cohort study. *Caries Res.* 2009;43(5):345–353

14. Oliveira AF, Chaves AM, Rosenblatt A. The influence of enamel defects on the development of early childhood caries in a population with low socioeconomic status: a longitudinal study. *Caries Res.* 2006;40(4):296–302

15. Seow WK, Clifford H, Battistutta D, Morawska A, Holcombe T. Case-control study of early childhood caries in Australia. *Caries Res.* 2009;43(1):25–35

16. Targino AG, Rosenblatt A, Oliveira AF, Chaves AM, Santos VE. The relationship of enamel defects and caries: a cohort study. *Oral Dis.* 2011;17(4):420–426

17. Psoter WJ, Spielman AL, Gebrian B, St Jean R, Katz RV. Effect of childhood malnutrition on salivary flow and pH. *Arch Oral Biol.* 2008;53(3):231–237

18. Johansson I, Saellstrom AK, Rajan BP, Parameswaran A. Salivary flow and dental caries in Indian children suffering from chronic malnutrition. *Caries Res.* 1992;26(1):38–43

19. Clarke M, Locker D, Berall G, Pencharz P, Kenny DJ, Judd P. Malnourishment in a population of young children with severe early childhood caries. *Pediatr Dent.* 2006;28(3):254–259

20. Schroth RJ, Levi J, Kliewer E, Friel J, Moffatt ME. Association between iron status, iron deficiency anaemia, and severe early childhood caries: a case-control study. *BMC Pediatr.* 2013;13:22

21. Schroth RJ, Levi JA, Sellers EA, Friel J, Kliewer E, Moffatt ME. Vitamin D status of children with severe early childhood caries: a case-control study. *BMC Pediatr.* 2013;13:174

22. Baume LJ, Franquin JC, Korner WW. The prenatal effects of maternal vitamin A deficiency on the cranial and dental development of the progeny. *Am J Orthod.* 1972;62(5):447–460

VI

23. Berdal A, Hotton D, Pike JW, Mathieu H, Dupret JM. Cell- and stage-specific expression of vitamin D receptor and calbindin genes in rat incisor: regulation by 1,25-dihydroxyvitamin D3. *Dev Biol.* 1993;155(1):172–179

24. Schroth RJ, Lavelle C, Tate R, Bruce S, Billings RJ, Moffatt ME. Prenatal vitamin D and dental caries in infants. *Pediatrics.* 2014;133(5):e1277–1284

25. Hujoel PP. Vitamin D and dental caries in controlled clinical trials: systematic review and meta-analysis. *Nutr Rev.* 2013;71(2):88–97

26. Schroth RJ, Rabbani R, Loewen G, Moffatt ME. Vitamin D and dental caries in children. *J Dent Res.* 2016;95(2):173–179

27. Herzog K, Scott JM, Hujoel P, Seminario AL. Association of vitamin D and dental caries in children: Findings from the National Health and Nutrition Examination Survey, 2005–2006. *J Am Dent Assoc.* 2016;147(6):413–420

28. Moynihan P, Cappelli DP, Mobley C. Oral consequences of compromised nutritional well-being. In: Touger-Decker R, Mobley M, Epstein JB, editors. *Nutrition and Oral Medicine.* New York: Springer Science+Business Media; 2014

29. Liu YF, Kim Y, Yoo T, Han P, Inman JC. Burning mouth syndrome: a systematic review of treatments. *Oral Dis.* 2017

30. Akintoye SO, Greenberg MS. Recurrent aphthous stomatitis. *Dent Clin North Am.* 2014;58(2):281–297

31. Le Doare K, Hullah E, Challacombe S, Menson E. Fifteen-minute consultation: a structured approach to the management of recurrent oral ulceration in a child. *Arch Dis Child Educ Pract Ed.* 2014;99(3):82–86

32. Akikusa JD, Garrick D, Nash MC. Scurvy: forgotten but not gone. *J Paediatr Child Health.* 2003;39(1):75–77

33. Bacci C, Sivolella S, Pellegrini J, Favero L, Berengo M. A rare case of scurvy in an otherwise healthy child: diagnosis through oral signs. *Pediatr Dent.* 2010;32(7): 536–538

34. Weinstein M, Babyn P, Zlotkin S. An orange a day keeps the doctor away: scurvy in the year 2000. *Pediatrics.* 2001;108(3):E55

35. American Academy of Pediatric Dentistry. Guideline on use of nitrous oxide for pediatric dental patients. In: *Reference Manual;* 2016–2017. p. 211–215

36. Sanders RD, Weimann J, Maze M. Biologic effects of nitrous oxide: a mechanistic and toxicologic review. *Anesthesiology.* 2008;109(4):707–722

37. Aine L. Dental enamel defects and dental maturity in children and adolescents with coeliac disease. *Proc Finn Dent Soc.* 1986;82 Suppl 3:1–71

38. Bucci P, Carile F, Sangianantoni A, D'Angio F, Santarelli A, Lo Muzio L. Oral aphthous ulcers and dental enamel defects in children with coeliac disease. *Acta Paediatr.* 2006;95(2):203–207

39. de Carvalho FK, de Queiroz AM, Bezerra da Silva RA, Sawamura R, Bachmann L, Bezerra da Silva LA, et al. Oral aspects in celiac disease children: clinical and dental enamel chemical evaluation. *Oral Surg Oral Med Oral Pathol Oral Radiol.* 2015;119(6):636–643

40. Priovolou CH, Vanderas AP, Papagiannoulis L. A comparative study on the prevalence of enamel defects and dental caries in children and adolescents with and without coeliac disease. *Eur J Paediatr Dent*. 2004;5(2):102–106

41. Shteyer E, Berson T, Lachmanovitz O, Hidas A, Wilschanski M, Menachem M, et al. Oral health status and salivary properties in relation to gluten-free diet in children with celiac disease. *J Pediatr Gastroenterol Nutr*. 2013;57(1):49–52

42. Wierink CD, van Diermen DE, Aartman IH, Heymans HS. Dental enamel defects in children with coeliac disease. *Int J Paediatr Dent*. 2007;17(3):163–168

43. Sonora C, Arbildi P, Rodriguez-Camejo C, Beovide V, Marco A, Hernandez A. Enamel organ proteins as targets for antibodies in celiac disease: implications for oral health. *Eur J Oral Sci*. 2016;124(1):11–16

44. Campisi G, Di Liberto C, Carroccio A, Compilato D, Iacono G, Procaccini M, et al. Coeliac disease: oral ulcer prevalence, assessment of risk and association with gluten-free diet in children. *Dig Liver Dis*. 2008;40(2):104–107

45. Olszewska M, Sulej J, Kotowski B. Frequency and prognostic value of IgA and IgG endomysial antibodies in recurrent aphthous stomatitis. *Acta Derm Venereol*. 2006;86(4):332–334

46. Littleton NW, Carter CH, Kelley RT. Studies of oral health in persons nourished by stomach tube. I. Changes in the pH of plaque material after the addition of sucrose. *J Am Dent Assoc*. 1967;74(1):119–123

47. Littleton NW, McCabe RM, Carter CH. Studies of oral health in persons nourished by stomach tube. II. Acidogenic properties and selected bacterial components of plaque material. *Arch Oral Biol*. 1967;12(5):601–609

48. Hidas A, Cohen J, Beeri M, Shapira J, Steinberg D, Moskovitz M. Salivary bacteria and oral health status in children with disabilities fed through gastrostomy. *Int J Paediatr Dent*. 2010;20(3):179–185

49. Al-Nowaiser A, Roberts GJ, Trompeter RS, Wilson M, Lucas VS. Oral health in children with chronic renal failure. *Pediatr Nephrol*. 2003;18(1):39–45

50. Nunn JH, Sharp J, Lambert HJ, Plant ND, Coulthard MG. Oral health in children with renal disease. *Pediatr Nephrol*. 2000;14(10–11):997–1001

51. Wolff A, Stark H, Sarnat H, Binderman I, Eisenstein B, Drukker A. The dental status of children with chronic renal failure. *Int J Pediatr Nephrol*. 1985;6(2): 127–132

52. Andrade MR, Antunes LA, Soares RM, Leao AT, Maia LC, Primo LG. Lower dental caries prevalence associated to chronic kidney disease: a systematic review. *Pediatr Nephrol*. 2014;29(5):771–778

53. Peterson S, Woodhead J, Crall J. Caries resistance in children with chronic renal failure: plaque pH, salivary pH, and salivary composition. *Pediatr Res*. 1985;19(8):796–799

54. Al Nowaiser A, Lucas VS, Wilson M, Roberts GJ, Trompeter RS. Oral health and caries related microflora in children during the first three months following renal transplantation. *Int J Paediatr Dent*. 2004;14(2):118–126

VI

55. Dye BA, Thornton-Evans G, Li X, Iafolla TJ. Dental caries and sealant prevalence in children and adolescents in the United States, 2011–2012. *NCHS Data Brief*. 2015(191):1–8

56. Moynihan P. Sugars and dental caries: Evidence for setting a recommended threshold for intake. *Adv Nutr*. 2016;7(1):149–156

57. Sheiham A, James WP. Diet and dental caries: The pivotal role of free sugars reemphasized. *J Dent Res*. 2015;94(10):1341–1347

58. Featherstone JD. Dental caries: a dynamic disease process. *Aust Dent J*. 2008; 53(3):286–291

59. Marshall TA, Broffitt B, Eichenberger-Gilmore J, Warren JJ, Cunningham MA, Levy SM. The roles of meal, snack, and daily total food and beverage exposures on caries experience in young children. *J Public Health Dent*. 2005;65(3):166–173

60. Maintaining and improving the oral health of young children. *Pediatrics*. 2014; 134(6):1224–1229

61. Heyman MB, Abrams SA. Fruit juice in infants, children, and adolescents: current recommendations. *Pediatrics*. 2017

62. Sports drinks and energy drinks for children and adolescents: are they appropriate? *Pediatrics*. 2011;127(6):1182–1189

63. Snacks, sweetened beverages, added sugars, and schools. *Pediatrics*. 2015;135(3): 575–583

64. Promoting food security for all children. *Pediatrics*. 2015;136(5):e1431–1438

65. Pascoe JM, Wood DL, Duffee JH, Kuo A. Mediators and adverse effects of child poverty in the United States. *Pediatrics*. 2016;137(4)

66. Phipps KR, Ricks TL. The oral health of American Indian and Alaska Native children aged 1-5 years: results of the 2014 IHS oral health survey. In: Service IH, editor. *Indian Health Service data brief*. Rockville, MD; 2015

67. Early childhood caries in indigenous communities. *Pediatrics*. 2011;127(6): 1190–1198

68. Breastfeeding and the use of human milk. *Pediatrics*. 2012;129(3):e827–841

69. Avila WM, Pordeus IA, Paiva SM, Martins CC. Breast and bottle feeding as risk factors for dental caries: A systematic review and meta-analysis. *PLoS One*. 2015;10(11):e0142922

70. Tham R, Bowatte G, Dharmage SC, Tan DJ, Lau MX, Dai X, et al. Breastfeeding and the risk of dental caries: a systematic review and meta-analysis. *Acta Paediatr*. 2015;104(467):62–84

71. Hong L, Levy SM, Warren JJ, Broffitt B. Infant breast-feeding and childhood caries: a nine-year study. *Pediatr Dent*. 2014;36(4):342–347

72. Chaffee BW, Feldens CA, Vitolo MR. Association of long-duration breastfeeding and dental caries estimated with marginal structural models. *Ann Epidemiol*. 2014;24(6):448–454

73. Kato T, Yorifuji T, Yamakawa M, Inoue S, Saito K, Doi H, et al. Association of breastfeeding with early childhood dental caries: Japanese population-based study. *BMJ Open*. 2015;5(3):e006982

74. Nirunsittirat A, Pitiphat W, McKinney CM, DeRouen TA, Chansamak N, Angwaravong O, et al. Breastfeeding duration and childhood caries: A cohort study. *Caries Res.* 2016;50(5):498–507

75. Kramer MS, Kakuma R. Optimal duration of exclusive breastfeeding. *Cochrane Database Syst Rev.* 2012(8):CD003517

76. Featherstone JD. Prevention and reversal of dental caries: role of low level fluoride. *Community Dent Oral Epidemiol.* 1999;27(1):31–40

77. Hamilton IR. Biochemical effects of fluoride on oral bacteria. *J Dent Res.* 1990;69 Spec No:660–667; discussion 682–663

78. Nutrient Data Laboratory, Agricultural Research Service, U.S. Department of Agriculture. USDA national fluoride database of selected beverages and foods, release 2. Beltsville, MD; 2005

79. Centers for Disease Control and Prevention Division of Oral Health. Community water fluoridation. https://www.cdc.gov/fluoridation/statistics/2014stats.htm. Published 2016. Updated August 19, 2016. Accessed June 4, 2017

80. United States Department of Health and Human Services Federal Panel on Community Water Fluoridation. U.S. Public Health Service recommendation for fluoride concentration in drinking water for the prevention of dental caries. *Public Health Rep.* 2015;130(4):318–331

81. Clark MB, Slayton RL. Fluoride use in caries prevention in the primary care setting. *Pediatrics.* 2014;134(3):626–633

82. Salas MM, Nascimento GG, Vargas-Ferreira F, Tarquinio SB, Huysmans MC, Demarco FF. Diet influenced tooth erosion prevalence in children and adolescents: Results of a meta-analysis and meta-regression. *J Dent.* 2015;43(8):865–875

83. Taji S, Seow WK. A literature review of dental erosion in children. *Aust Dent J.* 2010;55(4):358–367

84. Habib M, Hottel TL, Hong L. Prevalence and risk factors of dental erosion in American children. *J Clin Pediatr Dent.* 2013;38(2):143–148

85. Gravelle BL, Hagen Ii TW, Mayhew SL, Crumpton B, Sanders T, Horne V. Soft drinks and in vitro dental erosion. *Gen Dent.* 2015;63(4):33–38

86. Reddy A, Norris DF, Momeni SS, Waldo B, Ruby JD. The pH of beverages available to the American Consumer *J Am Dent Assoc.* 2016;147(4):255–263

87. Harrington N, Prado N, Barry S. Dental treatment in children with asthma - a review. *Br Dent J.* 2016;220(6):299–302

88. Hermont AP, Pordeus IA, Paiva SM, Abreu MH, Auad SM. Eating disorder risk behavior and dental implications among adolescents. *Int J Eat Disord.* 2013;46(7):677–683

89. Mantegazza C, Angiero F, Zuccotti GV. Oral manifestations of gastrointestinal diseases in children. Part 3: Ulcerative colitis and gastro-oesophageal reflux disease. *Eur J Paediatr Dent.* 2016;17(3):248–250

90. Carvalho TS, Lussi A, Jaeggi T, Gambon DL. Erosive tooth wear in children. *Monogr Oral Sci.* 2014;25:262–278

VI

91. Linnett V, Seow WK. Dental erosion in children: a literature review. *Pediatr Dent.* 2001;23(1):37–43

92. Lightdale JR, Gremse DA. Gastroesophageal reflux: management guidance for the pediatrician. *Pediatrics.* 2013;131(5):e1684–1695

93. Rosen DS. Identification and management of eating disorders in children and adolescents. *Pediatrics.* 2010;126(6):1240–1253

94. Kantovitz KR, Pascon FM, Rontani RM, Gaviao MB. Obesity and dental caries—A systematic review. *Oral Health Prev Dent.* 2006;4(2):137–144

95. Hooley M, Skouteris H, Boganin C, Satur J, Kilpatrick N. Body mass index and dental caries in children and adolescents: a systematic review of literature published 2004 to 2011. *Syst Rev.* 2012;1:57

96. Hayden C, Bowler JO, Chambers S, Freeman R, Humphris G, Richards D, et al. Obesity and dental caries in children: a systematic review and meta-analysis. *Community Dent Oral Epidemiol.* 2013;41(4):289–308

97. Li LW, Wong HM, Peng SM, McGrath CP. Anthropometric measurements and dental caries in children: a systematic review of longitudinal studies. *Adv Nutr.* 2015;6(1):52–63

98. Golden NH, Schneider M, Wood C. Preventing obesity and eating disorders in adolescents. *Pediatrics.* 2016;138(3)

99. Daniels SR, Hassink SG. The role of the pediatrician in primary prevention of obesity. *Pediatrics.* 2015;136(1):e275–292

Nutrition and Public Health

Chapter 49

Preventing Food Insecurity—Available Community Nutrition Programs

The need for providers to become familiar with their local nutrition resources came into sharper focus when the American Academy of Pediatrics (AAP) published its policy statement on food insecurity in 2015.[1] A food-insecure household is one in which the "access to adequate food is limited by lack of money or other resources."[2,3] Rates of food insecurity in the United States vary year by year, but in most years, approximately one fifth of children are food insecure. Families living below the poverty level are not the only food-insecure US families; children of immigrant families, large families, and those headed by a single woman or experiencing parental separation or divorce are at greater risk.[3-5]

Food insecurity is an important risk factor for increased childhood illness, increased rates of hospitalization, developmental problems, dysregulated behavior, and reduced academic achievement.[6,7] Adolescents in food-insecure families are more likely to experience dysthymia and suicidal ideation.[8] Food insecurity is also associated with obesity.[9,10] Importantly, the health effects of food insecurity may persist beyond childhood, increasing the risk of diabetes, hyperlipidemia, and cardiovascular disease in adults.[11,12]

Because of the substantial impact of food insecurity on children and adults and the fact that it is not limited to traditional underserved neighborhoods, the AAP developed recommendations for screening at each annual health care visit using the Hunger Vital Sign to identify food insecurity.[13,14] The AAP recommendations are found in Table 49.1, and the Hunger Vital sign is found in Table 49.2.

The following chapter sections summarize the available community nutrition programs that provide food and nutrition assistance to children and their families.

Introduction

Promoting the nutritional health and wellness of children and their families is a common goal of the nutrition services offered by a wide variety of public and private agencies, organizations, and individuals in communities across the nation. These include federal government agencies; state health and education departments; local health agencies, such as city and county health departments; community health centers; health maintenance and preferred

Table 49.1.
Recommendations for Pediatricians[12]

Practice Level
1. A 2-question validated screening tool (Table 49.2) is recommended for pediatricians screening for food insecurity at scheduled health maintenance visits or sooner if indicated.
2. It is beneficial for pediatricians to familiarize themselves with community resources so that when children screen positively for food insecurity, referral mechanisms to WIC, SNAP, school nutrition programs, local food pantries, summer and child care feeding programs, and other relevant resources are accessible and expedient.
3. When advocating for programs targeted at families with food insecurity, it is important that pediatricians be aware of the nutritional content of food offered in supplemental programs.
4. In the office setting, pediatricians who are aware of the factors that may increase vulnerability of food-insecure populations to obesity and factors that disproportionately burden food-insecure households may address these issues at clinic visits.

System Level
1. Food insecurity, including screening tools and community-specific resource guides, can be incorporated into education of medical students and residents, to prepare future generations of physicians to universally screen for and address food insecurity.
2. Pediatricians can advocate for protecting and increasing access to and funding for SNAP, WIC, school nutrition programs, and summer feeding programs at the local, state, and national levels. Advocacy must also include keeping the food offered in these programs high in nutrient quality and based on sound nutritional science.
3. Pediatricians can strongly support interdisciplinary research that elucidates the relationship between stress, food insecurity, and adverse health consequences, the barriers to breastfeeding for women under stress in food-insecure households; and evidence-based strategies that optimize access to high-quality, nutritious food for families facing food insecurity.

provider organizations; hospital and ambulatory outpatient clinics; nutritionists and dietitians in public and private practice; voluntary health agencies, such as the American Diabetes Association and the American Heart Association; social service agencies; elementary and secondary schools; colleges and universities; and business and industry.

Table 49.2.
Screening for Food Security

For each statement, ask if it is "often true," "sometimes true," or "never true":
1. Within the past 12 months, we worried whether our food would run out before we had money to buy more.
2. Within the past 12 months, the food we bought just didn't last and we didn't have money to get more.

Adapted from Hager et al.[14] Although an affirmative response to both questions increases the likelihood of food insecurity existing in the household, an affirmative response to only 1 question is often an indication of food insecurity and should precipitate further questioning.

Nutrition Services Provided Through Federal, State, and Local Health and Nutrition Agencies

Each year, Congress appropriates funds for a variety of nutrition and health programs, many of which are targeted to low-income mothers and their children and families. Such programs are administered at the national level by the US Department of Agriculture (USDA) and the US Department of Health and Human Services (DHHS). USDA services include Child Nutrition Programs (National School Lunch Program, School Breakfast Program, Special Milk Program, Summer Food Service Program, Fresh Fruit and Vegetable Program, and the Child and Adult Care Food Program); the Special Supplemental Nutrition Program for Women, Infants, and Children (WIC); the Supplemental Nutrition Assistance Program (SNAP; formerly known as the Food Stamp Program); the Emergency Food Assistance Program; and the Food Distribution Program on Indian Reservations. Services of the DHHS include maternal and child health services block grant programs; preventive health services block grant programs; Early and Periodic Screening, Diagnostic, and Treatment (EPSDT) services under Medicaid; Indian Health Services, and programs from the Centers for Disease Control and Prevention (CDC). There are also programs such as community health centers and migrant health projects that serve at-risk populations.[15]

In addition to federal support, considerable state and local funds also support child health programs. An example of a local resource is community-based food programs that are nonprofit, nongovernmental, grass-roots, self-help community developmental programs. One such resource is Feeding America (formerly known as America's Second Harvest),

VII

which coordinates a vast network of local food pantries and meal programs across the country. Many of these food programs are tied to other services that low-income mothers and children may need.

Physicians and other primary health care professionals should be knowledgeable about local food and nutrition programs so they can assist families to become informed consumers and appropriate referrals can be made. An informed health care professional can also serve as an advocate to strengthen policy and budget decisions that guide the provision of quality, cost-effective nutrition programs focused on improving the health of the nation.

Although nutrition services were introduced into public health programs as early as the late 1920s, Title V of the Social Security Act of 1935 (Pub L No. 74-721) initiated the federal-state partnership for maternal and child health that served as the major impetus for the development of nutrition services for mothers and children.[16] A census of public health nutrition personnel in 1999–2000 showed that approximately 10 904 public health nutritionists are employed in federal, state, and local public health agencies.[17] Public health nutritionists provide a wide range of services related to core public health functions, including assessment, assurance (support to meet nutritional needs), and policy development. Public health nutritionists provide direct clinical services (eg, screening, assessment, nutrition counseling, monitoring); population-based research; development and implementation of nutrition services and policies that focus on disease prevention and health promotion; provision of technical assistance to a range of providers and consumers; collection and analysis of health-related data, including nutrition surveillance and monitoring; investigation and control of disease, injuries, and responses to natural disasters; protection of the environment, housing, food, water, and workplaces; public information, education, and community mobilization; quality assurance; training and education; leadership, planning, policy development, and administration; targeted outreach and linkage to personal services; and other direct clinical services.[18]

Many community nutrition services include screening, education, counseling, and treatment to improve the nutritional status of an individual or a population. These services are designed to meet the preventive, therapeutic, and rehabilitative health care needs of all segments of the population. The focus of nutrition services, including nutrition education, in an agency is based on several factors, including the mission of the agency, funding, analysis of data from a community-needs assessment, resources, and politics.[19] Public agencies provide nutrition services for individuals throughout the life cycle, provided in a variety of inpatient and outpatient settings. The broadest range of nutrition services may be most evident in community-based nutrition programs, in which services are based on core public health functions. It is important for physicians and other primary health care professionals to familiarize themselves with the location of these services in their communities. Professional and federal resources for nutrition services are listed in Table 49.3. The Maternal and Child Health (MCH) Library at Georgetown University maintains the MCH Organizations Database (https://library.tmc.edu/website/mch-library-maternal-child-health-library-at-georgetown-university/), which lists more than 2000 government, professional, and voluntary organizations involved in MCH activities, primarily at a national level. This is a useful resource for pediatricians and other primary care providers. Qualified providers of nutrition services include physicians, registered dietitian nutritionists (RDNs)/registered dietitians (RDs) and/or licensed dietitians, licensed nutritionists, nurses, and other qualified professionals. The Academy of Nutrition and Dietetics (AND), the largest organization of professional dietitians and nutritionists, has identified qualified providers as RDNs/RDs and other qualified professionals who meet licensing and other standards prescribed at the state level.[20]

VII

Table 49.3.
Selected Professional and Federal Resources for Nutrition Services

Selected Professional Nutrition Organizations
Academy of Nutrition and Dietetics (AND) 120 S. Riverside Plaza, Suite 2000 Chicago, IL 60606-6995 Phone: 800-877-1600; Consumer Nutrition Hot Line: 800-366-1655 www.eatright.org
School Nutrition Association (SNA) 700 S. Washington Street, Suite 300 Alexandria, VA 22314 Phone: 703-739-3900; Fax 703-739-3915 www.schoolnutrition.org
Association of State and Territorial Public Health Nutrition Directors PO Box 1001 Johnstown, PA 15907-1001 Phone: 814-255-2829 http://www.astphnd.org/
National WIC Association 2001 S Street, NW, Suite 580 Washington, DC 20009-3405 Phone: 202-232-5492; fax: 202-387-5281 http://www.nwica.org/
American Public Human Services Association (APHSA) 810 First Street, NE Suite 500 Washington, DC 20002 Phone: 202-682-0100 Fax: 202-289-6555 http://www.aphsa.org/Home/home_news.asp
Feeding America E. Wacker Drive, Suite 2000 Chicago, IL 60601 Phone: 800-771-2303 www.feedingamerica.org (Web site has a search function to locate local services)

Table 49.3. *Continued*

Selected Professional and Federal Resources for Nutrition Services

Selected Federal Resources
US Department of Agriculture Resources
US Department of Agriculture Food and Nutrition Service (FNS) 3101 Park Center Drive Alexandria, VA 22302 Phone: 703-305-2062 Information on USDA nutrition assistance programs including associated research, nutrition education initiatives, such as WIC Breastfeeding Campaign, Team Nutrition, Eat Smart Play Hard, State Nutrition Action Plans (SNAP), and Food Stamp Nutrition Education, are found at: http://www.fns.usda.gov/fns/ and www.wicworks.fns.usda.gov. US Department of Agriculture Center for Nutrition Policy and Promotion (CNPP) 3101 Park Center Drive Alexandria, VA 22302 Phone: 703-305-7600 The CNPP develops and promotes dietary guidance that links scientific research to the nutrition needs of consumers. For information on CNPP resources, the Dietary Guidelines for Americans, and MyPlate, see http://www.cnpp.usda.gov/ and http://www.choosemyplate.gov US Department of Agriculture Cooperative State Research, Education, and Extension Service (CSREES) 1400 Independence Avenue, SW, Stop 2201 Washington, DC 20250-2201 Phone: 202-720-7441 The CSREES provides linkages between federal and state components of a broad-based national agricultural higher education, research, and extension system designed to address national problems and needs related to agriculture, the environment, human health and well-being, and communities; see http://www.csrees.usda.gov/. National Agricultural Library (NAL) US Department of Agriculture Abraham Lincoln Building 10301 Baltimore Avenue Beltsville, MD 20705-2351 Phone: 301-504-5414 (for FNIC); Fax: 301-504-6409 (for FNIC) http://www.nal.usda.gov/ The NAL sponsors the Food and Nutrition Information Center (FNIC the Food Stamp Nutrition Connection Resource System, and the USDA/FDA Foodborne Illness Education Information Center. The FNIC/NAL also sponsors the "Nutrition.gov" Web site, which provides easy access to the best food and nutrition information from across the federal government.

VII

Continued

Table 49.3. *Continued*

Selected Professional and Federal Resources for Nutrition Services

US Department of Health and Human Services Resources
Centers for Disease Control and Prevention Division of Nutrition and Physical Activity 4770 Buford Highway, Mailstop K25 Atlanta, GA 30341 Phone: 770-488-6042 Information and resources on infant and child nutrition, physical activity, and the obesity epidemic are available from the CDC Web site at http://www.cdc.gov/nccdphp/dnpa. Food and Drug Administration 5600 Fishers Lane Rockville, MD 20857 For general inquiries: 1-888-INFO-FDA (1-888-463-6332) For Office of Public Affairs: 301-827-6250 This Web site is a central source of information about FDA activities and resources and includes a section on consumer advice and publications on food safety and nutrition: www.fda.gov. The National Center for Education in Maternal and Child Health (NCEMCH) Georgetown University Box 571272 Washington, DC 20057-1272 Phone: 202-784-9770; fax 202-784-9777 Funded by the Maternal and Child Health Bureau, Health Resources and Services Administration, Department of Health and Human Services, the NCEMCH Web site (www.ncemch.org) provides online access to NCEMCH initiatives, educational resources, and publications; a virtual MCH library and MCH databases; bibliographies; and knowledge paths.

Table 49.3. *Continued*

Selected Professional and Federal Resources for Nutrition Services

US Department of Health and Human Services Resources—*Continued*
US Department of Health and Human Services 200 Independence Avenue, SW Washington, DC 20201 For more information by mail, write: National Health Information Center PO Box 1133 Washington, DC 20013-1133 Phone: 301-565-4167 Toll Free: 1-800-336-4797 The HealthierUS initiative is a national effort, sponsored by the Department of Health and Human Services and the Executive Office of the President, to improve people's lives, prevent and reduce the costs of disease, and promote community health and wellness. See the Web site, which includes information on nutrition, physical activity, and healthy choices: www.HealthierUS.gov. National Heart, Lung, and Blood Institute PO Box 30105 Bethesda, MD 20824-0105 Phone: 301-592-8573 or toll-free 866-35-WECAN *We Can!* or "Ways to Enhance Children's Activity and Nutrition" is a national education program from the National Institutes of Health designed for families and caregivers to help children 8 to 13 years of age achieve a healthy weight. This program offers communities and families resources including materials for healthcare providers, physicians, and parents. See the Web site: http://wecan.nhlbi.nih.gov. Indian Health Service The Reyes Building 801 Thompson Avenue, Ste. 400 Rockville, MD 20852-1627 Phone: 301-443-1083 For information on how the Indian Health Service works to improve the health of patients with nutrition related diseases, and prevent these illnesses in future generations through interventions in schools, community health programs, and hospital and clinic based services, see the Web site: http://www.ihs.gov.

Health and Nutrition Agencies: A Nutrition Resource to Provide Services and Identify Qualified Providers

Federal, state, and local health and nutrition agencies, particularly those employing public health nutritionists, can be helpful resources for physicians and other primary health care professionals. Nutritionists provide extensive technical assistance to clients and their families and physicians, especially for children with special health care needs. One example is services for children with an inborn error of metabolism. The diet prescription includes special medical formulas and foods that are modified to meet medical and socioeconomic needs. The formulas and foods are expensive, and the costs are generally not reimbursed by insurance companies. Many states have provisions for coverage for special formulas and foods.[21] Physicians can contact the special needs program of their state health department for information about patient eligibility for coverage for these formulas and foods and procedures for obtaining them.

Another example in which a nutritionist and nutrition services are instrumental in supporting feeding and growth is an early intervention program. In an early intervention program, nutritionists work with the child's family, other team members, and the child's primary health care professional to optimize development from birth to 3 years of age.[22] This national early intervention program for infants and toddlers with disabilities and their families was created by Congress in 1986 under the Education for All Handicapped Children Act (Pub L No. 94-142 [1975]), which then became the Individuals with Disabilities Education Act (Pub L No. 101-476 [1990]), and is administered by states. To be eligible for services, children must be younger than 3 years and have a confirmed disability or established developmental delay as defined by the state, in 1 or more of the following areas of development: physical, cognitive, communication, social-emotional, and/or adaptive. A complete evaluation of the child and family must be conducted, at no cost to the family, to determine whether a child is eligible for this early intervention program. The evaluation would include an assessment of the child's nutritional history and dietary intake; anthropometric, biochemical, and clinical variables; feeding skills and feeding problems; and food habits and food preferences. If a child and family are found eligible for services, the parents and a team will develop a written plan (Individualized Family Service Plan [IFSP]) for providing early intervention services to the child and, as necessary, to the family. The child's and family's IFSP can include nutrition, or nutrition may be listed as another service that the child receives but is not provided or paid for by the early intervention program. Depending on the child's assessed nutritional needs, a qualified nutritionist, as a member of the IFSP team, would develop and monitor appropriate goals and objectives to address any nutritional needs and also make referrals to appropriate community resources to focus on nutrition goals, if needed. For more information on disabilities in infants, toddlers, children, and youth and the Individuals with Disabilities Education Act, which is the law authorizing special education and the early intervention program, see the website of the National Dissemination Center for Children with Disabilities (www.nichcy.org).

Other types of nutrition services provided by many state and local health agencies include nutrition counseling, classes on specific aspects of nutrition (eg, infant feeding, breastfeeding, diet and prevention of heart disease, and weight management), radio and cable television programs on nutrition topics, publications and educational materials on a wide range of topics for the lay public, and nutrition seminars and workshops. Local nutrition education resources are available from the USDA-funded Cooperative Extension Service. This service provides up-to-date information about the science of nutrition and its practical application in planning low-cost, nutritious meals. Many nutrition publications provided by the Cooperative Extension Service and other public health agencies are available in various foreign languages and for clients with low literacy skills.[19,23]

The National Institute of Food and Agriculture (formerly the Cooperative State Research, Education, and Extension Service) of the USDA operates the Expanded Food and Nutrition Education Program in all 50 states and in American Samoa, Guam, Micronesia, Northern Marianas, Puerto Rico, and the Virgin Islands. The Expanded Food and Nutrition Education Program is designed to assist limited-resource audiences in acquiring the knowledge, skills, attitudes, and behavior changes necessary to follow nutritionally sound diets and to contribute to their personal development and improvement of the total family diet and nutritional well-being (for more information, see https://nifa.usda.gov/program/expanded-food-and-nutrition-education-program-efnep).

The director of the nutrition department at the state health department is another excellent resource for identifying specific state, regional, or national resources and services. Similar information can be obtained from the Association of State and Territorial Public Health Nutrition Directors (Table 49.3). The state affiliate of the AND or the AND consultant directory

VII

can help identify an RDN/RD with specific clinical expertise (Table 49.3). Consumers may also call the AND consumer hotline number and speak directly to an RDN/RD who can assist them with answers to general questions ranging from food labeling to food sanitation and other topics.

In addition to federal, state, and local health agencies, agencies such as visiting nurse associations, the American Diabetes Association, the American Heart Association, health maintenance organizations, and hospital inpatient and outpatient departments frequently employ personnel with nutrition expertise. They usually provide technical consultation in nutrition to physicians and nurses and nutrition counseling to patients and other agencies in the community. An increasing number of RDNs/RDs have also established private or independent practices.

Nutrition-Assistance Programs

National policy has long provided for publicly supported nutrition-assistance programs to safeguard the health of individuals whose nutrition status is compromised because of poverty or complex physiologic, social, or other stressors. The National School Lunch Act of 1946 (Pub L No. 79-396) provided for a major federal role in food service for school children. The Food and Nutrition Service (FNS) and Center for Nutrition Policy and Promotion (CNPP) are agencies of the USDA's Food, Nutrition, and Consumer Services. FNS works to end hunger and obesity through the administration of 15 federal nutrition assistance programs, including WIC, Supplemental Nutrition Assistance Program (SNAP), and school meals. In partnership with state and tribal governments, FNS programs serve 1 in 4 Americans during the course of a year.

The CNPP was created within the US Department of Agriculture in 1994. The mission of the CNPP is to improve the health of Americans by developing and promoting dietary guidance that links scientific research to the nutrition needs of consumers. The CNPP carries out its mission to improve the health of Americans by (1) serving as the federal authority on evidence-based food, nutrition, and economic analyses to inform policy and programs; (2) translating science into actionable food and nutrition guidance for all Americans; and (3) leading national communication initiatives that apply science-based messages to advance consumers' dietary and economic knowledge and behaviors.

Supplemental Nutrition Assistance Program

SNAP—formerly known as the Food Stamp Program—is a nutrition-assistance program that enables people with low income to buy nutritious food and make healthy food choices within a limited budget.[24] It is the largest of the federal nutrition-assistance programs. States have the option to include nutrition education and obesity prevention activities to SNAP participants and eligible individuals as part of their administrative services through the SNAP Nutrition Education and Obesity Prevention Grant Program (SNAP-Ed). Every state now conducts SNAP-Ed, which works by building partnerships with community organizations. SNAP-Ed activities include social marketing campaigns, holding nutrition education classes, and improving policies, systems, and environments where people live, work, learn, eat, and play. The average monthly household benefit level in fiscal year 2015 was $254. SNAP benefits are provided on an electronic card that is used by participants at authorized retail stores to buy food. SNAP benefits redeemed at local stores not only provide nutrition benefits for the participants but also provide an economic boost to the local community. Every $5 in new SNAP benefits generates $9.00 in total community spending.[25]

SNAP is a federal program, but it is administered by state and local agencies. As an entitlement program, it is available to all who meet the eligibility standards. In 2015, the program served 83% of all individuals eligible for SNAP. Nearly two thirds of SNAP participants were children, elderly, or people with disabilities. Forty-four percent of participants were younger than 18 years, 11% were 60 years or older, and 10% were disabled nonelderly adults.[26] The FNS, which oversees SNAP, offers numerous resources and tools to help community and faith-based organizations, state and local offices, food retailers, and other health and social service providers teach their clients with low income about the nutrition benefits of food stamps and help them enroll. These materials are available free online (https://www.cbpp.org/research/policy-basics-the-supplemental-nutrition-assistance-program-snap).

To qualify for SNAP benefits, a person must apply through a local SNAP office and have income and resources under certain limits. The FNS Web site offers the "step 1" online prescreening tool (https://www.snap-step1.usda.gov/fns/) in English and Spanish, which privately tells users whether they may be eligible for benefits and how much they could receive. The FNS website also provides SNAP application and local office locators (https://www.fns.usda.gov/snap/state-directory).

VII

School Nutrition Programs *(See Also Chapter 9)*

The National School Lunch Program (NSLP), the School Breakfast Program (SBP), the Fresh Fruit and Vegetable Program (FFVP), and the Special Milk Program are administered in most states by the state education agency, which enters into agreements with officials of local schools or school districts to operate nonprofit food services. Most public and private schools in the United States participate in the NSLP. Participating schools can receive cash reimbursements and USDA Foods regardless of the number of children eligible for free lunch program. Any public or nonprofit private school of high school grade or less is eligible. Public and licensed, nonprofit, private residential child care institutions, such as orphanages, community homes for disabled children, juvenile detention centers, and temporary shelters for runaway children, are also eligible. For more information on USDA school meals programs, visit https://www.ers.usda.gov/topics/food-nutrition-assistance/child-nutrition-programs/.

Schools participating in the federal school meals programs agree to serve nutritious meals and offer them at a reduced price or free to children who are determined to be eligible on the basis of uniform national poverty guidelines, determined annually by the DHHS. A child's eligibility to receive reduced-price or free meals is based on their household size and income. Additionally, a child from a household currently certified to receive SNAP benefits or benefits under the Food Distribution Program on Indian Reservations (FDPIR) or Temporary Assistance to Needy Families (TANF) is categorically eligible for free benefits. Foster and homeless children are also categorically eligible to receive school meals. The school meals program provides some level of federal reimbursement for program meals served to children from all income levels; however, free and reduced-price meals served to children determined to be eligible by income criteria are subsidized at a higher rate.

The Healthy, Hunger-Free Kids Act (HHFKA) of 2010 (Pub L No. 111-296) required the Food and Nutrition Service to review and update the meal pattern requirements for the NSLP and SBP. Federal nutrition requirements are specified in program regulations to ensure that the nutrition goals of the school meal programs are met and are intended to enhance the diet of school children nationwide and help mitigate childhood obesity. They provide children daily access to fruits, vegetables, whole grains, and fat-free and low-fat fluid milk in school meals; limit sodium, saturated fat, and trans fat in school meals; and establish calorie ranges to ensure that children receive age-appropriate school meals. In 2012, the USDA updated the meal patterns and dietary specifications for the National School Lunch and School Breakfast Programs on the basis of recommendations from the Institute of Medicine (now the National Academy of Medicine) to align them with the latest Dietary Guidelines for Americans. The Dietary Guidelines for Americans (Dietary Guidelines) are the cornerstone of federal nutrition policy and nutrition education activities. They are jointly issued and updated every 5 years by the USDA and DHHS. The *MyPlate* food guidance system provides food-based guidance to help implement the recommendations of the Dietary Guidelines. The Dietary Guidelines provide authoritative advice for people 2 years and older about how good dietary habits can promote health and reduce risks of major chronic diseases. Note that dietary guidelines for pregnant women and children from birth to 2 years of age are expected with the 2020 Dietary Guidelines for Americans. For more information the Dietary Guidelines, see http://www.dietaryguidelines.gov and for more information on *MyPlate*, see http://www.choosemyplate.gov.

The new meal pattern requirements were phased in over multiple school years to facilitate implementation. The majority of the lunch meal pattern took effect in school year 2012–2013, and the breakfast meal pattern was implemented over school years 2013–2014 and 2014–2015. The USDA is continuing to provide guidance, training programs, and technical assistance resources to assist school nutrition operators in implementing the nutrition standards and offering healthy school meals.

The HHFKA of 2010 also directed the USDA to establish nutrition standards for all foods and beverages sold to students in school during the school day (ie, competitive foods, or foods sold in competition with school meals), including foods sold through school fundraisers. The Smart Snacks in School final regulation ensures that nutrition standards for competitive foods are consistent with those used for the NSLP and SBP, holding competitive foods to standards similar to those applied to other foods made available during the school day. These standards, combined with recent improvements in school meals, will help promote diets that contribute to students' long-term health and well-being. In addition, these standards continue to support a healthy school environment and the efforts of parents to promote healthy choices for children at home and at school. The competitive foods nutrition standards have been implemented in schools since July 1, 2014. The standards are designed to help schools to make the healthy choice the easy choice by offering students more of the foods and beverages that should be encouraged—whole grains, fruits, and vegetables; leaner

VII

protein; and lower-fat dairy—while limiting foods with higher levels of sugars, saturated and trans fats, and sodium. For more information, visit USDA's Smart Snacks website at https://www.fns.usda.gov/school-meals/tools-schools-focusing-smart-snacks.

The Special Milk Program reduces the cost of each half-pint of milk served to children by providing cash reimbursement at an annually adjusted rate. A school district can choose to provide milk free to children who meet the eligibility guidelines. This program is available only to schools, child care institutions, and summer camps that do not participate in other federal meal service programs. Schools in the NSLP or SBP may also participate in the Special Milk Program to provide milk to children in half-day pre-kindergarten and kindergarten programs where children do not have access to the school meal programs. At present, the Special Milk Program allows schools or institutions to offer only pasteurized fluid types of milk that are low-fat (1% milk fat or less, unflavored) or fat-free (unflavored or flavored). These milks must meet all state and local standards. All milk types offered are required to contain vitamins A and D at levels specified by the FDA.

Local School Wellness Policies

Under the Child Nutrition and WIC Reauthorization Act of 2004 (Pub L No. 108-265), each local educational agency participating in a program authorized by the National School Lunch Act or the Child Nutrition Act of 1966 (Pub L No. 89-642) was required to establish a local school wellness policy by school year 2006. The purpose of implementing local wellness policies is to create healthy school nutrition environments that promote healthy eating and physical activity for students. The HHFKA of 2010 expanded the scope of local school wellness policies to include goals for nutrition promotion and guidelines for all foods available on the school campus that are consistent with the updated school meal and competitive food nutrition standards. It also added requirements to existing wellness policy standards related to wellness committee participation and review and reporting of wellness policies. The final regulation on local school wellness policies, published in July 2016, requires all local educational agencies that participate in the NSLP and SBP to meet expanded local school wellness policy requirements consistent with the requirements set forth in the HHFKA. The final rule requires each local educational agency to establish minimum content requirements for the local school wellness policies, ensure stakeholder participation in the development and updates of such policies, and periodically assess and disclose to the public schools' compliance with the local school wellness policies. These regulations are intended to result in local school wellness policies that strengthen the ability of a local educational agency to create a school nutrition environment that promotes students' health, well-being, and ability to learn. In addition, these regulations will increase transparency for the public with regard to school wellness policies and therefore contribute to integrity in the school nutrition program.

The legislation placed the responsibility of developing and implementing a wellness policy at the local level so that the individual needs of each local educational agency can be addressed. Preventing childhood obesity is a collective responsibility requiring family, school, community, corporate, and governmental commitments. The key is to implement changes through coordinated and collaborative efforts from all sectors. For more information, and access to school wellness policy implementation resources, visit the USDA website at https://www.fns.usda.gov/tn/local-school-wellness-policy.

The AAP has encouraged its members to become involved in assisting their local school districts in developing and implementing school wellness policies. School districts are required to permit school health professionals and the general public to participate in the wellness policy committee; as such, AAP members are encouraged to seek out their local school districts' wellness committee and participate as they are able. The AAP and the AND are cooperating with the Action for Healthy Kids, a national nonprofit organization, to address the epidemic of overweight, undernourished, and sedentary youth through tangible changes in the school environment. Useful information for how pediatricians can become involved in school wellness policies is available (www.actionforhealthykids.org). The USDA School Nutrition Environment and Wellness Resources website includes many resources to support implementation of the school wellness policy process (http://healthymeals.fns.usda.gov/school-wellness-resources).

Child and Adult Care Food Program

The Child and Adult Care Food Program (CACFP) provides cash reimbursement and USDA Foods for the provision of meals and snacks to child and adult care institutions and family or group day care homes. Institutions eligible to participate include at-risk after-school care centers, adult day care centers, nonprofit child care centers, Head Start centers, family day care homes, and emergency shelters. Some for-profit child care centers and adult care centers serving children from families with low incomes may also be eligible to participate in the program.

Although federal subsidies continue to be provided for meals and snacks served to children from all income levels, program benefits are primarily directed to needy children. Children up to 18 years and younger are eligible to receive up to 2 meals and 1 snack or 2 snacks and 1 meal each day at an at-risk after-school care center, child care center, or day care home. Children who reside in emergency shelters may receive up to 3 meals each day. Migrant children 15 years and younger and people with disabilities, regardless of their age, are eligible to receive reimbursable meals. After-school care snacks and meals are available to children through 18 years of age. For more information on the Child and Adult Care Food Program, visit the website (https://www.fns.usda.gov/cacfp/child-and-adult-care-food-program).

The HHFKA of 2010 also required the USDA to update the CACFP meal patterns and make them more consistent with the most recent version of the Dietary Guidelines for Americans. The final regulation for the CACFP meal patterns, published in April 2016, helps ensure the most vulnerable citizens have access to the nutrition they need. Informed by evidence-based recommendations, this final regulation updates meal patterns in the CACFP using science-based standards to improve the nutritional quality of meals and snacks served to millions of children and adults every day and ensuring young children develop healthy habits from the start. This is the first major revision of the CACFP meal patterns since the program's inception in 1968. Since the beginning of the CACFP, nutrition-related health problems have greatly shifted from malnutrition to overconsumption of calories, saturated fats, added sugars, and sodium as well as underconsumption of fiber and other essential nutrients. Under the updated meal patterns, young children and adults in day care will receive meals with more whole grains, a greater variety of vegetables and fruits, and less added sugars and solid fats. The changes also improve access to healthy beverages, including low-fat and fat-free milk and water, and encourage breastfeeding among the youngest program participants. For more information, visit the USDA website on the nutrition standards for CACFP meals and snacks: https://www.fns.usda.gov/cacfp/meals-and-snacks.

Summer Food Service Program

The Summer Food Service Program (SFSP) provides nutritious meals for children 18 years and younger during school vacations at centrally located sites, such as schools or community centers in neighborhoods with low incomes, or at summer camps. Meals are served free to all children in eligible sites and must meet the nutritional standards established by the USDA. Sponsors of the program must be public or private nonprofit schools, public agencies, or private nonprofit organizations. For more information on the Summer Food Service Program, visit the website (https://www.fns.usda.gov/sfsp/summer-food-service-program).

Fresh Fruit and Vegetable Program

The Fresh Fruit and Vegetable Program (FFVP) is a federally assisted program providing free fresh fruits and vegetables to students in low-income elementary schools during the school day. The goal of the FFVP is to improve children's overall diet and create healthier eating habits to impact their present and future health. The FFVP helps schools create healthier school environments by providing healthier food choices, expanding the variety of fruits and vegetables children experience, and increasing children's fruit and vegetable consumption. The FFVP has been highly effective in increasing consumption of fruits and vegetables among low-income students. Studies have shown that children participating in the FFVP have statistically significant increased consumption of fruits and vegetables. The USDA FNS administers the FFVP at the federal level. At the state level, the FFVP is usually administered by the state education agency, which operates the program through agreements with school food authorities. The FFVP is targeted to elementary schools with the highest free and reduced price meals enrollment. The state agency decides the per-student funding amount for the selected schools based on total funds allocated to the state and the enrollment of applicant schools. With these funds, schools purchase additional fresh fruits and vegetables to serve free to students during the school day. They must be served outside of the normal time frames for the NSLP and SBP. The state agency or school food authority determines the best method to obtain and serve the additional fresh produce. Schools are also encouraged to develop partnerships to help implement the program, such as with local universities, extension services, and local grocers. Schools must also agree to widely publicize the availability of the program. For more information on the FFVP, visit the USDA website at https://www.fns.usda.gov/ffvp/fresh-fruit-and-vegetable-program.

Use of Local Foods in the Child Nutrition Programs

The USDA is committed to helping child nutrition program operators incorporate local foods in the school meal programs as well as the Summer Food Service Program and Child and Adult Care Food Program. This is

VII

accomplished through grants, training and technical assistance, and research. The USDA Farm to School Grant Program assists eligible entities in implementing farm to school programs that improve access to local foods in eligible schools. On an annual basis, the USDA awards competitive grants for training, supporting operations, planning, purchasing equipment, developing school gardens, developing partnerships, and implementing farm to school programs. For more information on the Farm to School Program, visit the USDA website at https://www.fns.usda.gov/farmtoschool/farm-school.

Team Nutrition Initiative

In June 1995, the USDA launched the Team Nutrition initiative, which continues to support the federal child nutrition programs through training and technical assistance for food service, nutrition education for children and their caregivers, and school and community support for healthy eating and physical activity. Team Nutrition is an integrated, behavior-based, comprehensive initiative for promoting the nutritional health of the nation's children. The funding supports the efforts of the USDA FNS to establish policy, develop materials and trainings that meet the needs of state and local partners, disseminate resources and materials in ways that meet state and local needs, and develop partnerships with other federal agencies and organizations. Team Nutrition provides resources to schools, child care settings, and summer meal sites that participate in federal child nutrition programs. Team Nutrition uses 3 strategies to change behavior: (1) provide training and technical assistance to child nutrition professionals to enable them to prepare and serve nutrition meals that appeal to children; (2) increase nutrition education through multiple communication channels to help children have the knowledge, skills, and motivation to make healthy food and physical activity choices as part of a healthy lifestyle; and (3) build support for healthy school and child care environments that encourage nutritious food choices and physically active lifestyles. Team Nutrition brings together public and private networks to promote food choices for a healthy diet and deliver consistent nutrition messages through multiple communication channels including food service initiatives, classroom and child care activities, school-wide events, home activities, community programs and events, and traditional and social media. Schools participating in the NLSP are invited to sign up as Team Nutrition Schools and join an important network of schools working towards healthier school nutrition and physical activity environments.

Team Nutrition funds a limited number of competitive grants to state agencies each year to help states establish or enhance sustainable infrastructures to achieve Team Nutrition's goals of improving children's lifelong eating and physical activity habits. The Team Nutrition Training Grants, authorized in 1978, are one of the anchor delivery systems for supporting the implementation of the USDA's nutrition requirements and the Dietary Guidelines for Americans in meals served in schools and child care institutions. Some efforts by state agencies receiving these grants have resulted in child nutrition program foodservice personnel receiving training and technical assistance that equips them to prepare and serve nutritious meals that appeal to students; providing mini grants to local school districts and child care institutions to enhance promotion of healthy eating and physical activity; nutrition education in schools and child care settings using many USDA-developed Team Nutrition materials; integrating nutrition education into students learning content standards, including trainings and workshops provided to teachers; and building community support for healthy eating and physical activity. More information on Team Nutrition Training Grants can be found at https://www.fns.usda.gov/tn/team-nutrition-training-grants.

Nutrition education resources are available from the USDA's Team Nutrition initiative. These Team Nutrition materials help schools and child care providers integrate nutrition education into classroom learning and also include materials for home, cafeteria, and community connections. In addition to the nutrition education materials for schools being standards-based, materials are child-, teacher-, and parent-tested through extensive research including focus group testing, in-depth interviews, and field-testing. Materials are based on the social cognitive theory, as this theory addresses personal, behavioral, and environmental factors that influence behavior. Team Nutrition materials also include curriculum kits, lesson plan posters, games, stickers, event planning guidebooks, brochures, and more for both schools and child care institutions.

Team Nutrition also has materials to help school nutrition professionals provide students with nutritious and delicious meals that meet meal pattern requirements. These resources provide guidance on using sound business practices to ensure continued availability of healthy meals as well as the financial viability and accountability of the school meal programs.

Team Nutrition print materials are available only to schools and child care institutions that participate in the federal child nutrition programs; all others are welcome to download Team Nutrition materials at http://team-nutrition.usda.gov. Many Team Nutrition publications are also available in Spanish, and a small selection of family newsletters are available in other languages.

Supplemental Food Programs

WIC

The WIC program is the premiere public health nutrition program serving low-income, nutritionally at-risk pregnant, breastfeeding, and nonbreast-feeding postpartum women, infants, and children up to 5 years of age. The WIC program is administered at the federal level by the FNS of the USDA and was created by Congress to serve as an adjunct to health care during critical times of growth and development. The legislative requirements for the WIC program are contained in section 17 of the Child Nutrition Act of 1966. Because WIC is a nondiscretionary program, each year Congress appropriates funds to support the program through an appropriation law. FNS then awards grants to state agencies (typically state health depart-ments) annually to fund the program in their states. The benefits of the WIC program include nutritious supplemental foods, nutrition educa-tion, and referrals for health and social services, which are all provided to participants at no cost. Many studies show that the WIC program has made many contributions toward improving maternal and child health and saving children's lives.[27-30]

The WIC program is available in all 50 states, 34 Indian Tribal Organizations, American Samoa, the District of Columbia, Guam, Puerto Rico, the Virgin Islands, and the Commonwealth of the Northern Marianas Islands. As of 2016, state agencies administered the WIC program through 1800 local agencies and 9000 clinic sites. Of the 7.7 million people who received WIC benefits each month in fiscal year 2016, approximately 51.7% were children, 24.4% were infants, and 23.9% were women. In 2013, 84% of infants eligible for WIC were participating in the program (2 387 233 infants).[31] Services under WIC are provided in county health departments, hospitals, mobile clinics (vans), community centers, schools, public housing sites, Indian reservations, migrant health centers and camps, and Indian Health Service facilities.

Since the piloting of the WIC program in 1972, the appropriated funding level has increased to approximately $6.35 billion annually. Program funds are allocated to state agencies according to a formula that considers both nutrition services and administration costs and supplemental food costs. The average monthly food package cost for fiscal year 2016 was $42.76.[32]

The food packages provided to WIC participants are scientifically based and intended to address the supplemental needs of pregnant, breastfeeding, and nonbreastfeeding postpartum women, infants, and children and provide nutrients frequently lacking in the diets of the target population. In 2014, the FNS published the final WIC Food Package Rule, which required all WIC state agencies to provide food packages that align with the Dietary Guidelines for Americans and infant feeding practice guidelines of the AAP. The final food package regulation represents the culmination of the first comprehensive revisions to the WIC food packages since 1980.

The WIC food packages provide breakfast cereals, eggs, milk and milk alternatives (including soy based beverage, cheese and tofu), whole wheat bread and other whole grains, fruit and vegetable cash value vouchers, peanut butter, legumes, canned fish, juice, infant foods, infant formula, exempt infant formula, and WIC-eligible nutritionals. For the complete provisions and requirements for foods in the WIC food packages, refer to the full regulation at www.fns.usda.gov/wic.

Although federal regulations specify the minimum nutritional requirements for the WIC foods, state agencies are responsible for using the federal regulations when determining the brands, types, and forms of foods authorized on state food lists. The process of food package design at the state level involves maximizing the nutritional value of WIC food packages while managing cost. Acceptability and availability of eligible foods to participants are also important considerations in designing state agency food lists.

WIC food packages promote and support the establishment of successful, long-term breastfeeding and provide WIC participants with a wide variety of foods, including fruits, and vegetables, and whole grains; provide less saturated fat and cholesterol and more fiber to women and children; reinforce the nutrition messages provided to participants; and provide WIC state agencies greater flexibility in prescribing food packages to accommodate the cultural food preferences of WIC participants. Nutrition education is an important benefit of the WIC program. Efforts are made to provide client-centered nutrition education that focuses on the individual participant's nutritional needs, cultural preferences, and education level. Breastfeeding promotion and support activities are an important component of WIC nutrition education. WIC supports breastfeeding mothers by

VII

providing: (1) information and support through counseling and educational materials; (2) a greater quantity and variety of foods than for mothers who formula feed their infants; (3) eligibility to participate in WIC longer than nonbreastfeeding mothers—up to 1 year postpartum; (4) mother-to-mother support through WIC breastfeeding peer counselors; and (5) breast pumps and other aids that are necessary to help support the initiation and continuation of breastfeeding.

The WIC Farmers' Market Nutrition Program provides additional coupons to WIC recipients that can be used to buy fresh fruits and vegetables from authorized farmers, farmers markets, or roadside stands.

For more information on the WIC program, see http://www.fns.usda.gov/wic.

Food Distribution Programs

USDA Foods Programs

USDA Foods are items that are 100% American grown and produced and purchased by the USDA to support nutrition assistance programs and domestic agriculture. These foods include fresh, frozen, canned, and dried fruits and vegetables; grains; proteins; and dairy products. The USDA purchases more than $2.2 billion of food annually to provide to food assistance programs such as schools, food banks, and Indian Tribal Organizations through a variety of programs, described below.

The Emergency Food Assistance Program

The Emergency Food Assistance Program is a federal program administered by the USDA that helps supplement the diets of low-income Americans by providing them with emergency food and nutrition assistance at no cost. Under the Emergency Food Assistance Program, the USDA makes USDA Foods available to state distributing agencies. States provide the food to local agencies that they have selected, usually food banks, which in turn distribute the food to soup kitchens and food pantries that directly serve the public. These organizations distribute the USDA Foods for household consumption or use them to prepare and serve meals in a congregate setting. Recipients of food for home use must meet income eligibility criteria set by the states. State agencies receive the food and supervise overall distribution. For more information on The Emergency Food Assistance Program, see https://www.fns.usda.gov/tefap/emergency-food-assistance-program.

Food Distribution Program on Indian Reservations

The Food Distribution Program on Indian Reservations provides USDA Foods to low-income households on Indian reservations and to American Indian households residing in approved areas near reservations or anywhere in Oklahoma. Many households participate in the Food Distribution Program on Indian Reservations as an alternative to the SNAP, because they do not have easy access to SNAP offices or authorized food stores. The program is administered at the federal level by the USDA FNS. The Food Distribution Program on Indian Reservations is administered locally by either Indian Tribal Organizations or an agency of a state government. As of 2017, there are approximately 276 tribes receiving benefits through 102 Indian Tribal Organizations and 3 state agencies. Average monthly participation for fiscal year 2017 is approximately 90 000 individuals.

Each month, participating households receive a food package to help them maintain a nutritionally balanced diet. Participants may select from more than 70 products, including: frozen ground beef, beef roast, and chicken; canned meats, poultry, and fish; fresh fruits and vegetables; canned fruits and vegetables, soups, and spaghetti sauce; macaroni and cheese, pastas, cereals, rice, and other grains; cheese, eggs, egg mix, nonfat dry and evaporated milk, and low-fat ultra-high temperature fluid milk; flour, cornmeal, low-fat bakery mix, and reduced sodium crackers; low-fat refried beans, dried beans, and dehydrated potatoes; canned juices and dried fruits; peanuts and peanut butter; and light buttery spread and vegetable oil. For more information on the Food Distribution Program on Indian Reservations, see https://www.fns.usda.gov/fdpir/food-distribution-program-indian-reservations.

Where to Seek Nutrition Assistance (Table 49.3)

VII

Nutrition-assistance programs are usually administered at the local level by the following agencies:

1. Local school food authority: National School Lunch Program, School Breakfast Program, Special Milk Program, and Fresh Fruit and Vegetable Program.
2. State and local health, social services, education, or agriculture agencies; public or private nonprofit health agencies; and Indian Tribal Organizations or groups recognized by the US Department of the Interior:

WIC; Food Distribution Program on Indian Reservations; Summer Food Service Program; Child and Adult Care Food Program; The Emergency Food Assistance Program.

3. Local social services, human services, or welfare department: SNAP.
4. Community or faith-based organizations.

Other Federal Agencies Providing Nutrition Services to Improve Pediatric Health and Well-Being

CDC Nutrition and Physical Activity Program to Prevent Obesity and Other Chronic Diseases

The CDC administers the state-based Nutrition and Physical Activity Program to Prevent Obesity and Other Chronic Diseases. This program is based on a cooperative agreement between the CDC Division of Nutrition and Physical Activity and Obesity and all 50 state health departments. The program was established in fiscal year 1999 to prevent and control obesity and other chronic diseases by supporting states in developing and implementing nutrition and physical activity interventions, particularly through population-based strategies (eg, policy-level changes, environmental supports).

States receive funding from the program to work to prevent and control obesity and other chronic diseases through these strategies: balancing caloric intake and expenditure, increasing physical activity, increasing consumption of fruits and vegetables, decreasing television-viewing and other screen time, and increasing breastfeeding. The program also helps states work to reduce soft-drink consumption and decrease portion size. States funded by the program partner with stakeholders in government, academia, industry, and other areas to create statewide health plans—one of the most important ways to help guide state efforts. State plans promote working with a variety of partners and using all available resources to prevent and control obesity and other chronic diseases. For more information on CDC programs and campaigns, research reports, surveillance data, training modules, nutrition education, and related resources, see the website (http://www.cdc.gov/nccdphp/dnpa).

Maternal and Child Health Services

The Title V MCH block grant program provides states with federal funds that support a wide variety of health services, including nutrition services. Title V seeks to improve the health of all mothers and children (including children with special health care needs) by assessing needs, setting priorities, and providing programs and services. Specifically, the Title V MCH program seeks to:

1. Ensure access to quality care, especially for those with low-incomes or limited availability of care;
2. Reduce infant mortality;
3. Provide and ensure access to comprehensive prenatal and postnatal care to women (especially low-income and at-risk pregnant women);
4. Increase the number of children receiving health assessments and follow-up diagnostic and treatment services;
5. Provide and ensure access to preventive and child care services as well as rehabilitative services for certain children;
6. Implement family-centered, community-based systems of coordinated care for children with special health care needs; and
7. Provide toll-free hotlines and assistance in applying for services to pregnant women with infants and children who are eligible for Medicaid.

On the basis of a comprehensive 5-year needs assessment, state Title V MCH programs identify their priority needs and develop a program plan and state performance measures to address these needs, to the extent that they are not addressed by the program's 18 national performance measures. Each state is unique in the type of services it provides under its Title V MCH block grant. The conceptual framework for the services of the Title V MCH block grant is a pyramid, which includes 4 tiers of services (ie, direct health care services, enabling services [such as coordination with Medicaid and WIC services], population-based services, and infrastructure building services). The MCH block grant program is the only federal program that provides services at all 4 levels, including state population-based capacity and infrastructure-building services and that targets the entire population and not only the low-income population.

In 2006, the Health Resources and Services Administration's Maternal and Child Health Bureau (MCHB) included a new national performance measure that addresses the "percentage of children, ages 2 to 5 years, receiving WIC services with a body mass index at or above the 85th percentile." Another national performance measure, which had previously focused on the "percentage of mothers who breastfeed their infants at hospital discharge," was revised to reflect the "percent of mothers who breastfeed their infants at 6 months of age."

VII

The Title V Information System electronically captures data reported in the annual Title V MCH block grant applications and reports on 59 states, territories, and jurisdictions. State-reported financial data, program data, and information on key measures and indicators of MCH in the United States are posted on the Title V Information System Web site (https://mchb.tvisdata.hrsa.gov).

In addition to the formula block grants to states, Title V supports activities under the Special Projects of Regional and National Significance grants and the Community Integrated Service Systems grants. Activities supported under Special Projects of Regional and National Significance include MCH research, training, breastfeeding promotion and support, nutrition services, and a broad range of other MCH initiatives and grant projects. The Community Integrated Service Systems program seeks to improve the health of mothers and children by funding projects for the development and expansion of integrated health, education, and social services at the community level. Additional information on MCHB-funded programs is available on the MCHB Web site (http://http://mchb.hrsa.gov/).

The Early and Periodic Screening, Diagnostic and Treatment (EPSDT) program is the child health component of Medicaid. The EPSDT program is required in every state and is designed to improve the health of low-income children by financing appropriate and necessary pediatric services. State Title V agencies can play an important role in fulfilling the potential of EPSDT services. Federal rules encourage partnerships between state Medicaid and Title V agencies to ensure better access to and receipt of the full range of screening, diagnostic, and treatment services.

Bright Futures, initiated in 1990, is a longstanding, major effort of the MCHB and its partners to improve the quality of health promotion and prevention for infants, children, and adolescents and their families. Over the years, Bright Futures has evolved to encompass a vision, a philosophy, and a set of expert guidelines, tools, and other resources to implement a practical developmental approach to providing health supervision for children of all ages, from birth through adolescence.

Recognizing the need for more in-depth materials in certain areas to complement the guidelines, the MCHB launched the Building Bright Futures Project to foster the implementation of the Bright Futures health supervision guidelines by publishing practical tools and materials and by providing technical assistance and training. Through a cooperative agreement between MCHB and the AAP, *Bright Futures: Guidelines for Health Supervision of Infants, Children, and Adolescents*, Fourth Edition[33] and *Bright Futures: Nutrition*, Third Edition[34] are available at https://brightfutures.aap.org.

Conclusion

As the key provider of child health care, the pediatrician has a major role in ensuring that nutrition services for children include assessment of nutritional status and provision of a safe food supply adequate in quality and quantity, nutrition counseling, and nutrition education for children and parents. This includes assessment and intervention for the presence of food insecurity. The pediatrician can, together with other school stakeholders, join the school or district wellness committee to contribute to and support the development and implementation of local school wellness policies. As the primary expert on health in the community and as a concerned citizen, the pediatrician, in coordination with other members of the health care team, including the nutritionist or dietitian and nurse, can provide meaningful leadership and advocacy in the formulation of sound nutrition policy that includes preventive measures for food insecurity, and the education of legislators, administrators, and others who influence the response of the community to the nutritional needs of its children. The pediatrician also has the responsibility to join with additional stakeholders to advocate for nutrition policy at the national, state, and local levels, working with the resources provided by the AAP Department of Federal Affairs and the AAP Division of State Government Affairs. Funding for the federal and state programs that support community nutrition services are renewed on a regular basis, and pediatricians have the responsibility and the opportunity to influence such legislation and its funding.

References

1. American Academy of Pediatrics, Council on Community Pediatrics, Committee on Nutrition. Policy statement: Promiting food security for all children. *Pediatrics.* 2015;136(5):e1431–e1438

2. Coleman-Jensen A, Gregory C, Singh A. Household food security in the United States in 2013. Publication No. ERR-173. September 2014; Available at: https://www.ers.usda.gov/webdocs/publications/45265/48787_err173.pdf?v=42265. Accessed May 2, 2019

3. Coleman-Jensen A, McFall W, Nord M. Food Insecurity in Households With Children: Prevalence, Severity, and Household Characteristics, 2010–11. Publication No. EIB-113. May 2013; Available at: https://www.ers.usda.gov/webdocs/publications/43763/37672_eib-113.pdf?v=41424. Accessed May 2, 2019

4. Gundersen C. Food insecurity is an ongoing national concern. *Adv Nutr.* 2013;4(1):36–41

5. Chilton M, Black, M.M., Berkowitz C, Casey PH, et al. Food insecurity and risk of poor health among US-born children of immigrants. *Am J Public Health.* 2009;99(3):556–562

6. Rose-Jacobs R, Black MM, Casey PH, et al. Household food insecurity: associations with at-risk infant and toddler development. *Pediatrics*. 2008;121(1): 65–72

7. Jyoti DF, Frongillo EA, Jones SJ. Food insecurity affects school children's academic performance, weight gain, and social skills. *J Nutr*. 2005;135(12): 2831–2839

8. Alaimo K, Olson CM, Frongillo EA. Family food insufficiency, but not low family income, is positively associated with dysthymia and suicide symptoms in adolescents. *J Nutr*. 2002;132(4):719–725

9. Institute of Medicine. *Hunger and Obesity: Understanding a Food Insecurity Paradigm: Workshop Summary*. Washington, DC: National Acadmies Press; 2011

10. Laraia BA. Food insecurity and chronic disease. *Adv Nutr*. 2013;4(2):203–212

11. Calkins K, Devaskar SU. Fetal origins of adult disease. *Adolesc Health Care*. 2011;41(6):158–176

12. Portrait F, Teeuwiszen E, Deeg D. Early life undernutrition and chronic diseases in older ages: The effects of the Dutch famine on cardiovascular diseases and diabetes. *Soc Sci Med*. 2011;73(5):711–718

13. Schwarzenberg SJ, Kuo AA, Linton JM, Flanagan P, American Academy of Pediatrics, Council on Community Pediatrics and the Committee on Nutrition. Promoting food security for all children. *Pediatrics*. 2015;136(5):e1431–e1438

14. Hager ER, Quigg AM, Black MM, et al. Development and validity of a 2-item screen to identify families at risk for food insecurity. *Pediatrics*. 2010;126(1): e26–e32

15. Eagan MC, Oglesby AC. Nutrition services in the maternal and child health program: a historical perspective. In: Sharbaugh CO, Egan MC, eds. *Call to Action: Better Nutrition for Mothers, Children, and Families*. Washington, DC: National Center for Education in Maternal and Child Health; 1991:73–92

16. US Department of Health and Human Services. *Healthy People 2010. With Understanding and Improving Health and Objectives for Improving Health*. 2nd ed. Washington, DC: US Government Printing Office; 2000

17. McCall M, Keir B. *Survey of the Public Health Nutrition Workforce 1999–2000*. Alexandria, VA: US Department of Agriculture; 2003

18. Institute of Medicine. *The Future of the Public's Health in the 21st Century*. Washington, DC: National Academies Press; 2003

19. Edelstein S. *Nutrition in Public Health: Handbook for Developing Programs and Services*. Sudbury, MA: Jones and Bartlett Publishers; 2005

20. American Dietetic Association. Position of the American Dietetic Association: cost-effectiveness of medical nutrition therapy. *J Am Diet Assoc*. 1995;95(1):88–91

21. An Act Further Regulating Insurance Coverage for Certain Inherited Diseases. Massachusetts Session Law. Chapter 384 §1-11 (1993). Available at: http://archives.lib.state.ma.us/actsResolves/1993/1993acts0384.pdf. Accessed January 19, 2013

22. Bayerl CT, Ries J, Bettencourt MF, Fisher P. Nutritional issues of children in early intervention programs: primary care team approach. *Semin Pediatr Gastrointest Nutr.* 1993;4:11–15

23. Owen AY, Splett PL, Owen GM, Frankle RT. *Nutrition in the Community. The Art and Science of Delivering Services.* Boston, MA: McGraw-Hill; 1999

24. US Department of Agriculture. Supplemental Nutrition Assistance Program Food and Nutrition Service. 2007; Available at: http://www.fns.usda.gov/supplemental-nutrition-assistance-program-snap. Accessed July 2017

25. Hanson K. The Food Assistance National Input-Output Multiplier (FANIOM) Model and Stimulus Effects of SNAP. Publication No. ERR-103. 2010; Available at: https://www.ers.usda.gov/publications/pub-details/?pubid=44749. Accessed May 2, 2019

26. US Department of Agriculture. Characteristics of Supplemental Nutrition Assistance Program Households: Fiscal Year 2015. Report No. SNAP-16-CHAR. 2016; Available at: https://fns-prod.azureedge.net/sites/default/files/ops/Characteristics2015.pdf. Accessed May 2, 2019

27. US General Accounting Office. *Early Intervention: Federal Investments Like WIC Can Produce Savings: Report to Congressional Requesters.* Publication No. GAO/HRD-92-18. Washington, DC: US General Accounting Office;1992

28. Mathematica Policy Research Inc. *The Savings in Medicaid Costs for Newborns and Their Mothers From Prenatal Participation in the WIC Program.* Alexandria, VA: Food and Nutrition Service, US Department of Agriculture; 1991

29. Bitler MP, Currie J. Does WIC work? The effects of WIC on pregnancy and birth outcomes. *J Policy Anal Manage.* 2005;24(1):73–91

30. Henchy W. WIC in the States: Thirty-One Years of Building a Healthier America. 2005; Available at: http://www.ncdsv.org/images/FRAC_WIC-in-the-State-31-years-of-building-a-healthier-America_2005.pdf. Accessed May 2, 2019

31. Johnson P, Huber E, Giannarelli L, Betson D. National and State-Level Estimates of Special Supplemental Nutrition Program for Women, Infants, and Children (WIC) Eligibles and Program Reach, 2013. 2015; Available at: https://fns-prod.azureedge.net/sites/default/files/ops/WICEligibles2013-Summary.pdf. Accessed May 2, 2019

32. US Department of Agriculture, Food and Nutrition Service. WIC Program Grant Levels by State agency. Available at: https://www.fns.usda.gov/wic/wic-funding-and-program-data. Accessed May 2, 2019

33. Hagan J, Shaw J, Duncan P. *Bright Futures. Guidelines for Health Supervision of Infants, Children, and Adolescents.* 4th ed. Elk Grove Village, IL: American Academy of Pediatrics; 2017

34. Holt K, Wooldridge N, Story M, Sofka D. *Bright Futures Nutrition.* 3rd ed. Elk Grove Village, IL: American Academy of Pediatrics; 2011

VII

Federal Regulation of Foods and Infant Formulas, Including Addition of New Ingredients: Food Additives and Substances Generally Recognized as Safe (GRAS)

Introduction

It is imperative that infants and children consume foods that are safe and nutritionally adequate for optimal health. In consuming a healthful diet, infants and children are exposed to food additives and generally recognized as safe (GRAS) substances. Such ingredients may be found in infant formulas, toddler foods, or foods that are marketed for the general population. The American Academy of Pediatrics (AAP) supports exclusive breastfeeding (in which all fluid, energy, and nutrients come from human milk, with the possible exception of small amounts of medicinal/nutrient supplements) for approximately 6 months, although it has acknowledged recent concerns about the timing of introduction of allergenic foods and the relationship to food allergy[1] (see Chapter 6: Complementary Feeding, and Chapter 34: Food Allergy). The US Department of Health and Human Services also recommends that infants be exclusively breastfed for the first 4 to 6 months of life, preferably for 6 months.[2] Similarly, the World Health Organization recommends exclusive breastfeeding for the first 6 months of life,[3] but for many reasons, including medical conditions, human milk may not be available to all infants. In the absence of human milk, iron-fortified infant formulas are the most appropriate substitutes for feeding healthy, full-term infants during the first year of life. By 3 months of age, despite the improving rates of breastfeeding initiation, nearly 40% of US infants are exclusively formula fed, and 65% are receiving some infant formula at 6 months of age.[4.]

Although infant formulas do not duplicate the composition of human milk, formulas are reformulated as new nutritional information, ingredients, and technology become available. Infant formula manufacturers often consider the composition of human milk in trying to improve their products. When used as the sole source of nourishment during the first 6 months of life, infant formulas meet all the energy and nutrient requirements of healthy, term infants. After 6 months of age, formulas complement the increasing variety of solid foods being introduced into the diet and continue to supply a significant part of the infant's nutritional requirements.[5,6].

Preterm infants consume infant formulas specially designed to meet their needs. These infants, typically defined as those born before 37 weeks of gestation, are at risk of medical complications attributable to their preterm births. Ordinarily, preterm infants are hospitalized in neonatal intensive care units (NICUs), where their care often includes nutrition via parenteral administration and specialized formulas.[7] Preterm infant formulas are higher in calories and provide additional vitamins and minerals relative to term infant formulas. Preterm follow-up formulas may be used at home after discharge from the NICU; such formulas are nutrient dense, being higher in protein and some vitamins and minerals. Multiple factors must be considered in determining the appropriate formula for an infant, including the infant's body weight and overall health status.

Complementary feeding is defined as providing nutrient- and energy containing solid, semi-solid, or liquid foods in addition to human milk or infant formula.[8] Complementary foods are generally introduced between 4 and 6 months of age. The age at which first foods are introduced to an infant and the type of food offered varies considerably and is largely determined by cultural practices and perceptions.

Beyond infancy, children may consume toddler foods for 1 or 2 years while learning to transition to foods that are marketed for the general population. Under its regulations, the US Food and Drug Administration (FDA) considers toddlers to be children from 12 months to 36 months of age

Federal Regulation of Ingredients Added to Food

The Center for Food Safety and Applied Nutrition of the FDA is responsible for promoting and protecting public health by making sure that the food supply is safe and wholesome. Its food safety mission is broad in scope and includes regulatory and research programs to address health risks associated with foodborne chemical and biological contamination, proper labeling of foods, including health claims, dietary supplements, food industry compliance, and international harmonization efforts. It provides oversight for more than 80% of the food in the US food supply (see Chapter 52: Food Safety). An important part of the Center for Food Safety and Applied Nutrition's mission is to review the safety of ingredients added to food, including infant formula and other foods developed for children. It also reviews substances contacting food, including materials used to package infant formula and baby food.

Food from plant or animal sources contains carbohydrates, proteins, lipids, vitamins, minerals, and other nutrients. As such, food is a complex mixture of hundreds or thousands of chemical substances. Under the Federal Food, Drug, and Cosmetic Act (FD&C Act),* whole foods are presumed to be safe on the basis of their history of common use. This presumption is not extended to ingredients added to food, which must undergo a safety assessment and meet the safety standard of "reasonable certainty of no harm."

The term "food ingredients," as used in this chapter, includes food additives, color additives, and other substances that are "generally recognized as safe" (GRAS) under specified conditions of use. These ingredients are intentionally added to food for technical reasons, including: (1) to maintain or improve safety and freshness; (2) to improve or maintain nutritional value or (3) to improve taste, texture, and appearance. In addition, some ingredients are added to conventional foods for their effects on the human body. It is important to understand that the regulatory framework for foods defines a standard of safety and not the efficacy of the food additive. Thus, the evaluation of ingredients by the FDA is limited to consideration of risks rather than benefits.

Materials used to package or transport food are called food contact substances. Although not intentionally added to food, food contact substances are subject to the same safety standard as food ingredients. Some food contact substances (eg, plastic packaging materials, can coatings, and sealants for lids and caps) are also relevant to the packaging of infant formula. In 2019, the FDA issued guidance for regulating food contact substances in contact with infant formula and human milk.[9] Consumer exposure to any one food chemical is expected to be relatively low in adults and children, as they eat of a variety of foods packaged in a variety of materials. However, infants 0 to 6 months of age typically consume human milk and/or infant formula exclusively and consume higher amounts of food in relation to their body weight than an adult. There are also clear differences in pharmacokinetic parameters in infants compared with adults, and infants also undergo distinctive periods of rapid growth and development of all organ systems. These factors must be considered when assessing the safety of food contact substances for infant foods. Further consideration of food contact substances is beyond the scope of this chapter, but this topic is reviewed in Chapter 52: Food Safety, as well as in a 2018 policy statement from the AAP.[10]

The FDA has several programs to ensure the safety of food ingredients, including a mandatory review processes for food and color additives and a voluntary notification program for GRAS substances. When a petition for GRAS status is filed for new food ingredients (eg, docosahexaenoic acid [DHA]), the notice of filing and the agency's final action on a petition

VII

---

* https://www.fda.gov/regulatory-information/laws-enforced-fda/federal-food-drug-and-cosmetic-act-fdc-act

are published in the *Federal Register*. An inventory of GRAS notices and the agency's response to those notices is posted on the FDA website: https://www.accessdata.fda.gov/scripts/fdcc/?set=GRASNotices.

Food Ingredients: Food Additive or GRAS Substance?

In 1958, Congress enacted the Food Additives Amendment to the FD&C Act. A food additive is broadly defined as a substance that, when added to food, becomes a component or otherwise affects the characteristics of food. Food additives must undergo premarket review and approval by the FDA to be added to foods. This includes a substance that imparts color to a food. In addition, a source of radiation is explicitly defined by the law as a food additive, thus, giving the FDA regulatory power over the use of irradiation of food. Of note, infant formulas are not irradiated and do not contain color additives.

On the other hand, the FD&C Act states that substances that are designated as GRAS for their intended use by experts qualified by scientific training and experience to evaluate their safety are excluded from the food additive definition. Put simply, GRAS substances are not "food additives" and do not require premarket review and approval by the FDA. As noted previously, irrespective of whether a substance is deemed to be GRAS or is a food additive, the safety determination is always limited to the substance's intended conditions of use, not its efficacy. In other words, the GRAS substance does not have to be shown to be beneficial to use in food but has to be shown not to be harmful.

For approval of a food additive, data and information, which may be proprietary, must be sent to the FDA to evaluate the safety of the additive. Thus, for a food additive, the FDA determines the safety of the ingredient, whereas a determination that an ingredient is GRAS can be made by any qualified experts, including those outside government.

A food substance may be GRAS either through scientific procedures or, for a substance used in food before passage of the FD&C Act, through experience based on common use in food prior to 1958. General recognition of safety for a GRAS substance through scientific procedures requires the same quantity and quality of scientific evidence required to obtain approval of the substance as a food additive and ordinarily is based on published studies, which may be corroborated by unpublished studies and other data and information. General recognition of safety through experience based on common use in foods prior to 1958 requires a substantial history of widespread consumption for food by a significant number of consumers.

Voluntary Submissions for GRAS Substances

A substance that will be added to food is subject to mandatory premarket review and approval by the FDA unless its use is determined by qualified experts to be GRAS. In August 2016, the FDA issued a final rule[11] to establish a voluntary notification procedure whereby any person may notify the FDA of a determination by that person that a particular use of a substance is GRAS. The FDA accepts voluntary GRAS notices for use in human food. Thus, submission of a GRAS notice is voluntary, and in the case of an ingredient intended for use in infant formula, establishing the safety prior to infant formula notification is advantageous to the industry and the FDA.

As described in the GRAS final rule,[11] the FDA evaluates whether each submitted notice provides a sufficient basis for a GRAS determination and whether information in the notice or otherwise available to the FDA raises issues that lead the agency to "question" whether use of the substance is GRAS. Following this evaluation, the FDA responds to the notifier by letter in 1 of 3 categories:

1. The agency does not question the basis for the notifier's GRAS conclusion;
2. The agency concludes that the notice does not provide a sufficient basis for GRAS conclusion; or
3. The response letter states that the agency has, at the notifier's request, ceased to evaluate the GRAS notice.

The first category, referred to as the "no questions letter," is often seen as an "approval by the FDA, but this is open for interpretation and does not necessarily mean approval on the part of the FDA.

Not surprisingly, the GRAS process has been the subject of controversy,[12] as noted in a recent AAP policy statement.[10] Although intended to be used in limited situations, it is now the way the majority of new ingredients get added to food, including infant formula. Concerns have been raised that the FDA may not able to ensure the safety of voluntary GRAS applications from various entities, as most submitters of which have potential conflicts of interest. More information about GRAS substance process can be found on the FDA website: https://www.federalregister.gov/documents/2016/09/08/C1-2016-19164/substances-generally-recognized-as-safe.

Ingredient Review Focuses on Safety

The term "safe," as it refers to food additives and ingredients (including food contact substances), is defined by legislation as a "reasonable certainty in the minds of competent scientists that a substance is not harmful under the intended conditions of use." The concept of safety involves the question of whether a substance is hazardous to the health of man or animal and takes into consideration that in reality it is impossible to establish with complete certainty the absolute harmlessness of the use of any substance.[13]

The safety data considered in reviewing a food ingredient include, at a minimum, chemical information and toxicologic data. Microbiologic information is also needed when a microorganism is used in the production of an ingredient. Clinical studies designed for purposes other than safety may still provide information pertaining to the safe use of an ingredient in infant formula.

Chemical Information

Information provided for the ingredient includes composition as well as information on the method of manufacture that allows identification and characterization of both the intended component(s) and any likely impurities (eg, residual starting materials, products of side reactions, and decomposition products of reactants or of the additive) in the food ingredient (Table 50.I.1). For food ingredients of natural origin that might contain

Table 50.I.1.

Types of Chemistry Data and Information Typically Evaluated for New Ingredients or New Uses of Ingredients

Identity	• Chemical name and CAS number • Structure and molecular weigh • Physical characteristics
Manufacturing process	• Full description of process • List of chemicals/reagents used
Specifications	• Typically proposed or references published specifications • Includes description of the ingredients, identification tests, purity assay, and limits for impurities/contaminants
Stability	• Data demonstrating the stability • Discussion of the fate of the ingredient
Technical effect and intended use	• Type of food and use level • Data to show that the use level accomplishes the technical effect
Analytical methodology	• If a use limitation of the additive is required for safe use, the petition must include a method able to quantify the substance for the purpose of enforcing the limit

known toxicants, consideration of the ability of the manufacturing process to control, reduce, or concentrate toxicant levels is important. In addition, food grade specifications include identification and quantification of components of the ingredient as well as limitations for impurities or contaminants if needed (eg, lead, residual solvents, microorganisms).

As part of the chemist's evaluation of the intended use of an ingredient, the dietary exposure is estimated by considering the amount of a substance added to various foods and the amount of such foods generally consumed by the population at large on a daily basis over a lifetime.

Toxicologic Information

For a safety assessment, the types and number of safety studies needed depends primarily on the chemical nature of the substance being evaluated and the dietary exposure estimated from the conditions of intended use. The fate of the substance in the gut and other metabolic considerations (ie, absorption, distribution, metabolism, and elimination) are important as well. Toxicologic studies play a prominent role. Other specialized studies may be needed as determined on a case-by-case basis. Types of toxicologic studies typically evaluated for new ingredients or new uses of ingredients are listed in Table 50.I.2. The FDA has provided guidance documents to assist individuals who wish to submit data for the safety assessment of a food ingredient: https://www.fda.gov/downloads/food/guidanceregulation/ucm222779.pdf.

Table 50.I.2.

Type of Toxicological Studies Typically Evaluated for New Ingredients or New Uses of Ingredients

- Short-term tests for genetic toxicity (in vivo and in vitro testing)
- Metabolism and pharmacokinetic studies
- Subchronic feeding studies (at least 90 days) in a rodent (eg, rat) and nonrodent (eg, dog) species
- Two-generation reproduction study with a teratology phase (developmental toxicity study) in a rodent (eg, rat)
- Chronic feeding studies (at least 1 year) in a rodent (eg, rat) and nonrodent (eg, dog) species (may be conducted as a component of a lifetime carcinogenicity study in rodents)
- Two-year carcinogenicity studies in two rodent species (eg, rats and mice). The rat carcinogenicity study should also include an in utero phase
- Other studies as needed (eg, neurotoxicity and immunotoxicity) on the basis of available data and information about the substance

VII

Microbiological Information

Microorganisms used in the production of ingredients should be taxonomically identified and shown to be nonpathogenic and nontoxigenic. However, certain strains of microorganisms normally considered to be nontoxigenic may be capable of producing toxins when cultured under certain conditions. When such microorganisms are used as sources of ingredients, the fermentation conditions should be adjusted to prevent toxin synthesis, and appropriate tests should be conducted to ensure that the final ingredients do not contain toxins at unsafe levels. Alternatively, such microorganisms may be genetically modified to inactivate biochemical pathways involved in toxin synthesis. All the information relevant to the identity and safety of the microorganisms used as sources of ingredients should be described, including current and previous uses in food or in the production of food ingredients, if applicable. Microbiological considerations relevant to an ingredient safety assessment are discussed further by Mattia and Merker.[14]

Other Information, Including Human Studies

Scientific reviewers at the Center for Food Safety and Applied Nutrition do not use a checklist of required studies for a given food ingredient safety review. Although general guidelines exist, all safety reviews are approached on a case-by-case basis. In evaluating the safety of any ingredient, all scientific issues relevant to the intended use of the ingredient must be resolved. Therefore, a wide variety of study types could be included in an ingredient data package. Some additional examples of the types of studies that may bear on the safe use of an ingredient in foods include epidemiologic and clinical studies as well as specialized studies in well-defined scientific disciplines. Human studies that are not conducted for safety assessment per se may be relevant sources of information for safety evaluations. For example, efficacy studies of food ingredients conducted primarily for substantiating claims may contain relevant safety information.

For infant formula, human studies are often conducted to determine whether the formula supports normal physical growth when the formula is fed as the sole source of nutrition. Such testing is discussed by a 1998 report of the Life Sciences Research Organization.[15] Although growth studies are not safety studies, they are evaluated as part of the safety assessment of an ingredient added to infant formula.

"Functional Foods" and Provisions for Claims

In recent years, the food industry has been developing and marketing foods that it refers to as "functional foods." Although there is no formal definition of what the industry means by functional food, one report defines functional foods as "foods and food components that provide a health benefit beyond basic nutrition (for the intended population)".[16] These substances provide essential nutrients often beyond quantities necessary for normal maintenance, growth, and development and/or other biologically active components that impart health benefits or desirable physiological effects.

Currently, the FDA has neither a definition nor a specialized regulatory rubric for foods being marketed as "functional foods." Rather, the FDA regulates foods that are marketed as "functional foods" under the same regulatory framework as other conventional foods. Thus, any ingredient in a "functional food" needs to be safe and lawful, in accordance with the existing provisions of the FD&C Act.[16] As with a safety assessment for any food ingredient, the purported benefits of a "functional" ingredient are not relevant, except to the extent that such effects might negatively affect health.

In the FD&C Act, a food is misbranded if its labeling is false or misleading in any way. The FD&C Act also lays out the statutory framework for the use of labeling claims that characterize the level of a nutrient in a food or that characterize the relationship of a nutrient to a disease or health-related condition. If products bear any claims on the label or in labeling, those claims are the purview of the Office of Nutrition, Labeling, and Dietary Supplements. See the FDA website for more information on claims: https://www.fda.gov/Food/GuidanceRegulation/GuidanceDocumentsRegulatoryInformation/LabelingNutrition/default.htm.

Another type of claim is a structure/function claim, which historically has appeared on products including conventional foods. The FDA defines structure/function claims as claims that describe the role of a food or food component (such as a nutrient) that is intended to affect the structure or function of the human body (eg, "builds stronger bones"). There is a regulatory process for structure/function claims for dietary supplements; however, there is no process for structure/function claims made for food ingredients or conventional foods, including infant formula. Examples of structure/function claims on infant formulas include "easy-to-digest comfort proteins," "calcium for stronger bones," and "proven to build a stronger immune system." Draft guidance for the substantiation of structure/function claims for infant formula labels has recently been proposed[17] (see also Chapter 50.II: Federal Regulation of Food Labeling).

VII

Regulation of Infant Formula

In the United States, infant formula is regulated as food by the FDA. Therefore, the laws and regulations governing all foods also apply to infant formula. The FD&C Act defines infant formula as "a food which purports to be or is represented for special dietary use solely as food for infants by reason of its simulation of human milk or its suitability as a complete or partial substitute for human milk." Infant formulas are formulated to meet the differing nutritional needs of term infants, preterm infants, and infants with inborn errors of metabolism or other medical or dietary problems.

Infant formula is subject to specific additional statutory and regulatory requirements, because it often provides the sole source of nutrition during a critical period of growth and development. For this reason, infant formula is manufactured using specific standards and critical measures to ensure the safety and nutritive value of the product. Prior to marketing, infant formula manufacturers must notify the FDA of a change in formulation or processing (eg, addition of new ingredients, changes in packaging, a new manufacturing plant, etc).

The Center for Food Safety and Applied Nutrition is responsible for regulation of infant formula. Within the Center for Food Safety and Applied Nutrition, 2 offices share the responsibility for evaluating information regarding infant formula. The Office of Nutrition, Labeling, and Dietary Supplements has program responsibility for infant formula, and the Office of Food Additive Safety has program responsibility for the safety of food ingredients added directly to formula as well as substances used in the packaging of infant formula. The Office of Nutrition, Labeling, and Dietary Supplements evaluates whether the infant formula manufacturer has met the requirements of the FD&C Act. It consults with the Office of Food Additive Safety regarding the safety of ingredients in infant formula and packaging materials for infant formula. Together, the regulatory programs of the 2 offices ensure that infant formulas available in the United States have adequate nutritional quality and are safe. For additional information on the FDA's regulation of infant formula, see https://www.fda.gov/Food/GuidanceRegulation/GuidanceDocumentsRegulatoryInformation/InfantFormula/default.htm.

Infant Formula Ingredients, Including New Ingredients

It is estimated that 40% of infants in the United States are exclusively formula fed by 3 months of age.[4] As the sole source of nutrition, infant formula, by itself, must provide adequate nutrition. Serious adverse effects can result in infants who do not receive adequate nutrition. On the basis of these considerations, infant formula is more highly regulated than other types of foods.

The need for greater regulatory oversight of infant formula became apparent after a reformulation error caused hypochloremic metabolic alkalosis in infants fed chloride-deficient soy formulas.[18] Following this incident, Congress passed the Infant Formula Act (IFA) of 1980 (Pub L No. 96-359), which amended the FD&C Act. The FDA's implementing regulations set out recall procedures, quality-control procedures, and labeling and nutrient requirements. In 1986, Congress again amended the FD&C Act, among other things, to specify that an infant formula is adulterated unless it provides certain required nutrients and unless it meets quality factor requirements. The regulations implementing the IFA are consistent with the general food provisions of the FD&C Act. Any ingredient added to infant formula must be GRAS (see previous discussion) or covered by a food additive regulation for this intended use. The entire formulation must be suitable for its intended use as a sole source of nutrition to support the healthy growth of infants. If this is not the case, the FDA has the authority to remove the product from the marketplace.

In 2014, the FDA published a final rule that included provisions for good manufacturing practices, quality-control procedures, quality factors, notification requirements, and reports and records for the production of infant formula.[19] The final rule requires that all infant formulas support normal physical growth, that infant formulas be tested for nutrient content in the final product stage, and that all formulas be tested for harmful pathogens including *Salmonella* and *Cronobacter* organisms.

Since the IFA was enacted, manufacturers' changes to infant formula formulations first focused on changes in macronutrients. Subsequently, the changes have focused more on the addition of substances with the intention of more closely mimicking the advantages associated with consumption of human milk. Other changes focus on new sources of ingredients. As previously noted in the section on Voluntary Submissions for GRAS Substances (see previous discussion), in the case of an ingredient intended for use in infant formula, establishing the safety prior to infant formula notification is advantageous to the industry and the FDA. A way to establish the safety of an ingredient intended for use in infant formula prior to the submission to Office of Nutrition, Labeling, and Dietary Supplements is to submit a GRAS notice to the Office of Food Additive Safety.[11] Examples of substances intended for use in infant formula that have been evaluated in the GRAS notification program and received a "no questions" letter regarding the

GRAS status from the FDA include docosahexaenoic acid (DHA), various probiotic bacteria (eg, *Bifidobacterium lactis*), and galacto-oligosaccharide. Recent GRAS filings for infant formulas includes fructo-oligosaccharides. An up-to-date website of GRAS notices is available at: https://www.accessdata.fda.gov/scripts/fdcc/index.cfm?set=GRASNotices&sort=GRN_No&order=DESC&showAll=true&type=basic&search=

Required Nutrients

According to the FD&C Act, infant formula must provide infants with 30 essential substances, which include macronutrients, vitamins, and minerals (Table 50.I.3). This includes minimum levels of required nutrients

Table 50.I.3.

Recommended Nutrient Levels of Infant Formulas (per 100 kcal)[a]

Nutrient	Range	
	Minimum	*Maximum*
Protein, g	1.8[b]	4.5[b]
Fat, g Linoleic acid (18:2 ω6), mg	3.3 (30% of kcal) 300 (2.7% of kcal)	6.0 (54% of kcal)
Vitamins		
A, IU	250 (75 µg)[c]	750 (225 µg)[c]
D, IU	40 (1 µg)[d]	100 (2.5 µg)[d]
K, µg[e]	4	...
E, IU	0.7 (0.5 mg)[f] at least 0.7 IU (0.5 mg)/g linoleic acid	...
C (ascorbic acid), mg	8	...
B₁ (thiamine), µg	40	...
B₂ (riboflavin), µg	60	...
B₆ (pyridoxine), µg	35[g]	...
B₁₂, µg	0.15	...
Niacin, µg	250 (or 0.8 mg niacin equivalents)	...
Folic acid, µg	4	...

Table 50.I.3. *Continued*

Recommended Nutrient Levels of Infant Formulas (per 100 kcal)[a]

Nutrient	Range Minimum	Range Maximum
Pantothenic acid, μg	300	...
Biotin, μg	1.5[h]	...
Choline, mg	7[h]	...
Inositol, mg	4[h]	...
Minerals		
Calcium, mg	60[i]	...
Phosphorus, mg	30[i]	...
Magnesium, mg	6	...
Iron, mg[j]	0.15	3.0
Zinc, mg	0.5	...
Manganese, μg	5	...
Copper, μg	60	...
Iodine, μg	5	75
Selenium, μg[a]	2	7
Sodium, mg	20 (0.9 mEq)	60 (2.6 mEq)
Potassium, mg	80 (2.1 mEq)	200 (5.1 mEq)
Chloride, mg	55 (1.6 mEq)	150 (4.2 mEq)

[a] From the US Infant Formula Act of 1980 (Pub L No. 96-359), amended 1986 (Pub L No. 99-570) and Infant Formula: The addition of minimum and maximum levels of selenium to infant formula and related labeling (Document number 2015-15394)

[b] Biologically equivalent to or better than casein. If protein of lower quality used, minimum is increased in proportion. In no case, protein with biological value <70%.

[c] Retinol equivalents

[d] Cholecalciferol.

[e] Any vitamin K added shall be in the form of phylloquinone.

[f] All rac-a-tocopherol equivalents.

[g] At least 15 μg for each g protein in excess of 18 g/100 kcal.

[h] Naturally present in cow milk-based formulas; addition required only in non-cow milk-based formulas.

[i] Calcium-to-phosphorus ratio should be no less than 1.1 and more than 2.

[j] If contains ≥1 mg/100 kcal, must be labeled as formula "with iron."

and maximum levels that cannot be exceeded in all infant formula products. If these nutrient requirements are not met, the infant formula would be considered adulterated, unless the infant formula is classified as "exempt." Requirements for selenium where added to the list of required nutrients in 2015.[20]

An exempt infant formula is "any infant formula which is represented and labeled for use by an infant who has an inborn error of metabolism or low birth weight, or who otherwise has an unusual medical or dietary problem." This includes preterm infant formulas and human milk fortifiers used for preterm infants.[21] Thus, the FDA recognizes that exempt formulas may need to differ from nonexempt infant formulas because of the specific medical condition for which the exempt formula is used but also recommends that manufacturers follow, to the extent practical, the published recommendations for nonexempt formulas.[22]

Other Added Ingredients
Compositional analyses have shown that human milk contains nutrients already required in infant formula manufacturing, such as carbohydrates, fats, proteins, vitamins, and minerals[22] as well as other components not required by the IFA. Human milk contains bioactive components, such as enzymes, antibodies, white blood cells, prebiotics, and microorganisms. These substances are thought to be important in the early stages of development of the gastrointestinal tract and immune systems (see Chapter 3: Breastfeeding, Table 3.1). Manufacturers now add the following categories of ingredients to infant formula: lipids (docosahexaenoic acid [DHA] and arachidonic acid [ARA]), carotenoids, probiotics and prebiotics, and most recently, human milk fat globule membranes (MFGMs). MFGMs and probiotics and prebiotics are discussed in the following sections. For additional information, see Chapter 4: Formula Feeding of Term Infants.

Milk Fat Globular Membranes
The MFGM is a very complex structure that includes a number of phospholipids, glycolipids, proteins, and glycoproteins. Not a quantitatively significant ingredient of milk, MFGMs contribute little to energy production, although the constituents may play important roles in the development of the brain, intestinal tract, and other organs. Phospholipids constitute 30% of the total lipid weight of the MFGM, including sphingomyelin, phosphatidylcholine, phosphatidylethanolamine; taken together, the MFGM phospholipids account for 60% to 70% of the phospholipids in milk.[23] Almost

all of the milk gangliosides in human milk are located in MFGMs and are important in cell membranes, most prominently within the brain. In addition to lipids, the outer layer of MFGMs contain hundreds of glycosylated and nonglycosylated proteins.[24] These only account for 1% to 2% of the total milk protein content but are bioactive components believed to have health benefits.[25] Historically, MFGMs surrounding the milk fat globule are largely removed from cow milk in the formula manufacturing process when the fat fraction is replaced with vegetable oils. However, recent advances in dairy science have allowed for separation of MFGMs from fat globules, allowing bovine MFGMs to be added in concentrated form to infant formulas.[26] (A recent report has found that the phospholipid content of MFGM-fortified infant formula is in the range of that found in human milk.[27])

There are 3 small randomized controlled trials (RCTs) evaluating MFGMs in formula-fed infants.[28–30] In first of these trials from Indonesia (29–30 infants per group), infants were randomly assigned between 2 and 8 weeks of age to receive formula with or without added bovine gangliosides in a mixture of other complex milk lipids, which was continued until 6 months of age.[28] The primary outcome was the Griffiths Mental Developmental Scale at 24 weeks. The authors concluded the ganglioside supplement may have provided some advantages in cognitive skill development, particularly related to motor skills.[28] In the second of these developmental/behavioral RCTs from Sweden (about 70 infants per group), the experimental group was fed a formula supplemented with MFGMs, providing 4% of the total protein content as MFGM protein, between <2 and 6 months of age.[29] Primary outcome was the Bailey Scales of Infant and Toddler Development III at 12 months of age. The MFGM-fed infants had a statistically higher mean cognitive score than the control group (105.8 vs 101.8, respectively; $P < .008$), with no differences in motor or verbal domain scores. In yet a third noninferiority developmental/behavioral RCT from France and Italy (about 50 infants per group), a control group was compared with either a protein-rich or a lipid-rich MFGM-fortified formula, starting at 2 weeks of age and continuing until 4 months of age.[30] The primary outcome was weight gain at 4 months, and there were no differences between the 3 groups. Unexpectedly, however, the protein-rich MFGM group had a higher rate of eczema than the lipid-rich MFGM group (13.9% vs 1.4%). A combined review of these 3 studies with small numbers of subjects concluded that although the interventions were safe, these studies were not comparable given their heterogeneity, especially for the type and amount MFGM used.[31]

VII

Thus, despite the fact the MFGMs have been introduced into US formulas, evidence in support of this is very limited at this time, and a general recommendation cannot be made.

New Ingredients: Probiotics and Prebiotics

Probiotics are viable, nonpathogenic microorganisms, usually bacteria, added to food for their effects on the human intestinal tract; prebiotics are carbohydrates known to encourage the grown of certain commensal microorganisms. Since the previous edition of this book was published, an increasing number of probiotics and prebiotics have qualified for GRAS status and are being added to infant formula.

Technically speaking, the regulation of these products by the FDA depends on how these products are to be used. Thus, they can be regulated as foods (as in yogurt or kimchi), dietary supplements/food ingredients (as infant formula), cosmetics, or drugs/biologics when used to cure a disease (eg, antibiotic-associated diarrhea).[32,33] The FDA's Center for Food Safety and Applied Nutrition (CFSAN) regulates probiotics and prebiotics when they are added as food ingredients to infant formulas. Thus, probiotics and prebiotics can now be added to infant formula utilizing the GRAS process as described previously.

The gastrointestinal tract of the human body represents a complex ecosystem, and current evidence suggests that the microflora may be altered by diet and certain diseases as well as obesity.[34,35] The intestine is relatively sterile prior to birth; after birth, inoculation occurs quite rapidly with microorganisms from both the mother and the environment. The relative proportions of microorganisms in infants vary depending on the type of birth (vaginal vs cesarean delivery) and source of nutrition (human milk vs different types of infant formula).[36] In newborn infants, the immune system develops tolerance as a result of its interactions with the commensal microorganisms in the infant's gut[36] (see also Chapter 2: Development of the Gastrointestinal Tract).

The consumption of microorganisms in food dates back thousands of years; fermented foods and beverages have been consumed throughout history. In comparison, the science of microbiology is relatively new, and the microorganisms involved in these food fermentations were not identified until the early 20th century.[37] Today, many believe that by altering the microbial content of the gut, either through consuming foods containing certain microorganisms (ie, probiotics) or foods containing ingredients intended to encourage growth in the gut of certain microorganism (ie, prebiotics), a variety of potential health benefits can be added. The composition of the fecal microflora in infants fed formula with added bifidobacteria compares favorably to infants fed human milk with no differences in prevalence of diarrhea between groups.[38]

Most organisms commonly considered to be probiotics are lactic acid bacteria of the genera *Bifidobacterium* (*Bifidobacterium lactis*, *Bifidobacterium longum*) and *Lactobacillus* (*Lactobacillus reuteri*, *Lactobacillus rhamnosus*), although particular strains of *Bacillus coagulans* and a single yeast, *Saccharomyces boulardii*, have been described in the literature as probiotics.[39] Bibliographies in the GRAS notices on various probiotics in FDA's Inventory of GRAS Notices (http://www.fda.gov/grasnoticeinventory) provide a wealth of references on these topics.

Aureli et al reviewed various mechanisms by which purported probiotics may promote human health.[34] One proposed mechanism is that the absorption of organic acids, produced as end-products of anaerobic fermentation of carbohydrates by probiotic bacteria, influence human mood, energy level, and even cognitive abilities. Other possible mechanisms are competition by probiotic bacteria with pathogens, directly or by providing incompatible conditions for their growth, and stimulating host immune responses by producing specific polysaccharides. In general, although the consumption of probiotic bacteria is thought to stimulate the immune system, any specific effects are believed to be strain based, with differences even among related organisms, and dependent on the levels of microorganisms added (see also Chapter 1: Nutrition for the 21st Century—Integrating Nutrigenetics, Nutrigenomics, and Microbiomics).

Currently, labels on food products marketed as probiotic rarely specify the minimum levels of the organism that should be present. However, a review of GRAS notices indicates that use levels are based on the numbers of viable bacteria, typically expressed as colony-forming units (CFUs); the use levels in most notices is for a maximum level of 10^8 CFUs/g of powdered infant formula. As noted previously, the FDA's authority is limited to consideration of safety. For microorganisms, the major safety considerations focus on the lack of pathogenicity and absence of toxin production in the microorganisms. Clear identification of the species and strain using molecular techniques is also extremely important. Many of the genomes of these microorganisms have been sequenced, and comparisons with known pathogens can be made. Animal feeding studies, tolerance studies in humans, and efficacy studies also provide relevant safety data. In infants, growth studies may be used to confirm the absence of adverse effects predicted using preclinical data. Many uses of microorganisms in the production of various foods are considered GRAS on the basis of history of use prior to 1958. Currently, the FDA is developing improved methodology for determining purity of probiotic products.[40]

Prebiotics are typically carbohydrate compounds that are have been shown to enhance the growth of beneficial bacteria, such as *Bifidobacterium* and *Lactobacilli* species, in the gastrointestinal tract. Prebiotics were first described by Gibson and Roberfroid in 1995.[41] In a publication in 2007, Roberfroid revisited prebiotics and offered the following definition: "A prebiotic is a selectively fermented ingredient that allows specific changes, both in the composition and/or activity in the gastrointestinal microflora that confers benefits upon host well-being and health."[42]

Complex carbohydrates (oligosaccharides) that encourage growth of bifidobacteria and other resident microorganism are present in human milk. To emulate the function of these carbohydrates in human milk, infant formula manufacturers have begun adding prebiotics to infant formula. However, commercially available prebiotics for inclusion in infant formula are limited and are of a much simpler structure than most of those found in human milk. There have been no head-to-head RCTs of these products, although their effects on cultures of infant microflora have been compared in vitro.[43] The addition of prebiotics to infant formula has appeared to bring the microbiota of formula-fed infants closer to those of breastfed infants, but there is no convincing evidence to date that they effect infant immune function.[38,44] Thus, the addition of prebiotics to infant formula cannot be generally recommended at this time. However, prebiotics with GRAS status are now being added to infant formula, including fructo-oligosaccharides and galacto-oligosaccharides. Most recently, 2'-fucosylactose has received GRAS status for addition to infant formula (see previous discussion).

Newer Food Ingredients for the Pediatric Population

Once infants and toddlers transition away from infant formula and toddler foods, they consume food intended for the general population and are exposed to the same food additives and GRAS substances that older children and adults consume. This section is limited to a discussion of probiotics, prebiotics, and nonnutritive sweeteners, which have been addressed in a number of AAP reports.[45,46]

Probiotics and Prebiotics

Industry has been eager to add probiotics and prebiotics to food. The inclusion of certain species of bacteria in yogurt is a common example of probiotics in food. FDA food regulations for various types of yogurt state that yogurt must be fermented by *Lactobacillus delbrueckii* subspecies *bulgaricus* (formerly *Lactobacillus bulgaricus*) and *Streptococcus thermophilus*. Most yogurt manufacturers also add *Lactobacillus acidophilus*, and some manufacturers add *Bifidobacterium* species, *Lactobacillus casei*, and *Lactobacillus rhamnosus* as well. These additional cultures are also added for purported probiotic effects and are regulated under food ingredients with GRAS status. Such yogurt products are formulated for consumers of all ages, although some are specifically targeted for consumption by young children. Prebiotic ingredients for use in foods generally include fructo-oligosaccharides, galacto-oligosaccharides, fibers from various plant sources (ie, oats, potato, carrot, wheat, and barley), a wheat bran extract composed largely of xylo- and arabino-galactans, and yeast beta glucan. The combined use of prebiotics and probiotics, such as in some yogurt products containing additional fiber, is becoming commonplace. The industry has submitted many GRAS notices for probiotic ingredients or prebiotic ingredients for which the FDA has issued response letters.

Nonnutritive Sweeteners

The use of nonnutritive sweeteners (NNSs) in children has recently been reviewed by the AAP.[46] Currently FDA-approved NNSs range from 180 to 20 000 times sweeter than table sugar. Therefore, it takes a smaller amount to create the same sweetness as sugar, with negligible calories (Table 50.I.4). To date, 8 sugar substitutes have been approved by the FDA for use in a variety of foods: saccharin, sucralose, aspartame, acesulfame K, neotame, advantame, Siraitia grosvenorii fruit extract (SGFE), and Stevia (plant extract of *Stevia rebaudiana*). SGFE and stevia were approved under GRAS status, the remaining NNSs being classified as food additives (Table 50.I.4). Sucralose has become the most commonly used NNS (most baked goods), while other sweeteners (eg, aspartame used in diet soda) are becoming less popular. On the other hand, the use of the natural sweetener stevia is increasing.[47]

As of July 12, 2015, 12 291 food products contained NNSs. The actual amount of consumption of NNSs by children and adolescents is unknown in that food labels in the United States do not include information on the amount of NNS contained.[46] From the National Health and Nutrition Examination Survey (NHANES), the percentage of children consuming

VII

Table 50.I.4.
Food and Drug Administration (FDA) Approved NNSs

Type (Approval Distinction)	Commercial Name	Kcal/g	Sweetness Compared with Sucrose	Introduction/ FDA Approval	Heating Reduces Sweetness	Contraindication/ Safety Issues
Saccharin (1, 2-benzisothiazolin-3-one, 1, 1-dioxide (food additive)	Sweet'N Low; Sugar Twin; Necta Sweet	0	200 to 700	Introduced in 1879; FDA approved for use.	No	None
Aspartame (N-(l-alpha-Aspartyl)-L-phenylalanine, 1-methyl ester) (food additive)	NutraSweet; Equal; Sugar Twin	4[a]	180	Approved for limited use (ie, table top sweetener) by the FDA in 1981 and approved for general use in 1996.	Yes	Phenylketonuria (PKU); reported cases of thrombocytopenia (78)
Acesulfame-potassium/ acelsulfame-k (Potassium 6 –methyl-2,2-dioxo-oxathiazin-4-folate) (food additive)	Sunett; Sweet One	0	300	Discovered 1967. FDA approved limited use 1988, general use (exceptions: meat and poultry) 2003.	No	Associated with cancer in animals at high dose. No known association in humans.
Sucralose (1,6-Dichloro-1, 6-dideoxy-Beta-D-fructofuranosyl-4-chloro-4-deoxy-alpha-D-galactopyranoside) (food additive)	Splenda	0	600	Discovered in 1976. FDA approved for limited use in 1998 and for general use in 1999.	No	None

Neotame (N-(N-(3,3-dimethylbutyl)-L-alpha-aspartyl-L-phenylalanine 1-methyl ester) (food additive)	Newtame	0	7000 to 13 000	FDA approved for general use 2002 (exceptions: meat and poultry).	No	Contains phenylalanine and aspartic acid and is therefore contraindicated in those with PKU.
Stevia (1,1-dioxo-1,2-benzothiazol-3-one) GRAS	Truvia; Pure Via; Enliten	0	200 to 400	Accepted as GRAS 4/20/2015.	Yes	None
Advantame ((N-(3-(3-hydroxy-4-methoxyphenyl))-propyl-alpha-aspartyl]-L-phenylalanine 1-methyl ester)	None	3.85	20 000	FDA approved for general use 2014 (exceptions: meat and poultry).	No	Determined to be safe for use in children.
Luo han guo fruit extract (GRAS)	Monk Fruit in the Raw; PureLo Lo Han Sweetener		600	GRAS 1/15/2010; intended for use as a table top sweetener, food ingredient and additional sweetening agent.	Unknown	

Reprinted from Baker-Smith et al.[46]

[a] Although aspartame contains 4 kcal/g, very little is used, and therefore, it essentially provides no extra calories.

GRAS indicates generally recognized as safe.

VII

NNSs increased from 8.7% in 1999–2000 to 15.0% in 2007–2008.[47] Similar estimates from NHANES data from 2003 to 2010 estimated NSS intake in children increased from 7.8% to 18.9% over this time period. The most recent NHANES estimate of NSS intake from 2009–2010 cross-sectional data is 25.1% of children vs 44% adults reported consumption of NNS.[48] Most of this increase was attributable to reduced-calorie beverages (fruit drinks and sport drinks) and did not result from an increase in diet soda intake.[47]

There has been much controversy about the potential adverse effects of NNSs in both adults and children, as noted in the AAP report.[46] There are hundreds of published studies that have evaluated the safety issues of NNSs,[46] but only 5 randomized controlled trials in children.[49–53] These studies evaluate the effects on weight control/obesity, and 1 study[49] evaluated the effects on behavior and cognitive performance in children. There are also no long-term follow-up studies of intakes in children. The following concerns have been raised regarding the possible effects of nonnutritive sweeteners: (1) increased cancer risk; (2) attention-deficit disorders and autism; (3) appetite and taste preference; (4) childhood obesity; and (5) metabolic syndrome and diabetes.[46] It is generally agreed that NNSs do not increase the risk of cancer or increase the rate of attention-deficit disorders or autism in children. Research on appetite and taste preference has been performed in animals and adolescents/adults. The effects of NNSs on weight loss and the metabolic syndrome remain poorly defined in both children and adults. An RCT in children 4 to 11 years of age with normal weight who consume beverages containing NNSs experience less weight gain over an 18-month period compared with those who consume sugar-sweetened beverages.[53] The difference between the 2 cohorts was 2.2 pounds. A second RCT in overweight and at-risk children found that, combined with additional changes in lifestyle, use of NNSs may contribute to slowed weight gain over a 6-month study period.[51] A third trial found that in children with obesity, use of NNSs contributed to a slower weight gain over the first year, but the difference in weight was not maintained during the subsequent year.[50]

New High-Intensity Sweeteners From the Stevia Plant

The leaves of the stevia plant (*S rebaudiana*) contain a class of compounds, steviol glycosides, that are known for their intense sweet taste. In fact, steviol glycosides are about 200-fold sweeter than table sugar. Since 2008, the FDA has responded to a number of GRAS notices on the highly purified components of the leaves of the stevia plant (rebaudiosides). These notices provided data and information supporting the conclusion of the notifiers that rebaudiosides are GRAS for use as a sweetener in various foods.[54] Among the information provided by the notifiers were published scientific studies and the conclusions of various panels that, although the data were incomplete regarding the safety of whole leaf stevia, the data were adequate to establish the safety of preparations of highly purified steviol glycosides.[54] However, it is important to note that an import alert originally issued by the FDA in 1991 and revised in 2010 prohibits the entry of stevia leaves and crude stevia extracts that do not meet the specifications for highly purified steviol glycosides into the United States for use as a food additive or GRAS substance.[55] The import alert does not prohibit the importation of stevia leaves for use solely as a dietary ingredient in the manufacture of a dietary supplement product. At the present time, steviol glycosides are in chocolate milk, soft drinks, many baked goods, and multivitamins targeted at the pediatric population. Their use continues to increase.

Biotechnology in the Development of New Food Ingredients—Bioengineered Foods

Biotechnology is a field of applied biology that uses a variety of scientific techniques, such as cross-breeding, molecular cloning, genetic engineering, and now genomic editing, to modify living organisms (both plants and animals) to produce new food ingredients. Since the 1990s, genetic engineering utilizing recombinant DNA (rDNA) techniques have been used to introduce new genes or to modify the expression of genes in plants used as food, as well as in microorganisms used in food for fermentation, sources of food ingredients, or as processing aids. This generally allows for the introduction of new DNA or rDNA into an organism's genome but generally without control of the location in the genome. Genetic engineering of food animals includes goats, cattle, pigs, cows, chickens, salmon, trout, carp, and catfish.[56] More recently, the term "genomic editing" has been introduced to describe a new set of technologies that can be used to introduce, remove, or substitute one or more specific nucleotides at a specific site in the DNA of an organism's genome, in both plants and animals. This is achieved with the use of protein-nucleotide complexes, including zinc-finger nucleases (ZFNs) and "cluster regulatory interspersed short palindromic repeat associated nucleases" (CRISPR). Genomic editing has now been accomplished in cattle, goats, pigs, chicken, and sheep.[57] However, none of these potential food products have been approved in the United States, although genetically

engineered salmon has been approved in Canada (http://futurism.com/
you-can-now-buy-genetically-engineered-salmon-in-canada/).

Genetically engineered plant varieties intended for food use include corn,
soybean, cotton (used for cottonseed oil and animal feed), wheat, sugar
beet, and most vegetable oils (canola, corn, cotton, soybean).[58] According
to a 2018 US Department of Agriculture (USDA) survey, 94% of soybean
and 92% of corn grown in the United States were bioengineered varieties.[59] Fruits and vegetables that have been genetically modified include
papaya, potato, zucchini, pineapple, plums, and apples.[59] As of 2011, the
most common traits in these bioengineered varieties were for agronomic
enhancement (ie, herbicide tolerance, pest resistance, prolongation of shelf
life; Table 50.I.5). These crops are generally handled as bulk commodities, and consequently, conventional varieties and bioengineered varieties
are not segregated, except when intended for use in products certified by
the USDA organic program[60] (see Chapter 13: Fast Foods, Organic Foods).
Consequently, corn-, cotton-, and soy-derived ingredients added to processed foods are largely derived from bioengineered varieties. The composition of ingredients from bioengineered, agronomically enhanced crops is

Table 50.I.5.

**Food Crops With New Traits Introduced by Recombinant DNA Technology
That Have Been the Subject of 85 Biotechnology Consultations With the
FDA Through 2011**

Crops	Trait
Alfalfa, canola, corn, cotton, soybean, sugar beet, creeping bent grass, flax, rice	Herbicide tolerance
Squash, plum, papaya	Virus resistance[a]
Corn, cotton, potato, soybean, tomato	Insect resistance[a]
Soybean, canola	Altered composition oils, 3 consultations to date
corn, canola, radicchio	Male sterility
Tomato, cantaloupe	Delayed ripening
Corn (increased lysine), canola (reduced phytate)	Altered composition, 2 consultations to date
Corn	Drought tolerance

[a]Regulated as a pesticide by the United States Environmental Protection Agency.

comparable to those produced from conventional varieties. Genomic editing of plants potentially used for food now includes various brassicas, corn, barley, soybean, sorghum, and rice. The number of plants is expanding rapidly, and transmissions to the next generation have been demonstrated.[61]

The FDA regulates food derived from genetically engineered plants for use in both humans and animals like it regulates all foods.[62] However, federal regulations of genetically modified animals used as food for humans is more complex (see below).

A 1992 FDA policy document applied to foods derived from all new plant varieties, including varieties developed using recombinant deoxyribonucleic acid (rDNA) that allowed for the expression of nonnative proteins by recipient plants.[62] The FDA considers DNA as GRAS on the basis of its consumption as a component of most whole foods and that the vast majority of proteins are neither toxins nor food allergens. The FDA considered that the characteristics of the food should be the focus of the FDA's safety evaluation rather than the method used to impart those characteristics. In the 1992 policy document, the FDA offered developers guidance on food safety and nutritional concerns for new plant varieties, including decision trees that indicate when developers should consult the FDA. In 1996, the FDA developed a voluntary consultation program and released guidance for industry regarding consultations under its 1992 policy. Through 2018, the FDA had evaluated more than 150 genetically engineered plant varieties through this program.[62] The traits addressed in these consultations are summarized in Table 50.I.4.

In January 2017, to inform its regulatory guidelines for the new genome editing techniques, the FDA published a docket to receive public comments on the use of these techniques to produce new plant varieties that are used for either human or animal food.[63] In this document, the FDA acknowledged that genomic editing has potential risks ranging from how the technology effects individual genomes to its potential environmental and ecosystem effects. Additionally, genome editing has raised fundamental ethical question about human (and animal) life.

As noted, the regulation of animals altered genetically for use as food is more complex. The FDA issued guidance for industry for regulation of genetically engineered animals containing heritable recombination DNA constructs in June 2009.[64] Expanding the scope of the 2009 guidelines, the FDA subsequently published a request for comments for regulation of intentionally altered genomic DNA in animals potentially used as food in January 2017.[65] Note that genetically modified biopharma animals that produce human biologics (ie, a genetically engineered goat that produces a human biologic in its milk) are regulated as a drug. Animals bioengineered to produce heathier meats (pigs that contain more omega-3 fatty acids) or for faster growth of meat (salmon) are more problematic. To date, only a single genetically modified animal for food production has made it through the FDA approval process—AquAdvantage salmon.[66] This may be partially explained by the fact the that the concept of "generally recognized as safe" or GRAS has not been applied to the regulation of genetically engineered animals. Unlike the FDA's process for regulation of genetically engineered food crops, the FDA's process for animals is mandatory.[67]

In December 2018, the FDA published its final rule for disclosure of bioengineered food (either or plant or animal origin) on all food labels. The definition of a bioengineered food is any food that contains genetic material that has been modified through in vitro recombination deoxyribonucleic acid (rDNA) techniques and for which the modification could not otherwise be obtained through conventional breeding or found in nature.[68] As of January 1, 2020, all bioengineered food labels must display the symbol depicted in Figure 50.I.1.

Products of Bioengineered Microorganisms Reviewed by the FDA

Enzymes are proteins used by food processors to confer chemical changes to foods or ingredients, including ingredients used in infant formula and other foods consumed by infants and children. Examples of enzymes used in food processing include amylases, glycosidases, and lipases.

Many enzymes currently used in food processing are derived from recombinant microorganisms. Food enzyme manufacturers commonly introduce genes encoding well-known enzymes from microorganisms into host organisms considered safe for enzyme production. The FDA has evaluated the safety of enzymes and other products produced by microorganisms modified through rDNA techniques in a number of GRAS notices and, prior to the GRAS notification program, in GRAS affirmation petitions that resulted in regulations.

Microbial enzymes used in food processing are sold as enzyme preparations that contain in addition to the desired enzyme activity other metabolites of the production strain as well as added materials such as preservatives and stabilizers. Thus, safety evaluation of food enzyme preparations poses special challenges that are not typically encountered with other food ingredients. The food safety assessments of enzyme preparations focus on the safety of the host organism and the safety of the expressed protein.[69]

Figure 50.I.1.
Disclosure symbol for bioengineered foods

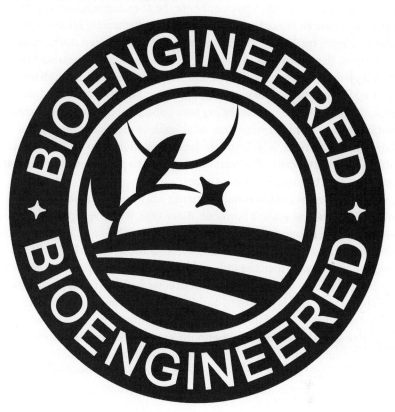

The host organism should not produce toxic substances related to patho-genic strains. Frequently used hosts for enzyme production include bacteria (eg, *Bacillus subtilis*) and fungi (eg, *Aspergillus niger* and *Aspergillus oryzae*). Because fungal strains are known to produce mycotoxins, most commercial fungal strains (*Aspergillus* species and *Trichoderma reesei*) have been modified to block mycotoxin production.[70] Pariza and Johnson[71] provided a strategy for toxicity testing of proteins produced by a bioengineered microorganism.

Bioengineered microorganisms can be used directly in food fermenta-tions or used to produce nonprotein substances used in food. For example, several yeast varieties with modified traits primarily for use in winemaking have been developed. Also, a strain of the yeast *Yarrowia lipolytica* was geneti-cally augmented with a number of genes derived from a variety of organ-isms to produce eicosenoic acid-rich triglyceride oil for use in food.

Hormones Used in Animal Production

Hormones used in animal production are also regulated by the FDA. Most of these are sex steroids. Such hormones may be of endogenous or exogenous origin and have been used as growth stimulants to increase lean muscle mass. Animals treated with these sex steroids have included steers, heifers, veal calves, sheep, swine, and poultry.[72] At present, steroid implants have been approved for use in beef cattle and sheep by the FDA, although they have not been approved for growth enhancement in dairy cows, veal calves, pigs, or poultry.[73] Although there has been concern about the relative contribution of meat from hormone-treated animals to the total consumption of hormones in humans, it is clear that the contribution from meat of treated animals is insignificant when hormones have been properly used and must be considered biologically without effect.

One of the most controversial hormones has been bovine somatotropin (BST), or bovine growth hormone. Since 1994, it has been possible to synthesize the hormone using rDNA technology with genetically engineered *Escherichia coli* to create recombinant bovine somatotropin (rBST). rBST is injected into cows to increase milk yield. There is no evidence that the composition of milk is altered by treatment of cows with rBST.[74] Approximately 90% of the hormone is destroyed during pasteurization, and there is also no evidence that the milk of treated cows has a significantly increased amount of bovine growth hormone. Furthermore, growth hormone is destroyed in the gastrointestinal tract when consumed orally and must be injected to retain biologic activity. Bovine growth hormone is very specific and is biologically inactive in humans. Thus, any bovine growth hormone present in food products has no physiological effect on humans, and its safety in humans has been reconfirmed by the FDA.[75]

Conclusions

The definition of food is broad and includes infant formula. Any ingredient added to food in the United States must be approved by the FDA for such use, or the intended use of the ingredient must be GRAS. Over many years, the FDA has gained much experience in conducting safety assessments for a variety of ingredients to provide safe and wholesome foods. Although chemical, toxicologic, and microbiological studies are typically reviewed, a variety of types of studies, including studies conducted in humans and specialized studies, may be used to address all of the issues that arise in conducting a safety evaluation.

No area of ingredient testing or safety assessment is more critical to public health than assessing the safety of ingredients added to infant formula or, for that matter, for foods specifically marketed to young children. Infants may rely on infant formula as their sole source of nutrition, and young children who are transitioning to eating adult foods cannot choose from the full range of dietary products available. Both infants and young children have high energy demands to support their rapid growth and development. Poor nutrition or unsafe foods could have adverse health effects that persist throughout life. As science and technology change over time, it will be important to refine toxicity testing paradigms with infants and children in mind to ensure the safety of the products they consume; likewise, refined methods for estimating dietary exposure in infants and children will be needed. As manufacturers continue to research and to develop new ingredients for use in foods for consumers of all ages, regulatory agencies will need to keep pace with developments to continually improve their assessments to protect and promote public health.

To emulate the functionality of human milk, manufacturers of infant formulas are adding ingredients that are present in human milk including prebiotics, probiotics, and milk fat globule membranes. What is contentious is whether the addition of these ingredients confers additional benefits, beyond ordinary nutrition, to infants who consume them. In evaluating the safety of ingredients added to foods, the FDA does not consider benefits. However, with the advent of "functional ingredients" and "functional foods," risk assessment strategies for the future may be designed to more directly address purported beneficial effects on the human body. In other words, assessments may need to consider the risk of adding a new ingredient relative to the risk of not adding it, if a benefit has been convincingly demonstrated in infants, children, or adults.

Many of the ingredients that have been added to foods in recent years are common components of food with new uses. As a result, use of these ingredients falls under the GRAS provisions of the FD&C Act. Some of the more interesting ingredients to enter the market place through the GRAS process include long-chain polyunsaturated fatty acids, probiotics and prebiotics, carotenoids, steviol glycosides, and milk fat globule membranes. These are components of foods that generally are present in the diet; however, their intended uses in foods have changed. For example, certain bacteria have been used in fermentation processes for millennia, but the addition of these microorganisms directly to food to transiently inhabit the gut is relatively new. Innovations in the sourcing of ingredients and the methods of manufacture of ingredients have also changed in the last decade. For example, oils previously obtained from marine sources are now produced by culturing single-cell organisms, such as algae or fungi. It is now commonplace to produce enzymes using bioengineered microorganisms and biotechnology has moved forward using new genetic engineering techniques to modifying food crops to enhance their agronomic and nutritive value. On the other hand, the use of genetic engineering to modify animals used for food is very limited at present. As food science continues to evolve, the FDA will continue to ensure the safety and wholesomeness of foods and food ingredients in the US marketplace.

References

1. American Academy of Pediatrics, Section on Breastfeeding. Policy statement: Breastfeeding and the use of human milk. *Pediatrics.* 2012;129(3):e827–e841

2. Department of Health and Human Services. HHS Blueprints and Breastfeeding Policy Statements. Available at: http://www.womenshealth.gov/breastfeeding/government-in-action/hhs-blueprints-and-policy-statements. Accessed November 15, 2012

3. World Health Organization. The World Health Organization's infant feeding recommendation. Available at: http://www.who.int/nutrition/topics/infantfeeding_recommendation/en/index.html. Accessed November 15, 2012

4. Grummar-Strawn LM, Scanlon KS, Fein SB. Infant feeding and feeding transitions during the first year of life. *Pediatrics.* 2008;122(Suppl 2):S36–S42

5. Roess AA, Jacquier EF, Catellier DJ, et al. Food consumption patterns of infants and toddlers: findings from the Feeding Infants and Toddlers Study (FITS) 2016. *J Nutr.* 2018;148(Suppl 3):1525S–1535S

6. Jun S, Catellier DJ, Eldridge AL, Dwyer JT, Eicher-Miller HA, Bailey RL. Usual nutrient intakes from the diets of US children by WIC participation and income: findings from the Feeding Infants and Toddlers Study (FITS) 2016. *J Nutr.* 2018;148(9 Suppl):1567S–1574S

7. Institute of Medicine, Committee on Understanding Premature Birth and Assuring Healthy Outcomes. *Preterm Birth: Causes, Consequences, and Prevention.* Behrman RE, Butler AS, eds. Washington, DC: National Academies Press; 2007

8. English LK, Obbagy JE, Wong YP, et al. Timing of introduction of complementary foods and beverages and growth, size, and body composition: a systematic review. *Am J Clin Nutr.* 2019;109(Suppl):935S–955S

9. US Department of Health and Human Services, US Food and Drug Administration, Center for Food Safety and Applied Nutrition. Preparation of food contact notifications for food contact substances in contact with infant formula and/or human milk: guidance for industry. Available at: https://www.fda.gov/media/124714/download. Accessed June 2, 2019

10. Trasande L, Shaffer RM, Sathyanarayana S, American Academy of Pediatrics, Council on Environmental Health. Policy statement: Food additives and child health. *Pediatrics*. 2018;142(2):e20181408

11. Substances generally regarded as safe. US Food and Drug Administration final rule. *Fed Regist*. 2916;81(159):54960–55055

12. Government Accountability Office. Food safety: FDA should strengthen it oversite of food ingredients determined to be generally recognized as safe (GRAS). 2010; Available at: https://www.gao.gov/new.items/d10246.pdf. Accessed August 24, 2018

13. *Scott v FDA*, (728 F 2d 322, 6th Cir 1984)

14. Mattia A, Merker R. Regulation of probiotic substances as ingredients in foods: premarket approval or "generally recognized as safe" notification. *Clin Infect Dis*. 2008;46(Suppl 2):S115–S118

15. Raiten DJ, Talbot JM, Waters JH. LSRO Report: Assessment of nutrient requirements for infant formulas. *J Nutr*. 1998;128(Suppl 1):2200S–2201S

16. Institute of Food Technologists. Functional Foods: Opportunities and Challenges. Washington, DC: Institute of Food Technologists; 2005. Available at: http://www.ift.org/knowledge-center/read-ift-publications/science-reports/expert-reports/~/media/Knowledge%20Center/Science%20Reports/Expert%20Reports/Functional%20Foods/Functionalfoods_expertreport_full.pdf. Accessed November 15, 2012

17. Draft guidance for industry: Substantiation for structure/function claims made in infant formula labels and labeling. *Fed Regist*. 2016;81(175):62509–62511

18. Linshaw MA, Harrison HL, Gruskin AB, et al. Hypochloremic alkalosis in infants associated with soy protein formula. *J Pediatr*. 1980;96(4):635–640

19. US Food and Drug Administration. Current good manufacturing practice, quality control procedures, quality factors, notification requirements, and records and reports, for the production of infant formula. *Fed Regist*. 2014;79(111): 33057–33072

20. Infant formula: the addition of minimum and maximum levels of selenium to infant formula and related labeling requirements. *Fed Regist*. 2015;80(120): 35834–35841

21. Guidance for industry: Exempt infant formula production: Current good manufacturing practices (CGMPS), quality control procedures, conduct of audits, and records and reports. *Fed Regist*. 2016;81(73):22174–22175

22. Institute of Medicine, Committee on the Evaluation of the Addition of Ingredients New to Infant Formula. *Infant Formula: Evaluating the Safety of New Ingredients*. Washington, DC: National Academies Press; 2004

23. Gallier S, Gragson D, Jimenez-Flores R, Everett D. Using confocal laser scanning microscopy to probe the milk fat globule membrane and associated proteins. *J Agric Food Chem*. 2010;58(7):4250–4257

VII

24. Lopez C, Menard O. Human milk fat globules: polar lipid composition and in situ structural investigations revealing the heterogeneous distribution of proteins and the lateral segregations of sphingomyelin in the biological membrane. *Colloids Surf B Biointerfaces.* 2011;83:29–41

25. Reinhardt TA, Lippolis JD. Bovine milk fat globule membrane proteome. *J Dairy Res.* 2006;73:406–416

26. Dewettinck K, Rombaul R, Thienpont N, Le TT, Messens K, Van Camp J. Nutritional and technologica. Aspects of milk fat globule membrane material. *Int Dairy J.* 2008;18(5):436–457

27. Claumarchirant L, Cilla A, Matencio E, et al. Addition of milk fat globule membranes as an ingredient of infant formulas for resembling the polar lipids of human milk. *Int Dairy J.* 2016;61:228–238

28. Gurnida DA, Rowan AM, Idjradinata J, Muchtadi D, Sekarwana N. Association of complex lipids containing gangliosides with cognitive development of 6-month-old infants. *Early Hum Dev.* 2012;88(8):595–601

29. Timby N, Domellof E, Hernell O, Lönnerdal B, Domellöf M. Neurodevelopment, nutrition, and growth until 12 months of age in infants fed a low-energy, low protein formula supplemented with bovine milk fat globule membranes. *Am J Clin Nutr.* 2014;99(4):860–868

30. Billeaud C, Puccio G, Saliba E, et al. Safety and tolerance evaluation of milk fat globule membrane-enriched infant formulas: a randomized controlled multicenter noninferiority trial in healthy term infants. *Clin Med Insights Pediatr.* 2014;8:51–60

31. Timby N, Domellöf M, Lönnerdal B, Hernell O. Supplementation of infant formula with bovine fat globule membranes. *Adv Nutr.* 2017;8(2):351–355

32. Venugopalan V, Shriner KA, Wong-Beringer A. Regulatory oversight and safety of probiotic use. *Emerg Infect Dis.* 2010;16(11):1661–1665

33. Vaillancourt JV. Regulation pre- and pro-biotics: a US FDA perspective. Available at: http://www.nationalacademies.org/hmd/~/media/9CBB573341634F789FB36 AF1D1C3EF4A.ashx. Accessed September 7, 2018

34. Aureli P, Capurso L, Castellazzi AM, et al. Probiotics and health: an evidence-based review. *Pharmacol Res.* 2011;63(5):366–376

35. O'Connor EM. The role of gut microbiota in nutritional status. *Curr Opin Clin Nutr Metab Care.* 2013;16(5):509–516

36. Tanaka M, Nakayama J. Development of the gut microbiota in infancy and its impact on health in later life. *Allergol Int.* 2017;66(4):515–522

37. Figueroa-Gonzalez I, Quijano G, Ramirez G, Cruz-Guerrero A. Probiotics and prebiotics—perspectives and challenges. *J Sci Food Agric.* 2011;91(8):1341–1348

38. Baglatzi L, Gavrili S, Stamouli K, et al. Effect of formula containing a low dose of the probiotic Bifiobacterium lactis CNCM 1-3446 on immune and gut functions in C-section delivered babies: a pilot study. *Clin Med Insights Pediatr.* 2016;10:11–19

39. Saxelin M. Probiotic formulations and applications, the current probiotics market, and changes in the marketplace: a European perspective. *Clin Infect Dis.* 2008;46(Suppl 2):S76–S79

40. US Food and Drug Administration. FDA developing improved methodology for determining purity of probiotic products. Available at: https://www.fda.gov/biologicsbloodvaccines/scienceresearch/ucm493702.htm. Accessed September 7, 2018

41. Gibson GR, Roberfroid MB. Dietary modulation of the human colonic microbiota: introducing the concept of prebiotics. *J Nutr.* 1995;125(6):1401–1412

42. Roberfroid MB. Prebiotics: the concept revisited. *J Nutr.* 2007;137(3 Suppl 2): 830S–837S

43. Stiverson J, Chen J, Adams S, et al. Prebiotic oligosaccharides: comparative evaluation using in vitro cultures of infants' fecal microbiomes. *Appl Environ Microbiol.* 2014;80(23):7388–7397

44. Vandenplas Y, Zakharova I, Dmitrieva Y. Oligosaccharides in infant formula; more evidence to validate the role of prebiotics. *Br J Nutr.* 2015;113(9):1339–1344

45. Thomas DW, Greer FR. Clinical report: Probiotics and prebiotics in pediatrics. *Pediatrics.* 2010;126(6):1217–1231

46. Baker-Smith CM, de Ferranti SD, Cochran AJ, American Academy of Pediatrics, Committee on Nutrition, Section on Gastroenterology Hepatology and Nutrition. Policy statement: The use of nonnutritive sweeteners in children. *Pediatrics.* 2019;in press

47. Sylvetsky AC, Rother KI. Trends in the consumption of low-calorie sweeteners. *Physiol Behav.* 2016;164(Pt B):446–450

48. Sylvetsky AC, Brown RJ, Bau JE, Welsh JA, Rother KI, Talegawkar SA. Consumption of low-calorie sweeteners among children and adults in the United States. *J Acad Nutr Diet.* 2017;117(3):441–448

49. Wolraich ML, Lindgren SD, Stumbo PJ, Stegink LD, Appelbaum MI, Kiritsy MC. Effects of diets high in sucrose or aspartame on the behavior and cognitive performance of children. *N Engl J Med.* 1994;330(5):301–307

50. Ebbeling CB, Feldman HA, Chromitz VR, et al. A randomized trial of sugar-sweetened beverages and adolescent body weight. *N Engl J Med.* 2012;367(15): 1407–1416

51. Rodearmel SJ, Wyatt HR, Stoebele N, Smith SM, Ogden LG, Hill JO. Small changes in dietary sugar and physical activity as an approach to preventing excessive weight gain: the America on the Move family study. *Pediatrics.* 2007;120(4):e869–e879

52. Ebbeling CB, Feldman HA, Osganian SK, Chomitz VR, Ellenbogen SJ, Ludwig DS. Effects of decreasing sugar-sweetened beverage consumption on body weight in adolescents: a randomized controlled pilot study. *Pediatrics.* 2006;117(3):673–680

VII

53. de Ruyter JC, Olthof MR, Seidel JC, Katan MB. A trial of sugar-free or sugar-sweetened beverages and body weight in children. *N Engl J Med*. 2012;367(15): 1397–1406

54. US Food and Drug Administration. GRAS Notice No GRN 000780. Available at: https://www.fda.gov/downloads/Food/IngredientsPackagingLabeling/GRAS/NoticeInventory/UCM616345.pdf. Accessed September 10, 2018

55. US Food and Drug Administration. Additional information about high-intensity sweeteners permitted for use in food in the United States Available at: https://www.fda.gov/food/ingredientspackaginglabeling/foodadditivesingredients/ucm397725.htm#Steviol_glycosides. Accessed September 4, 2018

56. Van Eenennaam AL. Genetic modification of food animals. *Curr Opin Biotechnol*. 2017;44:27–34

57. Bhat SA, Malik AA, Ahmad SM, et al. Advances in genome editing for improved animal breeding: a review. *Vet World*. 2017;10(11):1361–1366

58. Domingo JL. Safety assessment of GM plants: an updated review of the scientific literature. *Food Chem Toxicol*. 2016;95:12–18

59. Johnson D, O'Connor S. These charts show every genetically modified food people already eat in the U.S. *Time*. April 30, 2015. Available at: http://time.com/3840073/gmo-food-charts/ Accessed September 25, 2018

60. US Department of Agriculture. Organic 101: Can GMO's be used in organic products? May 17, 2013; Available at: https://www.usda.gov/media/blog/2013/05/17/organic-101-can-gmos-be-used-organic-products. Accessed May 1, 2019

61. Georges F, Ray H. Genome editing of crops: a renewed opportunity for food security. *GM Crops Food*. 2017;8(1):1–12

62. US Food and Drug Administration. How FDA regulates food from genetically engineered plants. Available at: https://www.fda.gov/food/ingredientspackaginglabeling/geplants/ucm461831.htm. Accessed September 25, 2018

63. US Food and Drug Administration. Genome editing in new plant varieties used for foods; Request for comments. January 19, 2017

64. US Food and Drug Administration. Guidance for industry. Regulation of genetically engineered animals containing heritable recombinant DNA constructs. Available at: https://www.fda.gov/downloads/AnimalVeterinary/GuidanceComplianceEnforcement/GuidanceforIndustry/UCM052463.pdf. Accessed September 25, 2018

65. US Food and Drug Administration. Guidance for industry. Regulation of intentionally altered genomic DNA in animals. Draft guidance. Available at: https://www.fda.gov/downloads/AnimalVeterinary/GuidanceComplianceEnforcement/GuidanceforIndustry/ucm113903.pdf. Accessed September 25, 2018

66. US Food and Drug Administration. AquAdvantage salmon approval letter and appendix. 2015; Available at: https://www.fda.gov/AnimalVeterinary/DevelopmentApprovalProcess/BiotechnologyProductsatCVMAnimalsand AnimalFood/AnimalswithIntentionalGenomicAlterations/ucm466214.htm. Accessed September 26, 2018

67. Murray JD, Maga EA. Opinion: A new paradigm for regulating genetically engineered animals that are used as food. *Proc Natl Acad Sci U S A*. 2016;113(13): 3410–3413

68. US Department of Agriculture, Agriculture Marketing Service. National bioengineered food disclosure standard. December 2018; Available at: https://www.federalregister.gov/documents/2018/12/21/2018-27283/national-bioengineered-food-disclosure-standard. Accessed January 30, 2019

69. Pariza MW. The safety of microbial enzymes used in food processing. 101 Toxic Food Ingredients. 2016; Available at https://www.progressivegardening.com/food-poisoning/the-safety-of-microbial-enzymes-used-in-food-processing. html. Accessed September 25, 2018

70. Olempska-Beer ZS, Merker RI, Ditto MD, DiNovi MJ. Food-processing enzymes from recombinant microorganisms—a review. *Regul Toxicol Pharmacol*. 2006;45(2):144–158

71. Pariza MW, Johnson EA. Evaluating the safety of microbial enzyme preparations used in food processing: update for a new century. *Regul Toxicol Pharmacol*. 2001;33(2):173–186

72. Velle W. The Use of Hormones in Animal Production. Available at: http://www.fao.org/DOCREP/004/X6533E/X6533E01.htm. Accessed November 15, 2012

73. US Food and Drug Administration. Steroid hormone implants used for growth in food-producing animals. 2017; Available at: https://www.fda.gov/animalveterinary/safetyhealth/productsafetyinformation/ucm055436.htm. Accessed September 25, 2018

74. American Academy of Pediatrics, Committee on Environmental Health. Food safety. In: Etzel RA, Balk SJ, eds. *Pediatric Environmental Health*. Elk Grove Village, IL: American Academy of Pediatrics; 2012:247–267

75. US Food and Drug Administration. Bovine Somatotropin (BST). 2018; Available at: https://www.fda.gov/animalveterinary/safetyhealth/productsafetyinformation/ucm055435.htm. Accessed September 25, 2018

VII

Food Labeling

Introduction

In 1990, the Nutrition Labeling and Education Act (NLEA [Pub L No. 101-535]) was enacted, mandating numerous changes in food labeling. Before that time, nutrition labeling on food products was voluntary, except for those that contained added nutrients or carried nutrition claims. As Americans became more interested in nutrition, food label regulations were revised to provide nutrition information that would help consumers make more informed food choices to meet national dietary recommendations.

The US Food and Drug Administration (FDA) published final rules implementing the NLEA in 1993. The labels of most packaged foods were required to feature the new "Nutrition Facts" panel.[1] Labeling is voluntary for fresh fruits and vegetables and raw meat, poultry, and seafood. For these raw foods, nutrition information may be printed on the package or on pamphlets or posters displayed near the food in the supermarket. Food labeling is regulated by the FDA, with the exception of meat and poultry products, which are regulated by the US Department of Agriculture (USDA).

In 2016, the FDA published regulations revising the Nutrition Facts label format, updating the Daily Values, modifying requirements for determining serving sizes, and updating the mandatory declared nutrients taking into consideration nutrients of public health significance and information to help inform dietary choices. Compliance with the new regulations is enforced as of January 1, 2020. These regulations constitute the most significant changes to the Nutrition Facts label since it was developed in 1993.

Ingredient Labeling

Ingredient labeling is an important source of information for consumers about the composition of packaged foods. Both FDA and USDA regulations require that food products with 2 or more ingredients provide a listing of ingredients in descending order of their prominence by weight.[2-4] There are exemptions for declaration of certain minor ingredients. Preservatives and color additives, when used, must be labeled as such, and certified color additives must be listed by name (eg, Blue 1 or Yellow 5).

In January 2006, food allergen labeling requirements of the Food Allergen Labeling and Consumer Protection Act (FALCP [Pub L No. 108-282]) became effective on FDA-regulated food and beverage products.[5] The Act defined the 8 major food allergens (milk, egg, wheat, soy, peanuts, tree nuts, fish, and crustacea) and requires 1 of 2 options for ingredient labeling of food products:

1. Immediately following the ingredient listing, the label states "Contains:" followed by the name of the food source from which the major food allergen is derived (eg, "Contains: milk, egg, walnuts."). In the case of tree nuts, fish, or shellfish, each specific food in these classes that is an ingredient in the food must be declared (ie, salmon, cod, crab, pecan, hazelnut) rather than the group listing.

2. Within the ingredient listing, in parentheses following the common or usual name of the allergenic ingredient, the label presents the name of the food source from which the major food allergen is derived—for example, "...whey (milk)..."

For families with food allergies, it is essential to read the ingredient listings on food labels to determine the presence of the 8 major allergens. Because food and beverage manufacturers are continually making ingredient and recipe changes, food-allergic individuals and their caregivers should read the ingredient declaration and check the "Contains..." statement on the food label of every product purchased, each time it is purchased and consumed (or served). It is important to remember that the "Contains" allergen statement is optional. If a product label does not have a "Contains" allergen statement, consumers or their caregivers should read the list of ingredients and not assume that no allergens are present in the food. There are currently no regulations for "May Contain" allergen statements that also appear on many food labels. "May Contain" allergen statements are often used by manufacturers when controls and cleaning are not adequate to ensure that allergen containing foods or ingredients do not come into contact with foods that do not contain the allergen as part of the recipe.

THE NUTRITION FACTS PANEL

The Nutrition Facts panel includes information on the quantity of nutrients in a food as well as how much the nutrient contributes to the established Daily Value for that nutrient (Fig 50.II.1, Fig 50.II.2, and Fig 50.II.3). The nutrients and percent Daily Values required on the label were revised by FDA in 2016 and manufacturers are in the process of revising labels for their products (https://www.fda.gov/regulatory-information/search-fda-guidance-documents/guidance-industry-food-labeling-guide). Simplified or shortened formats may be used for products that contain insignificant

Fig 50.II.1.
Nutrition Label Format, Food for Children and Adults 4 Years and Older

Nutrition Facts

8 servings per container

Serving size   **2/3 cup (55g)**

Amount per serving

Calories   **230**

	% Daily Value*
Total Fat 8g	**10%**
Saturated Fat 1g	**5%**
Trans Fat 0g	
Cholesterol 0mg	**0%**
Sodium 160mg	**7%**
Total Carbohydrate 37g	**13%**
Dietary Fiber 4g	**14%**
Total Sugars 12g	
Includes 10g Added Sugars	**20%**
Protein 3g	
Vitamin D 2mcg	10%
Calcium 260mg	20%
Iron 8mg	45%
Potassium 240mg	6%

* The % Daily Value (DV) tells you how much a nutrient in
a serving of food contributes to a daily diet. 2,000 calories
a day is used for general nutrition advice.

amounts (an amount declarable as zero in labeling; generally less than 0.5 g) of certain mandatory label nutrients. Package size constraints may also dictate different formats.

The following provides more details about the various features of the Nutrition Facts panel for foods for adults and children 4 years and older (Fig 50.II.1):

1. Serving size: Serving sizes are determined based on FDA-defined reference amounts for different food categories. The reference amounts represent the amount of food typically eaten at one time, using data from national food consumption surveys. Because serving sizes are based

Fig 50.II.2.

Nutrition Label Format, Food for Children Younger Than 12 Months

Nutrition Facts	
4 servings per container	
Serving size	**1 pack (70g)**

Amount per serving

Calories	25

	% Daily Value
Total Fat 0g	**0%**
Saturated Fat 0g	
Trans Fat 0g	
Cholesterol 0mg	
Sodium 74mg	
Total Carbohydrate 5g	**5%**
Dietary Fiber 1g	
Total Sugars 3g	
Includes 0g Added Sugars	
Protein 0g	**0%**
Vitamin D 0mcg	0%
Calcium 10mg	4%
Iron 1mg	10%
Potassium 230mg	35%

on consumption, they do not always correspond to an amount of food that is recommended as part of a healthy balanced diet. The serving size typically includes both a common household measure and a metric amount (eg, 1 muffin [42 g]).

2. Calories: Total calories in one serving are identified. In the FDA revised Nutrition Facts format, the type size required for declaration of calories has increased substantially, which may benefit consumers in weight control and maintenance.

3. Nutrients: Information about the content of nutrients most related to today's health concerns must be listed. For the new Nutrition Facts panel, in addition to calories, these nutrients include total fat, saturated fat, trans fat, cholesterol, sodium, total carbohydrate, dietary fiber, total sugars, added sugars, protein, vitamin D, calcium, iron, and potas-

Fig 50.II.3.

Nutrition Label Format, Food for Children 1 Through 3 Years

Nutrition Facts

1 serving per container
Serving size   1 container (85g)

Amount per serving
Calories   **70**

% Daily Value*

Total Fat 1.5g	**4%**
Saturated Fat 0.5g	**5%**
Trans Fat 0g	
Cholesterol 10mg	**3%**
Sodium 240mg	**16%**
Total Carbohydrate 11g	**7%**
Dietary Fiber 1g	**7%**
Total Sugars 1g	
Includes 1g Added Sugars	**4%**
Protein 3g	**23%**
Vitamin D 0mcg	0%
Calcium 40mg	6%
Iron 0.6mg	8%
Potassium 30mg	0%

* The % Daily Value (DV) tells you how much a nutrient in a serving of food contributes to a daily diet. 1,000 calories a day is used for general nutrition advice.

sium. Mandatory declaration of vitamins A and C is no longer required, because the FDA determined them to no longer be of public health significance. These and other nutrients are listed voluntarily, unless they are added to the food, such as a fortified food, or a claim is made about the nutrient on the label or in labeling. If a food contains an insignificant amount of certain required nutrients, these may be omitted from the label or declared in a footnote as "not a significant source…" Nutrient amounts on the new labels are listed in both quantitative amounts (grams, milligrams, or micrograms) and for those nutrients with defined daily values, in percent Daily Value. When label space is limited, quantitative amounts of micronutrients may be omitted from the label (Fig 50.II.1).

VII

4. Daily Values: The "% Daily Value" characterizes how the amount of a nutrient in a food or beverage contributes to a moderate, varied, and balanced diet. The term Daily Value is an umbrella term for 2 sets of reference values: Daily Reference Values (DRVs) and Recommended Daily Intakes (RDIs). The DRVs are set for total fat, saturated fat, cholesterol, total carbohydrate, dietary fiber, added sugars, sodium, and protein. They are established for adults and children 4 years or older on the basis of current nutrition recommendations. DRVs have been established for total fat, saturated fat, total carbohydrate, dietary fiber, and protein on the basis of a 2000-kcal reference diet; DRVs for cholesterol and sodium are not based on caloric intake. Actual dietary need for nutrients that are based on caloric intake may be higher or lower depending on the calorie needs of the individual (Fig 50.II.1). There is no defined Daily Value for trans fat or total sugars for any age group. Declaration of percent Daily Values for nutrients with a DRV is required except for protein.

5. Added sugars: With the revisions to the food label, the FDA now requires mandatory declaration of "added sugars" in the Nutrition Facts panel. Added sugars are included in the amount listed for total sugars. Added sugars include sugars (free, monosaccharides, and disaccharides) as well as sugars from syrups, honey, molasses, and concentrated fruit juices and vegetable juices. Juice that is not concentrated (single strength juice) and concentrated juice sold to consumers for the purposes of making single strength juice are not considered "added sugars."

Current Dietary Reference Intakes are listed in Appendix E.

Nutrition Facts Panels for Infants Younger Than 12 Months and Children Between 1 and 3 Years of Age

Nutrition Facts panels on food labels on products specifically marketed to infants through 12 months of age and children 1 through 3 years of age are different from those for children and adults 4 years of age and older. Protein is listed in grams per serving and as a percentage of the Daily Value on foods for children between 1 and 3 years of age (Fig 50.II.3). Other than on labels for foods specifically marketed for infants and children 3 years or younger, percent Daily Value for protein is not required to be included on the food label unless the label includes a claim made for protein content. For children 1 through 3 years of age, DRVs have been established for total fat, saturated fat, total carbohydrate, dietary fiber, and added sugars on the basis of a 1000-kcal diet (Fig 50.II.3). For infants, protein is a Reference Daily Intake and not a DRV. DRVs for infants through 12 months are only defined for total fat and total carbohydrate (Fig 50.II.2). The Daily Value used to calculate other nutrient percentages are calculated based on the RDI for each population (Table 50.II.1).

Serving sizes of foods for infants and children 1 through 3 years are based on government-defined reference amounts that have been determined on the basis of consumption data. These reference amounts are typically

Table 50.II.1.

Daily Values Used to Calculate % Daily Value for Nutrition Facts Panel[a]

Food Component	Adults and Children 4 Years and Older	Children 1 Through 3 Years	Infants Through 12 Months
Daily Reference Value			
Total fat	65 g[b]	39 g[c]	30 g
Saturated fat	20 g[b]	10 g[c]	
Cholesterol	300 mg	300 mg	
Sodium	2400 mg	1500 mg	
Total carbohydrate	300 g[b]	150 g[c]	95 g
Dietary fiber	25 g[d]	14 g[c]	
Protein	50 g[b]	13 g[c]	11 g[e]
Added sugars	50 g[b]	25 g[c]	
Reference Daily Intake			
Potassium	4700 mg	3000 mg	700 mg
Reference Daily Intake			
Potassium	4700 mg	3000 mg	700 mg

[a] Based on a 2000-kcal diet for adults and children older than 4 years.
[b] Daily value based on a 2000-kcal reference diet.
[c] Based on a 1000 calorie diet.
[d] Daily value based on 11.5 g/1000 kcal.
[e] Protein is an RDI for infants.

smaller than those established for adults and children 4 years and older. Many young children consume the same foods as the rest of the family. Percent daily values on labels of foods not specifically marketed to young children, represent the contribution to an adult diet and not the contribution to the diet of an infant or toddler. This is particularly important for children younger than 3 years who consume foods not specifically marketed (or labeled) for young children. For example, a 15-g serving of crackers labeled with a daily value for sodium of 6% DV (150 mg of sodium) would actually contribute 10% DV for a child 1 through 3 years of age. Another example would be a ready-to-eat "all family" breakfast cereal with 6 g of added sugar per serving (12% of the DV), which would contribute 24% DV for a child 1 through 3 years for the same serving size.

Nutrition Claims
Nutrient content claims are those that characterize the amount of a nutrient in a food, using terms such as free, low, reduced, less, more, added, good source, and high. Using these terms in connection with a specific nutrient is strictly defined (Table 50.II.2).

Table 50.II.2.
Nutrition Claims

	Definition, per Serving
Calories	
Calorie free	<5 kcal
Low calorie	≤40 kcal
Reduced or fewer calories	At least 25% fewer calories[a]
Light or lite	One third fewer calories or 50% less fat[a]
Sugar	
Sugar free	<0.5 g
Reduced sugar or less sugar	At least 25% less sugars
No added sugar; without added sugar; no sugar added	No sugars added during processing or packaging, including ingredients that contain sugars, such as juice or dry fruit

Table 50.II.2. *Continued*
Nutrition Claims

	Definition, per Serving
Fat	
Fat free	<0.5 g
Low fat	≤3 g
Reduced or less fat	At least 25% less fat[a]
Light or lite	One third fewer calories or 50% less fat[a]

Saturated fat
   Saturated fat free
   Low saturated fat
 	
   Reduced or less saturated fat
	
	<0.5 g
	≤1 g saturated fat and no more than 15% of calories from saturated fat
	At least 25% less saturated fat[a]

Cholesterol	
Cholesterol free	<2 mg cholesterol and <2 g fat
Low cholesterol	≤20 mg cholesterol and <2 g saturated fat
Reduced or less cholesterol	At least 25% less cholesterol[a] and <2 g saturated fat
Sodium	
Sodium free	<5 mg
Very low sodium	≤35 mg
Low sodium	≤140 mg
Reduced or less sodium	At least 25% less sodium[a]
Light in sodium	50% less sodium[a]
Fiber	
High fiber	≥5 g[b]
Good source of fiber	2.5 to 4.9 g
More or added fiber	At least 2.5 g more or added[a]

Continued

VII

Table 50.II.2. *Continued*
Nutrition Claims

	Definition, per Serving
Other Claims	
High, rich in, excellent source of [name of nutrient]	≥20% of daily value[a]
Good source of, contains, provides [name of nutrient]	10% to 19% of daily value[a]
More, enriched, fortified, added [name of nutrient]	≥10% or more of daily value more or added[a]
Lean[c]	<10 g fat, (<4.5 g saturated fat, and <95 mg cholesterol)
Extra lean[c]	<5 g fat, <2 g saturated fat, and <95 mg cholesterol
Healthy	Meets standards for "low" fat and saturated fat; contains ≤480 mg sodium; ≤60 mg cholesterol; and contains at least 10% daily value for vitamin A, vitamin C, calcium, iron, protein, or fiber

[a] Compared with a standard serving size of the traditional food.
[b] Must also meet the definition for low fat, or the level of fat must appear next to the high-fiber claim.
[c] On meat, poultry, seafood, and game meats.

Infant food labels may carry claims for vitamins and minerals. Claims about protein, total fat, saturated fat, cholesterol and sodium are not currently allowed on products intended for infants younger than 1 year.

Ingredient absence claims (eg, no preservatives) or ingredient presence claims (eg, made with apples) are permitted if they are truthful and not misleading. Claims that address a product's taste such as unsweetened or unsalted are also permitted.

Juice Labeling
There are specific labeling requirements for juice. Since 1994, the percentage of juice must be specified on the food label if a beverage claims to contain fruit or vegetable juice.[6] Label statements must be declared using the language, "Contains [x] percent [name of fruit or vegetable] juice," "[x] percent

juice," or a similar phrase (eg, Contains 50% apple juice"). If a beverage contains minor amounts of juice for flavoring, the product may use the term "flavor," "flavored," or "flavoring" with a fruit or vegetable name, as long as the product does not bear the term "juice" (other than in the ingredient declaration) and does not visually depict the fruit or vegetable from which the flavor is derived. If the beverage contains no juice, but appears to contain juice, the label must state, "Contains no [name of fruit or vegetable] juice," or similar statements. These percentage juice statements appear near the top of the information panel of the beverage label.

Gluten-Free Labeling

In August 2013, the FDA published its final rule to define the term "gluten free" for voluntary use in labeling of foods. The rule allows manufacturers to label a food gluten free if the food does NOT contain any of the following[7,8]:

1. An ingredient that is any type of wheat, rye, barely, or crossbreeds of these grains.
2. An ingredient derived from these grains and that has not been processed to remove gluten.
3. An ingredient derived from these grains and that has been processed to remove gluten, if it results in the food containing 20 or more parts per million (ppm) of gluten.
4. 20 ppm or more gluten.

"Gluten-free" is a voluntary claim that can be used at the manufacturer's discretion provided the product complies with the defined regulatory requirements. There is no third-party certification required to make a gluten free claim and no FDA established iconography.

Health Claims

In addition to nutrient content claims, a food label may bear claims about the health benefits of the food or a component of the food. Products must meet strict nutrition requirements before they can carry these claims associating foods, nutrients, or substances with reduced risk of a disease or health related condition.

Health claims are based on significant scientific agreement and to date, the FDA has authorized 12 health claims.[9] Although the wording on packages may differ, all health claims must include both a substance and the name of the disease or health related condition. The following summarizes the allowed claims that describe the link between reduced risk of disease or health related condition and a substance:

VII

1. Calcium and osteoporosis: Physical activity and a calcium-rich diet may reduce the risk of osteoporosis, a condition in which the bones become soft or brittle.
2. Fat and cancer: A diet low in total fat may reduce the risk of some cancers.
3. Saturated fat and cholesterol and heart disease: A diet low in saturated fat and cholesterol may reduce the risk of heart disease.
4. Fiber-containing grain products, fruits, and vegetables, and cancer: A low-fat diet rich in fiber-containing grain products, fruits, and vegetables may reduce the risk of some cancers.
5. Fruits, vegetables, and grain products that contain fiber and heart disease: A diet low in saturated fat and cholesterol and rich in fruits, vegetables, and grain products that contain some types of dietary fiber may reduce the risk of heart disease.
6. Sodium and high blood pressure: A low-sodium diet may reduce the risk of high blood pressure, which is a risk factor for heart attacks and strokes.
7. Fruits and vegetables and some cancers: A low-fat diet rich in fruits and vegetables (foods that are low in fat and may contain dietary fiber, vitamin A, or vitamin C) may reduce the risk of some cancers.
8. Folic acid and neural tube birth defects: Women who consume 0.4 mg of folic acid daily may reduce their risk of giving birth to a child affected with a neural tube defect.
9. Noncariogenic carbohydrate sweeteners (sugar alcohols, sucralose) and dental caries: Frequent eating of foods high in sugars and starches as between-meal snacks can promote tooth decay. The [name of sugar alcohol, or sucralose] used to sweeten this food may reduce the risk of dental caries.
10. Soluble fiber from certain foods and risk of coronary heart disease: Soluble fiber from [name of food (eg, oat bran, psyllium. or barley fiber)], as part of a diet low in saturated fat and cholesterol, may reduce the risk of heart disease.
11. Soy protein and risk of coronary heart disease: Diets low in saturated fat and cholesterol that include 25 g of soy protein a day may reduce the risk of heart disease. One serving of [name of food] provides [x] g of soy protein.
12. Plant sterol or stanol esters and risk of coronary heart disease: Diets low in saturated fat and cholesterol that include 2 servings of foods

that provide a daily total of at least 1.3 g of vegetable oil sterol esters in 2 meals may reduce the risk of heart disease. A serving of [name of the food] supplies [x] g of vegetable oil sterol esters. Diets low in saturated fat and cholesterol that include 2 servings of foods that provide a daily total of at least 3.4 g of vegetable oil stanol esters in 2 meals may reduce the risk of heart disease. A serving of [name of the food] supplies [x] g of vegetable oil stanol esters.

To bear a health claim, each food must not exceed (unless exempted by FDA) specified levels of fat, saturated fat, cholesterol, and sodium.

Claims that describe the link between a substance and a disease that have not reached a level of significant scientific agreement are referred to as "qualified health claims." The qualification of the claim reflects the level of scientific evidence supporting the disease-substance relationship. There are currently 17 qualified health claims that can be used without objection from FDA. Included in this category are claims for the benefits of nuts and heart disease; calcium and hypertension, pregnancy induced hypertension and preecalmpsia; and tomatoes and cancer risk; and the recent qualified health claim for peanut introduction and reduce risk of developing peanut allergy. The complete list of qualified health claims is available on the FDA website.

In addition to the above health claims, the FDA Modernization Act of 1997 (FDAMA [Pub L No. 105-115]) established an additional route to establish health claims as well as nutrient content claims. FDAMA procedures allow a health claim to be made if it is based on a published authoritative statement, currently in effect, about the relationship between a nutrient and a disease or health-related condition to which the claim refers, issued by a scientific body of the US government with official responsibility for public health protection or research directly relating to human nutrition (eg, *Dietary Guidelines for Americans* from USDA and the Department of Health and Human Services; DRI reports from the National Academy of Sciences).

In July 1999, the first such health claim was established related to whole-grain foods and reduced risk of heart disease and cancer. The health claim states: Diets rich in whole-grain foods and other plant foods and low in total fat, saturated fat, and cholesterol, may help reduce the risk of heart disease and certain cancers. To qualify for the claim, a food must contain 51% or more whole-grain ingredients per serving, be low in fat, and meet other general criteria for health claims.

In October 2000, a second FDAMA health claim was established related to potassium-containing foods and reduced risk of high blood pressure and stroke. The health claim states: Diets containing foods that are good sources of potassium and low in sodium may reduce the risk of high blood pressure and stroke. To qualify for the claim, a food must be a good source of potassium and low in sodium, total fat, saturated fat, and cholesterol (see "Nutrition Claims").

In December 2003, a third FDAMA health claim was established related to whole-grain foods with moderate fat content and reduced risk of heart disease. The health claim states: Diets rich in whole-grain foods and other plant foods may help reduced the risk of heart disease. To qualify for the claim, a food must contain 51% or more grain ingredients as whole grain and meet other FDA-specified criteria. These foods do not have to be low fat (<3 g per serving) but must contain <6 g of fat per serving and must meet other criteria for saturated fat, cholesterol, and sodium and have <0.5 g of trans fat per serving.

Health claims for nutrient deficiency diseases (eg, iron and reduced risk of iron deficiency anemia) are permitted and do not follow the same process for other health claims. Claims for reduced risk of nutrient deficiency diseases should include reference to the occurrence of the nutrient deficiency disease in the United States. Health claims are also permitted on exempt infant formulas and medical foods.

Structure/Function Claims

A food label may also include a structure/function claim that describes the role of a nutrient or dietary ingredient and its effect on the normal structure or function of the body. Structure/function claims can be used on FDA-regulated foods and dietary supplements. The FDA published final regulations defining the types of structure or function claims permitted on dietary supplement labels in February 2000.[10] Structure/function claims may be based on well-known and established nutrition science or they may be based on modest levels of evidence. Companies are not required to notify FDA before making structure function claims on foods or presubmit labels for approval; however, for a structure/function claim made for a dietary supplement, notification must be submitted to the FDA no later than 30 days after marketing. The FDA can take action against a structure/function claim if the claim is false or misleading. For a comparison of structure/function claims and health claims, see Table 50.II.3.

Structure/function claims typically include the name of the nutrient or substance as well as the function or structure of the body affected.

Table 50.II.3.

Structure/Function Claims Versus Health Claims on Food Labels

Structure/Function Claim Language	Health Claim Language
Supports the immune system	Reduces risk of colds
Builds strong bones	Reduces risk of fractures
Helps promote softer stools	Reduces risk of chronic constipation
Promotes digestive health	Reduces risk of diverticulitis

Additional examples of structure/function claims that have been found on food label marketed for children are as follows:

- Vitamin C proven to help build a strong immune system
- Vitamin E and calcium to support healthy growth and development
- Prebiotics to support digestive health
- Calcium for strong bones
- Nucleotides, prebiotics, and carotenoids for immune support
- Reduced lactose formula for fussiness and gas
- Docosahexaenoic acid (DHA) to help support brain and eye development
- Good bacteria/probiotics to help strengthen an infant's digestive system
- Antioxidants vitamin C to help maintain cell integrity
- Iron to help support learning ability

Structure/function claims have been used frequently on infant formula labels, and in 2016, the FDA issued a proposed draft of voluntary guidance for industry for substantiation of structure/function claims made in infant formula labels and labeling. This was published in the *Federal Register* but remains in the draft stage.[11]

Package Dating

Package dating on labels provides a measure of a product's freshness. Although the FDA does not regulate most package dating, FDA food labeling law and regulations require that such information is truthful and not misleading. *Open dates* are calendar dates that are imprinted or stamped on a food label that indicate to the consumer the freshness and safety of the product. Open dates are stated alphanumerically (eg, October 15) or numerically (eg, 10–15 or 1015). An open date might be featured as:

1. Pull or "sell by" date: This is the last day that the manufacturer recommends sale of the product. Usually, the date allows for additional storage and use time at home.
2. Freshness or quality assurance date: This date suggests how long the manufacturer believes the food will remain at peak quality. The label might read, "Best if used by October 2007." However, the product may still be used safely after this date. A "freshness date" has a different meaning than the word "fresh" printed on the label, which often suggests that a food is raw or unprocessed.
3. Pack date: The date when the food was packaged or processed.
4. Expiration date: The last day the product should be eaten. State governments regulate these dates for perishable foods, such as milk and eggs. The FDA requires expiration dates on infant formula.

Front-of-Package Nutrition Rating Systems and Symbols

Over the past 40 years, there has been substantial growth in the number of front-of-package (FOP) symbols and rating systems designed to summarize nutritional profiles of food products for the consumer. In response to this, Congress in 2009 directed the Centers for Disease Control and Prevention (CDC) to undertake a study with the Institute of Medicine (IOM) to examine and provide recommendations regarding FOP nutrition rating systems and symbols.[12] In 2010, Congress directed the CDC to continue the study, for which the FDA and later the USDA Center of Nutrition Policy and Promotion provided support.[13] This has resulted in 2 reports from the IOM on FOP labeling.[12,13] The 2010 IOM report reviewed 20 representative systems that had been introduced into the marketplace.[12] They had been developed by the food industry, governments, and nonprofit organizations to encourage healthier food choices and purchase decisions.[13]

As many consumers have difficulty in evaluating product healthfulness on the Nutrition Facts panel, a well-designed and simplified FOP labeling system would more likely be used by consumers unable to understand or are less motivated to use the Nutrition Facts panel, given time constraints at the point of purchase. Therefore, the 2012 IOM report,[13] which extended the 2010 IOM report[12] on FOP labeling systems, recommended that the FDA develop, test, and implement a single, standardized FOP system to appear on all food and beverage products, consistent with 2010 *Dietary Guidelines for Americans*. Implementation of this system will require further modifications and/or exemptions to current FDA regulations and development of both new regulations and food group specifications for establishing evaluative criteria.

In the meantime, a voluntary FOP labeling program, "Facts Up Front," was adopted by the Grocery Manufacturers Association and the Food Marketing Institute in 2011. It includes 4 basic icons on the principal display panel that provide information on calories, saturated fat, sodium, and total sugar content.[14] In a letter to the Grocery Manufacturers Association and the Food Marketing Institute in December 2011, the FDA viewed the "Facts Up Front" and basic icons as nutrient content claims subject to all the requirements of the Agency's regulations.[15] However, the FDA recognized that the standardized, nonselective presentation of the 4 basic icons on a company's product line would alleviate some of its concerns regarding the potential for product labeling to mislead consumers by presenting only the "good news" about nutrient content of the front of the package (selecting only the favorable nutrient information for the label). The FDA also acknowledged in its letter that, if the "Facts Up Front" program were uniformly adopted by the food industry, it may contribute to the FDA's public health goals by fostering public awareness of the nutrient content of foods in the marketplace and the ability to make healthy food choices. The FDA agreed to work with industry to evaluate the "Facts Up Front" system to ensure that it promotes public health and is useful to consumers.[15] However, it is important to point out that the Facts Up Front program does not specifically apply to infants and young children.

Conclusion

Food labeling helps consumers and parents make food choices to meet dietary recommendations by providing specific information about the content of certain nutrients in the product. This information currently contained in the recently revised nutrition facts panel on the back of the package may be used to compare foods, to choose foods that help provide a balance of recommended nutrients, and to build meals and a total diet that is moderate, varied, and balanced. In addition, ingredient declarations are useful for consumers to make food choices based on health, or food allergy concerns. The new Nutrition Facts panel which is currently appearing in the marketplace, also helps consumers and caregivers make more informed

VII

choices about the foods they select, while informing them about elements of public health significance.

Food labels may contain both health claims and structure/function claims, but these are not without controversy and have been reviewed here. There are no FDA guidelines for FOP nutrition rating systems and symbols, and there is currently no timetable for instituting a national FOP labeling system as recommended by the IOM.

References

1. US Food and Drug Administration. *Focus on Food Labeling: An FDA Consumer Special Report*. Washington, DC: Government Printing Office; 1993

2. US Food and Drug Administration. Food; designation of ingredients, 21 CFR §101.4 (2012)

3. US Department of Agriculture, Food Safety and Inspection Service. Labels: definition; required features, 9 CFR §317.2c (2008)

4. US Food and Drug Administration. Ingredients statement, 9 CFR §381.118 (2008)

5. Food Allergen Labeling and Consumer Protection Act. Pub L No. 108-282 (2006)

6. US Food and Drug Administration. Percentage juice declaration for foods purporting to be beverages that contain fruit or vegetable juice., 21 CFR §101.30 (2011)

7. US Food and Drug Administration. Gluten Allergy Labeling. Available at: https://www.fda.gov/food/food-labeling-nutrition/gluten-free-labeling-foods. Accessed March 1, 2018

8. US Food and Drug Administration. Food Labeling; Gluten-Free Labeling of Foods; Reopening of comment period. *Fed Regist*. 2011;76(149):46671–46677

9. US Food and Drug Administration. Health claims: calcium, vitamin D, and osteoporosis., 21 CFR §101.72–§101.83 (2012)

10. US Food and Drug Administration. Structure/Function Claims Dietary Supplements/Conventional Foods. Available at: http://www.fda.gov/Food/LabelingNutrition/LabelClaims/StructureFunctionClaims/default.htm. Accessed March 1, 2018

11. US Food and Drug Administration. Draft guidance for industry: Substantiation for structure/function claims made in infant formula labels and labeling. Available at: http://www.fda.gov/downloads/Food/GuidanceRegulation/GuidanceDocumentsRegulatoryinformation/UCM514642.pdf. Accessed March 1, 2018

12. Institute of Medicine. *Examination of Front-of-Packaging Nutrition Rating Systems and Symbols: Phase I Report*. Washington, DC: National Academies Press; 2010

13. Institute of Medicine. *Front-of-Packaging Nutrition Rating Systems and Symbols: Promoting Healthier Choices*. Washington, DC: National Academies Press; 2012

14. News Release. GMA and FMI Announce 'Facts Up Front' as Theme for Front-of-Pack Labeling Program Consumer Education Campaign. 2011; Available at: http://www.gmaonline.org/news-events/newsroom/gma-and-fmi-announce-facts-up-front-as-theme-for-labeling-program-consumer-/. Accessed March 1, 2018

15. US Food and Drug Administration. FDA Letter of Enforcement Discretion to GMA/FMI re "Facts Up Front." 2011; Available at: http://www.fda.gov/Food/LabelingNutrition/ucm302720.htm. Accessed March 1, 2018

VII

Chapter 51

Food Safety: Infectious Disease

Introduction

In the United States, an estimated 48 million cases of foodborne illness occur every year, resulting in approximately 128 000 hospitalizations and 3000 deaths.[1] More than 200 infectious and noninfectious agents have been associated with foodborne and waterborne illness with a wide range of clinical manifestations; these agents include bacteria, viruses, parasites and their toxins, marine organisms and their toxins, and chemical contaminants including heavy metals.[2–6] Infants, children, pregnant women, the elderly, and immunocompromised people are particularly vulnerable to more severe forms of foodborne illnesses.[7,8]

Prevention of foodborne illness remains a continuing challenge. As more people live with immunocompromising conditions, the risks of infection and severe illness from foodborne pathogens may increase. Furthermore, identification of new pathogens and established pathogens in unexpected food vehicles will continue to occur.[9] Increased importation of food and international travel increases the potential for exposure to novel or rare pathogens, and centralization of food processing in the United States and widespread distribution of commercial products increases the risk of large, national foodborne illness outbreaks if a problem occurs.[10–12] In addition, antibiotic resistance in some foodborne pathogens, such as nontyphoidal *Salmonella* and *Campylobacter*, has been increasing.[13]

Because primary care practitioners are often the first to be contacted by people with foodborne illness, an understanding of the possible causes, spectrum of illness, diagnostic methods, and public health importance of foodborne infections is crucial, not only for initial patient treatment but also to ensure timely reporting to public health authorities for accurate surveillance. Understanding the diversity and nature of foodborne pathogens and associated vehicles of transmission is crucial to recognize, control, and prevent foodborne disease outbreaks. This chapter will focus on: (1) the epidemiology of infectious foodborne disease; (2) the clinical manifestations, testing, and management of foodborne illness; (3) foodborne disease surveillance; (4) control and prevention; and (5) resource materials available.

Epidemiology of Foodborne Disease

Although foodborne illness can be caused by many pathogens, several pathogens have been recognized as frequent or severe causes of foodborne disease. It is estimated that 59% of foodborne illness in the United States is caused by viruses, 39% by bacteria, and 2% by parasites.[1] Norovirus is the leading cause of foodborne illness (58%) in the United States from known pathogens, followed by nontyphoidal *Salmonella* species (11%), *Clostridium perfringens* (10%), and *Campylobacter* species (9%). However, nontyphoidal *Salmonella* species are the leading cause of foodborne illness hospitalizations (35%) and deaths (28% [Table 51.1]).[1] Although less common, *Listeria monocytogenes*, *Clostridium botulinum*, and *Toxoplasma gondii* can also cause serious foodborne illness.

Most cases of foodborne illness are sporadic and are not part of recognized outbreaks. Investigations of foodborne disease outbreaks provide critical information about food vehicles, emerging pathogens, and food production and preparation practices associated with illness. Of the 902 foodborne outbreaks reported to the Centers for Disease Control and Prevention (CDC) through the National Outbreak Reporting System (NORS) in 2015, 443 (49%) were caused by a single laboratory-confirmed etiologic agent, of which bacteria accounted for 54%, viruses for 38%, chemicals for 7%, and parasites for 1% (Table 51.2).[14] Among outbreaks with a single,

Table 51.1.

Estimated Number of Foodborne Illnesses, Hospitalizations, and Deaths from the Major Pathogens Transmitted Commonly by Foods, United States, 2011[1]

Pathogen	Estimated Number of Foodborne Illnesses	Estimated Number of Foodborne Hospitalizations	Estimated Number of Foodborne Deaths
Norovirus	5 461 731	14 663	149
Salmonella, nontyphoidal	1 027 561	19 336	378
Clostridium perfringens	965 958	438	26
Campylobacter species	845 024	8463	76
Staphylococcus aureus	241 148	1064	6
Toxoplasma gondii	86 686	4428	327
Escherichia coli O157, Shiga toxin-producing	63 153	2138	20
Listeria monocytogenes	1591	1455	255

Table 51.2.

Confirmed and Suspected Causes of Single-Etiology Foodborne Outbreaks Reported to the National Outbreak Reporting System, CDC, 2015[14]

Etiology	Etiology Confirmed	Etiology Suspected	Total
Bacterial			
Salmonella	149	9	158
Clostridium perfringens	17	21	38
Escherichia coli, Shiga toxin-producing	27	7	34
Campylobacter	21	12	33
Staphylococcus enterotoxin	5	8	13
Bacillus cereus	2	6	8
Shigella	4	2	6
Vibrio parahaemolyticus	4	2	6
Clostridium botulinum	4	—	4
Staphylococcus species	1	3	4
Listeria	2	—	2
Vibrio vulnificus	—	1	1
Escherichia coli, enteropathogenic	1	—	1
Streptococcus, group A	—	1	1
Yersinia enterocolitica	1	—	1
Other bacterial	0	6	6
Total	**238**	**78**	**316**
Chemical and toxin			
Ciguatoxin	19	2	21
Scombroid toxin/histamine	9	1	10
Puffer fish tetrodotoxin	1	0	1
Other	4	3	7
Total	**33**	**6**	**39**

Continued

Table 51.2. *Continued*

Confirmed and Suspected Causes of Single-Etiology Foodborne Outbreaks Reported to the National Outbreak Reporting System, CDC, 2015[14]

Etiology	Etiology Confirmed	Etiology Suspected	Total
Parasitic			
Cryptosporidium species	2	—	2
Cyclospora species	1	—	1
Trichinella species	1	—	1
Total	**4**	**—**	**4**
Viral			
Norovirus	164	147	311
Hepatitis A	3	—	3
Sapovirus	1	1	2
Total	**168**	**148**	**316**
Known etiology	**443**	**232**	**675**
Unknown etiology[a]	**—**	**209**	**209**
Multiple etiologies	**8**	**10**	**18**
Total	**451**	**451**	**902**

[a] An etiologic agent was not confirmed or suspected based on clinical, laboratory, or epidemiologic information.

laboratory-confirmed etiology, norovirus was the most common pathogen, causing 37% of outbreaks, followed by *Salmonella* species, which caused 34% of outbreaks.

Infectious and noninfectious agents of foodborne disease can be acquired from a variety of sources, with some linked more frequently with specific foods (see also Chapter 52: Food Safety: Pesticides, Industrial Chemicals, Toxins, Antimicrobial Preservatives, Irradiation, Food Contact Substances). For instance, outbreaks of *Salmonella* serotype Enteritidis infections are commonly associated with eggs and poultry meat, and *Escherichia coli* O157:H7 outbreaks are frequently associated with ground beef, leafy greens, and unpasteurized dairy products. Listeriosis is frequently associated with consuming produce and dairy products.[15] *Salmonella* and *Campylobacter* infections in infants and children have been associated with riding in a shopping cart next to raw meat or poultry products.[16–18]

A wide variety of contaminated foods have caused foodborne illness outbreaks. In 2015, the most commonly implicated food categories in foodborne disease outbreaks were fish, chicken, pork, and dairy.[14] However, new foods continue to be identified as causes of outbreaks, including flour, soy nut butter, chia powder, and caramel apples.[19–21] Table 51.3 lists examples of recent foodborne disease outbreaks in the United States by location, food vehicle, and etiology, indicating the diversity in vehicles and pathogens. Several recent outbreaks have predominantly affected children and adolescents, including an *E coli* O157:H7 outbreak associated with consumption of a soy nut butter and an outbreak of *Salmonella* Wandsworth and Typhimurium infections associated with consumption of a vegetable-coated snack food.[22,23]

Animal contact can also cause illnesses from pathogens usually transmitted through foods. Poultry including baby chicks, turtles and other reptiles, amphibians such as aquatic frogs, and animals in petting zoos have been implicated in *Salmonella* and *E coli* O157:H7 outbreaks.[24–28] Although illness can be acquired through direct animal contact (ie, touching or petting the animal), animals can also be an indirect source of infection through cross-contamination, when food or food-preparation surfaces become contaminated with feces from an infected animal.[29] This may occur when cages or aquariums are cleaned in the kitchen (in the sink or on surfaces), when pets carrying pathogens are allowed to roam in the house, and when proper handwashing or surface cleaning is not performed before food preparation after contact with the animal, animal's environment, or pet food.

In addition, person-to-person contact is a recognized mode of transmission for some pathogens that can be transmitted through foods, including norovirus, *Shigella* species, and *Salmonella* species. Institutional settings may be especially relevant to illnesses from person-to-person contact. Among 6587 outbreaks of acute gastroenteritis transmitted by person-to-person contact or environmental contamination during 2009–2013, most occurred in an institution—4726 (72%) in long-term acute care facilities, 530 (8%) in schools, 438 (7%) in child care facilities, and 243 (4%) in hospitals.[30] Some foodborne pathogens exhibit seasonality, such as illnesses from *Campylobacter*, *Cyclospora*, nontyphoidal *Salmonella*, and *Vibrio* species being more common during summer months.[31]

VII

Table 51.3.

Examples of Recent Foodborne Outbreaks in the United States by Location, Vehicle, and Cause

Pathogen	Food Vehicle	Where	Year	No. Cases	Ref.
Clostridium botulinum	Illicit alcohol brewed in prison	Mississippi	2016	31	75
Salmonella Virchow	Organic shake and meal products	Multistate	2016	33	76
Escherichia coli O121 and O26	Flour	Multistate	2016	63	20
Clostridium botulinum	Potato salad made from home-canned potatoes	Ohio	2015	29	77
Escherichia coli O157:H7	Rotisserie chicken salad	Multistate	2015	19	78
Listeria monocytogenes	Ice cream	Multistate	2015	10	79
Salmonella Poona	Cucumbers	Multistate	2015	907	80
Listeria monocytogenes	Commercially produced, prepackaged caramel apples	Multistate	2014	35	19
Salmonella Newport, Hartford, and Oranienburg	Organic sprouted chia powder	Multistate	2014	31	21

Cryptosporidium	Unpasteurized goat milk	Idaho	2014	11	81
Hepatitis A	Frozen pomegranate arils	Multistate	2013	165	82
Cyclospora	Fresh cilantro	Multistate	2013	546	83
Salmonella Saintpaul	Cucumbers	Multistate	2013	84	84
Vibrio parahaemolyticus	Raw shellfish	Multistate	2013	104	85
Escherichia coli O26	Raw clover sprouts	Multistate	2012	29	86
Listeria monocytogenes	Ricotta salata cheese	Multistate	2012	22	87
Salmonella Bredeney	Peanut butter	Multistate	2012	42	88
Salmonella Heidelberg	Ground turkey	Multistate	2011	136	89
Listeria monocytogenes	Cantaloupe	Multistate	2011	147	90
Escherichia coli O145	Shredded romaine lettuce	Multistate	2010	33	91
Salmonella Montevideo	Pepper-coated salami products	Multistate	2009	272	92
Salmonella Saintpaul	Alfalfa sprouts	Multistate	2009	228	93

VII

Clinical Manifestations

Table 51.4 describes 5 clinical/epidemiologic profiles into which illnesses caused by most foodborne agents can be categorized. These profiles were derived from national data on foodborne outbreaks including incubation period, duration of illness, percentage of affected people with vomiting or fever, and vomiting-to-fever ratio.[32] These syndromes are vomiting toxin, diarrhea toxin, diarrheagenic *E coli* syndrome, norovirus syndrome, and *Salmonella*-like syndrome. Although there may be some overlap between these syndromes, the profiles can be used to help classify outbreaks and guide laboratory testing. For example, sudden onset of nausea and vomiting after a meal should prompt suspicion of an illness from an enterotoxin, such as *Staphylococcus aureus* or *Bacillus cereus*. Most foodborne illness is self-limited and results in gastrointestinal tract symptoms, such as vomiting, diarrhea, and abdominal cramps.[3,6] Neurologic manifestations are less common but may include paresthesia (fish, shellfish, and monosodium glutamate); cranial nerve palsies, hypotonia, and descending paralysis (*Clostridium botulinum*); and a variety of other neurologic signs and symptoms (fish, shellfish, mushrooms). Systemic manifestations are varied and are associated with a variety of etiologies, including *Brucella* species, *Listeria* species, *Toxoplasma* species, *Trichinella* species, *Vibrio* species, and hepatitis A virus. Pregnant women with listeriosis typically experience a mild flu-like illness, but the infection usually results in miscarriage, stillbirth, preterm delivery, or severe illness in the newborn infant.[33] Other complications or sequelae of enteric illnesses include hemolytic-uremic syndrome (HUS) associated with *E coli* O157:H7 and other Shiga toxin-producing *E coli* (STEC) infections, reactive arthritis following *Campylobacter* and *Salmonella* enteritis, Guillain-Barré syndrome after *Campylobacter* infection, *Salmonella* meningitis in infants, and *Salmonella* osteomyelitis in patients with sick cell disease.[34–40]

Laboratory Testing

Because the presenting signs and symptoms are common to many causes, many infectious and noninfectious agents must be considered in people suspected of having foodborne illness, and establishing an etiologic diagnosis may be difficult on clinical grounds alone. Testing clinical specimens is often the only way to establish a diagnosis, but specimens are often not obtained for laboratory testing. For individual cases of illness, collecting specimens for laboratory diagnosis should be considered for the following conditions: (1) in patient populations more likely to develop severe illness,

Table 51.4.
Distinct Foodborne Pathogen Syndromes[32]

Syndrome	Incubation Period (h)	Duration (h)	Vomiting (%)	Fever (%)	Vomiting/ Fever Ratio[a]	Main Causative Agents[b]
Vomiting-toxin	1.5–9.5	6.3–24	50–100	0–28	0–4.3	Chemical *Bacillus cereus* *Staphylococcus aureus* *Clostridium perfringens*
Diarrhea-toxin	10–13.0	12–24	3.6–20	2.3–10	0.40–1.3	*Bacillus cereus* *Clostridium perfringens*
Escherichia coli-like	48–120	104–185	3.1–37	13–25.3	0.25–1.1	*E coli*
Norovirus-like	34.5–38.5[c]	33–47	54–70.2	37–63	0.70–1.7	Norovirus
Salmonella-like	18.0–88.5	63–144	8.9–51	31–81	0.20–1.0	*Campylobacter* Norovirus *Salmonella* *Shigella*

Table adapted from: Hall JA, Goulding JS, Bean NH, Tauxe RV, Hedberg CW. Epidemiologic profiling: evaluating foodborne outbreaks for which no pathogen was isolated by routine laboratory testing: United States, 1982–9. *Epidemiol Infect.* 2001;127(3):381–387

[a] Ratio of proportion vomiting to proportion with fever.

[b] Viral and bacterial pathogens were listed as a main causative agent of each syndrome if ≥25% of the foodborne outbreaks included in the Hall et al study fit the clinical/epidemiologic syndrome.

[c] More recent reports estimate the typical norovirus incubation period to be 12–48 hours.[54]

VII

including infants, children, the elderly, pregnant women, and immuno-compromised hosts; (2) in patients with underlying gastrointestinal tract disease that might increase the risk of enteric infection and serious illness, such as inflammatory bowel disease, malignancy, prior gastrointestinal tract surgery, or radiation; use of gastric acid inhibitors; malabsorption syndromes; and other structural or functional conditions; (3) in the presence of specific signs and symptoms that are more consistent with bacterial infection or severe illness, including bloody diarrhea; severe abdominal pain and fever; sudden onset of nausea, vomiting or diarrhea; dehydration associated with diarrhea; neurologic involvement including cranial nerve palsies, motor weakness, or paresthesia; and evidence of HUS; and (4) under circumstances raising public health issues, such as travel, hospitalization, occupation, child care or nursing home attendance, or when an illness outbreak is suspected. The occurrence of neurologic signs and symptoms and HUS are particularly worrisome because of the potential for life-threatening complications.

Laboratory testing of stool specimens may include culture for bacteria; culture-independent diagnostic test (CIDT) assays for viruses, bacteria, or parasites; microscopic examination for parasites, and direct antigen detection tests of culture broths. CIDTs detect antigens, nucleic acid sequences, or toxins of pathogens. Use of CIDTs on stool specimens has been increasing.[41] These tests, which may be available in clinical and public health laboratories, may yield results quicker than cultures but have varying sensitivities and specificities compared with culture and do not generate an isolate. CIDTs available today do not provide information about subtype and antimicrobial susceptibility. Collaboration and communication with clinical microbiology laboratory personnel and local public health officials can improve laboratory testing, because a search for some organisms may not be part of routine testing procedures and may require special requests. Other tests may be available only through public health laboratories or large commercial laboratories. For example, the CDC recommends that all stool specimens submitted for routine enteric pathogen testing from patients with acute community-acquired diarrhea be cultured for *E coli* O157 and tested simultaneously for non-O157 STEC by an assay that detects Shiga toxins or the genes encoding these toxins. However, not all clinical laboratories routinely perform both tests. Testing should be performed regardless of whether blood or white blood cells are present or absent in the stool, because not all patients with STEC infection have bloody diarrhea or fecal leukocytes.[42] Serologic testing can be useful in the diagnosis of some foodborne diseases, such as trichinosis and toxoplasmosis. Diagnostic methods for norovirus focus on detecting viral RNA or viral antigen. Most public health and clinical virology laboratories test for norovirus by using quantitative reverse transcriptase-polymerase chain reaction (RT-qPCR) assays. These assays are very sensitive and can detect as few as 10 to 100 norovirus copies per reaction. They use different oligonucleotide primer sets to differentiate genogroup I and genogroup II norovirus. RT-qPCR assays are also quantitative and can provide estimates of viral load. The assays may be used to detect norovirus in stool, vomitus, foods, water, and environmental specimens. Several recent commercial molecular assays are designed to detect many gastrointestinal pathogens simultaneously, including norovirus. The sensitivity of these assays for norovirus is in the same range as RT-qPCR. More detailed information on laboratory procedures for identification of foodborne pathogens can be obtained from clinical and microbiology specialists and local or state public health personnel.

For suspected outbreaks of foodborne disease involving gastrointestinal tract symptoms, stools should always be collected for laboratory testing when possible. Important clues for investigating and determining the etiology of an outbreak of foodborne illness include obtaining information about the incubation period, duration of illness, and clinical signs and symptoms. If a foodborne disease outbreak is suspected, appropriate clinical specimens should be submitted for laboratory testing, and the local public health authorities should be notified.

Management

Enteric infections generally are self-limited conditions that resolve with supportive care and fluid and electrolyte therapy (see also Chapter 28: Oral Therapy for Acute Diarrhea). Patients should be monitored for signs and symptoms of dehydration. When possible, oral rehydration solutions should be used for fluid replacement in children with mild to moderate dehydration; severely dehydrated patients require intravenous fluids.[43] Antimotility agents should be avoided in children with bloody diarrhea.[39] Routine use of antimicrobial agents is not indicated for the treatment of acute, community-acquired diarrheal illness in the United States, because most illnesses are caused by viruses, are self-limited, and are not shortened by antimicrobial therapy.[3] Depending on the etiology, antimicrobial therapy might be indicated for patients at higher risk of severe or invasive illness

VII

(eg, patients with immunocompromising conditions, infants, pregnant women). In some instances, it may eradicate fecal shedding of the causative organism, prevent transmission of the enteropathogen, abbreviate clinical symptoms, or prevent future complications. However, antimicrobial therapy can prolong the duration of *Salmonella* excretion into the stool and has been identified as a risk factor in *E coli* O157:H7 infection for progression to HUS.[44–46] Antibiotic treatment may also disrupt the normal gut flora and exacerbate diarrhea, particularly because some pathogens have developed resistance to certain antibiotics. Therefore, careful consideration of the illness etiology and the medical history of the patient are important before treatment.

Botulism is a medical and public health emergency. Health care providers should immediately report any suspected case of botulism to their local or state health department. To assist health care providers in the diagnosis and management of botulism, the California Infant Botulism Treatment and Prevention Program provides emergency consultations for suspected infant botulism cases. For suspected botulism cases in people older than 1 year, the Alaska Department of Health and Social Services and California Department of Public Health provide emergency consultations for cases in Alaska and California, respectively. The CDC (770-488-7100) and health department staff provide emergency consultations for suspected cases in the remaining states. Administration of botulinum antitoxin early in the course of illness can prevent the progression of neurologic dysfunction. Heptavalent botulinum antitoxin, an equine-derived antitoxin, is available through the CDC to treat noninfant botulism.[47] Botulism Immune Globulin (BabyBIG) is available through the California Infant Botulism Treatment and Prevention Program to treat infant botulism.[48]

Several resources are available to guide clinicians in the prevention, evaluation, and management of gastroenteritis and foodborne illnesses. Guidelines endorsed by the American Academy of Pediatrics (AAP) for the management of acute gastroenteritis in children are available.[6,43,49] The 2001 Infectious Diseases Society of America (IDSA) guidelines on infectious diarrhea provide recommendations on a variety of topics, including rehydration, laboratory testing, antibiotics, and public health reporting.[6] A primer on foodborne diseases contains information about causes of foodborne illness, clinical considerations, patient scenarios, and patient handout material and resources.[3] DPDx is a website (http://www.dpd.cdc. gov/dpdx/Default.htm) developed by the CDC Division of Parasitic Diseases to aid diagnosis of parasitic diseases; diagnostic help through telediagnosis is available.[50] The AAP *Red Book* also provides additional clinical, diagnostic, and treatment information for specific pathogens.[39] Health care providers should ensure hospitalized patients are placed under the appropriate isolation precautions (eg, contact precautions) and notify their local or state health department of reportable illnesses.[51] Vaccines are not available for most foodborne illnesses, but the hepatitis A vaccine is safe, effective, and recommended by the Advisory Committee on Immunization Practices (ACIP) for all children and for people at increased risk of hepatitis A, including travelers to areas with high or intermediate endemicity of hepatitis A infection. Typhoid fever vaccines are also available for travelers to areas where there is an increased risk of exposure to *Salmonella serotype* Typhi.

Surveillance for Foodborne Diseases

The CDC collects information on foodborne disease outbreaks through the Foodborne Disease Outbreak Surveillance System, with reporting through NORS. This surveillance system is passive in that it relies on state health departments reporting outbreaks to the CDC. The data collected help monitor foodborne disease outbreak etiologies, types of implicated food vehicles, and contributing factors (eg, factors that resulted in contamination of a food vehicle). Data from this surveillance system need to be interpreted with caution, because many outbreaks are not detected, investigated, or reported by local or state health departments because of variations in patient care, clinical diagnostic capabilities and practice, public health reporting, and public health resources. The surveillance system is important for monitoring trends in foodborne disease outbreaks, describing the various types of foodborne pathogens, determining the risk of exposure from different types of foods, and summarizing factors that contributed to the outbreaks.

PulseNet USA, the national molecular subtyping network for bacterial foodborne disease surveillance, was started in 1996 to enhance foodborne disease outbreak detection and investigation.[52] More than 80 public health and food regulatory laboratories, including all state health departments, participate in PulseNet USA and perform pulsed-field gel electrophoresis (PFGE) on clinical isolates of *Campylobacter* species, *Cronobacter zakazakii*, *Listeria monocytogenes*, *Salmonella enterica*, STEC, *Shigella* species, *Vibrio cholerae*, and *Vibrio parahaemolyticus* using standardized methods. The resulting PFGE pattern is a molecular "fingerprint" of the bacteria. The PFGE patterns are shared electronically in real time, allowing PulseNet-affiliated public health laboratories and CDC to compare the patterns of bacteria from ill people; epidemiologists use this information to determine whether they are likely from a common source (ie, part of the same outbreak). In addition to PFGE, the CDC and partners now use whole genome sequencing (WGS) results from clinical, food, and environmental samples in outbreak investigations of illness from pathogens commonly transmitted by food, livestock, or companion animals. WGS enables high resolution characterization of isolates.[53] For example, compared with PFGE, after implementation of WGS for *L monocytogenes*, PulseNet detected more clusters and epidemiologists solved more outbreaks (ie, linking more outbreaks to specific foods) than was occurring when only PFGE was used.[15]

Because of the extensive food distribution system in the United States, contaminated foods may be distributed to people in many locations, with few ill people in a specific location. PulseNet is extremely useful at detecting foodborne disease outbreaks, including widely dispersed outbreaks, by quickly compiling information on genetic profiles of bacterial isolates from ill people and food specimens across the country.[10,52] However, an inherent limitation of PulseNet is that laboratory confirmation of infection and a bacterial isolate are required for case detection, thus emphasizing the importance of appropriately culturing clinical, food, or environmental samples when patients present with gastrointestinal illness. Together, the real-time acquisition of PFGE patterns and WGS from PulseNet and the routine reporting of enteric disease outbreaks through NORS allow for more thorough outbreak detection and control.

Similarly, surveillance for norovirus involves epidemiologic data from NORS and laboratory data from CalciNet. Launched in 2009, CalciNet is an electronic norovirus outbreak surveillance network consisting of 33 local, state, and federal public health and regulatory laboratories.[54] CalciNet-certified laboratories perform genotyping of norovirus using RT-PCR and share the resulting sequences electronically. CalciNet aims to track circulating norovirus strains, identify emerging strains, and identify links between norovirus outbreaks that may suggest a common source. To improve the timeliness of norovirus outbreak reporting and better integrate outbreak epidemiologic data from NORS with laboratory data from CalciNet, the CDC launched Norovirus Sentinel Testing and Tracking (NoroSTAT) in 2012.[55] This network has decreased reporting time of norovirus outbreaks to the CDC, increased the number of outbreaks linked in NORS and CalciNet, and improved completeness of submitted data.

In 1996, the CDC, in collaboration with participating state health departments, the USDA/Food Safety and Inspection Service (FSIS), and the FDA, started the Foodborne Diseases Active Surveillance Network (FoodNet) to track infections commonly transmitted through food.[56,57] FoodNet conducts active, population-based surveillance for laboratory-confirmed infections caused by 9 pathogens, including the bacterial pathogens *Campylobacter* species, *Listeria monocytogenes*, *Salmonella* species, *Shigella* species, STEC including *E coli* O157:H7, *Vibrio* species, *Yersinia* species excluding *Yersinia pestis*, and the parasitic organisms *Cryptosporidium* species and *Cyclospora* species. FoodNet operates in 10 sites covering approximately 15% of the US population (an estimated 49 million people in 2015) and collects data from more than 650 clinical laboratories that test specimens from people who reside in the FoodNet sites. Because of the increasing use of CIDTs by clinical laboratories to detect enteric pathogens, FoodNet added CIDT-positive infections to surveillance in 2012. FoodNet also conducts active surveillance for physician-diagnosed pediatric post-diarrheal HUS, a serious complication of STEC infection, by review of hospital discharge data through a network of nephrologists and infection preventionists.

Bacterial pathogens including *Campylobacter*, *Salmonella*, and *Shigella* species are the most frequently identified causes of laboratory-diagnosed infections in FoodNet.[57] Table 51.5 shows the incidence by age group, total number of cases, and death rate among people infected with specific pathogens under surveillance in 2016. Pathogens with the highest incidence in children younger than 5 years are *Salmonella* species, *Campylobacter* species, *Shigella* species, STEC, and *Cryptosporidium* species.[58] Compared with 2006–2008, the overall incidence of culture-confirmed or CIDT-positive *Campylobacter*, *Salmonella*, *Vibrio*, and *Yersinia* species has increased.[57] These increases may be attributable to increasing use of CIDTs, which may indicate increased testing and varying test sensitivity, a true increase in infections, or a combination of these reasons. Fig 51.1 shows trends in incidence of infection by selected FoodNet pathogens in 2016 compared with the 2006–2008 baseline. Using FoodNet data from 2005 through 2008, Scallan et al estimated the actual number of illnesses from bacterial enteric pathogens among US children <5 years old by incorporating steps required for an illness to be laboratory-confirmed (eg, patient evaluated by a health care provider, enteric disease suspected, stool culture submitted). Nontyphoidal *Salmonella* species was the leading pathogen (42%), followed by *Campylobacter* species (28%), *Shigella* species (21%), *Yersinia enterocolitica* (5%), and *Escherichia coli* O157 (3%).[59]

Table 51.5.

Incidence of Laboratory-Diagnosed Infection by Age Group, Total Cases, and Deaths, FoodNet, 2016[a,b,31,57]

Pathogen	Incidence Rate[c] by Age Group (y)					Total Cases		Total Deaths	
	<5	5–9	10–19	20–59	≥60	No.	Rate	No.	CFR[d]
Bacteria									
Campylobacter species	28.9	11.8	9.9	17.6	16.6	8547	17.4	26	0.3
Listeria species	0.3	0	0.1	0.1	0.8	127	0.3	17	13.4
Salmonella species	63.9	18.4	10.4	12.7	16.3	8172	16.7	40	0.5
Shigella species	20.5	16.4	3.8	5.0	2.1	2913	5.9	2	0.1
STEC[e]	16.1	5.2	5.0	2.4	2.3	1845	3.8	3	0.2
Vibrio species	0.2	0.2	0.4	0.5	0.8	252	0.5	4	1.6
Yersinia species	1.1	0.4	0.2	0.5	0.9	302	0.6	3	1.0
Parasites									
Cryptosporidium species	8.8	5.4	3.5	3.4	2.5	1816	3.7	3	0.2
Cyclospora species	0.0	0.0	0.0	0.2	0.1	55	0.1	0	0.0

Adapted from: Centers for Disease Control and Prevention. FoodNet Fast. Atlanta, Georgia: U.S. Department of Health and Human Services. Available at: http://wwwn.cdc.gov/foodnetfast. Accessed July 5, 2017; and Marder EP, Cieslak PR, Cronquist AB, et al. Incidence and trends of infections with pathogens transmitted commonly through food and the effect of increasing use of culture-independent diagnostic tests on surveillance—Foodborne Diseases Active Surveillance Network, 10 U.S. Sites, 2013–2016. *MMWR Morb Mortal Wkly Rep.* 2017;66(15):397–403

[a] Laboratory-diagnosed infections include culture-confirmed and culture-independent diagnostic test (CIDT)-positive results.

[b] Data are preliminary.

[c] Per 100 000 population for FoodNet areas.

[d] Case fatality ratio (CFR) = number of deaths/total cases.

[e] Shiga toxin-producing *Escherichia coli*.

Fig 51.1.

Trends in selected pathogens in Foodborne Diseases Active Surveillance Network (FoodNet) sites. Relative rates of culture-confirmed or culture-independent diagnostic test (CIDT)-positive infections with *Campylobacter, Salmonella, Shigella, Vibrio,* and *Yersinia* organisms, compared with 2006–2008 baseline rates, by year.[a,57]

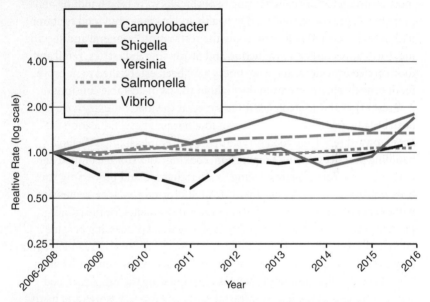

From: Marder EP, Cieslak PR, Cronquist AB, et al. Incidence and trends of infections with pathogens transmitted commonly through food and the effect of increasing use of culture-independent diagnostic tests on surveillance—Foodborne Diseases Active Surveillance Network, 10 U.S. Sites, 2013–2016. *MMWR Morb Mortal Wkly Rep.* 2017;66(15):397–403.

[a] The position of each line indicates the relative change in the incidence of that pathogen compared with 2006–2008. The absolute incidences of these infections cannot be determined from this graph. Data for 2016 are preliminary.

Through active surveillance and additional studies, FoodNet produces estimates of the burden of foodborne diseases in the United States, providing information that can help target, develop, and evaluate foodborne illness prevention and control strategies. For example, after prevention measures, such as the Hazard Analysis and Critical Control Point (HACCP) measures, have been implemented, FoodNet measures changes in bacterial and parasitic infection rates to track progress toward reducing foodborne illness. The CDC maintains interactive online tools enabling users to search and download data from FoodNet (FoodNet Fast — https://wwwn.cdc.gov/foodnetfast/) and Foodborne Disease Outbreak Surveillance System (FOOD Tool — https://wwwn.cdc.gov/foodborneoutbreaks/).

Food Safety and Prevention of Foodborne Illness

From 1993 through 1997, the most commonly reported food preparation practices that contributed to foodborne disease were improper holding temperatures of food and poor personal hygiene of preparers of food.[60] In restaurant-associated foodborne disease outbreaks during 1998–2013, the most common factors contributing to outbreaks were food handling and preparation practices, food worker health and hygiene, and food contamination that occurred before reaching the restaurant.[61] General and specific measures aimed at food production and processing industries, retail and food service providers, and consumers have been established to improve foodborne disease prevention throughout the farm-to-table continuum.

Prevention and control measures aimed at the food industry have been broadly implemented to prevent foodborne illness. Education targeted toward retail and food service operators emphasizing safe food handling practices during preparation, cooking, and storage of food and pathogen-control measures during food production and processing have been implemented.[62] In 1996, the USDA FSIS introduced comprehensive pathogen-reduction and HACCP systems requirements for meat and poultry processors. HACCP regulations for seafood processing became effective in 1997. The FDA Food Code, last updated in 2013, is a model regulatory code that provides local, state, and tribal food regulatory authorities with scientifically rigorous guidelines for regulating the retail and food service segment of the industry (restaurants and grocery stores and institutions such as nursing homes).[63] In 2010, the FDA created the Reportable Food Registry program, which requires the food industry to report to FDA food items that have a "reasonable probability" of causing serious adverse health consequences or death to humans or animals. In 2011, the Food Safety Modernization Act (Pub L No. 111-353) was signed into law. The Act gives FDA new enforcement authorities designed to achieve higher rates of compliance with prevention- and risk-based food safety standards, including for foreign food producers. It also gives new authorities in response to food contamination events, such as mandatory recall of foods, and focuses on enhanced surveillance and outbreak detection and response.

Measures have been enacted that are specific for defined food products, and these have been associated with a decline in the incidence of foodborne infections.[57,64] These measures have included increased attention to good agriculture practices aimed at fresh fruit and vegetables, increased regulation of imported foods, food safety education, pasteurization of dairy products, new egg safety regulations, and the use of technology during food production to prevent or mitigate food contamination.[62,64,65] Information about these and other measures enacted to reduce foodborne disease can be found at various websites shown in the directory of resources (Table 51.6).

Table 51.6.
Directory of Online Resources for Prevention of Foodborne Illness

Surveillance, Reporting, and Outbreaks
Estimates of Foodborne Illness in the United States (CDC): http://www.cdc.gov/foodborneburden/
Nationally Notifiable Conditions: https://wwwn.cdc.gov/nndss/conditions/notifiable/2017/
CSTE's Index of State Reportable Conditions list: http://www.cste.org/?page=StateReportable
CDC's OutbreakNet/Outbreak Response Team: https://www.cdc.gov/foodsafety/outbreaks/index.html
Diagnosis and Management of Suspected Foodborne Illness
Diagnosis and Management of Foodborne Illnesses: A Primer for Physicians and Other Health Care Professionals (CDC): http://www.cdc.gov/mmwr/PDF/rr/rr5304.pdf
Managing Acute Gastroenteritis Among Children: Oral Rehydration, Maintenance, and Nutritional Therapy (CDC): http://www.cdc.gov/mmwr/PDF/RR/RR5216.pdf
CDPH Infant Botulism Treatment and Prevention Program: http://www.infantbotulism.org/
Updated Norovirus Outbreak Management and Disease Prevention Guidelines (CDC): http://www.cdc.gov/mmwr/preview/mmwrhtml/rr6003a1.htm?s_cid=rr6003a1_w
CDC Parasites Transmitted by Food: http://www.cdc.gov/parasites/food.html
CDC DPDx (for parasites): http://www.dpd.cdc.gov/dpdx/Default.htm
Recommendations for Diagnosis of Shiga Toxin-Producing *Escherichia coli* Infections by Clinical Laboratories: http://www.cdc.gov/mmwr/preview/mmwrhtml/rr5812a1.htm

VII

Continued

Table 51.6. *Continued*

Directory of Online Resources for Prevention of Foodborne Illness

Food Safety
CDC Food Safety: http://www.cdc.gov/foodsafety/
FDA Food Safety: https://www.fda.gov/food/
USDA/FSIS: https://www.fsis.usda.gov/wps/portal/fsis/home
Food Safety Modernization Act (2011): https://www.fda.gov/food/guidanceregulation/fsma/
FDA Food Code: https://www.fda.gov/Food/GuidanceRegulation/RetailFoodProtection/FoodCode/
FDA Reportable Registry for Industry: https://www.fda.gov/Food/ComplianceEnforcement/RFR/default.htm
Compendium of Measures to Prevent Disease Associated with Animals in Public Settings, 2009: http://www.cdc.gov/mmwr/preview/mmwrhtml/rr5805a1.htm
Food Safety Consumer Education Resources
FoodSafety.gov: http://www.foodsafety.gov/
The Basics: Clean, Separate, Cook, and Chill: http://www.foodsafety.gov/keep/basics/index.html
Safe Minimum Cooking Temperatures: http://www.foodsafety.gov/keep/charts/mintemp.html
Fight BAC! Partnership for Food Safety Education campaign: http://www.fightbac.org/
CDC Food Safety and Raw Milk: http://www.cdc.gov/foodsafety/rawmilk/raw-milk-index.html
CDC Reptiles, Amphibians, and *Salmonella*: http://www.cdc.gov/Features/SalmonellaFrogTurtle/

Food safety in the home is also critical for preventing foodborne illness. Cleanliness is a major factor in preventing foodborne illness. Hands should be washed with warm, soapy water for 20 seconds before preparing any foods and after handling uncooked eggs or raw meat, poultry, seafood, and their juices. The cleaning of surfaces in the kitchen is also important to preventing cross-contamination during food preparation. Microorganisms can be transmitted in the kitchen via hands, cutting boards, utensils, and countertops. Cross contamination from one food item to another is a major problem when handling raw meat, poultry, seafood, and eggs. In addition to hand washing, cutting boards, utensils, and countertops should be washed with hot, soapy water after preparing each food item. Contamination of foods with viruses is particularly easy when preparing food. Any contact of bare, contaminated hands with food then eaten without heating has the potential to transmit pathogens and cause infection. Individuals who have had vomiting or diarrhea within the past 48 hours should refrain from preparing or serving food.[66] Food preparation surfaces can become contaminated; this contamination can be unapparent and may resist disinfection with common products. A solution of 1 teaspoon liquid chlorine bleach per quart of clean water can sanitize surfaces; to be effective, the solution should be left on for about 10 minutes, then the surface rinsed clean. Replace cutting boards after they become excessively worn or develop hard-to-clean grooves. Hands should always be washed after people using the bathroom; changing diapers; tending to a sick person; blowing one's nose, coughing, or sneezing; or handling pets or their food or cages to prevent contamination of foods or preparation surfaces.

Normal cooking will kill most pathogens that cause foodborne illness (Table 51.7). Eggs should be cooked until both yolk and white are firm; all poultry (ground, whole, parts) should be cooked until it has an internal temperature of 165°F. As measured with a food thermometer placed in the thickest part of the food, whole cuts of meat, such as pork, steaks, roasts, and chops, should be cooked to an internal temperature of 145°F; fish should be cooked to 145°F (and until it is opaque and flakes easily with a fork); ground meat, especially hamburger meat, should be cooked to 160°F. Because bacteria grow at room temperature, hot foods should be maintained at 140°F or higher and cold foods at 40°F or lower. Perishables, prepared foods, and leftovers should be refrigerated or frozen within 2 hours of preparation with minimal handling. Foods should be defrosted in the refrigerator, under cold running water or in a microwave, not at room temperature; similarly, foods should be marinated in the refrigerator.

These measures are especially relevant for people at high risk, including infants, children, the elderly, immunocompromised people, and pregnant women.[8] High-risk people should avoid eating or drinking raw (unpasteurized) milk or raw milk products, raw or partially cooked eggs or raw egg products, raw or undercooked meat and poultry, raw or undercooked fish and shellfish, raw flour and dough, unpasteurized juice, and raw sprouts. Honey should not be fed to infants younger than 12 months because of

VII

Table 51.7.

Safe Minimum Cooking Temperatures

Food	Minimum Internal Temperature
Ground beef, ground pork, ground veal, ground lamb	160°F
Ground turkey, ground chicken	165°F
Beef, lamb, and veal steaks and roasts	145°F and allow to rest at least 3 minutes
Poultry, including chicken and turkey (ground, whole, or parts), duck, and goose	165°F
Pork chops, ribs, and roasts	145°F and allow to rest at least 3 minutes
Eggs	Until yolk and white are firm
Egg dishes	160°F
Fish	145°F
Stuffing, casseroles, and leftovers	165°F

Adapted from http://www.foodsafety.gov/keep/charts/mintemp.html (Accessed May 11, 2017) and https://www.fsis.usda.gov/wps/portal/fsis/topics/food-safety-education/teach-others/fsis-educational-campaigns/is-it-done-yet/thermometer-placement-and-temperatures/ct_index (Accessed May 11, 2017).

the risk of infant botulism. Physicians and parents should be aware that powdered infant formulas, although heat-treated during processing, are not sterile, in contrast to liquid formulas.[67] Before mixing the powdered infant formula with water, the person preparing the formula should wash their hands and the bottles, bottle nipples, and other equipment used to make the formula with soap and water.[68] "Transition" infant formulas that are generally used for preterm or low birth weight infants after hospital discharge are available in both nonsterile powder form and commercially sterile liquid form. Because of the risk of *C sakazakii* infection (formerly *Enterobacter sakazakii*), which can cause meningitis, sepsis, and necrotizing enterocolitis in infants, the FDA recommends that powdered infant formulas not be used in neonatal intensive care settings unless no alternative is available.[67,69–71] Parents should be encouraged to separate infants and children from raw meat and poultry products while shopping and to place children in the shopping cart child seats rather than the baskets.[18]

Food safety education materials aimed at consumers are available online through several organizations (Table 51.6, Food Safety Consumer Education Resources). Current consumer messaging from the Partnership for Food Safety Education emphasizes 4 simple steps that can be taken when preparing food to help prevent food poisoning—clean, separate, cook, and chill—which focus on hand washing and surface cleaning, prevention of cross contamination, cooking of food at proper temperatures, and prompt and appropriate refrigeration of food before and after cooking or preparation.[72] However, consumers cannot eliminate all foodborne illness risks. For example, no consumer-level method of washing fruits and vegetables has consistently been shown to fully eliminate pathogens associated with foodborne illnesses (eg, *L monocytogenes*).[73,74]

References

1. Scallan E, Hoekstra R, Angulo F, et al. Foodborne illness acquired in the United States—major pathogens. *Emerg Infect Dis.* 2011;17(1):7–15
2. Bryan F. Diseases Transmitted by Foods (A Classification and Summary). 2nd ed. Atlanta, GA: US Department of Heath and Human Services, Centers for Disease Control; 1982
3. Centers for Disease Control and Prevention. Diagnosis and management of foodborne illnesses: a primer for physicians and other health care professionals. *MMWR Recomm Rep.* 2004;53(RR-4):1–33
4. Beer KD, Gargano JW, Roberts VA, et al. Surveillance for waterborne disease outbreaks associated with drinking water—United States, 2011–2012. *MMWR Morb Mortal Wkly Rep.* 2015;64(31):842–848
5. Pickering L. Approach to the diagnosis and management of gastrointestinal tract infections. In: Long S, Pickering L, Prober C, eds. *Principles and Practice of Pediatric Infectious Diseases.* 3rd ed: Churchill Livingstone Elsevier; 2008
6. Guerrant RL, Van Gilder T, Steiner TS, et al. Practice guidelines for the management of infectious diarrhea. *Clin Infect Dis.* 2001;32(3):331–351
7. Koehler KM, Lasky T, Fein SB, et al. Population-based incidence of infection with selected bacterial enteric pathogens in children younger than five years of age, 1996–1998. *Pediatr Infect Dis J.* 2006;25(2):129–134.
8. Gerba CP, Rose JB, Haas CN. Sensitive populations: who is at the greatest risk? *Int J Food Microbiol.* 1996;30(1):113–123
9. Tauxe RV. Emerging foodborne pathogens. *Int J Food Microbiol.* 2002;78(1–2):31–41
10. Sobel J, Griffin P, Slutsker L, Swerdlow D, Tauxe R. Investigation of multistate foodborne disease outbreaks. *Public Health Rep.* 2002;117(1):8–19

11. Gould LH, Kline J, Monahan C, Vierk K. Outbreaks of disease associated with food imported into the United States, 1996–2014. *Emerg Infect Dis.* 2017;23(3): 525–528

12. Behravesh C, Williams I, Tauxe R. *Emerging Foodborne Pathogens and Problems: Expanding Prevention Efforts Before Slaughter or Harvest Improving Food Safety Through a One Health Approach: Workshop Summary.* Washington, DC: National Academies Press; 2012

13. Centers for Disease Control and Prevention. Antibiotic Resistance Threats in the United States, 2013. Available at: https://www.cdc.gov/drugresistance/pdf/ ar-threats-2013–508.pdf. Accessed July 21, 2019

14. Centers for Disease Control and Prevention. *Surveillance for Foodborne Disease Outbreaks, United States, 2015, Annual Report.* Atlanta, GA: Centers for Disease Control and Prevention; 2017

15. Jackson BR, Tarr C, Strain E, et al. Implementation of nationwide real-time whole-genome sequencing to enhance listeriosis outbreak detection and investigation. *Clin Infect Dis.* 2016;63(3):380–386

16. Fullerton KE, Ingram LA, Jones TF, et al. Sporadic *Campylobacter* infection in infants: a population-based surveillance case-control study. *Pediatr Infect Dis J.* 2007;26(1):19–24

17. Jones TF, Ingram LA, Fullerton KE, et al. A case-control study of the epidemiology of sporadic *Salmonella* infection in infants. *Pediatrics.* 2006;118(6):2380–2387

18. Patrick M, Mahon B, Zansky S, Hurd S, Scallan E. Riding in shopping carts and exposure to raw meat and poultry products: prevalence of, and factors associated with, this risk factor for *Salmonella* and *Campylobacter* infection in children younger than 3 years. *J Food Protect.* 2010;73:1097–1100

19. Angelo KM, Conrad AR, Saupe A, et al. Multistate outbreak of *Listeria monocytogenes* infections linked to whole apples used in commercially produced, prepackaged caramel apples: United States, 2014–2015. *Epidemiol Infect.* 2017;145(5):848–856

20. Gieraltowski L, Schwensohn C, Meyer S, et al. Notes from the field: multistate outbreak of *Escherichia coli* O157:H7 infections linked to dough mix—United States, 2016. *MMWR Morb Mortal Wkly Rep.* 2017;66(3):88–89

21. Harvey RR, Heiman Marshall KE, Burnworth L, et al. International outbreak of multiple *Salmonella* serotype infections linked to sprouted chia seed powder— USA and Canada, 2013–2014. *Epidemiol Infect.* 2017;145(8):1535–1544

22. Centers for Disease Control and Prevention. Multistate outbreak of Shiga toxin-producing *Escherichia coli* O157:H7 infections linked to I.M. Healthy Brand SoyNut Butter (final update). 2017. Available at: https://www.cdc.gov/ecoli/2017/ o157h7-03-17/index.html. Accessed August 4, 2017

23. Sotir MJ, Ewald G, Kimura AC, et al. Outbreak of *Salmonella* Wandsworth and Typhimurium infections in infants and toddlers traced to a commercial vegetable-coated snack food. *Pediatr Infect Dis J.* 2009;28(12):1041–1046

24. Harris J, Neil K, Behravesh C, Sotir M, Angulo F. Recent multistate outbreaks of human *Salmonella* infections acquired from turtles: a continuing public health challenge. *Clin Infect Dis.* 2010;50(4):554–559

25. Gambino-Shirley K, Stevenson L, Wargo K, et al. Notes from the field: four multistate outbreaks of human *Salmonella* infections linked to small turtle exposure—United States, 2015. *MMWR Morb Mortal Wkly Rep.* 2016;65(25): 655–656

26. Laughlin M, Gambino-Shirley K, Gacek P, et al. Notes from the field: outbreak of *Escherichia coli* O157 infections associated with goat dairy farm visits—Connecticut, 2016. *MMWR Morb Mortal Wkly Rep.* 2016;65(5051):1453–1454

27. Centers for Disease Control and Prevention. Multistate outbreak of human *Salmonella* Typhimurium infections associated with aquatic frogs—United States, 2009. *MMWR Morb Mortal Wkly Rep.* 2011;58(51):1433–1436

28. Basler C, Nguyen TA, Anderson TC, Hancock T, Behravesh CB. Outbreaks of human Salmonella infections associated with live poultry, United States, 1990–2014. *Emerg Infect Dis.* 2016;22(10):1705–1711

29. Mermin J, Hoar B, Angulo F. Iguanas and *Salmonella marina* infection in children: a reflection of the increasing incidence of reptile-associated salmonellosis in the United States. *Pediatrics.* 1997;99(3):399

30. Wikswo ME, Kambhampati A, Shioda K, Walsh KA, Bowen A, Hall AJ. Outbreaks of acute gastroenteritis transmitted by person-to-person contact, environmental contamination, and unknown modes of transmission—United States, 2009–2013. *MMWR Surveill Summ.* 2015;64(12):1–16

31. Centers for Disease Control and Prevention. FoodNet Fast. 2017. Available at: https://wwwn.cdc.gov/foodnetfast/. Accessed July 5, 2017

32. Hall JA, Goulding JS, Bean NH, Tauxe RV, Hedberg CW. Epidemiologic profiling: evaluating foodborne outbreaks for which no pathogen was isolated by routine laboratory testing: United States, 1982–9. *Epidemiol Infect.* 2001;127(3):381–387

33. Jackson KA, Iwamoto M, Swerdlow D. Pregnancy-associated listeriosis. *Epidemiol Infect.* 2010;138(10):1503–1509

34. Brooks JT, Sowers EG, Wells JG, et al. Non-O157 Shiga toxin-producing *Escherichia coli* infections in the United States, 1983–2002. *J Infect Dis.* 2005;192(8):1422–1429

35. Griffin PM, Tauxe RV. The epidemiology of infections caused by *Escherichia coli* O157:H7, other enterohemorrhagic *E. coli*, and the associated hemolytic uremic syndrome. *Epidemiol Rev.* 1991;13:60–98

36. Hannu T, Mattila L, Rautelin H, et al. *Campylobacter*-triggered reactive arthritis: a population-based study. *Rheumatology.* 2002;41(3):312–318

37. Warren CP. Arthritis associated with *Salmonella* infections. *Ann Rheum Dis.* 1970;29(5):483

38. Mishu B, Ilyas AA, Koski CL, et al. Serologic evidence of previous *Campylobacter jejuni* infection in patients with the Guillain-Barre syndrome. *Ann Intern Med.* 1993;118(12):947–953

VII

39. Kimberlin D, Brady M, Jackson M, Long S, eds. *Red Book: 2018 Report of the Committee on Infectious Diseases*. 31st ed. Elk Grove Village, IL: American Academy of Pediatrics; 2018

40. Burnett MW, Bass JW, Cook BA. Etiology of osteomyelitis complicating sickle cell disease. *Pediatrics*. 1998;101(2):296–297

41. Huang JY, Henao OL, Griffin PM, et al. Infection with pathogens transmitted commonly through food and the effect of increasing use of culture-independent diagnostic tests on surveillance—Foodborne Diseases Active Surveillance Network, 10 U.S. Sites, 2012–2015. *MMWR Morb Mortal Wkly Rep*. 2016;65(14):368–371

42. Gould LH, Bopp C, Strockbine N, et al. Recommendations for diagnosis of shiga toxin—producing Escherichia coli infections by clinical laboratories. *MMWR Recomm Rep*. 2009;58(RR-12):1–14

43. Centers for Disease Control and Prevention. Managing acute gastroenteritis among children: oral rehydration, maintenance, and nutritional therapy. *MMWR Recomm Rep*. 2003;52(RR-16):1–16

44. Acheson D, Hohmann EL. Nontyphoidal Salmonellosis. *Clin Infect Dis*. 2001;32(2):263–269

45. Freedman SB, Xie J, Neufeld MS, et al. Shiga toxin–producing *Escherichia coli* infection, antibiotics, and risk of developing hemolytic uremic syndrome: a meta-analysis. *Clin Infect Dis*. 2016;62(10):1251–1258

46. Mody RK, Griffin PM. Editorial commentary: increasing evidence that certain antibiotics should be avoided for Shiga toxin–producing *Escherichia coli* infections: more data needed. *Clin Infect Dis*. 2016;62(10):1259–1261

47. Centers for Disease Control and Prevention. Investigational heptavalent botulinum antitoxin (HBAT) to replace licensed botulinum antitoxin AB and investigational botulinum antitoxin E. *MMWR Morb Mortal Wkly Rep*. 2010;59(10):299

48. Arnon SS, Schechter R, Maslanka SE, Jewell NP, Hatheway CL. Human botulism immune globulin for the treatment of infant botulism. *N Engl J Med*. 2006;354(5):462–471

49. American Academy of Pediatrics. Statement of endorsement: managing acute gastroenteritis among children: oral rehydration, maintenance, and nutritional therapy. *Pediatrics*. 2004;114(2):507

50. Centers for Disease Control and Prevention. DPDx - Laboratory Identification of Parasitic Diseases of Public Health Concern. Available at: https://www.cdc.gov/dpdx/az.html. Accessed August 8, 2017

51. Centers for Disease Control and Prevention. 2007 Guideline for Isolation Precautions: Preventing Transmission of Infectious Agents in Healthcare Settings. 2007. Available at: https://www.cdc.gov/niosh/docket/archive/pdfs/NIOSH-219/0219-010107-siegel.pdf. Accessed July 21, 2019

52. Gerner-Smidt P, Hise K, Kincaid J, et al. PulseNet USA: a five-year update. *Foodborne Pathog Dis*. 2006;3(1):9–19

53. Carleton HA, Gerner-Smidt P. Whole-genome sequencing is taking over foodborne disease surveillance. *Microbe.* 2016;11(7):311–317

54. Centers for Disease Control and Prevention. Updated norovirus outbreak management and disease prevention guidelines. *MMWR Recomm Rep.* 2011;60(3):1–15

55. Shah MP, Wikswo ME, Barclay L, et al. Near real-time surveillance of U.S. norovirus outbreaks by the Norovirus Sentinel Testing and Tracking Network—United States, August 2009–July 2015. *MMWR Morb Mortal Wkly Rep.* 2017;66(7):185–189

56. Henao OL, Jones TF, Vugia DJ, Griffin PM. Foodborne Diseases Active Surveillance Network—2 decades of achievements, 1996–2015. *Emerg Infect Dis.* 2015;21(9):1529–1536

57. Marder EP, Cieslak PR, Cronquist AB, et al. Incidence and trends of infections with pathogens transmitted commonly through food and the effect of increasing use of culture-independent diagnostic tests on surveillance—Foodborne Diseases Active Surveillance Network, 10 U.S. Sites, 2013–2016. *MMWR Morb Mortal Wkly Rep.* 2017;66(15):397–403

58. Centers for Disease Control and Prevention. Incidence and trends of infection with pathogens transmitted commonly through food—Foodborne Diseases Active Surveillance Network, 10 U.S. sites, 1996–2012. *MMWR Morb Mortal Wkly Rep.* 2013;62(15):283–287

59. Scallan E, Mahon BE, Hoekstra RM, Griffin PM. Estimates of illnesses, hospitalizations and deaths caused by major bacterial enteric pathogens in young children in the United States. *Pediatr Infect Dis J.* 2013;32(3):217–221

60. Bryan F, Guzewich J, Todd E. Surveillance of foodborne disease III. Summary and presentation of data on vehicles and contributory factors; their value and limitations. *J Food Protect.* 1996;60(6):701–714

61. Angelo KM, Nisler AL, Hall AJ, Brown LG, Gould LH. Epidemiology of restaurant-associated foodborne disease outbreaks, United States, 1998–2013. *Epidemiol Infect.* 2016;145(3):523–534

62. Tauxe RV. Food safety and irradiation: protecting the public from foodborne infections. *Emerg Infect Dis.* 2001;7(3 Suppl):516

63. US Food and Drug Administration. FDA Food Code 2013. Available at: https://www.fda.gov/food/guidanceregulation/retailfoodprotection/foodcode/default.htm. Accessed May 24, 2017

64. Centers for Disease Control and Prevention. Achievements in public health, 1990–1999: safer and healthier foods. *MMWR Morb Mortal Wkly Rep.* 1999;48(40):905–913

65. Billy TJ, Wachsmuth IK. Hazard analysis and critical control point systems in the United States Department of Agriculture regulatory policy. *Revue Scientifique et Technique.* 1997;16(2):342–348

VII

66. Hall AJ, Wikswo ME, Pringle K, Gould LH, Parashar UD. Vital signs: foodborne norovirus outbreaks—United States, 2009–2012. *MMWR Morb Mortal Wkly Rep.* 2014;63(22):491–495

67. US Food and Drug Administration. Health Professionals Letter on Enterobacter sakazakii Infections Associated With Use of Powdered (Dry) Infant Formulas in Neonatal Intensive Care Units. Available at: https://www.fda.gov/Food/RecallsOutbreaksEmergencies/SafetyAlertsAdvisories/ucm111299.htm. Accessed May 24, 2017

68. American Academy of Pediatrics. Sterilizing and Warming Bottles. 2011. Available at: https://www.healthychildren.org/English/ages-stages/baby/feeding-nutrition/Pages/Sterilizing-and-Warming-Bottles.aspx. Accessed 09/21/2017

69. Bowen AB, Braden CR. Invasive *Enterobacter sakazakii* disease in infants. *Emerg Infect Dis.* 2006;12(8):1185–1189

70. van Acker J, de Smet F, Muyldermans G, Bougatef A, Naessens A, Lauwers S. Outbreak of necrotizing enterocolitis associated with *Enterobacter sakazakii* in powdered milk formula. *J Clin Microbiol.* 2001;39(1):293–297

71. Jason J. Prevention of invasive *Cronobacter* infections in young infants fed powdered infant formulas. *Pediatrics.* 2012;130(5):e1076–e1084

72. Partnership for Food Safety Education. The Core Four Practices. Available at: http://www.fightbac.org/food-safety-basics/the-core-four-practices/. Accessed August 4, 2017

73. Fishburn J, Tang Y, Frank J. Efficacy of various consumer-friendly produce washing technologies in reducing pathogens on fresh produce. *Food Protect Trends.* 2012;32(8):456–466

74. Pezzuto A, Belluco S, Losasso C, et al. Effectiveness of washing procedures in reducing *Salmonella enterica* and *Listeria monocytogenes* on a raw leafy green vegetable (*Eruca vesicaria*). *Front Microbiol.* 2016;7:1663

75. McCrickard L, Marlow M, Self JL, et al. Notes from the field: botulism outbreak from drinking prison-made illicit alcohol in a federal correctional facility—Mississippi, June 2016. *MMWR Morb Mortal Wkly Rep.* 2017;65(52):1491–1492

76. Centers for Disease Control and Prevention. Multistate outbreak of *Salmonella* Virchow infections linked to Garden of Life RAW Meal Organic Shake & Meal Products (final update). 2016. Available at: https://www.cdc.gov/salmonella/virchow-02-16/index.html. Accessed June 21, 2017

77. McCarty CL, Angelo K, Beer KD, et al. Large outbreak of botulism associated with a church potluck meal—Ohio, 2015. *MMWR Morb Mortal Wkly Rep.* 2015;64(29):802–803

78. Centers for Disease Control and Prevention. Multistate outbreak of Shiga toxin-producing *Escherichia coli* O157:H7 infections linked to costco rotisserie chicken salad (final update). 2015. Available at: https://www.cdc.gov/ecoli/2015/o157h7-11-15/index.html. Accessed June 21, 2017

79. Centers for Disease Control and Prevention. Multistate outbreak of *Listeriosis* linked to Blue Bell Creameries products (final update). 2015. Available at: https://www.cdc.gov/listeria/outbreaks/ice-cream-03-15/index.html. Accessed June 21, 2017

80. Centers for Disease Control and Prevention. Multistate outbreak of *Salmonella* Poona infections linked to imported cucumbers (final update). 2016. Available at: https://www.cdc.gov/salmonella/poona-09-15/index.html. Accessed June 21, 2017

81. Rosenthal M, Pedersen R, Leibsle S, Hill V, Carter K, Roellig DM. Notes from the field: cryptosporidiosis associated with consumption of unpasteurized goat milk—Idaho, 2014. *MMWR Morb Mortal Wkly Rep.* 2015;64(7):194–195

82. Collier MG, Khudyakov YE, Selvage D, et al. Outbreak of hepatitis A in the USA associated with frozen pomegranate arils imported from Turkey: an epidemiological case study. *Lancet Infect Dis.* 2014;14(10):976–981

83. Centers for Disease Control and Prevention. Outbreaks of cyclosporiasis—United States, June–August 2013. *MMWR Morb Mortal Wkly Rep.* 2013;62(43):862

84. Centers for Disease Control and Prevention. Multistate outbreak of *Salmonella* Saintpaul infections linked to imported cucumbers (final update). 2013. Available at: https://www.cdc.gov/salmonella/saintpaul-04-13/index.html. Accessed June 21, 2017

85. Newton AE, Garrett N, Stroika SG, Halpin JL, Turnsek M, Mody RK. Increase in *Vibrio parahaemolyticus* infections associated with consumption of Atlantic Coast shellfish—2013. *MMWR Morb Mortal Wkly Rep.* 2014;63(15):335–336

86. Centers for Disease Control and Prevention. Multistate outbreak of Shiga toxin-producing *Escherichia coli* O26 infections linked to raw clover sprouts at Jimmy John's restaurants (final update). 2012. Available at: https://www.cdc.gov/ecoli/2012/O26-02-12/index.html. Accessed June 21, 2017

87. Heiman KE, Garalde VB, Gronostaj M, et al. Multistate outbreak of listeriosis caused by imported cheese and evidence of cross-contamination of other cheeses, USA, 2012. *Epidemiol Infect.* 2015;144(13):2698–2708

88. Viazis S, Beal JK, Monahan C, et al. Laboratory, environmental, and epidemiologic investigation and regulatory enforcement actions in response to an outbreak of Salmonella Bredeney infections linked to peanut butter. *Open Forum Infect Dis.* 2015;2(3):ofv114

89. Routh JA, Pringle J, Mohr M, et al. Nationwide outbreak of multidrug-resistant *Salmonella* Heidelberg infections associated with ground turkey: United States, 2011. *Epidemiol Infect.* 2015;143(15):3227–3234

90. McCollum JT, Cronquist AB, Silk BJ, et al. Multistate outbreak of listeriosis associated with cantaloupe. *N Engl J Med.* 2013;369(10):944–953

91. Taylor EV, Nguyen TA, Machesky KD, et al. Multistate outbreak of *Escherichia coli* O145 infections associated with romaine lettuce consumption, 2010. *J Food Protect.* 2013;76(6):939–944

VII

92. Gieraltowski L, Julian E, Pringle J, et al. Nationwide outbreak of *Salmonella* Montevideo infections associated with contaminated imported black and red pepper: warehouse membership cards provide critical clues to identify the source. *Epidemiol Infect.* 2012;FirstView:1–9

93. Centers for Disease Control and Prevention. *Salmonella* Montevideo infections associated with salami products made with contaminated imported black and red pepper—United States, July 2009–April 2010. *MMWR Morb Mortal Wkly Rep.* 2010;59(50):1647–1650

Chapter 52

Food Safety: Pesticides, Industrial Chemicals, Toxins, Antimicrobial Preservatives, Irradiation, and Food Contact Substances

Introduction

Foods available in the United States are among the safest found in the world. Nonetheless, there are a wide variety of nonnutritive chemical substances found in the food supply that may have health and safety implications for infants and children. As the United States continues to import significant amounts of food and food products, a rising challenge has been the monitoring of foods imported from more than 150 countries and territories. Imported foods now constitute 15% of the US food supply, including 70% of fresh fruits and vegetables and 80% of seafood.[1]

In contrast to the illnesses associated with microbial contamination of foods (see also Chapter 51: Food Safety: Infectious Disease), the safety issues related to chemical substances in foods are less well understood and result in effects that may be subclinical and, thus, difficult to document. However, contamination from naturally occurring and synthetic substances have occurred resulting in alarm given the unknown effect that they have on children's health. For example, in 2012, the Food and Drug Administration (FDA) suggested that some rice containing infant/toddler foods and snacks had higher concentrations of inorganic arsenic than others.[2] Although studies are ongoing to understand the implications of this finding, the American Academy of Pediatrics (AAP) recognized the difficulties this placed on families regarding food choices for these age groups and published recommendations for pediatricians and families to limit infants' exposure to arsenic in rice.[3] For many contaminants and additives, few or no data are available regarding safe levels of intake for infants and children.

The chronic effects of chemical substances in foods are generally more significant for the fetus and young child than for adults because of potential neurotoxic and developmental effects. Infants and children are often more sensitive than adults to environmental chemicals for a number of reasons.[4] Increased susceptibility may result from the greater intake of foods per unit of body weight. This is especially true for foods that are routinely consumed by most infants and young children. The immaturity of developing organ systems is another potential hazard, especially for the nervous, immune, and endocrine systems, and particularly during sensitive periods of development when relatively brief insults may result in long-term effects. The pharmacokinetic properties of chemical substances in foods can vary greatly because of the immaturity of organs, such as the liver and kidneys, and the changes in the amounts of body fat and extracellular water. These properties can lead to differential and often higher-dose exposures for children as compared with adults. For chronic effects, prevention of exposure is more important than most treatments.

US Food Safety Regulations Including Ingredients and Contaminants Advertently or Inadvertently Added to Food

The safety and quality of food involves 16 federal agencies with the primary responsibility for food safety in the United States residing within the FDA and the US Department of Agriculture (USDA) Food Safety and Inspection Service (FSIS). The FSIS regulates meat, poultry, catfish, and processed egg products. The FDA has jurisdiction over 80% of the food supply, including seafood, dairy, and produce and all other products not regulated by the FSIS. The Environmental Protection Agency (EPA) also plays a role in food safety as it is responsible for setting limits (tolerances) on pesticide residues in food and animal feed. The CDC has responsibility for ongoing surveillance; response to; and detection, investigation, and monitoring of foodborne and waterborne illness, including emerging pathogens and antimicrobial resistance patterns (see also Chapter 51: Food Safety: Infectious Disease). Multiple other agencies also have limited roles, including the National Marine Fisheries Service (NMFS) in the Department of Commerce, which conducts voluntary, fee-for-service inspections of seafood safety and quality, and the Department of Homeland Security, which coordinates agencies' food security activities. Food safety is supplemented by local, state, tribal, and territory laws and agencies with more than 3000 nonfederal agencies performing the large majority of food safety oversight.[5,6]

Regulation protecting food and drink from being misbranded and adulterated was first passed by Congress in 1906 and significantly expanded in the Federal Food, Drug, and Cosmetic Act of 1938 (Pub L No. 75-717). A major amendment, the Food Quality and Protection Act of 1996 (Pub L No. 104-170), changed how pesticides in foods are regulated and increased attention to pesticide-related food safety issues for infants and children (see text box). Until the Food Quality and Protection Act was passed, the allowable levels of pesticide residues in food were intended to protect adult health. This law was unique in that it explicitly required that the EPA ensure a "reasonable certainty that no harm will result in infants and children"

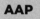

Food Quality Protection Act of 1996

- Established single health-based standards for all pesticides in food. Benefits, in general, cannot override the health-based standard.
- Prenatal and postnatal effects are to be considered.
- In the absence of data confirming the safety to infants and children, because of their special sensitivities and exposures, an additional uncertainty factor of up to 10X can be added to the safety values.
- Aggregate risk (the sum of all exposures to the chemical) and cumulative risk (the sum of all exposures to chemicals with similar mechanisms of action) must be considered in establishing safe levels.
- Risks are to be determined for both 1 year and lifetime exposure.
- Endocrine disrupters are to be included in the evaluation of safety.
- All existing pesticide registrations are to be reviewed by 2006. Expedited review is possible for safer pesticides.

Food Safety Modernization Act of 2011

- Gave the FDA authority to order a recall of food products, whereas in the past, the FDA could only issue recalls of infant formula and all other recalls were voluntarily issues by food manufacturers and distributors.
- Calls for more frequent inspections and for those inspections to be based on risk.
- Increases FDA's ability to oversee food produced in foreign countries and imported into the United States. Allows the FDA to prevent a food from entering this country if the facility has refused US inspection.
- Mandates that food facilities must have a written plan identifying possible safety issues of their products and further to outline steps that would help prevent those problems from occurring.
- Establishes science-based standards for the safe production and harvesting of fruits and vegetables.
- Allows exemptions from the produce safety standards for small farms that sell directly to consumers (eg, roadside stand or farmer's market).

VII

from exposure to pesticides and that the effects of chemicals that have the same mechanism of action be considered cumulatively. In response to Act requirements, by 2006, the EPA had established regulatory limits ("tolerances") on more than 9500 pesticides and pledged to reevaluate every active ingredient of pesticides every 15 years. The tolerance limits represent the maximum amount of pesticides that may legally remain in or on food and animal feed. When the tolerance is exceeded in foods, the FDA can take action to remedy the situation. For more details on federal food regulation, see Chapter 50.I.

Regulation of Ingredients Added to Food and Food Contact Material

The FDA provides oversight of more than 80% of the food supply in the United States and, within the Agency, the Center for Food Safety and Applied Nutrition (CFSAN), which includes the Office of Food Additive Safety, reviews the safety of food ingredients and packaging.[7] Today, more than 10 000 chemicals are allowed to be added to food and food contact materials in the United States, either directly or indirectly, under the 1958 Food Additives Amendment to the 1938 Federal Food, Drug, and Cosmetic (FD&C) Act. Additives are a fundamental part of the work of CFSAN, when a compound or a substance is evaluated by the FDA and is determined to, directly or indirectly, become a component or effect a component of a food.[8]

The FD&C Act allows for the use of chemical preservatives in foods if (1) it is "generally recognized as safe" (GRAS); (2) it is not used in a way to conceal damage or make the food appear better than it is; and (3) is properly declared on the label.[9] The Food Additive Status List omits certain categories, including those that are GRAS, certain synthetic flavorings, indirect food additives such as a pesticide chemical, and color additives. Substances are determined to be GRAS under the conditions of its intended use by the FDA. For more details on the GRAS process, see Chapter 50.I. For AAP concerns and suggestions for improving the GRAS process, see the AAP policy statement on food additives and child health.[10]

Sources of Chemical Substances of Concern for Food Safety

Chemical substances that are potentially toxic may occur in foods. Contaminants enter the food supply in a variety of ways, including: residues of substances (eg, pesticides) deliberately applied to food during agricultural practices; contaminants from industrial practices (eg, dioxins, metals, flame retardants, and perchlorates); contaminants that are naturally occurring toxins (eg, aflatoxin, vomitoxin); chemicals, such as colorings and flavorings and preservatives deliberately added to food during processing; and substances used in food contact materials or food processing byproducts (eg, adhesives, paper, plastics). This chapter presents an overview of this topic; for additional information, see the AAP manual *Pediatric Environmental Health*, published in 2018.[4]

Pesticides

Pesticides represent a broad classification of chemicals that are applied to kill or control insects, unwanted plants, molds, or unwanted animals (eg, rodents). Pesticides include insecticides, herbicides, fungicides, rodenticides, and fumigants. Although these products can increase both yield and quality of produce, pesticide residues are found on many foods, and chronic low-level exposure is common.

The quantity of specific residues an individual ingests from various foods is determined by the amount of pesticide applied to the crop; the time between application and harvesting, processing, or storage; the type of processing; the treatment of the food in the home; and the amount of the food ingested. Pesticide exposures have been linked to a wide variety of acute and chronic effects.[4]

Under the FD&C Act, the USDA and FDA have the responsibility to assess pesticide residues on foods sold (imported and domestic) in the United States. The USDA operates the Pesticide Data Program, which evaluates a wide variety of foods for pesticide residues and notifies the FDA and EPA if exceedances are found. Results of this program provide statistically representative data on pesticides in the US food supply. Rotating panels of commodities are selected for testing, which, in 2015, included analysis of 10 187 samples of 19 types of fruits and vegetables (96.9% of samples) and samples of peanut butter. Domestic samples accounted for 76.1% of the samples tested. In 2009, pesticide residues exceeding the established tolerance were detected in 0.53% (54 samples) of samples tested, and residues with no established tolerance were found in 3.9% of samples.[11] Of the samples analyzed, 15.5% of samples had no detectable pesticides, 11.5% had 1 pesticide, and 73% of the samples had more than 1 pesticide. Among the various fruits and vegetables selected for testing, more than 90% of apples, grapes, strawberries, cilantro, potatoes, and oranges contained pesticide residues, but nearly all were below the tolerance level.

The FDA provides an annual summary of its pesticide-monitoring program.[12] FDA sampling strategies include focused sampling and targeted sampling of food that may be suspect for violations. In 2014, 6638 samples (22% from domestically grown foods) were collected and analyzed by the FDA program. Pesticide residues were detected in 29.1% of domestic samples and in 47.1% of imported samples. Residues in violation of allowed tolerances were found in 1.4% of the domestic samples and 11.8% of the imported samples (see Table 52.1); 6.5% of the violations were for levels

VII

exceeding tolerance limits and 93.5% were for detection of residue for pesticides lacking tolerance limits representing a violative level.

In addition, the FDA reports data from the Total Diet Study, which, in 2014, evaluated approximately 800 table-ready foods for more than 200 different components, including toxic and nutrient elements, (pesticide residues, industrial chemicals, volatile organic compounds, radionuclides, and folate), and includes an analysis of approximately 30 infant and toddler foods. Nearly all table-ready foods analyzed have undetectable or very low pesticide levels.[11]

Pesticide Exposures From Foods

In a national sample of individuals ages 6 to 59 years, among 56 pesticide metabolites examined, 29 were detectable in most people; organophosphate and organochlorine insecticides were the most prevalent.[13] The food supply is the most important source of exposure for these insecticides, as organophosphates were banned for use in the home in 2000, and organochlorines (eg, p,p'-dichlorodiphenyltrichloroethane [DDT], dieldrin, and chlordane) were banned in the United States 20 to 30 years earlier.[14,15] Pyrethroids, which have replaced organophosphates for most uses, are now detectable in 75% of the national sample.[16] Food residues and residential use are the most important sources of exposure to pyrethroids for children and adolescents.

The FDA does not monitor pesticide usage in home gardens or enforce appropriate use in that setting. Excessive applications or too short a time between application and harvesting can result in greater residue levels than are tolerated in commercially produced foods. For detailed information on pesticides in foods, see the AAP statement on pesticide exposure in children.[14]

Effects of Pesticides in Children

Acute pesticide poisoning in US children is rarely seen, but chronic low-level exposures are common. Serious acute poisoning from pesticides most often follows unintentional ingestion.[15] Although pesticides in the food chain are not the major source for acute pesticide exposure in infants and children, such events do occur.

Of the pesticides, the insecticides are most likely to cause acute illness. Pyrethroids commonly in use have features at presentation that are similar to organophosphates and carbamates, both of which are acetylcholinesterase inhibitors, but pyrethroid symptoms dissipate with only supportive care in approximately 24 hours.[14] Organophosphates have greatest toxicity of the 3 types because of irreversible binding of the acetylcholinesterase inhibitor.

Table 52.1.

**US Food and Drug Administration Pesticide Residue Monitoring Program,
Fiscal Year 2014[7]**

	Without residues %	*Violative Samples %*
Totals – All Samples	**53.3**	**1.9**
Origin of Sample		
Domestic	52.3	0.9
Import	54.7	3.4
Commodity		
Grains and grain products	72.2	1.7
Mixed livestock food rations	30.2	4.2
Medicated livestock food rations		
Milk/dairy products/eggs	0	0
Fish/shellfish/other aquatic products/ aquaculture seafood group	0	0
Fruits	0	4.8
Vegetables	1.7	4.4
Other[a]	2.6	8.3

[a] Mostly nuts, seeds, oils, honey, candy, spices, multiple food products, and dietary supplements.

Treatment varies according to which type of pesticide has been ingested, so obtaining an accurate history is key.[14] Additional details on differentiating the pesticides and their treatments are found in AAP statements from the Committee on Environmental Health.[14,15]

Recent prospective cohort observational studies have correlated adverse effects of early-life exposure to organophosphates and organochlorine pesticides on neurodevelopment and behavior. Several papers have reviewed the evidence.[17–20] Ongoing studies have enrolled pregnant women living in urban or rural areas, objectively assessed their routinely encountered chronic exposures during pregnancy, and evaluated their children into the preschool ages. These studies report significant associations of higher levels of pesticide exposures with children's poorer cognitive development and increased scores on measures assessing pervasive developmental disorder,

VII

inattention, and attention-deficit/hyperactivity disorder. In the National Health and Nutrition Examination Survey (NHANES) sample of US children 8 to 15 years of age, those with higher urinary concentrations of organophosphate metabolites more often had a diagnosis of attention-deficit/hyperactivity disorder.[21] Studies are underway to elucidate genetic risks for pesticide effects in children and to further identify mechanistic pathways of neurodevelopment and other metabolic effects in animal models. These studies are evaluating effects at levels of pesticide exposure commonly encountered in samples from urban and rural settings in the United States.[22–24]

In general, one can assume that exposure in utero and early in infancy would be more harmful to the developing nervous system than exposure later in childhood.

Reducing Pesticide Exposure From Foods

People can reduce their pesticide exposures by purchasing organic foods.[25] A study in low-income Mexican American children placed on an organic diet for 7 consecutive days demonstrated a marked decrease in their urinary excretion of metabolites of organophosphate insecticides during the organic diet phase.[26] In 2002, the USDA defined organically grown food as food grown and processed using no synthetic fertilizers or pesticides. Producers and handlers must be certified by a USDA-accredited certifying agent to sell, label, or represent their product as "100% organic" or "organic" (at least 95% organic).[27] Organic food sales account for approximately 4% of all food sales in the United States with fresh fruits and vegetables accounting for more than 40% of the sales[28]; organic products cost up to 40% more than conventionally grown products.[29] According to the AAP statement on organic foods, organically grown fruits and vegetables have not been shown to have higher nutritional value.[25]

Food-preparation measures can also reduce pesticide residue on food. Measures that can be recommended to parents include (https://www.epa.gov/safepestcontrol/pesticides-and-food-healthy-sensible-food-practices):

- Thoroughly wash and scrub fresh fruits and vegetables with cold or warm running tap water to remove bacteria and traces of chemicals from the surface before consumption. However, not all pesticides can be removed by washing.
- Peel fruits and vegetables when possible. Discard the outer leaves of leafy vegetables, such as lettuce and cabbage.
- Trim the fat from meats and the skin and fat from poultry and fish.
- Select a variety of foods from a variety of sources.

Industrial Chemicals

Another source of contaminants is chemicals dispersed in the environment from industrial processes that have entered the food chain. These chemicals may precipitate from the atmosphere into water, onto soil, or directly onto food crops and contaminate underground or surface waters that may, in turn, affect the water supply for irrigation or consumption. Industrial chemicals that contaminate food during processing are termed "food contact substances" and are covered in a separate section.

The most ubiquitous group of compounds resulting from industrial production is termed "persistent toxic substances," which includes a class of compounds known as persistent organic pollutants (POPs). A wide variety of persistent toxic substances are encountered in the environment, more than 50 of which are monitored in the US National Health and Nutrition Examination Survey. Many of these substances are present in measurable levels in the majority of individuals tested in the United States.[13]

There were 12 original POPs—all chlorinated compounds—but additional, diverse compounds have been added to the list. POPs include polychlorinated biphenyls (PCBs), polychlorinated dibenzofurans (PCDFs), polychlorinated dibenzo-p-dioxins (PCDDs, including tetrachlorodibenzo-p-dioxin [TCDD], a particularly potent dioxin), organochlorines (eg, chlordane, heptachlor, DDT and its derivatives), polybrominated biphenyls (PBB), polybrominated diphenyl ethers (PBDEs), and a host of others (aldrin, dieldrin, endrin, hexachlorobenzene, mirex and toxaphene). The ongoing use of many of these chemicals has been extensively curtailed by international treaties. Information on these chemicals to supplement what is presented below is found in the 2018 edition of *Pediatric Environmental Health* from the AAP.[4]

PCBs were originally used by the electrical industry as insulators and dielectrics; PCDFs appear as contaminants after extreme heating of PCBs. PCDDs were formed as contaminants in the production of hexachlorophene, pentachlorophenol, and several herbicides, including Agent Orange (a defoliant during the Vietnam War). Organohalogen chemicals have been used as flame retardants and are present in more than 97% of the US population.[13] These chemicals have been found in human milk, which can be the sole source of nutrition for many infants. In September 2017, the Consumer Product Safety Commission voted to begin rulemaking on the removal of organohalogen flame retardants as a class from children's products, upholstered furniture, mattresses, and mattress pads and plastic casings on electronic devices.

VII

Another commonly encountered persistent toxic substance is perchlorate. Perchlorate is used in solid rocket fuel, propellants, and explosives. It is a contaminant of drinking water and is associated with elevated thyroid-stimulating hormone concentrations when iodine concentration is low.[30] Women with lower iodine and higher perchlorate concentrations have higher concentrations of thyroid-stimulating hormone.

Persistence in the Environment

These toxic chemicals persist in the environment and accumulate in produce grown in contaminated soils. Because of their lipophilic nature, they bioaccumulate in the fat tissue of many animal-based foods, including meat, eggs, dairy products, and fish (both saltwater and freshwater varieties), with sport fish from contaminated waters generally being the most concentrated food source of such chemicals. When ingested by humans in food, these toxicants bioaccumulate in human fat. Persistent toxic substances that are often acquired over many years, are transferred like those acutely ingested to the fetus from maternal stores and appear in human milk, because they are fat soluble and are not significantly metabolized. Thus, nursing infants are exposed to these chemicals. The combination of sources has resulted in exposures to infants and toddlers above the EPA's reference doses.[31,32]

Effects

In addition to the child developmental and behavioral effects of organohalogen flame retardant exposures discussed in the previous section, many of these compounds are thought to have endocrine-disrupting properties.[33] A prospective cohort study in children ages 7 to 9 years suggested that exposure to persistent organic pollutants such as PCBs affected insulin secretory function and was associated with an increased risk of diabetes.[34] Among women recruited from a prospective population-based birth cohort, those with higher levels of pesticides and PCBs in cord blood were more likely to have babies with increased levels of sex hormone-binding globulin and anti-Müllerian hormone and a decrease in free testosterone and aromatase index.[35] Furthermore, the presence of multiple chemicals such as PCBs and dioxins is associated with higher incidence of cryptorchidism and increased anogenital distances in neonates and infants.[36,37] In addition, higher PBDE blood concentrations were associated with reduced fertility.[38] PBDEs have direct toxic effects in laboratory studies on the developing nervous system and impair the thyroid hormone system, which is a critical component of early brain development.[39,40] In a study of 210 children in Mexico, after adjusting for potential confounders, higher cord blood PBDE concentrations were associated with lower developmental scores at 12, 24, and 36 months of age and lower IQ scores at 48 and 72 months of age.[41]

The carcinogenic potential of the dioxins has also been recognized by the EPA and CDC. TCDD, which causes chloracne in humans, is classified as a known human carcinogen.[42] Food, particularly fat-containing animal products (including seafoods), are the major sources of these organic pollutants.[42] Using NHANES dietary consumption data and the EPA's Stochastic Human Exposure and Dose Simulation (SHEDS) dietary exposure model, older age groups had higher levels of PCBs in their blood in patterns fairly consistent with fish consumption and exposure patterns.[43] Compared with a previous survey in the mid-1990s, the basic congenerous profiles for each animal type were fairly constant and the overall levels of these substances may have decreased, but changes in analytic methods may also play a role in reported findings. In the recent survey, the USDA tested fat samples in cattle, hogs, young chickens, and young turkeys and found relatively higher levels of these compounds in cattle and turkeys compared with chickens and hogs. However, dioxin results, overall, were lower in the 2013 survey compared with previous years.[44]

No specific treatments are known, and the prevention of excessive intake is the only therapeutic approach. To reduce food-related exposures, reducing the ingestion of the fats found in animals, dairy products, and fish are the basis of the recommendations currently proposed. Because these persistent toxic substances are minimally metabolized and excreted, intakes are cumulative over years. Fish vary in their fat content by species, and the level of contamination varies with species, location, body size, and the type of feeding, especially in farmed fish.[45] Because of the variation in the contamination in fresh water fish, states in which contaminated fish may be found publish fish advisories about where such fish may exist, with recommendations on their consumption by pregnant women, lactating mothers, and young children. Recommendations to reduce the intake of dioxin-like compounds in the diet, especially for children, young women, women who may become pregnant, and lactating mothers include:

- Choose lean cuts of meat and trim all visible fat before cooking.
- Choose fish for 1 to 2 meals per week. Avoid eating shark, swordfish, king mackerel, and tilefish, and check with the state or local health department to see if there are special advisories on fish caught from freshwater lakes and streams in the local area.

VII

- Use low-fat or fat-free dairy products routinely.
- Reduce the amount of butter or lard used in the preparation of foods.
- Cook meats and fish by broiling, grilling, or other methods that allow fat to be drained away.
- Do not save or reuse rendered fats.
- Wash fruits and vegetables and thoroughly peel root and waxy coated vegetables.

Metal Compounds

Another group of compounds that may contaminate food are metals. The metals of concern in food are mercury, lead, and arsenic.

Mercury

Mercury is primarily released into the environment by natural and industrial processes, particularly the burning of fossil fuels.[4] Coal-burning power plants remain the largest single source of mercury emissions in the United States, although emissions from artisanal or small-scale mining remains the primary source globally. Mercury-containing rains go into lakes, rivers, and oceans, where the mercury is biotransformed by bacteria to methylmercury. Methylmercury, a potent neurodevelopmental toxicant, is bioconcentrated up the aquatic food chain. Methylmercury has also been used as a fungicide on seed grains. Consumption of mercury-treated seed grains had caused widespread mercury poisoning among people in Iraq and China.[46]

Fish consumption is the source of most human mercury exposure in the United States. Chronic effects of methylmercury ingestion have been noted in the offspring of mothers who had elevated concentrations in their bodies. The EPA has determined that the chronic oral consumption of methylmercury be limited to 0.1 µg/kg/day to protect the fetal brain from damage. Analysis of data from adult women gathered in the National Health and Nutrition Examination Surveys since 2001 identified 3.7% of women with a mercury concentration above 5.8 µg/L.[47] Subsequent years (2009–2010) have shown a slight decrease (2.3%) in the total blood mercury geometric mean, although non-Hispanic black females had higher levels than Mexican-American or non-Hispanic white females.[13] Mercury concentrations in many ocean fish and shellfish have been evaluated.[48] Predatory fish generally have the highest mercury levels. Mercury concentrations in freshwater fish vary by location, and many fish are also highly contaminated. States' fish consumption advisories include data on mercury as well as PCBs with guidance on which fish to limit intakes and which to avoid either because of mercury and/or PCBs and other POPs. A national listing of fish advisories is available on the EPA website. (http://water.epa.gov/scitech/swguidance/fishshellfish/fishadvisories/index.cfm). Updated information can be obtained from state EPA offices.

Marine and freshwater fish and shellfish are important components of a balanced, healthy diet. Fish is high in protein and low in saturated fat and contains essential vitamins and minerals and long-chain omega-3 fatty acids (see Chapter 17: Fats and Fatty Acids). Unfortunately, fish are vulnerable to contamination by toxic industrial pollutants, such as mercury, as well as lipophilic chemicals including PCBs, dioxins, flame retardants, and others. These pollutants accumulate in fish flesh (as in the case of methylmercury) or fatty tissue (as in the case of PCBs), exposing people who eat them. Mothers can pass on these pollutants to their offspring both in utero and via human milk, and children may also be exposed to these harmful chemicals directly through eating fish. For some populations, locally caught fish may be the only good alternative for a nutritious diet. Finding the balance between acquiring the nutritional benefits from adequate fish consumption and avoiding the toxicity from consumption of polluted fish is a challenge. The suggested potential beneficial effects on child IQ from fish intake (>2 meals/week) during pregnancy must be weighed against negative effects from mercury in the fish. For example, a 2016 study has shown a strong association with maternal fish consumption during pregnancy and improved neurocognitive outcomes in children.[49]

The FDA has set a regulatory upper limit for methylmercury in commercial fish of 1 part per million (ppm; 1 μg/g). The FDA has issued an advisory to pregnant women, women of childbearing age, nursing mothers, and young children to avoid consumption of shark, king mackerel, swordfish, marlin, orange roughy, bigeye tuna, and tilefish. For other types of fish, including canned light tuna, the FDA has advised that consumption by children, pregnant women, and those who may become pregnant be kept below 12 ounces per week.[50] (Canned albacore and fresh tuna have approximately 3 times higher methylmercury concentration than canned light tuna.) Mercury content of many various commercial seafood varieties can be found on the FDA website (see Table 52.2 for a partial list).

The federal government does not regulate the levels of mercury or other contaminants, such as PCBs or dioxins, in fish caught for sport. Because of the potential contamination, states have issued advisories recommending public limits or the avoidance of consuming certain fish caught for sport from specific bodies of water. These include freshwater species, such

VII

<table>
<tr><td>

AAP

</td></tr>
</table>

Fish Recommendations
(see new FDA/EPA guidance)

Advice from the EPA on selecting healthier varieties of fish:

- **Do Not Eat (high mercury content)**: shark, king mackerel, swordfish, marlin, orange roughy, bigeye tuna, and tilefish
- **Eat up to 12 oz (2 average meals)** of fish and shellfish weekly.
  - o   Eat 2 to 3 servings per week of fish in the "Best Choices" category, based on a serving size of 4 ounces, in the context of a total healthy diet. Eat 1 serving a week of fish in the "Good Choices" category.
  - o   Do not eat fish in the "Choices to Avoid" category or feed them to young children. However, if you do, eat fish with lower mercury levels in the following weeks.
- **Check local advisories about the safety of sport fish.** If no advice is available, eat up to 6 oz (1 average meal) per week of fish you catch from local waters, but do not consume any other fish during that week. Because the EPA Fish Advisory website is not updated regularly, state fish advisories are more likely to provide accurate information.

as catfish, carp, bass, and sturgeon, which may have concentrations of mercury that would result in substantial exposure.

In general, guidelines for selecting safer fish focus on several major points. Women of childbearing age and all children should (1) avoid varieties of fish known to be highly contaminated with mercury; (2) know and follow local and federal fish consumption guidelines; (3) eat a wide variety of the "best choice" fish; and (4) limit weekly fish meals depending on which varieties are chosen. In general, leaner, smaller, and younger wild fish are least likely to be heavily polluted.

Lead

Although most lead exposure in the United States is not from food sources, there are many foods that can sometimes be identified as contributing to a child's lead burden, including ethnic spices, imported candy, and water. Additionally, a recent study by the Environmental Defense Fund (EDF) found that roughly 20% of baby food samples analyzed by the FDA contained detectable levels lead, compared with 14% of other foods assessed.[51] Root vegetables and fruit juices were more likely to have higher concentrations of lead. The FDA has multiple standards for lead depending on the food and the feasibility for achieving a certain standard. For example, the current

Table 52.2.

Mercury Concentration in Selected Commercial Seafood (1990–2010)[a]

Seafood	Mean Mercury Concentration (ppm)
	Highest Levels
Tilefish (Gulf of Mexico)	1.450
Shark	0.979
Swordfish	0.995
Mackerel king	0.730
	Moderate Levels
Orange roughy	0.571
Grouper (all species)	0.448
Bass Chilean	0.354
Tuna (fresh/frozen, yellowfin)	0.354
Tuna (canned, albacore)	0.350
Monkfish	0.181
	Lowest Levels
Tuna (canned, light)	0.128
Trout, freshwater	0.071
Crab	0.065
Scallops	0.003
Catfish	0.025
Pollock	0.031
Salmon (fresh/frozen)	0.022
Tilapia	0.013
Clams	0.009
Salmon (canned)	0.008
Shrimp	0.009

[a] Selected data from FDA.[48] Other contaminants, such as PCBs, may alter the safety of eating particular fish.

VII

guidance level for lead in fruit juices is 50 parts per billion (ppb), and the allowable limit in bottled water is 5 ppb. In 1993, the FDA established the maximum daily intake level at 6 mcg/dL; however, this is based on the CDC's previous action level of 10 mcg/dL and has not been updated since a reference level of 5 mcg/dL was established[52] (see *Pediatric Environmental Health* from the AAP[4] for additional details).

In June 2010, the Joint Food and Agriculture Organization of the United Nations and World Health Organization Expert Committee on Food Additives rejected its prior provisional tolerable weekly intake of lead of 25 µg/kg and recommended limiting lead intake to <0.3 µg/kg per day for a child and 1.2 µg/kg per day for an adult. These new recommendations were shown to be associated with negligible change to child IQ (0.5 IQ point loss).[53] Additionally, they adopted a recommendation that no more than 0.01 ppm of lead should be permitted in infant formula as consumed, recognizing that levels of lead in infant formula can be controlled by sourcing raw materials from areas where lead is less present.[54] Lead is taken up by growing plants, with highest concentration in the root and lowest in the fruit. Measurable amounts of lead in edible roots and shoots have been identified in urban gardens.[55]

Arsenic

Children can be exposed to arsenic in a number of different ways. Because it is a metal that is ubiquitously found in the soil, children playing in bare soil may be exposed. However, the primary source of arsenic is through ingestion of water and/or food. On a global scale, water is the most common source of arsenic in humans. However, in the United States, where municipal water must meet federal standards, food is the most common source in adults and children.

Rice and seafood are the most commonly ingested foods known to have contamination with arsenic. Inorganic arsenic is the more toxic form and is found in rice, with concentrations dependent on its growing conditions in the United States and around the world. Organic arsenic is found in seafood and is much less toxic. Most testing does not differentiate between inorganic and organic arsenic. Using data from the NHANES study, researchers found that total urinary arsenic concentration increased 14.2% with each 0.25-cup increase in cooked rice consumption.[56] The FDA suggests a voluntary approach for industry to decrease arsenic levels in foods consumed by infants and toddlers to below 50 mcg/kg, a level higher than most adult food products. However, in a study that assessed arsenic content of common infant and toddler rice cereals in US supermarkets, the average total arsenic and inorganic arsenic concentrations in infant rice cereal were 174.4 and 101.4 mcg/kg.[57] In response to these findings, the AAP suggested that cereals from other grains such as oatmeal and wheat as well as other pureed foods (eg, finely chopped meats and vegetable purees) are equally acceptable as rice cereal for introduction as first foods. Other thickeners, such as finely ground oats, could be considered in children with swallowing difficulty.[3]

Toxins

A wide variety of toxins are found in various foods. These toxins may be endogenously produced or the product of other organisms or bacteria that inhabit the food product.

Various varieties of seafood can produce toxins. In recent years, the presence of new compounds with high toxicity have been found and have been linked to warming oceans.[58] Tetrodotoxin is one of the most toxic biologic toxins known and is produced by puffer fish and the blue-ringed octopus. Because of this high toxicity, any puffer fish exported from Japan must be negative for the presence of the toxin on 2 tests prior to export. Several deaths from respiratory failure occur annually from the improper preparation and inexperienced chefs.

The most frequently reported seafood-toxin illness, globally and in the United States, is that of ciguatera caused by eating fish contaminated with ciguatera toxin. More than 500 fish species have caused human cases of ciguatera poisoning, including barracuda, sea bass, red snapper, grouper, kingfish, and sturgeon. The common factor is large size fish that ingest a toxin-producing algae. *Gambierdiscus toxicus* and other bacteria within dinoflagellates are the origins of ciguatera and the main nutritional source for small herbivorous fish, which in turn are the nutritional source for larger fish. Over time, the concentration of ciguatera increases in the adipose tissue of the large fish, resulting in toxicity to humans consuming those fish.[59] Symptoms of ciguatera poisoning include diaphoresis, headaches, abdominal pain with or without vomiting, profuse watery diarrhea, and a constellation of neurologic effects including paresthesia and reversal of temperature discrimination. The gastrointestinal tract symptoms usually last up to 48 hours, but the neurologic symptoms may persist for months.

Recent "red tides" have occurred in the Gulf of Mexico and Atlantic Ocean off the coast of the United States. Dinoflagellates such as *Karenia brevis* are a major source of food for mollusks and other shellfish during the

VII

"non-R" months (May through August) in the northern hemisphere. When the number of dinoflagellates producing brevetoxin becomes excessive, it results in the death of large numbers of birds and fish as well as respiratory symptoms in humans from the aerosolized brevetoxin. Neurologic symptoms may also occur.[60] Other seafood toxins that result in neurologic symptoms are found in Table 52.3.

Cooking does not remove seafood toxins. These toxins are generally found among seafood varieties in certain geographic areas, whereas the same varieties of seafood in other geographic areas lack toxins. The following general suggestions are available to limit risk of exposures to seafood toxins[61]:

- Do not use any seafood (fish or shellfish) that looks, smells, or tastes odd. However, ciguatera toxins do not affect the texture, taste, or smell of fish.
- Buy seafood from reputable sources.
- Avoid purchasing shellfish in areas during or shortly after algal blooms, locally referred to as "red tides" or "brown tides" (amnesic shellfish poisoning resulting from domoic acid contamination).
- Buy only fresh seafood that is refrigerated or properly iced.
- Do not buy cooked seafood if displayed in the same case as raw fish.
- Do not buy frozen seafood with torn, open, or crushed package edges.
- Keep seafood refrigerated immediately after buying it.

Naturally occurring toxins also can be found with a wide variety of other foods, including mushrooms, grains, and honey, either as a product within another food or by contamination of the food. More than 6000 calls to the US Poison Control Centers in 2015 were regarding mushroom ingestions, with the majority occurring in children younger than 5 years.[62] Mushrooms are categorized in 10 groups representing clinical symptoms caused by more than 15 toxins. The most common scenario is a person who mistakes a toxic mushroom for an edible mushroom in the wild. Worldwide, most fatalities are associated with the cyclopeptide-containing species such as *Amanita*. Early diagnosis is difficult, because symptoms of nausea, vomiting, and diarrhea do not occur until 6 hours after ingestion and may be mistaken for gastroenteritis. Liver injury can result in death in up to 30% of patients. Mistaken identity is common during the spring when individuals looking for the edible *Morchella esculenta* (morel) harvest the similar looking *Gyromitra esculenta* (false morel). Similar to the cyclopeptides, delayed gastrointestinal symptoms can occur followed by seizures in severe cases.

Table 52.3.
Toxins in Seafoods[61]

Organism Producing Toxin	Toxin	Seafood Affected	Health Effects
Marine bacteria	Tetrodotoxin	Puffer fish, blue-ringed octopus, horseshoe crab	Parasthesias, respiratory depression, hypotension
Gambierdiscus species	Ciguatera	Barracudas, groupers, snappers, jacks, mackerel, triggerfish	Acute symptoms of the gastrointestinal tract, central nervous system, and cardiovascular system; self-limited; usually subsides in several days
Many dinoflagellates	Saxitoxin derivatives Polyethers Brevetoxins Domoic acid	Mussels, clams, cockles, scallops Mussels, oysters, scallops Shellfish from the Florida coast Mussels	Paralytic shellfish poisoning Diarrheic shellfish poisoning Neurotoxic shellfish poisoning Amnesic shellfish poisoning
Marine bacteria	Histamine, also called scombrotoxin	Tuna, mahi mahi, bluefish, sardines, mackerel, amberjack, abalone Note: may also be in Swiss cheese	Burning mouth, upper body rash, hypotension, headache, pruritus, vomiting, and diarrhea

VII

Asking questions about mushroom consumption is key in the diagnosis as is using the mycologists associated with poison control centers to help identify the mushroom.

Mycotoxins produced by fungi on foods and foodstuffs result in food safety risks and health problems worldwide. Fungi such as *Claviceps purpura*, *Aspergillus flavus*, *Fusarium verticillioides*, and *Fusarium graminearum* can infect the seeds of grains such as corn, wheat, and barley. The toxins, ergot alkaloids, aflatoxin, fumonisins, and trichothecenes result in human toxicity and outbreaks in communities ingesting the grains. Ergot alkaloids were the first mycotoxin recognized to cause epidemic disease in humans. In 994 AD, 40 000 people in Aquitania, France, died from consuming rye contaminated with *C purpura* and the resulting convulsions.[63] Since that time, it has been implicated in other outbreaks of disease including the behaviors in Salem, Massachusetts, that resulted in the witch trials in 1692. Aflatoxin is produced by *Aspergillus* species and is a common contaminant of peanuts, soybeans, and grains, usually in tropical areas. Acutely, it has been associated with vomiting, abdominal pain, hepatitis, and death. However, aflatoxin B_1 is most commonly associated with hepatocellular cancer and has been implicated in the widespread deaths from liver cancer in China.[64] Fumonisins are mycotoxins isolated from corn contaminated with *Fusarium* species. Investigations have documented contaminated corn products to have resulted in fatal diseases in farm animals from the feed. Fumonisin contamination has been associated with birth defects as it has been shown to interfere with cellular folate uptake resulting in neural tube defects in some populations around the world.[65] Trichothecene mycotoxins are formed by *Fusarium* and *Stachybotrys* species. When ingested, these mycotoxins may result in alimentary toxic aleukia toxicosis, which is characterized by nausea, vomiting, diarrhea, leukopenia, hemorrhaging, skin inflammation, and in severe cases, death.[66] Both drought and flooding contribute to the problems with mycotoxins. Whereas fungi are normally unable to penetrate the intact seeds, drought may weaken the plant, resulting in the ability of the fungus to enter the seed. Consumers should avoid eating visibly moldy foods, but contaminated processed grains are not detectable. Mycotoxins are not destroyed by heating. The FDA has established Good Manufacturing Practice Guidelines for industry to eliminate the presence of fungi and their mycotoxins. This includes adequate irrigation schedules, pest management, breeding cultivars to resistant pest damage, and timely harvest. In addition, chemical/thermal inactivation, electronic sorting, and irradiation are recommended prior to processing and storage.[67] Additionally, guidance on aflatoxin B_1 and fumonisin levels have been established by the FDA.[68,69]

Antimicrobial Preservatives

The use of chemical agents exhibiting antimicrobial activity is one of the approaches used to preserve foods. The addition of food preservatives is intended to reduce the risk of foodborne infections, decrease microbial spoilage, and preserve the nutritional quality of the food. Although there are physical techniques used for food preservation—dehydration, freezing, refrigeration, freeze-drying, canning, curing, and pickling—chemical preservatives are used more often commercially. These chemicals may be either synthetic compounds intentionally added to foods or naturally occurring, biologically derived substances. A pesticide chemical as a residue in or on a food is not considered a food additive, but, instead, must comply with tolerances as regulated by the EPA but regulated by the FDA.[70]

Thus, antimicrobial preservatives in general are not considered food additives, even though the intended effects are on edible food or in water that comes in contact with food, but instead are regulated by the GRAS classification. Antimicrobial preservatives prevent the degradation of the food from the bacteria present on the food or packaging. Depending on the food, the range of chemicals includes, but is not limited to, lactic acid, sorbic acid (sodium sorbate), benzoic acid (sodium benzoate), sulfites, nitrites/nitrates, and propionic acid.[71] Although toxicities can occur with these chemicals, these have been more apparent when used in medications rather than food and at higher doses. Some consumers prefer (demonstrated by their buying habits) "preservative free" or "natural preservatives" in the foods purchased. At the same time, consumers wish for increased safety and shelf-life of the products they purchase. Given this dilemma, pediatricians may have a difficult time in weighing potential risks versus benefits of the addition of antimicrobial preservatives to food.

Food Irradiation

Food irradiation is a process by which food is exposed to a controlled source of ionizing radiation to prolong shelf-life and reduce food losses, to improve microbiologic safety, and/or to reduce the use of chemical fumigants and additives. The dose of the ionizing radiation determines the effects of this process on foods. Low-dose irradiation (up to 1 kGy) is used primarily to

VII

delay ripening of produce or to kill or render sterile insects and other higher organisms that may infest fresh food. Medium-dose irradiation (1–10 kGy) reduces the number of pathogens and other microbes on food and prolongs shelf-life. High-dose irradiation (>10 kGy) sterilizes food and is subject to more stringent regulations.

The sources of irradiation for treatment of foods is regulated by the FDA as a food additive. The USDA also has regulatory responsibilities for some types of foods irradiated for defined purposes. All petitioners for FDA approval of food irradiation must complete a process that ensures that food irradiated for a specific purpose under precise conditions will remain radiologically, toxicologically, and microbiologically safe and nutritionally adequate.[72]

Currently, all irradiated food sold in the United States must be labeled with the international sign of irradiation, the radura (Figure 52.1) and the statement "treated with radiation" or "treated by irradiation." Manufacturers may optionally add a statement with the purpose for irradiation (eg, "to control spoilage"). Current rules do not require food services to identify irradiated foods they serve.

Fig 52.1.
The radura is the international symbol indicating that a food has been irradiated.

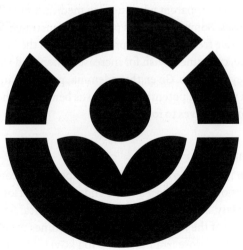

Radiologic Safety

Neither the food nor the packaging materials become radioactive as a result of food irradiation.[72,73] The radiation dose, the physical state of food (eg, fresh, frozen, or dried), and the packaging may alter the radiation of a given food and should be considered. Irradiated food should only receive the minimum radiation dose reasonably required to achieve the technical effect desired and must conform to a scheduled process.

Toxicologic Safety

Radiation absorbed by food causes a number of chemical reactions proportional to the dose of radiation applied. The desired reactions involve disrupting the DNA of spoilage and disease causing microbes and pests. Undesired reactions could involve creation of toxic compounds. A number of approaches involving hundreds of studies have been used over decades to determine whether such toxic compounds are created during irradiation and, if created, whether they are unique to the irradiation process (versus canning, freezing, drying, etc) or created in amounts large enough to cause harm. Previous studies have suggested that irradiation of lipids may result in fatty acids, esters, aldehydes, ketones, alkanes, alkenes, and other hydrocarbons; however, greater amounts of these products have been found in foods simply after heating. One product, 2-alkylcyclobutanone, is specific to the irradiation of lipids, but the low levels produced do not present any safety concerns at this time. Nonetheless, multigenerational animal feeding studies and analytical chemical modeling studies have failed to identify any unusual toxicity associated with consumption of irradiated foods.[74] However, food may be irradiated within the packaging, which may result in changes because of contact with the food (see below).

Microbiologic Safety

Irradiation kills microbes primarily by fragmenting DNA. The sensitivity of microorganisms increases with the complexity of the organism. Thus, viruses are most resistant to destruction by irradiation, and insects and parasites are most sensitive. Spores, cysts, toxins, and prions are quite resistant to the effects of irradiation, because they are in highly stable resting states or are not living organisms. The conditions under which irradiation takes place (ie, temperature, humidity, and atmospheric content) can affect the dose required to achieve the food-processing goal. Regardless, the quality of the food to be irradiated must be high, without heavy microbial contamination, for irradiation to achieve food-processing goals at any level.[74]

VII

When irradiation is used at nonsterilizing doses, the possibility of persistent pathogens is always present. Although it is true that pathogen loads can be substantially reduced using this technique, it is always possible for foods to become recontaminated. Irradiation does not obviate the need for strict application of safe food handling techniques including adequate storage, hygienic preparation and complete cooking, particularly of high-risk foods, such as foods of animal origin, precooked processed foods, or imported foods.[73,75]

Nutritional Value

As with any food-processing technique, irradiation can have a negative effect on some nutrients. It does not significantly damage carbohydrates, proteins, or fats at the doses recommended.[72] Certain vitamins may decrease in levels after irradiation with the extent dependent on the vitamin, the type of food and conditions of irradiation. Not all vitamin loss is nutritionally significant and depends on the specific food's contribution to the recommended daily requirements of that vitamin. When studied in pure solution, the water-soluble vitamins most sensitive to irradiation are thiamine (B_1), pyridoxine (B_6), and riboflavin (B_2).

Thiamine loss can be 50% or more under some conditions in some foods.[72] Loss is enhanced with increased irradiation doses, increased storage time after irradiation and cooking after irradiation. Rich sources of thiamine include whole-grain cereals, legumes, nuts, pork, brown rice, milk, and other foods that have been fortified. If all sources of thiamine come from irradiated products, a deficiency condition could develop, but this is unlikely in the United States. Although vitamin E loss can be significant when assessed in pure solution, many of the foods containing vitamin E are unlikely to be treated with radiation.

Although a few vitamins are significantly affected by irradiation, in general, irradiated food is quite nutritious. As long as a diet is balanced and food choices are varied, deficiency states are unlikely to develop.

Palatability

Taste, texture, color, and smell are all components that determine the palatability of foods. Some foods, particularly foods with high fat content, could suffer unacceptable changes in these qualities when irradiated. However, modified conditions, such as excluding oxygen from the atmosphere (oxidation can make food rancid), lowering the temperature, excluding light, reducing water content, or lowering the radiation dose can minimize or eliminate these changes. Use of low-dose radiation can reduce chemical changes to food to the point where only chemical analysis could detect a change. A welcome consequence of modifying irradiation conditions to preserve palatability is that the same modifications can also minimize vitamin loss.

Food-Contact Substances

Food-contact substances are defined by the FDA as substances used in food-contact materials, including adhesives, dyes, coatings, paper, paperboard, and polymers (plastics), that may come into contact with food as part of packaging or processing equipment but are not intended to be added directly to food.[76] The FDA maintains a list of more than 3000 approved food contact substances.[77] Approvals under this process are proprietary; thus, they are specific to the manufacturer identified and under the conditions stated in the application.

Although direct food additives undergo toxicologic testing prior to approval based on structure/activity relationships as well as anticipated human exposure levels,[78] testing of indirect food additives, such as food contact substances, is based primarily on anticipated exposure levels. The complexities of testing of food contact substances and other indirect food additives to meet FDA guidelines is available elsewhere.[78–81] It is of note that many common packaging materials were approved for use prior to the 1958 Food Additives Amendment to the FD&C Act (Pub L No. 85-929) and were, thus, "grandfathered in" for continued use as "prior approved" substances. Some of these substances are plasticizers like the phthalate esters (used in polyvinyl chloride [PVC] plastics, inks, dyes, and adhesives in food packaging), nonyl phenol (used in PVC, juice boxes, and lid gaskets), and bisphenol A (BPA).

There have been significant concerns regarding the endocrine disrupting potential of plasticizers such as phthalates and bisphenol A at the exposure levels that occur with food contact substances.[82] These chemicals can mimic or antagonize the actions of naturally occurring estrogens and may interact with nuclear estrogen receptors, the most common form of endocrine disruptor activity. In laboratory experiments, fetal, newborn, and young animals are very sensitive to even very low doses (sometimes picomolar to nanomolar) of chemicals having estrogenic effects.[83] BPA has been the focus of research that has found associations with various endocrinologic and other effects in adults and children.[4,84] Nonhuman laboratory studies and human epidemiologic studies suggest an association between BPA exposure and endocrine-related endpoints such as decreased fertility and early onset of puberty, although cause and effect has not been demonstrated and additional research is needed.

An observational study in preschool children verified that BPA could be found in more than 50% of solid food and liquid food samples and suggested that 99% of exposures of preschool children originated in the diet.[85] The NHANES examined children as young as 6 years and found that urinary BPA was detectable in 93% of individuals sampled, with concentrations highest in children.[86] The AAP has expressed concerns regarding BPA, with research showing that it has been associated with various endocrinologic and other effects in adults and children.[4,84] The FDA's working group on this subject has maintained that the current amounts of bisphenol A exposure through food contact substances are safe based on the current level of evidence but points to ongoing animal research in its report that may resolve this issue.[87] It is of note, however, that BPA has been removed by an FDA directive from baby bottles, sippy cup, and infant formula packaging, although it continues to be used in some water bottles and can liner enamels.[88] Plasticisers are still necessary to manufacture the products that are in use. The BPA, in many cases, has been replaced with closely related alternatives such as bisphenol S (BPS). These emerging alternatives have already been found in human urine.[89] The few studies focused on evaluating BPS have identified similar estrogenic activity but greater resistance to environmental degradation compared with BPA.[90]

BPA and phthalate exposures can be modified by attention to use of plastics with foods and drinks. Routine use of polycarbonate containers for cold beverages for 1 week was found to increase urinary BPA concentration by 69%,[91] whereas a 3-day intervention during which individuals ate "fresh food" (those with limited packaging) and avoided use of plastic cookware reduced BPA and phthalate urinary excretion by more than 50%.[92] A study of 455 commercially available plastic products found that most (even those labeled as BPA free) had some estrogenic activity; however, release of such chemicals was higher when the products were placed under stress conditions (eg, microwaving, ultraviolet radiation, hot water).[93] It is difficult to discern types of plastics, because labeling is not required by federal law. Food-handling recommendations that could potentially reduce exposures to plastics are discussed in "Reducing Exposures."

Housewares
In the past, the FDA typically has not required review of food-contact articles used exclusively in the home or in restaurants. Many such articles have

short contact times or are made of materials such as alloys and ceramics, so they are deemed to pose little likelihood of migration to food.[80] However, several chemicals sometimes found on products in the home that can be transferred to foods have important health concerns.

The FDA began regulating lead in glazes used on dishes made in the United States in the 1980s and further strengthened regulations in the 1990s. Dishes made in the United States before these regulations took effect may contain lead. Some imported ceramics contain lead. Of particular concern have been pottery from Mexico and ceramic ware from China. As the dishes wear or become chipped or cracked, lead can leach from the dishes into foods. Hot foods or acidic foods or drinks stored in such glazed containers may more rapidly leach metals from the glaze. Even some imported dishes labeled as "lead free" have been found to contain unsafe amounts of lead.[94] There are many safe alternatives, so using such dishes should be avoided. Lead contamination of drinking water represents another source for some children. As evident in municipalities around the United States, lead can leach into water from service pipes, solder, and fixtures. An increased number of children were recently found to have elevated blood concentrations in Flint, Michigan, when the source of water was changed to the Flint River. Additionally, schools across the country have found elevated levels of lead in water fountains. The only way to tell whether water has lead is to test it. The concentration of lead in drinking water can sometimes be reduced by flushing the system, but the time needed for this varies by locale, so local authorities should be consulted. Cold tap water, rather than hot tap water, should always be used for cooking and drinking. Most water filters remove lead.[4,95]

Since its creation in the 1970s, the use of the nonstick surfaced cooking pan has been a major contributor to substantial human exposure of perfluoroalkyl and polyfluoroalkyl substances (PFASs), particularly perfluorooctanoic acid (PFOA), which had been found in nonstick surfaced cooking pans and impregnated paper products (food and nonfood items), along with many other widely used household products.[96] Exposures became apparent not only in humans but also in wildlife and the environment, and US producers began to voluntarily phase out specific PFASs in the early 21st century. However, smaller-chain PFASs that have less persistence in the environment and do not bioaccumulate continue to be produced outside of the United States. The most common source of PFASs and related chemicals today is contaminated drinking water sources secondary to industrial pollution, uncontrolled run-off, and soil application of contaminated

VII

biosolids.[4] PFAS measurements have been included in the NHANES study since 1999 and have declined substantially for many of those tested, with the exception of perfluorononanoic acid (PFNA), which has increased in the same timeframe. Polyfluoroalkyl chemicals bioaccumulate, but blood serum concentrations in children are generally higher than those in adults.[97] This discrepancy may be attributable to the presence of PFASs in indoor dust and the transfer of the chemicals in pregnancy and human milk. A large epidemiologic study found an association between older age at onset of puberty and higher blood cholesterol concentrations with higher exposures than the general population.[98] Studies associating perfluoroalkyl chemicals with fetal outcomes (such as birth defects, preterm birth and low birth weight, and miscarriage and stillbirth) are mixed.[99] The EPA states that the risk for cancer is suggestive for PFOA and perfluorooctyl sulfonate, given the animal and human epidemiologic studies.[100]

Reducing Exposures

Chemicals can and will migrate from processing equipment, packaging materials, and storage containers into foods. A reasonable approach is to develop food preparation and storage practices that will minimize exposures, although it is difficult to know how to reduce exposures to many of these chemicals. The following suggestions should help to minimize unnecessary exposure to indirect food contaminants.[10] However, it is acknowledged that these suggestions can pose additional cost barriers particularly for low-income families and pediatricians may wish to tailor guidance in the context of practicality for cleaning plastics used for infants and children.

- Avoid routine use of single-serving packaging when possible. Such packaging maximizes contact between food and the packaging materials.
- When possible, consume fresh or frozen fruits and vegetables to minimize exposures to packaging materials and maximize nutrition. Wash fruits and vegetables that cannot be peeled.
- Use heat-safe glass or crockery when cooking or reheating food in the microwave. Heat increases migration of many contaminants into food, particularly foods containing fats. Do not use plastic in the microwave.
- Make sure a generous air space separates the surface of stored food from cling wraps used to seal containers. Avoid using cling wraps when microwaving foods.
- Encourage the use of stainless steel cookware. If using nonstick cookware products, new cookware should be used in well-ventilated envi-

ronments until it "ages" sufficiently to have minimal emission when
heated.[4]
- Be aware of the recycling codes on products to avoid plastics with recycling codes 3 (phthalates), 6 (styrene), and 7 (bisphenols).
- Wash hands prior to handling foods and/or drinks.

Finally, pediatricians are in an ideal position to provide important input
and continued encouragement to regulatory agencies to ensure that the
special exposures and vulnerabilities of children to toxic exposures remain
under consideration as food-related materials and processes are developed,
reviewed, and revised.

Chemical Byproducts From Food Processing

Food-processing technologies include many processes, such as drying,
salting, fermentation, acidification, freeze-drying, freezing, irradiation,
pasteurization, canning, pulsed electric field, ohmic heating (the process
by which an electric current is passed through the food), high-hydrostatic
pressure treatment, and others. All of these approaches are used to increase
safety while maintaining palatability and nutrient value. In addition, these
approaches also have the capacity to create chemical changes in the food
that may be detrimental. As analytical technology has improved, so has the
ability to identify more chemical byproducts in processed foods.

Acrylamide and furan are common byproducts that occur in food
processing and are more likely to occur after heat treatments of food.
Acrylamide, a known neurotoxicant and possible human carcinogen and
reproductive toxicant, is one such food processing chemical byproduct.[101]
Once thought to be only of significance in the occupational setting, in 2002
acrylamide was found in carbohydrate-containing foods treated with high
heat through frying, roasting, or baking but not boiling or steaming. It is a
product of the incomplete combustion of organic matter. It is mainly found
in foods made from plants, such as potatoes (French fries, potato chips),
grains (crackers, cereals, corn chips), or coffee. Furans are another group of
chemicals identified in 2004 in a wide range of foods, particularly formed
during traditional processing like canning, and have been measured in
commercially available foods, such as soups, sauces, beans, pasta meals, and
baby foods and also foods like crackers, potato chips, and tortilla chips.[102]
The risk posed by dietary exposure to these possible human carcinogens is
not yet well understood, and therefore, they are not regulated.

VII

Conclusion

Although many parents believe all foods are required to have no contaminants, this is not the case. Certain contaminants can be present, as long as they are below the standards set by the FDA and USDA. Food is just one source of exposures to heavy metals and chemicals. However, exposures can occur from multiple source resulting in an increased dose and cumulative effects over time of environmental toxins. Food contributes to the total exposure, but for some of these, other sources are more important to consider (eg, lead in paint chips and house dust). However, foods as a source of contaminants is important, and significant exposures from indirect and direct additives in foods may occur. Pediatricians should advocate and provide important input to regulatory agencies to ensure that the special exposures and vulnerabilities of children to toxic exposures remain under consideration as food-related materials and processes are developed, reviewed, and revised.

References

1. US Department of Agriculture, Economic Research Service. American diet includes many high-value imported products; Available at: https://www.ers. usda.gov/data-products/chart-gallery/gallery/chart-detail/?chartId=58398. Accessed August 17, 2017

2. Pediatric Environmental Health Specialty Units. Information on Arsenic in Food. Available at: http://www.pehsu.net/_Library/facts/Arsenic_in_Food.pdf. Accessed August 17, 2017

3. American Academy of Pediatrics, Arsenic in Rice Expert Working Group. AAP group offers advice to reduce infants' exposure to arsenic in rice. *AAP News.* 2014;35(11):13

4. American Academy of Pediatrics, Council on Environmental Health. *Pediatric Environmental Health.* Etzel RA, Balk SJ, eds. 4th ed. Elk Grove Village, IL: American Academy of Pediatrics; 2018

5. United States Government Accountability. Office Report to Congressional Requestors. Food Safety: A National Strategy is Needed to Address Fragmentation in Federal Oversight. Available at: http://www.gao.gov/ assets/690/682095.pdf. Accessed August 17, 2017

6. US Food and Drug Administration. The FDA Food Safety Modernization Act (FSMA). 2011; Available at: https://www.fda.gov/food/guidance-regulation-food-and-dietary-supplements/food-safety-modernization-act-fsma. Accessed October 27, 2017

7.   US Food and Drug Administration. Center for Food Safety and Applied Nutrition (CFSAN). Available at: https://www.fda.gov/about-fda/office-foods-and-veterinary-medicine/center-food-safety-and-applied-nutrition-cfsan. Accessed April 30, 2019

8.   Center for Food Safety and Applied Nutrition (CFSAN). What we do at CFSAN. Available at: https://www.fda.gov/AboutFDA/CentersOffices/OfficeofFoods/CFSAN/WhatWeDo/default.htm. Accessed November 14, 2018

9.   US Food and Drug Administration. About the GRAS Notification Program. Available at: https://www.fda.gov/food/generally-recognized-safe-gras/about-gras-notification-program. November 14, 2018

10. Trasande L, Shaffer RM, Sathyanarayana S, American Academy of Pediatrics, Council on Environmental Health. Policy statement: Food additives and child health. *Pediatrics.* 2018;142(2):e20181408

11. US Department of Agriculture. Pesticide Data Program. 2011; Available at: https://www.ams.usda.gov/sites/default/files/media/2015PDPAnnualSummary.pdf. Accessed August 17, 2017

12. US Food and Drug Administration. Residue Monitoring Reports. Available at: https://www.fda.gov/downloads/Food/FoodborneIllnessContaminants/Pesticides/UCM546325.pdf. Accessed September 20, 2017

13. Centers for Disease Control and Prevention, National Center for Environmental Health, Division of Laboratory Sciences. *National Report on Human Exposure to Environmental Chemicals.* NCEH Pub No. 05-0570. Atlanta, GA: Centers for Disease Control and Prevention; 2009

14. Roberts JR, Karr CJ, American Academy of Pediatrics, Council on Environmental Health. Technical report: Pesticide exposure in children. *Pediatrics.* 2012;130(6):e1765–e1788

15. American Academy of Pediatrics, Council on Environmental Health. Policy statement: Pesticide exposure in children. *Pediatrics.* 2012;130(6):e1757–e1763

16. Riederer AM, Bartell SM, Barr DB, Ryan PB. Diet and non-diet predictors of urinary 3-phenoxybenzoic acid in NHANES 1999–2002. *Environ Health Perspect.* 2008;116(8):1015–1022

17. Rowe C, Gunier R, Bradman A, et al. Residential proximity to organophosphate and carbamate pesticide use during pregnancy, poverty during childhood, and cognitive functioning in 10-year old children. *Environ Res.* 2016;150:128–137

18. Millenson ME, Braun JM, Calafat AM, et al. Urinary organophosphate insecticide metabolite concentrations during pregnancy and children's interpersonal, communication, repative and stereotypic behaviors at 8 years of age: The Home Study. *Environ Res.* 2017;157:9–16

19. Gunier RB, Bradman A, Harley KG, Koqut K, Eskenazi B. Prenatal residential proximity to agricultural pesticide use and IQ in 7-year-old children. *Environ Health Perspect.* 2017;125:057002

VII

20. Butler-Dawson J, Galvin K, Thorne PS, Rohlman D. Organophosphorus pesticide exposure and neurobehavioral performance in Latino children living in an orchard community. *Neurotoxicology.* 2016;53:165–172

21. Bouchard MF, Bellinger DC, Wright RO, Weisskopf MG. Attention-deficit/hyperactivity disorder and urinary metabolites of organophosphate pesticides. *Pediatrics.* 2010;125(6):e1270–e1277

22. Hertz-Picciotto I, Sass JB, Engel S, et al. Organophosphate exposures during pregnancy and child neurodevelopment: recommendations for essential policy reforms. *PLoS Med.* 2018;15(10):e1002671

23. Katsikantami I, Colosio C, Alegakis A, et al. Estimation of daily intake and risk assessment of organophosphorus pesticides based on biomonitoring data: the internal exposure approach. *Food Chem Toxicol.* 2018;123:57–71

24. Huen K, Solomon O, Kogut K, Eskenazi B, Holland N. PON1 DNA methylation and neurobehavior in Mexican-American children with prenatal organophosphate exposure. *Environ Int.* 2018;121(Pt 1):3140

25. Silverstein J, Foreman J, American Academy of Pediatrics, Committee on Nutrition, Council on Environmental Health. Organic foods: health and environmental advantages and disadvantages. *Pediatrics.* 2012;130(5): e1406–e1415

26. Bradman A, Quiros-Alcala L, Castrina R, et al. Effect of organic diet intervention on pesticide exposures in young children living in low-income urban and agricultural communities. *Environ Health Perspect.* 2015;123(1086–1093)

27. US Department of Agriculture, National Organic Program. Organic Labeling and Marketing Information. April 2008; Available at: https://www.ams.usda.gov/rules-regulations/organic/labeling . Accessed September 22, 2017

28. US Department of Agriculture. Organic Economic and Market Information: Economic Research Service. May 2017; Available at: https://www.ers.usda.gov/topics/natural-resources-environment/organic-agriculture.aspx. Accessed September 22, 2017

29. US Department of Agriculture. Organic Prices. Available at: https://www.ers.usda.gov/data-products/organic-prices/. Accessed September 22, 2017

30. Rogan WJ, American Academy of Pediatrics, Council on Environmental Health. Iodine deficiency, pollutant chemicals, and the thyroid: new information on an old problem. *Pediatrics.* 2014;133(6):1163–1166

31. Abdallah MA, Harrad S. Polybrominated diphenyl ethers in UK human milk: implications for infant exposure and relationship to external exposure. *Environ Int.* 2014;63(130–136)

32. Labunska I, Harrad S, Wang M, Johnston P. Human dietary exposure to PBDEs around e-waste recycling sites in Eastern China. *Environ Sci Technol.* 2014;48: 5555–5564

33. Russ K, Howard S. Developmental exposures to environmental chemicals and metabolic changes in children. *Curr Probl Pediatr Adolesc Health Care.* 2016;46 (255–285)

34. Park SH, Ha E, Hong YS, Park H. Serum levels of persistent organic pollutants and insulin secretion among children age 7-9 years: A prospective cohort study. *Environ Health Perspect.* 2016;124(1924–1930)

35. Warembourg C, Debost-Legrand A, Bonvallot N, et al. Exposure of pregnant women to persistent organic pollutants and cord sex hormone levels. *Hum Reprod.* 2016;31:190–198

36. Koskenniemi JJ, Vertanen HE, Kiviranta H, et al. Associationn between levels of persistent organic pollutants in adipose tissue and cryptorchidism in early childhood: a case-control study. *Environ Health* 2015;14:78

37. Rignell-Hydbom A, Lindh CH, Dillner J, Johnsson BA, Rylander L. A nested case-control study of intrauterine exposure to persistent organochlorine pollutants and the risk of hypospadias. *PLoS One.* 2012;7:e44767

38. Harley K, Marks A, Chevrier J, Bradman A, Sjödin A, Eskenazi B. PBDE concentrations in women's serum and fecundability. *Environ Health Perspect.* 2010;118(5):699–704

39. Dingemans MM, van den Berg M, Westerink RH. Neurotoxicity of brominated flame retardants: (in)direct effects of parent and hydroxylated polybrominated diphenyl ethers on the (developing) nervous system. *Environ Health Perspect.* 2011;119(7):900–907

40. Schreiber T, Gassmann K, Götz C, et al. Polybrominated diphenyl ethers induce developmental neurotoxicity in a human in vitro model: evidence for endocrine disruption. *Environ Health Perspect.* 2010;118(4):572–578

41. Herbstman JB, Sjödin A, Kurzon M, et al. Prenatal exposure to PBDEs and neurodevelopment. *Environ Health Perspect.* 2010;118(5):712–719

42. National Toxicology Program, Department of Health and Human Services. 2,3,7,8-Tetrachlorodibenzo-p-dioxin. Available at: https://ntp.niehs.nih.gov/ntp/roc/content/profiles/tetrachlorodibenzodioxin.pdf Accessed September 25, 2017

43. Xue J, Liu SV, Zatarian VG, Geller AM, Schultz BD. Analysis of NHANES measured blood PCBs in the general US population and application of SHEDS model to identify key exposure factors. *J Expo Sci Environ Epidemiol.* 2014;24: 615–621

44. US Department of Agriculture. DIOXIN 13 Survey: Dioxins and Dioxin-Like Compounds in the U.S. Domestic Meat and Poultry Supply. May 2015; Available at: https://www.fsis.usda.gov/wps/wcm/connect/da1d623d-3005-4116-bef7-2a61d1ebd543/Dioxin-Report-FY2013.pdf?MOD=AJPERES. Accessed September 25, 2017

45. Institute of Medicine and National Research Council. Dioxins and Dioxin-like Compounds in the Food Supply: Strategies to Decrease Exposure. Washington, DC: National Academies Press; 2003: Available at: https://doi.org/10.17226/10763. Accessed September 25, 2017

46. Clarkson TW, Magos L, Myers GJ. Human exposure to mercury: the three modern dilemmas. *J Trace Elem Exp Med.* 2003;16(18):321–343

VII

47. Environmental Protection Agency. Trends in blood mercury concentrations and fish consumption among U.S. women of childbearing age. NHANES 1999–2010. Final Report. July 2013. EPA-823-R-13-002. Available at: https://nepis. epa.gov/Exe/ZyPDF.cgi/P100LP7Q.PDF?Dockey=P100LP7Q.PDF. Accessed September 25, 2017

48. US Food and Drug Administration. Mercury Levels in Commercial Fish and Shellfish (1990–2012). Available at: https://www.fda.gov/food/ foodborneillnesscontaminants/metals/ucm115644.htm. Accessed September 25, 2017

49. Julvez J, Mendez M, Ferandez-Barres S, et al. Maternal consumption of seafood in pregnancy and child neuropsychological development: a longitudinal study based on a population with high consumption levels. *Am J Epidemiol.* 2016;183: 169–182

50. US Food and Drug Administration. Eating Fish: What pregnant women and parents should know. 2017; Available at: https://www.fda.gov/downloads/ Food/FoodborneIllnessContaminants/Metals/UCM537120.pdf. Accessed September 25, 2017

51. Neltner T, Environmental Defense Fund. Lead in food: A hidden health threat. 2017; Available at: https://www.edf.org/health/lead-food-hidden-health-threat. Accessed September 25, 2017

52. US Food and Drug Administration. Questions and Answers on Lead in Food. 2017; Available at: https://www.fda.gov/food/foodborneillnesscontaminants/ metals/ucm557424.htm. Accessed September 25, 2017

53. Food and Agricultural Organization of the United Nations and World Health Organization. Joint FAO/WHO Expert Committee on Food Additives: Summary and Conclusions, 73rd meeting, June 2010. Available at: http://www.who.int/ foodsafety/publications/chem/summary73.pdf. Accessed September 27, 2017

54. Food and Agricultural Organization of the United Nations and World Health Organization. General Standard for Contaminants and Toxins in Food and Feed. Codex Stan 193–1995. 2015

55. Spliethoff HM, Mitchell RG, Shayler H, et al. Estimated lead (Pb) exposures for a population of urban community gardeners. *Environ Geochem Health.* 2016;38 (955–971)

56. Davis MA, Mackenzie TA, Cottingham KL, Gilbert-Diamond D, Punshon T, Karagas MR. Rice consumption and urinary arsenic concentrations in U.S. children. *Environ Health Perspect.* 2012;120(10):1418–1424

57. Juskelis R, Li W, Nelson J, Cappozzo JC. Arsenic speciation in rice cereals for infants. *J Agric Food Chem.* 2013;61(45):10670–10676

58. Botana LM. Toxicological Perspective on Climate Change: Aquatic Toxins. *Chem Res Toxicol.* 2016;29:619–625

59. Friedman MA, Fernandez M, Backer LC, et al. An updated review of ciguatera fish poisoning: clinical, epidemiological, environmental and public health management. *Marine Drugs.* 2017;15(3):e72

60. Fleming LE, Backer LC, Baden DG. Overview of aerosolized Florida red tide toxins: exposures and effects. *Environ Health Perspect.* 2005;113(5):618–620

61. Ansdell VE. The pretravel consultation: food poisoning from toxins. *CDC Health Information for International Travel.* 2018; Available at: https://wwwnc.cdc.gov/travel/yellowbook/2018/the-pre-travel-consultation/food-poisoning-from-marine-toxins. Accessed October 4, 2017

62. Mowry JB, Spyker DA, Brooks DE, Zimmerman A, Schauben JL. 2015 Annual report of the American Association of Poison Control Centers' National Poison Data System (NPDS): 33rd Annual Report. *Clin Toxicol (Phila).* 2016;54(10): 924–1109

63. Leschke E. *Clinical Toxicology: Modern Methods in the Diagnosis and Treatment of Poisoning.* Baltimore, MD: William Wood; 1934

64. Sun XN, Su P, Shan H. Mycotoxin contamination of rice in China. *J Food Sci.* 2017;82(3):573–584

65. Suarez L, Felkner M, Brender JD, Canfield M, Zhu H, Hendricks KA. Neural tube defects on the Texas-Mexico border: what we've learned in the 20 years since the Brownsville cluster. *Birth Defects Res A Clin Mol Teratol.* 2012;94(11):882–892

66. Marin S, Ramos AJ, Cano-Sancho G, Sanchis V. Mycotoxins: occurrence, toxicology, and exposure assessment. *Food Chem Toxicol.* 2013;60:218–237

67. US Food and Drug Administration. GMPs – Section Two: Literature Review of Common Food Safety Problems and Applicable Controls. 2004; Available at: https://www.fda.gov/Food/GuidanceRegulation/CGMP/ucm110911.htm. Accessed October 5, 2017

68. US Food and Drug Administration. Guidance for Industry: Fumonisin Levels in Human Foods and Animal Feeds. 2001; Available at: https://www.fda.gov/regulatory-information/search-fda-guidance-documents/guidance-industry-fumonisin-levels-human-foods-and-animal-feeds. Accessed October 5, 2017

69. US Food and Drug Administration. CPG Sec. 555.400 Foods - Adulteration with Aflatoxin. 2005; Available at: https://www.fda.gov/ICECI/ComplianceManuals/CompliancePolicyGuidanceManual/ucm074555.htm. Accessed October 5, 2017

70. US Food and Drug Administration. CPG Sec. 562.600 Preservatives; Use in nonstandardized foods; label declaration. 1989; Available at: https://www.fda.gov/regulatory-information/search-fda-guidance-documents/cpg-sec-562600-preservatives-use-nonstandardized-foods-label-declaration. Accessed October 5, 2017

71. US Food and Drug Administration. Guidance for Industry: Antimicrobial Food Additives. 1999; Available at: https://www.fda.gov/regulatory-information/search-fda-guidance-documents/guidance-industry-antimicrobial-food-additives. Accessed October 5, 2017

72. US Food and Drug Administration. Irradiation in the production, processing, and handling of food. *Fed Regist.* 2014;79(71):20771–20779

VII

73. US Food and Drug Administration. Subchapter B. Radiation and radiation sources. Irradiation in the production processing and handling of food. Available at: https://www.accessdata.fda.gov/scripts/cdrh/cfdocs/cfcfr/cfrsearch.cfm?fr=179.26. Accessed April 30, 2019

74. Shahbaz HM, Akram K, Ahn JJ, Kwon JH. Worldwide status of fresh fruits irradiation and concerns about quality, safety and consumer appearance. *Crit Rev Food Nutr.* 2016;56(11):1790–1807

75. World Health Organization. WHO 5 Keys to Safer Food Programme. Available at: http://www.who.int/foodsafety/consumer/5keys/en/index.html. Accessed October 27, 2017

76. US Food and Drug Administration. List of Indirect Food Additives Used in Food Contact Substances. 2010; Available at: https://www.accessdata.fda.gov/scripts/fdcc/?set=IndirectAdditives. Accessed October 27, 2017

77. US Food and Drug Administration. Inventory of Effective Food Contact Substance (FCS) Notifications. Available at: https://www.accessdata.fda.gov/scripts/fdcc/?set=fcn. Accessed October 29, 2017

78. US Food and Drug Administration. Guidance for Industry and Other Stakeholders. Toxicological Principles for the Safety Assessment of Food Ingredients. Redbook 2000. Available at: https://www.fda.gov/Food/GuidanceRegulation/GuidanceDocumentsRegulatoryInformation/IngredientsAdditivesGRASPackaging/ucm2006826.htm. Accessed October 29, 2017

79. US Food and Drug Administration. Guidance for Industry: Preparation of Food Contact Notifications for Food Contact Substances: Toxicology Recommendations. Available at: https://www.fda.gov/regulatory-information/search-fda-guidance-documents/guidance-industry-preparation-food-contact-notifications-food-contact-substances-toxicology. Accessed October 29, 2017

80. US Food and Drug Administration. Guidance for Industry: Submitting Requests under 21 CFR 170.39 Threshold of Regulation for Substances Used in Food-Contact Articles. Available at: https://www.accessdata.fda.gov/scripts/cdrh/cfdocs/cfCFR/CFRSearch.cfm?fr=170.39. Accessed October 29, 2017

81. US Food and Drug Administration. Threshold of Regulation Exemptions. Available at: https://www.fda.gov/Food/IngredientsPackagingLabeling/PackagingFCS/ThresholdRegulationExemptions/default.htm. Accessed October 29, 2017

82. Vandenberg LN, Maffini MV, Sonnenschein C, Rubin BS, Soto AM. Bisphenol-A and the great divide: a review of controversies in the field of endocrine disruption. *Endocr Rev.* 2009;30(1):75–95

83. vom Saal FS, Nagel SC, Timms BG, Welshons WV. Implications for human health of the extensive bisphenol A literature showing adverse effects at low doses. *Toxicology.* 2005;212(2-3):244–252

84. Trasande L, Shaffer RM, Sathyanarayana S, American Academy of Pediatrics, Council on Environmental Health. Technical report: Food additives and child health. *Pediatrics.* 2018;142(2):e20181410

85. Wilson NK, Chuang JC, Morgan MK, Lordo RA, Sheldon LS. An observational study of the potential exposures of preschool children to pentachlorophenol, bisphenol-A, and nonylphenol at home and daycare. *Environ Res.* 2007;103(1): 9–20

86. Calafat AM, Ye X, Wong Y-L, Reidy JA, Needham LL. Exposure of the U.S. Population to Bisphenol A and 4-tertiary-Octylphenol:2003–2004. *Environ Health Perspect.* 2008;116(1):39–44

87. Bisphenol A (BPA) Joint Emerging Science Working Group to FDA Chemical and Environmental Science Council (CESC). Updated review of literature and data on Bisphenol A 2014; Available at: https://www.fda.gov/downloads/Food/IngredientsPackagingLabeling/FoodAdditivesIngredients/UCM424071.pdf. Accessed November 27, 2018

88. US Food and Drug Administration. Indirect food additives: polymers. *Fed Regist.* 2012;77(137):41899–41902

89. Liao C, Liu F, Alomirah H, et al. Bisphenol S in urine from the United States and seven Asian countries: occurrence and human exposures. *Environ Sci Technol.* 2012;46(12):6860–6866

90. Danzl E, Sei K, Soda S, Ike M, Fujita M. Biodegradation of bisphenol A, bisphenol F and bisphenol S in seawater. *Int J Environ Res Public Health.* 2009;6(4): 1472–1478

91. Carwile JL, Luu HT, Bassett LS, et al. Polycarbonate bottle use and urinary bisphenol A concentrations. *Environ Health Perspect.* 2009;117(9):1368–1372

92. Rudel RA, Gray JM, Engel CL, et al. Food packaging and bisphenol a and bis(2-ethyhexyl) phthalate exposure: findings from a dietary intervention. *Environ Health Perspect.* 2011;119(7):914–920

93. Yang CZ, Yaniger SI, Jordan VC, Klein DJ, Bittner GD. Most plastic products release estrogenic chemicals: a potential health problem that can be solved. *Environ Health Perspect.* 2011;119(7):989–996

94. US Food and Drug Administration. Guidance for industry: the safety of imported traditional pottery intended for use with food and the use of the term 'lead free' in the labeling of pottery; and proper identification of ornamental and decorative ceramicware. 2010; Available at: https://www.fda.gov/regulatory-information/search-fda-guidance-documents/guidance-industry-safety-imported-traditional-pottery-intended-use-food-and-use-term-lead-free. Accessed April 30, 2019

95. American Academy of Pediatrics, Council on Environmental Health. Policy statement: Prevention of childhood lead toxicity. *Pediatrics.* 2016;138(1):e20161493

96. Kotthoff M, Muller J, Juriling H, Schlummer M, Fiedler D. Perfluoroalkyl and polyfluoroalkyls substances in consumer products. *Environ Sci Pollut Res Int.* 2015;22:14546–14559

VII

97. Toms LL, Calafat AM, Kato K, et al. Polyfluoroalkyl chemicals in pooled blood serum from infants, children, and adults in Australia. *Environ Sci Technol.* 2009;43(11):4194–4199

98. Nelson J, Hatch E, Webster T. Exposure to polyfluoroalkyl chemicals and cholesterol, body weight, and insulin resistance in the general U.S. population. *Environ Health Perspect.* 2010;118(8):197–202

99. Olsen GW, Butenhoff JL, Zobel LR. Perfluoroalkyl chemicals and human fetal development: an epidemiologic review with clinical and toxicological perspectives. *Reprod Toxicol.* 2009;27(3-4):212–230

100. US Environmental Protection Agency. Basic information about Per- and Polyfluoroalkyl substances (PFASs). Available at: https://www.epa.gov/pfas/basic-information-about-and-polyfluoroalkyl-substances-pfass#tab-3. Accessed October 27, 2017

101. US Food and Drug Administration. Acrylamide Guidance for Industry: Acrylamide in Foods. Available at: https://www.fda.gov/Food/GuidanceRegulation/GuidanceDocumentsRegulatoryInformation/ucm374524.htm. Accessed October 27, 2017

102. US Food and Drug Administration. Questions and answers on the occurrence of furan in food. Available at: https://www.fda.gov/food/foodborneillnesscontaminants/chemicalcontaminants/ucm078451.htm. Accessed October 27, 2017

Appendices

Composition of Human Milk

Table 1.
Nutrient Content of Human Milk[a]

Nutrients (per Liter)[b]	Early Milk (0–0.5 mo)	Mature Milk (0.5–1.5 mo)
Energy (kcal)		650–700
Carbohydrate		
Lactose (g)	20–30	67–70
Glucose (g)	0.2–1.0	0.2–0.3
Oligosaccharides (g)	22–24	12–14
Nitrogen/Protein		
Total nitrogen (g)	3.05 ± 0.59	1.93 ± 0.24
Nonprotein nitrogen (g)	0.53 ± 0.09	0.45 ± 0.03
Protein nitrogen[c] (g)	2.52	1.48
True protein[d] (g)	15.75 ± 4.2	9.25 ± 1.8
Casein (g)	3.8	5.7
ß-casein (g)	2.6	4.4
κ-casein (g)	1.2	1.3
α-Lactalbumin (g) (present in whey fraction)	3.62 ± 0.59	3.26 ± 0.47
Lactoferrin (g) (present in whey fraction)	3.53 ± 0.54	1.94 ± 0.38
Serum albumin (g)	0.39 ± 0.06	0.4 ± 0.07
sIgA (g)	2.0	1.0
IgM (g)	0.12	0.2
IgG (g)	0.34	0.05

Continued

APP

Table 1. *Continued*
Nutrient Content of Human Milk[a]

Nutrients (per Liter)[b]	Early Milk (0–0.5 mo)	Mature Milk (0.5–1.5 mo)
Lipids		
Total lipids (g)	20	35
Triglyceride (% total lipid)	97–98	97–98
Cholesterol[e] (% total lipids)	0.7–1.3	0.–0.5
Phospholipids (% total lipids)	1.1	0.6–0.8
Fatty acids (weight %)	88	88
Total saturated (weight %)	43–44	44–45
C12:0 Lauric acid		5
C14:0 Myristic acid		6
C16:0 Palmitic acid		20
C18:0 Stearic acid		8
Monounsaturated (weight %)		40
C18:1n-9 Oleic acid	32	31
Polyunsaturated (PUFA) (weight %)	13	14–15
Total n-3 (weight %)	1.5	1.5
C18:3n-3 Linolenic acid	0.7	0.9
C22:5n-3 Eicosapentaenoic acid	0.2	0.1
C22:6n-3 Docosahexaenoic acid	0.5	0.2
Total n-6 (weight %)	11.6	13.06
C18:2n-6 Linoleic acid	8.9	11.3
C20:4n-6 Arachidonic acid	0.7	0.5
C22:4n-6 Docosatetraenoic acid	0.2	0.1

Nutrients (per Liter)[b]	Early Milk (0–0.5 mo)	Mature Milk (0.5–1.5 mo)
Water-soluble vitamins		
Ascorbic Acid (mg)		100
Thiamin (μg)	20	200
Riboflavin (μg)		400–600
Niacin (mg)	0.5	1.8–6.0
Vitamin B_6 (mg)		0.09–0.31
Folate (μg)		80–140
Vitamin B_{12} (μg)		0.5–1.0
Pantothenic Acid (mg)		2–2.5
Biotin (μg)		5–9
Fat-soluble vitamins		
Retinol (mg)	2	0.3–0.6
Carotenoids (mg)	2	0.2–0.6
Vitamin K (μg)	2–5	2–3
Vitamin D (μg)		0.33
Vitamin E (mg)	8–12	3–8
Major minerals		
Major minerals		
Calcium (mg)	250	200–250
Magnesium (mg)	30–35	30–35
Phosphorus (mg)	120–160	120–140
Sodium (mg)	300–400	120–250
Potassium (mg)	600–700	400–550
Chloride (mg)	600–800	400–450

Continued

APP

Table 1. *Continued*
Nutrient Content of Human Milk[a]

Nutrients (per Liter)[b]	Early Milk (0–0.5 mo)	Mature Milk (0.5–1.5 mo)
Trace minerals		
Iron (mg)	0.5–1.0	0.3–0.9
Zinc (mg)	8–12	1–3
Copper (mg)	0.5–0.8	0.2–0.4
Manganese (µg)	5–6	3
Selenium (µg)	40	7–33
Iodine (µg)		150
Fluoride (µg)		4–15

[a] Data from: Jensen RG, ed. Handbook of Milk Composition. New York, NY: Academic Press; 1995; and Picciano MF. Appendix: Representative values for contituents of human milk. *Pediatr Clin North Am*. 2001;48(1):263-264.

[b] All values are expressed per liter of milk with the exception of lipids that are expressed as a percentage of weight of total lipids. All values are expressed as a mean or a range of concentrations.

[c] Protein nitrogen = Total nitrogen (g) minus nonprotein nitrogen (g).

[d] Total (true) protein = total protein nitrogen x 6.25.

[e] The cholesterol content of human milk ranges from 100 to 200 mg/L in most samples of human milk after day 21 of lactation.

Table 2.

Influence of Maternal Status and Maternal Diet on Breast Milk Nutrients

	Infant reliance on BM	Concentrations trend	Affected by maternal status	Affected by maternal diet	Affected by maternal supplementation	Maternal factors influencing BM concentrations	Comments
Thiamin	+	Increases over first several months	−	+	+/− (+ in case of maternal dietary insufficiency)	Insufficient data	The body does not store thiamin so continuous supply is needed to mother
Vitamin B-6	+/−	Increases during first weeks postpartum, followed by gradual decline	+	+	+	Insufficient data	Gestational reserves help support infant vitamin B-6 needs through first months of lactation; after 6 mo, BM alone may be insufficient to meet infant needs (1)
Vitamin B-12	+	Decreases during first 3–4 mo of lactation	+	+	+/−	Veganism/ vegetarianism/ low consumption of animal source foods (−), pernicious anemia (−)	Limited infant reserves at birth

Continued

APP

Table 2. *Continued*

Influence of Maternal Status and Maternal Diet on Breast Milk Nutrients

	Infant reliance on BM	Concentrations trend	Affected by maternal status	Affected by maternal diet	Affected by maternal supplementation	Maternal factors influencing BM concentrations	Comments
Folate	+	Peaks at 2–3 mo of lactation	–	–	–	Insufficient data	Supplemental folate may affect BM folate concentrations in undernourished women (2); more data are needed; only severe maternal deficiency compromises BM concentrations
Choline	+	Increases rapidly from 7 to 22 d postpartum and remains stable in mature milk	+	+	+	SNPs in MTHFR (–), preterm delivery (–), inflammation (+), hormones (+/–)	Gene polymorphisms may explain variation in BM choline concentrations in women with similar intakes (3)

Vitamin C	+	Highest in colostrum, decreases with progression of lactation	–	+/–	+/–	Preterm delivery (+), smoking (–), diabetes (–)	Greater effect of diet and supplementation in women with poor status; the body does not store vitamin C so continuous supply is needed to mother and infant
Vitamin A	+	Highest in colostrum, stabilizes in mature milk	– (unless maternal reserves are depleted)	+/– (if maternal reserves are inadequate)	+	Preterm delivery (–), adolescence (–), parity (+)	BM vitamin A derived from circulating as well as dietary retinol (4)
Vitamin D	+/– [vitamin D_3, but not active 25(OH)D]	Little 25(OH)D in BM	+/– (conflicting data)	+/– [diet may affect BM vitamin D_3, but not active 25(OH)D]	+	Season, sun exposure (+), obesity (–)	Primary form passed from maternal circulation to BM is vitamin D_3, the biological precursor of 25(OH)D (5, 6)

Continued

APP

Table 2. *Continued*

Influence of Maternal Status and Maternal Diet on Breast Milk Nutrients

	Infant reliance on BM	Concentrations trend	Affected by maternal status	Affected by maternal diet	Affected by maternal supplementation	Maternal factors influencing BM concentrations	Comments
Vitamin E	+	Decreases from colostrum to mature milk, then stable	–	–	+	Preterm delivery (–)	Limited infant reserves at birth; Greater increase in BM vitamin E concentrations with natural (RRR-α-tocopherol) vs. synthetic all-rac-α-tocopherol) supplementation (7)
Vitamin K	–	Low concentrations in BM	–	–	+	Insufficient date	—
Iron	–	Low concentrations in BM, declines through first year of lactation	–	–	–	No consistent evidence	Infants depend on hepatic reserves to meet iron needs (8)

Copper	−	Low concentrations in BM, declines as lactation progresses	—	—	—	BM selenium concentrations (+)	Hepatic reserves protect infants from deficiency in early infancy (9)
Zinc	+/− (in early lactation)	Sharp initial decrease followed by gradual decline	—	—	—	Age (−), parity (−), iron deficiency (−)	Infant zinc stores are limited (9)
Calcium	+	Increases in first week, subsequent gradual decline for duration of lactation	—	+/− (where habitual calcium intake is low)	—	Adolescence (−), iron deficiency anemia (−)	—
Phosphorus	+	Increases in first week, subsequent gradual decline for duration of lactation	+/− (only in case of genetic anomalies)	—	No data	Familial hypophosphatemia (−), hyperparathyroidism (−)	BM phosphorus is tightly regulated (10)
Magnesium	+	Stable during lactation	—	—	—	Adolescence (−)	—

Continued

Table 2. *Continued*

Influence of Maternal Status and Maternal Diet on Breast Milk Nutrients

	Infant reliance on BM	Concentrations trend	Affected by maternal status	Affected by maternal diet	Affected by maternal supplementation	Maternal factors influencing BM concentrations	Comments
Iodine	+	Initial decline, stable after 1 mo	–	–	–	Smoking (–)	Influenced by environment (soil iodine, salt iodization, etc.); infants are born with limited reserves
Selenium	+	Decreases throughout lactation	+/– (weak correlation, if present)	+	+	No consistent evidence	Influenced by environment (soil selenium); infants are born with limited reserves
Protein	+	Brief, sharp decrease, then stable from 2 to 6 mo until weaning	–	+/– (amino acid composition varies by maternal intake)	N/A	Milk volume (–)	Similar concentrations in BM of well-nourished and undernourished mothers

Lipids	+	Sharp increase in first week, then stable	+	+/– (FA composition varies by maternal intake)	N/A	%IBW (+), milk volume (–)	Large intraindividual CV
Carbo-hydrates	+	Lactose is lowest in colostrum, stabilizes as milk matures	–	–	N/A	BMI (–), milk volume (+), preterm delivery (–)	Non-nutritive HMOs decrease from colostrum to mature milk

[1] BM, breast milk; HMO, human-milk oligosaccharide; IBW, ideal body weight; MTHFR, methylenetetrahydrofolate reductase; N/A, Not available; SNP, single nucleotide polymorphism; 25(OH)D, 25-hydroxyvitamin D; +, Yes; –, No.

Reprinted with permission from Dror DK, Allen LH. Overview of nutrients in human milk. *Adv Nutr.* 2018;9(Suppl 1):278S–294S

Infant Formula Act Regulations and Expert Recommendations for Term US Infant Formulas[a]

(All values listed from vitamin A down are expressed in units/100 Kcal)

Nutrient	Units	IFA[1] Min	IFA[1] Max	LSRO[2] Min	LSRO[2] Max	Upper Limits[3]
Protein[b]	g	1.8	4.5	1.7	3.3	3.2–3.5
Fat	g	3.3	6.0	4.4	6.4	6.0
LA	% FA	9[c]		8	35	30
ALA	% FA			1.75	4	3
DHA	% FA					0.5
EPA	% FA					0.8
Vitamin A	IU	250	750	200	500	750–1000
Vitamin D	IU	40	100	40	100	100
Vitamin E	IU	0.7		0.75	7.5	15
Vitamin K	mcg	4		1	25	20
Thiamin	mcg	40		30	200	200
Riboflavin	mcg	60		80	300	300
Pyridoxine	mcg	35		30	130	175
Vitamin B_{12}	mcg	0.15		0.08	0.7	0.75
Niacin	mcg	250		550	2000	1250
Folic acid	mcg	4		11	40	20
Pantothenate	mcg	300		300	1200	1500
Biotin	mcg	1.5		1	15	7.5
Vitamin C	mg	8		6	15	40
Choline	mg	7		7	30	
Inositol	mg	4		4	40	
Calcium	mg	60		50	140	89[d]

Continued

APP

Appendix B. *Continued*

Nutrient	Units	IFA[1] Min	IFA[1] Max	LSRO[2] Min	LSRO[2] Max	Upper Limits[3]
Phosphorus	mg	30		20[e]	70[e]	67–93[d]
Magnesium	mg	6		4	17	18
Iron	mg	0.15	3	0.2	1.65	3
Zinc	mg	0.5		0.4	1	1.5
Manganese	mcg	5		1	100	50
Copper	mcg	60		60	160	200
Iodine	mcg	5	75	8	35	75
Selenium	mcg	2	7	1.5	5	4[c]
Sodium	mg	20	60	25	50	
Potassium	mg	80	200	60	160	
Chloride	mg	55	150	50	160	
Taurine	mg			0	12	
Nucleotides	mg			0	16	
Fluoride	mcg			0	60	
Carbohydrate	g			9	13	

FA indicates fatty acids; IU, International Units, LSRO Life Sciences Research Organization.

[a] See original sources for additional specific details

[b] Assumes protein source with biologic value of at least casein.

[c] Value extrapolated from original source

[d] Applies to cow milk protein formulas. Soy may need to be higher.

[e] Available phosphorus. Phytate phosphorus is considered unavailable.

References

1. Infant Formula: The Addition of Minimum and Maximum Levels of Selenium to Infant Formula and Related Labeling. 2015. Available at: https://www.federalregister.gov/documents/2015/06/23/2015-15394/infant-formula-the-addition-of-minimum-and-maximum-levels-of-selenium-to-infant-formula-and-related. Accessed June 29, 2017

2. Assessment of nutrient requirements for infant formulas. *J Nutr.* 1998;128 (11 Suppl):2059S–2293S

3. Upper limits of nutrients in infant formulas. *J Nutr.* 1989;119(12 Suppl):1763–1873

Appendix C

Increasing the Caloric Density of Infant Formula

Using Concentrated Liquid:

Most concentrated liquids contain 40 kcal/fl oz and when diluted 1:1, produce a formula that contains 20 kcal/fl oz. If a more concentrated final formula is desired using these products, use the upper part of the Table. For the few concentrated liquid products that contain 38 kcal/fl oz and normally produce a formula with 19 kcal/fl oz, more concentrated formulas can be made using the lower part of the Table.

Concentrated Liquid One Can	Added Water	Approximate Yield fl oz	Approximate Final Caloric Density - kcal/fl oz
Using Concentrated Liquid That Normally Produces a Formula With 20 kcal/fl oz			
13 fl oz	13 fl oz	26 fl oz	20
13 fl oz	11 fl oz	24 fl oz	22
13 fl oz	9 fl oz	22 fl oz	24
13 fl oz	6 fl oz	19 fl oz	27
13 fl oz	4.5 fl oz	17.5 fl oz	30
Using Concentrated Liquid That Normally Produces a Formula With 19 kcal/fl oz			
13 fl oz	13 fl oz	26 fl oz	19
13 fl oz	10 fl oz	23 fl oz	21
13 fl oz	8 fl oz	21 fl oz	24
13 fl oz	5 fl oz	18 fl oz	27
13 fl oz	4 fl oz	17 fl oz	29

APP

Using Powder:

Because of the variability of scoop sizes for different formulas from different manufacturers and the variability of household measures, no single set of recipes can be provided that is safe for all products. Some manufacturers provide recipes for their specific products on their websites. In the absence of such information, contact the manufacturer directly.

Increasing Caloric or Protein Density Using Additives:

- Vegetable oils provide 40 kcal per teaspoon.
- Microlipid water miscible safflower oil provides 22.5 kcal per teaspoon.
- Medium-chain triglyceride (MCT) oil provides 7.7 kcal/mL and 38 kcal per teaspoon.
- Liquigen water miscible MCT oil provides 4.5 kcal/ per teaspoon.
- Polycose liquid provides 10 kcal per teaspoon; Polycose powder provides 8 kcal per teaspoon.
- Solucarb maltodextrin powder provides 7.7 kcal per teaspoon.
- Duocal powder contains cornstarch and vegetable oils and provides 14 kcal per teaspoon.
- Beneprotein whey powder provides 6 g protein/25 kcal per enclosed scoop (7g).
- Complete Amino Acid Mix powder provides 2.38 g protein and 9.5 kcal per teaspoon.
- Benecalorie liquid provides 37.5 kcal and 0.8 g protein per teaspoon from high-oleic sunflower oil and casein.

Note that increasing caloric density using fat and/or carbohydrate should be performed with caution, because the additional energy (calories) effectively decreases the density (amount per 100 kcal) of all other nutrients.

D-1: Formulas for Low Birth Weight and Preterm Infants
and
D-2: Human Milk Fortifiers for Preterm Infants Fed Human Milk

APPENDIX D-1
Formulas for Low Birth Weight and Preterm Infants (per L)

	Similac Special Care 24[a] Liquid (Abbott Nutrition, Columbus, OH)	Enfamil Premature 24[a] Fe & (low Fe) Liquid (Mead Johnson, Evansville, IN)	GoodStart Premature 24[a] cal Liquid (Nestle, Fremont, MI)	Similac Special Care 24[a] HP Liquid (Abbott Nutrition, Columbus, OH)	Enfamil Premature High Protein 24[a] Liquid (Mead Johnson, Evansville, IN)	GoodStart Premature 24[a] High Protein Liquid Nestle, Fremont, MI)
Energy, kcal	806	810	812	812	811	812
Protein, g	22[b]	24[b]	24.3[c]	26.8[b]	28[b]	29.2[c]
Fat, g	43.8	41	42.2	44.1	40.8	42.2
Polyunsaturated, g	8.3	10.3	9.3			9.3
Monounsaturated, g	3.5	4.5	12			13
Saturated, g	32	26.2[d]	18.5	50%	40%	15.7
Linoleic acid, g	5.7	8.5	8.0	30%		8.0
MCT	50%	40%	40%			40%
Soy	30%	40%	29%	18%		29%
Safflower	—	—	29%	0.25%	0.32% FA	29%
Coconut	20%	20%	—	0.40%	0.64% FA	0.32%
DHA	0.25%	0.32% FA	0.32% FA			0.64%
ARA	0.40%	0.64% FA	0.64% FA			
Carbohydrate, g	86.1	90	85.2	81	85	78.7
Lactose %	50%	40%	50%	50%		50%
Glucose polymers %	50%	60%	50% (malto-dextrin)	50%		50% (malto-dextrin)
Mineral						
Calcium, mg	1460	1340	1331	1461	1340	1331
Phosphorus, mg	730	670	690	812	670	690
Magnesium, mg	100	73	81	97.4	73	81
Iron, mg	3.0	14.6 (4.1)	14.6	14.6	14.6	14.6
Zinc, mg	12.2	12.2	10.6	12.2	12.2	10.6
Manganese, μg	100	51	56.8	97	51	56.8
Copper, μg	2030	1010	1217	2029	970	1217
Iodine, μg	50	200	284	49	200	284
Sodium, mEq	15	13.9	20.4	15.2	13.9	20.4
Potassium, mEq	27	21	25	26.8	21	25
Chloride, mEq	19	19.4	19.7	18.6	19.4	19.7

Similac Special Care 30 Cal Liquid (Abbott Nutrition, Columbus, OH)	Enfamil Premature 30 cal Liquid, Mead Johnson, Evansville, IN)	Neosure 22 Cal Liquid (Abbott Nutrition, Columbus, OH)	Enfacare 22 Cal Liquid, Mead Johnson, Evansville, IN)	GoodStart Nourish 22 cal Liquid (Nestle, Fremont, MI)	Similac Special Care 20 Liquid (Abbott Nutrition, Columbus, OH)	Enfamil Premature 20 Fe & (low Fe) Liquid, Mead Johnson, Evansville, IN)	GoodStart, 20 cal premature Liquid (Nestle, Fremont, MI)
1014	1010	746	740	744	676	676	676
30.4[b]	30[b]	20.8[b]	21[b]	20.8[c]	20.3[b]	20[b]	20.3[c]
67.1	52	41	39	38.7	36.7	34	35.2
				8.2			7.7
				20.6			10
50%	40%	—		10	50%	8.5	15.4
30%		5.6	7.1	6.7	30%	40%	6.7
		25%		20%		40%	40%
18%		45%		18%	18%	20%	29%
0.21%	32% FA	29%		60%	0.25%	0.32% FA	29%
0.33%	64% FA	0.25%	0.32%	0.32%	0.40%	0.64% FA	0.32% FA
		0.40%	0.64%	0.64%			0.64% FA
78.4	112	75.1	79	78.1	69.7	74	71
50%				60%	50%	40%	50%
50%				40%	50%	60%	50%
				(malto-dextrin)			(malto-dextrin)
1826	1670	781	890	893	1217	1120	1109
1014	840	461	490	484	676	560	575
122	91	67.0	59	74	81	61	67.6
18.3	18.3	13.4	13.3	13.4	12	12.2 (3.4)	12.2
15.22	15.2	8.9	9.0	8.9	10.1	10.1	8.8
122	64	74	111	52	81	43	47.3
2536	1220	893	890	893	1691	810	1015
61	250	112	111	149	41	169	237
19.0	25.7	10.7	11.3	11.3	12.6	16.7	16.2
33.5	26.3	27.0	20.2	20	22.3	16.9	20.8
23.2	24.2	15.7	16.5	15.7	15.5	17.2	16.2

Continued

APP

	Similac Special Care 24[a] Liquid (Abbott Nutrition, Columbus, OH)	Enfamil Premature 24[a] Fe & (low Fe) Liquid (Mead Johnson, Evansville, IN)	GoodStart Premature 24[a] cal Liquid (Nestle, Fremont, MI)	Similac Special Care 24[a] HP Liquid (Abbott Nutrition, Columbus, OH)	Enfamil Premature High Protein 24[a] Liquid (Mead Johnson, Evansville, IN)	GoodStart Premature 24[a] High Protein Liquid Nestle, Fremont, MI)
Vitamin						
A, USP Units	10 081	10 100	8116	10 144	10 100	8116
D, USP Units	1210	1950	1461	1217	1950	1461
E, USP Units	32.3	51	48.7	32.5	51	48.7
K, μg	97	65	65	97.4	73	65
Thiamine (B$_1$), μg	2016	1620	1623	2029	1620	1623
Riboflavin (B$_2$), μg	5000	2400	2435	5032	2400	2435
Pyridoxine (B$_6$), μg	2016	1220	1623	2029	1220	1623
B$_{12}$, μg	4.4	2	2	4.5	2	2
Niacin (B$_3$), mg	40.3	32	32.5	40.6	32	32.5
Folic acid (B$_9$), μg	298	320	365	300	320	365
Pantothenic acid (B$_5$), mg	15.3	9.7	11.4	15.4	9.7	11.4
Biotin (B$_7$), μg	298	32	40.6	300	32	40.6
C (ascorbic acid), mg	298	162	243	300	162	243
Choline, mg	81	162	122	81	162	122
Inositol, mg	48.4	360	284	325	360	284

MCT indicates medium-chain triglyceride; DHA, docosahexaenoic acid; ARA, arachidonic acid; FA, fatty acid.

[a] 24 kcal/oz; 81 kcal/dL.

[b] Nonfat milk, whey protein concentrate.

[c] Partially hydrolyzed whey protein.

[d] Included 17.4 g MCT oils.

Similac Special Care 30 Cal Liquid (Abbott Nutrition, Columbus, OH)	Enfamil Premature 30 cal Liquid, Mead Johnson, Evansville, IN)	Neosure 22 Cal Liquid (Abbott Nutrition, Columbus, OH)	Enfacare 22 Cal Liquid, Mead Johnson, Evansville, IN)	GoodStart Nourish 22 cal Liquid (Nestle, Fremont, MI)	Similac Special Care 20 Liquid (Abbott Nutrition, Columbus, OH)	Enfamil Premature 20 Fe & (low Fe) Liquid, Mead Johnson, Evansville, IN)	GoodStart, 20 cal premature Liquid (Nestle, Fremont, MI)
12 681	12 700	2604	3330	3348	8454	850	6764
1522	2400	521	520	595	1014	1620	1217
40.6	64	26.8	30	30	27	43	40.6
122	91	81.8	59	60	81	54	54
2536	2000	1302	1480	1116	1691	1350	1353
6290	3000	1116	1480	1488	4193	2000	2029
2536	2000	744	740	744	1691	1010	1353
5.58	2.5	2.9	2.2	1.9	3.7	1.7	1.7
50.7	41	14.5	14.8	11.2	33.8	27.0	27.1
375	410	186	192	186	250	270	304
19.2	12.2	6.0	6.3	7.4	12.8	8.1	9.5
375.3	41	67	44	22	250	27	33.8
375	200	112	118	149	250	135	203
101	200	119	178	179	68	135	101
406	450	260	220	223	271	300	237

APP

APPENDIX D-2
**Human Milk Fortifiers for Preterm Infants Fed Human Milk
(Nutrients Added for 100 mL of Human Milk)**

Nutrient	Enfamil Powder Human Milk Fortifier (4 pkt), Mead Johnson, Evansville, IN	Similac Powder Human Milk Fortifier (4 pkt), Abbott Nutrition, Columbus, OH	Prolacta/HMF (20 mL), Prolacta Bioscience, Monrovia, CA
Energy (kcal)	14	14	28
Protein (g)	1.1	1.0	1.2
Fat (g)	1	0.36	1.8
Linoleic acid (mg)	140	0	?
α-Linolenic acid (mg)	17	0	?
Carbohydrate (g)	<0.4	1.8	1.8
Minerals			
Calcium (mg)	90	116	103
Phosphorus (mg)	50	64	53.8
Magnesium (mg)	1	6.8	4.7
Iron (mg)	1.44	0.32	0.1
Zinc (mg)	0.72	1	0.7
Manganese (μg)	10	7.2	<12
Copper (μg)	44	172	64
Sodium (mEq)	0.7	0.64	1.61
Potassium (mEq)	0.74	1.6	1.28
Chloride (mEq)	0.37 (13 mg)	1.08	0.82 (29 mg)

Similac Human Milk Fortifier Hydrolyzed Protein Concentrated Liquid (4pkts), Abbott Nutrition, Columbus, OH	Similac Liquid Human Milk Fortifier Concentrated Liquid, Abbott Nutrition, Columbus, OH	Enfamil Human Milk Fortifier Acidified Liquid (4 vials), Mead Johnson, Evansville, IN
28	28	30
2	1.4	2.2
0.84	1.08	2.3
54	4	230
?	?	?
3	3.24	<1.2
120	140	116
68	80	63
8.4	8.8	1.84
0.44	0.44	1.76
1.24	1.2	0.96
8.8	8.4	10
60	60	60
0.8	0.92	1.18
2	2.12	1.16
1.6	1.52	0.79 (28 mg)

Continued

APP

Nutrient	Enfamil Powder Human Milk Fortifier (4 pkt), Mead Johnson, Evansville, IN	Similac Powder Human Milk Fortifier (4 pkt), Abbott Nutrition, Columbus, OH	Prolacta/HMF (20 mL), Prolacta Bioscience, Monrovia, CA
Vitamins			
A (IU)	950	620	61
D (IU)	150	120	26
E (IU)	4.6	3.2	0.4
K (μg)	4.4	8.4	<0.2
Thiamine (B_1) (μg)	150	232	4
Riboflavin (B_2) (μg)	220	416	15
Niacin (B_3) (mg)	3	3.59	52.4
Pantothenate (B_5) (mg)	0.73	1.5	74.8
Pyridoxine (B_6) (μg)	115	212	4.1
Biotin (B_7) (μg)	2.7	26	?
Folate (B_9) (μg)	25	23	5.4
B_{12} (μg)	0.18	0.64	0.05
C (ascorbate) (mg)	12	25.2	<0.2

ARA indicates arachidonic acid; DHA, docosahexaenoic acid.

? = no value available

Data from the following websites:

https://www.meadjohnson.com/pediatrics/us-en/product-information/products/premature/enfamil-human-milk-fortifier-powder#nutrients

https://abbottnutrition.com/similac-human-milk-fortifier-powder

http://www.prolacta.com/Data/Sites/14/media/PDF/mkt-180-prolact-hmf-nutrition-labels.pdf

https://static.abbottnutrition.com/cms-prod/abbottnutrition-2016.com/img/Similac-Human-Milk-Fortifier-Hydrolyzed-Protein-Concentrated-Liquid.pdf

https://static.abbottnutrition.com/cms-prod/abbottnutrition-2016.com/img/Infant-and-New-Mother.pdf

https://www.meadjohnson.com/pediatrics/us-en/product-information/products/premature/enfamil-human-milk-fortifier-acidified-liquid

https://abbottnutrition.com/liquid-protein-fortifier

Similac Human Milk Fortifier Hydrolyzed Protein Concentrated Liquid (4pkts), Abbott Nutrition, Columbus, OH	Similac Liquid Human Milk Fortifier Concentrated Liquid, Abbott Nutrition, Columbus, OH	Enfamil Human Milk Fortifier Acidified Liquid (4 vials), Mead Johnson, Evansville, IN
788	788	1160
140	140	188
4	4	5.6
9.6	9.6	5.7
192	192	184
296	492	260
3.92	4.16	3.7
1.24	1.236	0.92
200	196	140
23.2	30.4	3.4
28	28	31
.52	0.32	0.64
30.8	30.8	15.2

folic acid

pantothenic acid

mEq

http://www.nafwa.org/convert2.php?name=Calcium+%28Ca%29&oneserving=&milligrams=0&name=Chlorine+%28Cl%29&oneserving=&milligrams=0&name=Magnesium+%28Mg%29&oneserving=&milligrams=0&name=Phosphorus+%28P%29&oneserving=&milligrams=0&name=Potassium+%28+K+%29&oneserving=&milligrams=0&name=Sodium+%28Na%29&oneserving=.48&milligrams=0&name=Sulfur+%28S%29&oneserving=&milligrams=0&name=Sulfate+%28SO4%29&oneserving=&milligrams=0&name=Zinc+%28Zn%29&oneserving=&milligrams=0

APP

Appendix E

E-1: Dietary Reference Intakes: Recommended Intakes for Individuals and

E-2: Dietary Reference Intakes (DRIs): Tolerable Upper Intake Levels (ULs)

APP

APPENDIX E-1
Dietary Reference Intakes: Recommended Intakes for Individuals

	Infants 0-6 mo	Infants 7-12 mo	Children 1-3 y	Children 4-8 y	Males 9-13 y	Males 14-18 y	Females 9-13 y	Females 14-18 y	Pregnancy ≤18 y	Lactation ≤18 y
Carbohydrate (g/day)	60*	95*	130	130	130	130	130	130	175	210
Total Fiber (g/day)	ND	ND	19*	25*	31*	38*	26*	26*	28*	29*
Fat (g/day)	31*	30*	ND	ND	ND	ND	ND	ND	ND	ND
n-6 Polyunsaturated Fatty Acids (g/day) (Linoleic Acid)	4.4*	4.6*	7*	10*	12*	16*	10*	11*	13*	13*
n-3 Polyunsaturated Fatty Acids (g/day) (α-Linolenic Acid)	0.5*	0.5*	0.7*	0.9*	1.2*	1.6*	1.0*	1.1*	1.4*	1.3*
Protein (g/day[a], g/kg/d)	9.1* 1.5*	11.0 1.5*	13 1.1	19 0.95	34 0.95	52 0.85	34 0.95	46 0.85	71 1.31	71 1.31
Vitamin A (µg/d)[b]	400*	500*	300	400	600	900	600	700	750	1200
Vitamin C (mg/d)	40*	50*	15	25	45	75	45	65	80	115
Vitamin D (IU/d)[c,d]	400*	400*	600	600*	600	600*	600	600	600	600
Vitamin E (mg/d)[e]	4*	5*	6	7	11	15	11	15	15	19
Vitamin K (mg/d)	2.0*	2.5*	30*	55*	60*	75*	60*	75*	75*	75*
Thiamin (mg/d)	0.2*	0.3*	0.5	0.6	0.9	1.2	0.9	1.0	1.4	1.4
Riboflavin (mg/d)	0.3*	0.4*	0.5	0.6	0.9	1.3	0.9	1.0	1.4	1.6

Nutrient										
Niacin (mg/d)[f]	2*	4*	6	8	12	16	12	14	18	17
Vitamin B6 (mg/d)	0.1*	0.3*	0.5	0.6	1.0	1.3	1.0	1.2	1.9	2.0
Folate (µg/d)[g,h,i]	65*	80*	150	200	300	400	300	400[g]	600[h]	500
Vitamin B12 (µg/d)	0.4*	0.5*	0.9	1.2	1.8	2.4	1.8	2.4	2.6	2.8
Pantothenic acid (mg/d)	1.7*	1.8*	2*	3*	4*	5*	4*	5*	6*	7*
Biotin (µg/d)	5*	6*	8*	12*	20*	25*	20*	25*	30*	35*
Choline (mg/d)[j]	125*	150*	200*	250*	375*	550*	375*	400*	450*	550*
Calcium (mg/d)	200*	260*	700	1000	1300	1300	1300	1300	1300	1300
Chromium (µg/d)	0.2*	5.5*	11*	15*	25*	35*	21*	24*	29*	44
Copper (µg/d)	200*	220*	340	440	700	890	700	890	1000	1300
Fluoride (mg/d)	0.01*	0.5*	0.7*	1*	2*	3*	2*	3*	3*	3*
Iodine (µg/d)	110*	130*	90	90	120	150	120	150	220	290
Iron (mg/d)	0.27*	11	7	10	8	11	8	15	27	10
Magnesium (mg/d)	30*	75*	80	130	240	410	240	360	400	360
Manganese (mg/d)	0.003*	0.6*	1.2*	1.5*	1.9*	2.2*	1.6*	1.6*	2.0*	2.6*
Molybdenum (µg/d)	2*	3*	17	22	34	43	34	43	50	50
Phosphorus (mg/d)	100*	275*	460	500	1250	1250	1250	1250	1250	1250
Selenium (µg/d)	15*	20*	20	30	40	55	40	55	60	70

Continued

APP

APPENDIX E-1 (Continued)

Dietary Reference Intakes: Recommended Intakes for Individuals

	Infants 0–6 mo	Infants 7–12 mo	Children 1–3 y	Children 4–8 y	Males 9–13 y	Males 14–18 y	Females 9–13 y	Females 14–18 y	Pregnancy ≤18 y	Lactation ≤18 y
Zinc (mg/d)	2*	3	3	5	8	11	8	9	12	13
Potassium (g/d)	0.4*	0.86*	2.0*	2.3*	2.5*	3.0*	2.3*	2.3*	2.6*	2.5*
Sodium (g/d)	0.11*	0.37*	0.8*	1.0*	1.2*	1.5*	1.2*	1.5*	1.5*	1.5*
Chloride (g/d)	0.18*	0.57*	1.5*	1.9*	2.3*	2.3*	2.3*	2.3*	2.3*	2.3*

NOTE: This table (adapted from the DRI reports, see www.nap.edu) presents Recommended Dietary Allowances (RDAs) in **bold type** and Adequate Intakes (AIs) in ordinary type followed by an asterisk (*). An RDA is the average daily dietary intake level sufficient to meet the nutrient requirements of nearly all (97–98%) healthy individuals in a group. It is calculated from an Estimated Average Requirement (EAR). If sufficient scientific evidence is not available to establish an EAR, and thus calculate and RDA, an AI is usually developed. For healthy breastfed infants, the AI is the mean intake. The AI for other life stage and gender groups is believed to cover needs of all individuals in the groups, but lack of data or uncertainty in the data prevent being able to specify with confidence the percentage of individuals covered by this intake.

a Based on g protein per kg of body weight for the reference body weight. Reference weights for g/kg/d taken from: Dietary Reference Intakes: The essential guide to nutrient requirements divided into smaller groupings. Based on NCHS/CDC 2000 Growth Charts. Institute of Medicine, 2006.

b As retinol activity equivalents (RAEs). 1 RAE = 1 μg retinol, 12 μg β-carotene, 24 μg α-carotene, or 24 μg β-cryptoxanthin in foods. The RAE for dietary provitamin A carotenoids is twofold greater than retinol equivalents (REs), whereas the RAE for preformed vitamin A is the same as RE.

c As cholecalciferol. 1 μg cholecalciferol = 40 IU vitamin D.

d Under the assumption of minimal sunlight.

e As α-tocopherol. α-Tocopherol includes RRR-α-tocopherol, the only form of α-tocopherol that occurs naturally in foods, and the 2R-stereoisomeric forms of α-tocopherol (RRR-, RSR-, RSR-, RRS-, and RSS-α-tocopherol) that occur in fortified foods and supplements. It does not include the 2S-stereoisomeric forms of α-tocopherol (SRR-, SSR-, SRS-, and SSS-α-tocopherol), also found in fortified foods and supplements.

f As niacin equivalents (NE). 1 mg of niacin = 60 mg of tryptophan; 0–6 months = preformed niacin (not NE).

g As dietary folate equivalents (DFE), 1 DFE=1 μg food folate = 0.6 μg of folic acid from fortified food or as a supplement consumed with food = 0.5 μg of a supplement taken on an empty stomach.

[h] In view of evidence linking folate intake with neural tube defects in the fetus, it is recommended that all women capable of becoming pregnant consume 400 µg from supplements or fortified foods in addition to intake of food folate from the diet.

[i] It is assumed that women will continue consuming 400 µg from supplements or fortified food until their pregnancy is confirmed and they enter prenatal care, which ordinarily occurs after the end of the periconceptional period-the critical time for formation of the neural tube.

[j] Although AIs have been set for choline, there are few data to assess whether a dietary supply of choline is needed at all stages of the life cycle, and it may be that the choline requirement can be met by endogenous synthesis at some of these stages.

Adapted from https://ods.od.nih.gov/Health_Information/Dietary_Reference_Intakes.aspx. Accessed May 30, 2017. Reference data for sodium and potassium accessed June 13, 2019.

APPENDIX E-2
Dietary Reference Intakes (DRIs): Tolerable Upper Intake Levels (UL[a])

	Infants 0-6 mo	Infants 7-12 mo	Children 1-3 y	Children 4-8 y	Males/Females 9-13 y	Males/Females 14-18 y	Pregnancy ≤18 y	Lactation ≤18y
Vitamin A (µg/d)[b]	600	600	600	900	1700	2800	2800	2800
Vitamin C (mg/d)	ND[f]	ND	400	650	1200	1800	1800	1800
Vitamin D (IU/d)	1000	1520	2520	3000	4000	4000	4000	4000
Vitamin E (mg/d)[c,d]	ND	ND	200	300	600	800	800	800
Vitamin K (µg/d)	ND	ND	ND	ND	ND	ND	ND	ND
Thiamin (mg/d)	ND	ND	ND	ND	ND	ND	ND	ND
Riboflavin (mg/d)	ND	ND	ND	ND	ND	ND	ND	ND
Niacin (mg/d)[d]	ND	ND	10	15	20	30	30	30
Vitamin B6 (mg/d)	ND	ND	30	40	60	80	80	80
Folate (µg/d)[d]	ND	ND	300	400	600	800	800	800
Vitamin B12 (mg/d)	ND	ND	ND	ND	ND	ND	ND	ND

Pantothenic Acid (mg/d)	ND	ND	ND	ND	ND	ND	ND	ND
Biotin (μg/d)	ND	ND	ND	ND	ND	ND	ND	ND
Choline (mg/d)	ND	ND	1.0	1.0	2.0	3.0	3.0	3.0
Carotenoids[e]	ND	ND	ND	ND	ND	ND	ND	ND
Arsenic[g]	ND[f]	ND	ND	ND	ND	ND	ND	ND
Boron (mg/d)	ND	ND	3	6	11	17	17	17
Calcium (mg/d)	1000	1500	2500	2500	3000	3000	3000	3000
Chromium	ND	ND	ND	ND	ND	ND	ND	ND
Copper (μg/d)	ND	ND	1000	3000	5000	8000	8000	8000
Fluoride (mg/d)	0.7	0.9	1.3	2.2	10	10	10	10
Iodine (μg/d)	ND	ND	200	300	600	900	900	900
Iron (mg/d)	40	40	40	40	40	45	45	45
Magnesium (mg/d)[h]	ND	ND	65	110	350	350	350	350
Manganese (mg/d)	ND	ND	2	3	6	9	9	9
Molybdenum (mg/d)	ND	ND	300	600	1100	1700	1700	1700
Nickel (mg/d)	ND	ND	0.2	0.3	0.6	1.0	1.0	1.0

Continued

APP

APPENDIX E-2 *(Continued)*
Dietary Reference Intakes (DRIs): Tolerable Upper Intake Levels (UL^a)

	Infants 0-6 mo	Infants 7-12 mo	Children 1-3 y	Children 4-8 y	Males/Females 9-13 y	Males/Females 14-18 y	Pregnancy ≤18 y	Lactation ≤18y
Phosphorus (mg/d)	ND	ND	3	3	4	4	3.5	4
Selenium (μg/d)	45	60	90	150	280	400	400	400
Silicon^i	ND	ND	ND	ND	ND	ND	ND	ND
Vanadium (mg/d)^j	ND	ND	ND	ND	ND	ND	ND	ND
Zinc (mg/d)	4	5	7	12	23	34	34	34
Sodium (g/d)	ND	ND	1.5	1.9	2.2	2.3	2.3	2.3
Chloride (g/d)	ND	ND	2.3	2.9	3.4	3.6	3.6	3.6

https://ods.od.nih.gov/Health_Information/Dietary_Reference_Intakes.aspx
Accessed 5/30/2017

^{a} UL = The highest level of daily nutrient intake that is likely to pose no risk of adverse health effects to almost all individuals in the general population. Unless otherwise specified, the UL represents total intake from food, water, and supplements. Due to lack of suitable data, ULs could not be established for vitamin K, thiamin, riboflavin, vitamin B$_{12}$, pantothenic acid, biotin, or carotenoids. In the absence of a UL, extra caution may be warranted in consuming levels above recommended intakes. Members of the general population should be advised not to routinely exceed the UL. The UL is not meant to apply to individuals who are treated with the nutrient under medical supervision or to individuals with predisposing conditions that modify their sensitivity to the nutrient.

^{b} As preformed vitamin A only.

^{c} As α-tocopherol; applies to any form of supplemental a-tocopherol.

^{d} The ULs for vitamin E, niacin, and folate apply to synthetic forms obtained from supplements, fortified foods, or a combination of the two.

e β-Carotene supplements are advised only to serve as a provitamin A source for individuals at risk of vitamin A deficiency.

f ND = Not determinable due to lack of data of adverse effects in this age group and concern with regard to lack of ability to handle excess amounts. Source of intake should be from food only to prevent high levels of intake.

g Although the UL was not determined for arsenic, there is no justification for adding arsenic to food or supplements.

h The ULs for magnesium represent intake from a pharmacological agent only and do not include intake from food and water.

i Although silicon has not been shown to cause adverse effects in humans, there is no justification for adding silicon to supplements.

j Although vanadium in food has not been shown to cause adverse effects in humans, there is no justification for adding vanadium to food and vanadium supplements should be used with caution. The UL is based on adverse effects in laboratory animals and this data could be used to set a UL for adults but not children and adolescents.

APP

Appendix F

ChooseMyPlate

Fig F.1.
ChooseMyPlate

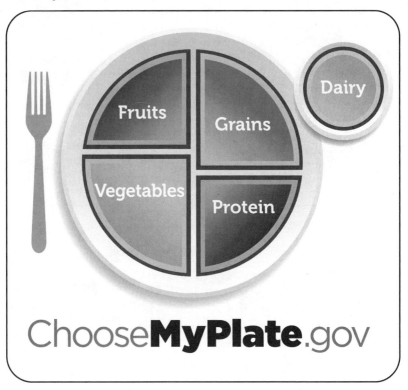

Fig F.2.
Healthy Eating for Preschoolers

United States Department of Agriculture

Get your child on the path to healthy eating.

Offer a variety of healthy foods.
Choose foods from each MyPlate food group. Pay attention to dairy foods, whole grains, and vegetables to build healthy habits that will last a lifetime.

Be mindful of sweet drinks and other foods.
Offer water instead of sugary drinks like regular soda and fruit drinks. Other foods like hot dogs, burgers, pizza, cookies, cakes, and candy are only occasional treats.

Focus on the meal and each other.
Your child learns by watching you. Let your child choose how much to eat of foods you provide. Children copy your likes, dislikes, and your interest in trying new foods.

Be patient with your child.
Children enjoy food when eating it is their own choice. Some new foods take time. Give a taste at first and wait a bit. Let children serve themselves by taking small amounts. Offer new foods many times.

Cook together.
Eat together.
Talk together.
Make meal time family time.

FNS-451
Revised December 2016

Healthy Eating for Preschoolers

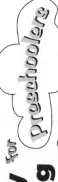
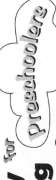
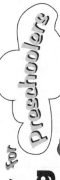

Dairy

Grains

Protein

Fruits

Vegetables

ChooseMyPlate.gov

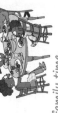

Food and Nutrition Service
USDA is an equal opportunity provider and employer.

Based on the Dietary Guidelines for Americans.

Healthy *for* Eating *preschoolers* Daily Food Checklist

Use this Checklist as a general guide.

- This food checklist is based on average needs. Do not be concerned if your child does not eat the exact amounts suggested. Your child may need more or less than average. For example, food needs increase during growth spurts.

- Children's appetites vary from day to day. Some days they may eat less than these amounts; other days they may want more. Let your child choose how much to eat. Throughout a day, offer amounts shown below.

Food group	2 year olds	3 year olds	4 and 5 year olds	What counts as:
Fruits Focus on whole fruits	1 cup	1 – 1½ cups	1 – 1½ cups	**½ cup of fruit?** ½ cup mashed, sliced, or chopped fruit ½ cup 100% fruit juice ½ small banana 4-5 large strawberries
Vegetables Vary your veggies	1 cup	1 – 1½ cups	1½ – 2 cups	**½ cup of veggies?** ½ cup mashed, sliced, or chopped vegetables 1 cup raw leafy greens ½ cup vegetable juice 1 small ear of corn
Grains Make half your grains whole grains	3 ounces	3 – 5 ounces	4 – 5 ounces	**1 ounce of grains?** 1 slice bread 1 cup ready-to-eat cereal flakes ½ cup cooked oatmeal, rice, or pasta 1 tortilla (6" across)
Protein Foods Vary your protein routine	2 ounces	2 – 4 ounces	3 – 5 ounces	**1 ounce of protein foods?** 1 ounce cooked meat, poultry, or seafood 1 egg 1 Tablespoon peanut butter ¼ cup cooked beans or peas (kidney, pinto, lentils)
Dairy Choose low-fat or fat-free milk or yogurt	2 cups	2 – 2½ cups	2½ cups	**½ cup of dairy?** ½ cup milk 4 ounces yogurt ¾ ounce cheese

Some foods are easy to choke on while eating. Children need to sit when eating. Foods like hot dogs, grapes, and raw carrots need to be cut into small pieces the size of a nickel. Be alert if serving 3- to 5-year-olds foods like popcorn, nuts, seeds, or other hard foods.

There are many ways to divide the Daily Food Checklist into meals and snacks. View the 'Meal and Snack Patterns and Ideas' to see how these amounts might look on your preschooler's plate at www.ChooseMyPlate.gov/preschoolers-meal-and-snack-patterns.

APP

Fig F.3.
MyPlate Daily Checklist

United States Department of Agriculture

MyPlate Daily Checklist

Find your Healthy Eating Style

Everything you eat and drink matters. Find your healthy eating style that reflects your preferences, culture, traditions, and budget—and maintain it for a lifetime! The right mix can help you be healthier now and into the future. The key is choosing a variety of foods and beverages from each food group—*and making sure that each choice is limited in saturated fat, sodium, and added sugars*. Start with small changes—**"MyWins"**—to make healthier choices you can enjoy.

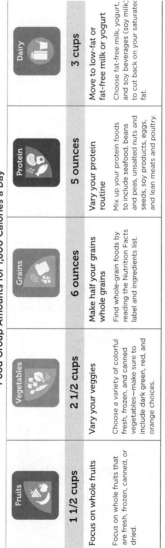

Food Group Amounts for 1,800 Calories a Day

Fruits	Vegetables	Grains	Protein	Dairy
1 1/2 cups	**2 1/2 cups**	**6 ounces**	**5 ounces**	**3 cups**
Focus on whole fruits	Vary your veggies	Make half your grains whole grains	Vary your protein routine	Move to low-fat or fat-free milk or yogurt
Focus on whole fruits that are fresh, frozen, canned, or dried.	Choose a variety of colorful fresh, frozen, and canned vegetables—make sure to include dark green, red, and orange choices.	Find whole-grain foods by reading the Nutrition Facts label and ingredients list.	Mix up your protein foods to include seafood, beans and peas, unsalted nuts and seeds, soy products, eggs, and lean meats and poultry.	Choose fat-free milk, yogurt, and soy beverages (soy milk) to cut back on your saturated fat.

Limit

Drink and eat less sodium, saturated fat, and added sugars. Limit:
- Sodium to **2,300 milligrams** a day.
- Saturated fat to **20 grams** a day.
- Added sugars to **45 grams** a day.

Be active your way: Children 6 to 17 years old should move **60 minutes** every day. Adults should be physically active at least **2 1/2 hours** per week.
Use SuperTracker to create a personal plan based on your age, sex, height, weight, and physical activity level.
SuperTracker.usda.gov

Pediatric Nutrition, 8th Edition

MyPlate Daily Checklist

Write down the foods you ate today and track your daily MyPlate, MyWins!

Food group targets for a 1,800 calorie* pattern are:

	Write your food choices for each food group	Did you reach your target?

Fruits

1 1/2 cups

1 cup of fruits counts as
- 1 cup raw or cooked fruit; or
- 1/2 cup dried fruit; or
- 1 cup 100% fruit juice.

[Y] [N]

Vegetables

2 1/2 cups

1 cup vegetables counts as
- 1 cup raw or cooked vegetables; or
- 2 cups leafy salad greens; or
- 1 cup 100% vegetable juice.

[Y] [N]

Grains

6 ounce equivalents

1 ounce of grains counts as
- 1 slice bread; or
- 1 ounce ready-to-eat cereal; or
- 1/2 cup cooked rice, pasta, or cereal.

[Y] [N]

Protein

5 ounce equivalents

1 ounce of protein counts as
- 1 ounce lean meat, poultry, or seafood; or
- 1 egg; or
- 1 Tbsp peanut butter; or
- 1/4 cup cooked beans or peas; or
- 1/2 ounce nuts or seeds.

[Y] [N]

Dairy

3 cups

1 cup of dairy counts as
- 1 cup milk; or
- 1 cup yogurt; or
- 1 cup fortified soy beverage; or
- 1 1/2 ounces natural cheese or 2 ounces processed cheese.

[Y] [N]

MyWins Track your MyPlate, MyWins

Limit:
- Sodium to **2,300 milligrams** a day.
- Saturated fat to **20 grams** a day.
- Added sugars to **45 grams** a day.

[Y] [N]

Be active your way:

Adults:
- Be physically active at least 2 1/2 hours per week.

Children 6 to 17 years old:
- Move at least **60 minutes** every day.

[Y] [N]

* This 1,800 calorie pattern is only an estimate of your needs. Monitor your body weight and adjust your calories if needed.

Center for Nutrition Policy and Promotion
January 2016
USDA is an equal opportunity provider and employer.

Fig F.4.
Eat Smart To Play Hard

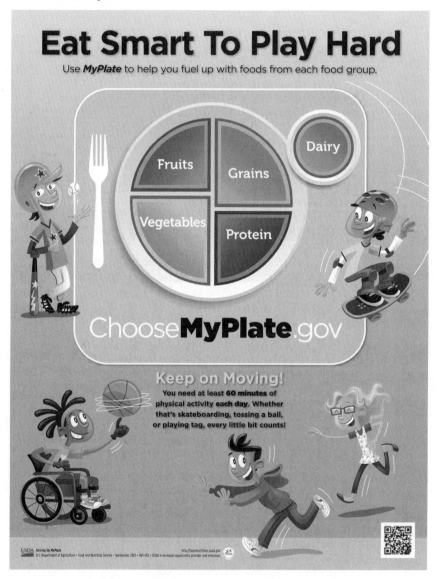

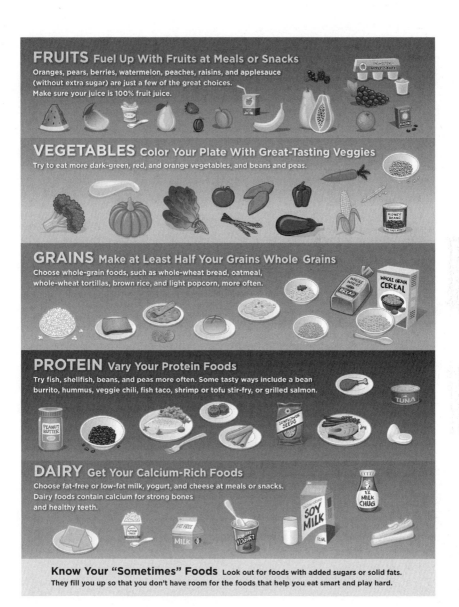

FRUITS Fuel Up With Fruits at Meals or Snacks

Oranges, pears, berries, watermelon, peaches, raisins, and applesauce (without extra sugar) are just a few of the great choices. Make sure your juice is 100% fruit juice.

VEGETABLES Color Your Plate With Great-Tasting Veggies

Try to eat more dark-green, red, and orange vegetables, and beans and peas.

GRAINS Make at Least Half Your Grains Whole Grains

Choose whole-grain foods, such as whole-wheat bread, oatmeal, whole-wheat tortillas, brown rice, and light popcorn, more often.

PROTEIN Vary Your Protein Foods

Try fish, shellfish, beans, and peas more often. Some tasty ways include a bean burrito, hummus, veggie chili, fish taco, shrimp or tofu stir-fry, or grilled salmon.

DAIRY Get Your Calcium-Rich Foods

Choose fat-free or low-fat milk, yogurt, and cheese at meals or snacks. Dairy foods contain calcium for strong bones and healthy teeth.

Know Your "Sometimes" Foods Look out for foods with added sugars or solid fats. They fill you up so that you don't have room for the foods that help you eat smart and play hard.

APP

Appendix G

Food-Drug Interactions

Drug-drug interactions are frequently known and evaluated appropriately if significant. Drug-food, also known as drug-nutrient, interactions are less recognized with few exceptions. Food-drug interactions are significant if they affect nutritional status or alter a response to a medication. Additionally, supplements and herbals can affect drug absorption or metabolism.

Nutritional status such as obesity or malnutrition can alter drug distribution and clearance and even affect drug concentration.

Foods that affect drugs and decrease bioavailability can lead to treatment failure. If bioavailability is increased, then there can be adverse effects and associated toxicities.

Drugs can affect food intake. Some medications lead to altered sense of taste or smell, which can cause one to change eating habits. Other drugs may cause nausea, vomiting, anorexia, diarrhea, and constipation, all of which may lead to malnutrition.

Drug inactivation can occur when drugs and nutrients are both given intravenously. To avoid this, it is best to administer drugs via a different intravenous line or at a different time then the IV nutrition. Most oral drugs should not be mixed with enteral nutrition formulas. If medications are administered via tubes, the tube should be flushed before and after medication administration. Some medications need to be separated from tube feeds by 1 to 3 hours. Many medications should not be crushed if administered via tubes, because they can clog the tube. In general, long-acting preparations cannot be crushed for tube administration. For some medications, absorption is affected by site of administration, and thus, consideration of gastrostomy versus jejunostomy tube needs to be considered. There are also some liquid medications that contain ethyl alcohol, which can alter food intake and tastes.

Many foods can affect cytochrome P450 enzyme, which metabolizes many drugs. The discovery that grapefruit juice affects this enzyme system more than 20 years ago has led to much more attention paid to these interactions.

Recently, it has been discovered that other foods can affect the cytochrome P450 system. These include pomegranates, Seville oranges, black pepper, cranberry juice, grape juices, black tea, cruciferous vegetables, lava, licorice root, wine, and olive oil. The amounts needed to be consumed are unknown, but if ingested in usual dietary quantities, these are not currently considered problematic.

APP

There are many articles describing tyramine with monoamine oxidase inhibitors (MAOIs), the combination of which can increase blood pressure. Giving blood thinners with vitamin K-rich foods will cause the blood thinners to be less active or even inactive.

Grapefruit juice and medication interactions are drug not class specific. One grapefruit, or 240 mL (8oz), can cause reduction in CYP450 system for up to 4 days. Specifically, the CYP3A4 is affected. Additionally, even if medication is taken 24 hours after grapefruit ingestion, absorption of the drug will still be increased.

It is important to be aware of foods that can have an effect on specific medications.

Bananas are rich in potassium, as are some salt substitutes. Kale, green leafy vegetables including spinach, Brussel sprouts, and broccoli contain potassium. Care should be taken if combined with diuretics that are potassium sparing.

Some foods are rich in vitamin K and should be avoided if using blood thinners such as warfarin. This combination will affect the amount of blood thinning that occurs. It is best to avoid kale, broccoli, cabbage, and spinach.

Black licorice is uncommon in the United States. Licorice flavor does not impact these medications. It can make some drugs less effective, including oral contraceptive pills. Licorice root, an herbal remedy for some gastrointestinal ailments, should be avoided if using oral contraceptive pills. According to Drugs.com (2017), there are 198 moderate drug interactions with licorice root.

Milk contains calcium, as do other dairy products. Dairy products with calcium can interact with tetracyclines and quinolones.

Grapefruit interaction was discovered more than 20 years ago. 85 drugs and probably more are known to interact with grapefruit. Approximately ½ of these interactions are of a serious nature. As new drugs are brought to market the number of interactions is expected to rise. One 8 oz glass (240 mL) of grapefruit juice can significantly impact bioavailability of drugs. Repeated ingestion of grapefruit juice is additive. While it's best to avoid grapefruit juice and grapefruits while on many medications if it can't be avoided it's best to allow maximal time between the medication and the grapefruit juice.

Many foods contain tyramine, including salami, cheese, avocados, chocolate, red wine, and anchovies. These can cause BP to increase when combined with MAOIs.

APPENDIX G-1:
Food-Drug Interactions by Class

Class	Drug	Interaction
Analgesics		
Anti-inflammatory miscellaneous	Acetaminophen	Food delays absorption but not extent. Food may decrease GI upset.
	Salsalate, sulfasalazine	Take with food.
Nonsteroidal anti-inflammatory		Take with food and a full glass of water to minimize GI side effects.
	Ibuprofen, naproxen, diclofenac, indomethacin	If on high dose, may need extra vitamin C, vitamin K, and folic acid.
	Aspirin	Avoid products that can affect blood coagulation (garlic, ginger). Salicylate accumulation can occur if combined with tea, raisins, or prunes. Fresh fruit can increase the excretion of aspirin. Curry powder, paprika, and licorice contain a small amount of salicylate and intake should be limited.
Narcotic analgesics		Take with food.
Angiotensin-converting enzyme inhibitors (ACE-I)		Take on an empty stomach as food can decrease absorption. Avoid salt, calcium, and natural licorice.
	Captopril	Zinc deficiency with long-term use, which can alter taste perception.
	Quinapril	High-fat meals decrease absorption.

Continued

APPENDIX G-1: *Continued*
Food-Drug Interactions by Class

Class	Drug	Interaction
Anticonvulsants	Carbamazepine	Take with food or milk. Avoid grapefruit juice and other citrus fruits. May need vitamin D and calcium supplementation. Absorption decreased by fiber.
	Valproic acid, divalproex	May administer with food to decrease GI adverse effects.
Anti-arrhythmic	Digoxin	Fiber may decrease absorption. Food delays but does not decrease extent of absorption.
Anticoagulant	Warfarin	Limit foods containing vitamin K. High doses of vitamin E may increase risk of bleeding. Avoid garlic and ginger.
Antidepressant		
Benzodiazepines	Lorazepam, diazepam, alprazolam	Limit grapefruit juice and citrus consumption. Can take with or without food.
Monoamine oxidase inhibitors	Phenelzine, tranylcypromine	Follow physician's directions regarding diet exactly. Fatal blood pressure increase can occur. The following should be avoided while on these medications and for 2 weeks after discontinued. Avoid alcohol and tyramine-containing foods. Avoid aged cheese, aged meat, soy sauce, tofu, miso, fava beans, snow peas, sauerkraut, avocadoes, bananas, yeast extracts, raisins, ginseng, licorice, chocolate, and caffeine.
	Lithium	To decrease gastrointestinal adverse effects, may administer with food.

Tricyclic antidepressants	Trazodone	Short acting: give after a meal or snack to reduce postural hypotension, sedation. Extended release: take on an empty stomach.
	Amitriptyline, doxepin, imipramine	Fiber may decrease blood levels.
Antidiabetic	Metformin, glyburide	Fiber may reduce absorption.
	Glipizide	Extended release take with breakfast. Immediate release. Take 30 minutes before a meal (usually breakfast).
Antihistamine		Take with food if GI distress.
	Fexofenadine	Avoid grapefruit, orange, and apple juice as they decrease bioavailability.
Anti-infectives		Some can reduce effectiveness of oral contraceptives.
HIV	Amprenavir	Bioavailability decreased if administered with high fat meal
	Didanosine	Best if taken 30 minutes before or 2 hours after a meal.
	Efavirenz	Take on an empty stomach. Food may cause adverse effects and increase drug concentration.
	Indinavir	Take 1 hour before or 2 hours after a meal. If combined with ritonavir may take with food.
	Nelfinavir	To improve bioavailability, take with food. Tablets can be dissolved in water, or crushed and administered in pudding or other nonacidic foods.
	Ritonavir	Give with meals to improve palatability. Liquid is highly concentrated and tastes poorly. Best to save for patients on tube feedings.

Continued

APP

APPENDIX G-1: *Continued*
Food-Drug Interactions by Class

Class	Drug	Interaction
HIV *Continued*	Saquinavir	To increase absorption, should give within 2 hours of a meal.
	Tenofovir disoproxil fumarate	Powder must be administered with food, applesauce, baby food, yogurt. Does not dissolve in liquid. Tablets can be taken regardless of meals.
Antiprotozoal	Atovaquone	Administer with a high-fat meal.
Penicillins	Penicillin, amoxicillin, ampicillin	Take on an empty stomach, but if upsets take with food. Avoid guar gum fiber as it may reduce penicillin absorption.
	Amoxicillin and clavulanate (Augmentin)	Can give regardless of meals. To decrease gastrointestinal adverse effects, take at the start of a meal. May mix with milk, formula, or juice.
	Cloxacillin, dicloxacillin	Take 1 hour before or 2 hours after a meal
Cephalosporins	Cephalexin, cefaclor, cefixime, cefprozil, cefadroxil	Take on an empty stomach unless upsets stomach. Take medicine 1 hour before antacids.
	Ceftibuten	Capsule administer with/without food. Suspension: administer 2 hours before or 2 hours after a meal.
	Cefpodoxime	Food increase absorption
	Cefuroxime	Suspension take with food. Tablet can take with food if gastrointestinal upset.

Macrolides	Azithromycin, clarithromycin, erythromycin	Take with food if stomach upset. Azithromycin should be taken on an empty stomach. Avoid carbonated drinks and citrus. Avoid antacids with all except for extended-release azithromycin.
	Metronidazole	Avoid alcohol, take with food to decrease gastrointestinal upset but extended-release preparation should be taken on an empty stomach.
Quinolones	Ciprofloxacin, levofloxacin	Preferably take on an empty stomach, but taking with food will minimize gastrointestinal distress. Do not take with dairy or calcium-fortified products or fruit juices fortified with calcium. Can increase levels of caffeine causing excitability and nervousness.
Sulfonamides	Sulfamethoxazole	Take with food and lots of water.
Tetracyclines	Tetracycline, doxycycline, minocycline	Take on an empty stomach. Avoid dairy products, antacids, iron, and multivitamins containing iron as they can interfere with medications effectiveness.
Antifungals	Amphotericin B	May decrease availability of magnesium, potassium, sodium, and liposomal amphotericin B. May also cause hyperglycemia.
	Fluconazole, ketoconazole	Take with food to increase absorption.
	Griseofulvin	Administer with a fatty meal to increase absorption and to avoid gastrointestinal upset.
	Itraconazole	Do not take with grapefruit juice. Do not administer with antacids. Capsule and tablet should be taken with food but solution should be taken on an empty stomach.
	Ketoconazole	Take 2 hours before antacids to avoid decreasing absorption.

Continued

APP

APPENDIX G-1: *Continued*
Food-Drug Interactions by Class

Class	Drug	Interaction
Miscellaneous		
	Chloroquine hydroxychloroquine	To decrease gastrointestinal upset, can administer with food. The chloroquine phosphate tablets have a bitter taste that can be masked by mixing in chocolate syrup.
	Ethambutol	May take with food to decrease gastrointestinal irritation.
	Isoniazid	Take on an empty stomach as food will decrease bioavailability.
	Nitrofurantoin	Administer with food to reduce gastrointestinal distress. Suspension may be mixed with formula, milk, water, or fruit juice
	Rifampin	Administer 1 hour before or 2 hours after meals on an empty stomach to increase absorption.
Beta Blockers	Atenolol, carvedilol, metoprolol, propranolol	Take with food to increase bioavailability. Food may also decrease the risk of orthostatic hypotension. Avoid natural licorice; take 2 hours before or 6 hours after calcium supplement. Do not take with orange juice.
Bronchodilators		
	Albuterol	Take with food if GI distress. May cause hyperglycemia and hypokalemia
	Theophylline	High-fat meals increase levels and high carbohydrate meals may decrease drug level. Avoid or limit caffeine intake .
	Zafirlukast	Administer 1 hour before or 2 hours after meals. Bioavailability reduced 40% by food.

Calcium channel blockers	Diltiazem	Take before meals.
	Nifedipine	Can be administered with or without food.
Corticosteroids	Fludrocortisone, hydrocortisone, prednisone, prednisolone	Take with food or milk to decrease upset stomach. May want to decrease sodium intake. Limit grapefruit juice.
	Spironolactone, triamterene	Potassium sparing diuretics avoid potassium-rich foods.
Cholesterol-lowering agents	Simvastatin	Take with food, avoid grapefruit juice. Best taken with evening meal to increase absorption.
	Cholestyramine	May require supplementation of folic acid, iron, as well as vitamins A, D, E, and K, with long-term use or high doses. Powder must be mixed in a liquid. Do not sip or hold in mouth as it can discolor teeth or cause decay of enamel.
Diuretics	Furosemide, hydrochlorothiazide	Food reduces bioavailability but if gastrointestinal distress, take with food. May need supplemental potassium, calcium, and magnesium. Avoid natural licorice.
	Triamterene, spironolactone, amiloride	Avoid eating foods containing lots of potassium.
Electrolytes	Potassium–all salts	Administer with meals and a full glass of water

Continued

APP

APPENDIX G-1: *Continued*
Food-Drug Interactions by Class

Class	Drug	Interaction
Gastrointestinal		
H2 blockers	Famotidine	May administer with antacids, iron, and food.
Proton pump inhibitors (PPI)	Lansoprazole, omeprazole	Take 30 minutes before meals.
Immunosuppresants		
	Mycophenolate	Take 1 hour before or 2 hours after meals.
	Tacrolimus	Can be taken with or without food. Extended-release prop should be taken on an empty stomach.
Miscellaneous		
Iron salts	Ferrous sulfate, gluconate	Take on empty stomach, 2 hours before or 4 hours after antacids.
Alendronate		Take with plain water 30 minutes before a morning meal.
Allopurinol		Take after meals with plenty of fluids.
Sevelamer		Give with food. Give 1 hour before or 3 hours after other medications.

APPENDIX G-2:
Grapefruit-Drug Interactions

Drug or Drug Class	Effect of Grapefruit Juice on Drug Level	Implications/Significance	Specific Medications Within a Class
Acetbutolol	Can decrease area under the curve (AUC)	Separate by 4 hours but may not be clinically significant	
Aliskiren	Decrease in AUC by up to 60%	Separate by 4 hours	
Amlodipine	Increase levels	Moderate effect, monitor blood pressure	
Amiodarone	Bioavailability increased by 50%	Avoid grapefruit juice	
Atorvastatin	Can increase serum concentration	Avoid quantities >1 qt/day	
Apixaban	Increase	May increase bleeding; drink grapefruit juice with caution	
Budesonide oral tablet or capsule	Increase significantly	Avoid grapefruit juice	
Buspirone	Increase drug levels	Avoid >1 qt per day of grapefruit juice, increase risk of sedation or dizziness	

Continued

APP

APPENDIX G-2: *Continued*
Grapefruit-Drug Interactions

Drug or Drug Class	Effect of Grapefruit Juice on Drug Level	Implications/Significance	Specific Medications Within a Class
Calcium channel blockers	Increase levels with some but varies	Can develop tachycardia, severe hypotension, flushing; current opinion is to avoid grapefruit juice with all	Amlodipine, diltiazem, felodipine, nicardipine, nifedipine, nimodipine, nisoldipine, verapamil
Carbamazepine	Increase levels	Avoid grapefruit juice	
Clomipramine	Increase level and perhaps toxicity	Avoid grapefruit juice	
Cilostazol	Increase levels and toxicity	Avoid grapefruit juice	
Clopidogrel	Reduce effectiveness	600 mL grapefruit juice reduces effectiveness of clopidogrel; avoid or minimal consumption	
Colchicine	Increase	Avoid grapefruit juice	
Cyclosporine	Increases	Avoid grapefruit juice	
Dronedarone	Increase significantly	Avoid grapefruit juice	
Erythromycin	Possibly increase in AUC and peak	Avoid grapefruit juice or choose a different antibiotic	
Fentanyl oral, transmucosal	Peak effects delayed	Avoid grapefruit juice with Actiq or Lazanda	
Fexofenadine	Decrease bioavailability	Avoid grapefruit juice	

3-hydroxy-3-methyl-glutaryl-coenzyme A (HMG-CoA) reductase inhibitors	Absorption and drug levels increased for many in this class	Headache, gastrointestinal complaints and muscle pain can occur; avoid grapefruit juice; pravastatin, rosuvastatin and fluvastatin are not affected by grapefruit juice	Atorvastatin, lovastatin, simvastatin,
Itraconazole	Increase	Avoid grapefruit juice	
Levothyroxine	Decrease absorption	Avoid grapefruit juice	
Methadone	Increase	Avoid grapefruit juice	
Midazolam but not other benzodiazepines	Increase	Avoid grapefruit juice	Other benzodiazepines are not affected Diazepam
Pimozide	Increase	Avoid grapefruit juice	
Primaquine	Increase in AUC and peak level	Avoid grapefruit juice; risk of myelotoxicity	
Quinidine	Decreased rate of absorption	Avoid grapefruit juice	
Rilpivirine	Increase	Avoid grapefruit juice as increased risk of toxicity	
Sildenafil	Increase serum level	Avoid grapefruit juice, may increase risk of toxicity	
Sirolimus	Decrease clearance	Avoid grapefruit juice	
Tacrolimus	Increase level	Avoid grapefruit juice; if used concomitantly, monitor for toxicity	
Zolpidem	Increase level	Avoid grapefruit juice	

APP

References

1. Lexi-Comp Online. Pediatric & Neonatal Lexi-Drugs online. Hudson, OH: Lexi-Comp Inc; May 2017

2. Boullata JJ. Drug and nutrition interactions: not just food for thought. *J Clin Pharm Ther.* 2013;38:269–271

3. Genser D. Food and drug Interactions: consequences for the nutrition/health status. *Ann Nutr Metab.* 2008;52(Suppl 1):29–32

4. Webb D. When food and drugs collide-studies expose interactions between certain foods and medications. *Today's Dietitian.* 2010;12(12):26–31

5. Bailey DG. Grapefruit – medication interactions: forbidden fruit or avoidable consequences. *Can Med Assoc J.* 2013;185(4):309–316

6. Potential drug interactions with grapefruit. *Pharmacist's Letter.* 2013;29(1):290101

Calories and Electrolytes in Beverages

Beverages Calories and Selected Electrolytes (per fl oz)[a]				
Beverage	Energy, kcal	Sodium, mg	Potassium, mg	Phosphorous, mg
Regular Soft Drinks				
Cola or pepper cola	13	1–3	0–2	3
Decaffeinated cola	13	1	2	3
Lemon-lime (clear)	12	3	0	0
Orange	15	4	1	0
Grape	13	5	0	0
Root beer	13	4	0	0
Ginger ale	10	2	0	0
Tonic water	10	2	0	0
Diet Soft Drinks				
Diet cola or pepper cola	1	1–2	2	3
Decaffeinated diet cola or pepper cola	0	1	2	3
Diet lemon-lime	0	2	1	0
Diet root beer Club soda, seltzer, and sparkling water	0 0	5 6	3 1	1 0
Juices				
Apricot nectar, canned	18	1	36	3
Apple juice, unsweetened	14	1	31	2
Cranberry juice cocktail, bottled Cranberry juice (100% juice) Cranberry juice, diet Fruit Punch	17 14 1 15	1 2 2 12	4 23 2 10	0 2 0 1
Grape juice, canned, unsweetened	19	2	33	4

Continued

Calories and Electrolytes in Beverages

Beverages Calories and Selected Electrolytes (per fl oz)[a]			
Beverage	**Energy, kcal**	**Sodium, mg**	**Potassium, mg**	**Phosphorous, mg**
---	---	---	---	---
Grapefruit juice, canned, unsweetened	12	0	47	3
Orange juice, with or without pulp	15	1	55	15
Pear nectar, canned	19	1	4	1
Peach nectar, canned	17	2	12	2
Pineapple juice, canned, unsweetened Pomegranate juice Strawberry & Watermelon blend Juicy Juice	17 17 15	1 3 2	41 67 34	3 3 0
Tomato juice, canned, without salt added	5 7	3 12	70 5	5 3
Sports (electrolyte) Drinks	10 2	13 13	5 4	0 2
Gatorade Powerade G2 Powerade Zero Vitamin Water Zero Pedialyte	0 0 3 0 0 20	13 0 32 1 1 10	3 44 24 15 11 45	0 0 3 1 0 20
Caffeinated Drinks	0	1	0	0
Coffee Tea Iced coffee (mocha, milk-based) Iced tea, bottled, unsweetened Iced tea, sweetened Sweetened tea beverage (Arizona, Arnold Palmer) Energy drink	0 11 12 14 13 24 64	1 6 1 3 1 1 0	0 6 3 1 8 29 1	0 8 0 0 4 6 1
Alcohol Beer Wine Gin, rum, vodka, whiskey (80 proof)				

[a] From US Department of Agriculture, Agricultural Research Service, Nutrient Data Laboratory. USDA National Nutrient Database for Standard Reference, Release 28. September 2015; Revised May 2016. Available at: https://ndb.nal.usda.gov/ndb/search/list. Accessed April 19, 2017

Relevant AAP Policy Statements/Clinical Reports:

Policy Statement: Fruit Juice in Infants, Children and Adolescents: Current Recommendations. *Pediatrics*. 2017;139(6):e20170967

Clinical Report: Sports Drinks and Energy Drinks for Children and Adolescents: Are They Appropriate? *Pediatrics*. 2011;127(6):118201189 (Reaffirmed July 2017)

Clinical Report: Nonnutritive Sweeteners in Children
Committee on Nutrition, Section on Gastroentrology, Hepatology and Nutrition
Approved and in press; expected fall 2019

Policy Statement: Public Policy to Protect Children from the Health Effects of Added Sugars
Section on Obesity, Committee on Nutrition, American Heart Association
Intent Stage

APP

Dietary Fiber: Food Sources Ranked by Amounts of Dietary Fiber and Energy per Standard Food Portions and per 100 g of Foods

Food	Standard Portion Size	Calories in Standard Portion[a]	Dietary Fiber in Standard Portion (g)[a]	Calories per 100 g[a]
High fiber bran ready-to-eat cereal	⅓–¾ cup	60–81	9.1–14.3	200–260
Navy beans, cooked	½ cup	127	9.6	140
Small white beans, cooked	½ cup	127	9.3	142
Yellow beans, cooked	½ cup	127	9.2	144
Shredded wheat ready-to-eat cereal (various)	1–1 ¼ cup	155–220	5.0–9.0	321–373
Cranberry (roman) beans, cooked	½ cup	120	8.9	136
Adzuki beans, cooked	½ cup	147	8.4	128
French beans, cooked	½ cup	114	8.3	129
Split peas, cooked	½ cup	114	8.1	116
Chickpeas, canned	½ cup	176	8.1	139
Lentils, cooked	½ cup	115	7.8	116
Pinto beans, cooked	½ cup	122	7.7	143
Black turtle beans, cooked	½ cup	120	7.7	130

Continued

APP

Appendix I *Continued*

Dietary Fiber: Food Sources Ranked by Amounts of Dietary Fiber and Energy per Standard Food Portions and per 100 g of Foods

Food	Standard Portion Size	Calories in Standard Portion[a]	Dietary Fiber in Standard Portion (g)[a]	Calories per 100 g[a]
Mung beans, cooked	½ cup	106	7.7	105
Black beans, cooked	½ cup	114	7.5	132
Artichoke, globe or French, cooked	½ cup	45	7.2	53
Lima beans, cooked	½ cup	108	6.6	115
Great northern beans, canned	½ cup	149	6.4	114
White beans, canned	½ cup	149	6.3	114
Kidney beans, all types, cooked	½ cup	112	5.7	127
Pigeon peas, cooked	½ cup	102	5.6	121
Cowpeas, cooked	½ cup	99	5.6	116
Wheat bran flakes ready-to-eat cereal (various)	¾ cup	90–98	4.9–5.5	310–328
Pear, raw	1 medium	101	5.5	57
Pumpkin seeds, whole, roasted	1 ounce	126	5.2	446
Baked beans, canned, plain	½ cup	119	5.2	94
Soybeans, cooked	½ cup	149	5.2	173
Plain rye wafer crackers	2 wafers	73	5.0	334
Avocado	½ cup	120	5.0	160

Food	Standard Portion Size	Calories in Standard Portion[a]	Dietary Fiber in Standard Portion (g)[a]	Calories per 100 g[a]
Broadbeans (fava beans), cooked	½ cup	94	4.6	110
Pink beans, cooked	½ cup	126	4.5	149
Apple, with skin	1 medium	95	4.4	52
Green peas, cooked (fresh, frozen, canned)	½ cup	59–67	3.5–4.4	69–84
Refried beans, canned	½ cup	107	4.4	90
Chia seeds, dried	1 Tbsp	58	4.1	486
Bulgur, cooked	½ cup	76	4.1	83
Mixed vegetables, cooked from frozen	½ cup	59	4.0	65
Raspberries	½ cup	32	4.0	52
Blackberries	½ cup	31	3.8	43
Collards, cooked	½ cup	32	3.8	33
Soybeans, green, cooked	½ cup	127	3.8	141
Prunes, stewed	½ cup	133	3.8	107
Sweet potato, baked in skin	1 medium	103	3.8	90
Figs, dried	¼ cup	93	3.7	249
Pumpkin, canned	½ cup	42	3.6	34
Potato, baked, with skin	1 medium	163	3.6	94
Popcorn, air-popped	3 cups	93	3.5	387
Almonds	1 ounce	164	3.5	579

Continued

APP

Appendix I *Continued*

Dietary Fiber: Food Sources Ranked by Amounts of Dietary Fiber and Energy per Standard Food Portions and per 100 g of Foods

Food	Standard Portion Size	Calories in Standard Portion[a]	Dietary Fiber in Standard Portion (g)[a]	Calories per 100 g[a]
Pears, dried	¼ cup	118	3.4	262
Whole wheat spaghetti, cooked	½ cup	87	3.2	124
Parsnips, cooked	½ cup	55	3.1	71
Sunflower seed kernels, dry roasted	1 ounce	165	3.1	582
Orange	1 medium	69	3.1	49
Banana	1 medium	105	3.1	89
Guava	1 fruit	37	3.0	68
Oat bran muffin	1 small	178	3.0	270
Pearled barley, cooked	½ cup	97	3.0	123
Winter squash, cooked	½ cup	38	2.9	37
Dates	¼ cup	104	2.9	282
Pistachios, dry roasted	1 ounce	161	2.8	567
Pecans, oil roasted	1 ounce	203	2.7	715
Hazelnuts or filberts	1 ounce	178	2.7	628
Peanuts, oil roasted	1 ounce	170	2.7	599
Whole wheat paratha bread	1 ounce	92	2.7	326
Quinoa, cooked	½ cup	111	2.6	120

[a] Source: US Department of Agriculture, Agricultural Research Service, Nutrient Data Laboratory. 2014. USDA National Nutrient Database for Standard Reference, Release 27. Available at: http://www.ars.usda.gov/nutrientdata.

Approximate Calcium Contents of 1 Serving of Some Common Foods That Are Good Sources of Calcium

Food	Serving Size	Calcium Content, mg	No. of Servings to Equal Calcium Content in 1 Cup of Low-Fat Milk
Dairy foods			
Whole milk	1 cup (244 g)	276	1.1
Low-fat (1%) milk	1 cup (244 g)	305	—
Nonfat milk Lactose free, skim milk	1 cup (245 g) 1 cup (240 mL)	299 300	1.02 1.02
Yogurt, nonfat, fruit variety	6 oz (170 g)	258	1.2
Frozen yogurt, vanilla, soft serve	1/2 cup (72 g)	103	3.0
Cheese, cheddar Cheese, cottage low fat 2% Cheese, mozzarella part-skim	1 oz (28 g) 1 cup (226g) 1 oz (28 g)	201 251 222	1.5 1.2 1.4
Cheese, pasteurized, processed, American	1 slice 3/4-oz (21 g)	219	1.4
Cheese, ricotta, part skim milk Ice cream, vanilla	1/2 cup (124 g) 1/2 cup (66g)	337 84	0.9 3.6
Nondairy foods			
Salmon, sockeye canned, drained, with bones Sardines, canned in olive oil	3 oz (85 g) 2.8 oz (79g)	203 200	1.5 1.5

Continued

APP

Appendix J. *Continued*

Approximate Calcium Contents of 1 Serving of Some Common Foods That Are Good Sources of Calcium

Food	Serving Size	Calcium Content, mg	No. of Servings to Equal Calcium Content in 1 Cup of Low-Fat Milk
Tofu, firm, prepared with calcium sulfate and magnesium chloride	1/2 cup (126 g)	253	1.2
White beans, cooked, boiled	1 cup (179 g)	131	2.3
Broccoli, cooked, boiled, drained	1 cup, chopped (156 g)	62	4.9
Collards, cooked, boiled, drained	1 cup, chopped (190 g)	266	1.1
Baked beans, canned	1 cup (253 g)	126	2.4
Kale, cooked, boiled, drained	1 cup (130 g)	94	3.3
Rhubarb, frozen, cooked with sugar	1 cup (240 g)	348	0.9
Spinach, cooked, boiled, drained	1 cup (180 g)	245	1.3
Tomatoes, canned, stewed	1 cup (255 g)	87	3.5
Foods fortified with calcium			
Calcium-fortified orange juice	1 cup (240 mL)	500	0.6
Selected calcium-fortified cereal	3/4 cup (30 g)	1000	0.3
Instant oatmeal, fortified, plain, prepared with water	1/2 cup (117 g)	94	3.2
English muffin, plain, enriched, with calcium propionate	1 muffin (57 g)	93	3.3

Food	Serving Size	Calcium Content, mg	No. of Servings to Equal Calcium Content in 1 Cup of Low-Fat Milk
Soy milk[a] (all flavors) low fat with added calcium, vitamins A and D	1 cup (243 g)	199	1.5
Almond milk, sweetened	1 cup (240 mL)	451	0.7

[a] Native soy milk contains 63 mg of calcium per cup (240 mL).

Source: US Department of Agriculture, Agricultural Research Service, Nutrient Data Laboratory. USDA National Nutrient Database for Standard Reference, Release 28. Version Current: September 2015. Revised May 2016. Available at: https://ndb.nal.usda.gov/ndb/search/list. Accessed May 19, 2017

Iron Content of Selected Foods

Food	Portion	Iron, mg
Apricots, raw	3 medium	0.41
Apricots, dried halves	10 each	0.93
Avocado, California	1 medium	0.83
Banana, raw	1 medium	0.31
Black-eyed peas, boiled	½ cup	2.5
Bread, white	1 slice	1.05
Bread, whole wheat	1 slice	0.79
Bread, gluten-free whole grain, Udi's	1 slice	0.18
Broccoli, boiled	½ cup	0.52
Brussels sprouts, cooked	½ cup	0.94
Butter	1 tsp	0.00
Cheddar cheese	1 oz	0.04
Chicken, light and dark, without skin, roasted	3.5 oz	1.20
Chocolate, dark (60%–69% cacao solids)	1 ox	1.79
Chocolate, semisweet	1 oz	0.89
Chocolate, sweet	1 oz	0.78
Chili, Amy's organic	1 cup	1.80
Clams, raw	3 oz	1.38
Cream of wheat, instant, cooked	¾ cup	9.54
Egg, white	1 large	0.03
Egg, whole, fried	1 large	0.87
Egg, yolk	1 large	0.46
Frankfurter, beef	1 frank, 8/lb	0.59
Frankfurter, turkey	1 frank, 10/lb	0.66
Garbanzos, canned	½ cup	0.74
Grape juice, canned or bottle	8 oz	0.63
Grapes, red or green, raw	1 cup	0.54
Halibut, cooked	3 oz	0.17
Ham, 95% lean meat	1 oz	0.42

Continued

APP

Appendix K: *Continued*
Iron Content of Selected Foods

Food	Portion	Iron, mg
Hamburger, extra lean, broiled, medium	3 oz	2.45
Lettuce, iceberg	1 leaf	0.06
Lettuce, romaine, shredded	½ cup	0.23
Liver (beef)	3 ½ oz	6.5
Liver (pork)	3 ½ oz	17.77
Milk, 2%	8 oz	0.05
Molasses	1 tbsp	0.94
Navy beans, canned	½ cup	2.42
Oatmeal, cooked with water	¾ cup	1.57
Orange juice, includes concentrate	8 oz	0.32
Oysters, raw (Eastern, wild-farmed)	6 medium	3.87-4.86
Papaya nectar, canned	8 oz	0.85
Peanut butter, smooth	1 tbsp	0.28
Potato, baked with skin	1 med.	1.11
Prune juice, canned	½ cup	1.51
Prunes, dehydrated, stewed	½ cup	1.64
Raisins, seedless	⅔ cup	1.83
Rice, brown, cooked, medium grain	1 cup	1.03
Rice, white, enriched, cooked, medium grain	1 cup	2.77
Soybeans, green, boiled	½ cup	2.25
Spinach, boiled	½ cup	3.21
Tomato juice, no added salt	½ cup	0.47
Tortilla, corn	1 (1 oz)	0.35
Original Vegan Burgers, Boca Yeast, baker's	1 patty 1 oz	2.90 0.62
Yogurt, low fat (12 g protein per 8-oz serving)	8 oz	0.18

[a] From US Department of Agriculture, Agricultural Research Service, Nutrient Data Laboratory. USDA National Nutrient Database for Standard Reference, Release 28. Version Current: September 2015, slightly revised May 2016. Internet: /nea/bhnrc/ndl
https://ndb.nal.usda.gov/ndb/search/list Accessed April 19 & May 25, 2017
http://udisglutenfree.com/product-category/breads-rolls-buns/ Accessed April 19, 2017.

Zinc Content of Common Household Portions of Selected Foods

Food	Portion	Zinc, mg
Fish (flounder, tuna, salmon)	3 oz	0.33–0.65
Oysters, Eastern, wild, raw	6 medium	33.01
Crab	3 oz	3.24
Poultry 　Dark meat 　Light meat	 3 oz 3 oz	 2.48 1.23
Beef, tenderloin	3 oz	3.43
Pork, loin	3 oz	2.46
Bologna	3 oz	0.40
Liver (pork), cooked	3 oz	5.71
Whole egg	1 large	0.65
Lentils, cooked	1cup	2.51
Milk, whole	1 cup	0.90
Cheese (cheddar)	1 oz	1.03
Bread 　White 　Wheat	 1 slice 1 slice	 0.21 0.57
Rice, medium grain, enriched 　White 　Brown	 ½ cup ½ cup	 0.39 0.60
Cornmeal (cooked)	½ cup	0.52
Oatmeal (cooked)	½ cup	1.17
Bran flakes, enriched 　Unenriched	1 oz 1 oz	16.8 1.5–2.5
Corn flakes	1 oz	0.17

From US Department of Agriculture, Agricultural Research Service, Nutrient Data Laboratory. USDA National Nutrient Database for Standard Reference, Release 28. Version Current: September 2015, slightly revised May 2016. Available at: https://ndb.nal.usda.gov/ndb/search/list. Accessed May 19, 2017

Appendix M

M-1: Selected Enteral Products for Special Indications
and
M-2: Enteral Products Grouped by Usage Indication
and
M-3: Sources of Medical Food Modules and Modified Low-Protein Foods for Treatment of Inborn Errors of Metabolism

APPENDIX M-1.
Selected Enteral Products for Special Indications[a]

Product	Energy, kcal/L	Protein Source, g/L	
Alfamino Junior (Nestle)	1000	Free amino acids	33
Benecalorie (Nestle)	330/41.3 g (1.5 oz)	Ca caseinate	7
Beneprotein (Nestle)	25/7 g (1 scoop)	Whey protein isolates	6
Boost Breeze (Nestle)	1054	Whey protein isolate	38
Boost (Nestle)	1012	Milk & soy protein concentrates	42
Boost Glucose Control (Nestle)	1060	Sodium and Calcium Caseinates (milk), L-arginine	58.2
Boost High Protein (Nestle)	1000	Na and Ca caseinate, milk protein concentrate, soy protein isolate	63
Boost Plus (Nestle)	1500	Milk protein concentrate, Na and Ca caseinate, soy protein isolate	59
Boost Kids Essentials 1.0 (Nestle)	1000	Milk protein concentrate	30

Carbohydrate Source, g/L		Fat Source, g/L		Fiber g/L	Purpose
Corn syrup solids, potato starch, maltodextrin	122	MCT, soybean oil	44		Nutritionally complete hypoallergenic amino acid formula; 65% fat MCT, used in malabsorptive issues and multiple food allergies,
None	0	High-oleic sunflower oil	33		High-calorie protein/ fat-based liquid modular supplement, nutritionally incomplete
None	0	None	0		Protein powder modular supplement, nutritionally incomplete
Sugar, corn syrup	228	None	0		Fat-free clear liquid oral supplement, incomplete nutrition
Corn syrup, sucrose	173	Canola, high-oleic sunflower, and corn oils	17		Nutritionally complete, lactose-free oral supplement
Tapioca dextrin, fructose, corn syrup Fiber: FOS, partially hydrolyzed guar gum; soy fiber	84	Canola oil	49.4	12.6	Adult formula specifically formulated for use in the dietary management of diabetes mellitus
Corn syrup, sucrose	139	Canola, high-oleic sunflower, and corn oils	25		High-protein, nutritionally complete oral supplement
Corn syrup, sucrose Fiber: FOS, inulin, gum acacia	190	Canola, high-oleic sunflower and corn oils	59	12.6	High-calorie nutritionally complete oral supplement
Brown rice syrup, sucrose	135	Canola oil	38		Complete formula for children 1–13 y

Continued

APP

APPENDIX M-1. *Continued*
Selected Enteral Products for Special Indications[a]

Product	Energy, kcal/L	Protein Source, g/L	
Boost Kids Essentials 1.5 (Nestle)	1500	Na and Ca caseinate, whey protein concentrate	42
Boost Kids Essentials 1.5 w/ fiber (Nestle)	1500	Milk protein concentrate	42
Carnation Breakfast Essentials Ready-to-Drink (Nestle)	1000	Milk protein concentrate, soy protein isolate	42
Carnation Breakfast Essentials Ready-to-Drink High Protein (Nestle)	900	Milk protein concentrate, Ca and Na caseinates, soy protein isolate	63
Compleat (Nestle)	1060	Milk protein concentrate, dehydrated chicken powder	48
Compleat Pediatric (Nestle)	1000	Milk protein concentrate, dehydrated chicken powder, pea protein isolate	38

Carbohydrate Source, g/L		Fat Source, g/L		Fiber g/L	Purpose
Brown rice syrup, sucrose	165	Canola oil and soybean oils, MCT	76		High-calorie complete formula for children 1–13 y
Brown rice syrup, sucrose Fiber: gum acacia, pea fiber	165	Canola oil & soybean oils, MCT	76	8.4	High-calorie complete formula for children 1–13 y with soluble and insoluble fiber
Corn syrup, sucrose	170	Canola, high-oleic sunflower and corn oils	17		Lactose-free, gluten-free, low-residue oral supplement
Corn syrup solids, sucrose Fiber: gum acacia, FOS, inulin	118	Canola, high-oleic sunflower and corn oils	25.3	12.6	High-protein, lactose-free, gluten-free oral supplement
Brown rice syrup, tomato paste, peach puree, green bean powder, carrot powder, cranberry juice concentrate Fiber: pea fiber, pea powder, FOS, gum acacia, inulin	136	Canola oil	40	8	Blenderized tube feed formulated from traditional foods
Brown rice syrup, tomato paste, peach puree, green bean powder, carrot powder, cranberry juice concentrate Fiber: pea fiber, pea powder, FOS, gum acacia, inulin	136	Canola oil, MCT	38	8	Intact protein, formulated from traditional foods including meats, vegetables, and fruit; for children 1–10 y

Continued

APP

APPENDIX M-1. *Continued*
Selected Enteral Products for Special Indications[a]

Product	Energy, kcal/L	Protein Source, g/L	
Compleat Pediatric Organic Blends Chicken-Garden Blend (Nestle)	1200	Organic cooked dark meat chicken, organic hydrolyzed pea protein, organic brown rice flower	43
Compleat Pediatric Organic Blends Plant-Based Blend (Nestle)	1200	Organic hydrolyzed pea protein, organic rice protein concentrate, organic sweet potato puree, organic brown rice flour	43
Compleat Pediatric Reduced Calorie (Nestle)	600	Dehydrated chicken powder, milk protein concentrate, pea protein isolate	30
Diabeti-Source AC (Nestle)	1200	Soy protein, L-arginine	60

Carbohydrate Source, g/L		Fat Source, g/L		Fiber g/L	Purpose
Organic ingredients: Mango puree, butternut squash puree, brown rice flour, organic beet puree, spinach puree	137	Organic extra virgin olive oil, organic canola oil	53	10	Complete blenderized organic, non-GMO whole foods formula; Fiber from fruit, vegetables & grain, Gluten-free, Soy, dairy, corn-free
Organic ingredients: Sweet potato puree, pear puree, brown rice flour, blueberry puree, kale puree	137	Organic extra virgin olive oil, organic canola	53	16	Complete blenderized organic, non-GMO whole foods formula; Fiber from fruit, vegetables & grain, Gluten-free, Soy, dairy, corn-free
Green bean powder, tomato paste, peach puree, cranberry juice concentrate, carrot powder, brown rice syrup Fiber: pea fiber, pea powder, gum acacia, FOS, inulin	88	Canola oil, MCTs (20%)	20	10	Reduced energy density formula formulated from traditional foods including meats, vegetables, and fruit
Corn syrup, fructose, tapioca dextrin, green pea, green bean puree, peach puree, orange juice concentrate Fiber: soy fiber, FOS, partially hydrolyzed guar gum	100	Refined fish oil	59	15.2	Traditional food ingredients, designed for abnormal glucose tolerance and stress-induced hypoglycemia No dairy protein

APP

Continued

APPENDIX M-1. *Continued*
Selected Enteral Products for Special Indications[a]

Product	Energy, kcal/L	Protein Source, g/L	
Duocal (Nutricia)	492/100 g powder	None	0
EleCare Jr. (1 kcal/mL) (Abbott)	1000	Free L-amino acids	31
Ensure (Abbott)	1060	Milk protein concentrate, soy protein isolate, nonfat milk	38
Ensure Clear (Abbott)	1012	Whey protein isolate	33.7
Ensure Enlive (Abbott)	1466	Whey protein concentrate, milk protein concentrate, Na caseinate, soy protein isolate	84
Ensure High Protein (Abbott)	875	Milk protein concentrate, soy protein isolate, Ca caseinate, whey protein concentrate	104
Ensure Plus (Abbott)	1476	Milk protein concentrate, soy protein isolate, nonfat milk	55
Neocate Splash (Nutricia)	1000	Free amino acids	30
Glucerna 1.0 (Abbott)	928	Na and Ca caseinate	41.7

Carbohydrate Source, g/L		Fat Source, g/L		Fiber g/L	Purpose
Hydrolyzed cornstarch	72.7	Refined vegetable oils (corn & coconut), MCT (coconut, palm kernel)	22.3		Carbohydrate and fat calorie modular supplement, nutritionally incomplete 35% MCT
Corn syrup solids	107	High-oleic safflower oil, MCT (33%) and soy oils	49		Nutritionally complete elemental formula children 1 y and older who require an amino acid-based medical food
Sucrose, corn maltodextrin Fiber: scFOS	173	Canola & corn oils	25	12.6	Nutritionally complete oral formula
Sugar, corn syrup solids	219.4	none	0	0	Clear liquid, high protein, fat free; Fruit flavored
Corn syrup, sucrose	186	Canola & corn oils	25	12.6	High-calorie, fat-free, clear liquid oral supplement, nutritionally incomplete 1.5 gm HMB per serving
Sucrose, corn maltodextrin	96	Canola oil	10	12	High-protein, low-fat, low-sugar oral formula with prebiotic fiber
Corn maltodextrin, sucrose Fiber: scFOS	211	Corn & canola oils	46	12.5	High-calorie, complete oral supplement
Maltodextrin, sucrose	105	Refined vegetable oils (high-oleic sunflower oil & canola oil), MCT (modified palm kernel and/or coconut oil) oil	51		Elemental, flavored, oral formula for children >1 y with severe gastrointestinal tract (GI) impairment
Corn maltodextrin, fructose Fiber: corn & soy fibers, scFOS	96.2	Canola oil	54.4	14.3	Complete oral or tube feeding for patients with diabetes mellitus

Continued

APP

APPENDIX M-1. *Continued*
Selected Enteral Products for Special Indications[a]

Product	Energy, kcal/L	Protein Source, g/L	
Glucerna 1.5 (Abbott)	1500	Na and Ca caseinate, soy protein isolate	82.7
Impact (Nestle)	1000	Na and Ca caseinate, L-arginine	56
Impact Advanced Recovery (Nestle)	1125	Calcium and sodium caseinates, L-arginine	101
Impact Peptide 1.5 (Nestle)	1500	Hydrolyzed casein, L-arginine	94
Isosource HN (Nestle)	1200	Soy protein isolate, Na & Ca caseinates	54
Isosource 1.5 (Nestle)	1500	Na & Ca caseinates, soy protein isolates,	68
Jevity 1 Cal (Abbott)	1060	Na and Ca caseinate, soy protein isolate	44.3

Carbohydrate Source, g/L		Fat Source, g/L		Fiber g/L	Purpose
Corn maltodextrin, isomaltulose, fructose, sucromalt Fiber: scFOS, soy fiber	132.9	High-oleic safflower oil, canola oil, soy oil	75	16.1	High-calorie, high-protein complete oral or tube feeding for patients with diabetes or altered glucose metabolism due to illness or trauma
Maltodextrin	132	Palm kernel, safflower, high-oleic sunflower, and refined fish oils	28		Designed for metabolically stressed patients without high energy needs
Sugar, maltodextrin	84	Refined fish oil, corn oil, MCTs	45		Contains increased amounts of arginine, omega-3 fatty acids and nucleotides for immune system support to reduce the risk of postsurgical infections
Maltodextrin, corn starch	140	MCT (50%), fish oil, soybean oil	63.6		High-calorie, high-protein formula with arginine, omega-3 fatty acids, and nucleotides designed for critically ill patients
Corn syrup, maltodextrin	156	Canola and MCT oils	40		High-nitrogen, high-calorie soy protein formula
Maltodextrin, corn syrup Fiber: pea fiber, gum acacia, FOS, inulin	176	Canola, soybean, and MCT oils	59.2	15.2	High-nitrogen, high-calorie complete formula with fiber
Corn maltodextrin, corn syrup solids, Fiber: soy fiber	154	Canola, corn, and MCT oils	34.7	14.4	Isotonic, fiber-containing nutritionally complete tube feeding formula

Continued

APP

APPENDIX M-1. *Continued*
Selected Enteral Products for Special Indications[a]

Product	Energy, kcal/L	Protein Source, g/L	
Jevity 1.2 Cal (Abbott)	1200	Na and Ca caseinate, soy protein isolate	56
Jevity 1.5 Cal (Abbott)	1500	Na and Ca caseinate, soy protein isolate	63.8
Kate Farms Standard 1.0 (Kate Farms)	1000	Organic pea protein	49.2
Kate Farms Pediatric Standard 1.2 (Kate Farms)	1200	Organic pea protein	48
Kate Farms Pediatric Peptide 1.5 (Kate Farms)	1500	Organic hydrolyzed pea protein	52

Carbohydrate Source, g/L		Fat Source, g/L		Fiber g/L	Purpose
Corn maltodextrin, corn syrup solids Fiber: scFOS, soy & oat fibers	170	Canola, corn, and MCT oils	35	18	Higher-calorie, high-protein, fiber-containing tube feeding formula
Corn maltodextrin, corn syrup solids Fiber: scFOSsoy & oat fibers	215.7	Canola, corn, and MCT oils	49.8	22	High-calorie, high-protein, fiber containing tube feeding formula
Organic agave syrup, organic brown rice syrup solids, organic quinoa flour	116.9	Organic high-linoleic sunflower oil, organic coconut oil, organic flax seed oil	36.9	15.3	Certified organic & non-GMO plant based formula, contains "superfood blend"; Gluten-free, plant-based, vegan, whey-free, casein-free, soy-free, nut-free, corn-free *some herbs & spices may not be suitable for certain medical conditions
Organic brown rice syrup solids, organic agave syrup, organic quinoa flour	144	Organic coconut oil, organic high-linoleic sunflower oil, organic flax seed oil, organic sunflower lecithin	48	12	Certified organic & non-GMO plant based formula, contains "superfood blend"; Gluten-free, plant-based, vegan, whey-free, casein-free, soy-free, nut-free, corn-free *some herbs & spices may not be suitable for certain medical conditions
Organic brown rice syrup solids, organic agave syrup, organic quinoa flour	160	Organic coconut oil, organic high-linoleic sunflower oil, organic flax seed oil, organic sunflower lecithin	68	12	Certified organic & non-GMO plant based formula, contains "superfood blend"; Gluten-free, plant-based, vegan, whey-free, casein-free, soy-free, nut-free, corn-free *some herbs & spices may not be suitable for certain medical conditions

APP

Continued

APPENDIX M-1. *Continued*

Selected Enteral Products for Special Indications[a]

Product	Energy, kcal/L	Protein Source, g/L	
MCT oil (Nestle)	116 kcal/ tbsp 8.3 kcal/g	None	0
Microlipid (Nestle)	67.5 kcal/ tbsp	None	0
Neocate Jr. (Nutricia)	1000	Free amino acids	31
Neocate Jr. with Prebiotics (Nutricia)	1000	Free amino acids	31
Nepro (Abbott)	1800	Ca, Mg, and Na caseinate, milk protein isolate	81
NovaSource Renal (Nestle)	2000	Na and Ca caseinate, isolated soy protein	74
Nutren 1.0 (Nestle)	1000	Na & Ca caseinates, soy protein isolate	40
Nutren 1.0 With fiber (Nestle)	1000	Na & Ca caseinates, soy protein isolate	40

Carbohydrate Source, g/L		Fat Source, g/L		Fiber g/L	Purpose
None	0	Coconut oil and/or palm kernel oil	14 g/tbsp		Modular fat supplement or substitute for patients with long-chain fatty acid malabsorption – directly absorbed into portal vein, nutritionally incomplete
None	0	Safflower oil; polyclycerol esters of fatty acids	7.5 g/tbsp		Modular fat emulsion (50%) for special use in oral or tube feeding formulas, nutritionally incomplete
Corn syrup solids, maltodextrin	107	MCT (palm and/or coconut oils), high oleic sunflower, sunflower, & canola oils	50		Nutritionally complete elemental formula for children 1–10 y with severe GI tract impairment
Corn syrup solids, maltodextrin Fiber: FOS, inulin	114	MCT (palm and/or coconut oils), high oleic sunflower, sunflower, & canola oils	47	4.2	Nutritionally complete elemental formula with prebiotic fiber for children 1–10 y with severe GI tract impairment
Corn syrup solids, sucrose, corn maltodextrin Fiber: scFOS	161	High-oleic safflower oil and canola oil	96		Very high-calorie, complete oral or tube feeding designed for patients on dialysis
Corn syrup, fructose	200	Canola oil	100		Very high-calorie, -vitamin and -mineral profile specifically formulated for dialysis patients
Maltodextrin, corn syrup	136	Canola, MCT soy lecithin	34		Complete liquid nutrition for patients with normal calorie and protein needs
Maltodextrin, corn syrup Fiber: pea fiber, FOS, inulin	148	Canola, MCT corn oils, soy lecithin	34	15.2	Complete liquid nutrition with fiber

APP

Continued

APPENDIX M-1. *Continued*
Selected Enteral Products for Special Indications[a]

Product	Energy, kcal/L	Protein Source, g/L	
Nutren 1.5 (Nestle)	1500	Na & Ca caseinates, soy protein isolate	68
Nutren 2.0 (Nestle)	2000	Ca and Na caseinate, soy protein isolate	84
Nutren Jr (Nestle)	1000	Casein, whey (50%), milk protein concentrate	30
Nutren Jr With fiber (Nestle)	1000	Casein, whey (50%); milk protein concentrate	30
Nutren Pulmonary (Nestle)	1500	Ca and K caseinate	68
Osmolite 1 Cal (Abbott)	1060	Na and Ca caseinates, soy protein isolate	44.3
Osmolite 1.2 Cal (Abbott)	1200	Na and Ca caseinates	55.5
Osmolite 1.5 Cal (Abbott)	1500	Na and Ca caseinates, soy protein isolate	63
Oxepa (Abbott)	1500	Na and Ca caseinates	62.7

Carbohydrate Source, g/L		Fat Source, g/L		Fiber g/L	Purpose
Maltodextrin, corn syrup	176	MCT (50%), canola,	60		Complete high-calorie liquid nutrition for high calorie needs or limited volume tolerance, 50% MCT oil
Corn syrup, maltodextrin	216	MCT (50%), canola oil	92		Very high-calorie, severe fluid restriction, 50% MCT oil
Maltodextrin, sucrose	112	MCT (20%), canola, soybean oils	48		Balanced formula designed to meet needs of children 1–10 y; oral or enteral
Maltodextrin, sucrose, Fiber: pea fiber, FOS, inulin	116	MCT (20%), canola, and soybean oils	48	6	Balanced formula with prebiotic fiber designed to meet needs of children 1–10 y; oral or enteral
Maltodextrin, sucrose	100	Canola, MCT (40%), corn oils, soy lecithin	94.8		High fat content, designed to reduce CO_2 production for use in pulmonary patients
Corn maltodextrin, corn syrup solids	143.9	Canola, corn, and MCT oils	34.7		Isotonic, nutritionally complete, high-nitrogen, formula for oral or tube feeding
Corn maltodextrin	157.5	High-oleic safflower, canola, and MCT oils	39.3		Higher-calorie, high-nitrogen, low-residue complete oral or tube feeding
Corn maltodextrin	203	High-oleic safflower, canola, and MCT oils	49		High-calorie, high-protein, low-residue complete nutrition for oral or tube feeding use
Sucrose, corn maltodextrin	105.3	Canola, MCT, marine, and borage oils, soy lecithin	93.8		High-calorie, complete tube feeding formula for critically ill patients with acute lung injury, acute respiratory distress syndrome, and systemic inflammatory response syndrome

Continued

APPENDIX M-1. *Continued*
Selected Enteral Products for Special Indications[a]

Product	Energy, kcal/L	Protein Source, g/L	
Pediasure Grow & Gain (Abbott)	1000	Milk protein concentrate, nonfat milk, soy protein isolate	30
Pediasure and Pediasure Enteral, with fiber (Abbott)	1000	Milk protein concentrate	29.5
Pediasure 1.5 Cal (Abbott)	1500	Milk protein concentrate	59
Pediasure 1.5 Cal with Fiber (Abbott)	1500	Milk protein concentrate	59
Pediasure Peptide	1000	Whey protein hydrolysate, hydrolyzed Na caseinate	30
Pediasure Peptide 1.5 (Abbott)	1500	Whey protein hydrolysate, hydrolyzed Na caseinate	45
Pediasure Sidekicks 0.63 kcal (Abbott)	633	Milk protein concentrate, soy protein isolate, whey protein concentrate	29.5
Peptamen (Nestle)	1000	Enzymatically hydrolyzed whey	40
Peptamen with Prebio (Nestle)	1000	Enzymatically hydrolyzed whey	40
Peptamen 1.5 (Nestle)	1500	Enzymatically hydrolyzed whey	68

Carbohydrate Source, g/L		Fat Source, g/L		Fiber g/L	Purpose
Sucrose, corn maltodextrin	139	Canola, corn, & tuna oils	38		Complete oral or tube feeding formula designed for patients 1-13 years
Sucrose, corn maltodextrin Fiber: scFOS, oat & soy fibers	139.2	High-oleic safflower, soy, MCT	38	13	Complete oral or tube feeding formula with fiber designed for patients 1–13 y
Corn maltodextrin	160.3	High-oleic safflower, soy, MCT	67.5		High-calorie complete oral or tube feeding formula designed for patients 1–13 y
Corn maltodextrin, Fiber: scFOS, oat & soy fiber	166	High-oleic safflower, soy, MCT	68	13	High-calorie complete oral or tube feeding formula with fiber designed for patients 1–13 y
Corn maltodextrin, sucrose Fiber: scFOS	134	Structured lipid (interesterified canola/MCT), MCT, canola, tuna oils	41	3	Peptide-based complete oral or tube feeding formula for patients 1–13 y with malabsorption
Corn maltodextrin, Fiber: scFOS	201	Structured lipid (interesterified canola/MCT), MCT, canola, tuna oils & soy lecithin	61	5	Nutritionally complete, peptide based for those with malabsorption or other GI conditions requiring higher caloric density
Sucrose Fiber: scFOS	88.6	Soy oil	21	12.6	Nutritionally complete w/ less calories & fat; for children requiring lower calorie feedings
Maltodextrin, corn starch	128	MCT (70%), soybean oil, soy lecithin	40		Peptide-based, isotonic, designed for general malabsorption
Maltodextrin, corn starch, Fiber: FOS, inulin	128	MCT (70%), soybean oil, soy lecithin	40	4	Peptide-based, isotonic formula with fiber designed for general malabsorption
Maltodextrin, corn starch, sucrose	188	MCT (70%), soybean oil	56		High-calorie, peptide-based, high percentage MCT oil designed for malabsorption

APP

Continued

APPENDIX M-1. *Continued*
Selected Enteral Products for Special Indications[a]

Product	Energy, kcal/L	Protein Source, g/L	
Peptamen AF (Nestle)	1200	Enzymatically hydrolyzed whey	76
Peptamen, Jr. (Nestle)	1000	Enzymatically hydrolyzed whey	30
Peptamen, Jr. Fiber (Nestle)	1000	Enzymatically hydrolyzed whey	30
Peptamen Jr. HP (Nestle)	1200	Enzymatically hydrolyzed whey protein	48
Peptamen, Jr. Prebio (Nestle)	1000	Enzymatically hydrolyzed whey	30
Peptamen, Jr. 1.5 (Nestle)	1500	Enzymatically hydrolyzed whey	46

Carbohydrate Source, g/L		Fat Source, g/L		Fiber g/L	Purpose
Maltodextrin, corn starch Fiber: FOS, inulin	112	MCT (50%), soybean, refined fish oils, soy lecithin	54	6	High-protein, peptide-based, high percentage MCT oil designed for general malabsorption and higher-calorie needs 2.4 g EPA & DHA/L
Maltodextrin, sucrose, Cornstarch Flavored: monk fruit juice concentrate	136	MCT (60%), soybean, and canola oils	38		Designed for children 1–10 y, peptide-based, 60% of fat from MCT oil
Maltodextrin, sucrose Cornstarch, monk fruit juice concentrate Fiber: partially hydrolyzed guar gum, pea fiber	144	MCT (60%), soybean, and canola oils	38	8	Peptide-based complete formula with fiber and 60% of fat from MCT oil, designed for children 1–10 y
Maltodextrin, sucrose, corn starch, monk fruit juice concentrate Fiber: partially hydrolyzed guar gum	152	MCT, soybean & canola oils, soy lecithin	48	4	Nutritionally complete enzymatically hydrolyzed why protein, 60% fat MCT, used for impaired GI function
Maltodextrin, sucrose, Cornstarch, monk fruit juice concentrate Fiber: FOS, inulin	140	MCT (60%), soybean, and canola oils	38	4	Peptide-based complete formula with prebiotics and 60% of fat from MCT oil, designed for children 1–10 y
Maltodextrin, Cornstarch, Fiber: partially hydrolyzed guar gum	184	MCT (60%), soybean, and canola oils, soy lecithin, refined fish oil	68	6	High-calorie, complete peptide based formula designed for children 1–13 y, 60% of fat from MCT oil, and contains fish oil

Continued

APP

APPENDIX M-1. *Continued*
Selected Enteral Products for Special Indications[a]

Product	Energy, kcal/L	Protein Source, g/L	
Perative (Abbott)	1300	Hydrolyzed Na caseinate, whey protein hydrolysate, L-arginine	66.7
Promod Liquid Protein (Abbott)	100/30 mL	Hydrolyzed beef collagen, L-tryptophan	10
Promote (Abbott)	1000	Sodium caseinate, soy protein isolate	63
Promote with fiber (Abbott)	1000	Sodium and calcium caseinate, soy protein isolate	62.5
Pulmocare (Abbott)	1500	Na and Ca caseinates	62.4
Renalcal (Nestle)	2000	Essential and select nonessential amino acids, whey protein concentrate	34
ReSource 2.0 (Nestle)	2000	Ca and Na caseinates	84.3
Suplena with Carb Steady (Abbott)	1800	Milk protein isolates, Na caseinate	45
Tolerex (Nestle)	1000	Free amino acids	20.5

Carbohydrate Source, g/L		Fat Source, g/L		Fiber g/L	Purpose
Corn maltodextrin, Fiber: scFOS	180.3	Canola, MCT (40%), and corn oils	37.3	6.5	Higher-calorie complete tube feeding formula designed for metabolically stressed patients with wounds, burns, or a postoperative state 8 g Arginine/L
Glycerine	14	None	0		Protein calorie supplement, nutritionally incomplete
Corn maltodextrin, sucrose	130	MCT and safflower oils, soy lecithin, soy oil	26		Very high-protein complete oral or tube feeding formula
Corn maltodextrin, sucrose Fiber: soy fiber	138.3	Soy, MCT, and safflower oils	28.2	14.4	Very high-protein complete oral or tube feeding formula with fiber
Sucrose, corn maltodextrin	105.4	Canola, MCT (20%), high-oleic safflower and corn oils, soy lecithin	93.2		High-calorie, high-fat, low-carbohydrate complete oral or tube feeding designed for pulmonary patients
Maltodextrin, corn starch	292	MCT (70%), canola, and corn oils, soy lecithin	82		Very high-calorie, low-protein for patients with renal failure designed to maintain positive nitrogen balance, added histidine, negligible electrolytes
Corn syrup, sucrose, maltodextrin	219.4	Canola and MCT (20%) oils	88		Very high-calorie, high-protein oral beverage, pouch pak
Corn maltodextrin, isomaltulose, sucrose, glycerin Fiber:scFOS	196	High-oleic safflower, canola oil, soy lethicin	96	12.7	Very high-calorie, low-protein, complete formula for patients with renal failure
Maltodextrin, modified corn starch	226	Safflower oil	2		Complete, low-fat, elemental formula for those >3 years of age

Continued

APPENDIX M-1. *Continued*
Selected Enteral Products for Special Indications[a]

Product	Energy, kcal/L	Protein Source, g/L	
TwoCal HN (Abbott)	2000	Na and Ca caseinates	84
Vital 1.0 Cal (Abbott)	1000	Whey protein hydrolysate, partially hydrolyzed Na caseinate	40
Vital AF 1.2 Cal (Abbott)	1200	Whey protein hydrolysate, hydrolyzed Na caseinate	75
Vital 1.5 Cal (Abbott)	1500	Whey protein hydrolysate, partially hydrolyzed Na caseinate	67.5
Vital HP (Abbott)	1000	Whey protein hydrolysate, hydrolyzed Na caseinate	87.5
Vivonex Pediatric (Nestle)	800	Free amino acids	24
Vivonex Plus (Nestle)	1000	Free amino acids	43
Vivonex T.E.N. (Nestle)	1000	Free amino acids	38.3

[a] Sources: Abbott Nutrition Division, Abbott Laboratories, Columbus, OH (www.abbottnutrition.com); information obtained via manufacturer website 9/3/19

Kate Farms, Santa Barbara, CA (www.katefarms.com); information obtained via manufacturer website 9/3/19

Carbohydrate Source, g/L		Fat Source, g/L		Fiber g/L	Purpose
Corn syrup solids, corn maltodextrin, sucrose Fiber:scFOS	218.5	High-oleic safflower, and canola oils, soy lecithin	90.7	5	Complete very high-calorie feeding with fructo-oligosaccharides
Corn maltodextrin, sucrose Fiber: scFOS	130	Structured lipid (interesterified canola/ MCT), canola oil, MCT	38.1	4.2	Complete, peptide-based formula for patients with impaired GI tract function
Corn maltodextrin, Fiber: scFOS	110.6	Structured lipid (interesterified marine oil/MCT), MCT, canola and soy oils	53.9	5.1	Higher-calorie nutritionally complete, peptide based formula for patients with impaired GI tract function; with fish-oil based structured lipid and prebiotic 3.8 g DHA/EPA per L
Corn maltodextrin, sucrose Fiber: scFOS	187	Structured lipid (interesterified canola/ MCT), canola oil, MCT	57.1	6	High-calorie nutritionally complete, peptide-based formula for patients with impaired GI tract function
Corn maltodextrin, sucrose	112	MCT, Marine oil	23.2		Nutritionally complete, peptide-based elemental, low-fat, added fish oil to help modulate inflammation 3.8 g DHA/EPA per L
Maltodextrin, modified starch	128	MCT (70%) and soybean oils	23.2		Nutritionally complete, elemental formula for children, unflavored, may use flavor packets Ages 1-13 yo
Corn maltodextrin, modified corn starch	193	Soybean oil	6.7		High-nitrogen, low-fat elemental diet; additional glutamine arginine and branched-chain amino acids For ages >3 yo
Corn maltodextrin, modified corn starch	206	Safflower oil	3		Free amino acids plus additional glutamine, low fat, designed for GI tract impairment For ages >3 yo

Nestle Clinical Nutrition, Glendale, CA (www.nestlehealthscience.us); information obtained via manufacturer website 9/3/19

Nutricia North America Advanced Medical Nutrition, Scientific Hospital Supplies North America, Gaithersburg, MD (www.nutricia-na.com); information obtained via manufacturer website 9/3/19

APP

Appendix M-2
Enteral Products Grouped by Usage Indication

Indication	Product
Standard adult oral	Boost, Ensure, Carnation Breakfast
Standard adult tube feeding	Jevity 1 cal, Nutren 1.0, Osmolite
High-protein oral	Boost High Protein, Ensure High Protein, Ensure Muscle Health, Ensure Clinical Strength
High-protein tube feeding	FiberSource HN, Isosource HN, Jevity 1.2 cal, Osmolite 1 cal, Osmolite 1.2 cal, Promote, Nutren Replete, Vital HN
1.5 kcal/mL	Boost Plus, Ensure Plus, Carnation Breakfast Plus, Nutren 1.5, Isosource 1.5, Jevity 1.5, Osmolite 1.5
2.0 kcal/mL	Carnation Breakfast VHC, Nutren 2.0, ReSource 2.0, TwoCal HN
Standard pediatric (>1 y)	Nutren Jr., Pediasure (1.0, 1.5), Boost Kids Essentials (1.0, 1.5)
Blenderized	Compleat, Compleat Pediatric, Compleat Pediatric Reduced Calories, Kate Farms Komplete, Liquid Hope, Nourish
Clear fortified liquid	Enlive, Boost Breeze
Peptide-based adult	Peptamen, Peptamen 1.5, Peptamen AF, Perative, Vital HN, Vital (1.0, 1.5)
Peptide-based pediatric	Pepdite Jr., Peptamen Jr. (1.0, 1.5), Pediasure Peptide
Free amino acid adult	Tolerex, Vivonex T.E.N., Vivonex Plus
Free amino acid pediatric (>1 y)	Elecare Junior, Neocate Junior, Neocate Splash, Vivonex Pediatric
Immune enhancing	Impact (1.0, 1.5), Impact Advanced Recovery, Pivot 1.5
Wound healing	Crucial, Isosource HN, Nutren Replete, Impact (1.0, 1.5), Perative
Diabetes	Boost Glucose Control DiabetiSource AC, Glucerna, Nutren Glytrol, ReSource Diabetishield

Indication	Product
Kidney disease	Nepro, NovaSource Renal, Renalcal, Suplena
Liver disease	NutriHep
Pulmonary disease	NovaSource Pulmonary, Nutren Pulmonary, Oxepa, Pulmocare
Inflammatory bowel disease	Optimental, Peptamen AF, Vital AF 1.2
Carbohydrate modulars	Polycal
Protein modulars	Beneprotein, Promod, Complete Amino Acid Mix
Calorie enhancers	Duocal, Benecalorie
Fat modulars	MCT oil, Microlipid, Liquigen

APP

Table M-3.

Sources of Medical Food Modules and Modified Low-Protein Foods for Treatment of Inborn Errors of Metabolism

Company	Medical Food Module	Modified Low-Protein Modules
Abbott Nutrition Metabolic Products (Inherited Metabolic Disorders) 3300 Stelzer Road Columbus, OH 43219-3034 Tel: (800) 986-8755 (for health care professionals) Website: www.abbottnutrition.com	Medical formulas for inherited disorders involving protein, fat, or carbohydrate metabolism; protein-free formula	
Applied Nutrition 10 Saddle Road Cedar Knolls, NJ 07927 Tel: (800) 605-0410 FAX: (973) 734-0029 Website: www.medicalfood.com/products.php	Medical protein formulas for PKU, MSUD, and GA1; medical protein bars for PKU and MSUD, LNAA powder and tablets for PKU; single amino acids	Baking mixes, cereal, snacks, sweets
Cambrooke Foods, Inc. 4 Copeland Drive Ayer, MA 01432 Tel: (866) 4-LOW-PRO (456-9776) FAX: (978) 443 1318 Website: www.cambrookefoods.com/	Medical protein formula for PKU, ready-to-drink medical beverages for PKU and MSUD, medical protein formula with Glytactin for PKU	Baking mixes, breads, breakfast cereal, cheeses, desserts, meat alter-natives, rice and pasta, snacks, seasonings, premade frozen items

Canbrands Specialty Foods PO BOX 117 Gormley, Ontario LOH 1GO Tel: (905) 888-5008 FAX: (905) 888-5009	Cookies, gelatin desserts, egg replacer
Dietary Specialties 8 South Commons Road Waterbury, CT 06704 Tel: (888) 640-2800 FAX: (973) 884-5907 Website: www.dietspec.com/	Baking mixes, pasta entrees, soups, pasta, rice and porridge, sauce mixes, cake mixes, peanut butter spread, egg replacer, breads, rolls, bagels, frozen premade foods
Ener-G Foods 5960 1st Avenue South Seattle, Washington 98108 Tel: (800) 331-5222 FAX: (206) 764-3398 Website: www.ener-g.com	Breads, crackers and snacks, cookies, egg replacer, baking mixes
Mead Johnson Medical Department (Products) 2400 West Lloyd Expressway Evansville, IN 47721 Tel: (812) 429-6399 Website: www.mjn.com/app/iwp/ hcp2/content2.do?dm=mj&id=- 12490&iwpst=HCP&ls=0&csred= 1&r=3508098857	Medical formulas for inherited disorders involving protein, fat, or carbohydrate metabolism; protein-free formula

Continued

APP

Table M-3. *Continued*

Sources of Medical Food Modules and Modified Low-Protein Foods for Treatment of Inborn Errors of Metabolism

Company	Medical Food Module	Modified Low-Protein Modules
Nutricia North America – United States PO Box 117 Gaithersburg, MD 20884 Tel: (800) 365-7354 FAX: (301) 795-2301 Website: www.shsna.com/index.htm	Medical formulas for inherited disorders involving protein, fat, or carbohydrate metabolism; protein-free formula, vitamin modules; ketogenic formula	Baking mixes, pasta, and rice, cereals, crackers, drink mix, energy bars, snacks
Nutricia North America - Canada 4517 Dobrin Street St. Laurent, QC H4R 2L8 Phone: (877) 636-2283 FAX: (514) 745-6625 Website: www.shsna.com/index.htm	Medical formulas for inherited disorders involving protein, fat, or carbohydrate metabolism; protein-free formula, vitamin modules; ketogenic formula	Baking mixes, pasta, and rice, cereals, crackers, drink mix, energy bars, snacks
Solace Nutrition 10 Alice Court Pawcatuck, CT 06379 Tel: (888) 876-5223 FAX: (401) 633-6066 Website: www.solacenutrition.com	Medical formulas for inherited disorders involving protein metabolism; supplements for mitochondria and cholesterol disorders	

Company	Products	
Taste Connections 612 Meyer Lane #13 Redondo Beach, CA 90278 Telephone: (310) 798-1935 FAX: (310) 971-8861 Website: www.tasteconnections.com/		Baking mixes, premade baked items, snacks
Vitaflo USA 211 N Union St Suite 100 Alexandria, VA 22314 Tel: (888) 848-2356 FAX: (631) 693-2002 Website: www.vitaflousa.com/default.aspx	Ready-to-drink medical protein beverages for inherited disorders involving protein metabolism; formulas and supplements for fatty acid oxidation disorders, protein-free medical formulas, single amino acid and essential fatty acid supplements, energy supplements	

PKU indicates phenylketonuria; MSUD, maple syrup urine disease; GA1, glutaric acidemia type 1; LNAA, large neutral amino acids.

Sports/Nutrition Bars

APPENDIX N.
Sports/Nutrition Bars

Product (weight, g) (Manufacturer)	Calories	Protein	Fat (Saturated Fat)	Fiber	Sodium	Calcium (% DV)	Iron (% DV)
Atkins Harvest Trail Bar (38 g) (ANI, New York, NY) – average of 5 flavors	162	8 g	11.2 g (3.1 g)	9.6 g	162 mg	5.6%	9.6%
Atkins Lift Protein Bar (60 g) (ANI, New York, NY)	200	20 g	5 g (2.5 g)	16 g	170 mg	10%	2%
Balance Nutrition Bar (50 g) (The Balance Bar Co, Tarrytown, NY)	200	14 g	7 g (4 g)	2 g	190 mg	15%	30%
Balance Nutrition Energy Bar (34 g)	160	4 g	8 g (1.5 g)	3 g	110 mg	2%	2%
Clif (68 g) (Clif Bar Inc, Berkeley, CA)	235	10 g	4 g (1 g)	5 g	133 mg	25%	25%
Clif's Luna Bar (48 g)	193	10 g	5.9 g (2.7 g)	2.1 g	185 mg	43%	38%
Clif's Luna High Protein Bar (45 g)	170	12 g	5 g (3.5 g)	3 g	250 mg	25%	15%
Clif Mojo Trail Mix Bar (45 g) – average of 4 flavors	202.5	7.5 g	10.75 g (2.88 g)	2.5 g	205 mg	5.5%	28%
Clif Mojo Fruit & Nut Trail Mix Bar (40 g) – average of 3 flavors	187	5 g	11 g (1.83 g)	4 g	115 mg	5.3%	5.3%
Clif Mojo Sweet & Salty Trail Mix Bar (45 g) – average of 2 flavors	190	8.5 g	9 g (1.75 g)	2 g	210 mg	6%	7%
Clif Builder's Protein Bar (68 g)	280	20 g	10 g (5 g)	2 g	320 mg	30%	0%
Clif Kid Zbar Protein (36 g)	130	5 g	2.5 g (1 g)	3 g	95 mg	20%	10%

Product							
EAS – Advantage Bar (50 g) (Abbott Laboratories, Columbus, OH)	190	15 g	7 g (4 g)	4 g	140 mg	0%	0%
Essential Everyday Chewy Protein Bar (40 g) (SuperValu, Eden Prairie, MN)	190	10 g	12 g (3 g)	5 g	180 mg	6%	4%
GeniSoy (56 g) (GeniSoy Food Co, Tulsa, OK) – average of 2 flavors	215	10 g	5.3 g (3 g)	2.5 g	168 mg	21.5%	20%
Health Warrior SuperFood Protein Bar (50 g) (Health Warrior, Richmond, VA)	210	10 g	9 g (1 g)	5 g	170 mg	15%	15%
Kashi GoLean Plant-Powered Bar (78 g) (Kashi Co, La Jolla, CA)	304	13 g	6 g (3 g)	6 g	250 mg	8%	7%
Kashi Chewy Nut Butter Bar (35 g)	150	3 g	7 g (2.5 g)	3 g	140 mg	2%	4%
Kashi Savory Bars (30 g)	130	3 g	5 g (1 g)	4 g	160 mg	4%	6%
Kashi Chewy Granola Bar (35 g)	140	5 g	5 g (0 g)	3 g	55 mg	2%	4%
Kashi Layered Granola Bar (32 g)	130	3 g	4.5 g (1 g)	3 g	65 mg	0%	4%
Kashi Crunchy 7 Grain Bars (40 g)	180	3 g	6 g (1 g)	3 g	110 mg	2%	4%
Kellogg Special K Protein Bar (45 g) (Kellogg Company, Battle Creek, MI)	180	12 g	6 g (3.5 g)	5 g	210 mg	20%	20%
Kind – Strong an Kind Bar (45 g) (Kind, LLC, New York, NY)	230	10	16 g (1.5 g)	3 g	115 mg	8%	10%
Larabar Alt Protein Bar (60 g) (General Mills, Golden Valley, MN)	270	10 g	13 g (3.5 g)	4 g	10 mg	2%	8%

Continued

APP

APPENDIX N. *Continued*
Sports/Nutrition Bars

Product (weight, g) (Manufacturer)	Calories	Protein	Fat (Saturated Fat)	Fiber	Sodium	Calcium (% DV)	Iron (% DV)
Met-Rx Big 100 Colossal Meal Replacement Bar (100 g) (Met-Rx USA, Bohemia, NY)	410	32 g	14 g (6 g)	3 g	410 mg	20%	25%
Muscle Milk High Protein Bar (73 g)	310	25 g	11 g (6 g)	5 g	220 mg	10%	15%
Nature's Path Organic Qi'a Superfood Snack Bar (38 g) (Nature's Path Foods, Richmond, British Columbia, Canada)	190	5 g	11 g (5 g)	4 g	10 mg	2%	6%
Nature's Path Organic Envirokidz Crispy Rice Bar (28 g)	110	1 g	3 g (0.5 g)	1 g	70 mg	0%	4%
Odwalla Chewy Nut Bar (45 g) (Odwalla, Half Moon Bay, CA)	180	3 g	4 g (1.5 g)	2 g	125 mg	25%	4%
Odwalla Nourishing Bar (56 g)	220	4 g	5 g (0.5 g)	5 g	105 mg	25%	6%
Odwalla Original Superfood Bar (56 g)	210	4 g	4.5 g (2 g)	3 g	105 mg	25%	8%
Odwalla Super Protein Bar (56 g)	210	14 g	4.5 g (1 g)	4 g	150 mg	25%	10%
Odwalla Protein Bar (56 g)	230	7 g	8 g (1.5 g)	4 g	170 mg	25%	8%
PowerBar Performance Energy Bar (65 g) (Premier Nutrition Corporation, part of Post Holdings, Saint Louis, MO)	230	10 g	4 g (0.5 g)	2 g	200 mg	2%	10%

Product							
PowerBar Plant Protein Bar (50 g)	230	10 g	13 g (2.5 g)	8 g	190 mg	6%	10%
PowerBar Protein Plus 30g (93 g)	370	30 g	13 g (5 g)	5 g	390 mg	6%	6%
PowerBar Protein Plus 20g (60 g)	200	20 g	7 g (3.5 g)	5 g	210 mg	10%	0%
Probar Bite (46 g) (Probar LLC, Park City, UT)	190	6 g	7 g (1.5 g)	3 g	45 mg	2%	10%
Probar Meal Bar (85 g)	380	11 g	19 g (3.5 g)	6 g	35 mg	8%	20%
Probar Bolt Chews (30 g)	90	0 g	0 g (0 g)	0 g	60 mg	0%	0%
Probar Fuel (51 g)	200	3 g	7 g (1 g)	6 g	55 mg	6%	6%
Probar Base (53 g)	220	15 g	7 g (4.5 g)	3 g	10 mg	6%	10%
Promax Original Protein Bar (75 g) (Promax Nutrition, Concord, CA)	290	20 g	6 g (3.5 g)	4 g	250 mg	25%	40%
PureFit Premium Nutrition Bar (57 g) (PureFit Inc, Irvine, CA)	220	18 g	7 g (1 g)	4 g	160 mg	6%	25%
SoLo Bar (50 g) (Solo GI Nutrition, Edmonton, Alberta, Canada)	200	11 g	7g (3 g)	4 g	120 mg	20%	10%
Original Protein Nut Bar (38 g) (Think Products, San Francisco, CA)	190	9 g	12 g (1.5 g)	3 g	115 mg	6%	15%
ThinkThin High Protein Bar (60 g)	230	20	8 g (3 g)	1 g	210 mg	10%	10%
Tiger's Milk Protein Rich Nutrition Bar (35g) (Weider Health & Fitness, Woodland Hills, CA)	140	6 g	5 g (2 g)	1 g	60 mg	15%	20%

Continued

APP

APPENDIX N. *Continued*
Sports/Nutrition Bars

Product (weight, g) (Manufacturer)	Calories	Protein	Fat (Saturated Fat)	Fiber	Sodium	Calcium (% DV)	Iron (% DV)
Tiger's Milk America's Original Nutrition Bar (55 g) (Schiff Nutrition Group, Salt Lake City, UT)	220	10 g	8 g (3 g)	1 g	100 mg	25%	30%
Vega Sport Protein Bar (60 g) (Whitewave Foods, Denver, CO)	260	15 g	11 g (3 g)	3 g	150 mg	0%	4%
Worldwide Sport Nutrition Bar (78 g) (Worldwide SportNutrition, Bohemia, NY)	310	31 g	10 g (4.5 g)	2 g	310 mg	35%	15%
Zone Perfect Nutrition Bar (50 g) (Abbott Nutrition, Columbus, OH)	200	14 g	6 g (4 g)	3 g	200 mg	20%	10%
Zone Perfect Classic Crunch Bar (50 g)	211	15 g	7 g (2.3 g)	1 g	260 mg	10%	10%
Zone Perfect Kidz Nutrition Bar (35 g) – average of 2 flavors	145	5 g	5.3 g (3 g)	3 g	105 mg	10%	15%

NOTE: All values may vary slightly according to flavor.

DV indicates daily value. (*Guidance for Industry: A Food Labeling Guide. US Department of Health and Human Services, FDA, Center for Food Safety and Applied Nutrition; January 2013.*)

US Department of Agriculture, Agricultural Research Service, Nutrient Data Laboratory. USDA Branded Food Products Database. Version Current: January 2017. Available at: http://ndb.nal.usda.gov. Accessed June 16, 2017.

Sodium Content of Foods, mg per Serving

>400 mg	251-400 mg	141-250 mg	51-140 mg	50 mg or less
⅛ tsp salt	½ cup regularly seasoned spinach, beets, beet greens	1 slice regular bread	½ cup of the following unsalted vegetables: frozen mixed peas and carrots, beets, spinach	½ cup of the following fresh, frozen, or canned vegetables, canned without salt: 1 artichoke (edible base and leaves), carrots, celery, dandelion greens, kale, mustard greens, peas (black-eyed), succotash, turnip greens, turnip (white), lima beans
¾ tsp monosodium glutamate	1 hard roll	½ cup canned carrots	¾ cup milk (6 oz)	
1 bouillon cube	½ cup rice cooked in salted water	or seasoned vegetables not listed elsewhere	½ cup pasta cooked in salted water	
1 average serving ea: ½ cup of cooked rice, spaghetti, noodles, hominy, seasoned with salt	2 thin slices bacon, crisp and drained	1 cup pasta cooked in salted water	1 oz tuna, drained (not rinsed)	
½ cup drained sauerkraut	3 oz canned sardines or salmon	1 oz natural cheddar cheese	1 tsp or 1 packet yellow mustard	
1 average frankfurter (1½ oz)	1 oz plain, salted, hard pretzels	1 tbsp catsup	1 round slice kosher or dill pickle	
1 oz salami	½ cup grits cooked in salted water	1 oz plain potato chips	5 saltine crackers	
3 oz shrimp (frozen, treated and thawed), cooked	½ cup tomato juice	1 Tbsp of BBQ sauce	3 oz shrimp (fresh), cooked	1 oz fresh, cooked fish fillet (cod or pollock)
1 tsp soy sauce	3 oz fish fillets, previously frozen, cooked (cod, pollock)	1 oz low sodium turkey deli meat		
	1 oz turkey deli meat			

From US Department of Agriculture, Agricultural Research Service, Nutrient Data Laboratory. USDA National Nutrient Database for Standard Reference, Release 28. Version Current: September 2015, slightly revised May 2016. Available at: https://ndb.nal.usda.gov/ndb/search/list. Accessed May 25, 2017.

To help maintain a lower-sodium diet, on food labels, select items with 140 mg or less per serving size, and avoid foods with visible salt, such as potato chips, pretzels, or salted nuts.

APP

Saturated and Polyunsaturated Fat and Cholesterol Content of Common Foods

Appendix P
Saturated and Polyunsaturated Fat and Cholesterol Content of Common Foods

Foods	Quantity	Saturated Fat, g	Polyunsaturated Fat, g	Cholesterol, mg	kcal
Almonds (roasted, salted, shelled)	1 oz	1.2	3.7	0	170
Avocado	1 cup	3.0	2.7	0	240
Bacon (cured, cooked)	2 slices	2.3	0.8	17	89
Beef, lean, choice	3 oz	2.9	0.4	76	175
Bread, white	1 slice	0.2	0.5	0	77
Butter	1 tbsp	7.3	0.4	31	102
Cheese					
Cheddar	1 oz	5.4	0.4	28	115
Cottage, creamed	1/2 cup	1.9	0.1	19	111
Cream or spread	2 tbsp	5.9	0.4	29	102
Chicken (breast meat, without skin)	3.5 oz	1.0	0.8	84	164
Coconut (dried, sweetened)	¼ cup	7.3	0.1	0	116
Canola oil	1 tbsp	1.0	3.9	0	124
Coconut oil	1 tbsp	11.2	0.2	0	121
Corn oil	1 tbsp	1.8	7.4	0	122
Egg					
Whole, hard-boiled	1 large	1.6	0.7	186	78
White	1 large	0	0	0	17
Yolk	1 large	1.6	0.7	184	55

Food	Serving				
Fish (fillet or flounder, sole)	3 oz	0.5	0.4	48	73
Hamburger (85% lean)	3 oz	5.0	0.4	75	212
Ice cream (light) vanilla	½ cup	2.2	0.2	21	137
Lamb (lean leg)	3 oz	2.4	0.4	76	162
Lard	1 tbsp	5.0	1.4	12	115
Liver (beef)	3.5 oz	2.9	1.1	393	192
Margarine					
Regular (hydrogenated)	1 tbsp	2.4	3.0	0	101
Tub	1 tbsp	2.0	3.8	0	101
Smart Beat Smart Squeeze	1 tbsp	0.04	0.17	0	7
Pam Cooking Spray	3 second spray	0.05	0.2	0	7
Milk					
Whole	1 cup	4.6	0.5	24	149
2%	1 cup	3.1	0.2	20	122
Skimmed	1 cup	0.1	0	5	83
Almond milk, sweetened	1 cup	0	0.5	0	91
Soy milk, fortified	1 cup	0.5	2.1	0	104
Olive oil	1 tbsp	1.9	1.4	0	119
Oysters (Eastern, wild-farmed)	6 medium	0.4–0.4	0.4–0.5	34–21	43–50
Peanut oil	1 tbsp	2.3	4.3	0	119
Pork (lean, loin)	3.5 oz	3.4	0.7	78	202

Continued

APP

Appendix P *Continued*
Saturated and Polyunsaturated Fat and Cholesterol Content of Common Foods

Foods	Quantity	Saturated Fat, g	Polyunsaturated Fat, g	Cholesterol, mg	kcal
Safflower oil	1 tbsp	0.8	10.2	0	120
Salmon, pink (canned)	3 oz	0.8	1.3	71	117
Shrimp (canned)	3 oz	0.2	0.6	214	85
Soybean oil	1 tbsp	2.1	7.9	0	120
Tuna fish, white, canned in vegetable oil	3 oz	1.1	2.5	26	158
Turkey (breast, roasted)	3 oz	0.5	0.5	68	125

Source: US Department of Agriculture, Agricultural Research Service, Nutrient Data Laboratory, USDA National Nutrient Database for Standard Reference, Release 28. Version Current: September 2015, Revised May 2016. Available at: https://ndb.nal.usda.gov/ndb/search/list. Accessed May 26, 2017

Growth Charts

Table of Contents

Q-7.5   WHO Growth Velocity Standards: 2-month weight increments (g) BOYS Birth to 24 months (percentiles) (reprinted with permission from World Health Organization; https://www.who.int/childgrowth/standards/en/; accessed June 6, 2019; © World Health Organization)

Q-7.6   WHO Growth Velocity Standards: 6-month weight increments (g) BOYS Birth to 24 months (percentiles) (reprinted with permission from World Health Organization; https://www.who.int/childgrowth/standards/en/; accessed June 6, 2019; © World Health Organization)

Q-7.7   WHO Growth Velocity Standards: 2-month length increments (cm) GIRLS Birth to 24 months (percentiles) (reprinted with permission from World Health Organization; https://www.who.int/childgrowth/standards/en/; accessed June 6, 2019; © World Health Organization)

Q-7.8   WHO Growth Velocity Standards: 6-month length increments (cm) GIRLS Birth to 24 months (percentiles) (reprinted with permission from World Health Organization; https://www.who.int/childgrowth/standards/en/; accessed June 6, 2019; © World Health Organization)

Q-7.9   WHO Growth Velocity Standards: 2-month length increments (cm) BOYS Birth to 24 months (percentiles) (reprinted with permission from World Health Organization; https://www.who.int/childgrowth/standards/en/; accessed June 6, 2019; © World Health Organization)

Q-7.10   WHO Growth Velocity Standards: 6-month length increments (cm) BOYS Birth to 24 months (percentiles) (reprinted with permission from World Health Organization; https://www.who.int/childgrowth/standards/en/; accessed June 6, 2019; © World Health Organization)

Q-7.11   WHO Growth Velocity Standards: 2-month head circumference increments (cm) GIRLS Birth to 12 months (percentiles) (reprinted with permission from World Health Organization; https://www.who.int/childgrowth/standards/en/; accessed June 6, 2019; © World Health Organization)

Q-7.12   WHO Growth Velocity Standards: 6-month head circumference increments (cm) GIRLS Birth to 24 months (percentiles) (reprinted with permission from World Health Organization; https://www.who.int/childgrowth/standards/en/; accessed June 6, 2019; © World Health Organization)

APP

Q-7.13   WHO Growth Velocity Standards: 2-month head circumference increments (cm) BOYS Birth to 12 months (percentiles) (reprinted with permission from World Health Organization; https://www.who.int/childgrowth/standards/en/; accessed June 6, 2019; © World Health Organization)

Q-7.14   WHO Growth Velocity Standards: 6-month head circumference increments (cm) BOYS Birth to 24 months (percentiles) (reprinted with permission from World Health Organization; https://www.who.int/childgrowth/standards/en/; accessed June 6, 2019; © World Health Organization)

Q-8.1   Arm circumference-for-age GIRLS 3 months to 5 years (percentiles) (reprinted with permission from World Health Organization; https://www.who.int/childgrowth/standards/en/; accessed June 6, 2019; © World Health Organization)

Q-8.2   Arm circumference-for-age BOYS 3 months to 5 years (percentiles) (reprinted with permission from World Health Organization; https://www.who.int/childgrowth/standards/en/; accessed June 6, 2019; © World Health Organization)

Q-8.3   Mid upper arm circumference for age percentiles (reprinted with permission from Addo OY, Himes JH, Zemel BS. Reference ranges for midupper arm circumference, upper arm muscle area, and upper arm fat area in US children and adolescents aged 1-20 y. *Am J Clin Nutr*. 2017;105(1):111-120. © American Society for Nutrition)

Q-9.1   Triceps skinfold-for-age GIRLS 3 months to 5 years (percentiles) (reprinted with permission from World Health Organization; https://www.who.int/childgrowth/standards/en/; accessed June 6, 2019; © World Health Organization)

Q-9.2   Triceps skinfold-for-age BOYS 3 months to 5 years (percentiles) (reprinted with permission from World Health Organization; https://www.who.int/childgrowth/standards/en/; accessed June 6, 2019; © World Health Organization)

Q-1.1.
Birth to 24 months: Girls: Length-for-age and Weight-for-age percentiles

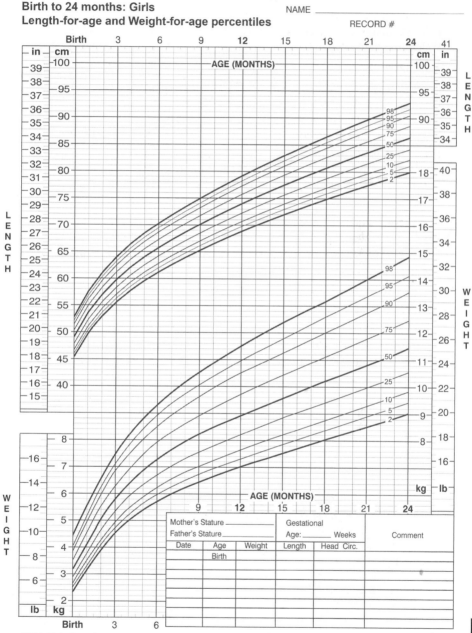

Birth to 24 months: Girls
Length-for-age and Weight-for-age percentiles

NAME _____

RECORD # _____

Published by the Centers for Disease Control and Prevention, November 1, 2009
SOURCE: WHO Child Growth Standards (http://www.who.int/childgrowth/en)

Q-1.2

Birth to 24 months: Girls: Head circumference-for-age and Weight-for-length percentiles

Birth to 24 months: Girls
Head circumference-for-age and
Weight-for-length percentiles

NAME _____

RECORD # _____

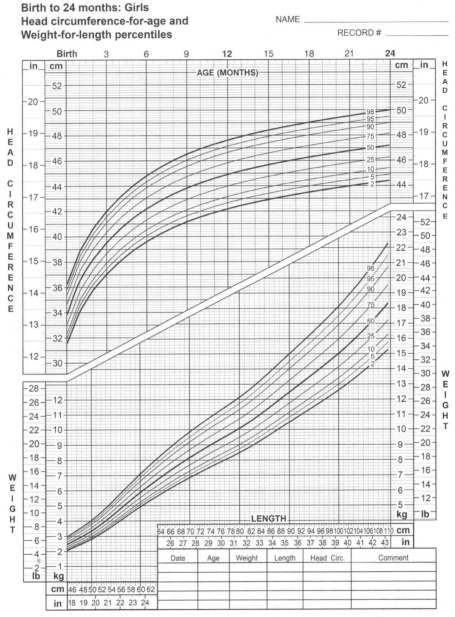

Published by the Centers for Disease Control and Prevention, November 1, 2009
SOURCE: WHO Child Growth Standards (http://www.who.int/childgrowth/en)

Q-1.3

Birth to 24 months: Girls: BMI-for-age percentiles

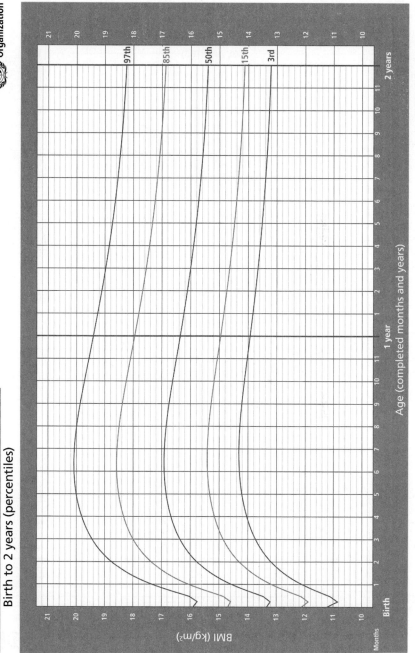

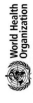

World Health Organization

WHO Child Growth Standards

BMI-for-age GIRLS

Birth to 2 years (percentiles)

BMI (kg/m²)

Age (completed months and years)

Months Birth

97th
85th
50th
15th
3rd

1 year

2 years

APP

Q-1.4

Birth to 24 months: Boys: Length-for-age and Weight-for-age percentiles

Birth to 24 months: Boys
Length-for-age and Weight-for-age percentiles

NAME _____

RECORD # _____

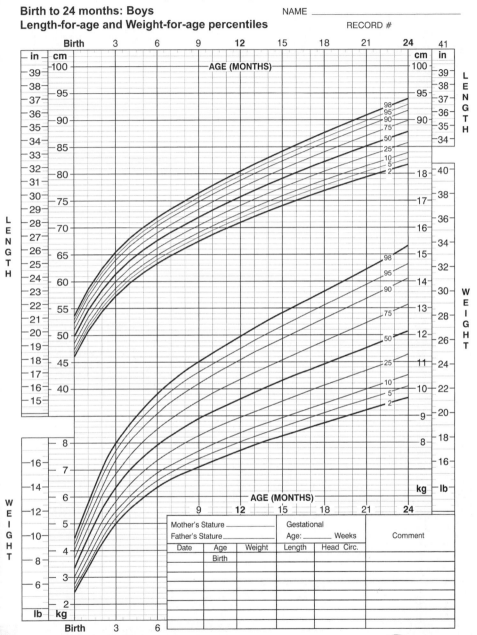

Published by the Centers for Disease Control and Prevention, November 1, 2009
SOURCE: WHO Child Growth Standards (http://www.who.int/childgrowth/en)

SAFER·HEALTHIER·PEOPLE™

Q-1.5

Birth to 24 months: Boys: Head circumference-for-age and Weight-for-length percentiles

Birth to 24 months: Boys
Head circumference-for-age and
Weight-for-length percentiles

NAME _____

RECORD # _____

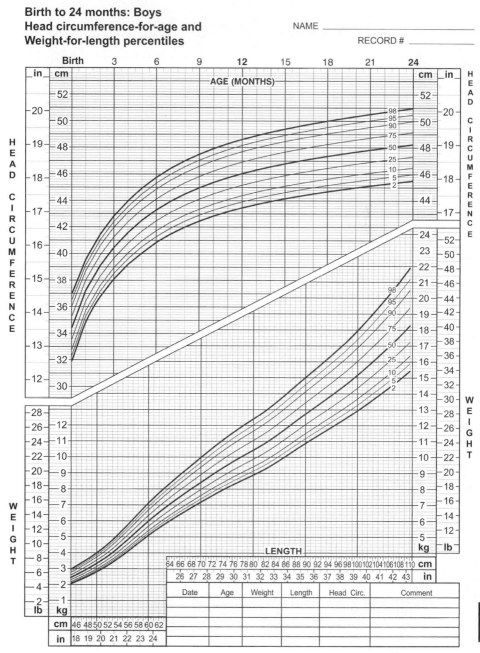

Published by the Centers for Disease Control and Prevention, November 1, 2009
SOURCE: WHO Child Growth Standards (http://www.who.int/childgrowth/en)

Q-1.6

Birth to 24 months: Boys: BMI-for-age percentiles

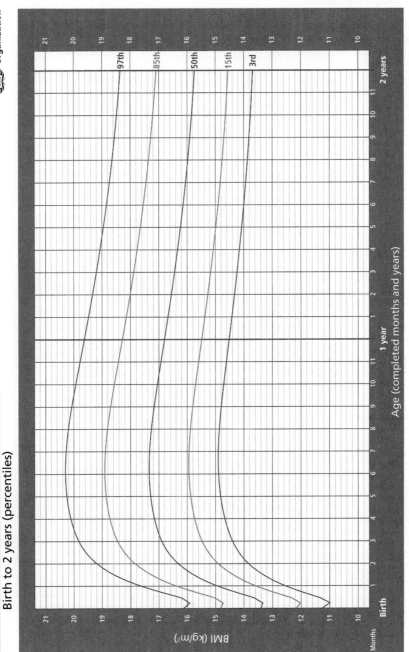

Q-1.7

2 to 20 years: Girls: Stature-for-age and Weight-for-age percentiles

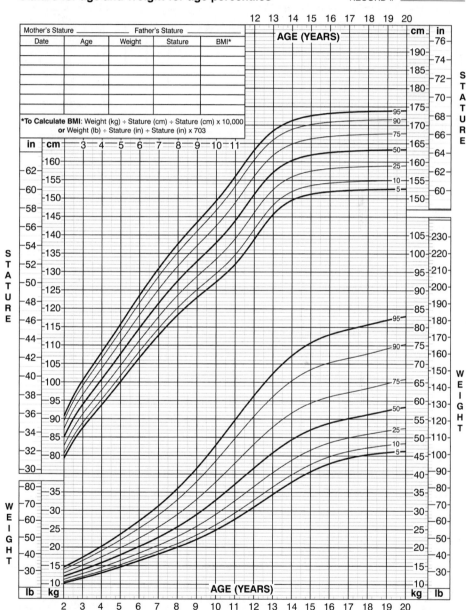

2 to 20 years: Girls
Stature-for-age and Weight-for-age percentiles

NAME _____

RECORD # _____

Mother's Stature _____ Father's Stature _____

Date	Age	Weight	Stature	BMI*

*To Calculate BMI: Weight (kg) ÷ Stature (cm) ÷ Stature (cm) x 10,000
or Weight (lb) ÷ Stature (in) ÷ Stature (in) x 703

AGE (YEARS)

STATURE

WEIGHT

Published May 30, 2000 (modified 11/21/00).
SOURCE: Developed by the National Center for Health Statistics in collaboration with
the National Center for Chronic Disease Prevention and Health Promotion (2000).
http://www.cdc.gov/growthcharts

CDC

APP

SAFER · HEALTHIER · PEOPLE™

Q-1.8

2 to 20 years: Girls: Body mass index-for-age percentiles

2 to 20 years: Girls
Body mass index-for-age percentiles

NAME _____

RECORD # _____

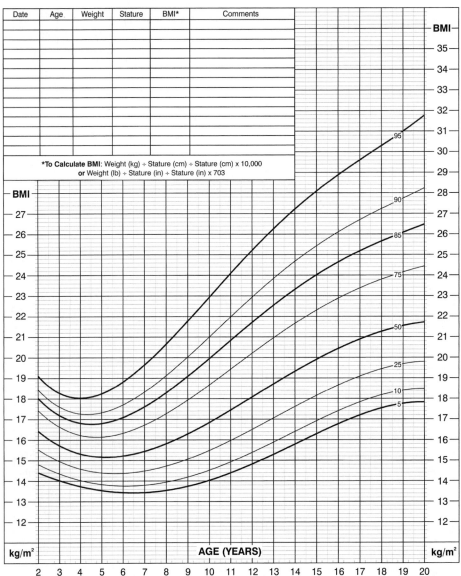

Published May 30, 2000 (modified 10/16/00).
SOURCE: Developed by the National Center for Health Statistics in collaboration with
the National Center for Chronic Disease Prevention and Health Promotion (2000).
http://www.cdc.gov/growthcharts

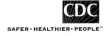

Q-1.9

2 to 20 years: Boys: Stature-for-age and Weight-for-age percentiles

2 to 20 years: Boys
Stature-for-age and Weight-for-age percentiles

NAME _____

RECORD # _____

Mother's Stature _____ Father's Stature _____

Date	Age	Weight	Stature	BMI*

*To Calculate BMI: Weight (kg) ÷ Stature (cm) ÷ Stature (cm) x 10,000
or Weight (lb) ÷ Stature (in) ÷ Stature (in) x 703

AGE (YEARS)

STATURE

WEIGHT

Published May 30, 2000 (modified 11/21/00).
SOURCE: Developed by the National Center for Health Statistics in collaboration with
the National Center for Chronic Disease Prevention and Health Promotion (2000).
http://www.cdc.gov/growthcharts

CDC
SAFER · HEALTHIER · PEOPLE™

APP

Q-1.10

2 to 20 years: Boys: Body mass index-for-age percentiles

2 to 20 years: Boys
Body mass index-for-age percentiles

NAME _____

RECORD # _____

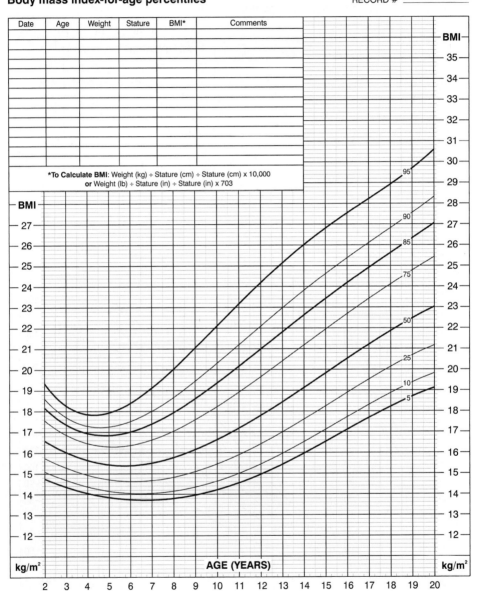

*To Calculate BMI: Weight (kg) ÷ Stature (cm) ÷ Stature (cm) x 10,000
or Weight (lb) ÷ Stature (in) ÷ Stature (in) x 703

Published May 30, 2000 (modified 10/16/00).
SOURCE: Developed by the National Center for Health Statistics in collaboration with
the National Center for Chronic Disease Prevention and Health Promotion (2000).
http://www.cdc.gov/growthcharts

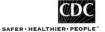

SAFER · HEALTHIER · PEOPLE™

Q-2.1

Fenton preterm growth chart: Girls: Weight, Length, and Head Circumference

(reprinted with permission from University of Calgary. © University of Calgary)

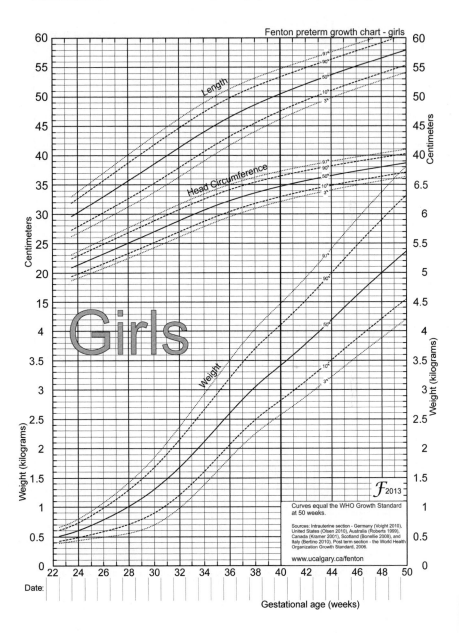

APP

Q-2.2

Fenton preterm growth chart: Boys: Weight, Length, and Head Circumference

(reprinted with permission from University of Calgary. © University of Calgary)

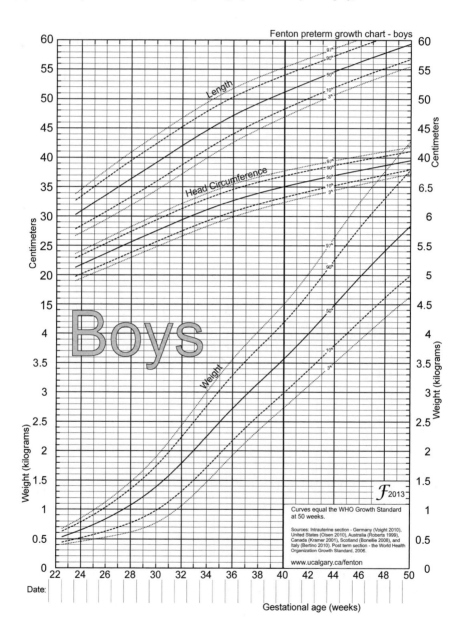

Q-3.1
Intrauterine growth curves: Females: Birth weight for Gestational age

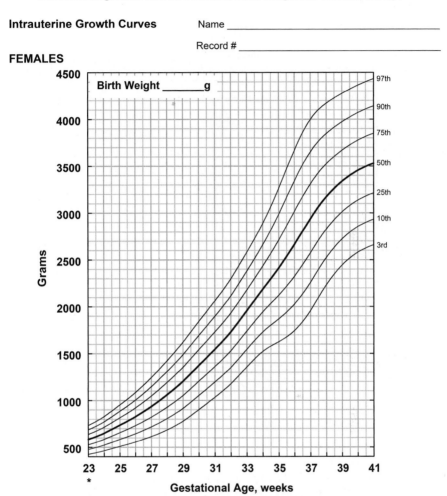

Intrauterine Growth Curves   Name _____

Record # _____

FEMALES

Reproduced with permission from: Olsen IE, Groveman S, Lawson ML, Clark R, Zemel B. New intrauterine growth curves based on U.S. data. *Pediatrics*, Volume 125, Pages e214-e244. Copyright 2010 by the American Academy of Pediatrics. Data source: Pediatrix Medical Group

BIRTH SIZE ASSESSMENT

Date of birth: / / (wks GA)	Select one
Large-for-gestational age (LGA) >90th percentile	☐
Appropriate-for-gestational age (AGA) 10-90th percentile	☐
Small-for-gestational age (SGA) <10th percentile	☐

* 3rd and 97th percentiles on all curves for 23 weeks should be interpreted cautiously given the small sample size.

APP

Q-3.2

Intrauterine growth curves: Females: Length and Head circumference for Gestational age

Page 2   Name _____

                                                 Record # _____

FEMALES

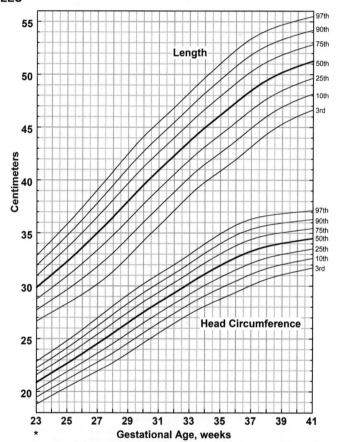

Reproduced with permission from: Olsen IE, Groveman S, Lawson ML, Clark R, Zemel B. New intrauterine growth curves based on U.S. data. *Pediatrics*, Volume 125, Pages e214-e244. Copyright 2010 by the American Academy of Pediatrics. Data source: Pediatrix Medical Group

Date																
GA (wks)																
WT (g)																
L (cm)																
HC (cm)																

* 3rd and 97th percentiles on all curves for 23 weeks should be interpreted cautiously given the small sample size.

Q-3.3

Intrauterine growth curves: Females: BMI for Gestational age

BMI Females

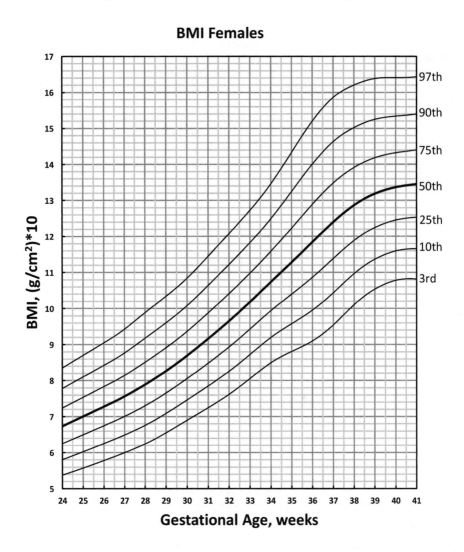

Olsen IE et al. BMI curves for preterm infants. Pediatrics. 2015;135:e572-e581. Reproduced with permission.
The authors specifically grant to any health care provider or related entity a perpetual, royalty free license to use and reproduce these BMI growth curves (Figure 2) as part of treatment and care protocol.

APP

Q-3.4

Intrauterine growth curves: Males: Birth weight for Gestational age

Intrauterine Growth Curves

Name _____

Record # _____

MALES

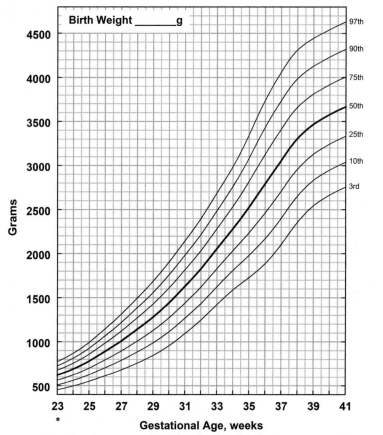

Reproduced with permission from: Olsen IE, Groveman S, Lawson ML, Clark R, Zemel B. New intrauterine growth curves based on U.S. data.
Pediatrics, Volume 125, Pages e214-e244. Copyright 2010 by the American Academy of Pediatrics. Data source: Pediatrix Medical Group

BIRTH SIZE ASSESSMENT:

	Select one
Date of birth: / / (wks GA)	
Large-for-gestational age (LGA) >90th percentile	☐
Appropriate-for-gestational age (AGA) 10-90th percentile	☐
Small-for-gestational age (SGA) <10th percentile	☐

* 3rd and 97th percentiles on all curves for 23 weeks should be interpreted cautiously given the small sample size.

Q-3.5

Intrauterine growth curves: Males: Length and Head circumference for Gestational age

Page 2   Name _____

                                        Record # _____

MALES

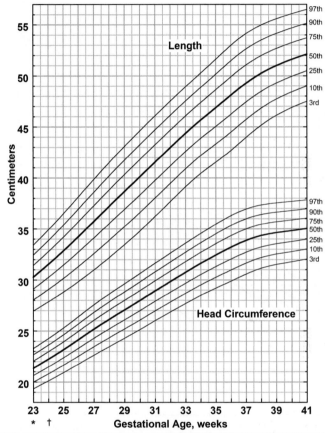

Reproduced with permission from: Olsen IE, Groveman S, Lawson ML, Clark R, Zemel B. New intrauterine growth curves based on U.S. data. *Pediatrics*, Volume 125, Pages e214-e244. Copyright 2010 by the American Academy of Pediatrics. Data source: Pediatrix Medical Group

Date																				
GA (wks)																				
WT (g)																				
L (cm)																				
HC (cm)																				

* 3rd and 97th percentiles on all curves for 23 weeks should be interpreted cautiously given the small sample size.
† Male head circumference curve at 24 weeks all percentiles should be interpreted cautiously as the distribution of data is skewed left.

APP

Q-3.6

Intrauterine growth curves: Males: BMI for Gestational age

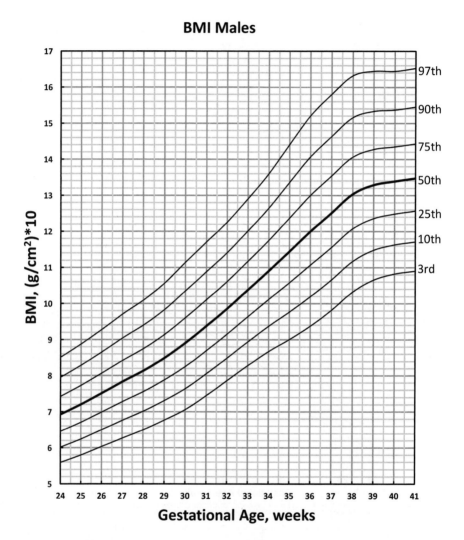

BMI Males

Olsen IE et al. BMI curves for preterm infants. Pediatrics. 2015;135:e572-e581. Reproduced with permission. *The authors specifically grant to any health care provider or related entity a perpetual, royalty free license to use and reproduce these BMI growth curves (Figure 2) as part of treatment and care protocol.*

Q-4.1
Female Growth Charts For Preterm Infants in NICU

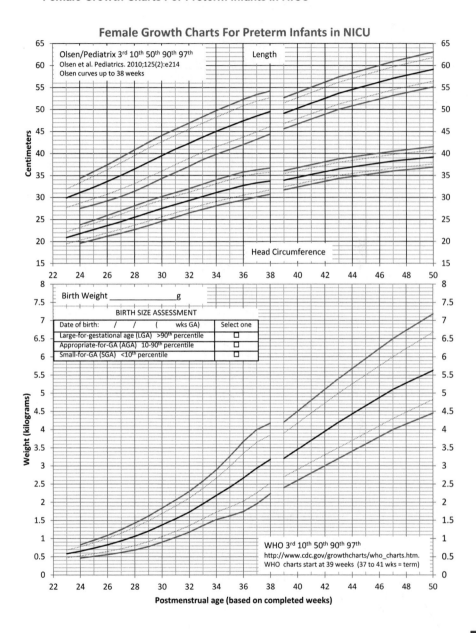

APP

Q-4.2
Male Growth Charts For Preterm Infants in NICU

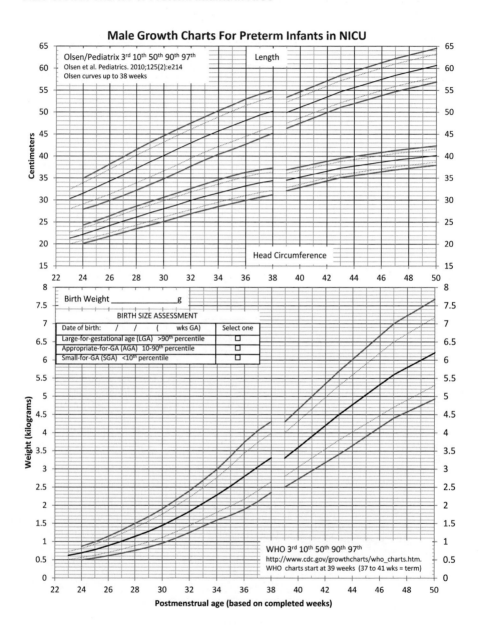

Q-5.1

Comparison of Olsen Intrauterine ("cross-sectional") and Postnatal ("longitudinal") Median BMI Growth Curves

Comparison of Olsen Intrauterine ("cross-sectional") and Postnatal ("longitudinal") Median Growth Curves

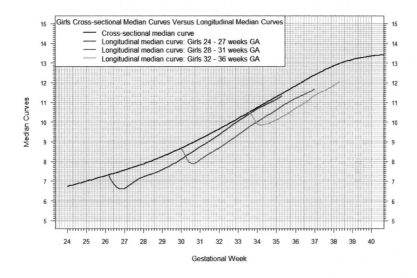

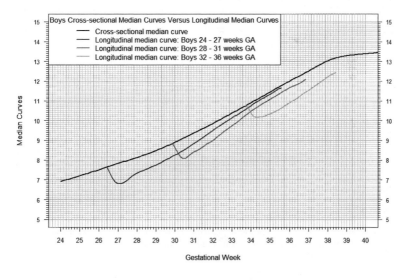

APP

Q-5.2

Postnatal Growth Curves Data: Mean BMI per Day by 3rd, 50th, and 97th Percentiles for Girls 28-31 Weeks GA at Birth

Postnatal Growth Curves Data: Mean BMI per Day by 3rd, 50th, and 97th Percentiles for Girls 28-31 Weeks GA at Birth

Days Since Birth	Birth Percentile Group 1			Birth Percentile Group 2			Birth Percentile Group 3			Birth Percentile Group 4			Birth Percentile Group 5		
	C3	C50	C97	C3	C50	C97	C3	C50	C97	C3	C50	C97	C3	C50	C97
0	6.378	7.336	8.054	7.451	8.148	8.921	8.018	8.693	9.473	8.854	9.233	9.594	9.308	10.202	11.466
1	6.214	7.217	8.105	7.205	7.936	8.744	7.728	8.437	9.256	8.255	8.985	9.672	8.834	9.819	11.190
2	6.064	7.080	8.151	6.942	7.706	8.545	7.414	8.155	9.009	7.721	8.694	9.629	8.396	9.464	10.908
3	5.949	6.962	8.183	6.741	7.543	8.419	7.186	7.965	8.862	7.401	8.475	9.553	8.066	9.201	10.685
4	5.885	6.894	8.214	6.622	7.470	8.393	7.058	7.885	8.835	7.267	8.357	9.502	7.859	9.048	10.550
5	5.888	6.906	8.282	6.590	7.492	8.472	7.018	7.903	8.914	7.251	8.344	9.541	7.771	9.008	10.522
6	5.948	6.992	8.399	6.626	7.587	8.634	7.041	7.989	9.070	7.298	8.414	9.677	7.773	9.054	10.581
7	6.033	7.111	8.537	6.686	7.704	8.821	7.087	8.101	9.251	7.371	8.513	9.843	7.810	9.129	10.669
8	6.113	7.226	8.669	6.736	7.803	8.989	7.126	8.201	9.414	7.438	8.600	9.978	7.836	9.188	10.738
9	6.187	7.334	8.793	6.782	7.889	9.141	7.157	8.289	9.558	7.498	8.677	10.093	7.855	9.237	10.795
10	6.257	7.439	8.911	6.836	7.978	9.297	7.189	8.373	9.691	7.554	8.758	10.218	7.884	9.294	10.860
11	6.322	7.541	9.026	6.901	8.074	9.460	7.223	8.456	9.820	7.609	8.847	10.360	7.928	9.367	10.941
12	6.380	7.635	9.139	6.968	8.169	9.618	7.260	8.537	9.941	7.665	8.936	10.497	7.980	9.446	11.034
13	6.432	7.719	9.253	7.031	8.256	9.764	7.299	8.616	10.056	7.723	9.020	10.615	8.033	9.527	11.135
14	6.480	7.798	9.371	7.091	8.340	9.901	7.342	8.695	10.171	7.782	9.102	10.724	8.087	9.609	11.244
15	6.531	7.879	9.495	7.156	8.428	10.038	7.394	8.781	10.290	7.840	9.188	10.840	8.142	9.693	11.360
16	6.587	7.966	9.622	7.225	8.525	10.177	7.454	8.872	10.417	7.896	9.280	10.971	8.201	9.780	11.484
17	6.650	8.057	9.752	7.297	8.625	10.312	7.519	8.967	10.546	7.950	9.375	11.107	8.262	9.871	11.615
18	6.719	8.151	9.881	7.367	8.727	10.442	7.586	9.063	10.675	8.003	9.472	11.244	8.326	9.967	11.750
19	6.790	8.250	10.014	7.437	8.831	10.566	7.654	9.158	10.804	8.058	9.572	11.379	8.391	10.066	11.888
20	6.860	8.352	10.157	7.507	8.937	10.688	7.722	9.254	10.931	8.119	9.678	11.514	8.455	10.164	12.023
21	6.926	8.457	10.306	7.577	9.045	10.808	7.791	9.351	11.060	8.185	9.787	11.646	8.518	10.262	12.154
22	6.987	8.564	10.443	7.644	9.149	10.922	7.862	9.450	11.190	8.251	9.893	11.769	8.581	10.358	12.279
23	7.043	8.672	10.556	7.707	9.249	11.029	7.934	9.551	11.322	8.315	9.992	11.880	8.647	10.453	12.398
24	7.098	8.780	10.653	7.770	9.349	11.134	8.006	9.652	11.453	8.383	10.087	11.980	8.713	10.546	12.513
25	7.160	8.885	10.747	7.838	9.454	11.246	8.077	9.749	11.582	8.465	10.184	12.073	8.779	10.638	12.626
26	7.234	8.989	10.848	7.913	9.566	11.365	8.146	9.842	11.707	8.558	10.283	12.160	8.843	10.728	12.742
27	7.320	9.091	10.965	7.989	9.675	11.483	8.214	9.931	11.830	8.645	10.375	12.244	8.904	10.819	12.867
28	7.413	9.193	11.105	8.062	9.779	11.595	8.283	10.016	11.951	8.713	10.454	12.326	8.963	10.910	13.004
29	7.508	9.292	11.251	8.136	9.878	11.703	8.354	10.100	12.073	8.771	10.530	12.415	9.018	10.999	13.144
30	7.599	9.389	11.384	8.212	9.976	11.812	8.428	10.184	12.196	8.832	10.614	12.522	9.070	11.081	13.275
31	7.684	9.483	11.496	8.293	10.073	11.924	8.504	10.269	12.319	8.900	10.709	12.642	9.120	11.155	13.393
32	7.763	9.573	11.596	8.378	10.170	12.038	8.580	10.354	12.439	8.971	10.804	12.759	9.166	11.224	13.503
33	7.839	9.661	11.694	8.466	10.266	12.152	8.655	10.437	12.553	9.038	10.893	12.863	9.211	11.291	13.606
34	7.917	9.746	11.796	8.553	10.357	12.262	8.731	10.524	12.665	9.099	10.981	12.966	9.256	11.357	13.700
35	8.002	9.831	11.903	8.636	10.441	12.363	8.811	10.617	12.780	9.149	11.073	13.085	9.306	11.421	13.782
36	8.094	9.914	12.012	8.715	10.518	12.456	8.893	10.717	12.894	9.192	11.168	13.214	9.363	11.485	13.851
37	8.186	9.993	12.110	8.794	10.594	12.548	8.969	10.812	12.998	9.240	11.256	13.322	9.432	11.552	13.908
38	8.273	10.067	12.189	8.878	10.675	12.644	9.034	10.896	13.085	9.304	11.331	13.388	9.513	11.625	13.959
39	8.356	10.138	12.256	8.963	10.757	12.740	9.093	10.974	13.163	9.377	11.397	13.431	9.598	11.705	14.018
40	8.437	10.211	12.324	9.047	10.838	12.832	9.152	11.053	13.240	9.450	11.458	13.477	9.676	11.795	14.101
41	8.516	10.286	12.398	9.126	10.915	12.916	9.211	11.132	13.319	9.522	11.520	13.536	9.742	11.893	14.209
42	8.593	10.359	12.476	9.198	10.985	12.988	9.265	11.205	13.390	9.603	11.583	13.600	9.794	11.992	14.325
43	8.668	10.429	12.558	9.260	11.045	13.045	9.310	11.267	13.448	9.696	11.648	13.664	9.835	12.088	14.436
44	8.744	10.499	12.644	9.315	11.100	13.093	9.351	11.323	13.502	9.785	11.714	13.741	9.864	12.177	14.530
45	8.823	10.570	12.738	9.370	11.155	13.138	9.397	11.385	13.562	9.850	11.779	13.845	9.886	12.254	14.596

C3, 3rd percentile; C50, 50th percentile; C97, 97th percentile. Birth Percentile Group based on BMI percentile at birth: Group 1, 0-20th percentile; Group 2, 20-40th percentile; Group 3, 40-60th percentile; Group 4, 60-80th percentile; Group 5, 80-100th percentile.

Reproduced with permission from: Williamson AL, Derado J, Barney BJ, Saunders G, Olsen IE, Clark RH, Lawson ML. Longitudinal BMI Growth Curves for Surviving Preterm NICU Infants Based on a Large US Sample. *Pediatrics* 2018;142(3):e20174169. Copyright 2018 by Williamson et al. The authors specifically grant to any health care provider or related entity a perpetual, royalty free license to use and reproduce these figures as part of treatment or care protocol.

Q-5.3
Postnatal Growth Curves Data: Mean BMI per Day by 3rd, 50th, and 97th Percentiles for Boys 28-31 Weeks GA at Birth

Postnatal Growth Curves Data: Mean BMI per Day by 3rd, 50th, and 97th Percentiles for Boys 28-31 Weeks GA at Birth

Days Since Birth	Birth Percentile Group 1			Birth Percentile Group 2			Birth Percentile Group 3			Birth Percentile Group 4			Birth Percentile Group 5		
	C3	C50	C97	C3	C50	C97	C3	C50	C97	C3	C50	C97	C3	C50	C97
0	6.557	7.494	8.291	7.710	8.354	9.181	8.117	8.865	9.616	9.071	9.457	9.852	9.765	10.459	12.099
1	6.387	7.353	8.303	7.464	8.136	9.002	7.857	8.643	9.434	8.494	9.240	10.025	9.194	10.112	11.719
2	6.229	7.209	8.322	7.184	7.880	8.781	7.550	8.369	9.195	8.011	8.937	9.931	8.605	9.785	11.319
3	6.114	7.100	8.354	6.988	7.715	8.658	7.319	8.176	9.043	7.703	8.707	9.801	8.150	9.536	11.054
4	6.055	7.052	8.408	6.892	7.660	8.655	7.188	8.091	9.011	7.542	8.584	9.733	7.909	9.383	10.926
5	6.064	7.084	8.504	6.885	7.703	8.762	7.154	8.115	9.097	7.499	8.567	9.760	7.843	9.333	10.912
6	6.130	7.187	8.639	6.939	7.814	8.943	7.191	8.216	9.270	7.532	8.630	9.874	7.877	9.366	10.976
7	6.218	7.317	8.778	7.010	7.942	9.141	7.244	8.332	9.457	7.594	8.721	10.020	7.952	9.438	11.069
8	6.298	7.438	8.897	7.062	8.048	9.309	7.272	8.415	9.604	7.644	8.799	10.149	8.019	9.510	11.152
9	6.374	7.548	9.006	7.101	8.135	9.453	7.288	8.479	9.726	7.685	8.865	10.259	8.072	9.577	11.221
10	6.453	7.654	9.125	7.142	8.223	9.594	7.318	8.555	9.857	7.730	8.930	10.357	8.111	9.642	11.282
11	6.539	7.758	9.257	7.189	8.315	9.736	7.367	8.649	10.005	7.783	9.001	10.454	8.143	9.708	11.344
12	6.626	7.856	9.394	7.235	8.405	9.873	7.423	8.745	10.154	7.839	9.079	10.560	8.175	9.775	11.416
13	6.707	7.948	9.525	7.276	8.488	9.998	7.474	8.832	10.288	7.895	9.165	10.684	8.218	9.846	11.506
14	6.778	8.034	9.650	7.316	8.568	10.116	7.526	8.916	10.417	7.947	9.256	10.822	8.272	9.922	11.610
15	6.834	8.114	9.773	7.361	8.652	10.236	7.586	9.007	10.553	7.995	9.348	10.968	8.335	10.003	11.724
16	6.879	8.194	9.896	7.411	8.743	10.361	7.658	9.109	10.699	8.042	9.440	11.115	8.404	10.090	11.845
17	6.923	8.278	10.025	7.463	8.835	10.484	7.738	9.218	10.853	8.094	9.536	11.255	8.471	10.183	11.973
18	6.975	8.372	10.165	7.515	8.926	10.603	7.822	9.332	11.011	8.159	9.637	11.384	8.530	10.282	12.109
19	7.036	8.474	10.316	7.572	9.022	10.727	7.906	9.444	11.164	8.228	9.744	11.514	8.588	10.386	12.253
20	7.105	8.581	10.478	7.643	9.133	10.867	7.984	9.547	11.306	8.287	9.854	11.661	8.651	10.495	12.407
21	7.179	8.691	10.647	7.725	9.256	11.020	8.056	9.643	11.436	8.338	9.967	11.821	8.723	10.605	12.566
22	7.256	8.800	10.815	7.808	9.377	11.170	8.128	9.738	11.563	8.398	10.080	11.966	8.797	10.713	12.726
23	7.331	8.907	10.974	7.883	9.486	11.304	8.205	9.838	11.693	8.481	10.190	12.076	8.868	10.814	12.881
24	7.405	9.011	11.119	7.952	9.586	11.427	8.287	9.944	11.827	8.575	10.296	12.168	8.937	10.909	13.028
25	7.478	9.116	11.247	8.022	9.685	11.549	8.371	10.052	11.961	8.656	10.397	12.265	9.005	10.998	13.168
26	7.551	9.221	11.361	8.095	9.786	11.672	8.455	10.161	12.093	8.720	10.496	12.375	9.075	11.083	13.296
27	7.626	9.328	11.465	8.171	9.888	11.796	8.537	10.267	12.221	8.777	10.595	12.492	9.145	11.167	13.405
28	7.705	9.433	11.566	8.248	9.991	11.921	8.615	10.369	12.342	8.836	10.698	12.612	9.216	11.255	13.492
29	7.789	9.537	11.664	8.327	10.093	12.046	8.691	10.468	12.458	8.898	10.803	12.729	9.284	11.344	13.570
30	7.876	9.638	11.756	8.406	10.195	12.171	8.764	10.564	12.571	8.960	10.906	12.842	9.346	11.434	13.656
31	7.966	9.736	11.847	8.486	10.295	12.296	8.834	10.658	12.681	9.023	11.006	12.946	9.401	11.524	13.755
32	8.055	9.833	11.941	8.565	10.392	12.419	8.901	10.749	12.787	9.085	11.099	13.042	9.456	11.615	13.861
33	8.140	9.928	12.042	8.644	10.486	12.540	8.965	10.835	12.889	9.148	11.187	13.127	9.516	11.706	13.970
34	8.221	10.025	12.146	8.723	10.580	12.664	9.026	10.918	12.987	9.216	11.272	13.209	9.579	11.790	14.077
35	8.296	10.126	12.249	8.808	10.676	12.792	9.085	10.999	13.084	9.293	11.360	13.292	9.646	11.859	14.177
36	8.368	10.230	12.346	8.895	10.774	12.925	9.144	11.079	13.180	9.378	11.446	13.376	9.715	11.912	14.271
37	8.442	10.332	12.434	8.980	10.868	13.054	9.204	11.161	13.279	9.459	11.519	13.448	9.788	11.958	14.362
38	8.523	10.432	12.513	9.059	10.952	13.172	9.267	11.244	13.380	9.529	11.573	13.505	9.866	12.005	14.453
39	8.610	10.526	12.591	9.131	11.029	13.282	9.331	11.330	13.484	9.589	11.623	13.575	9.949	12.059	14.543
40	8.701	10.615	12.679	9.200	11.102	13.385	9.395	11.416	13.589	9.643	11.690	13.693	10.038	12.121	14.626
41	8.790	10.698	12.780	9.267	11.172	13.484	9.458	11.501	13.691	9.703	11.776	13.853	10.127	12.193	14.694
42	8.875	10.778	12.891	9.332	11.242	13.580	9.517	11.582	13.788	9.789	11.867	14.006	10.204	12.269	14.735
43	8.954	10.856	13.010	9.397	11.312	13.675	9.568	11.656	13.876	9.908	11.953	14.112	10.258	12.347	14.745
44	9.029	10.934	13.134	9.460	11.380	13.766	9.614	11.722	13.954	10.025	12.031	14.203	10.286	12.427	14.742
45	9.105	11.012	13.260	9.519	11.444	13.851	9.653	11.783	14.026	10.098	12.101	14.329	10.287	12.510	14.745

C3, 3rd percentile; C50, 50th percentile; C97, 97th percentile. Birth Percentile Group based on BMI percentile at birth: Group 1, 0-20th percentile; Group 2, 20-40th percentile; Group 3, 40-60th percentile; Group 4, 60-80th percentile; Group 5, 80-100th percentile.

Reproduced with permission from: Williamson AL, Derado J, Barney BJ, Saunders G, Olsen IE, Clark RH, Lawson ML. Longitudinal BMI Growth Curves for Surviving Preterm NICU Infants Based on a Large US Sample. *Pediatrics* 2018;142(3):e20174169. Copyright 2018 by Williamson et al. The authors specifically grant to any health care provider or related entity a perpetual, royalty free license to use and reproduce these figures as part of treatment or care protocol.

APP

Q-6.1

International Newborn Size Standards: Weight (Girls)

(reprinted with permission from University of Oxford)

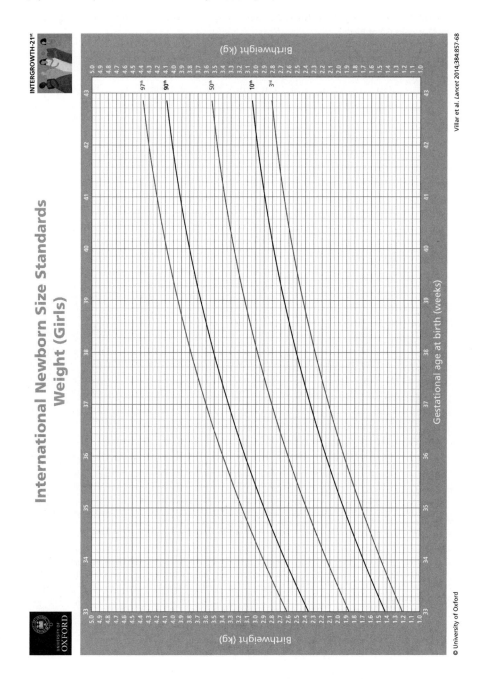

Q-6.2

International Newborn Size Standards: Length (Girls)

(reprinted with permission from University of Oxford)

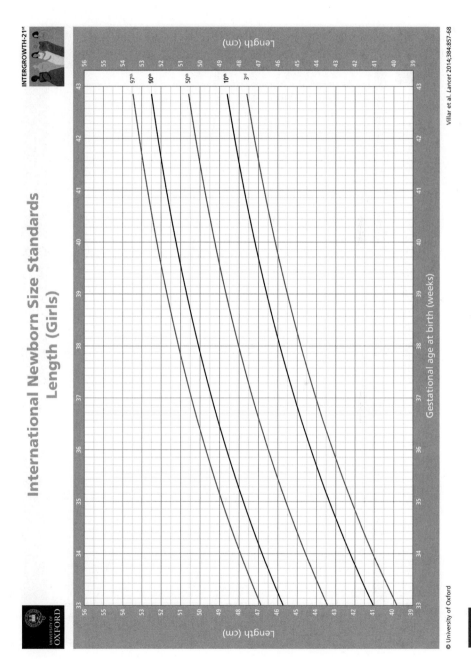

Q-6.3

International Newborn Size Standards: Head Circumference (Girls)

(reprinted with permission from University of Oxford)

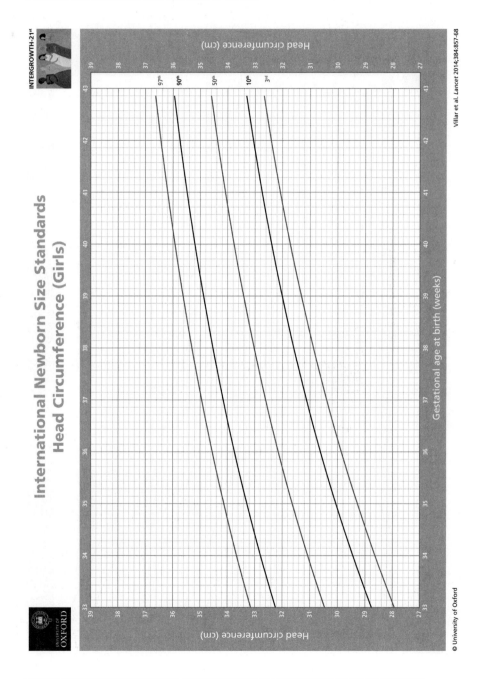

International Newborn Size Standards
Head Circumference (Girls)

INTERGROWTH-21st

Villar et al. *Lancet* 2014;384:857-68

© University of Oxford

Q-6.4
International Newborn Size Standards: Weight (Boys)
(reprinted with permission from University of Oxford)

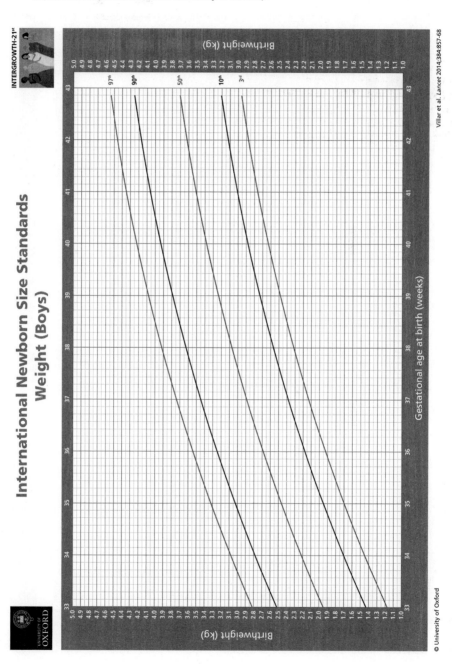

Q-6.5

International Newborn Size Standards: Length (Boys)

(reprinted with permission from University of Oxford)

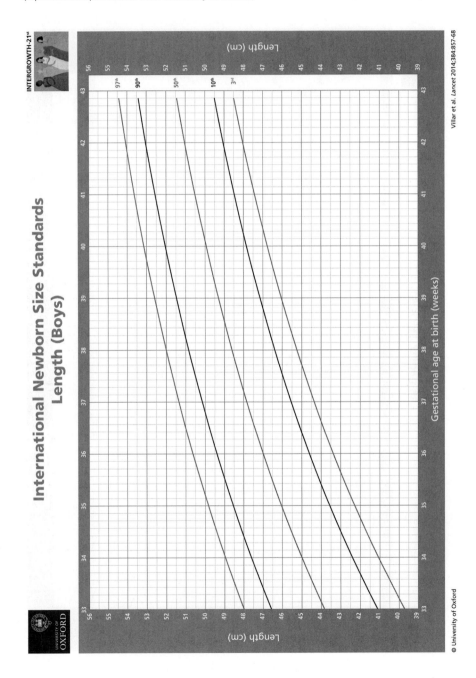

Q-6.6
International Newborn Size Standards: Head Circumference (Boys)

(reprinted with permission from University of Oxford)

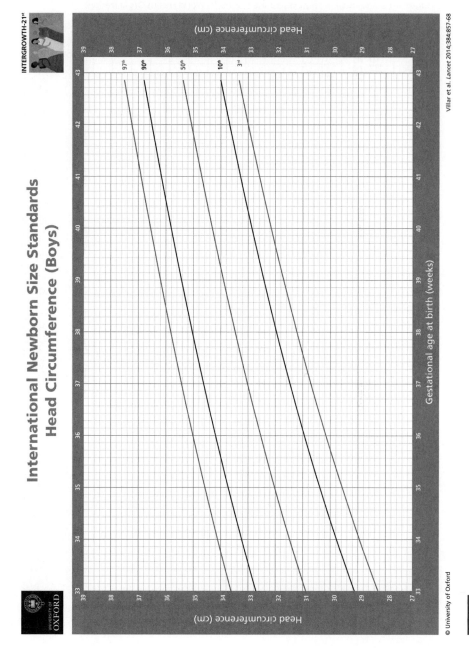

Q-7.1

WHO Growth Velocity Standards: 1-month weight increments (g) GIRLS Birth to 12 months (percentiles)

(reprinted with permission from World Health Organization; https://www.who.int/childgrowth/standards/en/; accessed June 6, 2019; © World Health Organization)

Simplified field tables

1-month weight increments (g) GIRLS
Birth to 12 months (percentiles)

Interval	1st	3rd	5th	15th	25th	50th	75th	85th	95th	97th	99th
0 - 4 wks	280	388	446	602	697	879	1068	1171	1348	1418	1551
4 wks - 2 mo	410	519	578	734	829	1011	1198	1301	1476	1545	1677
2 - 3 mo	233	321	369	494	571	718	869	952	1094	1150	1256
3 - 4 mo	133	214	259	376	448	585	726	804	937	990	1090
4 - 5 mo	51	130	172	286	355	489	627	703	833	885	983
5 - 6 mo	-24	52	93	203	271	401	537	611	739	790	886
6 - 7 mo	-79	-4	37	146	214	344	480	555	684	734	832
7 - 8 mo	-119	-44	-2	109	178	311	450	526	659	711	811
8 - 9 mo	-155	-81	-40	70	139	273	412	489	623	675	776
9 - 10 mo	-184	-110	-70	41	110	245	385	464	598	652	754
10 - 11 mo	-206	-131	-89	24	95	233	378	459	598	653	759
11 - 12 mo	-222	-145	-102	15	88	232	383	467	612	670	781

World Health Organization

WHO Growth Velocity Standards

Q-7.2
WHO Growth Velocity Standards: 2-month weight increments (g) GIRLS Birth to 24 months (percentiles)

(reprinted with permission from World Health Organization; https://www.who.int/childgrowth/standards/en/; accessed June 6, 2019; © World Health Organization)

Simplified field tables

2-month weight increments (g) GIRLS Birth to 24 months (percentiles)											World Health Organization
Interval	1st	3rd	5th	15th	25th	50th	75th	85th	95th	97th	99th
0-2 mo	968	1128	1216	1455	1604	1897	2210	2386	2696	2820	3062
1-3 mo	890	1030	1107	1317	1450	1714	2000	2163	2452	2569	2799
2-4 mo	625	740	804	978	1088	1307	1545	1681	1922	2020	2213
3-5 mo	451	556	615	773	874	1074	1290	1413	1632	1720	1894
4-6 mo	295	395	450	600	695	883	1085	1200	1403	1486	1646
5-7 mo	170	267	321	468	560	742	938	1048	1243	1321	1473
6-8 mo	76	175	229	377	469	651	846	955	1147	1223	1372
7-9 mo	3	103	157	306	399	581	775	883	1072	1147	1293
8-10 mo	-59	40	95	243	336	517	708	814	999	1073	1215
9-11 mo	-104	-3	53	203	297	478	670	776	960	1033	1174
10-12 mo	-135	-31	26	179	274	458	652	759	944	1018	1159
11-13 mo	-163	-57	1	157	254	441	637	745	932	1005	1147
12-14 mo	-185	-78	-19	140	238	428	626	736	924	999	1142
13-15 mo	-204	-95	-35	127	227	420	621	732	924	999	1144
14-16 mo	-219	-108	-47	118	220	416	622	735	930	1007	1154
15-17 mo	-231	-118	-55	112	216	418	627	743	943	1021	1172
16-18 mo	-243	-128	-64	106	212	417	631	750	954	1035	1189
17-19 mo	-255	-139	-75	97	205	413	631	751	959	1041	1199
18-20 mo	-267	-151	-86	88	196	407	628	751	962	1046	1206
19-21 mo	-279	-162	-97	79	188	402	626	750	965	1050	1213
20-22 mo	-291	-174	-109	67	178	393	620	745	963	1049	1214
21-23 mo	-305	-189	-124	53	164	381	608	735	954	1040	1207
22-24 mo	-318	-202	-137	39	150	367	596	723	942	1029	1197
WHO Growth Velocity Standards											

APP

Q-7.3

WHO Growth Velocity Standards: 6-month weight increments (g) GIRLS Birth to 24 months (percentiles)

(reprinted with permission from World Health Organization; https://www.who.int/childgrowth/standards/en/; accessed June 6, 2019; © World Health Organization)

Simplified field tables

6-month weight increments (g) GIRLS Birth to 24 months (percentiles)

Interval	1st	3rd	5th	15th	25th	50th	75th	85th	95th	97th	99th
0-6 mo	2701	2924	3049	3395	3620	4079	4597	4902	5462	5697	6170
1-7 mo	2174	2381	2498	2822	3033	3462	3946	4231	4753	4971	5409
2-8 mo	1684	1877	1985	2286	2480	2878	3324	3586	4063	4262	4660
3-9 mo	1279	1461	1563	1846	2030	2403	2821	3064	3506	3689	4054
4-10 mo	964	1140	1240	1514	1692	2052	2451	2682	3099	3271	3610
5-11 mo	725	900	999	1271	1446	1799	2186	2409	2807	2969	3288
6-12 mo	549	725	824	1097	1271	1618	1996	2211	2592	2746	3047
7-13 mo	425	603	702	975	1147	1489	1857	2065	2430	2577	2862
8-14 mo	340	519	619	891	1063	1400	1760	1962	2314	2454	2726
9-15 mo	284	465	565	838	1009	1343	1697	1895	2238	2375	2638
10-16 mo	249	431	532	805	975	1309	1660	1855	2194	2329	2588
11-17 mo	230	412	513	785	956	1288	1639	1834	2173	2307	2566
12-18 mo	221	401	501	772	942	1275	1627	1823	2163	2299	2560
13-19 mo	216	394	492	762	931	1264	1617	1815	2158	2296	2560
14-20 mo	211	386	484	751	920	1253	1608	1807	2155	2294	2563
15-21 mo	204	377	474	740	908	1242	1599	1800	2151	2292	2565
16-22 mo	193	365	461	726	894	1228	1586	1788	2143	2285	2561
17-23 mo	178	348	444	708	876	1210	1569	1772	2128	2271	2549
18-24 mo	161	330	425	689	857	1191	1551	1754	2111	2254	2533

World Health Organization

WHO Growth Velocity Standards

Q-7.4

WHO Growth Velocity Standards: 1-month weight increments (g) BOYS Birth to 12 months (percentiles)

(reprinted with permission from World Health Organization; https://www.who.int/childgrowth/standards/en/; accessed June 6, 2019; © World Health Organization)

Simplified field tables

1-month weight increments (g) BOYS
Birth to 12 months (percentiles)

Interval	1st	3rd	5th	15th	25th	50th	75th	85th	95th	97th	99th
0 - 4 wks	182	369	460	681	805	1023	1229	1336	1509	1575	1697
4 wks - 2 mo	528	648	713	886	992	1196	1408	1524	1724	1803	1955
2 - 3 mo	307	397	446	577	658	815	980	1071	1228	1290	1410
3 - 4 mo	160	241	285	403	476	617	764	845	985	1041	1147
4 - 5 mo	70	150	194	311	383	522	666	746	883	937	1041
5 - 6 mo	-17	61	103	217	287	422	563	640	773	826	927
6 - 7 mo	-76	0	42	154	223	357	496	573	706	758	859
7 - 8 mo	-118	-43	-1	111	181	316	457	535	671	724	827
8 - 9 mo	-153	-77	-36	77	148	285	429	508	646	701	806
9 - 10 mo	-183	-108	-66	48	120	259	405	486	627	683	790
10 - 11 mo	-209	-132	-89	27	100	243	394	478	623	680	791
11 - 12 mo	-229	-150	-106	15	91	239	397	484	635	695	811

World Health Organization

WHO Growth Velocity Standards

APP

Q-7.5

**WHO Growth Velocity Standards: 2-month weight increments (g) BOYS
Birth to 24 months (percentiles)**

(reprinted with permission from World Health Organization; https://www.who.int/
childgrowth/standards/en/; accessed June 6, 2019; © World Health Organization)

Simplified field tables

2-month weight increments (g) BOYS Birth to 24 months (percentiles)										**World Health Organization**
Interval	1st	3rd	5th	15th	25th	50th	75th	85th	95th	97th	99th
0-2 mo	1144	1338	1443	1720	1890	2216	2552	2737	3054	3179	3418
1-3 mo	1040	1211	1303	1549	1701	1992	2296	2463	2753	2868	3088
2-4 mo	675	810	884	1081	1202	1438	1685	1822	2059	2154	2336
3-5 mo	455	576	642	820	930	1145	1371	1496	1715	1802	1970
4-6 mo	291	404	466	634	738	941	1156	1277	1486	1569	1731
5-7 mo	165	271	330	487	585	778	982	1096	1294	1374	1528
6-8 mo	79	182	238	390	486	673	871	982	1175	1252	1402
7-9 mo	16	117	172	323	417	601	797	907	1098	1174	1322
8-10 mo	-41	60	115	266	360	544	739	848	1039	1115	1261
9-11 mo	-92	10	67	219	315	502	700	810	1003	1079	1227
10-12 mo	-132	-28	30	187	286	478	681	795	992	1070	1221
11-13 mo	-169	-62	-2	159	260	458	666	782	984	1064	1218
12-14 mo	-202	-92	-31	133	236	437	648	766	969	1050	1206
13-15 mo	-230	-119	-58	109	212	414	626	744	947	1028	1183
14-16 mo	-250	-138	-75	93	197	401	614	731	935	1016	1170
15-17 mo	-262	-148	-84	87	193	399	615	734	939	1020	1176
16-18 mo	-272	-155	-90	84	192	401	619	739	945	1027	1183
17-19 mo	-281	-162	-97	79	188	398	617	737	944	1025	1181
18-20 mo	-291	-170	-104	73	182	393	611	731	937	1018	1173
19-21 mo	-299	-178	-111	67	176	387	605	725	929	1010	1164
20-22 mo	-307	-185	-118	61	171	382	599	719	923	1003	1156
21-23 mo	-314	-191	-123	57	167	378	596	715	919	999	1151
22-24 mo	-320	-196	-128	53	164	376	594	713	917	997	1149
WHO Growth Velocity Standards										

Q-7.6

**WHO Growth Velocity Standards: 6-month weight increments (g) BOYS
Birth to 24 months (percentiles)**

(reprinted with permission from World Health Organization; https://www.who.int/
childgrowth/standards/en/; accessed June 6, 2019; © World Health Organization)

Simplified field tables

6-month weight increments (g) BOYS
Birth to 24 months (percentiles)

World Health
Organization

Interval	1st	3rd	5th	15th	25th	50th	75th	85th	95th	97th	99th
0-6 mo	2940	3229	3387	3810	4072	4580	5114	5412	5929	6136	6534
1-7 mo	2342	2611	2759	3157	3406	3893	4411	4701	5210	5413	5809
2-8 mo	1736	1968	2096	2443	2662	3093	3555	3816	4275	4461	4821
3-9 mo	1319	1523	1636	1945	2141	2530	2949	3188	3609	3779	4112
4-10 mo	1030	1217	1321	1607	1789	2152	2546	2771	3169	3331	3647
5-11 mo	806	982	1080	1351	1524	1871	2249	2465	2849	3005	3311
6-12 mo	642	813	909	1175	1346	1688	2062	2277	2658	2813	3116
7-13 mo	515	683	778	1042	1212	1553	1927	2141	2521	2675	2978
8-14 mo	415	582	676	938	1106	1445	1816	2028	2404	2557	2856
9-15 mo	341	506	599	858	1024	1359	1725	1934	2304	2453	2746
10-16 mo	291	455	547	805	970	1301	1662	1868	2232	2379	2665
11-17 mo	258	422	515	772	937	1267	1624	1827	2184	2329	2609
12-18 mo	236	400	493	750	914	1241	1593	1793	2143	2284	2558
13-19 mo	221	386	479	735	898	1222	1569	1765	2108	2246	2513
14-20 mo	212	377	470	725	887	1207	1549	1741	2077	2212	2472
15-21 mo	206	372	465	719	880	1196	1533	1721	2050	2182	2435
16-22 mo	202	368	460	713	872	1184	1515	1700	2021	2150	2397
17-23 mo	198	363	455	706	863	1171	1496	1677	1992	2117	2358
18-24 mo	195	360	451	700	855	1158	1478	1656	1964	2086	2321

WHO Growth Velocity Standards

APP

Q-7.7

WHO Growth Velocity Standards: 2-month length increments (cm) GIRLS
Birth to 24 months (percentiles)

(reprinted with permission from World Health Organization; https://www.who.int/ childgrowth/standards/en/; accessed June 6, 2019; © World Health Organization)

Simplified field tables

2-month length increments (cm) GIRLS
Birth to 24 months (percentiles)

World Health Organization

Interval	1st	3rd	5th	15th	25th	50th	75th	85th	95th	97th	99th
0-2 mo	5.3	5.8	6.1	6.7	7.1	7.9	8.7	9.1	9.7	10.0	10.5
1-3 mo	4.2	4.6	4.8	5.4	5.7	6.4	7.0	7.4	8.0	8.2	8.6
2-4 mo	3.0	3.4	3.7	4.2	4.5	5.2	5.8	6.1	6.7	6.9	7.3
3-5 mo	2.2	2.6	2.8	3.4	3.7	4.3	4.9	5.2	5.8	6.0	6.4
4-6 mo	1.6	2.0	2.2	2.7	3.0	3.6	4.2	4.5	5.0	5.2	5.6
5-7 mo	1.3	1.6	1.8	2.3	2.6	3.2	3.7	4.0	4.5	4.7	5.1
6-8 mo	1.1	1.4	1.6	2.1	2.4	3.0	3.6	3.9	4.4	4.6	4.9
7-9 mo	1.0	1.3	1.5	2.0	2.3	2.9	3.4	3.7	4.2	4.4	4.8
8-10 mo	0.9	1.2	1.4	1.9	2.2	2.7	3.3	3.6	4.1	4.3	4.6
9-11 mo	0.8	1.2	1.3	1.8	2.1	2.6	3.2	3.4	3.9	4.1	4.5
10-12 mo	0.7	1.1	1.3	1.7	2.0	2.5	3.1	3.3	3.8	4.0	4.3
11-13 mo	0.7	1.0	1.2	1.6	1.9	2.4	3.0	3.2	3.7	3.9	4.2
12-14 mo	0.6	0.9	1.1	1.6	1.8	2.4	2.9	3.2	3.6	3.8	4.2
13-15 mo	0.5	0.8	1.0	1.5	1.8	2.3	2.8	3.1	3.6	3.8	4.1
14-16 mo	0.4	0.7	0.9	1.4	1.7	2.2	2.8	3.0	3.5	3.7	4.1
15-17 mo	0.3	0.7	0.9	1.3	1.6	2.2	2.7	3.0	3.5	3.7	4.0
16-18 mo	0.3	0.6	0.8	1.3	1.6	2.1	2.7	2.9	3.4	3.6	4.0
17-19 mo	0.2	0.5	0.7	1.2	1.5	2.0	2.6	2.9	3.4	3.6	3.9
18-20 mo	0.1	0.5	0.7	1.2	1.4	2.0	2.5	2.8	3.3	3.5	3.8
19-21 mo	0.1	0.4	0.6	1.1	1.4	1.9	2.5	2.8	3.2	3.4	3.8
20-22 mo	0.0	0.4	0.6	1.0	1.3	1.9	2.4	2.7	3.2	3.4	3.7
21-23 mo	0.0	0.3	0.5	1.0	1.3	1.8	2.4	2.6	3.1	3.3	3.7
22-24 mo	0.0	0.3	0.5	0.9	1.2	1.8	2.3	2.6	3.1	3.3	3.6

WHO Growth Velocity Standards

Q-7.8

**WHO Growth Velocity Standards: 6-month length increments (cm) GIRLS
Birth to 24 months (percentiles)**

(reprinted with permission from World Health Organization; https://www.who.int/
childgrowth/standards/en/; accessed June 6, 2019; © World Health Organization)

Simplified field tables

6-month length increments (cm) GIRLS
Birth to 24 months (percentiles)

World Health Organization

Interval	1st	3rd	5th	15th	25th	50th	75th	85th	95th	97th	99th
0-6 mo	12.8	13.5	13.9	14.8	15.4	16.5	17.6	18.2	19.2	19.6	20.4
1-7 mo	10.5	11.1	11.5	12.3	12.9	13.9	14.9	15.5	16.4	16.8	17.5
2-8 mo	8.7	9.3	9.6	10.4	10.9	11.8	12.8	13.3	14.2	14.5	15.2
3-9 mo	7.4	8.0	8.3	9.0	9.5	10.3	11.2	11.7	12.6	12.9	13.5
4-10 mo	6.6	7.1	7.4	8.1	8.5	9.3	10.2	10.7	11.4	11.8	12.4
5-11 mo	6.0	6.5	6.8	7.5	7.9	8.7	9.5	9.9	10.7	11.0	11.6
6-12 mo	5.6	6.1	6.4	7.0	7.4	8.2	9.0	9.5	10.2	10.5	11.1
7-13 mo	5.4	5.8	6.1	6.7	7.1	7.9	8.7	9.1	9.8	10.1	10.7
8-14 mo	5.1	5.6	5.8	6.4	6.8	7.6	8.4	8.8	9.5	9.8	10.3
9-15 mo	4.9	5.3	5.6	6.2	6.6	7.3	8.1	8.5	9.2	9.5	10.0
10-16 mo	4.7	5.1	5.3	6.0	6.4	7.1	7.8	8.3	9.0	9.2	9.8
11-17 mo	4.5	4.9	5.2	5.8	6.2	6.9	7.6	8.0	8.7	9.0	9.5
12-18 mo	4.3	4.7	5.0	5.6	6.0	6.7	7.4	7.8	8.5	8.8	9.3
13-19 mo	4.1	4.6	4.8	5.4	5.8	6.5	7.2	7.6	8.3	8.6	9.1
14-20 mo	4.0	4.4	4.6	5.2	5.6	6.3	7.1	7.5	8.2	8.4	9.0
15-21 mo	3.8	4.2	4.5	5.1	5.4	6.1	6.9	7.3	8.0	8.2	8.8
16-22 mo	3.7	4.1	4.3	4.9	5.3	6.0	6.7	7.1	7.8	8.0	8.6
17-23 mo	3.5	4.0	4.2	4.8	5.1	5.8	6.5	6.9	7.6	7.9	8.4
18-24 mo	3.4	3.8	4.0	4.6	5.0	5.6	6.3	6.7	7.4	7.7	8.2

WHO Growth Velocity Standards

APP

Q-7.9

**WHO Growth Velocity Standards: 2-month length increments (cm) BOYS
Birth to 24 months (percentiles)**

(reprinted with permission from World Health Organization; https://www.who.int/
childgrowth/standards/en/; accessed June 6, 2019; © World Health Organization)

Simplified field tables

2-month length increments (cm) BOYS
Birth to 24 months (percentiles)   World Health Organization

Interval	1st	3rd	5th	15th	25th	50th	75th	85th	95th	97th	99th
0-2 mo	5.9	6.4	6.6	7.3	7.7	8.5	9.3	9.7	10.4	10.6	11.1
1-3 mo	4.7	5.2	5.4	6.0	6.3	7.0	7.7	8.0	8.6	8.9	9.3
2-4 mo	3.4	3.8	4.0	4.6	4.9	5.6	6.2	6.6	7.2	7.4	7.8
3-5 mo	2.3	2.7	3.0	3.5	3.9	4.5	5.1	5.5	6.1	6.3	6.7
4-6 mo	1.7	2.0	2.3	2.8	3.1	3.7	4.3	4.7	5.2	5.4	5.9
5-7 mo	1.3	1.6	1.8	2.3	2.7	3.2	3.8	4.1	4.7	4.9	5.3
6-8 mo	1.0	1.4	1.6	2.1	2.4	3.0	3.5	3.8	4.4	4.6	5.0
7-9 mo	0.9	1.3	1.5	2.0	2.3	2.8	3.4	3.7	4.2	4.4	4.8
8-10 mo	0.8	1.2	1.4	1.8	2.1	2.7	3.2	3.5	4.1	4.3	4.6
9-11 mo	0.7	1.1	1.3	1.7	2.0	2.6	3.1	3.4	3.9	4.1	4.5
10-12 mo	0.7	1.0	1.2	1.7	1.9	2.5	3.0	3.3	3.8	4.0	4.4
11-13 mo	0.6	0.9	1.1	1.6	1.8	2.4	2.9	3.2	3.7	3.9	4.3
12-14 mo	0.5	0.8	1.0	1.5	1.8	2.3	2.8	3.1	3.6	3.8	4.2
13-15 mo	0.4	0.7	0.9	1.4	1.7	2.2	2.8	3.1	3.5	3.7	4.1
14-16 mo	0.3	0.7	0.8	1.3	1.6	2.1	2.7	3.0	3.5	3.7	4.0
15-17 mo	0.3	0.6	0.8	1.2	1.5	2.1	2.6	2.9	3.4	3.6	4.0
16-18 mo	0.2	0.5	0.7	1.2	1.5	2.0	2.5	2.8	3.3	3.5	3.9
17-19 mo	0.2	0.5	0.7	1.1	1.4	1.9	2.5	2.8	3.3	3.5	3.9
18-20 mo	0.1	0.4	0.6	1.1	1.4	1.9	2.4	2.7	3.2	3.4	3.8
19-21 mo	0.0	0.4	0.5	1.0	1.3	1.8	2.4	2.7	3.2	3.4	3.8
20-22 mo	0.0	0.3	0.5	1.0	1.3	1.8	2.4	2.7	3.2	3.4	3.7
21-23 mo	0.0	0.3	0.4	0.9	1.2	1.8	2.3	2.6	3.1	3.3	3.7
22-24 mo	0.0	0.2	0.4	0.9	1.2	1.7	2.3	2.6	3.1	3.3	3.7

WHO Growth Velocity Standards

Q-7.10
**WHO Growth Velocity Standards: 6-month length increments (cm) BOYS
Birth to 24 months (percentiles)**

(reprinted with permission from World Health Organization; https://www.who.int/
childgrowth/standards/en/; accessed June 6, 2019; © World Health Organization)

Simplified field tables

6-month length increments (cm) BOYS
Birth to 24 months (percentiles)

World Health Organization

Interval	1st	3rd	5th	15th	25th	50th	75th	85th	95th	97th	99th
0-6 mo	13.8	14.5	14.9	15.9	16.5	17.7	18.8	19.4	20.4	20.8	21.6
1-7 mo	11.0	11.7	12.1	13.1	13.6	14.7	15.8	16.4	17.4	17.8	18.5
2-8 mo	8.8	9.5	9.8	10.7	11.3	12.3	13.3	13.9	14.8	15.2	15.9
3-9 mo	7.3	7.9	8.2	9.1	9.6	10.6	11.5	12.1	13.0	13.3	14.0
4-10 mo	6.3	6.9	7.2	8.0	8.5	9.4	10.3	10.8	11.7	12.0	12.6
5-11 mo	5.7	6.2	6.5	7.3	7.8	8.6	9.5	10.0	10.8	11.1	11.7
6-12 mo	5.3	5.8	6.1	6.8	7.3	8.1	8.9	9.4	10.2	10.5	11.0
7-13 mo	5.0	5.6	5.8	6.5	6.9	7.7	8.5	9.0	9.7	10.0	10.5
8-14 mo	4.8	5.3	5.6	6.3	6.7	7.4	8.2	8.6	9.3	9.6	10.1
9-15 mo	4.7	5.1	5.4	6.0	6.4	7.2	7.9	8.3	9.0	9.3	9.8
10-16 mo	4.5	4.9	5.2	5.8	6.2	6.9	7.6	8.0	8.7	9.0	9.4
11-17 mo	4.3	4.8	5.0	5.6	6.0	6.7	7.4	7.8	8.4	8.7	9.2
12-18 mo	4.1	4.6	4.8	5.4	5.8	6.5	7.2	7.6	8.2	8.4	8.9
13-19 mo	4.0	4.4	4.6	5.2	5.6	6.3	7.0	7.3	8.0	8.2	8.7
14-20 mo	3.8	4.3	4.5	5.1	5.4	6.1	6.8	7.1	7.8	8.0	8.5
15-21 mo	3.7	4.1	4.3	4.9	5.3	5.9	6.6	7.0	7.6	7.8	8.3
16-22 mo	3.6	4.0	4.2	4.8	5.1	5.8	6.5	6.8	7.4	7.7	8.1
17-23 mo	3.4	3.9	4.1	4.7	5.0	5.6	6.3	6.7	7.3	7.5	7.9
18-24 mo	3.3	3.7	4.0	4.5	4.9	5.5	6.2	6.5	7.1	7.3	7.8

WHO Growth Velocity Standards

APP

Q-7.11

WHO Growth Velocity Standards: 2-month head circumference increments (cm) GIRLS Birth to 12 months (percentiles)

(reprinted with permission from World Health Organization; https://www.who.int/childgrowth/standards/en/; accessed June 6, 2019; © World Health Organization)

Simplified field tables

Interval	1st	3rd	5th	15th	25th	50th	75th	85th	95th	97th	99th
0-2 mo	2.8	3.1	3.2	3.6	3.9	4.4	4.8	5.1	5.5	5.7	6.0
1-3 mo	1.9	2.1	2.3	2.6	2.8	3.1	3.5	3.6	4.0	4.1	4.3
2-4 mo	1.4	1.6	1.7	1.9	2.1	2.3	2.6	2.8	3.1	3.2	3.4
3-5 mo	1.1	1.2	1.3	1.6	1.7	2.0	2.2	2.4	2.6	2.7	2.9
4-6 mo	0.8	1.0	1.1	1.3	1.4	1.7	1.9	2.0	2.3	2.4	2.5
5-7 mo	0.6	0.8	0.8	1.0	1.2	1.4	1.6	1.8	2.0	2.1	2.2
6-8 mo	0.4	0.6	0.6	0.8	1.0	1.2	1.4	1.5	1.7	1.8	2.0
7-9 mo	0.3	0.4	0.5	0.7	0.8	1.0	1.2	1.3	1.5	1.6	1.8
8-10 mo	0.2	0.3	0.4	0.5	0.6	0.8	1.1	1.2	1.4	1.4	1.6
9-11 mo	0.1	0.2	0.3	0.4	0.5	0.7	0.9	1.1	1.2	1.3	1.5
10-12 mo	0.0	0.1	0.2	0.4	0.5	0.7	0.9	1.0	1.1	1.2	1.4

2-month head circumference increments (cm) GIRLS Birth to 12 months (percentiles) — World Health Organization

WHO Growth Velocity Standards

Q-7.12

WHO Growth Velocity Standards: 6-month head circumference increments (cm) GIRLS Birth to 24 months (percentiles)

(reprinted with permission from World Health Organization; https://www.who.int/childgrowth/standards/en/; accessed June 6, 2019; © World Health Organization)

Simplified field tables

6-month head circumference increments (cm) GIRLS
Birth to 24 months (percentiles) — World Health Organization

Interval	1st	3rd	5th	15th	25th	50th	75th	85th	95th	97th	99th
0-6 mo	6.2	6.6	6.8	7.3	7.6	8.3	8.9	9.3	10.0	10.2	10.7
1-7 mo	4.9	5.1	5.3	5.7	6.0	6.5	7.0	7.3	7.9	8.1	8.5
2-8 mo	3.8	4.1	4.2	4.6	4.8	5.2	5.7	5.9	6.4	6.5	6.9
3-9 mo	3.1	3.3	3.4	3.8	4.0	4.3	4.7	5.0	5.4	5.5	5.8
4-10 mo	2.5	2.7	2.9	3.1	3.3	3.7	4.0	4.2	4.6	4.7	5.0
5-11 mo	2.1	2.3	2.4	2.6	2.8	3.1	3.5	3.7	4.0	4.1	4.3
6-12 mo	1.7	1.9	2.0	2.2	2.4	2.7	3.0	3.2	3.5	3.6	3.8
7-13 mo	1.4	1.6	1.7	1.9	2.0	2.3	2.6	2.8	3.1	3.2	3.4
8-14 mo	1.2	1.3	1.4	1.6	1.8	2.0	2.3	2.5	2.7	2.8	3.0
9-15 mo	1.0	1.1	1.2	1.4	1.5	1.8	2.1	2.2	2.5	2.6	2.7
10-16 mo	0.8	0.9	1.0	1.2	1.4	1.6	1.9	2.0	2.2	2.3	2.5
11-17 mo	0.7	0.8	0.9	1.1	1.2	1.5	1.7	1.8	2.1	2.2	2.3
12-18 mo	0.5	0.7	0.8	1.0	1.1	1.3	1.6	1.7	1.9	2.0	2.2
13-19 mo	0.4	0.6	0.7	0.9	1.0	1.2	1.4	1.6	1.8	1.9	2.0
14-20 mo	0.4	0.5	0.6	0.8	0.9	1.1	1.4	1.5	1.7	1.8	1.9
15-21 mo	0.3	0.4	0.5	0.7	0.8	1.1	1.3	1.4	1.6	1.7	1.8
16-22 mo	0.2	0.4	0.5	0.6	0.8	1.0	1.2	1.3	1.5	1.6	1.7
17-23 mo	0.2	0.3	0.4	0.6	0.7	0.9	1.1	1.2	1.4	1.5	1.6
18-24 mo	0.1	0.3	0.4	0.5	0.6	0.8	1.1	1.2	1.3	1.4	1.5
WHO Growth Velocity Standards											

APP

Q-7.13

WHO Growth Velocity Standards: 2-month head circumference increments (cm) BOYS Birth to 12 months (percentiles)

(reprinted with permission from World Health Organization; https://www.who.int/childgrowth/standards/en/; accessed June 6, 2019; © World Health Organization)

Simplified field tables

2-month head circumference increments (cm) BOYS Birth to 12 months (percentiles)										World Health Organization
Interval	1st	3rd	5th	15th	25th	50th	75th	85th	95th	97th	99th
0-2 mo	3.0	3.3	3.5	3.9	4.2	4.7	5.2	5.5	5.9	6.1	6.5
1-3 mo	2.2	2.4	2.5	2.8	3.0	3.4	3.7	3.9	4.3	4.4	4.7
2-4 mo	1.6	1.8	1.9	2.1	2.2	2.5	2.8	3.0	3.2	3.3	3.6
3-5 mo	1.3	1.4	1.5	1.7	1.8	2.1	2.3	2.5	2.7	2.8	3.0
4-6 mo	1.0	1.1	1.2	1.4	1.5	1.7	2.0	2.1	2.3	2.4	2.6
5-7 mo	0.7	0.8	0.9	1.1	1.2	1.4	1.7	1.8	2.0	2.1	2.3
6-8 mo	0.5	0.6	0.7	0.9	1.0	1.2	1.4	1.5	1.8	1.8	2.0
7-9 mo	0.3	0.4	0.5	0.7	0.8	1.0	1.2	1.3	1.5	1.6	1.8
8-10 mo	0.2	0.3	0.4	0.6	0.7	0.9	1.1	1.2	1.4	1.5	1.6
9-11 mo	0.1	0.2	0.3	0.5	0.6	0.8	1.0	1.1	1.3	1.3	1.5
10-12 mo	0.0	0.1	0.2	0.4	0.5	0.7	0.9	1.0	1.2	1.2	1.4
WHO Growth Velocity Standards											

Q-7.14

WHO Growth Velocity Standards: 6-month head circumference increments (cm) BOYS Birth to 24 months (percentiles)

(reprinted with permission from World Health Organization; https://www.who.int/childgrowth/standards/en/; accessed June 6, 2019; © World Health Organization)

Simplified field tables

6-month head circumference increments (cm) BOYS
Birth to 24 months (percentiles)   **World Health Organization**

Interval	1st	3rd	5th	15th	25th	50th	75th	85th	95th	97th	99th
0-6 mo	6.8	7.1	7.3	7.9	8.2	8.9	9.5	9.9	10.6	10.8	11.3
1-7 mo	5.2	5.5	5.7	6.1	6.4	6.9	7.5	7.8	8.3	8.6	9.0
2-8 mo	4.0	4.3	4.4	4.8	5.1	5.5	6.0	6.2	6.7	6.9	7.2
3-9 mo	3.2	3.4	3.6	3.9	4.1	4.5	4.9	5.2	5.6	5.7	6.0
4-10 mo	2.6	2.8	2.9	3.2	3.4	3.8	4.2	4.4	4.8	4.9	5.2
5-11 mo	2.1	2.3	2.4	2.7	2.9	3.2	3.6	3.8	4.1	4.2	4.5
6-12 mo	1.7	1.9	2.0	2.3	2.4	2.7	3.1	3.2	3.6	3.7	3.9
7-13 mo	1.4	1.6	1.7	1.9	2.1	2.4	2.7	2.8	3.1	3.2	3.4
8-14 mo	1.1	1.3	1.4	1.6	1.8	2.0	2.3	2.5	2.8	2.9	3.1
9-15 mo	0.9	1.1	1.2	1.4	1.5	1.8	2.1	2.2	2.5	2.6	2.8
10-16 mo	0.8	0.9	1.0	1.2	1.3	1.6	1.8	2.0	2.2	2.3	2.5
11-17 mo	0.7	0.8	0.9	1.1	1.2	1.4	1.7	1.8	2.0	2.1	2.3
12-18 mo	0.5	0.7	0.8	0.9	1.1	1.3	1.5	1.6	1.8	1.9	2.1
13-19 mo	0.5	0.6	0.7	0.8	1.0	1.2	1.4	1.5	1.7	1.8	1.9
14-20 mo	0.4	0.5	0.6	0.8	0.9	1.1	1.3	1.4	1.6	1.7	1.8
15-21 mo	0.3	0.5	0.5	0.7	0.8	1.0	1.2	1.3	1.5	1.6	1.7
16-22 mo	0.3	0.4	0.5	0.6	0.8	0.9	1.1	1.3	1.4	1.5	1.7
17-23 mo	0.2	0.4	0.4	0.6	0.7	0.9	1.1	1.2	1.4	1.5	1.6
18-24 mo	0.2	0.3	0.4	0.6	0.7	0.9	1.0	1.2	1.3	1.4	1.5

WHO Growth Velocity Standards

APP

Q-8.1

Arm circumference-for-age GIRLS 3 months to 5 years (percentiles)

(reprinted with permission from World Health Organization; https://www.who.int/
childgrowth/standards/en/; accessed June 6, 2019; © World Health Organization)

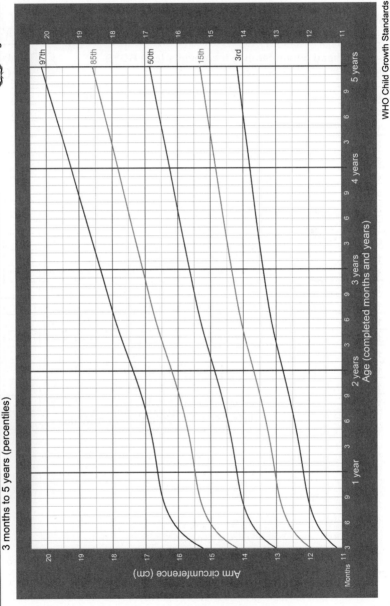

Q-8.2

Arm circumference-for-age BOYS 3 months to 5 years (percentiles)

(reprinted with permission from World Health Organization; https://www.who.int/childgrowth/standards/en/; accessed June 6, 2019; © World Health Organization)

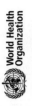

Arm circumference-for-age BOYS

3 months to 5 years (percentiles)

Arm circumference (cm)

Age (completed months and years)

WHO Child Growth Standards

World Health Organization

APP

Q-8.3

Mid upper arm circumference for Age percentiles

(reprinted with permission from Addo OY, Himes JH, Zemel BS. Reference ranges for midupper arm circumference, upper arm muscle area, and upper arm fat area in US children and adolescents aged 1-20 y. *Am J Clin Nutr.* 2017;105(1):111-120. © American Society for Nutrition)

TABLE 3. Mid Upper Arm Circumference for age percentiles.

Mid Upper Arm Circumference, cm

Age years	Males									Females								
	2nd	5th	10th	25th	50th	75th	90th	95th	98th	2nd	5th	10th	25th	50th	75th	90th	95th	98th
1.0	13.9	14.2	14.6	15.2	15.8	16.5	17.3	17.9	18.4	13.5	13.8	14.2	14.8	15.5	16.2	17.0	17.6	18.1
1.5	14.1	14.3	14.7	15.3	16.0	16.8	17.6	18.2	18.7	13.7	14.0	14.4	15.1	15.8	16.6	17.4	18.0	18.5
2.0	14.2	14.5	14.9	15.5	16.2	17.0	17.9	18.5	19.0	13.9	14.2	14.6	15.3	16.0	16.9	17.7	18.4	18.9
2.5	14.4	14.6	15.0	15.7	16.4	17.2	18.1	18.8	19.3	14.0	14.3	14.8	15.5	16.3	17.1	18.0	18.8	19.3
3.0	14.5	14.8	15.2	15.9	16.6	17.5	18.5	19.2	19.8	14.2	14.5	14.9	15.7	16.5	17.4	18.4	19.1	19.7
3.5	14.7	14.9	15.4	16.0	16.8	17.8	18.8	19.6	20.2	14.3	14.7	15.1	15.9	16.7	17.7	18.7	19.5	20.2
4.0	14.8	15.1	15.5	16.2	17.1	18.0	19.1	19.9	20.6	14.5	14.8	15.3	16.1	17.0	18.0	19.1	20.0	20.7
4.5	14.9	15.2	15.7	16.4	17.3	18.3	19.5	20.4	21.0	14.7	15.0	15.5	16.3	17.2	18.3	19.5	20.5	21.2
5.0	15.1	15.4	15.8	16.6	17.5	18.6	19.8	20.8	21.5	14.8	15.1	15.6	16.5	17.5	18.6	19.9	20.9	21.7
5.5	15.1	15.4	15.9	16.7	17.6	18.8	20.1	21.1	21.9	14.9	15.2	15.7	16.6	17.7	18.9	20.3	21.4	22.2
6.0	15.1	15.4	15.9	16.7	17.7	18.9	20.3	21.4	22.3	14.9	15.2	15.8	16.7	17.8	19.1	20.6	21.7	22.7
6.5	15.1	15.4	15.9	16.8	17.8	19.1	20.6	21.8	22.7	14.9	15.2	15.8	16.7	17.9	19.3	20.9	22.1	23.1
7.0	15.3	15.6	16.1	17.0	18.1	19.5	21.1	22.3	23.3	14.9	15.3	15.9	16.9	18.1	19.6	21.3	22.7	23.7
7.5	15.5	15.8	16.3	17.3	18.4	19.9	21.6	23.0	24.1	15.1	15.5	16.1	17.2	18.5	20.0	21.9	23.3	24.4
8.0	15.7	16.0	16.6	17.6	18.8	20.4	22.2	23.7	24.9	15.3	15.8	16.4	17.5	18.9	20.6	22.5	24.1	25.3
8.5	15.9	16.3	16.8	17.9	19.2	20.8	22.8	24.4	25.7	15.6	16.1	16.7	17.9	19.4	21.2	23.2	24.9	26.2
9.0	16.1	16.5	17.1	18.2	19.6	21.3	23.4	25.1	26.5	15.9	16.4	17.1	18.3	19.9	21.8	24.0	25.7	27.1
9.5	16.3	16.7	17.4	18.5	20.0	21.9	24.1	25.9	27.3	16.1	16.6	17.4	18.7	20.3	22.3	24.6	26.4	27.8
10.0	16.6	17.0	17.7	18.9	20.5	22.4	24.8	26.6	28.2	16.4	16.9	17.6	19.0	20.7	22.7	25.1	27.0	28.5
10.5	16.9	17.3	18.0	19.3	20.9	22.9	25.4	27.3	28.9	16.7	17.2	18.0	19.4	21.1	23.3	25.7	27.6	29.1
11.0	17.1	17.6	18.3	19.7	21.4	23.5	26.0	28.0	29.5	17.1	17.6	18.4	19.8	21.6	23.8	26.4	28.4	29.9
11.5	17.5	18.0	18.7	20.1	21.9	24.0	26.6	28.6	30.2	17.5	18.0	18.9	20.3	22.2	24.5	27.1	29.1	30.7
12.0	17.9	18.4	19.2	20.6	22.4	24.6	27.3	29.3	30.9	18.0	18.5	19.4	20.9	22.8	25.2	27.9	29.9	31.5
12.5	18.3	18.8	19.7	21.2	23.0	25.3	27.9	30.0	31.5	18.5	19.1	19.9	21.5	23.5	25.9	28.6	30.7	32.3
13.0	18.8	19.4	20.2	21.8	23.7	26.0	28.7	30.7	32.2	19.0	19.6	20.4	22.0	24.0	26.4	29.2	31.4	33.0
13.5	19.4	20.0	20.9	22.4	24.4	26.8	29.4	31.4	32.9	19.4	20.0	20.9	22.4	24.5	26.9	29.7	31.9	33.5
14.0	20.1	20.6	21.5	23.1	25.1	27.5	30.2	32.1	33.6	19.8	20.4	21.2	22.8	24.8	27.3	30.1	32.3	33.9
14.5	20.6	21.2	22.2	23.8	25.8	28.2	30.9	32.8	34.2	20.2	20.7	21.6	23.1	25.1	27.6	30.4	32.6	34.3
15.0	21.2	21.8	22.8	24.4	26.5	28.9	31.5	33.4	34.8	20.5	21.0	21.9	23.4	25.4	27.9	30.7	32.9	34.6

15.5	21.8	22.4	23.3	25.0	27.1	29.4	32.1	33.9	35.3	20.8	21.3	22.1	23.7	25.7	28.2	31.0	33.2	34.8
16.0	22.3	22.9	23.9	25.5	27.6	30.0	32.6	34.4	35.8	21.0	21.5	22.4	23.9	25.9	28.4	31.2	33.4	35.1
16.5	22.8	23.4	24.3	26.0	28.0	30.4	33.0	34.8	36.1	21.2	21.7	22.5	24.1	26.1	28.5	31.3	33.5	35.2
17.0	23.2	23.8	24.8	26.4	28.5	30.8	33.4	35.2	36.5	21.3	21.8	22.7	24.2	26.2	28.6	31.4	33.6	35.4
17.5	23.7	24.3	25.3	26.9	29.0	31.3	33.9	35.7	37.0	21.4	21.9	22.7	24.3	26.3	28.7	31.5	33.7	35.5
18.0	24.2	24.8	25.7	27.4	29.5	31.8	34.4	36.2	37.5	21.4	22.0	22.8	24.4	26.3	28.8	31.6	33.9	35.6
18.5	24.6	25.2	26.1	27.8	29.9	32.2	34.8	36.5	37.8	21.6	22.1	23.0	24.5	26.5	28.9	31.8	34.1	35.9
19.0	24.9	25.5	26.4	28.1	30.2	32.5	35.0	36.8	38.1	21.7	22.2	23.1	24.7	26.7	29.1	32.0	34.3	36.2
19.5	25.1	25.7	26.6	28.3	30.4	32.7	35.2	36.9	38.2	21.8	22.3	23.2	24.8	26.8	29.3	32.2	34.6	36.5
20.0	25.2	25.8	26.8	28.5	30.5	32.8	35.3	37.0	38.2	21.8	22.4	23.3	24.9	26.9	29.4	32.4	34.8	36.7

From: Addo OY, Himes JH, Zemel BS. Reference ranges for midupper arm circumference, upper arm muscle area, and upper arm fat area in US children and adolescents aged 1-20 y. Am J Clin Nutr. 2017;105(1):111-20.

APP

Q-9.1

Triceps skinfold-for-age GIRLS 3 months to 5 years (percentiles)

(reprinted with permission from World Health Organization; https://www.who.int/childgrowth/standards/en/; accessed June 6, 2019; © World Health Organization)

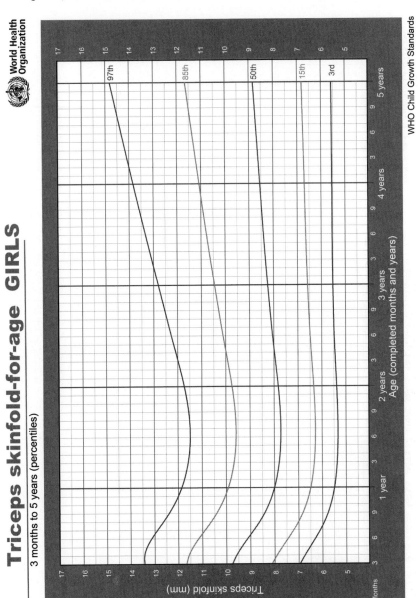

Q-9.2

Triceps skinfold-for-age BOYS 3 months to 5 years (percentiles)

(reprinted with permission from World Health Organization; https://www.who.int/childgrowth/standards/en/; accessed June 6, 2019; © World Health Organization)

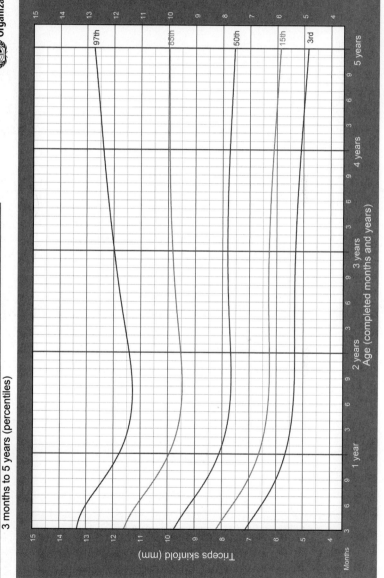

Hypermetabolism with trauma, 443
Hypernatremia and oral rehydration
   solutions, 824
Hyperoxaluria, 1127, 1129
Hypersensitivity (allergy), food,
   981–997
   clinical disorders in, 984–987
      mixed IgE-/non-IgE-associated,
         986–987
      non-IgE-mediated, 987
   common foods in, 982–983
   diagnosis of, 988–991
   gluten-free diet for, 398
   infant formula and, 101–102
   ingredient labeling and, 1415–1416
   introduction to, 981–982
   LC-PUFAs effects on, 525–527
   medical management of, 993–994
   natural resolution of, 994
   pathophysiology of, 982
   peanut, 174
   prevalence of, 984
   prevention of, 994–997
   school food service and, 264–266
   treatment of, 991–993
Hypertension, 1129–1131
   obesity and, 946
Hyperhomocysteinemia, 665
Hypoallergenic formulas, 101–102
Hypoglycemia, 887–905
   clinical manifestations of, 889–890
   diabetes mellitus and, 866–867
   differential diagnosis of, 896–900
   etiology of, 890–892
   evaluation of, 893–896
   introduction and definition of,
      887–889
   laboratory investigation of, 895–896
   treatment of, 901–905
Hypolactasia, 25
Hyponatremia, 122
Hypoprothrombinemia, 649
Hypothalamus and energy homeostasis, 929–932

I

Ileocecal valve, 1255
Illness. *See also* Acute illnesses;
   Chronic disease; Critically ill
   children
   feeding during, 205–206
   foodborne

clinical manifestations of, 1442
epidemiology of, 1435–1441
food safety and, 1452–1457
introduction to, 1435
laboratory testing of, 1442–1445,
   1450
management of, 1445–1447
surveillance for, 1447–1451
human immunodeficiency virus
   infection (*See* Human immunodeficiency virus infection)
vitamin K and risk of cancer, 650
Imaging technologies, 802–803,
   1163–1164
developmental disabilities and, 1051
nutritional status assessment using,
   753
Imerslund-Grasbeck syndrome, 666
Immunity, 1003–1031
   auto-, 1011
   copper deficiency and, 603
   developmental immunodeficiency,
      1015–1020
   foodborne illnesses and, 1447
   gut microbiome and
      microbiota, 1011–1012
      prebiotics, 1014–1015
      probiotics, 1012–1014
   HIV and (*See* Human immunodefi-
      ciency virus infection)
   human milk and, 52–53
   immunonutrition for, 1070–1071
   insufficient protein intake and,
      472–473
   interactions with
      fat-soluble vitamins, 1004–1005
      long-chain polyunsaturated fatty
         acids, 1009
      micronutrients, 1003–1004
      trace elements, 1006–1008
      water-soluble vitamins,
         1005–1006
   introduction to role of nutrition in,
      1003
   liver disease and, 1202
   neonatal intestine function in, 18
Immunoglobulin(s)
   A
      developmental immunodefi-
         ciency and, 1016
      in human milk, 31, 49